Cardiovascular Disorders

Pathogenesis and Pathophysiology

Cardiovascular Disorders

Pathogenesis and Pathophysiology

Michael B. Gravanis, M.D.

Professor of Pathology
Associate Professor of Cardiology
Emory University School of Medicine
Atlanta, Georgia

illustrated

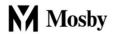 **Mosby**

St. Louis Baltimore Boston Chicago London Philadelphia Sydney Toronto

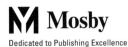

Mosby
Dedicated to Publishing Excellence

Editor: Susan M. Gay
Assistant Editor: Sandra E. Clark
Project Manager: Mark Spann
Production Editor: Jabari Asim
Book Designer: Julie Taugner
Cover Illustration: Dr. Michael B. Gravanis and Donald O'Connor

Printed in the United States of America.

Mosby–Year Book, Inc.
11830 Westline Industrial Drive
St. Louis, Missouri 63146

Library of Congress Cataloging-in-Publication Data
Cardiovascular disorders : pathogenesis and pathophysiology / [edited
  by] Micheal B. Gravanis.
     p. cm.
  ISBN 0-8016-6336-9
  1. Cardiovascular system—Diseases—Pathogenesis.
2. Cardiovascular system—Pathophysiology.   I. Gravanis, Michael
Basil, 1929-
  [DNLM: 1. Cardiovascular Diseases—etiology. 2. Cardiovascular
Diseases—physiopathology.   WG 142 C2631]
RC669.C283 1993
616.1'07—dc20
DNLM/DLC
for Library of Congress   92-48820
                                      CIP

96 95 94 93 92 CI/MY/MY/ 1 2 3 4 5 6 7 8 9 0

CONTRIBUTORS

Aftab A. Ansari, Ph.D.
Professor
Department of Pathology
Emory University School of Medicine
Atlanta, Georgia

Kenneth L. Baughman, M.D.
Associate Professor of Medicine
Chief, Division of Cardiology
Director, Cardiomyopathy Service
Johns Hopkins Medical Institutions
Baltimore, Maryland

Harisios Boudoulas, M.D.
Distinguished Senior Investigator
Central Ohio Chapter of the American Heart Association
Professor of Medicine and Pharmacy
Division of Cardiology
The Ohio State University College of Medicine
Columbus, Ohio

W. Virgil Brown, M.D.
Past President, American Heart Association, 1991-1992
Professor of Medicine
Director, Division of Arteriosclerosis and Lipid
  Metabolism
Emory University School of Medicine
Atlanta, Georgia

Stephen David Clements, Jr., M.D.
Professor of Medicine (Cardiology)
Emory University School of Medicine
Atlanta, Georgia

I. Sylvia Crawley, M.D.
Clinical Professor of Medicine
Emory University School of Medicine
Atlanta, Georgia

George C. Emmanouilides, M.D., M.S.
Professor of Pediatrics and Pediatric Cardiology
UCLA School of Medicine
Chief Division of Pediatric Cardiology
Harbor-UCLA Medical Center
Torrance, California

Robert H. Franch, M.D.
Professor of Medicine (Cardiology)
Emory University School of Medicine
Atlanta, Georgia

Gottlieb C. Friesinger, M.D.
Professor of Medicine
Division of Cardiology
Vanderbilt University Medical Center
Nashville, Tennessee

Michael B. Gravanis, M.D.
Professor of Pathology
Associate Professor of Cardiology
Emory University School of Medicine
Atlanta, Georgia

W. Dallas Hall, Jr., M.D.
Professor of Medicine
Director
Division of Hypertension
Emory University School of Medicine
Atlanta, Georgia

Ahvie Herskowitz, M.D.
Associate Professor of Medicine and Immunology
Division of Cardiology
Johns Hopkins Medical Institutions
Baltimore, Maryland

Gary L. Hertzler, M.D.
Assistant Professor of Pathology
Emory University School of Medicine
Atlanta, Georgia

Kirk R. Kanter, M.D.
Associate Professor of Surgery
Cardiothoracic Division
Emory University School of Medicine
Atlanta, Georgia

Ngoc-Anh Le, Ph.D.
Associate Professor of Medicine
Division of Arteriosclerosis and Lipid Metabolism
Emory University School of Medicine
Atlanta, Geogria

Angel R. Leon, M.D.
Assistant Professor of Medicine (Cardiology)
Department of Internal Medicine
Emory University School of Medicine
Crawford Long Hospital
Atlanta, Georgia

Celia M. Oakley, M.D. S.R.C.P., S.A.C.C., F.E.S.C.
Professor of Clinical Cardiology
Royal Postgraduate Medical School
Consultant Cardiologist
Hammersmith Hospital
London, England

Patricia A. O'Shea, M.D.
Associate Professor of Pathology
Department of Pathology and Laboratory Medicine
Emory University School of Medicine
Pediatric Pathologist
Egleston Children's Hospital
Atlanta, Georgia

Neal A. Scott, M.D., Ph.D.
Assistant Professor of Medicine
Division of Cardiology
Andreas Gruentzig Cardiovascular Center
Emory University School of Medicine
Atlanta, Georgia

Robert J. Siegel, M.D.
Associate Professor
Department of Pathology and Laboratory Medicine
Emory University School of Medicine
Grady Memorial Hospital
Atlanta, Georgia

Nanette Kass Wenger, M.D.
Professor of Medicine
Division of Cardiology
Emory University
School of Medicine
Director, Cardiac Clinics
Grady Memorial Hospital
Atlanta, Georgia

Sina Zaim, M.D.
Assistant Professor of Medicine (Cardiology)
Department of Internal Medicine
Emory University School of Medicine
Atlanta, Georgia

To
my parents,
teachers,
and my family
Lena, Katerina, and Basil.

FOREWORD

For almost 30 years, Dr. Michael B. Gravanis, a cardiac pathologist, has been closely associated with the cardiology division of our institution in the teaching and investigative arenas. He has spared no effort to explain to clinicians and trainees why cardiovascular disease is like it is—why it happens. His book, *Cardiovascular Disorders: Pathogenesis and Pathophysiology,* addresses the major cardiovascular problems in 17 chapters. Although a modest amount of text is devoted to cardiovascular diagnosis, treatment is not emphasized. Rather, a glance at the chapter titles suggests that the authors are looking at the problems from a different vantage point when compared with the usual approaches. This viewpoint is always useful because it forces a thought process that is different and often unconventional, but intriguing.

The book is dedicated to the inquisitive clinician and trainee who wants to know why the cardiovascular disorder occurred in the first place and why the structures are altered as they are. Dr. Gravanis and the contributors to the book discuss the genetic-molecular biologic-pathologic-physiologic information related to the major cardiovascular disorders.

As Dr. Gravanis writes in his preface, all of this new information is a part of the evolution of our knowledge about cardiovascular disease. Years ago we only correlated the clinical features of a disease with the pathologic findings. We then correlated the clinical features of disease with the altered anatomy and altered physiology. Now we must correlate the pathology and physiology with the emerging knowledge of molecular biology and genetics. Why should we?, you might ask. Because this new insight helps clinicians and trainees understand the value of a specific treatment and assists researchers in discovering new treatment modalities!

This extensively referenced book will meet many of the needs of students, house officers, fellows, and cardiologists who ask *why things are as they are.* Equally important, this first edition will serve as a foundation for subsequent editions because, it is clear, the type of information contained in this book will increase as time passes. This first edition places the reader in the vanguard of an era that is destined to be filled with change.

J. Willis Hurst, M.D.
Department of Medicine (Cardiology)
Emory University School of Medicine
Atlanta, Georgia

PREFACE

This volume on cardiovascular disorders was not designed to be either a book of cardiology or cardiovascular pathology. It was conceived, and we hope will be received, as primarily a book that focuses on pathogenetic mechanisms and pertinent pathophysiology of cardiac and vascular disease processes. The central concept for such presentation derives from our basic belief that, with only a few exceptions, structural changes correlate well with functional derangements, and that this correlative exercise creates an excellent foundation for studying and understanding disease processes. Moreover, the modest morphologic information incorporated in different chapters should serve to define the magnitude of the anatomic changes and enhance the appreciation of the level of functional derangements. A deliberate effort has been made, throughout the book, to bring to the bedside the molecular phenomena involved in the pathogenesis of cardiovascular disease. In doing so, we have cited investigative works from both humans and experimental models, as well as highlighted the difficulties in sorting out pathogenetic mechanisms in clinical heart disease.

Along with many other clinical investigators, we believe that application of molecular biology and related techniques holds great promise for the study of important clinical and experimental problems in cardiovascular medicine. Furthermore, we are convinced that we have entered an era in which medical therapy is no longer based on empirical observations, but on the clear understanding of molecular phenomena that control function.

As cardiology in the past moved from purely empiric treatments to those based on physiologic principles, it is widely expected that future steps would be towards strategies of therapy based on the fundamentals of molecular biology and molecular genetics. Similar to the demystification of hemodynamics of earlier decades, the goal of future practitioners of cardiology, as well as of academicians, should be familiarization of concepts of molecular cardiology.

The relevance of molecular biology in medicine has already become apparent in the utility of several drugs in our therapeutic armamentarium that are produced by genetic engineering and in the significant inroads that gene therapy is making in the practice of medicine.

Although this book covers in a comprehensive manner all pertinent cardiovascular diseases, the emphasis on selected disorders is designed to put into sharp focus present-day trends in the incidence and epidemiology.

Because this is a new book with no previous editions to confirm, we have had the opportunity to break new ground and be innovative without being iconoclastic, and to present new concepts without being dogmatic. We believe that this book is well suited to cardiologists and fellows in cardiology and should also be useful to cardiovascular pathologists engaged in the practice and teaching of this subspecialty.

ACKNOWLEDGMENTS

I am deeply indebted to
Sandra Estep for her assistance in library research and the preparation of many lengthy manuscripts.
Connie Wavrin for her most valuable contribution in the preparation of the pictorial material.

Many thanks to
Dr. Kenneth Dooley for his efforts in collecting the angiograms for the chapter on congenital heart disease.
Mosby, in particular Sandra Clark, also deserves our thanks for help and advice, commitment of resources, and determination to produce an attractive volume.

Last, but not least, I want to thank my thirteen-year-old son, Basil, for his undiminished enthusiasm in keeping my desk at home well supplied with writing material throughout the preparation of this book.

Michael B. Gravanis, M.D.
Editor

CONTENTS

Chapter 1

ATHEROGENESIS

W. Virgil Brown
Ngoc Anh Le
Michael B. Gravanis

Initiation
    Interactions of lipoproteins with endothelial cells
    Interaction of lipoproteins with monocytes
    Interactions of lipoproteins with smooth muscle cells
    Role of endothelial cell adhesion molecules
Proliferation
    Platelet-derived growth factor (PDGF)
    Transforming growth factor β (TCFβ)
    Interleukin-1 (IL-1)
    Tumor necrosis factor α (TNFα)
    Fibroblast growth factor (FGF)
    Colony-stimulating factor (CSF)
Hemodynamic factors in atherogenesis
Other theories of atherogenesis
    Tumor or monoclonal theory
    Viral theory

In spite of the steady decline in mortality rates from atherosclerosis, this vascular disorder remains the leading cause of death in the United States. Although much of the research focus has been on coronary atherosclerosis, it should be emphasized that the incidence of peripheral and cerebral atherosclerosis is just as high.[1,2] Atherosclerosis is a chronic disease that manifests itself as lipid deposits along the walls of blood vessels. Many morphologic studies have shown that the lesions of atherosclerosis begin as early as the second decade of life,[3] well before the onset of any clinically observable signs and symptoms. Atherosclerosis, which starts out as simple fatty lesions, is characterized by atheronecrosis, fibrosis, mineralization, hemorrhage, and/or ulceration.

The risk factors associated with atherosclerosis are numerous. Many risk factors, including serum cholesterol, cigarette smoking, obesity, and hypertension, have been demonstrated to have an effect on coronary heart disease mortality and morbidity.[4] When autopsy data from the 25-year follow-up of the Framingham Study were examined, serum cholesterol stood out as the only parameter that can be directly correlated to intimal involvement and/or luminal compromise.[4] Interestingly, correlation of systolic pressure with these two parameters characterizing the severity of the lesions could only be demonstrated in women.[4]

The direct link between serum cholesterol and atherosclerosis is further supported by a number of clinical trials and population-based epidemiologic studies, as well as metabolic and histologic investigations. Because 60% of the serum cholesterol is transported by the low density lipoproteins (LDL) it was not surprising when apoB, the primary protein component of LDL, was localized in arteriosclerotic plaques. The Collaborative Coronary Prevention Trial of the Lipid Research Clinics (CPPT-LRC) was one of the first multicenter primary prevention trials that was successful in demonstrating that a reduction in LDL-Cholesterol by 2 mg/dl can result in a 1% reduction in risk for coronary artery disease (CAD).[5] More recently, several clinical trials have been able to confirm this association. The Cholesterol Lowering Atherosclerosis Study (CLAS) went a step further when it reported that regression of the lesions could be demonstrated with aggressive cholesterol lowering therapy.[6]

Attention has also been directed in recent years to an antigenic variant of LDL, the lipoprotein Lp (a) also called apolipoprotein (a). Although this lipoprotein is present in

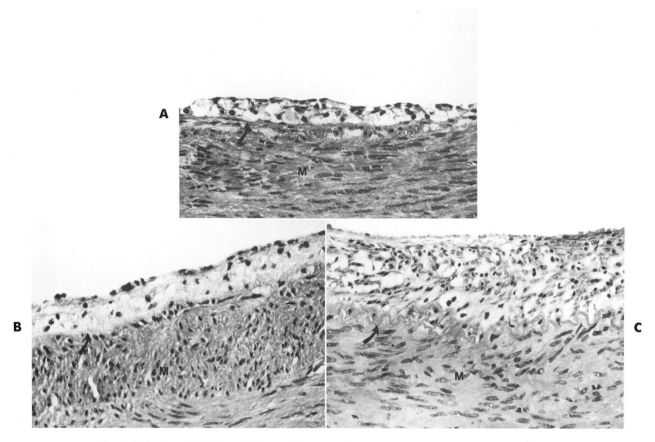

Fig. 1-1. A, B, and **C,** Several phases of fatty streak development. Note that the foamy cell accumulation is subendothelial, the endothelium is intact and the internal elastica well-preserved (arrow). The media (M) is uninvolved.

the plasma of most people, epidemiologic studies have shown that high levels of Lp (a) increase the risk of coronary artery disease and atherosclerosis in general. Blood levels of Lp (a) appear to be genetically determined. Molecular studies revealed that apo (a) resembles plasminogen; therefore it may be the missing link between lipoproteins and the coagulation system. It has been suggested that Lp (a) acts as a vehicle that delivers cholesterol to the vascular lesions, or perhaps acts as an inhibitor of plasminogen activator at a site of an evolving thrombus.[7] Lp (a) may interfere in the plasminogen plasmin conversion and thus prevent thrombolysis. However, the precise mechanism of action of this additional risk factor in atherosclerosis has not been clearly elucidated. Most of our information about its adverse effect on atherogenesis is derived from epidemiologic studies, although apo (a) and apo B have been detected in the wall of the coronary arteries.[8]

Although a number of factors are associated with the atherosclerotic process, the exact mechanism by which the fatty streak is actually initiated, evolves from the lipid deposition phase to an occluded vessel, and finally becomes an end-stage lesion, is not clearly understood.

In the following sections we will attempt to summarize some of the data regarding the cellular components that are known to be involved in this process, and their interactions and role in the development of this disorder.

INITIATION

Available data indicate that two processes are of paramount importance in the initiation of the atherogenic cascade: (1) increased endothelial transcytosis of plasma LDL, which accumulates in the proteoglycan-rich subendothelial space; and (2) preferential recruitment of blood monocytes to the intima, a process augmented by hyperlipidemia.[9]

Pinocytotic vesicles are the mechanism that in all likelihood accounts for the influx of LDL into the subendothelial space at lesion-prone sites.[10] The second process, monocyte recruitment to the intima of lesion-prone areas, is carried out by chemoattractants (MCP-1) secreted by both smooth muscle cells and endothelial cells.

The fatty streak is a lesion that appears in the aorta in the first decade of life and shows up somewhat later in the coronary and cerebral arteries. Fatty streaks may be seen by the naked eye as slightly raised, yellow lesions that are

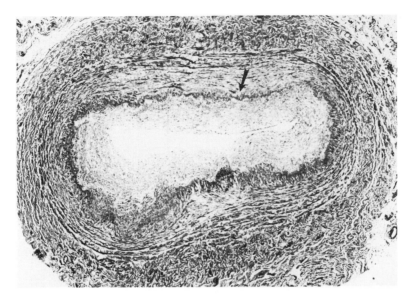

Fig. 1-2. Coronary artery from a young adult showing circumferential intimal hyperplasia with an intact internal elastica (arrow) and wide open lumen. Elastic stain.

relatively narrow and longitudinally-oriented.[11] Fatty streaks are characterized by subendothelial accumulation of foam cells, the cytoplasms of which contain cholesteryl esters and free cholesterol (Fig. 1-1). Studies using monoclonal antibodies reveal that a significant majority of the foam cells in fatty streaks are macrophages; only the minority of foam cells are of smooth muscle origin.[12] The recognized smooth muscle cells resemble the so-called secretory phenotype of arterial smooth muscle cells (dense bodies).[13]

In early phases of atherogenesis (young adults), which precede the development of the fibrous plaque, smooth muscle cells are known to acquire lipid. With progression of the fatty streak the smooth muscle cells increase in number (compared with macrophages) and finally become the dominant cell. The distribution of the two cellular populations (smooth muscle cells, macrophages) in the fatty streak is different, as has been shown with specific-antibodies. Macrophage-derived foam cells (identified by HAM56) are primarily located in the upper and middle layers of the lesion. However, contrary to previous studies, smooth muscle-derived foam cells (identified by HHF35) are found predominantly in the deeper layers of the lesion, next to the underlying media.[14] It appears, though, that the cellular composition in more advanced human lesions (fibrofatty plaque) might be different from that observed in the early lesions. Only a minimal amount of extracellular lipid is present in fatty streaks, along with some collagen fibrils, elastin, and proteoglycans. Currently, the fatty streak is widely thought to be the precursor of the fibrofatty plaque,[15] although not all fatty streaks necessarily progress into advanced fibrofatty plaques. Al-

though the fatty streaks are of universal occurrence and distribution, most of them, particularly those in the aorta, either remain harmless or disappear, although in certain arteries (coronary) they may evolve into fibrous plaques.

Perhaps it is important to stress that the fatty streak lesion develops under a structurally intact endothelium, although the endothelium has been described as thinned and attenuated, often revealing distortion and bulges caused by the underlying foam cells. This anatomic integrity of the endothelium in the fatty streak is obviously in conflict with the view, held widely for many years, that the initiating event in atherogenesis is loss of endothelial cells (endothelial injury hypothesis).[16] Alternative theories to the endothelial injury hypothesis have been proposed.[17] One such hypothesis stresses that the presence of macrophages under an intact endothelium poses a potential threat because these cells are known to possess and release cytotoxic factors (superoxide anion), and proteolytic and lipolytic enzymes that may damage the overlying endothelium. After this endothelial loss occurs, all the processes proposed by the endothelial injury hypothesis (e.g., adherence of platelets and release of PDGF) may begin to take place.[17]

Besides the fatty streak, other precursor lesions exist, particularly in childhood. Studies of the proximal portion of the left anterior descending (LAD) coronary artery in several hundred children and young adults have shown a lesion often referred to as diffuse intimal thickening.[18] At this site of the coronary artery, the intima early in life may be as thick as the media (Fig. 1-2). The increased thickness results from the presence of collagen, elastin, proteoglycans, and fibronectins. Cells present within the matrix are macrophages, T-lymphocytes, and smooth muscle

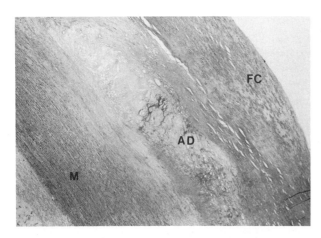

Fig. 1-3. Established atheromatous plaque. The fibrous cap (FC) contains numerous smooth muscle cells and collagen. The inner media (M) adjacent to the atheromatous debris (AD) appears fibrotic and distorted.

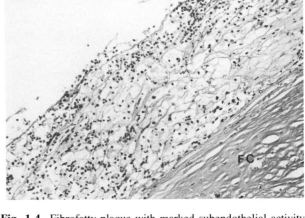

Fig. 1-4. Fibrofatty plaque with marked subendothelial activity. Note foamy cells and monocytes internal to an established fibous cap (FC).

cells. One may be tempted to interpret this intimal thickening as a normal response to hemodynamic or other stresses at certain anatomic sites of the coronary system. Occasionally, the intimal thickening is focal and cushion-like, suggesting a potential for later evolution into a fibrofatty plaque.[19]

Atheromatous plaques are rounded, raised lesions of various shapes and sizes: they also reveal certain histologic variability (Fig. 1-3). A typical fibrofatty plaque consists of a fibrous cap (which limits the lesion from the arterial lumen), and is composed of connective tissue containing elastin, collagen fibrils, proteoglycans, basement membrane, smooth muscle cells, and a few leukocytes (Fig. 1-4).[20,21] The area beneath and beside the cap (plaque shoulders) has a mixture of smooth muscle cells, T-lymphocytes, and macrophages; it is here that neovascularization is most obvious (Fig. 1-5).[22] The deep necrotic core of a fibrofatty plaque consists of cellular debris, extracellular lipid, cholesterol crystals, and numerous foam cells of the macrophage and smooth muscle type. The media of the vessel wall at the site of the plaque is thin, and calcium deposits are seen within the layers of the collagenous cap or in association with extracellular lipid. The adventitia appears fibrotic with areas of neovascularization and lymphocytic infiltration.

Interactions of lipoproteins with endothelial cells

The endothelium, in addition to serving as a barrier in the regulation of lipoprotein transport to the extravascular space and to the arterial subendothelial space, also provides support for lipoprotein lipase, which plays a central role in the distribution of dietary and endogenous triglycerides to the periphery (Fig. 1-6). Indirect toxic effects on the endothelium may be induced by excessively elevated

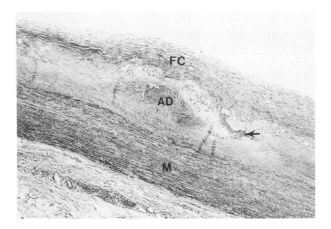

Fig. 1-5. Established atheromatous plaque. Note fibrous cap (FC), atheromatous debrib (AD), thinned out media (M) and neovascularization (arrow).

concentrations of the products of the hydrolysis of the triglyceride-rich lipoproteins, intestinally-derived chylomicrons, and hepatic very low-density lipoproteins. Elevated concentrations of triglyceride-poor and cholesterol-rich remnant lipoproteins (low-density lipoproteins, or LDL), such as those found in most common forms of hypercholesterolemia, have also been shown to damage endothelial cells in culture.[22,23] High-density lipoproteins (HDL), on the other hand, seem to have a protective effect on endothelial cell growth in culture.[24,25] This effect would be consistent with epidemiologic data on the antiatherogenic properties of HDL.

With respect to the triglyceride-rich chylomicrons of intestinal origin, which are present in the postprandial state, the endothelium appears to provide more than the supporting matrix for lipoprotein lipase. Studies both in the perfused heart and in cultured endothelial cells have shown that chylomicrons can bind to a specific surface receptor

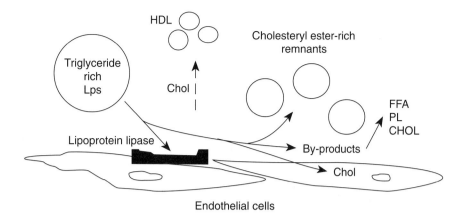

Fig. 1-6. Interactions of lipoproteins with endothelial cells. Triglyceride-rich lipoproteins se-creted by the intestine and by the liver interact with lipoprotein lipase, which is attached to the endothelial cells. The products of this hydrolytic action include free fatty acids, free glycerol, sur-face remnants composed of phospholipids and cholesterol, and lipoprotein particles enriched in cholesteryl esters. High density lipoproteins (HDL), serve as an acceptor for the surface remnants and may also mediate the efflux of cholesterol out of the cells.

on endothelial cells. This receptor has been demonstrated to be different from the LDL receptor. Cholesteryl esters from these intestinal lipoproteins are hydrolyzed with con-comitant degradation of the apoprotein component. The significance of this interaction in atherogenesis is yet to be examined, but excessive supply of free cholesterol to the endothelial cells could potentially lead to cell damage. The question of whether simple exposure to a high concentra-tion of cholesterol-rich lipoproteins will cause endothelial cells to release specific growth factors that may be in-volved in cell proliferation remains unanswered (see be-low).

It has also been suggested that platelet aggregation may be affected by interactions between plasma lipoproteins and endothelial cells as mediated via the prostacyclin path-way. Prostacyclin secreted by endothelial cells has been shown to inhibit platelet aggregation.[26] This process is be-lieved to be potentially important in preventing thrombosis and in suppressing the development of atherosclerotic le-sions. LDL has been reported to inhibit the conversion of arachidonic acid to prostacyclin,[27] whereas HDL appeared to stimulate the formation of prostacyclin in endothelial cells.[28] This dysfunction of cultured endothelial cells by LDL also included decreased membrane fluidity[29] and heightened endocytosis.

How do plasma lipoproteins exert their effect on endo-thelial cells? A high affinity receptor pathway in endothe-lial cells has been characterized specifically for LDL.[30] This uptake pathway for LDL, however, shows saturation at relatively low concentrations of LDL and thus may not contribute significantly to LDL accumulation. A second nonspecific pathway with 100-fold the capacity of the high affinity pathway is also available for the uptake and degra-dation of LDL, presumably via either absorptive endocyto-

sis or fluid-phase pinocytosis or both. Since the endothelial cell receptor appears to be saturated at LDL levels that are far below the plasma concentration, one would have to conclude that a large part of LDL transendothelial trans-port in vitro may occur via nonsaturable nonspecific path-ways.

By far, the most important interaction of endothelial cells with LDL in vitro would have to be the chemical modification of plasma LDL, which results in significant increases in the rate of uptake of these particles by macro-phages as compared with the metabolism of native LDL. Exposure of LDL to human cultured endothelial cells re-sulted in more dense particles of higher electrophoretic mobility, which are relatively poor in cholesterol. This modification is specific and limited to LDL only.[31] Avail-able data would suggest that EC-modified LDL is less ef-ficiently metabolized by cells expressing normal LDL re-ceptor activity but is preferentially metabolized by mono-nuclear phagocytes. Prolonged incubation of native LDL with cultured smooth muscle cells has also been shown to result in the formation of oxidized LDL, which is also rap-idly taken up by macrophages, with subsequent increases in the cholesterol content in the cell.

The possibility that the endothelium may restrict the transport of LDL from the subendothelial space back into plasma has not been adequately investigated.

Interactions of lipoproteins with monocytes

Although the mechanisms via which the cholesterol-rich LDL can be transported across the intact endothelium and accumulate within the subintimal space of an apparently normal artery[32,33] are still poorly understood, this process can be shown to occur in the rabbit model within days of initiating a high cholesterol regimen. Shortly after this ini-

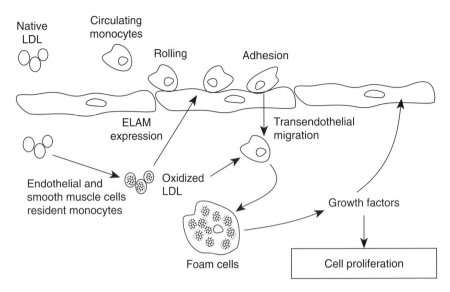

Fig. 1-7. Processes associated with the initiation of the atherosclerotic lesion. It has been postulated that as the functional integrity of the endothelial cells is altered, they become more permeable to LDL infiltration. These lipoproteins found in the subendothelial space are believed to be modified and are now capable of stimulating the expression of specific adhesion molecules on the surface of endothelial cells. With the expression of these adhesion molecules, the "rolling" monocytes adhere to the endothelial cells and monocyte transmigration is increased. Within the subendothelial space, the monocytes rapidly take up the modified lipoproteins via scavenger receptors, become foam cells, and begin releasing growth factors. These growth factors cause the expression and release of additional cytokines that further increase the transmigration of blood monocytes. The growth factors also initiate the proliferation process via their interactions with the smooth muscle cells in the supporting basement membrane. A recent report suggests that increased permeability to LDL may not be necessary for the expression of certain adhesion molecules.[36]

tial accumulation, circulating monocytes begin to adhere to the luminal surface of the overlying endothelium. Thus monocyte attachment to the endothelium is considered an important component in the atherogenic process.[34,35]

The linkage between LDL and endothelial cell binding of monocytes is still a mystery. As discussed above, low concentrations of biologically modified LDL or high concentrations of native LDL can affect the binding of monocytes to endothelial cells. A recent report indicated that at an LDL concentration of 240 mg/dl, the affinity of endothelial cells for monocytes can be demonstrated within 2 days.[36] These investigators also demonstrated that this effect is specific to LDL because incubation of HDL with endothelial cells did not increase monocyte adherence; neither did conditioned media from LDL-treated endothelial cells (Fig. 1-7).[37]

Regardless of whether the LDL-treated endothelial cells have been injured or have simply been activated, it has now been demonstrated that they express novel surface adhesion proteins: the endothelial cell-leukocyte adhesion molecules (ELAM) (see below). An excellent review of the role of ELAM in the development of atherosclerosis has recently been presented by Berman and Calderon.[38]

After monocytes become residents within the subintimal

space, their phenotypic expression is profoundly altered. The factors involved in these changes, however, have not been completely described. Regardless of what these mechanisms are, after the monocyte has changed to a macrophage, it begins to rapidly take up the cholesterol-rich LDL. This undoubtedly has to be the most damaging event in atherogenesis, ultimately resulting in the formation of foam cells within the subintimal space (Fig. 1-8). Although macrophages express the receptor for native LDL, the nonspecific scavenger receptors are believed to be the principal factor in foam cell formation. Data in support of this pathway came from several lines of research. As with other cell lines, the LDL receptor in macrophages is downregulated with exposure to high concentration of LDL in vitro; thus the formation of foam cells could not be achieved in vitro with native LDL alone. Furthermore, studies in patients with homozygote familial hypercholesterolemia as well as those in the receptor-deficient Watanabe Heritable Hyperlipidemic (WHHL) rabbit have documented a severe and rapid development of atherosclerosis despite a total lack of LDL receptors. The scavenger receptors have been shown to avidly take up chemically modified LDL via a saturable pathway which could not be downregulated. Several forms of chemically modified

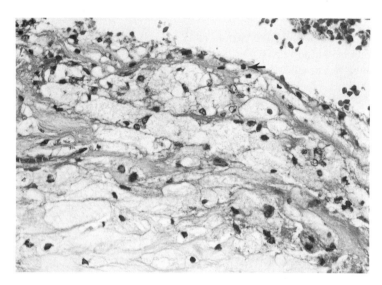

Fig. 1-8. Early phase of atherogenesis. Note subendothelial accumulation of foamy cells (macrophages and smooth muscle cells) and adherent monocytes *(arrow)* on the endothelium.

LDL have been shown to be taken up via this scavenger pathway, including acetylated LDL and malodialdehyde-conjugated LDL. Although data from in vitro studies were very convincing, there was little evidence that such chemical modifications occurred to any extent in vivo.

As discussed in the preceding sections, exposure of LDL to cultured endothelial cells was reported to generate a subpopulation of LDL particles that are taken up by macrophages at two to four times the rate seen with native LDL. Furthermore, this uptake process cannot be inhibited by the presence of excess native LDL in the medium. Several investigators were successful in demonstrating that the cell-induced modification of LDL was initiated as the result of peroxidation of polyunsaturated fatty acids present in the LDL lipids, and that this modification was inhibited by the presence of antioxidants in the medium, such as butylated hydroxytoluene (BHT) or vitamin E.[39,40,41]

Several lines of evidence have now been developed to support the hypothesis that oxidized LDLs not only occur in vivo but also are directly linked to the atherosclerotic process. LDL eluted from atherosclerotic lesions (but not from the normal arteries) have been shown to have many of the physical properties found in LDL oxidized in vitro.[42] Immunochemical localization of oxidized LDL has been demonstrated in lesions using monoclonal antibodies against oxidation-specific epitopes present in oxidized LDL but absent in native LDL.[43] Studies in WHHL rabbit treated with probucol, a lipid-lowering agent that has been shown to be a potent anti-oxidant,[44] indicated that the marked reduction observed in the atherosclerosis of the probucol-treated animals (as compared with the lovastatin-treated animals) could not be explained by the degree of cholesterol lowering.[45,46]

Preliminary data from Uhlinger and co-workers[47] seemed to suggest that certain plasma components present in the circulation during the postprandial period may increase the ability of leukocytes to generate superoxide in response to specific agonists by at least twofold. This increase in superoxide generation could be demonstrated within 4 hours of the consumption of a single fat-containing meal and remained in effect for up to 9 hours after the meal. Whether this burst of free radicals from neutrophils during the postprandial state could lead to the formation of oxidized LDL and thus contribute to the atherogenic role of postprandial lipemia is not clear.

Interactions of lipoproteins with smooth muscle cells

Smooth muscle cells (SMC) can chemically modify LDL by free radical oxidation and thus contribute directly to the generation of foam cells in the subintimal space.[40] Smooth muscle cells can also accumulate lipids and form foam cells.[9] As discussed in other sections, the contribution of smooth muscle cells to the atherosclerotic process is most apparent in the formation and secretion of a whole battery of growth factors by macrophages and endothelial cells. The resulting cell proliferation leads to progression and enlargement of the atherosclerotic lesion and ultimately to the occlusion of the artery.

Smooth muscle cells are present in both the fatty streak and the fibrofatty plaque, where they constitute the predominant cell type. Synthetic functions attributed to smooth muscle cells include connective tissue matrix, collagen, elastic tissue, and proteoglycans.[19,20]

Perhaps loss of an inhibitory mechanism in the arterial wall initiates smooth muscle proliferation in the media and intima. This function has been attributed to molecules secreted by endothelial cells[48] and by smooth muscle cells themselves.[49] Smooth muscle cells respond also to chemotactic factors and therefore migrate to the intima. Furthermore, smooth muscle cells involved in atherogenesis may express certain features of immature smooth muscle cells, as has been shown by a monoclonal antibody. This antibody (10F3) identifies a cell surface 90 kd protein present on smooth muscle cells of 7- to 8-week-old fetal human aorta. Although this antigen is lost during maturation of these mesenchymal cells, it is reexpressed in atherosclerotic lesions.[50] Expression of this antigen (ICAM-1, or intercellular adhesion molecule 1) was noted in both early and advanced atherosclerotic lesions. Inflammatory mediators such as interferon gamma, IL-1, and TNF may induce ICAM-1 expression in a wide variety of cell types, and increase binding of monocytes to mesenchymal cells.[51]

Role of endothelial cell adhesion molecules

Although the contribution of the cholesterol-rich lipoproteins in the formation of the fatty streak cannot be denied, several key events involving the circulating monocytes and the endothelium must occur for the atherogenic process to be initiated. One hypothesis has been that exposure of the endothelium to high levels of cholesterol may alter the metabolic function of endothelial cells. A number of cytokines and growth factors could also elicit a similar response from the endothelial cells. After endothelial cells have been injured, or activated, the ability of circulating hematopoietic elements to adhere to the surface of affected vessels is believed to play a key role in the development of atherosclerosis.[23,52] This increase in adhesion is mediated by the expression of specific adhesion molecules called endothelial cell adhesion molecules, or ELAMs. The genes for most of these adhesion proteins have been cloned, sequenced, and identified as members of two distinct families—the immunoglobulin gene superfamily, and the vascular selectins.[53,54]

As part of the activation of the endothelial cells, adhesion molecules are expressed on the membrane of endothelial cells concomitant with the expression of a matching series of adhesion molecules on the monocytes and T-lymphocytes. The casual reversible attachment of circulating leukocytes to the arterial wall has now become tight adherence. This is followed by transmigration of the monocytes into the subendothelial space of the intima. As the monocytes become transformed to foam cells, they elaborate a battery of cytokines that, in conjunction with other growth factors elaborated by endothelial and smooth muscle cells, are responsible for the cell proliferation associated with the early atherosclerotic lesions. As the lesions become complex plaques with the accumulation of foam cells, cholesterol, smooth muscle cells, and extracellular matrix, leukocytes continue to be recruited, and the secretion of a variety of cytokines is maintained.

PROLIFERATION

In spite of the fact that arteriosclerosis is the most common form of proliferative diseases, little is actually known regarding the rates of proliferation and the types of cells involved, as well as the interactions among the various cell types that ultimately are responsible for the progression of these lesions. As discussed in the preceding section, the fatty streak associated with the initial lesion of atherosclerosis consists primarily of lipid-filled, monocytes-derived macrophages, the so-called foam cells. The subsequent transformation to the fibrous plaque (the advanced form of the arteriosclerotic lesion) is dependent on the interplay of several growth-regulatory molecules. These molecules, which can both stimulate and/or inhibit cell proliferation, are key factors in determining whether the potentially occlusive fibrous plaque lesions will progress, regress, or remain unchanged.[55]

All through this growth process, it should be clear that leukocytes and monocytes continue to infiltrate the intima and could contribute significantly to the volume of the developing plaque.[56] A significant component of plaque growth could theoretically be accounted for by cellular migration into the intima without the need for cell proliferation. The identification of smooth muscle cell as the principal mesenchymal cell in human atherosclerotic plaques has generated a flurry of research to identify growth factors that can stimulate smooth muscle proliferation. The presence of alternating layers of leukocytes and smooth muscle cells in the intermediate developing lesion would suggest that the process of leukocyte infiltration and smooth muscle proliferation may be episodic or continuous, depending on the circumstances. The timing and relative contribution of these two processes are of extreme importance in understanding the progression of the atherosclerotic plaque.

One of the strongest suggestions that smooth muscle cell proliferation is integral to human plaque growth came from the studies of Benditt[57,58,59] and others, which demonstrated that most early plaques are monoclonal in nature. Data on the rate of cell growth in the atherosclerotic plaque had to wait until the development of proliferation-specific antibodies, e.g., antibodies to the proliferating cell nuclear antigen (PCNA).[60]

The primary growth factors include: platelet-derived growth factor (PDGF), fibroblast-derived growth factor (FGF), colony-stimulating factor (CSF), transforming growth factor β (TGFβ), interleukin-1 (IL-1), and tumor necrosis factor α (TNFα).

Platelet-derived growth factor

PDGF is a potent mitogenic and chemotactic factor for connective tissue cells such as smooth muscle cells. Several recent reviews that deal with the characteristics and action of PDGF are available.[61,62,63]

Of importance in understanding the physiologic action of PDGF is the fact that it is actually composed of two polypeptide chains (A and B) joined by disulfide bonds, and may occur in the form of a heterodimer (AB) or as homodimers of the A chain (AA) or B chain (BB). The A chain is coded on human chromosome 7, whereas the B chain has been localized to human chromosome 22. Although all three forms can induce similar chemotactic and proliferative responses, the receptors responsible for the recognition of PDGF have unique affinities for the different forms of PDGF. The A chain can only bind to one of the two receptor forms, the α-receptor subunit, whereas the B chain can bind to either the α- or the β-subunit.

The ability of PDGF to function as both a chemotactic and a mitogenic agent has been known for some time, but the direct presence of PDGF in human atherosclerotic lesions has only been demonstrated recently.[64] The source of this PDGF has now been identified in both human and nonhuman primate lesions as the monocyte-derived macrophages.[65]

Transforming growth factor β (TGFβ)

This molecule appears to have a dual function. At low concentrations TGFβ has been shown by Battegay[66] et al, to induce PDGF gene expression, specific for the A chain, PDGF-AA synthesis, and secretion and autocrine stimulation of connective tissue cells, including arterial smooth muscle cells. As the concentrations of TGFβ were increased, inhibition of smooth muscle proliferation was demonstrated.[66] This has been shown to result from the downregulation of the mRNA for the PDGF receptor.[66]

TGFβ is also a very potent catalyst of connective tissue synthesis. Thus TGFβ, which can be secreted by all of the cells known to be involved in the process of atherogenesis, can induce synthesis and secretion of various forms of collagen, proteoglycans, and elastic fiber macromolecules. Therefore in addition to its role in cell proliferation, TGFβ may be an important factor in the fibrosis associated with advance lesions. A number of reviews on the functions of TGFβ are available.[67,68]

Interleukin-1 (IL-1)

The cytokine IL-1 is one of the most widely known products of activated macrophages, which account for 80% to 90% of the cells identified in the initial lesion of atherosclerosis. In vitro studies have implicated IL-1 as a growth-regulatory molecule for smooth muscle cells and fibroblasts. IL-1 itself is not a direct mitogen but is believed to affect cell proliferation via secondary gene induction in a fashion similar to TGFβ.[69] IL-1 is similar to FGF in that it cannot be released from intact cells and is found in the medium following cell lysis. Several reviews on the functions and characteristics of IL-1 are available.[70,71]

Tumor necrosis factor α (TNFα)

TNFα, which is commonly associated with injury and inflammation,[72] is another of a group of cytokines which may play a role in the process of atherogenesis. Available evidence would suggest that TNFα, IL-1, and TGFβ do not act as direct initiators of cell proliferation but as effectors of secondary gene induction. Several cell types can release TNFα, including activated macrophages and endothelium. Hajjar et al[73] have reported that upon its binding to arterial endothelial cells, TNFα can induce secondary gene expression for PDGF B-chain and PDGF-BB synthesis and secretion by these cells. At the site of injury where TNFα is believed to be present as a product of activated macrophages, secondary gene expression, synthesis, and secretion of PDGF may occur.

Fibroblast growth factor

FGF consists of a single peptide and is recognized by a high-affinity cell-surface receptor that shares many of the characteristics of the PDGF receptors. Interactions of FGF with its receptor induces a series of mitogenic signals that are similar to those induced by PDGF. In contrast to PDGF, FGF appears to be localized within the macrophages, and can be released only if injury and lysis of these cells occur.[74] FGF has been suggested to play an important role in vivo in smooth muscle proliferative processes that occur after angioplasty in a rabbit model of balloon catheter deendothelialization.[75]

Colony-stimulating factor

The involvement of CSF (either monocyte CSF or granulocyte-monocyte CSF) in atherosclerotic lesions has been implied from a variety of experimental data demonstrating macrophage proliferation within the lesions of atherosclerosis in the rabbit[76] and nonhuman primate,[77] as well as in man.[78]

Although all of the cells that are potentially involved in atherogenesis, e.g., arterial endothelium, smooth muscle, macrophage, and T-lymphocytes, are capable of synthesizing and secreting CSF,[79,80] the nature of the stimulus in vivo is still not known.

HEMODYNAMIC FACTORS IN ATHEROGENESIS

Although atherogenesis arises from abnormal interactions between cellular elements in the vessel wall and blood-borne components, the entire process takes place in a milieu where hemodynamics play a central role. Atherosclerotic lesions are commonly found in the regions of arterial curvatures and branch orifices that have been reported to display increased intimal permeability.[81] At branch orifices, damage to endothelial cells can be seen in nontreated control animals. The severity of the damage can range from crateriform and balloon-like vesicular defects to focal areas of cellular desquamation.[82,83,84] Accumulation of platelet aggregates and deposition of leukocytes have also been reported to be predominant in the same sites.

Shear stress, which acts parallel to the axis of the blood vessel, represents the drag (or friction force) of the blood on the luminal surface and is independent of turbulence. It is proportional to the blood viscosity and rate of flow, and inversely proportional to the luminal radius. Shear stress is expected to be high in areas of arterial constriction, such as coarctation, arteriosclerotic stenosis, or arterial spasm. Ku et al[85] have suggested that atherosclerotic plaques tend to develop in those parts of the branch orifice where shear forces are relatively low. In other words, increased shear forces may exert a protective effect for the development of atherosclerotic lesions.

Lateral pressure force, commonly associated with hypertension, acts perpendicular to the axis of flow and is thought to facilitate the interaction of fluid and elements of the blood with the vascular wall. Studies with experimental hypertension have shown that elevated arterial pressure increases the permeability of the vessel wall to lipids.[86,87] Thus increased lateral pressure might alter lipid transport directly by pressure damage to the endothelial barrier, or indirectly through some form of minimal cellular damage that may interfere with normal metabolic processes.

One manifestation of the actions of different hemodynamic forces on the vascular wall in atherogenesis is commonly known as coronary vasospasm. Considerable evidence has accumulated implicating coronary vasospasm as a contributory factor to classic angina pectoris and acute myocardial infarction.[88,89,90] Coronary vasospasms, like atherosclerotic stenosis, may result in myocardial ischemia and/or infarction not only as a result of marked reduction in coronary flow but also as a result of endothelial damage. The possibility that coronary arterial spasm might itself contribute to the initiation of atherogenesis has been suggested on the basis of observations of endothelial damage and platelet attachment at these sites in experimental systems.[91] The endothelial damage at sites of spasm would be followed by platelet attachment to exposed subendothelial tissues, infiltration by lipoproteins and lipid-laden macrophages, and proliferation and intimal migration of arterial smooth muscle cells.[92]

Kawachi et al[93] examined the relationship between coronary hyperactivity and the presence of vascular changes induced by endothelial denudation and a high cholesterol diet in dogs. Although minimal differences could be noted between the denuded and the intact sites in the early stages, by 1 month the denuded sites constricted more than the intact sites. This was interpreted to suggest that functional changes had occurred locally that were reflected in modification of the response to vasoactive stimuli. From studies in minature pigs, a close correlation between spastic sites and histologically documented atheromatosis was observed, in spite of the absence of coronary lesions as as-

sessed by angiographic techniques.[94] Activation of multiple receptor-operated calcium channels has been proposed as the cause of coronary spasm in the atherosclerotic swine model.[95,96]

Clinical evidence for this pathogenetic relationship, however, is not very extensive.[97,98] In his review, Gutstein[99] emphasized that, in spite of the scarcity of clinical data, the wealth of experimental data supporting the relationship between coronary vasospasm and atherosclerosis justify a closer look at this hypothesis.

OTHER THEORIES OF ATHEROGENESIS

Up to now, we have not directly addressed the various hypotheses for the steps involved in the initiation of the fatty lesion. The view presented in the preceding section is based on the concept that some changes in the endothelium have occurred that facilitate the deposit of lipid-carrying particles, which in turn elicit a variety of responses from the surrounding cells. The insudation-inflammation theory, more commonly known as the injury hypothesis, holds that atherosclerosis is initiated by local intimal injury that is followed by the increased passage (imbibition or insudation) and accumulation of blood constituents (fluid and cellular) from the arterial lumen into the intima. This initial insudation results in an inflammatory process with edema, fatty degeneration of the intimal cells, and connective tissue proliferation in reaction to the degenerative mucoid pool. The so-called lipid hypothesis, on the other hand, would lead us to believe that abnormally elevated concentrations of extracellular lipids are themselves capable of contributing to the initiation of the atherogenic process. Several reviews addressing these more common views of the pathogenesis of atherosclerosis can be found. We will, however, focus the remainder of the discussion on two less well-known theories of atherogenesis.

Tumor or monoclonal theory

Although support for this theory is not widespread, it has yet to be disproved. Benditt and Benditt[57-58] suggested that individual atherosclerotic lesions are cloned from single smooth muscle cells that serve as progenitors for all subsequent cells. This was based on their observations that most individual atherosclerotic lesions from subjects with glucose-6-phosphate dehydrogenase (G6PD) deficiency contained either one or the other of the two isoenzymes. According to this theory, each atherosclerotic lesion represents a benign neoplasm derived from a cell that has been subjected to mutation by noxious agents, such as chemical or viral agents.[57]

Viral theory

A possible link between viral infection and atherosclerosis was first suggested by the observations of Paterson and Cottral[100] on the nature of the arteriosclerotic lesions in chicken infected by a viral agent and of Fabricant et al[101] on the formation of cholesterol crystal in cell cultures infected with a feline herpesvirus. These associations were extended to the case of human atherosclerotic plaques by the early work of Benditt and Benditt.[57-58] Support for this hypothesis also came from a series of reports from Fabricant and coworkers demonstrating the development of virus-induced atherosclerosis in the presence of normal cholesterol concentrations.[102,103]

Herpes viruses induce an arterial lesion characteristic of leukocytoclastic vasculitis. The lesion is associated with many events commonly associated with the classical atherosclerotic lesion, including granulocyte infiltration in the artery, thrombin formation, and fibrin deposition.[104] The finding that the virus can cause in animals a fatty proliferative lesion that occasionally contains microthrombin would support the hypothesis that surface expression of adhesion molecules and intimal hyperplasia may be initiated by a virally induced event.[105] This may in turn trigger cell proliferation by elaboration of growth factors and/or by release of cytokines from vascular cells and adherent monocytes.

A direct seroepidemiologic link between cytomegalovirus (CMV) infection and atherosclerosis has been suggested.[106] Epidemiologic link between infection with herpes viruses and atherosclerosis in humans could be demonstrated in the heart transplant population. Several studies have demonstrated a strong correlation between CMV infection and accelerated atherosclerosis.[107,108]

A vascular CMV infection may injure endothelial cells or reduce the anticoagulant properties of EC.[109] It has also been shown that CMV infection induces an upregulation of major histocompatibility (MHC) antigen expression by smooth muscle cells and endothelial cells.[110] MHC antigen upregulation is probably mediated by release of γ-interferon by activated T-lymphocytes in reaction to the viral infection.

Association of the herpes virus with atherosclerotic lesions has been demonstrated by a number of studies using a variety of tools, from the electron microscope[111] to in situ hybridization,[112] to polymerase chain reaction.[113] The presence of herpes viruses could also be demonstrated in the coronary arteries and the aorta of young trauma victims without clinical arteriosclerosis.[114]

The data above clearly indicate that some degree of immunologic activation is associated with human atherosclerosis. It does not, however, clarify whether the immune response plays a primary role or is merely a secondary phenomenon to antigenic stimuli arising within the plaque. Even though the answer to those speculations might not be forthcoming, the possibility still exists that immune mechanisms, even if secondary, contribute to atherogenesis.[115]

REFERENCES

1. Salonen R, Seppanne K, Rauramma R: Prevalence of carotid atherosclerosis and serum cholesterol levels in Eastern Finland, *Arteriosclerosis* 8:788, 1988.
2. Kannel WB, Wolf PE, Verter J: Manifestations of coronary disease predisposing to stroke, *JAMA* 250:2942, 1983.
3. Strong JP: Coronary atherosclerosis soldiers: a clue to the natural history of atherosclerosis in the young, *JAMA* 256:2863, 1986.
4. Kannel WB, Sorlie P, Brand F, et al: *Epidemiology of coronary atherosclerosis: postmortem vs clinical risk factor correlations. The Framingham Study.* In Gotto AM Jr, Smith LC, Allen B, eds: *Atherosclerosis V,* New York, 1979, Springer-Verlag.
5. Lipid Research Clinics Program. The Lipid Research Clinics Coronary Primary Prevention Trial results. II. The relationship of reduction in incidence of coronary heart disease to cholesterol lowering, *JAMA* 251:365, 1984.
6. Blankenhorn DH, Nessim SA, Johnson RL, et al: Beneficial effects of combined colestipol-niacin therapy on coronary atherosclerosis and coronary venous bypass grafts, *JAMA* 257:3233, 1987.
7. Hegele RA: Lipoprotein (a): a emerging risk factor for atherosclerosis, *Can J Cardiol* 5:263, 1989.
8. Rath M, Niendorf A, Reblin T, et al: Detection and quantification of lipoprotein (a) in the arterial wall of 107 coronary bypass patients, *Arteriosclerosis* 9:579, 1989.
9. Schwartz CJ, Valente AJ, Sprague EA, et al: The pathogenesis of atherosclerosis: an overview, *Clin Cardiol* 14:II, 1991.
10. Lin SJ, Jan K-M, Weinbaum S, et al: Transendothelial transport of low-density lipoprotein in association with cell mitosis in rat aorta, *Arteriosclerosis* 9:230, 1989.
11. Munro JM, Cotran RS: Biology of disease: the pathogenesis of atherosclerosis, atherogenesis and inflammation, *Lab Invest* 58:249, 1988.
12. Agel NM, Ball RY, Waldmann H, et al: Identification of macrophages and smooth cells in human atherosclerosis using monoclonal antibodies, *J Pathol* 146:197, 1985.
13. Chamley-Campbell J, Campbell GR, Ross R: The smooth muscle cell in culture, *Physiol Rev,* 59:1, 1979.
14. Katsuda S, Boyd HC, Flgner C, et al: Human atherosclerosis III. Immunohistochemical analysis of the cell composition of lesions in young adults, *Am J Pathol* 140:907, 1992.
15. Steinberg D, Witztum JL: Lipoproteins and atherogenesis, current concepts, *JAMA* 264:3047, 1990.
16. Ross R, Glomset JA: The pathogenesis of atherosclerosis, *N Engl J Med* 295:369;295:420, 1976.
17. Steinberg D: Metabolism of lipoproteins and their role in the pathogenesis of atherosclerosis, in Stokes J III, Macini M, eds: *Atherosclerosis Reviews* 18:1, 1988.
18. Stary HC, Letson GD: Morphometry of coronary components in children and young adults, *Arteriosclerosis* 3:485a, 1983.
19. Stary HC: Atheroma arises in eccentric intimal thickening from concurrent fatty streak lesions (abstr) *Fed Proc* 46:418, 1987.
20. Murata K, Motayama T, Katake C: Collagen types in various layers of the human aorta and their changes with the atherosclerotic process, *Atherosclerosis* 60:251, 1986.
21. Yla-Herttuala S, Sumuvuori H, Karkola K, et al: Glycosaminoglycans in normal and atherosclerotic human coronary arteries, *Lab Invest* 54:402, 1986.
22. Jonasson L, Holm J, Skalli O, et al: Regional accumulations of T-cells, macrophages, and smooth muscle cells in the human atherosclerotic plaque, *Arteriosclerosis* 6:131, 1986.
23. Ross R: Atherosclerosis: a problem of the biology of arterial wall cells and their interactions with blood components, *Arteriosclerosis* 1(5):293, 1981.
24. Ross R: The pathogenesis of atherosclerosis: an update, *N Engl J Med* 314:488, 1986.
25. Henriksen T, Evensen SA, Carlander SB: Injury to human endothelial cells in culture induced by low density lipoproteins, *Scand J Clin Lab Invest* 39:369, 1979.
26. Tauber JP, Cheng J, Gospodarowicz D: Effect of high and low density lipoproteins on proliferation of cultured bovine vascular endothelial cells, *J Clin Invest* 66:696, 1980.

27. Moncada S: *Prostacyclin and thromboxane A2 in platelet vessel wall interactions*. In Gotto AM Jr, Smith LC, Allen B, eds: *Atherosclerosis V* New York, 1979, Springer-Verlag.

28. Nordoy A: Lipids and thrombogenesis, *Ann Clin Res* 13:50, 1981.

29. Pritchard KA Jr, Schwarz SM, Medow MS, et al: Effect of low density lipoprotein on endothelial cell membrane fluidity and mononuclear cell attachment, *Am J Physiol* 260:C43, 1991.

30. Vlodavsky I, Fielding PE, Fielding CJ, et al: *Proc Natl Acad Sci USA* 75:356, 1978.

31. Henriksen T, Mahoney EM, Steinberg D: Interactions of plasma lipoproteins with endothelial cells, *Ann NY Acad Sci* 410:102, 1982.

32. Schwenke DC, Carew TE: Initiation of atherosclerotic lesions in cholesterol-fed rabbits. II. Selective retention of LDL vs selective increases in LDL permeability in susceptible sites of arteries, *Arteriosclerosis* 9:908, 1989.

33. Schwenke DC, Carew TE: Initiation of atherosclerotic lesions in cholesterol-fed rabbits. I. Focal increases in arterial LDL concentration precede development of fatty streak lesions, *Arteriosclerosis* 9:895, 1989.

34. Rosenfeld ME, Tsukada T, Gown AM, et al: Fatty streak initiation in Watanabe heritable hyperlipidemic and comparably hypercholesterolemic fat-fed rabbits, *Arteriosclerosis* 7:9, 1987.

35. DiCorleto PE, Chisolm GM: Participation of the endothelium in the development of the atherosclerotic plaque, *Prog Lipid Res* 25:365, 1986.

36. Pritchard KA Jr, Tota RR, Lin JHC, et al: Native low density lipoprotein endothelial cell recruitment of mononuclear cells, *Arterioscler Thromb* 11:1175, 1991.

37. Navab M, Imes SS, Hama SY, et al: Monocyte transmigration induced by modification of low density lipoprotein in co-cultures of human aortic wall cells is due to induction of monocyte chemotactic protein 1 synthesis and is abolished by high density lipoprotein, *J Clin Invest* 88:2039, 1991.

38. Berman JW, Calderon TM: The role of endothelial cell adhesion molecules in the development of atherosclerosis, Cardiovasc Pathol 1 (1):17, 1992.

39. Heinecke JW, Rosen H, Chait A: Iron and copper promote modification of low density lipoprotein by human arterial smooth muscle cells in culture, *J Clin Invest* 74:1890, 1987.

40. Morel DW, DiCorleto PE, Chisolm GM: Endothelial and smooth muscle cells alter low density lipoprotein in vitro by free radical oxidation, *Arteriosclerosis* 4:357, 1984.

41. Steinbrecher UP, Parthasarathy S, Leake DS, et al: Modification of low density lipoprotein by endothelial cells involves lipid peroxidation and degradation of low density lipoprotein phospholipids, *Proc Natl Acad Sci USA* 81:3383, 1984.

42. Yla-Herttula S, Palinski W, Rosenfeld ME, et al: Evidence for the presence of oxidatively modified low density lipoprotein in atherosclerotic lesions of rabbit and man, *J Clin Invest* 84:1086, 1980.

43. Rosenfeld ME, Palinski W, Yla-Herttula S, et al: Distribution of oxidized proteins and apoliprotein B in atherosclerotic lesions of varying severity from WHHL rabbits: immunocytochemical analysis using antibodies generated against modified and native LDL, *Arteriosclerosis* 10:336, 1990.

44. Parthasarathy S, Young SG, Witztum JL, et al: Probucol inhibits oxidative modification of low density lipoproteins, *J Clin Invest* 77:641, 1986.

45. Kita T, Nagano Y, Yokode M, et al: Probucol prevents the progression of atherosclerosis in WHHL rabbit, an animal model for familial hypercholesterolemia, *Proc Natl Acad Sci USA* 84:5928, 1987.

46. Carew TE, Schwenke, Steinbert D: Antiatherogenic effect of probucol unrelated to its hypocholesterolemic effect: evidence that an antioxidant in vivo can selectively inhibit low density lipoprotein degradation in macrophage-rich fatty streaks showing progression of atherosclerosis in the WHHL rabbit, *Proc Natl Acad Sci USA* 84:7725, 1987.

47. Uhlinger DJ, Burnham DN, Mullins RE, et al: Functional differences in human neutrophils isolated pre- and postprandially, *FEBS Lett* 286:28, 1991.

48. Castellot JJ Jr, Addonizio ML, Rosenberg R, et al: Cultured endothelial cells produce a heparin-like inhibitor of smooth muscle cell growth, *J Cell Biol* 90:372, 1982.

49. Fritze LM, Reilly CF, Rosenberg RD: An antiproliferative heparin sulfate species produced by post-confluent smooth muscle, *J Cell Biol* 100:1041, 1985.

50. Printseva OY, Peclo MM, Gown AM: Various cell types in human atherosclerotic lesions express 1CAM-1. Further immunocytochemical and immunochemical studies employing monoclonal antibody 10F3, *Am J Pathol* 140:889, 1992.

51. Springer TH: Adhesion receptors of the immune system, *Nature* 346:425, 1990.

52. Cybulsky MI, Gimbrone MA Jr: Endothelial expression of a mononuclear leukocyte adhesion molecule during atherogenesis, *Science* 251:788, 1991.

53. Simmons D, Makgoba MW, Seed B: ICAm an adhesion ligand of LFA-1 is homologous to the neural cell adhesion molecule NCAM, *Nature* 331:624, 1988.

54. Staunton DE, Martin SD, Stratowa C, et al: Primary structure of ICAM-1 demonstrated interaction between members of immunoglobulin and integrin supergene families, *Cell* 52:925, 1988.

55. Ross R: Polypeptide growth factors and atherosclerosis. *Trends Cardiovasc Med* 1 (7):277, 1991.

56. Gown AM, Tsukada T, Ross R: Human atherosclerosis. II. Immunocytochemical analysis of the cellular composition of human atherosclerotic lesions, *Am J Pathol* 125:191, 1986.

57. Benditt EP, Benditt JM: Evidence for a monoclonal origin of human atherosclerotic plaques, *Proc Natl Acad Sci USA* 7:1735, 1973.

58. Benditt EP: The monoclonal theory of atherogenesis, Atherogenesis *Atheroscler Rev* 3:77, 1978.

59. Pearson TA, Wang A, Solez K, et al: Clonal characteristics of fibrous plaques and fatty streaks from human aortas, *Am J Pathol* 81:379, 1975.

60. Bravo R: Synthesis of the nuclear protein cyclin (PCNA) and its relationship with DNA replication, *Exp Cell Res* 163:287, 1986.

61. Seifert RA, Hart CE, Phillips PE, et al: Two different subunits associate to create isoform-specific platelet-derived growth factor receptors, *J Biol Chem* 264:8771, 1989.

62. Heldin C-H, Westermark B: Platelet-derived growth factor: mechanism of action and possible in vivo function, *Cell Regul* 1:555, 1990.

63. Raines EW, Bowen-Pope DF, Ross R: *Platelet-derived growth factor*. In *Handbook of experimental pharmacology: peptide growth factors and their receptors*, New York, 1990, Springer-Verlag.

64. Barrett TB, Benditt EP: Platelet-derived growth factor gene expression in human atherosclerotic plaques and normal artery wall, *Proc Natl Acad Sci USA* 85:2810, 1988.

65. Ross R, Masuda J, Raines EW, et al: Localization of PDGF-B protein in macrophages in all phases of atherogenesis, *Science* 248:1009, 1990.

66. Battegay EJ, Raines EW, Seifert RA, et al: TGF- induces bimodal proliferation of connective tissue cells via complete control of an autocrine PDGF loop, *Cell* 63:515, 1990.

67. Roberts AB, Sporn MB: *The transforming growth factor- s*. In *Handbook of experimental pharmacology: peptide growth factors and their receptors*, New York, 1990, Springer-Verlag.

68. Lyons RM, Moses HL: Transforming growth factors and the regulation of cell proliferation, *Eur J Biochem* 187:467, 1990.

69. Raines EW, Dower SK, Ross R: IL-1 mitogenic activity for fibroblasts and smooth muscle cells is due to PDGF-AA, *Science* 243:393, 1989.

70. Dinarello CA: Biology of interleukin 1, *FASEB J* 2:108, 1988.

71. Dinarello CA, Savage N: Interleukin-1 and its receptors, *Crit Rev Immunol* 9:1, 1989.

72. Sherry B, Cerami A: Cachectin/tumor necrosis factor exerts endocrine, paracrine, and autocrine control of inflammatory responses, *J Cell Biol* 107, 1988.

73. Hajjar KA, Hajjar DP, Silverstein RL, et al: Tumor necrosis factor-mediated release of platelet-derived growth factor from cultured endothelial cells, *J Exp Med* 166:235, 1987.

74. Baird A, Mormede P, Bohlen P: Immunoreactive fibroblast growth factor in cells of peritoneal exudate suggests its identity with macrophage-derived growth factor, *Biochem Biophys Res Commun* 126:358, 1985.

75. Lindner V, Reidy MA: Proliferation of smooth muscle cells after vascular injury is inhibited by an antibody against basic fibroblast growth factor, *Proc Natl Acad Sci USA* 88:3739, 1991.

76. Rosenfeld ME, Ross R: Macrophage and smooth muscle cell proliferation in atherosclerotic lesions of WHHL and comparably hypercholesterolemic fat-fed rabbits, *Arteriosclerosis* 7:9, 1990.

77. Sasahara M, Fries JWU, Raines EW, et al: PDGF B-chain in neurons of the central nervous system, posterior pituitary, and in a transgenic model, *Cell* 64:217, 1991.

78. Gordon D, Reidy MA, Benditt EP, et al: Cell proliferation of human coronary arteries, *Proc Natl Acad Sci USA* 87:4600, 1990.

79. Metcalf D: The molecular control of cell division, differentiation commitment and maturation in haemopoietic cells, *Nature* 339:27, 1989.

80. Ralph P: *Colony stimulating factors.* In Zembala M, Asherson G, eds: *Human monocytes*, London, 1989, Academic Press.

81. Fry DL: *Hemodynamic forces in atherogenesis.* In Scheinberg P, ed: *Cerebrovascular diseases* New York, 1976, Raven Press.

82. Gertz SD, Forbes MS, Sunaga T, et al: Ischemic carotid endothelium: transmission electron microscopic studies, *Arch Pathol Lab Med* 100:522, 1976.

83. Nelson E, Gertz SD, Forbes MS, et al: Endothelial lesions in the aorta of egg yolk-fed minature swine: a study by scanning and transmission electron microscopy, *Exp Mol Pathol* 25:208, 1976.

84. Lewis JC, Kottke BA: Endothelial damage and thrombocyte adhesion in pigeon atherosclerosis, *Science* 196:1007, 1977.

85. Ku DN, Giddens DP, Zarins CK: Pulsatile flow and atherosclerosis in the human carotid bifurcation, positive correlation between plaque location and low and oscillating shear stress, *Arteriosclerosis* 5:293, 1985.

86. Bretherton KN, Day AJ, Skinner SL: Effect of hypertension on the entry of 125I-labeled low density lipoprotein into the aortic intima of normal-fed rabbits, *Atherosclerosis* 24:99, 1976.

87. Schwartz SM: Hypertension endothelial injury and atherosclerosis, *Trends Cardiovasc Med* 2:991, 1977.

88. Braunwald E: Coronary artery spasm as a cause of myocardial ischemia, *J Lab Clin Med* 97:299, 1981.

89. Hellstrom HR: The injury-spasm and vascular autoregulatory hypothesis of ischemic disease, *Am J Cardiol* 49:802, 1982.

90. Conti CR: Myocardial infarction: thoughts about pathogenesis and the role of coronary artery spasm, *Am Heart J* 110:187, 1985.

91. Gertz SD, Uretzky G, Wajnbert RS, et al: Endothelial cell damage and thrombus formation after partial arterial constriction: relevance to the role of coronary artery spasm in the pathogenesis of myocardial infarction, *Circulation* 63:476, 1981.

92. Betz E, Schlote W: Responses of vessel walls to chronically applied electrical stimuli, *Basic Res Cardiol* 74:10, 1979.

93. Kawachi Y, Tomoike H, Maruoka Y, et al: Selective hypercontraction caused by ergonovine in the canine coronary artery under conditions of induced atherosclerosis, *Circulation* 69:441, 1984.

94. Egashira K, Tomoike H, Yamamoto Y, et al: Histamine-induced coronary spasm in regions of intimal thickening in miniature pigs: roles of serum cholesterol and spontaneous or induced intimal thickening, *Circulation* 74:826, 1986.

95. Shimokawa H, Tomoike H, Nabayema S, et al: Coronary artery spasm induced in atherosclerotic miniature swine, *Science* 221:560, 1983.

96. Yamamoto Y, Tomoike H, Egashira K: Attenuation of endothelium-related relaxation and enhanced responsiveness of smooth muscle to histamine in spastic coronary arterial segments from miniature pigs, *Circ Res* 61:772, 1987.

97. Lown B, DeSilva RA: Is coronary arterial spasm a risk factor for coronary atherosclerosis? *Am J Cardiol* 45:901, 1980.

98. Dalen JE, Ochene IS, Alpert JS: Coronary spasm, coronary thrombosis and myocardial infarction: a hypothesis concerning the pathophysiology of acute myocardial infarction, *Am Heart J* 104:1119, 1982.

99. Gutstein WH: Coronary spasm and coronary arteriosclerosis, *Am J Cardiol* 48:389, 1981.

100. Paterson JC, Cottral GE: Experimental coronary sclerosis: III. Lymphomatosis as a cause of coronary sclerosis in chickens, *Arch Pathol* 49:699, 1950.

101. Fabricant CG, Krook L, Gillespie JH: Virus-induced cholesterol crystals, *Science* 181:566, 1973.

102. Fabricant CG, Fabricant J, Minick CR, et al: Herpes-virus induced atherosclerosis in chickens, *Fed Proc* 42:2476, 1983.

103. Hajjar DP, Fabricant CG, Minick CR, et al: Virus-induced atherosclerosis: herpes-virus infection alters aortic cholesterol metabolism and accumulation, *Am J Pathol* 122:62, 1986.

104. Vercellotti GM: Proinflammatory and procoagulant effects of herpes simplex injection on human endothelium, *Blood Cells* 16:209, 1990.

105. Minick CR, Fabricant CG, Fabricant J, et al: Atheroarteriosclerosis induced by infection with a herpesvirus, *Am J Pathol* 96:673, 1979.

106. Adam E, Melnick JL, Probesfield JL, et al: High levels of cytomegalovirus antibody in patients requiring vascular surgery for atherosclerosis, *Lancet* 2:291, 1987.

107. Grattan MT, Moreno-Cabral CE, Starnes VA, et al: Cytomegalovirus infection is associated with cardiac allograft rejection and atherosclerosis, *JAMA* 261:3561, 1989.

108. MacDonald K, Rector TS, Braulan EA, et al: Association of coronary artery disease in cardiac transplant recipients with cytomegalovirus infection, *Am J Pathol* 64:359, 1984.

109. Wu TC, Hruban RH, Ambinder RF, et al: Demonstration of cytomegalovirus nucleic acids in the coronary arteries of transplanted hearts, *Am J Pathol* 140:739, 1992.

110. Hosenpud JD, Chou S, Wagner CR: Cytomegalovirus (CMV) induced regulation of major histocompatibility complex class I antigen in human aortic smooth muscle cells, *J Heart Lung Transplant* 10:170, 1991.

111. Gyorkey F, Melnick JL, Guinn GA, et al: Herpes viridae in the endothelial and smooth muscle cells of the proximal aorta of atherosclerosis patients, *Exp Mol Pathol* 40:328, 1984.

112. Melnick JL, Petrie BL, Dreesman GR, et al: Cytomegalovirus antigen within human arterial smooth muscle cells, *Lancet* 2:644, 1983.

113. Hendricks MGR, Salimens MMM, Vanboven CPA: High prevalence of latently present cytomegalovirus in arterial walls of patients from grade III atherosclerosis, *Am J Pathol* 136:23, 1990.

114. Yamashiroya HM, Ghosh L, Yang R, et al: Herpes-viridae in the coronary arteries and aortas of young trauma victims, *Am J Pathol* 130:71, 1988.

115. Libby P, Hansson GK: Biology of disease involvement of the immune system in human atherosclerosis: current knowledge and unanswered questions, *Lab Invest* 64:359, 1984.

Chapter 2

ISCHEMIC HEART DISEASE

Harisios Boudoulas
Michael B. Gravanis

ANATOMY OF CORONARY ARTERIES

The left main coronary artery arises from the left sinus of Valsalva and divides into two major branches, the left anterior descending (LAD) and the circumflex (CX) arteries[1] (Fig. 2-1).

LAD coronary artery

The LAD coronary artery extends along the anterior interventricular sulcus, encircles the cardiac apex, and often ascends in the posterior interventricular sulcus to be distributed to the apical region of the posterior wall of both ventricles. The LAD supplies the anterior region of the left ventricular free wall and the interventricular septum. The number of septal branches (perforators) varies from three

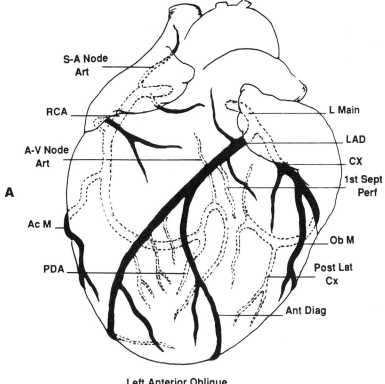

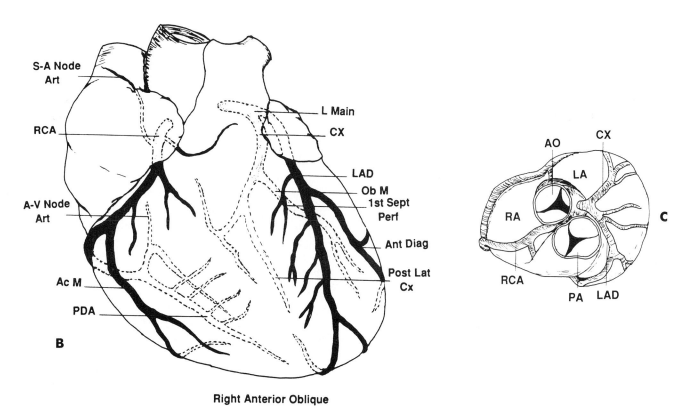

Fig. 2-1. A and **B,** Left and right anterior oblique views of coronary arteries and their distribution. **C,** Cephalad view of coronary artery distribution in relation to the great vessels. *S-A* = sinoatrial; *Art* = artery; *RCA* = right coronary artery; *A-V* = atrioventricular; *AcM* = acute marginal; *PDA* = posterior descending artery; *Ant* = anterior; *Post* = posterior; *Lat* = lateral; *Cx* = circumflex; *ObM* = obtuse marginal; *Sept* = septal; *Perf* = perforator; *LAD* = left anterior descending; *L* = left; *Ao* = aorta; *LA* = left atrium; *RA* = right atrium; *PA* = pulmonary artery.

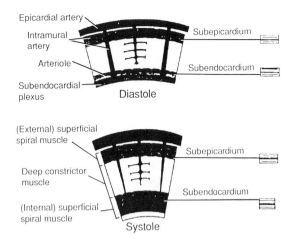

Fig. 2-2. Cross-section of the left ventricular wall in diastole and systole. Factors involved in the susceptibility of the subendocardium to the development of ischemia include the greater dependence of this region on diastolic perfusion and the greater degree of shortening, and therefore of energy expenditure, of this region during systole. (From Bell JR, Fox AC: Pathogenesis of subendocardial ischemia, *Am J Med Sci* 268:2, 1974.)

to five. They arise at a right angle from the LAD and run within the right half of the septum toward the posterior interventricular sulcus. The diagonal branches (1 to 3) may arise from the proximal LAD or the CX and only rarely from the left main coronary artery.

CX coronary artery

The CX coronary artery follows a horizontal course along the lateral and posterior atrioventricular sulcus, giving branches to the left atrium, several branches to the anterolateral region of the left ventricle, the obtuse marginal branches and finally, the posterolateral branch. In less than 50% of the cases, the CX coronary artery gives off the sinoatrial mode branch. In about 10% of the cases the CX coronary artery continues as the posterior descending artery after reaching the crux of the heart. This anatomic variance of the coronary artery system is referred to as *left dominant*. The artery to the atrioventricular node in a left dominant system is supplied by the CX coronary artery.

Right coronary artery (RCA)

This artery originates from the right sinus of Valsalva and runs along the anterior atrioventricular sulcus toward the crux of the heart (the point where the two atria meet with the two ventricles posteriorly) (Figure 2-1). The RCA at the crux gives off the atrioventricular node branch as it turns toward the apex and becomes the posterior descending artery (right preponderance). The posterior descending artery supplies the inferior surface of the interventricular sulcus, septum, and posterior left ventricle. The conus artery, which supplies the anterior portion of the pulmonary conus (right ventricular outflow tract), is the first branch of

the RCA. In approximately half of the cases the conus artery may arise from a separate ostium in the right sinus of Valsalva. The next branch of the RCA is the artery to the sinoatrial node. Beyond this branch the RCA gives off several branches to the anterior and posterior wall of the right ventricle, the largest of which is the acute marginal branch.

Penetrating vessels and capillaries

The epicardial coronary arteries give rise to smaller penetrating vessels approximately at right angles (Fig. 2-2). A large pressure drop occurs in these intramural vessels and in the coronary arterioles, hence their designation as resistance vessels.[2]

It has been estimated that the capillary density in the normal human heart is about 4000 capillaries per mm^2 cross section. Capillary density is not uniformly patent, because precapillary sphincters appear to serve a regulatory function, depending on the flow needs of the myocardium. The capillary density is equal in both ventricles and septum, but is somewhat reduced in the subendocardium. It is also reduced in the presence of ventricular hypertrophy.

CORONARY ARTERY STENOSES IN PATIENTS WITH ATHEROSCLEROTIC CORONARY ARTERY DISEASE (CAD)

Review of coronary artery cineangiograms from patients referred for evaluation of chest pain showed the following anatomic distribution of occlusive ($\geq 70\%$) atherosclerotic lesions[3]: 6% of the patients have left main coronary artery stenosis, 33% have three-vessel coronary artery stenosis, 17% have two-vessel coronary artery stenosis, and 27% have one-vessel coronary artery stenosis. The distribution of coronary stenoses in patients with one afflicted vessel is as follows: 51% LAD, 35% RCA, and 14% CX coronary artery. In patients with two-vessel disease, the CX coronary artery is involved in different combinations (either with LAD or RCA) only in 48% of cases, while the LAD and RCA are involved in 70% to 82%. The reason(s) for the low frequency of involvement of the CX coronary artery in atherosclerosis is not clear.

There are indications that atherosclerotic lesions in the coronary system do not develop randomly, but tend to localize at selected sites of the arterial tree. Branching sites and curved segments where there is blood disturbance, separation of streamlines, or eddies, are the areas that most often are associated with atheromatous plaques. Therefore, arterial hemodynamics play a crucial role in atherogenesis and progression of atherosclerosis.[4-6] Although distal segments of epicardial coronary arteries are not spared from atherosclerotic lesions, it is usually the proximal 3 cm to 5 cm of epicardial coronary arteries that are most often involved with atheroma.

NONATHEROSCLEROTIC CAUSES OF CORONARY ARTERY STENOSIS

Other causes besides coronary atherosclerosis may result in coronary artery disease. These causes are described briefly in the following passage.

The coronary ostia may become stenotic or completely occluded in inflammatory aortic conditions such as syphilis and Takayasu disease. In cases of Kawasaki disease (mucocutaneous lymph node syndrome), approximately 1% of the children affected develop coronary arteritis, resulting in aneurysms, mural thrombi, and myocardial infarction[7] (Fig. 2-3).

Some autoimmune vascular diseases such as systemic lupus erythematosus, systemic sclerosis, dermatomyositis, and mixed connective tissue disorders may reveal epicardial and/or intramyocardial coronary artery involvement. From those entities only systemic lupus erythematosus reveals actual arteritis of coronary vessels. Although coronary involvement in polyarteritis nodosa is relatively common, antemortem diagnosis is made only in a few cases. Rarely, the coronary arteries may be involved by giant cell arteritis.

Although atherosclerotic and congenital coronary aneurysms are rarely the cause of occlusion, a dissecting aneurysm may result in luminal occlusion. Coronary artery dissection is usually secondary to aortic dissection; a few spontaneous dissections of the coronary arteries have been reported in young women in the peripartum period. Iatrogenic causes of coronary artery dissection are usually associated with cardiac catheterization or coronary cannulation.

Embolic occlusion of coronary arteries is relatively uncommon, perhaps because of the protective shield of the aortic cusps. Most of the emboli, however, arise from vegetations in the left-sided valves or mural thrombi of the left atrium and ventricle (Fig. 2-4). Fragments of prosthetic valve material have been observed in the coronary tree, as

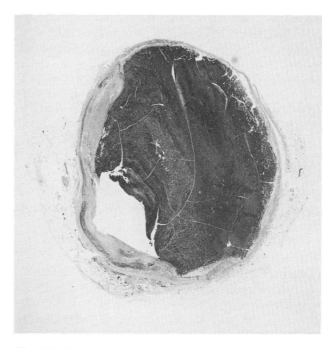

Fig. 2-3. Coronary artery aneurysm from a child with Kawasaki's disease. Note the occlusive mural thrombus.

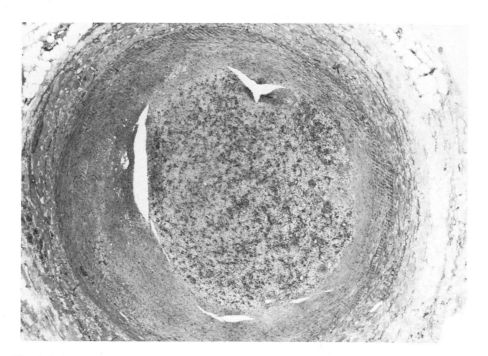

Fig. 2-4. Occlusive organized embolus in an epicardial coronary artery. The artery reveals mild intimal thickening.

well as fragments from a left atrial myxoma. It is not always easy to distinguish between an embolus and a locally formed thrombus in a coronary artery. Imperfect fit for the lumen of the occluding thrombus, evidence of a thrombus in a normal-appearing arterial branch, and the presence of bacteria or cholesterol crystals are all signs that favor an embolic episode.

Both penetrating and nonpenetrating blunt trauma may injure the epicardial coronary arteries, particularly the LAD because of its proximity to the anterior chest wall. Inadvertent ligation of a coronary artery during cardiac surgery, particularly when the artery has an anomalous course, is another rare cause of coronary artery occlusion.

COLLATERALS AND THEIR ROLE IN ISCHEMIC HEART DISEASE

Controversy regarding the clinical importance of coronary collateral circulation has subsided significantly over the last two decades. Initially it was thought that collaterals in humans are more an indication of severe regional ischemia than a sign of biologic "compensation" for a perfusion deficit.

There is now significant angiographic and histologic evidence that coronary collaterals develop as a sequence of chronic coronary artery disease, and that enlarged collaterals deliver blood to the region perfused by the occluded artery.[8-13] Studies of collateral circulation have demonstrated that for any given location of acute coronary occlusion, the degree of left ventricular function depends on the presence or absence of collaterals. They have also shown that there is an inverse quantitative relation between severity of stenosis and collateral function. As a general rule, no collaterals are visualized in patients with coronary artery stenosis of < 70%. Collaterals may be seen between segments of the same coronary artery (homocoronary), or between branches of different coronary arteries (intercoronary).

Several misconceptions about the great potential of collaterals or their inability to protect patients from ischemic episodes have confused the entire issue. Experimental work on collaterals was mostly carried out in the canine heart, which develops mainly subepicardial collaterals, whereas collaterals in the human heart develop primarily in the subendocardial plexuses. The latter process occurs when a dense subendocardial plexus develops after proximal coronary occlusion. Vessels from those plexuses are thin wall arteries, the largest of which reveal extensive subintimal proliferation. Over the years, physicians have learned that the pig heart is a much better model to study collateral circulation. We have also learned that angiography may not be the best method to study collaterals in humans. When appropriate methods become available, other variables such as measuring the regional blood flow on a quantitative basis and determining the amount of perfused myocardium may be more informative.

The concept that collaterals are present in some normal hearts (lucky ones) and open up wherever they are needed is still debated. Recent studies with experimental animals suggest that ischemic myocardium produces the biochemical signal for the proliferation of endothelial and smooth muscle cells in the development of collaterals. It is now accepted that collaterals result from growth adaptation of arterioles and capillaries that occurs in cases of slowly progressing coronary stenosis. Collateral circulation, however, may regress if the coronary artery obstruction is relieved.

The growth response of collaterals is probably caused by hormone-receptor interactions, because ischemia will lead to externalization of the growth receptors of endothelial and smooth muscle cells. The importance of coronary collaterals in the setting of reperfusion for acute myocardial infarction has been emphasized. The presence of coronary collaterals may extend the time window for the beneficial effect of thrombolysis and may facilitate thrombolysis because of the retrograde flow.

Existing evidence supports the protective role of collaterals in ischemic heart disease. There are indications that they may prevent myocardial infarction and left ventricular dysfunction. Studies have shown that in patients with good collaterals, the pressure distal to the inflated catheter used for coronary angioplasty could be up to 70% of the aortic pressure.[11]

SMALL VESSEL DISEASE

Any discussion about the pathophysiology of the coronary artery system will be incomplete without an insightful look into the structure and function of small coronary arteries in different disease entities.[14] Because technologic methods are improving rapidly and functional information can be obtained about the microcirculation, our ability to assess and appreciate the value of small vessel disease will significantly increase. It is important to understand that structural alterations in small coronary vessels revealing intimal and/or medial hypertrophy alter their luminal diameter; these structural changes may also affect the vessel's responsiveness to vasoactive influences and particularly their ability to dilate.

Disease processes that may primarily affect the media of small vessels are amyloidosis, scleroderma or fibromuscular dysplasia associated with Friedreich's ataxia. In these conditions luminal narrowing may be minimal but changes in the contractile capacity of the involved small arteries are significant. Vasomotive changes may result from structural or functional alterations in the endothelial cells of small vessels. This could be the underlying mechanism in pheochromocytoma, which may have a direct constrictive effect on small coronary vessels, along with widespread platelet aggregation.

Conditions that induce intimal thickening or inflammation of the wall of small coronary arteries, such polyarteritis, systemic lupus erythematosus or Whipple disease, may lead to luminal thrombosis.

Thrombosis of small coronary arteries may result from a number of causes although in the majority of circumstances the underlying mechanism for the thrombotic occlusion is embolization of debris from cardiac surgery (valve replacement), angioplasty, or bacterial endocarditis.

It can be concluded that either luminal narrowing or impaired vasoreactivity of a sufficient number of small coronary arteries may diminish the coronary reserve; the pathophysiologic mechanisms involved may differ according to the underlying disease.

CORONARY ARTERY SPASM

In discussing coronary arterial vasoreactivity it is important to appreciate that there is a spectrum of coronary vasoconstriction. At one end of the spectrum is the mild coronary constriction looked upon as a physiologic response to common vasoconstrictor stimuli. At the other end of the spectrum is the severe segmental constriction resulting in complete arterial occlusion, which is seen in patients who have variant angina. Naturally, other forms of nonocclusive constriction may fall between the two extremes described above.[15-20]

A dynamic increase in arterial tone at the site of coronary stenosis in patients with angina at rest has been proposed. Theoretically, even arteries without significant intimal atherosclerosis may exhibit occlusive spasm caused by strong stimuli or increased hyperactivity of a segment of the artery. The exact causes of such significant hyperactivity are still unknown. It is not exactly clear whether the segmental coronary spasm seen in patients with variant angina is the result of local hyperactivity alone.

In recent years adequate data have been accumulated indicating that coronary atherosclerosis is associated with abnormal vasodilatory function, probably due to deficiencies in the production and/or release of endothelium-derived relaxing factors. Paradoxic vasoconstriction has been produced by intracoronary administration of acetylcholine in patients who have coronary atherosclerosis. Data suggest that there is a progressive impairment in endothelium-mediated modulation of vasomotor tone of coronary arteries even in early stages of human atherosclerosis. Studies of patients who have angiographically normal coronary arteries but elevated plasma low-density lipoproteins, reveal endothelial dysfunction not only in the large epicardial vessels but also in the resistance vasculature. Vasodilatory response to increased coronary blood flow and to sympathetic stimulation in those vessels, is well-preserved, but in cases with angiographic evidence of coronary atherosclerosis the flow-mediated vasodilation is also impaired. Studies in experimental animals have revealed that atherosclerotic vessels exhibit increased vasoconstrictor response to serotonin and thromboxane A_2 and impaired vasodilatory reaction to adenosine diphosphate. When the vascular endothelium is intact and is functioning properly, serotonin has a vasodilating effect. However, when the endothelium is damaged, as in cases of coronary artery disease, serotonin has a direct, unopposed vasoconstricting effect. Infusion of serotonin in patients with atherosclerotic lesions may also cause reduction in coronary blood flow,

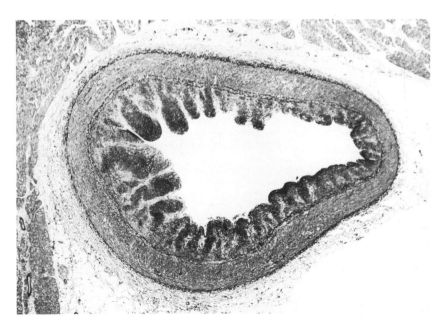

Fig. 2-5. Epicardial coronary artery (explanted heart). Note corrugated intimal proliferation. The corrugations probably reflect arterial spasm secondary to operative handling. Elastic stain.

probably resulting from a direct vasoconstricting effect on small resistance vessels, coronary arteries, or both. Infusion of serotonin in patients with stable angina causes vasoconstriction, the severity of which does not approach that observed during coronary spasm in patients who have variant angina.

It is entirely possible that in patients who have unstable angina, endothelial damage over an atherosclerotic plaque may provide an ideal site for platelet aggregation, release of vasoconstrictors such as serotonin (which may cause additional platelet aggregation), and vasoconstriction at the arterial site.

Studies have shown increased venous and coronary sinus levels of endothelin-1 in patients who have variant angina and provokable coronary vasospasm. Endothelin is one of the most potent vasoconstrictor substances known and is produced in the endothelium of the vessel wall. It has been suggested that endothelin-1 increases the calcium sensitivity of human arteries, interfering with a fundamental intracellular mechanism in the contractile process.

Although coronary artery spasm may exist (Fig. 2-5), it is not absolutely clear whether an atherosclerotic coronary artery can respond to vasoconstrictive stimuli by segmental occlusive spasm. Indeed, studies have suggested that "stiffness" and smooth muscle atrophy at the site of an atherosclerotic plaque have a negative effect on the degree of lumen reduction, since for the development of spasm a degree of smooth muscle contraction is required to overcome the rigidity of the plaque itself. It is likely, however, that abnormalities of coronary vasomotor response resulting

from the atherosclerotic plaque may play a modulatory, but not a major role, in impairing coronary blood flow.

ARTERIAL DISTENSIBILITY

Decreased vasodilatory capacity of nonstenotic arteries in animals with experimental atherosclerosis and in patients with coronary artery disease has been reported. Distensibility of the ascending aorta has been reported to be significantly decreased in patients with coronary artery disease and angiographically normal aorta. These changes are attributed to arterial wall intimal fibrosis and/or to abnormalities related to endothelium-derived relaxation factors. Vasa-vasorum flow also is an important factor that determines arterial distensibility; decreased vasa-vasorum flow has a negative effect on arterial distensibility.[21-24]

Arterial distensibility in humans can be calculated from changes in arterial diameter and arterial pressure (Fig. 2-6). Abnormal elastic properties of the coronary arteries certainly alter the response of arteries to different intrinsic stimulators and/or to therapeutic interventions. Additional abnormal elastic properties of the aorta may alter the ventricular-vascular coupling, which will result in a decrease in left ventricular performance.

FACTORS AS THEY AFFECT MYOCARDIAL OXYGEN SUPPLY AND DEMAND

Myocardial cells, even at rest, extract 75% to 80% of oxygen content in the blood. Thus, increased oxygen demand, such as with exercise, can only be supplied by increasing myocardial blood flow, which normally is regu-

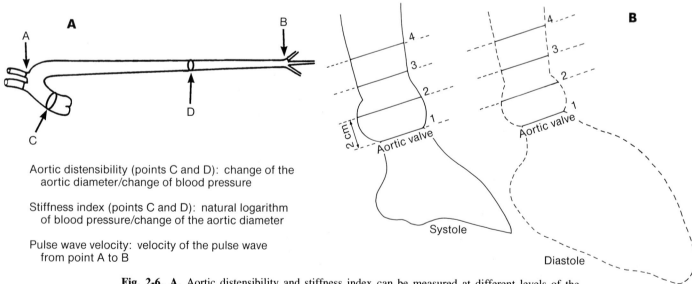

Aortic distensibility (points C and D): change of the aortic diameter/change of blood pressure

Stiffness index (points C and D): natural logarithm of blood pressure/change of the aortic diameter

Pulse wave velocity: velocity of the pulse wave from point A to B

Fig. 2-6. A, Aortic distensibility and stiffness index can be measured at different levels of the aorta (e.g., point C and D). Pulse wave velocity can be measured from the left carotid artery to the left femoral artery (from point A to B). (From Hirata K, et al: The Marfan syndrome: abnormal elastic properties, *J Am Coll Cardiol* 18:57-63, 1991). **B,** Left ventricular end-diastolic and end-systolic frames; the ascending aorta is also shown. Lines indicate the levels where aortic diameters are measured. (From Stefanadis C, et al: Aortic distensibility abnormalities in coronary artery disease, *Am J Cardiol* 59:1300-4, 1987.)

lated to maintain the metabolic demand of the heart.[25-26]

Myocardial ischemia occurs when myocardial oxygen demand exceeds the supply. The process begins when a significant obstruction in a coronary artery decreases myocardial blood flow, thereby decreasing myocardial oxygen supply.

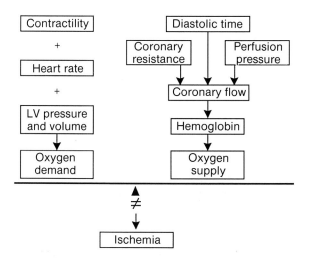

Fig. 2-7. Major factors determining myocardial oxygen supply and demand. (From Boudoulas H: *Coronary arteries: factors as they affect myocardial oxygen supply and demand.* In Leier CV, Boudoulas H, eds: *Cardiorenal Disorders and Diseases,* Mount Kisco, New York, 1992, Futura.)

Hemodynamic factors determining myocardial oxygen supply and demand are summarized[25-40] in Fig. 2-7.

Myocardial oxygen supply

Assuming normal hemoglobin levels, myocardial oxygen supply is directly related to coronary blood flow. Coronary perfusion pressure, diastolic time, and coronary artery resistance are the major factors determining coronary blood flow.

Coronary perfusion pressure. Coronary perfusion pressure during diastole is equal to coronary artery pressure minus left ventricular diastolic pressure[25-26] (Fig. 2-8). Coronary artery diastolic pressure distal to a significant obstruction is not only low but also does not change significantly with aortic pressure changes (Fig. 2-9). Thus only changes in left ventricular diastolic pressure can significantly alter coronary perfusion pressure.

Diastolic time. The majority of coronary blood flow occurs in diastole[37] (Fig. 2-10). Virtually all subendocardial flow is delivered during diastole; this is an especially important factor when left ventricular hypertrophy and/or coronary artery disease is present because left ventricular intramyocardial pressure during systole is equal to or greater than left ventricular systolic pressure in subendocardial muscle layers of the heart. In patients with severe obstructive coronary artery disease, systolic flow may be lost because the perfusion pressure distal to the obstructive lesions is less than the systolic ventricular wall pressure. Therefore subendocardial blood flow and flow distal

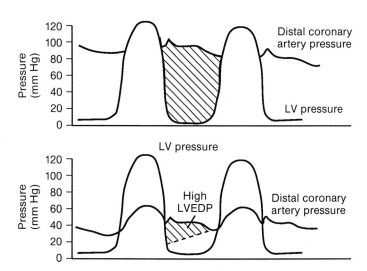

Fig. 2-8. Left ventricular (LV) pressure and coronary artery pressure in a coronary artery without obstruction (upper panel) and in a coronary artery with significant obstruction (lower panel). The cross-hatched areas indicate coronary perfusion pressure. Coronary perfusion pressure distal to a significant coronary artery lesion is low and depends largely on the LV diastolic pressure. Decreased LV diastolic pressure will result in an increase in coronary perfusion pressure (lower panel). *LVEDP* = left ventricular end diastolic pressure.(From Boudoulas H: *Coronary arteries: factors as they affect myocardial oxygen supply and demand.* In Leier CV, Boudoulas H, eds: *Cardiorenal Disorders and Diseases,* Mount Kisco, New York, 1992, Futura.)

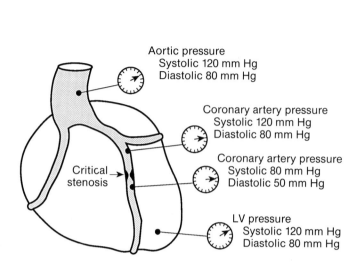

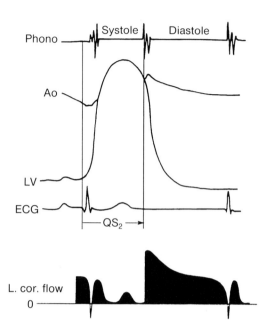

Fig. 2-9. Aortic pressure, left ventricular pressure, and coronary artery pressure proximal and distal to a significant obstruction, schematic presentation (See text for details). From Boudoulas H and Geleris P: *Coronary Artery Disease,* ed 2, Thessaloniki, Greece, 1990, University Studio Press.

Fig. 2-10. Schematic presentation of left coronary artery (L Cor) flow in relation to the cardiac cycle. Note that the greatest proportion of coronary flow occurs in diastole. The cross-hatched area represents the electromechanical delay. *Phono* = phonocardium; QS_2 = total electromechanical systole (total systolic time). Diastolic time begins after the end of QS_2 and ends with the beginning of the next QRS. (From Boudoulas H, et al.[37])

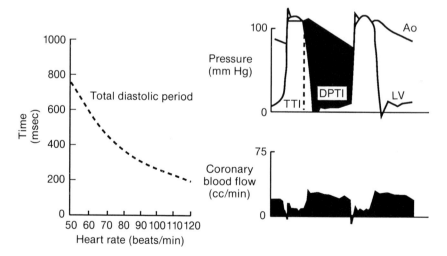

Fig. 2-11. Left panel: the relationship of heart rate to diastolic time is shown. Due to nonlinear relationship between heart rate and diastolic time, small changes in heart rate (particularly at slower rates) produce significant changes in diastolic time. Right panel: recordings of the aortic (Ao) pressure and left ventricular (LV) pressure. The tension time index (TTI) and diastolic time index (DPTI) are shown. Phasic coronary blood flow in relationship to DPTI is also shown.(From Boudoulas H, et al: Mitral valve prolapse and the mitral valve prolapse syndrome: A diagnostic classification and pathogenesis of symptoms, *Am Heart J* 118:796-818, 1989.)

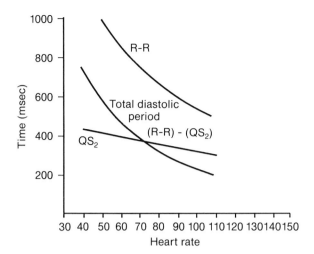

Fig. 2-12. Relationship between heart rate, total electromechanical systole (QS$_2$), RR interval, and total diastolic period. Two factors determine the duration of diastole: heart rate and duration of systole. Because of the nonlinear relationship of diastolic time and heart rate, small changes in heart rate produce significant changes in diastolic time. Diastolic time increases dramatically at heart rates less than 75 beats per minute. (From Boudoulas H, et al: Changes in diastolic time with various pharmacologic agents. Implications for myocardial perfusion, *Circulation* 60:164-169, 1979.)

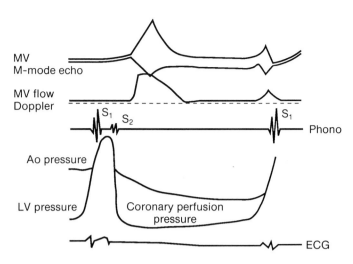

Fig. 2-13. Simultaneous recordings of the mitral valve (MV) opening, MV flow, phonocardiogram (phono), aortic (Ao) pressure, left ventricular (LV) pressure and electrocardiogram (ECG). Schematic presentation. During a long RR interval the MV stays open during diastole; the MV flow stops well before the end of diastole. The Ao pressure is greater than LV pressure throughout the diastole. Thus coronary flow is continued while flow through the mitral valve is terminated.

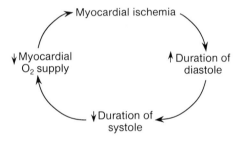

Fig. 2-14. Myocardial ischemia increases the duration of systole, abbreviates the duration of diastole, decreases myocardial oxygen supply and deteriorates the myocardial ischemia, leading to a vicious cycle (From Boudoulas H: Diastolic time: The forgotten dynamic factor. Implications for myocardial perfusion, *Acta Cardiol* 46:61-71, 1991.)

to a significant obstruction become dependent on the duration of diastole[27] (Fig. 2-11).

Diastolic time has a nonlinear relationship to heart rate. Thus small changes in heart rate produce significant changes in diastolic time. A decrease in heart rate below 75 beats per minute will produce a dramatic increase in diastolic time[34] (Fig. 2-12). Abrupt increase in heart rate may significantly decrease myocardial blood flow simply by decreasing diastolic time. Two factors determine the duration of diastolic time: heart rate and systolic time. A decrease in heart rate and/or shortening in systolic time will result in a prolongation of diastolic time and vice versa. Physiologic and/or pathologic states and pharmacologic agents can affect diastolic time by two means. One is by direct affect on heart rate; the other involves a fundamental change in heart rate-diastolic time relationship. Changes in heart rate alone produce movement along the curve. Shortening of the systolic time causes an upward shift of the curve; prolongation of the systolic time results in a downward shift.

In cases where diastolic time is prolonged, coronary blood flow continues throughout diastole while flow from the left atrium into the left ventricle stops in the middle portion of diastole (Fig. 2-13). Thus in cases involving extremely slow heart rates, myocardial blood flow will continue throughout diastole without increasing left ventricular diastolic volume and ventricular tension, i.e., without increasing myocardial oxygen consumption.

Studies of papillary muscle preparations and of patients who have coronary artery disease have shown that the duration of systole increased in the presence of myocardial ischemia. Thus at any given heart rate the duration of diastolic time during myocardial ischemia will be shorter compared with the diastolic time without myocardial ischemia. The decrease in diastolic time during myocardial ischemia will result in a decrease in myocardial oxygen supply with further deterioration of myocardial ischemia of systole, leading to a vicious cycle[38] (Fig. 2-14).

Coronary resistance. Factors determining coronary artery resistance include the metabolic rate of myocardial cells, autoregulation of the coronary system, mechanical compression of the intramyocardial coronary vessels, and the autonomic nervous system.

Metabolic rate of myocardial cells. Increased myocardial oxygen demand normally leads to arteriolar vasodilatation, decreased vascular resistance and increased myocardial flood flow, and therefore, myocardial oxygen supply.

In patients with coronary artery disease and significant coronary artery stenosis, coronary artery pressure distal to a significant obstruction is low[25-26] (Figures 2-8 and 2-9).

Autoregulation. The term *coronary autoregulation* pertains to the intrinsic ability of the heart to maintain its blood flow at a relatively constant level following changes in perfusion pressure when myocardial oxygen demands are constant.[32] Autoregulation obviously implies a local form of flow regulation and thus excludes effects of extrinsic nerves or circulating hormones as can be demonstrated in isolated, denervated hearts. Autoregulation is looked upon as a relatively rapid vascular adjustment that may also play a role in maintaining capillary hydrostatic pressure relatively constant over a wide range of systemic pressures and coronary artery pressures, preventing formation of tissue edema and damage to the microcirculation.

Most information about coronary autoregulation is derived from studies of left coronary circulation; only limited data exist about autoregulation in the right coronary circulation. Some studies suggest that the degree of autoregulation in the right coronary system is less than in the left. When a correction is made for myocardial oxygen consumption, however, autoregulation of coronary circulation in the right and left ventricles is similar.[30] Autoregulatory vasodilator reserve appears to be greater in the subepicardium than in the subendocardium. When coronary perfusion pressure is gradually reduced, autoregulation falls first in the subendocardium and then in the subepicardium. The reason for this may be caused by transmural differences in extravascular compressive forces, or by differences in myocardial oxygen consumption.

Theories proposed for autoregulation include, (1) the tissue pressure theory, (2) the myogenic theory and, (3) the metabolic theory.

The tissue pressure theory suggests that changes in perfusion pressure lead to similar changes in tissue pressure. Data of recent years, however, suggest that tissue pressure is probably not important in adjusting diastolic coronary resistance following changes in perfusion pressure.

The myogenic theory is based on the hypothesis that vascular resistance is proportional to transmural pressure at the microvascular level. Accordingly, a decrease in intravascular pressure will produce vasodilatation, and an increase in pressure will result in vasoconstriction.

The metabolic theory suggests that myocardial metabolism provides a focal feedback mechanism by which tissue oxygenation is maintained following changes in oxygen supply or demand. According to this hypothesis vascular resistance is controlled by tissue levels of a metabolic substrate or metabolite. Therefore a decrease in coronary pressure will reduce flow, which results in coronary vasodilatation by either decreasing myocardial substrate availability or increasing metabolite production. The degree of autoregulation, however, may depend more on the prevailing balance between myocardial oxygen supply and demand rather than on the absolute level of oxygen consumption. The metabolic theory is based on the premise that oxygen, through release of vasoactive metabolites, induces coronary vasodilatation when perfusion pressure and flow are reduced. Indeed, evidence indicates that coronary autoregulation is closely coupled to the prevailing coronary venous PO_2. It is not clear, however, if coronary autoregulation is the result of direct changes of myocardial PO_2, or occurs through the release of vasoactive metabolites. One of the proposed metabolites that may be involved in the autoregulatory phenomena is adenosine, which typically increases under hypoxic conditions. Studies using adenosine deaminase to destroy cardiac interstitial adenosine, however, have failed to demonstrate that adenosine plays a significant role in coronary autoregulation. A possible role for prostaglandins in coronary autoregulation cannot be excluded.

Mechanical compression of the coronary arteries. Myocardial contraction mechanically compresses intramyocardial vessels and facilitates forward blood flow. Such compression is primarily felt in the vessels of the left ventricle during systole but plays an insignificant or no important role in the right ventricle. The distribution of the compressive forces varies considerably from area to area within the myocardium, with their greater influence being applied in the subendocardium.

Autonomic nervous system. Coronary arteries respond to vasoconstriction of sympathetic α-receptor stimulation and vasodilatation to $β_2$-receptor stimulation. During rest the sympathetic stimuli create a low-grade vasoconstriction. During exercise the alpha-sympathetic action decreases but is not totally abolished.

Steal phenomenon, or proischemia

In patients with coronary artery disease and significant coronary artery stenosis, coronary artery pressure distal to a significant obstruction is low. When coronary artery pressure drops below a certain level, almost maximal vasodilatation takes place. Thus coronary artery resistance distal to a significant stenosis is low compared with normal coronary artery. Because the resistance distal to a significant obstruction is lower compared with normal coronary artery, coronary flow goes from the normal artery to stenotic coronary artery through collaterals. Potent arterial vasodilators will decrease the coronary artery resistance in normal coronary arteries much more than in the arterioles distal to a significant stenosis. This will result in a shift of coronary flow through collaterals from the stenotic to normal coronary artery (Fig. 2-15). This phenomenon is known as *steal phenomenon*. Steal phenomenon, or prois-

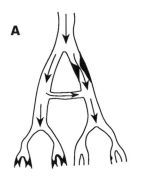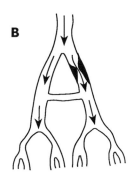

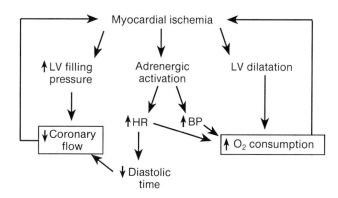

Fig. 2-15. A, Coronary artery resistance in a normal coronary artery and distal to a significant obstruction. Schematic presentation. Note that coronary artery resistance distal to a significant obstruction is decreased compared to normal coronary artery; thus flow through collaterals goes to the area perfused by the stenotic coronary artery. **B,** A potent arteriolar vasodilator will decrease significantly the resistance in the normal coronary artery but not the already low resistance, distal to coronary artery stenosis. Thus the resistance in the normal coronary artery and distal to a significant stenosis will become almost equal, with result cessation of flow through collaterals from the normal coronary to the stenotic coronary artery. This phenomenon is known as *steal phenomenon,* and this effect of the drugs can be considered a proischemic one.

Fig. 2-16. Myocardial ischemia is a dynamic condition, which if persists may lead to vicious cycles. *LV* = left ventricular, *HR* = heart rate, *BP* = blood pressure, ↑ = increased, ↓ = decreased.

chemia, may occur during therapy with dihydropyridine calcium channel blockers or sodium nitroprusside.[41]

Myocardial oxygen demand

Myocardial contractility, heart rate, and myocardial wall tension are the major determinants of myocardial oxygen demand. Left ventricular pressure and left ventricular volume are the major factors determining myocardial wall tension.

As was mentioned above, imbalance between myocardial oxygen consumption and demand will result in myocardial ischemia. It should be emphasized that myocardial ischemia is a dynamic process that can lead to vicious cycles if it is not treated appropriately or if it persists despite therapy (Fig. 2-16).

MORPHOLOGY AND PATHOLOGY OF CORONARY ARTERY LESIONS

Views about ischemic heart disease are constantly changing as we appreciate the dynamic nature of coronary atherosclerosis. To this end correlative studies of premortem and postmortem observations have been exceedingly helpful. Several angiographic and morphologic studies have shown that although there are multiple causes for luminal coronary artery stenosis, the overwhelming cause of coronary artery stenosis (over 90%) is atherosclerosis.[42-46]

The cardinal lesion in occlusive coronary artery disease is the atherosclerotic plaque, which may be concentric or eccentric (Fig. 2-17 and 2-18). This morphologic distinction into concentric and eccentric plaques has important functional and clinical implications (See Pathogenesis of

Acute Ischemic Syndromes later in this chapter). An eccentric plaque occupies only a segment of the arterial circumference. Therefore the remaining wall is either normal or reveals only a modest intimal thickening. The media of the normal segment is apparently responsive to vasoactive stimuli and may alter the cross-sectional area of the lumen. Concentric plaques are fixed and have no ability to alter the cross-sectional area of the lumen. This vascular rigidity of the concentric plaque is thought to be due to diffuse intimal fibrosis acting as a splinter and inducing extensive circumferential atrophy of the media.[42-46]

Atherosclerotic plaques, even from the same individual, vary considerably with regard to their different constituents. Generally, atherosclerotic plaques contain connective-tissue matrix proteins (collagen type I and III), elastin and proteoglycans. Plasma-derived lipids (cholesterol and its esters) are present in an atherosclerotic plaque intracellularly (foam cell), or are free in the intima. The size of the lipid pool in the center of the atheromatous plaque varies, as does the thickness of the cap. Our knowledge is rather limited regarding what factors determine the type of the plaque at different sites, and whether different types indicate evolution of one type of plaque to another.[47-55]

Correlative studies of coronary angiography and postmortem morphology have shown that in the overwhelming majority of cases the atheromatous plaque is the cause for the clinical syndromes of myocardial ischemia. One should be aware, however, that angiography is a luminogram by which comparisons are made between diseased segments and segments that are assumed to be normal. It is widely believed that coronary angiograms in patients with symptomatic ischemic heart disease often underestimate the degree of luminal narrowing. Equally important with angiographic underestimation, is the recognition that postmortem studies of coronary arteries tend to overestimate the degree of obstruction because of postmortem collapse of the vessels.

The relative lack of correlation between angiography

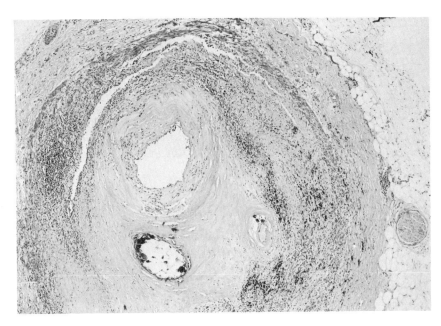

Fig. 2-17. Concentric atheromatous plaque in epicardial coronary artery.

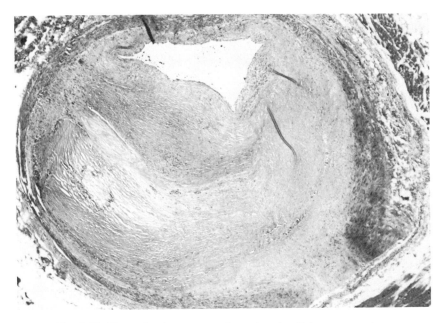

Fig. 2-18. Eccentric atheromatous plaque in epicardial coronary artery.

and postmortem findings are technical issues that are easy to explain. Most puzzling, however, is the lack of correlation that may exist between the extent and severity of fixed anatomic lesions in the coronary arteries and the development and severity of the various ischemic episodes, because acute ischemic syndromes may develop with any degree of fixed coronary artery narrowing. These findings stress that dynamic changes, most likely related to plaque rupture, may occur in the coronary arteries, and may convert an asymptomatic state into a chronic or acute ischemic episode.

PLAQUE RUPTURE AND INTRALUMINAL THROMBOSIS

Intimal injury at the site of an atheromatous lesion may be either superficial or deep. In the case of superficial injury denudation of endothelial cells occurs. With deep intimal injury a fissure is detected extending from the lumen into the plaque tissues. Plaque fissure or rupture may lead to an acute ischemic syndrome, chronic stable angina or may be totally asymptomatic[55] (if superficial, Fig. 2-19).

The precise pathogenesis of plaque rupture is not clear, although it is believed that soft, lipid-rich plaques exposed

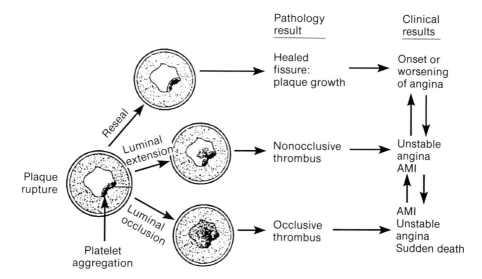

Fig. 2-19. Clinical manifestations of atherosclerotic plaque rupture in a coronary artery. Schematic presentation. *AMI* = acute myocardial infarction (From Davis MJ, Thomas AC: Plaque fissuring. The cause of acute myocardial infarction, sudden ischemic death and crescendo angina, *Br Heart J* 53:363-73, 1985.)

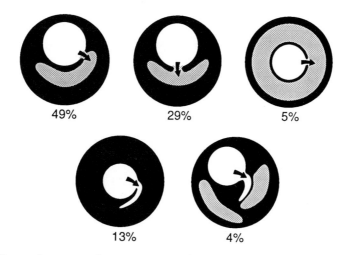

Fig. 2-20. Types of coronary plaque (seen in cross section) undergoing intimal tearing and sites of tearing (arrows). Percentages indicate proportion of plaques with various morphologies. Stippling, lipid; cross-hatching, calcification; black, fibrous tissue. (From Richardson PD, Davies MJ, Born GR: Influence of plaque configuration and stress distribution on fissuring of coronary atherosclerotic plaques, *Lancet* 2:941-944, 1989.)

to increased shear stress at the site of stenosis, or acute changes in coronary pressure or tone, may predispose to rupture[50] (Fig. 2-20). A computer modelling of different types of plaques revealed that at systole eccentric pools of lipids exerted stress on the cap near the edge of the plaque. However, when the lipid pool was relatively small (less than 15% of circumference) the point of maximum stress was over the center of the plaque and rupture occurred at that site. Focal accumulation of foam cells within the cap may weaken it, resulting in rupture without necessarily be-

ing the point of maximal stress (Fig. 2-21). Fibrous plaques exhibiting no lipid pool may also rupture, but the rupture is not followed by important clinical events (a large intraintimal thrombus cannot be formed in the absence of lipid pool). Similarly, rupture can occur in non-lipid plaques exhibiting a calcified plate within the intima that may subject adjacent areas to high shear stress. The possibility that increased interstitial free fluid pressure within an atheromatous plaque, due to filtered proteins, may exceed the tensile strength of the fibrous cap, leading to fissuring, must also be considered.[47-55]

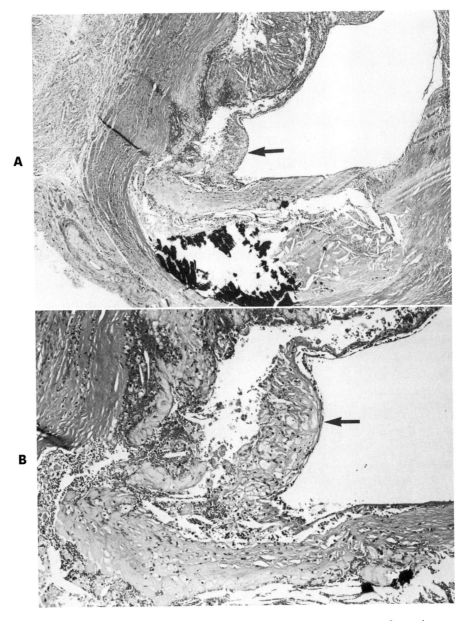

Fig. 2-21. A and **B,** Extensive foam cell infiltrate within the fibrous cap of an atheromatous plaque *(arrow).*

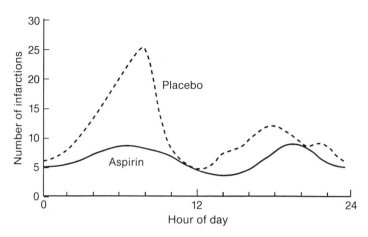

Fig. 2-22. The incidence of acute myocardial infarction (AMI) in the morning hours was greater in the placebo group than in the aspirin group. (From Ridker PM, et al: Circadian variation of acute myocardial infarction and the effect of low-dose aspirin in a randomized trial of physicians, *Circulation* 82:897-902, 1990.)

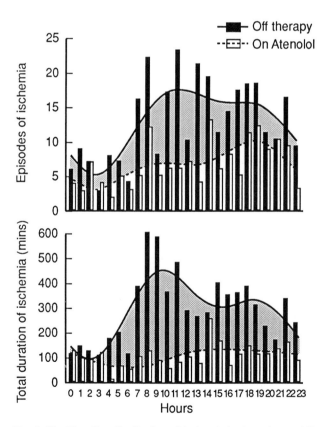

Fig. 2-23. Circadian distribution of ischemia in 41 patients while off and on atenolol. Top: Total ischemic episodes. Bottom: Total duration of ischemia. Bimodal fits are superimposed on each histogram.(From Mulcahy, et al: Circadian variation of total ischaemic burden and its alteration with anti-anginal agents, *Lancet* 2:755-58, 1988.)

One can justifiably state that stresses within the plaque are determined by the complex mechanical properties and variable mixture of plaque components. The stiffness of those components is an important determinant of the stress distribution and propensity to fissuring of atherosclerotic plaques. However, it has been postulated that stiffness of many biologic materials varies under conditions in which stress or strain varies with time, such as during a changing heart rate. It is believed that circadian variation of acute cardiovascular episodes is not a random process and that the increased frequency of ischemic episodes in the morning hours may be caused by increased aggregability of platelets and other components of the clotting system during this period[56] (Fig. 2-22). Similarly, increased sympathetic adrenergic activity in the morning hours may lead to an increase in blood pressure and heart rate with subsequent plaque rupture [57] (Fig. 2-23).

The above discussion about plaque rupture makes it clear that most of the proposed pathogenetic mechanisms are clearly speculative, and thus unproved. Perhaps we should look at this critical event of plaque fissuring as the end result of the culmination of several factors, some intrinsic to the atherosclerotic plaque (such as lipid pool-cap thickness), and some extrinsic, such as forces of turbulence, oscillations in shear stress, or flow instabilities distal to stenoses.

Deep intimal injury exposes significant amounts of collagen to platelets, resulting initially in the formation of a thrombus within the plaque (Fig. 2-24). Intraintimal thrombus may change the size and shape of the plaque and may induce an overlying luminal thrombosis (Fig. 2-25). Studies based on autopsy material have revealed different stages in the thrombosis associated with plaque fissuring. In the initial stage, the tear creates a communication between the lumen and the lipid-rich interior of the atheromatous plaque, leading to the formation of a platelet-rich thrombus within the intima. Later, a more fibrin-containing thrombus is formed over and within the fissure site. However, the intraintimal thrombotic mass may extend into the arterial lumen, thus establishing a mural component.

Angiographic studies have recognized intramural thrombi as filling defects with overhanging edges in patients with unstable angina and acute myocardial infarction. In the final stage an occlusive luminal thrombus may be formed composed mostly of fibrin, a few platelets, and only rare red blood cells. Several variables determine if the thrombus is labile or fixed, and therefore susceptible to either natural or iatrogenic thrombolysis. Intraluminal thrombi composed primarily of fibrin and some red cells are apparently labile. Major fissures and tears may result in a raised intimal flap, thus increasing the luminal impingement of the plaque. Furthermore, a large tear may facilitate luminal extrusion of cholesterol debris (crystals) and formation of a fixed thrombus resistant to lysis (Fig.

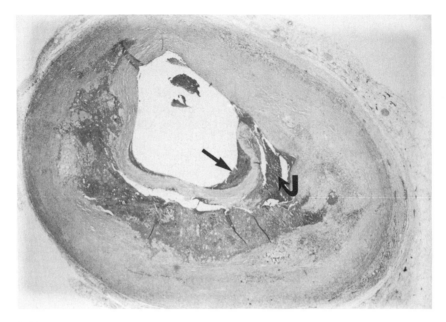

Fig. 2-24. Rupture of fibrous cap in an atheromatous plaque. Note thrombus formation within the plaque *(curved arrow)* and small intraluminal thrombus *(straight arrow)*.

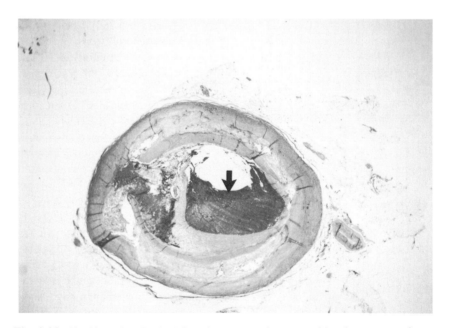

Fig. 2-25. Significant intraluminal thrombus *(arrow)* in an unstable atheromatous plaque.

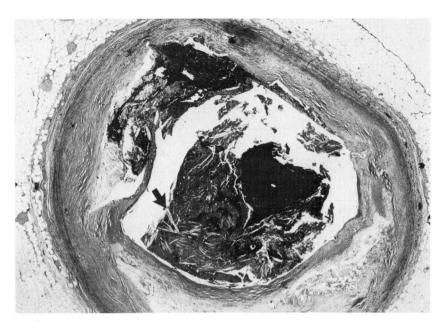

Fig. 2-26. Ruptured atheromatous plaque. Note intraluminal thrombus containing cholesterol debris, an indication of extrusion from the plaque atheroma.

2-26). In addition, angiographic studies have demonstrated transitions from mural to occlusive thrombi and vice versa in patients with developing infarction. A possible complication originating from the luminal thrombus is the emergence of platelet/fibrin microemboli in the microcirculation downstream from the occluded vessel. These microemboli have been found in hearts of patients that died as a result of a myocardial infarction. It has been suggested that these microemboli may contribute to the hemodynamic and/or electrical instability of such patients.

Intraluminal thrombi have been identified in many angiographic studies of patients with unstable angina and in cases of acute myocardial infarction. The incidence of such thrombi is related, at least in part, to the period between the onset of clinical symptoms and the performance of the angiography. A shorter period increases the likelihood of finding occlusive thrombi. It is believed that thrombotic occlusion in unstable angina is transient and is most likely the result of mild injury to the arterial wall. On the contrary, a deep intimal injury with rupture or ulceration of the plaque may lead to a persistent thrombotic occlusion and myocardial infarction. Factors such as the size of the involved artery, the status of the intrinsic fibrinolytic system, the adequacy of collateral flow, and changes in the vascular tone play an important role in the development of acute coronary syndromes.

Although different pathogenetic mechanisms are operational in the intimal tears, after balloon angioplasty the site of postangioplasty fissuring is identical to that seen in ischemic episodes, namely the junction of the plaque with the normal arterial segment. A possible explanation for the predilection of fissuring at this site is that the two segments (the plaque and normal wall) differ considerably in expansile strength.

MOLECULAR ALTERATIONS IN ACUTE MYOCARDIAL ISCHEMIA

An abrupt closure of a coronary artery eliminates the flow of oxygenated blood in the myocardial region that the artery supplies. Within 8 to 10 seconds oxygen trapped in the region will be consumed, leading to significant functional and metabolic changes that encompass cessation of contraction, electrocardiographic changes, and cellular injury leading to eventual myocardial necrosis (Fig. 2-27). Changes in the myocardium in cases of less than total ischemia (mild to moderate) are more difficult to characterize because of lack of uniformity. Note that observations about molecular alterations in the ischemic myocardium are primarily based on experimental animal studies.[58-89]

Following coronary occlusion, mitochondrial oxidative metabolism comes to a halt within a few seconds. Similarly, Krebs citric acid cycle and fatty acid oxidation are abolished. Then anaerobic glycolysis is accelerated and becomes the primary means of generating new high-energy phosphate. Anaerobic glycolysis is an inefficient source of high-energy phosphate and can provide only 7% of the high-energy phosphate needs of a contracting myocardium.[85] It is estimated that approximately 50% of the ATP stores are degraded within the initial 10 minutes of severe ischemia and that the remainder are degraded at slower rates. After the degradation of ATP to ADP, the ADP is converted to adenosine monophosphate (AMP) by the ade-

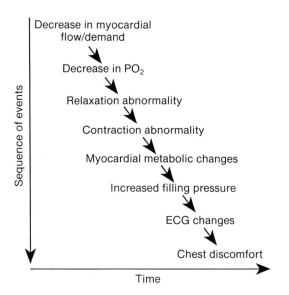

Fig. 2-27. Temporal sequence of events in myocardial ischemia. Note that electrocardiographic (ECG) changes and chest pain occur after the metabolic abnormalities.

nylate kinase reaction. Then the AMP is slowly degraded to adenosine, inosine, hypoxanthine and xanthine, which may accumulate at the site of the ischemic injury or wash away if the tissue is reperfused. Anaerobic glycolysis, which is high initially after the coronary occlusion, slows down in about 60 to 90 seconds, persists at this slow rate for about 40 to 60 minutes, and then ceases. Cessation of glycolysis is not due to exhaustion of substrate, but to low pH and high lactate levels.[84]

In addition to adverse effect of oxygen deprivation of the myocardium, other catabolic events may also contribute to the ischemic injury. Rapid accumulation of lactate, purine nucleotides, and bases occurs. Tissue acidosis may have deleterious consequences on the nuclear chromatin and mitochondria. The ischemic myocardium reveals an increased lipolysis, probably through a catecholamine-dependent mechanism.[85] Therefore there is increase of intracellular lipid in ischemic myocardium resulting from an increased uptake from plasma, reduced fatty acid oxidation, or both. It is believed that fatty acid esters such as lysophospholipids may act as detergents and disrupt cellular membranes, as is the case with arachidonic acid, which accumulates in the ischemic myocardium.[58-89]

Edema of myocytes observed in acute ischemia appears to be caused by the accumulation of osmotically active particles arising from ischemic metabolism. These metabolites (glycolytic intermediates, creatine ammonia, etc) increase the osmolar load; this increase will result in water accumulation in the myocytes and an immediate efflux of potassium ion. Myocyte potassium loss is one of the earliest events of ischemia, but its exact mechanism is not completely understood. Loss of intracellular potassium is

not coupled with intracellular sodium gain.[84] Thus, potassium loss is accompanied by cellular extrusion of other anions (such as phosphate and lactate) to maintain neutrality.[73] Loss of ion transport activity may also contribute to net influx of water and eventually to cell swelling. It should be emphasized that maintenance of electrolyte gradient is energy consuming; although it receives first priority of the available energy resources, it will eventually cease because of ATP depletion.

Increased cytosolic calcium also occurs in ischemia. This increase is related to enhanced influx from either extracellular tissues or sarcoplasmic reticulum, or to a lack of extrusion due to inadequate energy. Increased intracellular calcium may have a deleterious effect on the myocyte because calcium activates proteases, lipases, and phospholipases, enhances ATP depletion, and inhibits mitochondrial respiration.[74]

Changes in extracellular K^+ concentration cause a number of electrophysiologic changes to develop. These changes occur within 15 to 30 seconds after the initiation of ischemia. Ischemia induces shortening of the duration of action potential and slows intramyocardial conduction velocity. Although the molecular basis for the above changes is not well understood, it is most likely related to metabolic and electrolyte disturbances, including extracellular hyperkalemia, intracellular acidosis and/or cellular calcium overload.[71,75,87]

The intensity of alterations in the myocyte becomes more marked as the duration of ischemia increases. Yet, these changes are still considered reversible, even in the most ischemic zone. It has been shown that restoration of blood flow within 15 minutes after coronary occlusion results in rapid recovery of the myocytes. Longer duration of ischemia, however, will produce more pronounced changes. Additional ultrastructural alterations will appear in the myocytes, manifested as swollen mitochondria, disorganized cristae, and amorphous densities in their matrix. Further breaks in the membrane of the sarcolemma, particularly over areas of marked cellular edema, may occur. Changes in the mitochondria and sarcolemma will persist without reperfusion and will lead to coagulation necrosis. In the open-chest anesthetized dog, irreversibly injured myocytes are seen after 40 to 60 minutes of complete ischemia.[84]

Irreversibly injured myocardial cells release a number of enzymes into the circulation[90] (Fig. 2-28) where they can be measured by specific chemical reactions. Increased activities of many enzymes have been found in the serum or plasma of patients with acute myocardial infarction. Following experimental myocardial infarction, a small but significant myocardial venoarterial difference of enzyme activity can be measured, and elevated plasma levels of enzymes correlate with corresponding depletion of these same enzymes from infarcted tissue. Determinations of serum activity of creatine kinase (preferably its MB isoenzyme) and of lactate dehydrogenase are frequently used in the laboratory diagnosis of acute myocardial infarction.

Several hypotheses have been proposed for the pathogenesis of sarcolemmal disruption in ischemic injury. It has been suggested that during ischemia calcium-dependent endogenous phospholipases are activated that result in changes of sarcolemma phospholipids and increased permeability. If ischemia lasts more than 30 minutes, then arachidonate is released from phospholipids. Also contributing to membrane disruption is the fact that free radicals induce sarcolemma injury. However, although membrane injury by free radical peroxidation can occur with reperfusion, its role in membrane disruption in the initial ischemic injury has not been established. It is currently believed that during ischemia a number of processes may simultaneously contribute to the disruption of the sarcolemma membrane; therefore sarcolemma rupture has a multifactorial pathogenesis.[58-89]

Ultrastructural alterations secondary to ischemia are seen not only in the myocytes, but also in the microvasculature of the myocardium. Vascular injury may be mild, manifesting by increased capillary permeability, or severe, presenting by endothelial swelling and capillary obstruction. Reperfusion will result in necrosis of the microvasculature and extensive myocardial hemorrhage. Furthermore, capillary obstruction due to endothelial blebs, neutrophils, or microthrombi may be responsible for the "no-reflow phenomenon," despite the opening (spontaneous or iatrogenic) of the previous occluded coronary artery.[77]

The role of the neutrophil in the pathogenesis of acute myocardial ischemia and extension of myocardial injury has been only recently appreciated. Increased peripheral blood count and neutrophil activation correlates well with increased risk of ischemic events in humans.[78] Reports indicate that activated neutrophils will release arachidonic acid derivatives such as leukotrienes and thromboxane A_2 that affect the vasoreactivity of the endothelium. Activated neutrophils may also induce endothelial dysfunction and coronary vasoconstriction.[79] Neutrophils accumulated in the areas of ischemic injury may discharge oxygen-free radicals, proteolytic enzymes, granular constituents (elastase), and arachidonic acid, which may cause injury to cell membranes and mitochondria.[80] It is of considerable interest that oxygen-derived free radicals have been implicated in the pathogenesis of stunned myocardium and in the adverse effect on wall motion after reperfusion. Another potential risk from the activation of neutrophils is in situ activation of complement on an atherosclerotic plaque which may lead to membrane damage and tissue injury.

Increased sympathetic activity with high plasma catecholamines has been reported during myocardial ischemia. In addition to the high plasma norepinephrine levels in the circulation, there is a dramatic increase of norepinephrine in regional areas with myocardial ischemia, which may be more than 1000 times greater in concentration than the

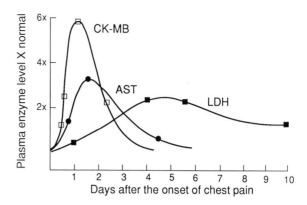

Fig. 2-28. Typical plasma profiles for the MB isoenzyme of creatine kinase (CK-MB), aspartate aminotransferase (AST), and lactate dehydrogenase (LDH) activities following onset of acute myocardial infarction. (Adapted from Hearse DJ: Myocardial enzyme leakage, *J Molec Med* 2:185, 1987.)

plasma norepinephrine.[67,81-83,88] Thus during myocardial ischemia there is increased concentration of plasma norepinephrine and local release of catecholamines (sympathetic neurons) in the ischemic myocardium, regardless of the systemic sympathetic nerve activity. Regional release of norepinephrine is seen after 10 minutes or less of complete ischemia. High concentrations of catecholamines during this ischemic period may produce myocardial damage. The combination of local excess of noradrenaline and enhanced tissue responsiveness may accelerate cell damage and permanently harm a previously reversible cell. This detrimental effect is probably due to catecholamine-induced increase in cellular energy demand and stimulation of calcium influx into the myocytes. The regional norepinephrine levels are further increased after reperfusion.

CORONARY ARTERY DISEASE: CLINICAL PRESENTATION

Patients with myocardial ischemia may be asymptomatic or exhibit symptoms of dyspnea, fatigue, and/or palpitations. Occasionally syncope and sudden death are the initial manifestations of ischemia. Up to 30% of patients with myocardial ischemia do not have chest pain. Painless ischemia may be more frequent in patients with diabetes mellitus, patients with chronic renal failure and elderly patients. Nevertheless, patients with coronary artery disease usually present with stable angina, unstable angina, or myocardial infarction. Fig. 2-29 schematically shows the pathologic conditions, the clinical manifestations, and the natural history of coronary artery disease.[26,39]

Chronic stable angina

Patients with chronic stable angina usually present with chest pain of short duration (5 to 15 minutes); the pain is reproducible under similar situations (physical or emotional stress), occurs with predictable frequency, and pre-

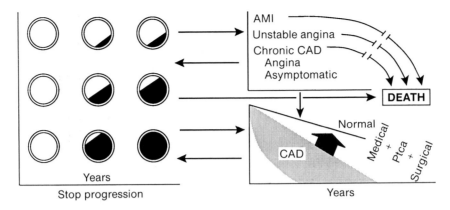

Fig. 2-29. Relation between coronary artery pathology, clinical manifestations of coronary artery disease (CAD), natural history, and therapy. The solid line represents survival in the general population. The shaded area represents survival in patients with CAD. Therapy (medical, percutaneous transluminal coronary angioplasty [PTCA], and surgery) may improve survival. Note the interrelationship between the clinical manifestations, natural history, and therapy. Coronary anatomy, however, usually is not altered by therapy.(See text for details, from Boudoulas H and Geleris P, Eds: *Coronary Artery Disease,* ed 2, Thessaloniki, Greece, 1990, University Press.)

dictably, responds to rest and/or nitrates. Stable angina is usually the result of increased myocardial oxygen demand and the inability of the stenosed arteries to increase oxygen delivery.

Unstable angina

Unstable angina is defined as recent onset angina, angina that now occurs with increasing frequency and severity, nocturnal angina, angina that occurs at rest, and angina developing within 4 weeks after acute myocardial infarction. *Crescendo angina, preinfarction angina,* or *intermediate syndrome* are terms that describe various subsets of symptoms falling within the category of unstable angina.

Acute myocardial infarction

Patients with myocardial infarction usually present with severe and persistent chest pain which does not respond to sublingual nitroglycerin administration or rest.

Myocardial ischemia related to coronary artery disease should be considered as a spectrum running from stable angina through unstable angina to myocardial infarction. Recognizing where an individual patient falls along that spectrum of coronary disease is essential to management. Patients with unstable angina and acute myocardial infarction are considered as having *acute ischemic syndrome*.

PATHOGENESIS OF ACUTE ISCHEMIC SYNDROMES

The underlying pathophysiology in acute ischemic syndromes (unstable angina, non-Q-wave myocardial infarction, Q-wave infarction), is usually the result of abrupt reduction or stoppage of coronary blood flow.

Several mechanisms may be involved in unstable an-

gina, including transient episodic thrombosis over injured plaque, release of vasoconstrictive substances (thromboxane A_2, serotonin) by platelets attached to damaged endothelium, or transient increase in myocardial oxygen demand (Fig. 2-30). Based on coronary arteriography, atherosclerotic plaques in patients with stable and unstable angina can be classified according to the following descriptions: (1) concentric, (2) eccentric type I (asymmetric narrowing with smooth borders and a broad neck), (3) eccentric type II (asymmetric with narrow neck or irregular borders or both), and (4) multiple irregular coronary narrowings in series.[44] Eccentric type II lesions are found in 54% of patients with unstable angina and in only 7% of patients with stable angina. In "angina-producing" arteries the frequency of eccentric type II lesions is seen in 71% of patients with unstable angina, and in only 16% of patients with stable angina. Coronary angiography in patients who progressed from stable to unstable angina has shown that progression of lesions is common in the latter. The eccentric type II lesion is the most frequently seen angiographic morphology.[89-100]

In about three fourths of cases, the underlying pathophysiology in non-Q-wave infarction is similar to that seen in unstable angina, i.e., plaque injury. In the remainder of the cases, a completely occluded infarct-related vessel may be found. However, the high rate of angiographic patency in non-Q-wave myocardial infarcts suggests complete occlusion followed by reperfusion or resolution of vasospasm as other possible mechanisms.

Deep intimal injury or ulceration which leads to formation of a fixed occlusive intraluminal thrombus is the most common underlying morphology in a Q-wave myocardial infarction. The lesion at the site of the thrombus formation may be modest, which indicates that the thrombus precip-

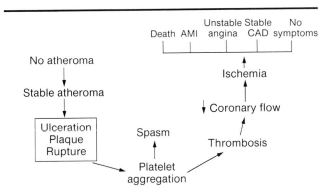

Fig. 2-30. The role of intravascular thromboses in coronary artery disease (CAD). Ulceration will result in platelet aggregation, arterial thrombosis and myocardial ischemia with the clinical manifestations of ischemia. *AMI* = acute myocardial infarction.

itates the acute episode. In cases with severely stenotic plaques, complete occlusion may occur without myocardial necrosis because of collaterals distal to obstruction. Patients with an acute myocardial infarction often reveal diffuse coronary atherosclerosis, although the site of the infarction is supplied by a single artery and in the majority of cases (80%), the cause of the occlusion is an intraluminal thrombus. However, other factors besides the thrombus may contribute to the complete arterial occlusion, such as platelet aggregation and/or coronary spasm.

The pathophysiologic mechanisms in sudden cardiac death may involve plaque rupture with subsequent thrombosis, myocardial ischemia and fatal ventricular arrhythmias. In deaths which occur several hours after the initiation of clinical symptoms, myocardial necrosis may be present.

SILENT MYOCARDIAL ISCHEMIA

Several recent studies have shown that patients with coronary artery disease may develop painless ischemia with little or no increase in myocardial oxygen consumption (i.e., minimal increased heart rate and/or arterial blood pressure). It appears, therefore, that patients with chronic stable angina may reveal variability of ischemic threshold; this variability may or may not be related to segmental coronary artery hyperactivity. This is in contrast to the hyperactivity and arterial occlusion observed in unstable angina and acute myocardial infarction.*

Reduction of coronary blood flow may also occur, even with small changes in heart rate during routine daily activities. This reduction occurs because small changes in heart rate produce significant changes in diastolic time (myocardial perfusion time); a decrease in diastolic time may result in a significant decrease in myocardial blood flow[27] (see

*References 17, 20, 27, 38, 57, 84, 87, 93, 98, 100-104.

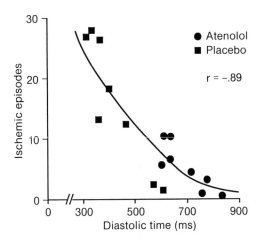

Fig. 2-31. Relationship between diastolic time and silent ischemic episodes in patients with coronary artery disease before and after therapy with atenolol. (Figure was constructed using data from Chierchia S, Glazier L: A model for the management of silent myocardial ischemia. Proceedings of a symposium. A quarter-century of β-blockade, *Postgrad Med* 2:120-122, 1988.)

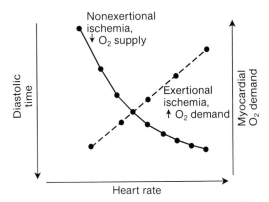

Fig. 2-32. Mechanisms of myocardial ischemia in patients with coronary artery disease. At fast heart rates (exertional angina), heart rate and myocardial oxygen consumption increase. At slow heart rates (non-exertional angina), small changes in heart rate will produce significant changes in diastolic time and myocardial blood flow but no or small changes in myocardial oxygen consumption. (From Boudoulas H: Diastolic time: The forgotten dynamic factor. Implications for myocardial perfusion, *Acta Cardiol* 46:61-71, 1991.)

Fig. 2-11). It is known that β-blockade therapy may prevent silent myocardial ischemia. This may be related to an increase in diastolic time. The relationship between diastolic time and silent ischemic episodes before and after β-blockade therapy is shown in Figure 2-31. It can be seen that an excellent nonlinear relationship exits between these two parameters. Silent ischemic episodes almost disappear when diastolic time is longer than 700 ms, and are dramatically increased when the diastolic time is shorter than 500 ms.[103]

Figure 2-32 shows schematically how myocardial ischemia can occur with insignificant changes of myocardial oxygen consumption due to alterations in diastolic time.[38] During exercise, the increase in heart rate may result in myocardial ischemia. At rest, small changes in heart rate may produce significant changes in diastolic time; these changes may lead to a significant decrease in myocardial blood flow, without or minimal changes in myocardial oxygen consumption. Thus, a decrease in diastolic time may produce myocardial ischemia. The fact that β-blocking drugs, which do not prevent coronary artery spasm, decrease the incidence of silent myocardial ischemia in patients with coronary artery disease supports the hypothesis that myocardial ischemia may result from a decrease in diastolic time. Further, the fact that calcium channel blocking drugs, which prevent coronary artery spasm, do not prolong survival in patients with coronary artery disease suggests that coronary artery spasm does not play a major role in the chronic phase of coronary artery disease.

SYNDROME X

Syndrome X has been defined as stress-induced angina and ST segment depression in patients who have angiographically normal coronary arteries without evidence of spasm of the epicardial arteries. Although the pathogenesis of syndrome X remains unknown, prearteriolar constriction has been postulated as the cause for the reduced vasodilator response and anginal pain observed after administration of dipyridamole in patients with this syndrome. A compensatory production of adenosine has also been suggested to explain the patchy distribution of myocardial ischemia in these patients.[105-107]

Earlier studies indicated that chest pain induced with rapid right atrial pacing, in patients with chest pain and normal coronary arteries, was associated with myocardial lactate production and ST segment depression. The degree of ST segment depression was directly related to amount of lactate production. More recent studies suggest that the metabolic pattern in these patients is different from that in patients with classic myocardial ischemia. Metabolic changes observed include greater myocardial extraction of glucose and glycerol and lower extraction of pyruvate. These changes are attributed to an increased fatty acid oxidation that inhibits pyruvate entry into the Krebs cycle. Small vessel disease has also been proposed as another factor responsible for the pathogenesis of syndrome X.[94,105-107]

MORPHOLOGIC RECOGNITION OF MYOCARDIAL INFARCTION: GROSS AND MICROSCOPIC FEATURES

Gross morphologic recognition of the exact age of an infarction is not an easy task. Several factors, including previous ischemic episodes in the vicinity of the new infarction, may alter the gross appearance of an infarction and make its precise morphologic dating difficult. Furthermore, gross identification of an infarction within the first few hours is not possible. The use of the nitro blue tetrazolium test on fresh slides of myocardium at autopsy usually discloses early infarction (3 to 4 hours) as pale areas in contrast to bright blue coloration of healthy myocardium.[108-116]

About 6 to 8 hours after myocardial infarction, the necrotic myocardium (coagulation necrosis) appears pale and swollen with a poorly defined border of hyperemia. The infarcted area becomes somewhat purplish after about 24 to 36 hours. Approximately 48 hours after myocardial in-

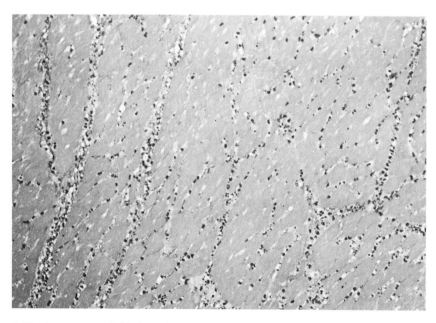

Fig. 2-33. Acute myocardial infarct (2-3 days). Significant numbers of polys are present, the myocytes have indistinct borders and their nuclei are lysed.

farction, it appears as a central gray area with a yellow border indicative of the neutrophilic influx. This peripheral yellow discoloration will extend over the entire infarcted area by the first week. During the second postinfarction week the infarcted area appears sunken (apparently due to loss of tissue); the yellow coloration will be replaced from the periphery into the central zone by purplish-red granulation tissue zone in 3 to 4 weeks. Beginning in the second month and continuing over the third month the infarction becomes pale-gray and has a gelatinous appearance. Beyond this period the infarction undergoes scarring and appears as a firm, white, slight depressed scar. Postischemic myocardial scars are usually smaller than the original mass that they replace.

Severe myocardial ischemia will cause clouding, swelling and hydropic degeneration of the myocytes; these ischemic myocytes, however, are considered potentially reversible. Enzymatic stains may facilitate the microscopic recognition of an infarcted area within 6 to 8 hours; hematoxylin and eosin stains, however, are quite adequate for histologic dating of an infarction. Perhaps one of the earliest tissue alterations within the infarcted area is interstitial edema, along with reactive hyperemia at the periphery. Neither of these two findings, however, is a reliable dating criterion. Approximately 6 hours after infarction, the cytoplasm of myocytes becomes intensely eosinophilic, while early mild changes (pyknosis) of the nuclei are observed. Nuclear changes reach a peak between 24 to 48 hours, and in about 2 to 3 days the nuclei are completely lysed and disappear (Fig. 2-33).

The myocardial fibers may appear somewhat stretched and wavy in patients who died from pump failure. In approximately 8 to 10 hours polymorphonuclear leukocytes appear in the interstitium while focal extravasation of erythrocytes is seen because of capillary rupture. The peak of polymorphonuclear leukocytes is reached between 48 to 70 hours postinfarction; this peak declines gradually over the next 2 weeks (Fig. 2-34). After about 24 hours the myocardial fibers lose their cross-striations, their cytoplasms become clumped, and focal hyalinization and irregular cross-bands appear. The peak of myocardial cell necrosis occurs around the fifth day, followed by the gradual disappearance of myocytes. The entrance of leukocytes from the periphery of the necrotic area towards the center of the lesion contributes to the myocyte breakdown. However, the rate of disappearance of myocytes depends on the size of the infarction. The center of a large infarction may be occupied by ghost myocardial cells for longer periods, or until neovascularization is completed and removal of necrotic cells is carried out. Lymphocytes, plasma cells , and macrophages appear at about the fourth or fifth day (the macrophages appear somewhat later), increase through the third week and may remain for several months in reduced numbers. In some infarctions, for reasons not very well understood, an influx of eosinophils is seen around the eighth postinfarction day to disappear by the second week.

Proliferation of fibroblasts is seen by the fourth day, with their numbers increasing through the first 3 weeks and gradually diminishing by the sixth week. Collagen fi-

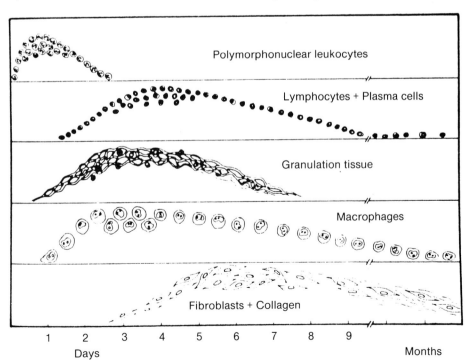

Fig. 2-34. Chronologic sequence of healing phenomena (dating) of an acute myocardial infarct. (From Gravanis MB, ed: *Cardiovascular pathophysiology.* NY, 1987, McGraw Hill. Used by permission.)

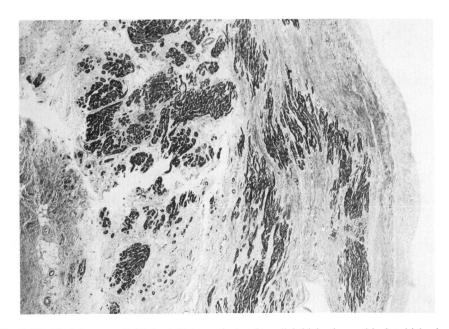

Fig. 2-35. Healed myocardial infarct. Note marked endocardial thickening and isolated islands of survived myocardium.

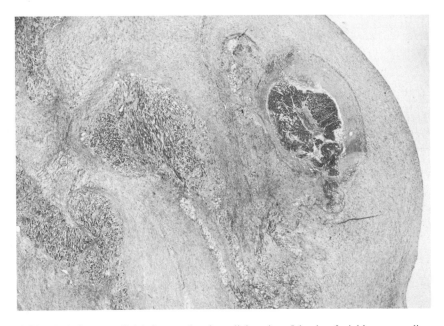

Fig. 2-36. Healed myocardial infarct, subendocardial region. Islands of viable myocardium are present in a sea of fibrosis.

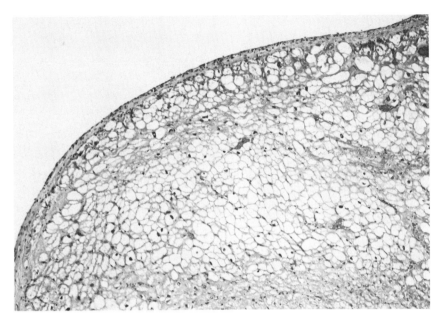

Fig. 2-37. Subendocardial zone showing severe myocytolysis (chronic hypoperfusion).

bers begin to appear by the ninth day along with significant proliferation of young blood vessels, which increase gradually and persist for several months. The final stage of this reparative process is the formation of a sclerotic, often acellular scar (Fig. 2-35).

The necrosis of myocytes in the central zone of an infarction, as was described above, is typical of *coagulation necrosis*. There is, however, an additional type of necrosis seen in the myocardium. This is the so-called *contraction band necrosis*. This is most often seen in areas of severe ischemia followed by reperfusion after thrombolytic therapy or spontaneous lysis of an occlusive thrombus. The involved myocytes in contraction band necrosis reveal, as the term denotes, cross densely eosinophilic amorphous lines interspersed by cleared areas in the sarcoplasm. The normal cross striations in these myocytes become blurred, and the nuclei lyse. Most contraction band infarctions become dark red and hemorrhagic as capillaries rupture and extravasation of red cells occurs. These types of necrosis are often seen in infarction and/or rupture of the posterior papillary muscle, which is commonly supplied by branches of both the circumflex and the right coronary arteries.

In myocardial infarctions the interface between the necrotic zone and spared myocytes is often irregular, presenting microscopically with islands of surviving myocytes interspersed with peninsulas of infarcted tissues that extend toward the epicardium. Although infarctions rarely involve the entire vascular areas at risk, the amount and location of surviving myocardium, in the area of distribution of the occluded vessel, is quite variable. Areas that usually survive the ischemic episode are variable in thickness in the subepicardial zone, at the lateral borders of the infarction, and in a thin rim of myocardium in the subendocardial area (Fig. 2-36). Diffusion of adequate oxygen and substrate from the ventricular cavity is most probably the reason for the survival of the thin strip of subendocardial myocardium. The narrow zones of surviving myocardium in the lateral borders of an infarction, and the thin rim of salvaged myocardium in the subendocardial zone both reveal hypoperfusion and subcellular changes (myocytolysis) after and beyond the establishment of infarction. These changes consist of cytoplasmic accumulation of neutral fat, which indicates a reduction of mitochondrial oxidation of fatty acids. Surviving subendocardial myocytes often reveal degenerative changes long after the acute ischemic episode and occasionally independently of such an event. These changes, which have been termed myocytolysis, are characterized by a clear vacuolated cytoplasm caused by loss of sarcoplasmic contractile elements. It is not clear, however, whether such myocytes remain in this degenerative condition indefinitely or become necrotic and disappear. Histopathologic evidence of necrosis of such myocytes with subsequent leukocytic reaction is insufficient.

Myocytolysis or colliquative necrosis is usually seen in chronic mild to moderate hypoperfusion of myocytes. This type of cellular injury is often observed at the border zones of an infarction or independent of an infarction in the subendocardium (Figure 2-37).

Distribution of the collateral blood flow in an ischemic region is uneven. This occurs because collateral flow is shunted preferentially to the subepicardial regions at the expense of the subendocardial zones. Collateral flow is to-

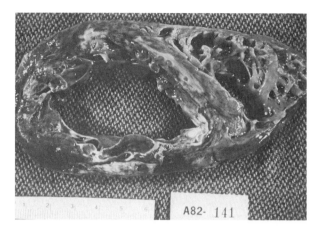

Fig. 2-38. Transmural, anteroseptal acute infarct (3-5 days), and posterior left ventricular wall healed infarct.

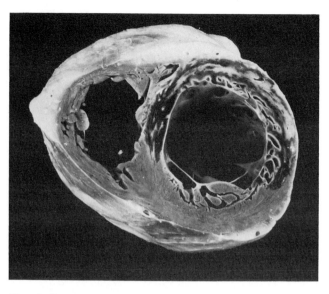

Fig. 2-40. Anteroseptal acute (3-5 days) myocardial infarct (Courtesy of Dr. William D. Edwards, Mayo Clinic).

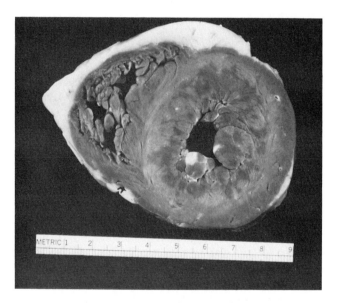

Fig. 2-39. Subendocardial circumferential acute infarct (3-5 days) (Courtesy Dr. William D. Edwards, Mayo Clinic).

tally diastolic, and the amount of collateral flow and especially subendocardial flow are related to the duration of diastole. Furthermore, there are regional differences in the metabolic activity of the myocardium, which are manifested with greater depletion of high energy phosphate, such as is seen in the subendocardial zone. The net result of the preferential distribution of the collateral blood flow and of the differences in regional metabolic activity is that irreversible myocyte ischemic injury occurs first in the subendocardial zone, gradually involving the middle myocardial regions and finally the subepicardial zone (Fig. 2-37). Infarctions in humans rarely involve the entire vascular area at risk. In ligation of a coronary artery in experimental animals (dogs), the transluminal wave front cell

death starts in the subendocardial zone in about 15 to 30 minutes after ligation, extends transmurally and establishes an infarction by 3 to 6 hours.

ANATOMIC DISTRIBUTION OF INFARCTIONS

Infarctions can be classified as transmural (Fig. 2-38) or nontransmural (subendocardial, Fig. 2-39). The latter may be focal or circumferential. There is fairly good correlation between the site of major coronary artery obstruction and the geographic location of a transmural myocardial infarction. Despite their name, transmural myocardial infarctions never involve the entire thickness of the left ventricular myocardium. Usually, one-fourth to one-fifth of the subepicardial myocardium, plus a thin rim of the subendocardial myocardium, is spared. Cavitary oxygen diffusion is perhaps responsible for the survival of the subendocardial layers of the myocardium; the explanation for the subepicardial myocardium salvage may be related to shunting of blood during ischemia to the subepicardial zones, and to direct supply of the subepicardial zones by short direct branches from the epicardial coronary arteries.[111-112,117-118]

Left ventricular infarction

Myocardial infarctions may involve the apical region, the middle portion, or the basal portion of the left ventricle or, as is the case in large infarctions, the entire region from apex to base. Posterior basal infarctions are considered in electrocardiographic terms as true posterior, while posterior midzonal infarctions are referred to as inferior. An anterior or anteroseptal myocardial infarction occurs after occlusion of the LAD coronary artery and tends to be more severe towards the apex (Fig. 2-40).

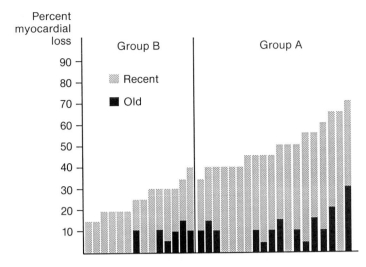

Fig. 2-41. Relationship between infarct size in patients dying after myocardial infarction with cardiogenic shock (group A) and without cardiogenic shock (group B). Patients dying with cardiogenic shock generally had greater than or equal to 40% of their ventricular muscle mass irreversibly damaged.(Page DL, et al: Myocardial changes associated with cardiogenic shock, *Eng J Med* 285:133, 1971.)

Occlusion of the RCA results in an inferior or inferior-posterior myocardial infarction of the left ventricle and, in approximately 25% of the cases, in right ventricular infarction.

As was stated earlier, the distribution of an acute transmural myocardial infarction corresponds in the majority of cases to the occluded artery supplying the area. In some cases, however, abrupt occlusion of a coronary artery may result in infarction of a distal region vascularized by collaterals from the acutely occluded artery. This is termed *infarction at a distance.*

Right ventricular infarction

Right ventricular infarction commonly occurs in association with acute inferior left ventricular myocardial infarction, rarely may occur with an anterior myocardial infarction, and occasionally may occur as an isolated infarction of the right ventricle. Isolated right ventricular infarction is estimated to be 1% to 2% of all myocardial infarctions involving the right ventricle. Patients with right ventricular infarction usually have occlusive coronary lesions of the right coronary artery and often multivessel disease. Reasons often mentioned for the protection of the right ventricle from ischemic events are the thin wall structure, the low pressures generated in the chamber, and therefore, the low oxygen consumption. In addition, because of low right ventricular systolic pressure, right ventricular blood flow is systolic and diastolic, while left ventricular blood flow is only diastolic. These protective factors account for the frequent absence of right ventricular infarction after occlusion of the right coronary artery. Whether or not right ventricular hypertrophy and pulmonary hypertension make

this chamber more susceptible to infarction remains a controversial issue.[117-119]

The most commonly mentioned complications of right ventricular infarction are hypotension and shock. Although the mortality rate is relatively high in patients with hemodynamically significant right ventricular infarction, patients surviving hospitalization generally have a good prognosis.

Atrial infarction

Atrial myocardial infarction may occur in combination with ventricular infarction. Right atrial ischemic injury is 6 times more common than left atrial ischemic injury. Regardless of the location, atrial myocardial infarctions are usually clinically inapparent because they are often overshadowed by the symptoms of the ventricular damage. Some atrial myocardial infarctions may be associated with mural thrombi or may involve the conduction system, particularly the sinoatrial mode.[120]

VENTRICULAR FUNCTION AFTER MYOCARDIAL INFARCTION: REMODELING, EXPANSION
Ventricular function

Acute myocardial infarction almost always induces some dysfunction of the left or right ventricle. The main determinant of the degree of ventricular dysfunction is the mass of the infarcted myocardium[121] (Fig. 2-41). The left ventricle after myocardial infarction can be considered as a two-component model. In this conceptual model the ventricle includes an infarcted segment that is noncontractile and less compliant, along with the noninfarcted segments

I   II   III   IV

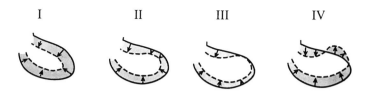

Fig. 2-42. Patterns of left ventricular contraction abnormalities in acute myocardial infarction: (I) normal, (II) hypokinesis, (III) akinesis, and (IV) dyskinesis.

that possess normal compliance and normal contractility.[121-130]

Although the two-component model ignores the transitional or border zones, which may have only mildly altered function, the model still explains adequately the pathophysiologic consequences of infarction. With this model in mind, it is accurate to state that the overall ventricular function depends on the size of the infarcted segment. In large myocardial infarctions where over 40% of the left ventricular myocardium has been damaged, the left ventricle cannot sustain cardiac function and leads to cardiogenic shock and death. Both left ventricular systolic and diastolic function are altered in myocardial infarction.

The end result of the ischemic insult is an uncoordinated ventricular contraction in which the necrotic region fails to contract (akinesis) or bulge passively during systole (dyskinesis). A somewhat decreased contractile function may be detected in the area peripheral to the infarction zones (hypokinesis) (Fig. 2-42). The passive bulging of the ischemic zone leads to an increase in end-diastolic volume, which in turn will increase the left ventricular wall tension and increase myocardial oxygen demand. These changes place an additional burden on the left ventricle as the passively bulging necrotic myocardium absorbs some kinetic energy allocated for pumping blood to the aorta.[130]

Ischemic myocardial necrosis also has a significant effect on left ventricular diastolic function. Repetitive stretching of the necrotic zones results initially in decreased myocardial diastolic stiffness (increased compliance). The increased ventricular compliance rapidly reverses (increased stiffness), however, probably due to sarcomere contracture and the accumulation of interstitial fluid. Decreased left ventricular compliance leads to increased ventricular filling pressure, which will be transmitted to the pulmonary capillaries, thus causing pulmonary congestion, fluid transudation, and dyspnea.

Recruitment of several compensatory mechanisms in myocardial infarction is a common event. Sympathetic stimulation results in increased contractile force, heart rate and cardiac output. Furthermore, the heart dilates as a means of maintaining adequate cardiac output. However, those compensatory mechanisms result in increased myocardial oxygen consumption and thus may aggravate the initial ischemic injury. Again, the size of the infarcted re-

gion dictates the beneficial or detrimental effect of the compensatory mechanisms. In small infarctions compensatory mechanisms are able to maintain circulatory homeostasis, while in large infarctions the opposite is true. Hemodynamic changes that accompany regional ischemia, such as alteration of preload, afterload, and coronary perfusion pressure, have an important influence on the function of the nonischemic myocardium.

Remodeling

There is strong evidence that large transmural myocardial infarctions precipitate changes in ventricular geometry involving both the infarcted and noninfarcted zones. These changes, termed *ventricular remodeling*, may have a significant effect on ventricular function and the patient's prognosis. Ventricular regions remote from the necrotic zone often reveal progressive increase in the end-diastolic myocardial lengths and greater relative shortening. These changes resemble compensatory responses seen in long-term volume overload.[124] This global ventricular enlargement is not due to acute distension and may continue long after complete healing of the infarction. Similar changes of cavity enlargement have been recognized in humans after myocardial infarction. These changes cannot be explained by elevated filling pressures.[125] Morphologic studies have concluded that the volume increase of the postinfarction ventricle is not the result of sarcomere stretching but the consequence of rearrangement of the myofibrils across the wall.[126] Increased left ventricular diastolic volume and pressure results in decreased myocardial blood flow in noninfarcted areas, especially in areas perfused from stenotic coronary arteries. This may produce contraction abnormalities in noninfarcted areas, even without worsening of coronary artery stenosis.[114,127,131]

Summarizing the changes stated above, it appears that although the early postinfarction findings involve thinning and lengthening of the infarction, dilatation and eccentric hypertrophy of the nonischemic myocardium starts early and continues long after healing of the infarction. Postinfarction ventricular enlargement is considered an initial compensation to maintain stroke volume after the loss of the contraction of the infarcted zone. Quite often, however, the extent of cavity dilatation is disproportionate to the augmentation in muscular mass. This finding may be associated with distinctly reduced survival.

Expansion

An important determinant of the clinical outcome of a patient immediately after an acute myocardial infarction is infarct expansion. This complication, which may occur as early as 24 hours after infarction, is characterized by a disproportionate regional thinning and dilatation of the infarct zone (without new necrosis), which is fixed and permanent. Obviously, infarct expansion will result in distortion of the left ventricular geometry; such distortion may cause ventricular dysfunction.

Although some degree of infarct expansion may be detected in about two thirds of transmural myocardial infarcts, moderate or severe expansion is seen in only one-third of the acute myocardial infarctions.

Morphologically, an expanded infarct is characterized by wall thinning, and marked cavity dilatation caused by an increase in regional segment length and regional radius curvature. Although infarct expansion is not associated with additional myocardial necrosis, it results in an increased percentage of left ventricular circumference to be involved by the infarct. Infarct expansion has more global effects on the left ventricle because it changes the overall geometry and alters the positions and relationships of different ventricular structures, including the papillary muscles. Increases of regional cavity size will increase the left ventricular cavity volume, the wall stress and oxygen consumption in the noninfarcted myocardium, and may result in additional ischemic injury.[132-138]

Two possibilities have been considered for the pathogenesis of thinning and dilatation related to myocardial expansion: cell stretch and cell slippage. In myocyte stretching, the cross-diameter of the cell is decreased while the length increases. The end-result is thinning and dilatation of the infarct zone. In cell slippage, the cross-cellular diameter remains constant, but myocytes or groups of myocytes rearrange in a way that reduces the total number of cells across the wall, resulting in thinning and dilatation. It seems that this latter mechanism of cell slippage is perhaps mostly responsible for the thinning and dilatation of expanded infarcts.

Early bulging of the infarcted zone is seen in almost all transmural myocardial infarctions during ventricular systole and diastole. However, as was stated above, not all transmural myocardial infarctions reveal fixed permanent expansion, which indicates that other additional factors play a role in determining whether this functional bulge will become a fixed structural change. These factors include infarct size, transmural versus nontransmural infarction, site of the infarction, early reperfusion, and ventricular loading conditions. Although a certain critical mass of acute necrosis is required for expansion to occur, the amount of necrosis is a poor predictive factor. Since only transmural myocardial infarctions show expansion, the pattern of transmural necrosis is important. The extent of expansion is inversely related to the thickness of surviving myocardium within the infarct zone.[134] Anterior and anteroseptal transmural myocardial infarctions are more prone to expansion because anterior infarctions are usually large, and the ventricular wall is normally thin in this location.

Changes in ventricular loading conditions, such as reduction of the afterload, may prevent or reverse expansion. The hypothesis for the beneficial effect of afterload reduction states that systolic stress on an ischemic segment contributes to cell slippage and expansion of the infarction.[138] Autopsy studies have confirmed what was suspected clinically by showing that infarct expansion precedes cardiac rupture and also plays a major role in the pathogenesis of left ventricular aneurysm.[135]

PRECONDITIONING, MYOCARDIAL HIBERNATION, MYOCARDIAL STUNNING, REPERFUSION
Myocardial preconditioning

It has been suggested in the past that brief repeated ischemic episodes might cumulatively cause infarction. However, recent evidence indicates that brief ischemic episodes increase the heart's tolerance to subsequent sustained periods of ischemia. Such tolerance has been called ischemic preconditioning. Preconditioning has been convincingly demonstrated in patients who have undergone elective angioplasty of the left anterior descending coronary artery. In this angioplasty setting, two 90-second coronary occlusions were separated by 5 minutes of reperfusion. The second ischemic episode created less chest pain, less ST segment elevation and less myocardial lactate production. The reduction of the coronary blood flow (as estimated from the blood flow from the accompanied cardiac vein) was similar both times, which suggests that the second, less severe ischemic episode was not due to increased collateral blood flow, but probably reflected the myocardial adaptation to ischemia.[140] An interesting observation was made from animal experiments in which the myocardial infarction size produced by a 40-minute coronary occlusion was reduced by 75% when the myocardium had first been subjected to four 5-minute episodes of coronary occlusion, each separated by 5 minutes of reperfusion. However, when the ischemic episode was allowed to extend beyond 3 hours, the preconditioning effect was abolished and the infarct size was no different from the control group. Morphologic studies have shown that preconditioning preserves the viability of both the myocytes and the microvasculature. Moreover, preconditioning reduces the susceptibility to ventricular fibrillation during subsequent ischemic episodes.[139-144]

A plethora of potential mechanisms for the pathogenesis of preconditioning have been suggested. It has been proposed that preconditioning significantly slows energy metabolism during ischemia. Thus ATP depletion occurs at a slower rate during the subsequent ischemic episodes. Similarly, both glycogenolysis and anaerobic glycolysis are slower; thus the accumulation of ischemic metabolite in the myocardium is substantially reduced.[141] Other investigators have stressed the potential role of the purine nucleoside adenosine in mediating preconditioning. Isolated blood-perfused rabbit hearts were used to evaluate the effects of adenosine receptor antagonists and agonists on infarct size in preconditioned and control hearts.[142] Proposed mechanisms regarding how adenosine might exert such an effect include preservation of ATP by enhancement of glycolytic flux and inhibition of reperfusion injury by activated neutrophils. Although the exact pathogenetic mechanism of preconditioning is not yet clear, it appears that preservation of ATP indicates a reduction in energy demand during ischemia.

Myocardial hibernation, myocardial stunning

Less than 2 decades ago, contractile dysfunction of the myocardium in patients with coronary artery disease was thought to be caused by either irreversible damage to myocytes due to myocardial infarction, or reversible ischemia. During the last 10 years, however, several studies have demonstrated that contractile dysfunction of the myocardium may occur in the absence of myocardial infarction or after an acute ischemic event. These phenomena are known as hibernating myocardium or stunned myocardium. Myocardial hibernation and myocardial stunning are conditions of chronic sustained abnormal contraction and decreased metabolism due to chronic underperfusion in patients with coronary artery disease. Myocardial hibernation and stunning are considered reversible when oxygen supply-demand ratio improves. Hibernation and myocardial stunning could occur separately or together during prolonged partial ischemia. However, the two conditions reveal some fundamental differences.[145-149]

Hibernating myocardium has been defined as the persistently impaired function of viable myocardium in the setting of reduced coronary blood flow. The term *hibernating* implies that myocardium reduces its function and metabolism to survive in the face of a reduction in oxygen supply. The concept of hibernating myocardium explains the reversal of long-standing segmental contraction abnormalities after coronary bypass surgery or coronary angioplasty. In myocardial hibernation, the contractile dysfunction is related to a decrease in Ca^{2+} transients while myofilament Ca^{2+} sensitivity and maximal Ca^{2+} activated pressure are normal.[146]

Stunned myocardium resembles hibernating myocardium in that both involve contractile dysfunction of potentially viable tissue. The difference between the two phenomena is the level of blood flow to the tissue. In stunned myocardium, however, reperfusion and relief of ischemia, the myocardial function remains depressed for hours, days, or even weeks afterward; in hibernating myocardium dysfunction of viable myocytes is present only during the period of reduced blood flow. Contractile dysfunction in stunned myocardium is related to decrease in myofilament Ca^{2+} sensitivity and maximal Ca^{2+} activated pressure, while the Ca^{++} transients are increased.[146]

In experiments with animals a 15-minute episode of coronary occlusion followed by reestablishment of blood flow results in increased tissue water and potassium content (lasting approximately 1 hour), substantial loss of adenine nucleotides, and postischemic contractile dysfunction that persists for 2 to 4 days.[143] The magnitude of blood flow reduction during the preceding period of ischemia and the duration of flow deprivation are important factors that determine the severity of myocardial stunning.[149] Other mechanisms that possibly contribute to myocardial stunning include the generation of oxygen radicals, calcium overload, and abnormalities in excitation-contraction uncoupling. Information gathered from clinical studies indicates that myocardial stunning is not merely a laboratory curiosity. Such studies have revealed that full recovery of contractile function is not immediate after successful reperfusion with thrombolytic agents. Another clinical example of stunned myocardium is the relatively prolonged left ventricular dysfunction that has been observed after coronary angioplasty, thrombolysis or coronary bypass surgery. The severity of stunning is greater in the inner layers of the left ventricular wall than in the outer layers.

Reperfusion injury

Thrombolytic therapy is based on the belief that early restoration of myocardial blood flow will reduce infarct size, limit left ventricular dysfunction and reduce early and late mortality. In essence, the basic premise is that reperfusion by thrombolysis may stop the march of the infarction process from the subendocardium to the subepicardium. This concept is based on the thought that within the ischemic zone there are severely injured cells that can be salvaged with timely restoration of blood flow. Reperfusion itself, however, may produce injury. *Reperfusion injury has been defined as cell injury caused by reperfusion itself, in contrast to cell injury caused by the preceding ischemia.* This definition in its broader interpretation includes mechanical dysfunction (myocardial stunning), cardiac arrhythmias (reperfusion arrhythmias), and vascular damage (no-reflow phenomenon). Whether reperfusion merely accelerates the damage that would have occurred during the initial ischemia, or whether there is a specific additional injury caused by reperfusion itself is still debated.[150-155]

The most commonly reported finding in patients that died after reperfusion is a hemorrhagic infarction. Hemorrhagic infarctions are exceedingly rare in nonreperfused myocardial ischemic events. In fact, in a large autopsy study of more than 200 cases of myocardial infarction, no hemorrhagic infarctions were found.[150] Recent morphologic studies comparing the healing sequences of acute myocardial infarction in patients who received early therapeutic coronary reperfusion (thrombolytic agents, angioplasty, bypass surgery) with those who received conventional therapy have revealed that for any given clinical age infarction, the reperfusion group was judged to have an older histologic age infarction than that of the control group (conventional therapy). Furthermore, the reperfusion group revealed, (for all ages of infarctions) more hemorrhage within the myocardial infarction area, more contraction band necrosis, less coagulative necrosis, nontransmural distribution of necrosis, and cellular response with more macrophages and less numbers of neutrophils. The degree of intramyocardial hemorrhage is greater in cases in which reperfusion occurs 4 to 6.5 hours after onset of symptoms. In myocardial infarction of less than 3 days, the cellular response is present throughout the myocardial infarction, in contrast to the distinct zones of demarcation seen in nonreperfused infarctions. In somewhat older infarctions (5 to 10 days), more active phagocytosis is noted in the reperfused myocardial infarctions. Older healing infarcts (10 to 40 days) exhibited scars that are patchy, more cellular and less vascular in reperfused patients, in contrast to confluent, acellular, revascularized scars in the control group.[151]

However, there are obvious differences between hemorrhagic infarctions in humans and those studied in experimental animals. Those differences reflect the type of occlusion (ligation or atheroma), collateral circulation, and rate of development of occlusion (slow or fast). In humans, hemorrhagic infarctions are transmural with some extension of the hemorrhagic process into the noninfarcted zones. Hemorrhagic infarctions are subendocardial in experimental animals.

Although the crucial role of reperfusion injury in revascularization procedures has been recognized, the etiology and pathogenesis of this phenomenon remains largely unknown. The possible role of reactive oxygen species in reperfusion injury has evolved from our knowledge that cells, in order to avert the formation of hydroxyl radicals, set in action elaborate enzyme systems that rapidly detoxify superoxide and peroxide. However, the metabolism of reactive oxygen (superoxide and peroxide) is not without additional, potentially damaging effects. Investigators have suspected that even physiologic quantities of peroxide may inhibit the aerobic oxidation of pyruvate within the cell and thus restrict cellular ATP formation.[151a]

Recent experimental work has suggested that reperfusion-generated peroxide does not have a direct toxic effect, but rather restricts mitochondrial ATP formation by inhibiting pyruvate dehydrogenase activity. Such an action of peroxide was demonstrated in isolated cardiac mitochondria and cultured myocytes. Furthermore, it is believed that peroxide-induced pyruvate dehydrogenase inhibition blocks the aerobic oxidation of glucose and leads to adenine nucleotide catabolism and release of adenosine and inosine, which may intensify cellular injury during reperfusion.[151a]

Recent reports indicate that endothelium-dependent relaxation of coronary microvessels is markedly impaired after ischemia with reperfusion. This microvascular endothelial dysfunction may be caused by blood products or myocardial metabolites that are released during the reperfusion period, or by oxygen free radicals. Impairment of endothelial-dependent relaxation is attributable to oxygen free radicals formed during myocardial reperfusion.[151b]

Endothelial-derived relaxing factor (EDRF) has been identified as nitric oxide (NO), although it is not certain whether EDRF is free NO, or whether the NO is transported from the endothelial cells to the smooth muscle cells of the arterial wall bound to an organic carrier molecule. There is no disagreement, however, that the site of action of NO is the smooth muscle cell. NO is a potent inhibitor of both platelet aggregation and neutrophil adherence. Animal experiments have demonstrated that the decrease in EDPF occurs soon after the generation of superoxide radicals by the reperfused vascular endothelium. Thus the early burst of superoxide radicals does not originate from neutrophils, because their accumulation does not occur until 3 to 4.5 hours after reperfusion. The sequence of events described above suggests that the most likely source of the superoxide radicals is the endothelium triggered by the introduction of molecular oxygen rather than vascular distention (reperfusion flow). After only 3 to 4.5 hours, at least in the experimental models, the endothelial dysfunction is amplified by neutrophil adherence and diapedesis into the infarcted area, enhancing postperfusion ischemic injury.[151c]

Somewhat different data have been reported by others regarding to the time course of neutrophil influx in the reperfused canine myocardium. According to these investigators, while neutrophils in nonreperfused model accumulate at the site of infarction after a period of 12 to 24 hours, in the reperfusion model there is an accelerated neutrophil accumulation within the ischemic region.[151d] Additional experimental data from reperfusion models indicate that the rate of neutrophil localization in the canine myocardium is greatest within the first hour after initiation of reperfusion, while localization is, at least in part, CD18-dependent for neutrophilic adherence. Moreover, neutrophils are preferentially localized within the subendocardial region.[151e]

From the discussion above, it appears that entrapped neutrophils can cause significant damage to the ischemic reperfused heart, but whether this injury is primarily mediated by free radicals or is due to capillary plugging and increased vascular resistance is not known.

The no-reflow phenomenon is considered a specific type of vascular damage after reperfusion. Explanations for this phenomenon include neutrophil plugging leading to endothelial cell edema, formation of microthrombi, and exces-

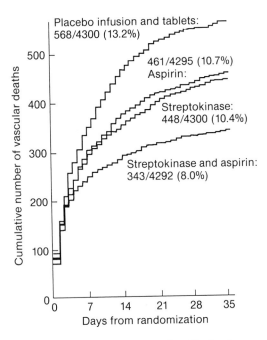

Fig. 2-43. Cumulative vascular mortality (deaths from cardiac, cerebral, hemorrhagic, or other known vascular disease) in days 0-35 of the Second International Study of Infarct Survival (ISIS-2). The four curves describe mortality for patients allocated (i) active streptokinase only, (ii) active aspirin only, (iii) both active treatments, and (iv) neither. Note that individually, aspirin and streptokinase have a favorable effect of similar magnitudes, and that together the benefits appear additive. (From ISIS-2 [Second International Study of Infarct Survival] Collaborative Group: Randomized trial of intravenous streptokinase, oral aspirin, both, or neither among 17,187 cases of suspected acute myocardial infarction: ISIS-2, *Lancet* 2:349, 1988.)

sive ischemic myocardial contracture with compression of the microvasculature.

One of the oldest hypotheses about reperfusion injury involves calcium overload. According to this theory, reperfusion causes a tenfold increase in calcium uptake by the myocyte, resulting in contraction band necrosis and intramitochondrial dense bodies. However, evidence indicates that under nonischemic conditions cellular calcium content can be increased at least fivefold above normal physiologic levels without inducing injury. Furthermore, it has been shown that upon reoxygenation, Ca^{2+} actually decreases at a time when hypercontracture is developing. This observation clearly refutes the concept that reoxygenation invariably produces further calcium overload.[151f]

Numerous events have been discussed with regard to reperfusion injury, including myocardial stunning, reperfusion arrhythmias, and vascular damage with no-reflow phenomenon. Whether reperfusion causes necrosis (contraction band necrosis) to viable or reversibly injured cells still remains controversial. Divergent results in several studies clearly indicate that the abrupt onset reperfusion in

animal models differs significantly from the situation in humans with thrombolysis.

Despite the controversial results from experimental studies, clinical studies have shown that reperfusion with thrombolytic agents up to 24 hours after the onset of symptoms may decrease mortality[155] (Fig. 2-43). Reperfusion may reduce ventricular dilatation and aneurysm formation, limit infarct expansion, and improve the electrical stability of the myocardium.[155-157]

Thrombolytic agents such as tissue plasminogen activators (t-PA), which produce early reopening of the occluded coronary artery, are not superior in reducing mortality compared to thrombolytic agents such as streptokinase, which do not quickly reopen the occluded coronary artery. It is possible that fast reperfusion may produce greater damage than does slow reperfusion. Thus the beneficial effect of fast recanalization may be offset by reperfusion injury.

COMPLICATIONS OF ACUTE MYOCARDIAL INFARCTIONS

A significant number of patients with acute myocardial infarction may die suddenly before arrival at the hospital. Fortunately, most patients with an acute myocardial infarction who reach the hospital will have an uncomplicated course. However, hospitalized patients may develop life-threatening complications or die during the hospitalization. The rate of complications and the in-hospital mortality depend on the type, location, and more importantly, the size of the infarction. For example, anterior myocardial infarctions have higher in-hospital mortality than do inferior myocardial infarctions because the former result in a greater loss of functioning myocardium.

Cardiac arrhythmias

The great majority of patients (approximately 95%) with acute myocardial infarction experience some disturbance of cardiac rhythm. The most common form of arrhythmias are premature ventricular beats, which are considered potentially dangerous because they can trigger ventricular tachycardia or ventricular fibrillation. Sustained episodes of ventricular tachycardia are often associated with circulatory collapse. Both anterior and inferior myocardial infarction reveal equal frequency of ventricular fibrillation, which may be primary or secondary. The latter usually occurs as a consequence of cardiogenic shock and is frequently the terminating event in this condition.[158-160]

Certain information from animal experiments may be applicable to ventricular arrhythmias in humans occurring during and after the ischemic episodes. **Phase I** of enhanced ventricular vulnerability occurs in the first 5 minutes after the onset of ischemia and lasts approximately 30 minutes. After an arrhythmia-free period, **phase II** occurs about 2 to 3 hours after the onset of ischemia and lasts about 24 hours. The late arrhythmias of **phase III** develop days or weeks after the onset of infarction. It is speculated that the pathogenetic mechanisms of ventricular arrhythmias are different in those three phases. The underlying mechanism in phase I is believed to be reentry within the still viable, although acutely anoxic, myocardium. In phase II, when most, if not all, myocytes at risk have died and, therefore, are nonelectrogenic, ventricular arrhythmias are probably due to enhanced automaticity of surviving border cells such as subendocardial Purkinje's cells. Phase III arrhythmias are thought to result from reentry, although some may be due to enhanced automaticity. Reentry usually occurs at the junction of regions of reversible myocyte injury and preserved muscle. Similar correlates may apply to reentry circuits resulting from healed myocardial infarction and ventricular aneurysms.[85]

Atrioventricular block is associated in general with unfavorable prognosis, although it is recognized that prognosis depends on the extent and location of the infarction. For example, although atrioventricular conduction abnormalities are frequent, they are usually transient in cases of inferior myocardial infarction. Histopathologic studies in patients with transient atrioventricular conduction disturbances have disclosed no structural abnormalities of the proximal conduction system, contrary to those patients with persistent conduction abnormalities in which damage to the conduction system proximal and distal has been demonstrated. Most of the inferior, posterior or inferoposterior myocardial infarctions are caused by occlusion of the right coronary artery, which supplies the atrioventricular node in about 90% of the hearts. For this reason, even a small inferior myocardial infarction may produce atrioventricular block because of the susceptibility of the conduction fibers as they are channeled into a rather narrow tract in the region of the atrioventricular junction. In contrast, the LAD coronary artery supplies the distal conduction system below the bundle of His. Therefore, an anterior myocardial infarction must be very extensive to produce a complete atrioventricular block able to affect the widely dispersed conducting fibers below the bundle of His. The right coronary artery almost never supplies the conduction system below the bundle of His.

Sudden cardiac death

Although the World Health Organization defines sudden death as one occurring within 24 hours, several authors limit this time period to 6 hours after onset of symptoms. The most common cause of sudden cardiac death in the United States is atherosclerotic coronary artery disease. The cause of sudden death in the majority of the cases is secondary to tachyarrhythmia (mostly ventricular), less often is related to atrioventricular block, and rarely involves ventricular rupture.

Cardiogenic shock

Cardiogenic shock is the condition characterized by acute, severe and persistent decrease of tissue perfusion secondary to primary failure of the heart. The arterial pressure is low, (usually less than 90 mmHg) or at least 30 mmHg lower compared to baseline levels. Note that cardiogenic shock may exist without arterial hypotension and that arterial hypotension is not always associated with cardiogenic shock. Acute myocardial infarction is the most common cause of cardiogenic shock. Cardiogenic shock most often occurs in cases involving left ventricular myocardial infarction, but may also occur in patients with right ventricular myocardial infarction.[121,161-166]

During the last decade the frequency of cardiogenic shock has been decreased. Admission of the patient into the coronary care unit early after the onset of symptoms, and the introduction of thrombolytic therapy were the two major factors resulting in decreased incidence of cardiogenic shock. Although the incidence of cardiogenic shock has decreased over the last decade, its incidence in patients with acute myocardial infarction is 7% to 10% and is responsible for the majority of deaths in hospitalized patients with acute myocardial infarction.[165]

Large myocardial infarction results in significant decrease in left ventricular ejection fraction. Decreased left ventricular ejection fraction will result in decreased stroke volume and increased left ventricular diastolic volume and pressure. The decreased stroke volume will result in decreased cardiac output, arterial pressure, and tissue hypoperfusion (Fig. 2-44). Patients with cardiogenic shock have symptoms secondary to pulmonary congestion and to severe decrease of tissue perfusion.

Studies have shown that it is possible to identify the high-risk patient who is most likely to develop cardiogenic shock. Risk factors include age greater than 65 years, left ventricular ejection fraction less than 35%, high MB isoenzyme of phosphocreatine kinase ($>$160 international units), diabetes mellitus, and history of previous myocardial infarction. The possibilities of a patient developing cardiogenic shock are 1.7%, 3.9%, 8.6%, 17.9%, 33.7% and 54.4%, respectively, when 0, 1, 2, 3, 4, and 5 of the risk factors mentioned are present.

Cardiogenic shock, less often, may occur in patients with right ventricular myocardial infarction. The pathophysiology of cardiogenic shock due to right ventricular myocardial infarction is different from that of patients with left ventricular myocardial infarction (Fig. 2-45). Large right ventricular myocardial infarction will result in right ventricular failure, decreased right ventricular stroke volume, decreased pulmonary venous return, decreased left ventricular preload and decreased left ventricular stroke volume resulting in tissue hypoperfusion. In addition, there is right-left ventricular interaction through the intra-

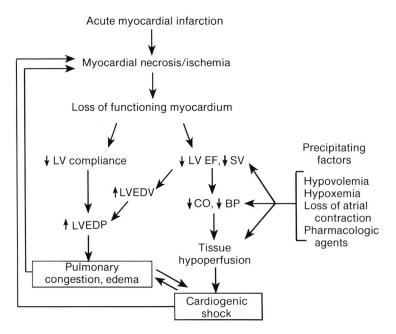

Fig. 2-44. Acute myocardial infarction will result in loss of functioning myocardium, decreased left ventricular (LV) compliance, LV ejection fraction (EF), and stroke volume (SV). Decreased LV compliance will result in increased LV end diastolic pressure (LVEDP) and pulmonary congestion. Decreased LVEF and SV will result in increased LV end diastolic volume (LVEDV), decreased cardiac output, blood pressure, tissue hypoperfusion and cardiogenic shock.

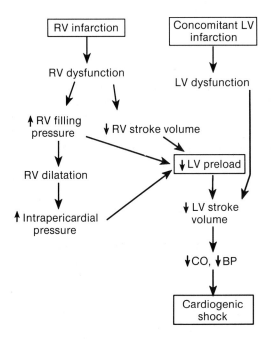

Fig. 2-45. Pathophysiologic mechanisms of cardiogenic shock in patients with right ventricular (RV) myocardial infarction. LV = left ventricle, CO = cardiac output, BP = blood pressure.

ventricular septum; the high right ventricular diastolic pressure may be transmitted to the left ventricle.

Cardiogenic shock also may occur in mechanical complications related to myocardial infarction such as papillary muscle rupture, ventricular septum rupture and free wall rupture.

Rupture of the free ventricular wall

Rupture of the free ventricular wall occurs in 1% to 3% of the cases with acute myocardial infarction and accounts for the 10% of deaths caused by the latter (Fig. 2-46). Free ventricular wall rupture occurs within 24 hours from the onset of symptoms in 30% of the cases, but most commonly occurs between the second and eighth day. Free ventricular wall rupture occurs within 4 days from the onset of symptoms in 50% of the cases and in 80% to 90% of the cases occurs between 7 and 14 days from the onset of symptoms. Rupture usually occurs in patients with transmural myocardial infarction and is much more common in the left ventricular compared to right ventricular infarction. Rupture is more common in patients with first myocardial infarction, in patients older than 70 years, in females, and in patients with history of arterial hypertension. Studies suggest that rupture may occur more often in patients with lateral myocardial infarction. Treatment with thrombolytic drugs within 7 hours of onset of symptoms decreases the incidence of free wall rupture. However, thrombolytic therapy increases the incidence of free wall rupture when it is administered 17 hours from the onset of

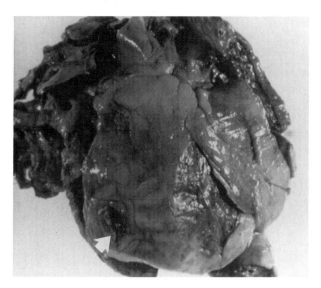

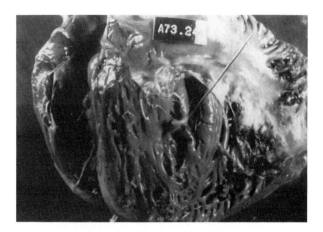

Fig. 2-47. Right ventricular view showing postinfarction rupture of the interventricular septum (probe).

Fig. 2-46. Postinfarction left anterior ventricular wall rupture (4-to 5 days).

symptoms. Therapy with β-blocking drugs immediately after the onset of symptoms decreases the incidence of free wall rupture.[167-169]

Morphologically, free wall ruptures may be divided into two categories: early (1 to 7 days) and late (14 to 21 days). The early ruptures are slit-like and usually occur near the junction of the necrotic myocardium and adjacent normal muscle. Late rupture, which is less frequent, usually occurs at the center of the infarct, particularly if there is infarct expansion. Some authors classify cardiac rupture as type I (early tear) occurring within 24 hours after onset of acute myocardial infarction, type II (slow erosion), and type III (early aneurysm formation). The latter two types are ruptures that occur after the first postinfarction week. Early rupture results in a rapid massive accumulation of blood in the pericardial sac and cardiac tamponade. Rapid extravasation of blood in the pericardial space may be prevented in late free wall rupture because pericardial layers may have become adherent to the epicardium. However, the adherent pericardium may slowly expand to form a pseudoaneurysm (false aneurysm). It is perhaps worth noting that pericarditis occurring a day or so before rupture may be a harbinger of the fatal event. The classic clinical clue of free wall rupture is electromechanic dissociation when electrical activity persists without detectable blood pressure and pulse.

Rupture of the ventricular septum

Rupture of the ventricular septum occurs in 0.5% to 1% of patients with acute myocardial infarction and accounts in 1% to 5% of deaths in patients with the same condition[170-173] (Fig. 2-47). Rupture of the ventricular septum will result in acute ventricular septal defect and shunt of large amounts of blood from left to right. This will result

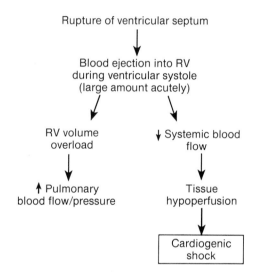

Fig. 2-48. Pathophysiologic mechanisms of cardiogenic shock in patients with rupture of the ventricular septum during the course of acute myocardial infarction.

in right ventricular failure. Large amounts of blood in the pulmonary circulation will increase the pulmonary venous return and increase left atrial pressure with resultant pulmonary congestion. Shunt from left to right will also result in tissue hypoperfusion and shock (Fig. 2-48). Tricuspid regurgitation occurs frequently with septal rupture and is due to high right ventricular pressure or right ventricular ischemia. Similar to free wall rupture, septal rupture is more likely to occur in elderly patients, patients with first myocardial infarction, and patients with a history of arterial hypertension. Shear and strain between the necrotic myocardium and the peri-infarct zone, and contraction of the adjacent healthy myocardium is probably responsible for the septal rupture. Junctional areas of discordant wall motion are also predisposed to rupture. The timing of sep-

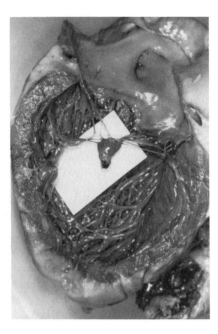

Fig. 2-49. Postinfarction rupture of anterolateral muscle. Note the hematoma at the site of the severed muscle. Left ventricular view.

tal rupture is from the third to twelfth postinfarction day with its peak between the fifth to seventh day. This serious complication of an acute myocardial infarction is usually heralded by sudden precordial pain and/or by the sudden development of heart failure and arterial hypotension. It is usually accompanied by a holosystolic murmur, which is often indistinguishable from the murmur of mitral insufficiency. Doppler color flow mapping superimposed on "real-time" two-dimensional echocardiographic images has been utilized for the precise diagnosis and evaluation of patients with septal rupture.[172] Cardiac catheterization is usually required for thorough hemodynamic assessment and for the definition of the coronary artery anatomy. Multiple sites of rupture and serpentine septal tears (tunnels) with openings at different left and right ventricular levels are not rare. Septal ruptures, unlike congenital septal defects, are not smooth, well-defined orifices.

Papillary muscle rupture

Papillary muscle rupture occurs in 1% of patients with acute myocardial infarction and accounts for the 5% of deaths in such cases. Papillary muscle rupture results in acute mitral regurgitation.[174] Severe acute mitral regurgitation results in pulmonary congestion and tissue hypoperfusion (see also mitral regurgitation, Chapter 3).

Partial or complete rupture of papillary muscles occurs in 0.3% to 0.95% of myocardial infarctions. Factors predisposing to papillary muscle rupture are quite similar to those enumerated for the septal and free wall ruptures, i.e., elderly individuals, patients with first myocardial in-

farction, and patients with a history of arterial hypertension. Recent reports also stress the frequent association of papillary muscle necrosis with cardiac hypertrophy, inferior-posterior myocardial infarction, or infarction that involves both ventricles and subendocardial infarctions.[174] Rupture usually occurs within the first week after the onset of the myocardial infarction and may involve one head of the papillary muscle, resulting in only modest mitral regurgitation amenable to surgical correction, or total rupture of a papillary muscle, leading to massive mitral regurgitation. Of the two papillary muscles, the posterior septal one is affected by rupture 6 to 12 times more often than the anterior lateral papillary muscle (Fig. 2-49). The explanation for this unequal involvement of the two papillary muscles lies in differences in blood supply; the posterior one receives blood from both the circumflex and right coronary arteries. Such an anatomic setting enhances the likelihood of reflow (and thus contraction band necrosis) in the infarcted posterior papillary muscle. The process that detaches the head of the papillary muscle appears to be the formation of a hematoma within the area of contraction band necrosis.

Papillary muscle dysfunction is much more common than rupture in patients with acute ischemic episodes. In fact, papillary muscle dysfunction is considered to be the most common cause of mitral regurgitation. The regurgitation may be mild or severe and may clear as the acute ischemia subsides, or may appear several months later due to residual scarring of the papillary muscle.

Extension of infarction

Extension of an infarct implies additional myocardial necrosis occurring after completion of the original infarct. Thus infarct extension results in a true increase in the total mass of infarcted myocardium, contrary to infarct expansion that increases the functional size of an infarct (see earlier). The reported frequency of infarct extension varies considerably from 10% to 80%. The highest frequency was reported in studies in which single criteria such as new angina, recurrent electrocardiographic changes, or new peak of creatine kinase were used to make the diagnosis.[174a] It appears that these single criterion studies probably overestimate the frequency of infarct extension. Therefore one needs the entire constellation of findings including recurrent angina, creatine kinase-MB isoenzyme elevation, and new electrocardiographic changes to arrive at a more definite diagnosis of infarct extension.[175]

The usual histoarchitectural findings in infarct extension involve a healing infarct with foci of recent necrosis at either the lateral borders of transmural or subendocardial infarcts, or a subepicardial extension of the previous infarct. These foci of recent infarction may reveal contraction band necrosis, which indicates either spontaneous reperfusion of these areas or intermittent flow through collateral channels. Extension of necrosis in the peri-infarct areas clearly indicates that the entire area at risk is usually not infarcted

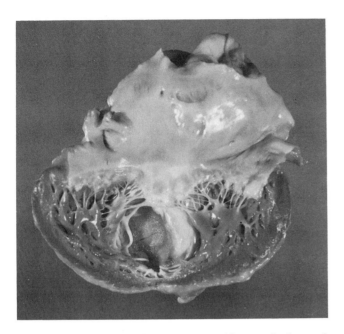

Fig. 2-50. Left ventricular aneurysm with organized mural thrombus.

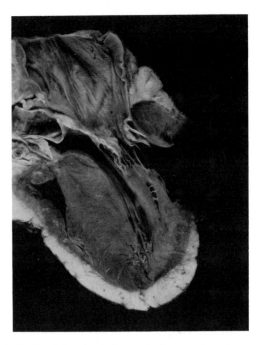

Fig. 2-51. Postinfarction left ventricular pseudoaneurysm (contained rupture) (Courtesy of Dr. William D. Edwards, Mayo Clinic).

and that borderline zones to the original infarct are at risk for new ischemic episodes. Non- Q-wave myocardial infarctions are often associated with incomplete arterial occlusions, recanalized arteries, or perfusion through collateral vessels. In time, the subtotal occlusion may become complete, or the efficacy of the collateral flow may diminish, resulting in new necrosis at the lateral border zones of a subendocardial infarct. Although clear risk factors for infarct extension have not been identified, it has been stated that patients with congestive heart failure, hypertension, diabetes mellitus, or episodic hypotension may be more prone to infarct extension. Patients with infarct extension have greater morbidity and mortality, present more often with congestive heart failure and dysrhythmias, and are more likely to die from cardiogenic shock.

Reinfarction

Reinfarction implies ischemic necrosis either adjacent to the original infarct or in regions remote from it after the acute hospital phase of an earlier infarct. Obviously, it is not easy to clinically distinguish it from infarct extension. Therefore other descriptive terms such as recurrent infarction are often used. Large clinical series indicate that reinfarction may occur in 10% to 20% of the cases.[138] Three-vessel disease appears to be a significant risk factor for reinfarction. The incidence of reinfarction is greatest in patients with early appearance of postinfarction angina.

Left ventricular aneurysm

The overall autopsy incidence of left ventricular aneurysms is estimated to be between 3% to 15% of patients with myocardial infarction (Fig. 2-50). A similar

range[176-178] (7.6%) was found in angiographic studies. The most common site is the anterior and anteroapical region. Although there is no uniformly accepted definition of a left ventricular aneurysm, the most widely used one for an anatomic aneurysm is abnormal diastolic contour of the left ventricle secondary to a localized cavitary protrusion of the free wall. In contrast to the anatomic aneurysm, a functional one is defined as a protrusion of the left ventricular wall that exists only during ventricular systole. There are distinct differences in both pathogenesis and morphology between a true and a false ventricular aneurysm. The true aneurysm has a mouth that is as wide as or wider than the maximal diameter of the aneurysm, and its wall consists of fibrous connective tissue with islands of viable or necrotic myocardium or both. In contrast, a false aneurysm has a mouth that is considerably smaller than the maximal diameter of the aneurysm (site of myocardial rupture), and its wall is composed of parietal pericardium without myocardial fibers (Fig. 2-51). For these reasons, true ventricular aneurysms usually do not rupture, and false aneurysms are susceptible to rupture. It has also been suggested that the prevalence of left ventricular aneurysm in patients with poor collateral circulation is much higher than those with significant collateral channels. The explanation given for the preventive role of collaterals is that well-developed collateral circulation increases the number of islands of viable heart muscle in the infarcted area, thereby enforcing its tensile strength and preventing the aneurysm formation.

A left ventricular aneurysm besides the localized geo-

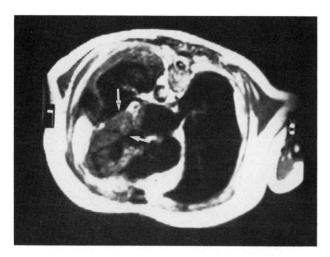

Fig. 2-52. Left ventricular mural thrombus (MRI).

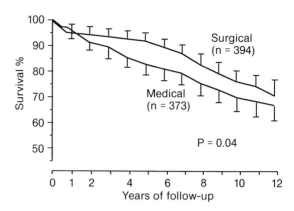

Fig. 2-53. Twelve years of survival in the surgical and medical groups. Note that the survival in the surgical group decreases and is parallel to the medical group 5 years following the coronary bypass surgery. (From Varnauskas E, et al: Twelve-year follow-up of survival in the randomized European Coronary Surgery Study, *N Engl J Med* 319:332-7, 1988.)

metric distortion produces a global cardiac remodeling with generalized dilatation. Furthermore, the efficiency of the left ventricular systolic work is decreased because a considerable amount is wasted by expansion of the aneurysm. Such altered mechanics may be the stimulus for the compensatory hypertrophy of the uninvolved by the infarct myocardium. A ventricle with an aneurysm is at mechanical disadvantage because changes in the curvature and thickness of the ventricular wall affect its performance.[132]

Clinical recognition of an aneurysm may be made by the persistent ST segment elevation on the electrocardiogram, or the presence of an abnormal bulge on the left ventricular contour on chest radiograph. However, a definite diagnosis is made by either contrast or radionuclide ventriculography, two-dimensional echocardiography, CT scan and magnetic resonance imaging. True left ventricular aneurysms usually are associated with large myocardial infarctions and left ventricular dilatation.

Studies applying cine-CT scans to reconstruct the three-dimensional geometry of the left ventricle with aneurysm indicated that reduced myocardial function extends beyond the anatomic border of the aneurysm. It is estimated that the size of the dysfunctioning zone is almost twice the size of the aneurysm. The pathogenesis for this phenomenon is not clear, although it is suggested that perhaps it is in part related to some geometric remodeling of the left ventricle. Data suggested that increased afterload is more likely to result in aneurysm formation than increased preload. Any factor that increases wall stress, such as arterial hypertension or exercise stress, may promote aneurysm formation in healed infarct scars.

Ventricular mural thrombi

Mural thrombi at the site of myocardial ischemic injury, according to data from autopsies, occur in 14% to 68% of such cases, although echocardiographic studies reveal a somewhat lower incidence.[177-179] The great majority of mural thrombi are found in association with anterior and anteroapical myocardial infarctions, large myocardial infarctions and in patients with concomitant congestive heart failure (Fig. 2-52). Mural thrombi are soft and shaggy early in their formation and, therefore, may break away and embolize, but later on (after 2 to 3 weeks) are organized, flatten and appear as an endocardial thickening with a pearly discoloration.

Postinfarction pericarditis and postinfarction syndrome

A transmural myocardial infarction may be associated with focal or diffuse pericardial inflammation in about 5% to 10% of the cases. This benign pericarditis develops within the first 5 days after the infarction; clinically it is manifested by pain, fever and supraventricular arrhythmias lasting for several days. This pericarditis appears as an incidental finding in the course of a more important illness. The postinfarction syndrome (Dressler's syndrome) usually appears between the second and tenth week after infarction, and is accompanied by pain, pericardial effusion, pleuritis with pleural effusion, pneumonitis and fever. Each such episode may persist for a week or two and usually subsides but may recur again. The pathogenesis of the postinfarction syndrome is thought to be an autoimmune response to antigenic changes in the damaged myocardium.[180-181]

COMPLICATIONS RELATED TO CORONARY BYPASS SURGERY

Discussion of medical or surgical therapy is beyond the scope of this chapter. However, brief reviews of selective topics regarding postoperative complications occurring af-

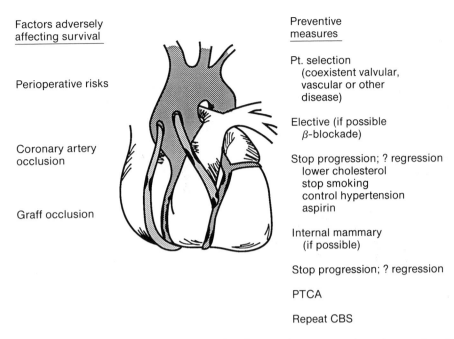

Factors adversely
affecting survival

Perioperative risks

Coronary artery
occlusion

Graff occlusion

Preventive
measures

Pt. selection
(coexistent valvular,
vascular or other
disease)

Elective (if possible
β-blockade)

Stop progression; ? regression
lower cholesterol
stop smoking
control hypertension
aspirin

Internal mammary
(if possible)

Stop progression; ? regression

PTCA

Repeat CBS

Fig. 2-54. Factors adversely affecting survival and preventive measures in patients undergoing coronary bypass surgery (CBS). Schematic presentation. *Pt* = patients, *PTCA* = percutaneous transluminal coronary angioplasty.

ter relevant established surgical or interventional procedures will be briefly presented.

Postpericardiotomy syndrome

This syndrome, which is diagnosed in about 20% to 30% of patients after cardiac surgery, usually occurs after the first postoperative week. It is characterized by a constellation of symptoms and signs, such as precordial discomfort, fever, and signs of pericardial and often pleural reactions, at times associated with effusions. Besides discomfort and the prolongation of the postoperative morbidity, this syndrome may be confused with other causes of postoperative fever such as endocarditis, sepsis, atelectasis or pneumonia. The cause of this usually self-limited but sometimes recurring illness is not known, although it is postulated that it represents an immunologic reaction to heart-reactive antibodies, such as in cases of Dressler's syndrome. The possibility of viral cause has also been suggested because some patients reveal significant titers of antibodies to one or more viral agents.[180-181]

Graft occlusion

Although surgical therapy has improved prognosis in high-risk patients, its advantage over medical therapy declines with longer follow-up[182-188] (Figure 2-53). Twelve-year follow-up studies have observed increasing mortality in the surgical group over time, with resultant convergence of the surgical and medical survival curves. One of the reasons for the decline in survival of bypassed patients with time is that saphenous vein grafts have a significant

incidence of acquired progressive stenosis[182-188] (Fig. 2-54). The status of the native coronary arteries after bypass surgery is another area of concern; follow-up studies have shown that patients with saphenous vein grafts at 10 years have a higher incidence of disease progression in native coronary arteries proximal to insertion of the graft, regardless of the graft patency.[188a]

Vein grafts resected from patients during surgery for repeated grafting have revealed some intriguing findings. Acute thrombosis can occur at any time in the life of the graft, from a few hours postoperatively to several months or years later (Fig. 2-55). While thrombus may be localized at any site of the graft, it occurs more often at the distal anastomosis. Saphenous grafts explanted within hours or days of insertion reveal fibrin deposits on the intima that may be circumferential, suggesting traumatic injury (Fig. 2-56). The role of these microthrombi in the later development of concentric fibrous intimal hyperplasia is not clear. Data indicate, however, that thrombosis and intimal fibroplasia are the most frequent causes of graft stenosis within the first 5 years after implantation; atherosclerosis assumes a steadily increasing role after 5 years.[183] The thickened intima of the vein graft contains numerous spindle cells embedded in a matrix of mucopolysaccharides and collagen. Rarely, a thin rim of calcium deposits is seen within the intima.[184]

Atherosclerosis of venous grafts has many similarities with the atheromatous lesions of arteries, although is more often concentric and diffuse. Venous graft atheromata have poorly developed fibrous caps, and contain plentiful

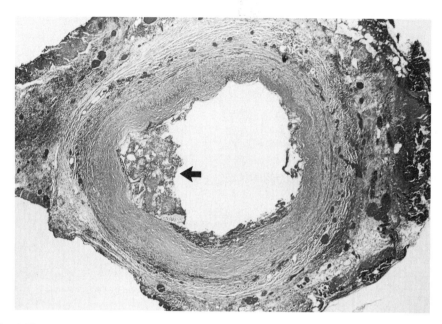

Fig. 2-55. Venous graft, approximately 2 years after bypass, showing intimal fibrosis and a small luminal thrombus.

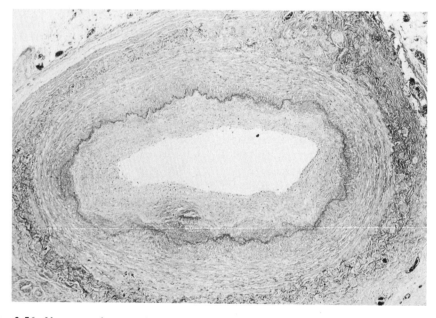

Fig. 2-56. Venous graft, approximately 1½ years after bypass, showing marked circumferential intimal proliferation. Elastic stain.

foam cells and lipid debris which may be directly exposed to the arterial lumen. Numerous inflammatory cells and lipid-laden multinucleate foreign body giant cells are often present in the intima. The inflammatory reaction may erode the media and extend into the adventitia. It has been suggested that the lack of a well-developed fibrous cap in these atheromatous plaques may be responsible for their fragility (rupture) and subsequent thrombosis.[184]

There are certain similarities between the saphenous vein graft atherosclerosis and the coronary atherosclerosis observed in transplanted hearts. Both develop relatively fast (3 to 5 years) and both tend to be concentric and diffuse. However, these morphologic similarities and the time frame of development may not necessarily denote similar pathogenetic mechanisms and/or etiology. Whether the stenotic lesions in vein grafts (intimal fibroplasia and atheroma) are the result of exposure of a delicate venous structure to systemic pressures, or some immunologic mechanism, is at present unclear. The higher long-term patency of the internal mammary artery has brought some new hopes for this revascularization technique.

COMPLICATIONS RELATED TO CORONARY ANGIOPLASTY

Percutaneous transluminal coronary angioplasty is being used with increasing frequency in the treatment of coronary artery disease. Initially used to treat proximal, noncalcified, short (< 5 mm), discrete obstructions in patients with single-vessel disease, the technique is now frequently used for patients with diffuse, multivessel disease including calcified and eccentric lesions. Depending on lesion morphology, angiographic immediate success is achieved in about 90% of the cases.[189-196]

Coronary angioplasty, however, has two largely unresolved problems: acute closure of the artery immediately or soon (< 48 hours) after the procedure, and late restenosis, a gradual process that has a peak incidence approximately 4 months after the procedure (Figs. 2-57 and 2-58). Acute closure occurs in about 2% to 10% of the patients, depending on the complexity of the lesion.[191] Late restenosis, which occurs in 20% to 30% of patients, is less predictable, but the possibility of its occurrence is increased in long, diffuse, eccentric and tortuous lesions. While restenosis can be successfully managed by repeat dilatation in the majority of patients, acute closure is responsible for the vast majority of complications of angioplasty including emergency bypass surgery, myocardial infarction and, rarely, death.

Postmortem studies of postangioplasty cases confirmed that in early deaths (within 24 hours after angioplasty) a recent thrombotic occlusion was present in one-third of the cases, although in only one-third of those was the thrombus completely occlusive. In all these cases, a certain degree of aneurysmal dilatation of the arterial wall at the site of angioplasty was detected. The dilatation was due primarily to stretching and thinning of the nonatheromatous segment of the arterial wall. Intimal splits were present in 75% of early cases. In eccentric plaques the intimal splits (cracks) occurred at the junction between the atheromatous plaque and the segment of the wall not involved or mini-

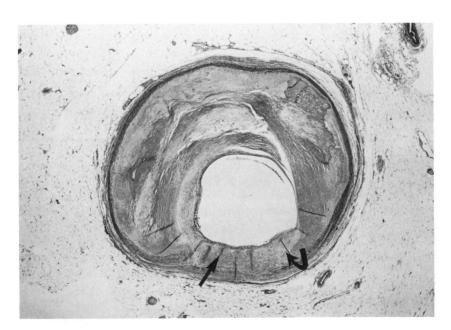

Fig. 2-57. Site of coronary angioplasty, approximately 4 months after PTCA. Note medial replacement by myofibroblastic proliferation at the nonatherosclerotic segment of the wall *(arrows)*.

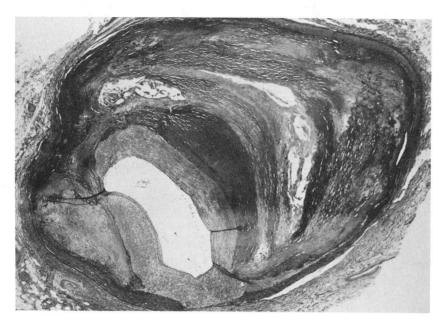

Fig. 2-58. Site of angioplasty (6½ months after PTCA) showing circumferential intimal proliferation. Elastic stain.

mally involved by atheroma. Only in concentric plaques did the intimal crack appear to involve the fibrous cap of the plaque at its most bulging portion.[196]

In cases in which the time interval between angioplasty and death was longer than 30 days (late causes), an intimal myoproliferative lesion was present, primarily over the nonatheromatous portion of the arterial circumference. Similar myloproliferative reaction was noted within crevices created from previous intimal disruptions. The main constituents of the intimal lesions were smooth muscle cells, fibroblasts, reticulum fibers, and elastic fibers. The media at the plaque-free segment of the arterial wall was partially or completely destroyed and was replaced by myofibroblastic tissue similar to the one observed in the intima. The internal elastica at the site of the dilatation was either disrupted or completely absent, while the externa elastica and adventitia were unaffected. These postmortem findings clearly indicate that improvement of the luminal diameter after angioplasty may result from expansion of the segment of the wall uninvolved by atheroma[196] (Fig. 2-59). However, while expansion of the normal portion of the wall contributes significantly to the primary success of this procedure, it also exposes the smooth muscle cells of the media to potential mechanical injury, the sequelae of which are marked intimal proliferation and possible restenosis. From several studies it appears that there is more than one mitogen released at the site of angioplasty. These mitogens are responsible for smooth muscle cell proliferation and migration into the intima.

Activated platelets are known to store and release platelet-derived growth factor (PDGF) which has both chemot-

actic and mitogenic properties and thus stimulates smooth muscle cell migration and proliferation. PDGF binds with high affinity to smooth muscle cells, inducing a sequence of cellular events culminating in DNA synthesis and cell replication. Activated platelets may also promote myoproliferation by releasing epidermal growth factor and transforming growth factor. However, the use of platelet inhibitors (aspirin, dipyridamole) has not reduced the rate of restenosis. Stretching of the medial layer of the vessel during balloon dilatation may trigger the release of endogenous mitogens similar to PDGF or block the release of substances which inhibit smooth muscle proliferation. Basic fibroblast growth factor (bFGF) may be involved in the development of stretch-induced smooth muscle proliferation. This factor is synthesized by endothelial and smooth muscle cells and may be released from these cells following vascular injury.

In addition, smooth muscle cell growth may be influenced by circulating proteins. One such protein is angiotensin II, a vasoactive serum protein, that may directly promote smooth muscle cell growth. Another serum protein, and potent cellular growth factor is insulin-like growth factor (IGF). One may justifiably state that at present our knowledge regarding the stimuli which initiate internal hyperplasia after angioplasty is only partial, and our understanding of the factors which may sustain a process is nonexistent. Atherectomy, a potential alternative to balloon angioplasty, does not appear to be free of the problem of restenosis. In fact, there are no appreciable differences in the intimal hyperplastic lesions seen in both procedures, a strong indication that the healing response of

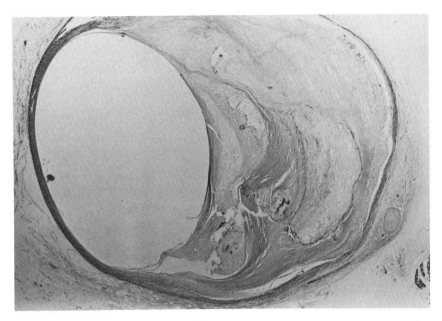

Fig. 2-59. Post-PTCA (24 hours) of an eccentric plaque. Note significant expansion of the non-atheromatous segment of the arterial wall.

the vessel is nonspecific and independent of the mechanism by which the artery is initially disrupted.

MANAGEMENT OF CORONARY ARTERY DISEASE BASED ON PATHOPHYSIOLOGY: GENERAL PRINCIPLES

After the onset of clinical manifestations of coronary artery disease, there is no definitive cure for the disease. The clinical picture and the natural history are related to the extent and severity of the underlying coronary pathologic conditions and the status of left ventricular function. Medical and/or surgical management may favorably alter the clinical manifestations and/or the natural history of the disease, but as a general rule, do not alter the underlying coronary artery pathologic conditions.

Coronary bypass surgery and angioplasty improve symptoms and in certain cases chances of survival by increasing blood flow. Pharmacologic agents improve symptoms and in certain cases may increase survival by reducing myocardial oxygen consumption, increasing myocardial oxygen supply, and/or by decreasing the incidence of plaque rupture or intravascular thrombosis. Further, therapeutic interventions that significantly decrease plasma cholesterol may stop the progression of atherosclerosis and/or in certain cases may produce regression of atherosclerosis.[107-203]

Management of coronary artery disease is not either medical or surgical but a combination of medical therapy, coronary bypass surgery, or coronary angioplasty. The different therapeutic interventions should represent a coordinated lifelong plan in which each is staged in relation to

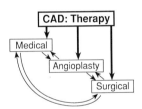

Fig. 2-60. Basic schema for management of patients with coronary artery disease (CAD). (From Boudoulas H: *Coronary artery disease: clinical presentation, diagnostic evaluations, and management.* In Leier CV, Boudoulas H, eds: *Cardiorenal Disorders and Diseases*, ed 2, Mount Kisco, New York, 1992, Futura.)

the patient's symptoms and certain objective findings[39] (Fig. 2-60).

Survival of patients with coronary artery disease is usually decreased compared to the general "normal" population. Therapy, medical, surgical, or coronary angioplasty, may improve survival in certain patients, but in general, survival is lower compared to a "normal" population.[197-203] Therapeutic interventions that may improve survival in patients with coronary artery disease are shown in Fig. 2-61. Thrombolytic therapy, β-blockade therapy, intravenous administration of nitroglycerin, aspirin administration and probably intravenous administration of heparin increase survival in patients with acute myocardial infarction.[203] Aspirin administered orally, heparin administered intravenously, and coronary bypass surgery (in selective cases) may increase survival in patients with unstable angina. Cessation of smoking, cholesterol reduction, aspirin administration, anticoagulation, β-blockade therapy, and

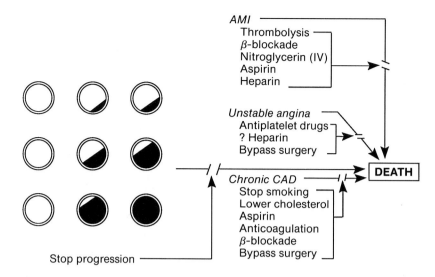

Fig. 2-61. Schematic presentation of coronary artery pathology, clinical manifestations and therapeutic intervention that increased survival in patients with acute myocardial infarction (AMI), unstable angina and chronic coronary artery disease. *IV* = intravenously.(From Boudoulas H: Therapeutic interventions which may improve survival in patients with coronary artery disease, *Acta Cardiol* 45:477-87, 1990.)

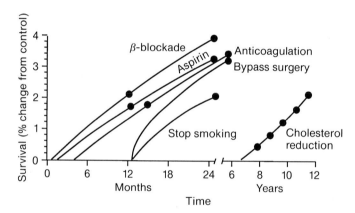

Fig. 2-62. Effect of therapeutic interventions on survival. On the vertical axis the change in survival compared with placebo administration is shown. On the horizontal axis, the time required from the initiation of therapeutic intervention to the time when the effect of therapeutic intervention on survival becomes obvious. β-blockade therapy and aspirin increased survival almost immediately after the initiation of therapy. The effect of smoking and coronary bypass surgery was obvious after 12 months. The effect of cholesterol became obvious after 6 or 7 years.(From Boudoulas H. and Geleris P eds: *Coronary Artery Disease,* ed 2, Thessaloniki, Greece, 1990, University Studio Press.)

coronary bypass surgery (in selective cases) improve survival in patients with chronic coronary artery disease.

The effect of therapeutic interventions on survival may become obvious immediately after therapy (e.g., thrombolysis), or long time after the initiation of therapy (e.g., cholesterol reduction). Fig. 2-62 shows the time required from the initiation of therapeutic intervention to the time when the effect of therapeutic intervention on survival becomes obvious.[26] The effect of β-blockade therapy and aspirin on survival becomes apparent early; the effect of coronary bypass surgery and cessation of smoking on survival

becomes obvious after the first 12 months; and the effect of cholesterol reduction on survival becomes obvious after several years.

REFERENCES

1. Walmsley R, Watson H: *Clinical anatomy of the heart.* New York, 1978, Churchill Livingstone.
2. Bell JR, Fox AC: Pathogenesis of subendocardial ischemia, *Am J Med Sci* 268:2, 1974.
3. Hillis LD, Winniford MD: Frequency of severe (70% or more) narrowing of the right, left anterior descending, and left circumflex arteries in right dominant circulations with coronary artery disease, *Am J Cardiol* 59:358-359, 1987.

4. Saner HE, Gobel FL, Salomonowitz E, et al: The free wall in coronary atherosclerosis: its relation to degree of obstruction, *J Am Coll Cardiol* 6:1096-1099, 1985.

5. Glagov S, Zarins L, Giddens et al: Hemodynamics and atherosclerosis. Insights and perspectives gained from studies of human arteries, *Arch Pathol Lab Med* 112:1018-1031, 1988.

6. Asakura T, Karino T: Flow patterns and spatial distribution of atherosclerotic lesions in human coronary arteries, *Circ Res* 66:1045-1066, 1990.

7. Kato H, Ichinose E, Kawaski T: Myocardial infarction in Kawasaki disease. Clinical analysis in 195 cases, *J Pediatr* 108:923-27, 1986.

8. Schwartz F, Wayner HD, Sesto M, et al: Native collaterals in the development of collateral circulation after chronic coronary stenosis in mongrel dogs, *Circulation* 66:303-308, 1982.

9. Epstein S: Influence of stenosis severity on coronary collateral development and importance of collaterals in maintaining left ventricular function during acute coronary occlusion, *Am J Cardio* 61:866-868, 1988.

10. Williams DO, Amsterdam EA, Miller RR, et al: Functional significance of coronary collateral vessels in patients with acute myocardial infarction: relation to pump performance, cardiogenic shock and survival, *Am J Cardiol* 37:345-351, 1988.

11. Probst P, Zangl W, Pachinser O: Relation of coronary arterial occlusion pressure during percutaneous transluminal coronary angioplasty to presence of collaterals, *Am J Cardiol* 55:1264-1269, 1985.

12. Topol EJ, Ellis SG: Coronary collaterals revisited. accessory pathway to myocardial preservation during infarction, *Circulation* 83:1084-86, 1991.

13. Hirai T, Fujita M, Nakajima H, et al: Importance of collateral circulation for prevention of left ventricular aneurysm formation in acute myocardial infarction, *Circulation* 79:791-6, 1989.

14. James TN: The spectrum of diseases of small coronary arteries and their physiologic consequences, *J Am Coll Cardiol* 15:763-74, 1990.

15. Factor SM, Cho S: Smooth muscle contraction bands in the media of coronary arteries: a postmortem marker of antemortem coronary spasm?, *J Am Coll Cardiol* 6:1329-1337, 1985.

16. MacAlpin RN. Relation of coronary arterial spasm to sites of organic stenosis, *Am J Cardiol* 46:143, 1980.

17. Yeung AC, Vekshtein VI, Krantz DS, et al: The effect of atherosclerosis on the vasomotor response of coronary arteries to mental stress, *N Engl J Med* 325:1551-6, 1991.

18. Lerman A, Edwards BS, Hallett JW, et al: Circulating and tissue endothelin immunoreactivity in advanced atherosclerosis, *N Engl J Med* 325:997-1001, 1991.

19. Matsuyama K, Yasue H, Okumura K, et al: Increased plasma level of endothelin-1-like immunoreactivity during coronary spasm in patients with coronary spastic angina, *Am J Cardiol* 68:991-5, 1991.

20. Maseri A, Davies G, Hackett D, et al: Coronary artery spasm and vasoconstriction. the case for a distinction, *Circulation* 81:1985-1991, 1990.

21. Stefanadis C, Wooley CF, Bush CA, et al: Aortic distensibility abnormalities in coronary artery disease, *Am J Cardiol* 59:1300-4, 1987.

22. Ross J: Is there a true increase in myocardial stiffness with acute ischemia?, *Am J Cardiol* 63:87E-91E, 1989.

23. Hirata K, Triposkiadis F, Sparks E, et al: The Marfan syndrome: abnormal elastic properties, *J Am Coll Cardiol* 18:57-63, 1991.

24. Stefanadis C, Stratos C, Boudoulas H, et al: Distensibility of the ascending aorta: Comparison of invasive and noninvasive techniques, *Eur Heart J* 11:990-6, 1990.

25. Boudoulas H: *Coronary arteries: factors as they affect myocardial oxygen supply and demand*. In Leier CV, Boudoulas H, eds: *Cardiorenal Disorders and Diseases*, ed 2, Mount Kisco, NY, 1992, Futura.

26. Boudoulas H, Geleris P, eds: *Coronary Artery Disease*, ed 2, Thessaloniki, Greece, 1990, University Studio Press.

27. Boudoulas H, Kolibash AJ, Baker P, et al: Mitral valve prolapse and the mitral valve prolapse syndrome: a diagnostic classification and pathogenesis of symptoms *Am Heart J*. 118:796-818, 1989.

28. Austin RE Jr, Aldea GS, Coggins DL, et al: Profound spatial heterogeneity of coronary reserve. Discordance between patterns of resting and maximal myocardial blood flow, *Circ Res* 67:319-331, 1990.

29. Dole WP: Autoregulation of the coronary circulation, *Prog Cardiovasc Dis* 29:293-323, 1987.

30. Yonekura S, Watanabe N, Caffrey JL, et al: Mechanism of attenuated pressure-flow autoregulation in right coronary circulation of dogs, *Circ Res* 60:133-141, 1987.

31. Marcus ML, Chilian WM, Kanatsuka H, et al: Understanding the coronary circulation through studies at the microvascular level, *Circulation* 82:1-7, 1990.

32. Feigl E: Coronary physiology, *Physiol Rev* 63:1-205, 1983.

33. Hanley FL, Grattan MT, Stevens MB, et al: Role of adenosine in coronary autoregulation, *Am J Physiol* 250:H558-H566, 1986.

34. Boudoulas H, Rittgers SE, Lewis RP, et al: Changes in diastolic time with various pharmacologic agents. Implications for myocardial perfusion, *Circulation* 60:164-169, 1979.

35. Boudoulas H, Lewis RP, Rittgers SE, et al: Increased diastolic time: a possible important factor in the beneficial effect of propranolol in patients with coronary artery disease, *J Cardiovasc Pharmacol* 1:503-513, 1979.

36. Boudoulas H, Karayannacos PE, Kein N, et al: *Noninvasive method of estimating relative subendocardial flow employing diastolic time*. In Diethrich EB, ed: *Noninvasive assessment of cardiovascular system*, Littleton, Massachusetts, 1982, John Wright.

37. Boudoulas H, Dervenagas S, Fulkerson PK, et al: *Effect of heart rate on diastolic time and left ventricular performance in patients with atrial fibrillation*. In Diethrich EG, ed: Noninvasive cardiovascular diagnosis, ed. 2, Littleton, Massachusetts, 1981, PSG.

38. Boudoulas H: Diastolic time: The forgotten dynamic factor. Implications for myocardial perfusion, *Acta Cardiol* 46:61-71, 1991.

39. Boudoulas H: *Coronary artery disease: clinical presentation, diagnostic evaluations, and management*. In Leier CV, Boudoulas H, eds: *Cardiorenal Disorders and Diseases*, Ed 2, Mount Kisco, NY, 1992, Futura.

40. Jan K: Distribution of myocardial stress and its influence on coronary blood flow, *J Biomech* 18:815-820, 1985.

41. Waters D: Proischemic complications of dihydropyridine calcium channel blockers, *Circulation* 84:2598-600, 1991.

42. Garratt KN, Edwards WD, Vlietstra RE, et al: Coronary morphology after percutaneous directional coronary atherectomy in humans: autopsy analysis of three patients, *J Am Coll Cardiol* 16:1432-6, 1990.

43. Sansa M, Cerbigliaro C, Bolognese L, et al: Angiographic morphology and response to therapy in unstable angina, *Clin Cardiol* 11:121-126, 1988.

44. Ambrose JA, Tannenbaum MA, Alexopoulos D, et al: Angiographic progression of coronary artery disease and the development of myocardial infarction, *J Am Coll Cardiol* 12:56-62, 1988.

45. Little WC, Constantinescu M, Applegate RJ, et al: Can coronary angiography predict the site of a subsequent myocardial infarction in patients with mild-to-moderate coronary artery disease?, *Circulation* 78:1157-66, 1988.

46. Mizuno K, Miyamoto A, Satomura K, et al: Angioscopic coronary macromorphology in patients with acute coronary disorders, *Lancet* 337:809-12, 1991.

47. Farb A, Virmani R, Atkinson JB, et al: Plaque morphology and pathologic changes in arteries from patients dying after coronary balloon angioplasty, *J Am Coll Cardiol* 16:1421-9, 1990.

48. Isner JM, Donaldson RF, Fortin AH, et al: Attenuation of media of coronary arteries in advanced atherosclerosis, *Am J Cardiol* 58:937-939, 1986.

49. Davies MJ: Pathology of atherosclerosis, plaque disruption, and thrombus formation, *Current Opinion in Cardiol* 4:464-467, 1989.

50. Richardson PD, Davies MJ, Born GVR: Influence of plaque configuration and stress distribution on fissuring of coronary atherosclerotic plaques, *Lancet* 2:941-944, 1989.

51. Lee RT, Grodzinsky AJ, Frank EH, et al: Structure-dependent dynamic mechanical behavior of fibrous caps from human atherosclerotic plaques, *Circulation* 83:1764, 1991.

52. Gotoh K, Minamino T, Hatoh O, et al: The role of intracoronary thrombus in unstable angina: angiographic assessment and thrombolytic therapy during ongoing anginal attacks, *Circulation* 77:526-534, 1988.

53. DeWood MA, Stiffer WF, Simpson CS, et al: Coronary arteriographic findings soon after non-Q-wave myocardial infarction, *N Engl J Med* 315:417-423, 1986.

54. Kragel AH, Reddy SG, Witles JT, et al: Morphometric analysis of the composition of atherosclerotic plaques in the four major epicardial coronary arteries in acute myocardial infarction and in sudden coronary death, *Circulation* 80:1747-56, 1989.

55. Davies MJ, Thomas AC: Plaque fissuring. The cause of acute myocardial infarction, sudden ischemic death and crescendo angina, *Br Heart J* 53:363-73, 1985.

56. Ridker PM, Manson JE, Buring JE, et al: Circadian variation of acute myocardial infarction and the effect of low-dose aspirin in a randomized trial of physicians, *Circulation* 82:897-902, 1990.

57. Mulcahy D, Cunningham D, Crean P, et al: Circadian variation of total ischaemic burden and its alteration with anti-anginal agents, *Lancet* 2:755-58, 1988.

58. Fink RJ, Rooney PA, Throwbridge JO, et al: Coronary thrombosis and platelet/fibrin microemboli in death associated with acute myocardial infarction, *Br Heart J* 49:196-200, 1988.

59. Fossel ET, Morgan HE, Ingwall JS: Measurement of changes in high-energy phosphates in the cardiac cycle by using gated ^{31}P nuclear magnetic resonance, *Proc Natl Acad Sci* USA 77:3654-58, 1980.

60. Bagchi D, Das DK, Engelman RM, et al: Polymorphonuclear leukocytes as potential source of free radicals in the ischemic-reperfused myocardium, *Eur Heart J* 11:800-813, 1990.

61. Jennings RB, Reimer KA, Steenbergen C: Myocardial ischemia revisited. The osmolar load, membrane damage and reperfusion, *J Mol Cell Cardiol* 18:769-780, 1986.

62. McCall T, Whittle BJR, Broughton-Smith NK, et al: Inhibition of FMLP-induced aggregation of rabbit neutrophils by nitric oxide, *Br J Pharmacol* 95:517P, 1988.

63. Chatelain P, Latour J, Tran D, et al: Neutrophil accumulation in experimental myocardium infarcts: Relation with extent of injury and effect of reperfusion, *Circulation* 75:1083, 1987.

64. Dreyer WJ, Michael LH, West MS, et al: Neutrophil accumulation in ischemic canine myocardium; insights into time course, distribution, and mechanism of localization during early reperfusion, *Circulation* 84:400, 1991.

65. Jennings RB, Ganote C: Mitochondrial structure and function in acute myocardial ischemic injury, *Circ Res* 38(suppl I):I80, 1976.

66. Quaife RA, Kohmoto O, Berry WH: Mechanisms of reoxygenation injury in cultured ventricular myocytes, *Circulation* 83:566, 1991.

67. Kranzhofer R, Haass M, Kurz T, et al: Effect of digitalis glycosides on norepinephrine release in the heart. Dual mechanism of action, *Circ Res* 68:1628-37, 1991.

68. Ward PA: Mechanisms of endothelial cell injury, *J Lab Clin Med* 118:421-26, 1991.

69. Sheridan FM, Dauber IM, McMurtry IF, et al: Role of leukocytes in coronary vascular endothelial injury due to ischemia and reperfusion, *Circ Res* 69:1566-1574, 1991.

70. Moore KH, Radloff JF, Hull FE, et al: Incomplete fatty acid oxidation by ischemic heart: B-hydroxy fatty acid production, *Am J Physiol* 239:H257, 1980.

71. Neely JR, Feuvray D: Metabolic products and myocardial ischemia, *Am J Pathol* 102:282, 1981.

72. Shine KJ: Ionic events in ischemia and anoxia, *Am J Pathol* 102:256, 1981.

73. Fozzard HA, Makielski JC: The electrophysiology of acute myocardial ischemia, *Annu Rev Med* 36:275, 1985.

74. Nayler WG: The role of calcium in the ischemic myocardium, *Am J Pathol* 102:262, 1981.

75. Kodama I, Wilde A, Janse MJ, et al: Combined effects of hypoxia, hyperkalemia and acidosis on membrane action potential and excitability of guinea-pig ventricular muscle, *J Mol Cell Cardiol* 16:247, 1984.

76. Freeman BA, Crapo JD. Biology of disease free radicals and tissue injury, *Lab Invest* 47:412-426, 1982.

77. Engler RL, Schmid-Schonbein GW, Palevec RS: Leukocyte capillary plugging in myocardial ischemia and reperfusion in the dog, *Am J Pathol* 111:98, 1983.

78. Ernest E, Hammerschmidt DE, Bagge V, et al: Leukocytes and the risk of ischemic heart disease, *JAMA* 257:2318-24, 1987.

79. Metha J, Nichols WW, Metha P: Neutrophils as potential participants in acute myocardial ischemia: relevance to perfusion, *J Am Coll Cardiol* 11:1309-16, 1988.

80. Werns SW, Lucchesi BR: Leukocytes, oxygen radicals, and myocardial injury due to ischemia and reperfusion, *Free Radic Biol Med* 4:31-37; 1988.

81. Rona G: Catecholamine cardiotoxicity, *J Mol Cell Cardiol* 17:291-306, 1985.

82. Schomig A: Catecholamines in myocardial ischemia: systemic and cardiac release, *Circulation* 82(suppl II):II13-II22, 1990.

83. Bilheimer DW, Buja LM, Parkey RW, et al: Fatty acid accumulation and abnormal lipid deposition in peripheral and border zones of experimental myocardial infarcts, *J Nucl Med* 19:276, 1978.

84. Jennings RB, Murray CE, Steenbergen C, et al: Development of cell injury in sustained acute ischemia, *Circulation* 82(suppl II):II2-II12, 1990.

85. Reimer KA, Ideker RE: Myocardial ischemia and infarction: anatomic and biochemical substrates for ischemic cell death and ventricular arrhythmias, *Hum Pathol* 18:462-475, 1987.

86. Connelly CM, McLaughlin RJ, Vogel WM, et al: Reversible and irreversible elongation of ischemic, infarcted and healed myocardium in response to increases in preload and afterload, *Circulation* 84:387, 1991.

87. Boudoulas H, Geleris P, Lewis RP, et al: Effect of increased adrenergic activity on the relationship between electrical (WT) and mechanical systole (QS$_2$). Relative prolongation of the electrial systole, *Circulation* 64:28, 1981.

88. Lewis RP, Boudoulas H, Forester WF, et al: Shortening of electromechanical systole as a manifestation of excessive adrenergic stimulation in acute myocardial infarction, *Circulation* 46:856, 1972.

89. Fuster V, Badimon L, Badimon JJ, et al: The pathogenesis of coronary artery disease and the acute coronary syndromes, *N Engl J Med* 326:242-50, 1992.

90. Hearse DJ: Myocardial enzyme leakage, *J Molec Med* 2:185, 1987.

91. Vrints CJM, Bult H, Hitter E, et al: Impaired endothelium-dependent coronary vasodilation in patients with angina and normal coronary arteries, *J Am Coll Cardiol* 19:21-31, 1992.

92. Boudoulas H, Lewis RP, Kates RE, et al: Hypersensitivity to adrenergic stimulation after propranolol withdrawal in normals, *Ann Intern Med* 87:433, 1977.

93. Fuster V, Badimon L, Cohen M, et al: Insights into the pathogenesis of acute ischemic syndromes, *Circulation* 77:1213-1220, 1988.

94. Golino P, Piscione F, Willerson JT, et al: Divergent effects of serotonin on coronary-artery dimensions and blood flow in patients with coronary atherosclerosis and control patients, *N Engl J Med* 324:641, 1991.

95. Muller JE, Toffer GH, Stone PH: Circadian variation and triggers of onset of acute cardiovascular disease, *Circulation* 79:733, 1989.

96. McCord JM: Oxygen-derived free radicals in postischemic tissue injury, *N Engl J Med* 312:159-163, 1985.

97. Methat JL, Lawson DL, Nichols WW: Attenuated coronary relaxation after reperfusion: effects of superoxide dismutase and TxA2 inhibitor V-63557, *Am J Physiol* 257:H1240, 1989.

98. Panza JA, Epstein SE, Quyyumi AA: Circadian variation in vascular tone and its relation to α-sympathetic vasoconstrictor activity, *N Engl J Med* 325:986-90, 1991.

99. Sherman CT, Litvack F, Grundfest W, et al: Coronary angioscopy in patients with unstable angina pectoris, *N Engl J Med* 315:913-9, 1986.

100. Chester AH, O'Neil GS, Moncada S, et al: Low basal and stimulated release of nitric oxide in atherosclerotic epicardial coronary arteries, *Lancet* 336:897-900, 1990.

101. Deedwania PC, Carbajal EV: Silent ischemia during daily life is an independent predictor of mortality in stable angina, *Circulation* 81:748-56, 1990.

102. Carbajal EV, Deedwania PC: Silent myocardial ischemia: mechanisms, diagnosis, prevalence, *Primary Cardiology* 17:30-40, 1991.

103. Chierchia S, Glazier L: A model for the management of silent myocardial ischemia. Proceedings of a symposium. A quarter-century of β-blockade, *Postgrad Med* 2:120-122, 1988.

104. Rozanski A, Berman DS: Silent myocardial ischemia. I. Pathophysiology, frequency of occurrence, and approaches toward detection, *Am Heart J* 114:615-26, 1987.

105. Boudoulas H, Cobb TC, Leighton RF, et al: Myocardial lactate production in patients with angina-like chest pain, angiographically normal coronary arteries and left ventricular function, *Am J Cardiol* 34:501, 1974.

106. Camici PG, Marraccini P, Lorenzoni R, et al: Coronary hemodynamics and myocardial metabolism in patients with syndrome X: response to pacing stress, *J Am Coll Cardiol* 17:1461, 1991.

107. Ishihara T, Seki I, Yamada Y, et al: Coronary circulation, myocardial metabolism and cardiac catecholamine flux in patients with syndrome X, *J Cardiol* 20:267-74, 1990.

108. Timmis AD, Griffin B, Crick JCP, et al: The effects of early coronary patency on the evolution of myocardial infarction: a prospective angiographic study, *Br Heart J* 58:345-351, 1987.

109. Lee JT, Ideker RE, Reimber KA: Myocardial infarct size and location in relation to the coronary vascular bed at risk in man, *Circulation* 64:526, 1981.

110. Jennings RB, Schaper J, Hill ML, et al: Effect of reperfusion late in the phase of reversible ischemic injury. Changes in cell volume, electrolytes, metabolites and ultrastructure, *Circ Res* 56:262, 1985.

111. Anderson HR, Falk E, Nielsen D: Right ventricular infarction: Frequency, size and topography in coronary artery disease: a prospective study comprising 107 consecutive autopsies from a coronary care unit, *J Am Coll Cardiol* 10:1223, 1987.

112. Gallagher KP, Gerren RA, Stirling MC, et al: The distribution of functional impairment across the lateral border of acutely ischemic myocardium, *Circ Res* 58:570-583, 1986.

113. Cabin HS, Roberts WC: Left ventricular aneurysm, intra-aneurysmal thrombus and systemic embolus in coronary heart disease, *Chest* 77:586-590, 1980.

114. Wickline SA, Verdonk ED, Wong AK, et al: Structural remodeling of human myocardial tissue after infarction. Quantification with ultrasonic backscatter, *Circulation* 85:259-68, 1992.

115. Herijgers P, Flameng W: Coronary artery thrombosis and thrombolysis in baboons: the effect of atenolol treatment on myocardial infarct size, *Eur Heart J* 12:1084-8, 1991.

116. Hori M, Kitakaze M, Sato H, et al: Staged reperfusion attenuates myocardial stunning in dogs. Role of transient acidosis during early reperfusion, *Circulation* 84:2135-45, 1991.

117. Kopelman HA, Forman MB, Wilson BH, et al: Right ventricular myocardial infarctions in patients with chronic lung disease. Possible role of right ventricular hypertrophy, *J Am Coll Cardiol* 5:1302, 1985.

118. Isner JM, Robert WC. Right ventricular infarction secondary to coronary artery disease: frequently location, associated findings and significance from analysis of 236 necropsy patients with acute or healed myocardial infarction, *Am J Cardiol* 42:885, 1978.

119. Goldstein JA, Vlahakes GJ, Verrier ED, et al: The role of right ventricular systolic dysfunction and elevated intrapericardial pressure in the genesis of low output in experimental right ventricular infarction, *Circulation* 65:513, 1982.

120. Fugiwara H, Saimyoji H, Kawai C, et al: Left atrial infarction with saddle embolism, *Jpn Heart J* 18:272, 1977.

121. Page DL, Caulfield JB, Kestor JA, et al: Myocardial changes associated with cardiogenic shock, *N Engl J Med* 285:133, 1971.

122. Aversano T, Marino PN: Effect of ischemic zones size on nonischemic zone function, *Am J Physiol* 258:H1786-H1795, 1980.

123. Buja LM, Willerson JT: Clinicopathologic correlates of acute ischemic heart disease syndromes, *Am J Cardiol* 47:343, 1981.

124. Theroux P, Rose J Jr, Franklin D, et al: Regional myocardial function and dimensions early and late after myocardial infarction in the unanesthetized dog, *Circ Res* 40:158-165, 1977.

125. Lamas GA, Pfeffer MA: Increased left ventricular volume following myocardial infarction in man, *Am Heart J* 111:30-35, 1986.

126. Linzbach AJ: Heart failure from the point of view of quantitative anatomy, *Am J Cardiol* 5:370-382, 1960.

127. Pfeffer MA, Braunwald E: Ventricular remodeling after myocardial infarction. Experimental observations and clinical implications, *Circulation* 81:1161-1172, 1990.

128. Weissler AM, Vohras, Sohn YH, et al: Left ventricular end-diastolic diameter as a risk indicator in coronary artery disease, *Am J Noninvas Cardiol* 1:268-74, 1987.

129. Boudoulas H, Leighton RF: Left ventricular pressure responses in post-angiographic angina, *Cathet Cardiovasc Diagn* 1:389, 1975.

130. Lew WYW, Chen Z, Guth B, et al: Mechanisms of augmented segment shortening in nonischemic areas during acute ischemia of the canine left ventricle, *Circ Res* 56:351-358, 1985.

131. Lessick J, Sideman S, Azhari H, et al: Regional three-dimensional geometry and functions of left ventricles with fibrous aneurysms, *Circulation* 84:1072, 1991.

132. Nicolosi AC, Spotnitz HM: Quantitative analysis of regional systolic function with left ventricular aneurysm, *Circulation* 78:856-862, 1988.

133. Whittaker P, Boughner DR, Kloner RA: Role of collagen in acute myocardial infarction expansion, *Circulation* 84:2123-34, 1991.

134. Pirolo JS, Hutchins GM, Moore GW: Infarct expansion: pathologic analysis of 204 patients with a single myocardial infarct, *J Am Coll Cardiol* 7:349-354, 1986.

135. Jugdutt BI: Identification of patients prone to infarct expansion by the degree of regional shape distortion on an early two-dimensional echocardiogram after myocardial infarction, *Clin Cardiol* 13:28-40, 1990.

136. Weiss JL, Marino PN, Shapiro EP: Myocardial infarct expansion: recognition, significance and pathology, *Am J Cardiol* 68:35D-40D, 1991.

137. Hutchins GM, Bulkley BH: Infarct expansion versus extension: two different complications of acute myocardial infarction, *Am J Cardiol* 41:1127, 1978.

138. Weisman HF, Healy B: Myocardial infarct expansion, infarct extension and reinfarction: pathophysiologic concepts, *Prog Cardiovasc Dis* 30:73-110, 1987.

139. Flack JE, Kimura Y, Engelman RM, et al: Preconditioning the heart by repeated stunning improves myocardial salvage, *Circulation* 84[suppl III]:III-369-III-374, 1991.

140. Deutsch E, Berger M, Kussmaul WG, et al: Adaptation to ischemia

during percutaneous transluminal coronary angioplasty: clinical, hemodynamic, and metabolic features, *Circulation* 82:2044, 1990.

141. Murry CE, Richard VJ, Reimer KA, et al: Ischemic preconditioning slows energy metabolism and delays ultrastructural damage during sustained ischemia, *Circ Res* 66:913, 1990.

142. Liu GS, Thornton J, Van Winkle DM, et al: Protection against infarction afforded by preconditioning is mediated by A1 adenosine receptors in the rabbit heart, *Circulation* 84:350, 1991.

143. Reimer KA, Murry CE, Jennings RB: Cardiac adaptation to ischemia. Ischemic preconditioning increases myocardial tolerance to subsequent ischemic episodes. *Circulation* 82:2266-68, 1990.

144. Hagar JM, Hale SL, Kloner RA: Effect of preconditioning ischemia on reperfusion arrhythmias after coronary artery occlusion and reperfusion in the rat, *Circ Res* 68:61-68, 1991.

145. Rahimtoola SH: The hibernating myocardium, *Am Heart J* 117:211, 1989.

146. Marban E: Myocardial stunning and hibernation. The physiology behind the colloquialisms. *Circulation* 83:681, 1991.

147. Przyklenk K, Kloner RA: What factors predict recovery of contractile function in the canine model of stunned myocardium? *Am J Cardiol* 64:18F-16F, 1989.

148. Kloner RA, Przyklenk K: Hibernation and stunning of the myocardium, *N Engl J Med* 325:1877-79, 1991.

149. Boli R: Mechanism of myocardial "stunning", *Circulation* 82:723-738, 1990.

150. Mathey DG, Schofer J, Kuck KH, et al: Transmural hemorrhagic myocardial infarction after intracoronary streptokinase. Clinical, angiographic, and necropsy finding, *Br Heart J* 48:546-551, 1982.

151. Cowan MJ, Reichenback D, Turner P, et al: Cellular response of the evolving myocardial infarction after therapeutic coronary artery reperfusion, *Hum Pathol* 22:154, 1991.

151a. Vlessis AA, Muller P, Bartos D et al: Mechanism of peroxide-induced cellular injury in cultured adult cardiac myocytes, *FASEB J* 5:2600, 1991.

151b. Quillen JE, Sellke FW, Brooks LA et al: Ischemia-reperfusion impairs endothelium-dependent relaxation of coronary microvessels but does not affect large arteries, *Circulation* 82:586, 1990.

151c. Lefer AM, Tsao PS, Lefer DJ et al: Role of endothelial dysfunction in the pathogensis of reperfusion injury after myocardial ischemia, *FASEB J* 5:2029, 1991.

151d. Chatelain P, Latour J, Tran D et al: Neutrophil accumulation in experimental myocardial infarcts: Relation with extent of injury and effect of reperfusion, *Circulation* 75:1083, 1987.

151e. Dreyer WJ, Michael LH, West MS et al: Neutrophil accumulation in ischemic canine myocardium; insights into time course, distribution and mechanism of localization during early reperfusion, *Circulation* 84:400, 1991.

151f. Quaife RA, Kohmoto O, Berry WH: Mechanisms of reoxygenation injury in cultured ventricular myocytes, *Circulation* 83:566, 1991.

152. Ganz W, Watanabe I, Kanamasa K, et al: Does reperfusion extend necrosis? A study in a single territory of myocardial ischemia - half reperfused and half not perfused, *Circulation* 82:1020-33, 1990.

153. Montrucchio G, Alloatti G, Mariano F, et al: Role of platelet-activating factor in the reperfusion injury of rabbit ischemic heart, *Am J Pathol* 137:71-83, 1990.

154. Ellis SG, Henschke CL, Sandor T, et al: Time course of functional and biochemical recovery of myocardium salvaged by reperfusion, *J Am Coll Cardiol* 1:1047-55, 1983.

155. Randomized trial of intravenous streptokinase oral aspirin, both, or neither among 17,187 cases of suspected acute myocardial infarction (ISIS-2), *Lancet* 2:349, 1988.

156. Hackett D, Davies G, Chierchia S, et al: Intermittent coronary occlusion in acute myocardial infarction: value of combined thrombolytic and vasodilator therapy, *N Engl J Med* 317:1055-59, 1987.

157. Gertz SD, Kragel AH, Kalan JM, et al: TIMI Investigators. Comparison of coronary and myocardial morphologic findings in patients with and without thrombolytic therapy during fatal first acute myocardial infarction, *Am J Cardiol* 66:904-9, 1990.

158. Janse MJ, Kleber AG: Electrophysiological changes and ventricular arrhythmias in the early phase of regional myocardial ischemia. *Circ Res* 49:1069, 1981.

159. Corr PB, Sobel VE: The importance of metabolites in the genesis of ventricular dysrhythmia induced by ischemia. I Electrophysiological considerations, *Mod Concepts Cardiovasc Dis* 28:43, 1979.

160. Lewis RP, Boudoulas H: Adrenergic activity and early arrhythmias in smokers and non-smokers with acute myocardial infarction, *Am Heart J* 88:526, 1974.

161. Nidorf SM, Thompson PL, de Klerk NH, et al: Prognostic significance of an early rise to peak creatine kinase after acute myocardial infarction, *Am J Cardiol* 61:1178-80, 1988.

162. Goldberg RJ, Gore JM, Alpert JS, et al: Cardiogenic shock after acute myocardial infarction. Incidence and mortality from a community-wide perspective, 1975-1988, *N Engl J Med* 325:1117-22, 1991.

163. Gunnar RM: Cardiogenic shock complicating acute myocardial infarction, *Circulation* 78:1508-10, 1988.

164. Hands ME, Rutherford JD, Muller JE, et al: The in-hospital development of cardiogenic shock after myocardial infarction: incidence, predictors of occurrence, outcome and prognostic factors. *J Am Coll Cardiol* 14:40-6, 1989.

165. Ratshin RA, Rackley CE, Russell RO Jr: Hemodynamic evaluation of left ventricular function in shock complicating myocardial infarction, *Circulation* 45:127, 1972.

166. Swan HJC, Forrester JS, Diamond G, et al: Hemodynamic spectrum of myocardial infarction and cardiogenic shock: a conceptual model, *Circulation* 45:1097, 1972.

167. Honan MB, Harrell FE, Reimer KA, et al: Cardiac rupture, mortality and the timing of thrombolytic therapy: a meta-analysis, *J Am Coll Cardiol* 16:359-67, 1990.

168. Julian D, Chamberlain D, Sandoe E, et al: Mechanisms for the early mortality reduction produced by beta-blockade started early in acute myocardial infarction: ISIS-1, *Lancet* 2:921-24, 1988.

169. Mann J, Roberts WC: Rupture of the left ventricular free wall during acute myocardial infarction: analysis of 138 necropsy patients and comparison with 50 necropsy patients with acute myocardial infarction without rupture, *Am J Cardiol* 63:847-859, 1988.

170. Bolooki H: Surgical treatment of complications of acute myocardial infarction, JAMA, 263:1237-40, 1990.

171. Radford MS, Johnson RA, Daggett WM, et al: Ventricular septal rupture: a review of clinical and physiologic features and analysis of survival. *Circulation* 65:545, 1981.

172. Helmcke F, Mahan EF, Nanda NC, et al: Two-dimensional echocardiography and Doppler color flow mapping in the diagnosis and prognosis of ventricular septal rupture, *Circulation* 81:1775-1783, 1990.

173. Fox AC, Glassman E, Isom OW: Surgically remediable complications of myocardial infarction, *Prog Cardiovasc Dis* 21:461-484, 1979.

174. Coma-Camella I, Gamalo L, Onsurbe PM, et al: Anatomic findings in acute papillary muscle necrosis, *Am Heart J* 118:188, 1989.

174a. Schuster EH, Bulkley BH: Early postinfarction angina: ischemia at a distance and ischemia in the infarct zone, *N Engl J Med* 305:1101, 1981.

175. Muller JE, Rude RE, Braunwald E, et al: Myocardial infarct extension: occurrence, outcome, and risk factors in the multicenter investigation of limitation of infarct size, *Ann Intern Med* 108:1-6, 1988.

176. Hochman JS, Bulkley BH: Pathogenesis of left ventricular aneurysms: an experimental study in the rat model, *Am J Cardiol* 50:83-8, 1982.

177. Stratton JR, Lighty GW, Pearlman AS, et al: Detection of left ven-

tricular thrombus by two-dimensional echocardiography: sensitivity, specificity, and causes of uncertainty, *Circulation* 66:156-66, 1982.

178. Visser CA, Kon G, Meltzer RS, et al: Embolic potential of left ventricular thrombus after myocardial infarction: a two-dimensional echocardiographic study of 119 patients, *J Am Coll Cardiol* 5:1276, 1985.

179. Asinger RW, Mikell FL, Elspenger J, et al: Incidence of left-ventricular thrombosis after acute transmural myocardial infarction. Serial evaluation by two-dimensional echocardiography, *N Engl J Med* 305:297-302, 1981.

180. Eagle MA, Zabriskie JB, Senterfit LB, et al: Viral illness and the postpericardiotomy syndrome: A prospective study in children, *Circulation* 62:1151, 1980.

181. Thadani V, Chopra MP, Aber CP, et al: Pericarditis after acute myocardial infarction, *BMJ* 2:135, 1971.

182. Varnauskas E, European Coronary Surgery Study Group: Twelve-Year follow-up of survival in the randomized European Coronary Surgery Study, *N Engl J Med* 319:332-7, 1988.

183. Smith SH, Geer JC: Morphology of saphenous vein coronary artery bypass grafts seven to 116 months after surgery, *Arch Pathol Lab Med* 107:13-18, 1983.

184. Ratliff NB, Myles JL: Rapidly progressive atherosclerosis in aorto-coronary saphenous vein grafts, *Arch Pathol Lab Med* 113:772-76, 1989.

185. Leimgruder PP, Roubin GS, Hollman J, et al: Restenosis after successful coronary angioplasty in patients with single-vessel disease, *Circulation* 73:710-17, 1986.

186. Boudoulas H, Snyder GL, Lewis RP, et al: Safety and rationale for continuation of propranolol therapy during coronary bypass operation, *Ann Thorac Surg* 26:222-27, 1978.

187. Boudoulas H, Lewis RP, Vasko JS, et al: Left ventricular function and adrenergic hyperactivity before and after saphenous vein bypass, *Circulation* 55:802, 1976.

188. Fitzgibbon GM, Leach AJ, Kafka HP, et al: Coronary bypass graft fate: long-term angiographic study, *J Am Coll Cardiol* 17:1075-80, 1991.

188a. Hwang MH, Meadows WR, Palec RT et al: Progression of native coronary disease at 10 years; insights from a randomized study of medical versus surgical therapy for angina, *J Am Coll Cardiol* 16:1066, 1990.

189. Sahni R, Maniet AR, Voci G, et al: Prevention of restenosis by lovastatin after successful coronary angioplasty, *Am Heart J* 121:1600-7, 1991.

190. Hirshfeld JW, Schwartz S, Jugo R, et al: Restenosis after coronary angioplasty: a multivariate statistical model to relate lesion and procedure variables to restenosis, *J Am Coll Cardiol* 18:647-56, 1991.

191. Ellis SG, Roubin GS, King SB, et al: Angiographic and clinical predictors of acute closure after native vessel coronary angioplasty, *Circulation* 77:372-79, 1988.

192. Bredlau CE, Roubin GS, Leimgruder PP, et al: In hospital morbidity and mortality in patients undergoing elective coronary angioplasty, *Circulation* 72:1044-1052, 1985.

193. Karas SP, Santoian EC, Gravanis MB: Restenosis following coronary angioplasty, *Clin Cardiol* 14:791, 1991.

194. Gajdusek EM, Carbon S: Injury-induced release of basic fibroblast growth factor from bovine aortic endothelium, *J Cell Physiol* 134:570, 1989.

195. Powell JS, Clozel JP, Muller RK, et al: Inhibitors of angiotensin converting enzyme prevent myointimal proliferation after vascular injury, *Science* 245:186, 1989.

196. Gravanis MB, Roubin GS: Histopathologic phenomena at the site of percutaneous transluminal coronary angioplasty: The problem of restenosis, *Hum Pathol* 20:477-85, 1989.

197. Hwang MH, Meadows WR, Palec RT, et al: Progression of native coronary disease at 10 years: Insights from a randomized study of medical versus surgical therapy for angina, *J Am Coll Cardiol* 16:1066-70, 1990.

198. De Vreede JJM, Gorgels APM, Verstraaten GMP, et al: Did prognosis after acute myocardial infarction change during the past 30 years? A meta-analysis, *J Am Coll Cardiol* 18:698-706, 1991.

199. Fiebach NH, Viscoli CM, Horwitz RI: Differences between women and men in survival after myocardial infarction. Biology or Methodology? *JAMA* 263:1092-6, 1990.

200. Pekkanen J, Linn S, Heiss G, et al: Ten-year mortality from cardiovascular disease in relation to cholesterol level among men with and without preexisting cardiovascular disease, *N Engl J Med* 322:1700-7, 1990.

201. Wong ND, Wilson PWFF, Kannel WB. Serum cholesterol as a prognostic factor after myocardial infarction: The Framingham Study, *Ann Intern Med* 115:687-93, 1991.

202. Kane JP, Malloy MJ, Ports TA, et al: Regression of coronary atherosclerosis during treatment of familial hypercholesterolemia with combined drug regimens, JAMA 264:3007-12, 1990.

203. Boudoulas H: Therapeutic interventions which may improve survival in patients with coronary artery disease, *Acta Cardiol* 45:477-87, 1990.

Chapter 3

VALVULAR HEART DISEASE

Harisios Boudoulas
Michael B. Gravanis

Structural and/or functional abnormalities of the cardiac valves are referred to as valvular heart disease. This general term includes a number of entities, each one with its own pathophysiologic presentation and natural history.

Valvular heart disease, more than any other facet of medicine, has changed dramatically in the last 30 to 40 years. The recognition of several nonrheumatic causes of valvular disease, and the significant reduction in the incidence of acute rheumatic fever and its sequelae are apparently responsible for the dramatic shift in the pathogenesis and etiology of valvular disorders. One should be aware though, that statistics regarding etiology are substantially dependent upon whether the data were derived from surgically excised diseased valves or at postmortem.

Disruption in the anatomic integrity of a valve may result in either stenosis or regurgitation. In conditions of mixed valvular disease (combined stenosis and regurgitation), one hemodynamic setting predominates pathophysiologically. Morphologic changes in size or shape in a ventricle or great vessel may precipitate functional, and eventually structural, alterations in the valves.

In aortic and pulmonary stenosis, the respective ventricles are subjected to pressure overload, resulting in muscular hypertrophy while the chamber size remains normal or even reduced (concentric hypertrophy). In aortic and mitral regurgitation the left ventricular chamber is subjected to volume overload. The left ventricle dilates in order to maintain a normal stroke volume, but the wall thickness is only slightly increased (eccentric hypertrophy). Of the two adaptive mechanisms, volume overload is less energy-consuming and therefore is tolerated for longer periods. Several clinical entities are often associated with valvular heart disease. These entities as they relate to valvular abnormalities are briefly described in this section.

CLINICAL ENTITIES ASSOCIATED WITH VALVULAR HEART DISEASE
Acute rheumatic fever

The incidence of acute rheumatic fever has declined in the last 30 to 40 years.[1-2] Factors responsible for the decline of acute rheumatic fever and consequently rheumatic valvular disease include socioeconomic improvements in many parts of the world, better medical conditions, and the use of antibiotics. However, a decline in the incidence of rheumatic fever was noted in the United States and other countries before the use of antibiotics, suggesting changes either in host susceptibility or changes in the virulence of the organisms involved, or both[1] (Fig. 3-1).

Recently, outbreaks of cases of rheumatic fever were reported in several areas of the United States. These clusters were reported from Salt Lake City, northeastern Ohio, the tri-state border of western Pennsylvania, and the naval

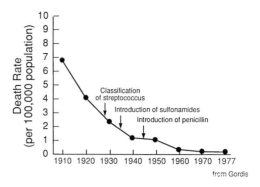

Fig. 3-1. Unadjusted rates of death due to rheumatic fever in the United States, 1910 through 1977. (Reprinted from Gordis L: The virtual disappearance of rheumatic fever in the United States; Lessons in the rise and fall of disease, *Circulation* 72:1155, 1985.)

training center in San Diego, California. In those reports the patients were usually white, middle class, and from nonurban areas.[3-5] Perhaps these outbreaks result from genetic predisposition of certain segments of the population, or the emergence of strains of group A streptococcus more likely to produce rheumatic fever.

Pathogenesis. It is widely accepted that changes in the biologic properties and particularly the virulence of streptococcal strains influence their potential to produce rheumatic fever. Indeed, M serotypes known to be highly virulent and commonly associated with acute rheumatic fever in the past were rarely isolated in the 1970s and 1980s, during which the incidence of acute rheumatic fever has declined. Group A streptococci can be classified into more than 70 nosologic types on the basis of M-protein, an antigen present in the cell surface. Its virulence is attributed primarily to its ability to form a capsule that protects the organism from phagocytosis, and to produce M-protein. Hemolysins S and O also contribute to the pathogenicity of group A streptococci by injuring the membrane of host cells and causing lysis of cytoplasmic granules.[6-12]

Many investigators have suggested that equally important are changes in patterns of host immunity to specific M serotypes. Thus the search for genetic markers of susceptibility to acute rheumatic fever has revealed an association between certain HLA class II antigens. A recent report from Brazil, which has a relatively high incidence of acute rheumatic fever, indicated that HLA-DR7 and HLA-DRw53 are markers for susceptibility to rheumatic fever.[6-7]

Rheumatic fever is a disease of the young (6 to 15 years old) but it may occur in adulthood.[9] It occurs as a delay sequela of pharyngeal infection with group A streptococci, but there is no antecedent streptococcal infection in about one-third of the patients. Rheumatic fever may affect the heart, joints, central nervous system, skin and subcutaneous tissues. The clinical presentation includes migratory arthritis, fever, subcutaneous nodules, erythema marginatum (a nonpruritic rash with sharp erythematous borders), chorea, and carditis.

Both humoral and cell-mediated immunologic responses are involved in acute rheumatic fever. Antigens in the cell membrane of the group A streptococcus share common antigenic determinants with the heart, as well as with other tissues in the body. The M-proteins are the most significant bacterial surface antigens. However, what are the actual specific cross reactive antigens in the heart is still unknown, although it is suspected that myosin, sarcolemma,

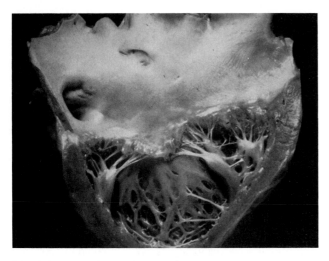

Fig. 3-2. Acute rheumatic valvulitis, mitral valve. Small verrucae are present along the line of closure of the leaflets.

and vascular intimal structures are probably involved in this cross reactivity. Two monoclonal antibodies against streptococci are specific for skeletal muscle and/or cardiac myosin and for some fragments of the myosin molecule.[12a]

Histopathology. Early myocardial lesions of acute rheumatic carditis are characterized by edema of the ground substance, fragmentation of collagen fibers, fibrinoid necrosis and reactive cellular infiltration. The diffuse cellular infiltrate is mostly composed of lymphocytes, polymorphonuclear leukocytes, histiocytes, and occasional eosinophils. It is believed that this interstitial myocarditis plays an important role during the acute phase of rheumatic carditis and may lead to heart failure. These changes may involve myocardial fibers that reveal degeneration and even actual necrosis. This phase of the exudative inflammatory process usually lasts 2 to 3 weeks, after which the most characteristic lesion of rheumatic carditis develops, namely the Aschoff nodule[7,13] (Figs. 3-2, 3-3).

The pathognomonic histologic lesion in rheumatic carditis is the Aschoff body, which is found most often in the interstitium of the myocardium, but occasionally seen in the endocardium and the valves. The Aschoff body is variable in size and may be round or elongated. It consists of a collection of large ill-defined cells with pink cytoplasm and prominent vesicular nuclei.[8] Some lymphocytes and plasma cells are also present. The Aschoff nodule may or may not have a central core of fibrinoid necrosis. The average measurement of an Aschoff body is 40×80 μ. Aschoff bodies often have been found in the auricular appendages of hearts with old rheumatic stigmata. Those Aschoff bodies are not considered to be indicative of continued rheumatic activity. The histogenesis of the Aschoff body has been controversial. Data suggest that the Aschoff

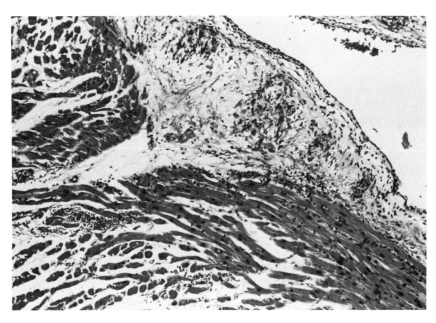

Fig. 3-3. Subendocardial Aschoff bodies.

and Anitschkow cells making up the Aschoff bodies are derived from histiocytes, although some cells may arise from blood monocytes. A relationship between myocardial Aschoff bodies and subcutaneous nodules of rheumatic fever has been suggested because both appear to have a histiocytic origin.[6-13]

During the acute phase of rheumatic carditis, the valves, particularly the left-sided ones, appear edematous and inflamed, and reveal a row of tiny verrucae 1 to 2 mm in diameter along the lines of closure (Figs. 3-4, 3-5). These verrucae are made up of platelets and fibrin and are usually attached to areas of necrosis of the underlying valve substance. At the base and edges of the valve leaflets, histiocytic cells line up and palisade at right angles to the base of the leaflet. Some of those histiocytic cells have elongated nuclei reminiscent of the Anitschkow cell. As the lesions progress, granulation tissue develops and progressive fibrosis takes place. Similar to the involvement of the valves, a lesion in the posterior wall of the left atrium is often seen in acute rheumatic fever, which in its healed stage reveals a thick, wrinkled and fibrotic endocardium known as MacCallum's patch.

The clinical presentation of acute valvulitis of the mitral valve is mitral regurgitation. The mechanism of mitral insufficiency in acute rheumatic fever is poorly defined. A study of 73 patients (age 7 to 27) with mitral regurgitation and active rheumatic carditis has been reported by Marcus, et al.[14] In this report, histologic findings from the involved valve removed at surgery revealed areas of fibrinoid necrosis in valve leaflets or annular tissues, polymorphonuclear leukocyte infiltrates, histiocytes and neovascularization of leaflets. According to these authors, rheumatic inflamma-

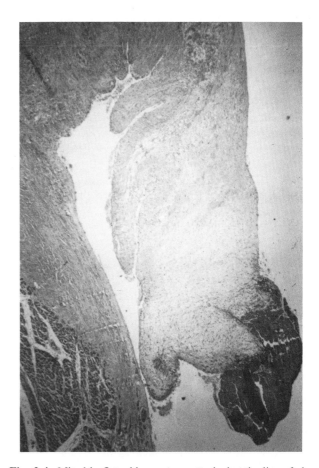

Fig. 3-4. Mitral leaflet with a verruca attached at the line of closure. Note the marked thickening of the leaflet due to inflammatory edema.

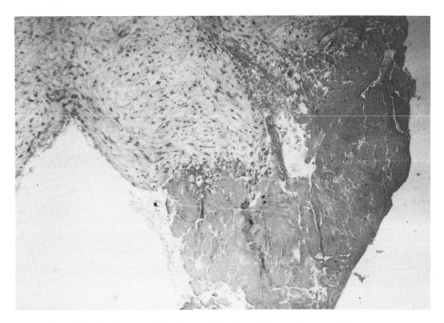

Fig. 3-5. Higher magnification at the site of the attachment of the verruca.

tion involves the connective tissue of the mitral valve apparatus (annulus, leaflets, and chordae). The inflammatory process of the annulus results in its dilatation, whereas increased tension on the chordae causes their elongation. These two changes, plus the inflammation of the leaflets, leads to anterior leaflet prolapse and mitral regurgitation. Perhaps the left atrial enlargement further aggravates the regurgitation.

Inflammation of the coronary arteries, particularly the intermyocardial ones, may also be an important factor in producing permanent myocardial injury. Thrombosis of large coronary arteries, however, is seldom seen in acute rheumatic carditis.

Seronegative spondylarthropathies

Entities such as ankylosing spondylitis, Reiter disease, psoriatic arthropathy, arthritis of inflammatory bowel disease, Whipple disease, and Behçet's disease are all grouped under the term seronegative spondyloarthropathies. They are characterized by absence of rheumatoid factor and the presence of HLA-B27. However, the precise role of the HLA-B27 antigen in the pathogenesis of the spondylarthropathies is not clear. Some investigators have suggested a pathogenetic mechanism based on an unknown antigen's molecular mimicry of the B27 antigen as the cause of the chronic inflammatory process.[15]

Ankylosing spondylitis. Valvular lesions described in this entity result from aortic regurgitation, aortic regurgitation and stenosis, and mitral regurgitation. Mitral valve regurgitation in ankylosing spondylitis is rather rare and has been attributed to a protrusion created by the extension of the fibrosis of the adventitia of the proximal aorta into the subaortic area adjacent to the base of the anterior mitral leaflet. However, another possible mechanism for the mitral regurgitation is the ventricular enlargement secondary to the aortic regurgitation.[16-18]

In the active phase of aortitis of ankylosing spondylitis, there is an endarteritis obliterans of small adventitial vessels which reveal perivascular cuffing by lymphocytes and plasma cells. The resulting fibrosis in the adventitia and media involves primarily the aorta behind the sinuses of Valsalva. Intimal fibrosis may extend over the coronary ostia. Grossly, the intima of the proximal aorta appears thickened and wrinkled and has gross similarities to intimal "tree barking" seen in syphilitic aortitis. The aortic ring is dilated; the cusps appear thickened at the base and at the free margins, where they appear to be somewhat rolled and inverted. The most significant morphologic changes are encountered in the proximal 3 cm to 4 cm of the aorta. Marked fibrosis and collagenization of the adventitia is seen extending into the groove between the anterior mitral leaflet and the aortic cusps, producing a fibrous ridge. Impingement of this fibrous process on the conduction system is not uncommon. The extent of the aortitis is variable. In some cases, the aorta may be alto-

gether spared, and the only morphologic changes are seen in the vicinity of the central fibrous body and the conduction system. There are some atypical cases of ankylosing spondylitis in which the disease may present as aortic arch syndrome, i.e., with one or more major branches of the aorta being partially or totally obstructed at their origins.

Although functional abnormalities of the myocardium have been described, the histopathologic findings in the myocardium of patients with ankylosing spondylitis are usually nonspecific and often minimal. Rarely, pericarditis, often adhesive but without clinical significance, is known to occur in ankylosing spondylitis. Some inflammatory cells may be present in the vicinity of the central fibrous body and the atrioventricular node. Another finding has been diffuse increase in myocardial interstitial connective tissue in some cases of ankylosing spondylitis. These changes may lead to atrioventricular block and other cardiac arrhythmias.

Heritable disorders of connective tissue origin

Connective tissue abnormalities are of etiologic importance in a broad spectrum of cardiovascular disorders. Marfan syndrome and Ehlers-Danlos syndrome, well-recognized heritable disorders of connective tissue, represent accepted examples of this association. It has also become apparent that there are many isolated cardiovascular abnormalities of connective tissue origin that do not fit within the currently recognized heritable connective tissue syndromes. Such isolated connective tissue abnormalities include isolated and combined valvular prolapse, annuloaortic ectasia, certain forms of isolated aortic regurgitation, and pulmonary artery dilatation[19-20] (see Box on p. 69).

Recognized heritable connective tissue syndromes with cardiovascular involvement

Marfan syndrome. Marfan syndrome is a heritable disorder of connective tissue with well-defined ocular, skeletal, and cardiovascular abnormalities. Although the precise biochemical defect is unknown, there is evidence that defective collagen crosslinking contributes to tissue weakness in Marfan syndrome. Abnormalities in elastin content and elastin cross-linking in aortic tissue have also been found. Recently, immunohistochemical studies have revealed that fibrillin, a connective tissue glycoprotein present in elastic tissue and periosteum, may be defective or deficient in cases of Marfan syndrome. A de novo missense mutation in the fibrillin gene (chromosome 15) in patients with sporadic Marfan syndrome has also been recently reported.[21-22]

Although inheritance is autosomal dominant, variability in penetrance leads to a wide spectrum of clinical expression, even within a given family. First-degree relatives of patients with Marfan syndrome have been found to have isolated cardiovascular involvement, with mitral valve pro-

---

Heritable connective tissue disorders* with cardiovascular involvement

Recognized syndromes	*Isolated abnormalities*
Marfan syndrome	Isolated valvular prolapse
Ehlers-Danlos syndrome	Combined valvular prolapse
Stickler syndrome	Annuloaortic ectasia
Adult polycystic kidney disease	Pulmonary artery aneurysm
Homocystinuria	
Osteogenesis imperfecta	
Pseudoxanthoma elasticum	
Mucopolysaccharidoses	

*From Bowen, et al: Cardiovascular disease of connective tissue origin, *Am J Med* 82:481, 1987.

---

lapse or aortic root dilatation, even in the absence of diagnostic features of the full syndrome. Ectopia lentis and myopia are related to laxity of the zonulas and increased axial globe length due to weakness of connective tissue. Skeletal manifestations include arachnodactyly, increased height, dolichostenomelia (long limbs relative to trunk), and thoracic skeletal deformities.[23]

Cardiovascular lesions include mitral, aortic, and tricuspid regurgitation, aortic root dilatation, and proximal aortic dissection. The severity of the cardiovascular lesions influences prognosis, and life expectancy is greatly reduced. The risk of aortic dissection during pregnancy appears to be greatest in patients with a dilated aortic root.

Ehlers-Danlos syndrome. Ehlers-Danlos syndrome refers to a group of disorders of collagen metabolism that share certain phenotypic expressions. At least nine separate types have been described to date, with cutaneous hyperextensibility, easy bruisability, and extreme tissue fragility as the most distinctive features. Inheritance of most of the Ehlers-Danlos types is autosomal dominant. X-linked forms of inheritance are also known to occur.[24] Cardiovascular aspects have been best described for type I (gravis form), type III (benign familial hypermobility syndrome), and type IV (ecchymotic or arterial form). Mitral valve prolapse, and enlargement of the aortic root or sinus of Valsalva are common abnormalities in patients with Ehlers-Danlos syndrome. Congenital defects, such as bicuspid aortic valve, atrial septal defect, and ventricular septal defect have also been described.

Stickler syndrome (hereditary arthroophthalmopathy). This is one of the most common of the hereditary disorders of connective tissue and is notably pleiotropic. The ocular features have been called Wagner syndrome by ophthalmologists. Preliminary evidence from studies of linkage between the Stickler phenotype and restriction site polymorphisms on candidate gene probes suggests that the basic defect lies in type II collagen. The skeletal features

are quite variable, and may be detectable only, or more reliably, by radiography.[20] Mild epiphyseal dysplasia produces prominence of large joints, generalized arthropathy, and precocious degenerative changes. The habitus is often slender and the joints hyperextensible, both reminiscent of Marfan syndrome. The facies may be characteristic, with hypognathism and a depressed midface. The only cardiovascular abnormality documented is mitral valve prolapse.

Adult polycystic kidney disease. The association between adult polycystic kidney disease and cardiovascular disease of connective tissue origin has been recognized for the last decade.[25] Patients have enlargement of the aortic root and mitral valvular regurgitation. Myxomatous degeneration with loss and disruption of collagen was found during histologic studies of aortic and mitral valvular tissue. The cardiac lesions could not be explained on any other etiologic basis such as systemic hypertension.

Homocystinuria. Homocystinuria is a disorder of methionine metabolism in which cystathionine synthetase activity is decreased.[19-20] Accumulation of homocysteine is thought to interfere with collagen crosslinking. The phenotype is similar to that of Marfan syndrome, with lens displacement and arachnodactyly. However, there is a marked thrombotic tendency, and arterial and venous thromboembolism are the dominant clinical cardiovascular features.

Osteogenesis imperfecta. Osteogenesis imperfecta is a generalized connective tissue disorder with cardiovascular manifestations. Six syndromes are recognized, with varying patterns of inheritance.[19-20] Fragile, brittle bones lead to pronounced skeletal deformities caused by repeated fractures and the stress of weight-bearing. Cardiovascular lesions are similar to those in cases of Marfan syndrome, with aortic regurgitation, aortic aneurysm, and valvular lesions occurring commonly.

Pseudoxanthoma elasticum. Pseudoxanthoma elasticum is a rare autosomal recessive disease with cardiovascular, eye, and skin manifestations.[19-20] There is a characteristic endocardial lesion with initial fibroelastic thickening and fragmentation of elastin fibers in deeper endocardial layers. Similar changes are seen in the elastic fibers of arteries. Clinical events include premature peripheral vascular and coronary occlusive disease.

The mucopolysaccharidoses. The mucopolysaccharidoses are a group of inherited metabolic disorders in which deficiency of lysosomal enzymes leads to intracellular accumulation of mucopolysaccharides (glycosaminoglycans) in many organs. In Hurler syndrome (the most completely studied example), the deficient enzyme is alpha-L-iduronidase.[19-20] Clinical features of Hurler syndrome include hepatosplenomegaly, skeletal deformities, and mental retardation. Glycosaminoglycan deposition occurs in cardiac valves, coronary arteries, and myocardium. Clinical expression may occur as aortic or mitral regurgitation, mitral stenosis, myocardial ischemia, or congestive heart failure.

Isolated cardiovascular connective tissue abnormalities[19]

Isolated valvular prolapse. The largest group of patients with connective tissue abnormalities of the cardiovascular system appears to be those with mitral valve prolapse (see mitral regurgitation, later in this chapter).

Combined valvular prolapse. The widespread use of echocardiography and Doppler echocardiography in the past decade has resulted in the increased recognition of valvular prolapse either as an isolated event or in combinations.[19] Coexisting aortic valve prolapse in patients with mitral valve prolapse, combined aortic, tricuspid, and mitral prolapse have been well documented.

Isolated aortic valvular regurgitation. Isolated aortic valvular regurgitation is frequently related to a disorder of connective tissue as the primary process. In the past, rheumatic heart disease and luetic aortitis were accepted as common causes of isolated aortic regurgitation. As these disorders became less frequent, other causes of aortic regurgitation were recognized.[19-20]

Annuloaortic ectasia. *Annuloaortic ectasia* is the term used to describe aneurysmal dilatation of the aortic annulus and ascending thoracic aorta in patients with pathologic evidence of cystic medial necrosis without evidence of connective tissue disease in other organ systems. Aortic regurgitation is usually present. Dissection is a common complication and cannot be predicted reliably from the size or configuration of the proximal aortic enlargement.[19-20]

Pulmonary artery aneurysm. Pulmonary artery aneurysm is a cardiovascular abnormality in which primary connective tissue disease may play a role.

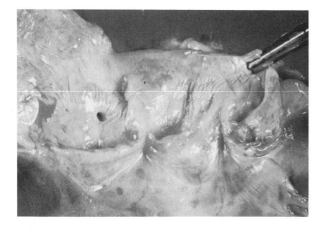

Fig. 3-6. Aortic valve and proximal aorta from a patient with tertiary syphilis. The cusps are thick and the free edges rolled, and the commissures are widened. The coronary ostia appear high above the sinuses (cuspal retraction) and the aortic intima reveals "tree barking."

Cardiovascular syphilis

Despite extensive public health educational efforts and effective antibiotic treatment, cases of cardiovascular syphilis still occur. If, according to the data from Centers for Disease Control, early syphilis is indeed increasing, then a parallel increase in cardiovascular syphilis is to be expected. Furthermore, according to many reports, the natural history of syphilis may be changing in the setting of HIV infection.[26-27]

Aortitis, which is a tertiary form of syphilis, occurs in 70% to 80% of patients with untreated syphilis. The treponemas lodge within the nutrient blood vessels (vasa vasorum) of the aortic adventitia and initiate the inflammatory process. Cuffing by plasma cells and lymphocytes leads to obliterative changes in those vasa vasorum, resulting in necrosis in the media, destruction of the elastic fibers, and finally scarring. Reactive intimal thickening which creates the so-called "tree barking" is usually present. All the above changes alter the elastic properties and strength of the aortic wall, leading to aortic root dilatation or aneurysm formation. Cardiovascular syphilis may present as aortic regurgitation, coronary ostial stenosis or aortic aneurysm (Fig. 3-6).

Aortic regurgitation is the most common complication of syphilitic aortitis and presents usually in the second or third decade after the infection and has a poor prognosis. About 20% of those patients may also have coronary ostial stenosis, but saccular aneurysms are rarely associated with aortic regurgitation. Coronary ostial stenosis is the second most common complication of syphilitic aortitis.

Syphilitic aortic aneurysms are the least common manifestation of aortitis. These aneurysms are usually saccular, rarely fusiform, and approximately 50% occur in the ascending aortic arch. When sizeable, they may compress the superior vena cava, right bronchus, and right pulmonary artery. Rupture of an aneurysm most often occurs into the pericardium. However, rupture into the right bronchus, right pleura, esophagus, mediastinum, or through the anterior chest wall may also occur. About 30% to 35% of the aneurysms occur in the transverse arch and are associated with hoarseness (involvement of recurrent laryngeal nerve) or dysphagia. Aneurysms in the descending arch (10% to 15% of the cases) occur in the proximity of the esophagus, vertebral column, and left bronchus. Infrequently (5%), aneurysms may occur in the abdominal aorta.

Gummatous myocarditis is rare. It may present with conduction abnormalities or myocardial infarction. The base of the interventricular septum is the most common location of gummata. A diffuse gummatous myocarditis is extremely rare.

Endocarditis

Nonbacterial thrombotic endocarditis (NBTE). Nonbacterial thrombotic endocarditis, also known as marantic endocarditis, is a verrucous valvular lesion seen in association with a wide spectrum of diseases. Although reports of echocardiographic recognition of NBTE have become more frequent, the great majority of cases are discovered only at autopsy. Statistics derived from postmortem studies give an incidence ranging from 0.3% to 9.3%. The prevalence of NBTE is often underestimated because of inadequate pathologic evaluation. Males and females are affected in approximately equal numbers, and patients are usually in their fourth to eighth decade.

A large study of consecutive autopsies has shown that three fourths of the cases of NBTE were associated with malignant neoplasms, more than half of which were adenocarcinomas. NBTE has also been observed in patients with disseminated intravascular coagulation (rapidly decreased platelet count, rising prothrombin time, hypofibrinogenemia) as may occur in severe infections or other fulminant disease, such as burns. NBTE may be responsible for cerebral and other embolic events.

Autoimmune diseases such as systemic lupus erythematosus or chronic rheumatic heart disease have also been associated with NBTE. Rare cases of NBTE associated with endocardial fibroelastosis, dehydration, chronic glomerulonephritis and aplastic anemia have also been reported. More recently, acquired immunodeficiency syndrome and bone marrow transplantation have emerged as predisposing conditions. NBTE involving the pulmonary valve has been attributed to cardiac catheterization.[28-30]

The symptoms and signs attributed to NBTE are not pathognomonic for the entity; therefore an antemortem diagnosis, even with echocardiography, may not be easy. The presence of a murmur in the setting of malignancy or disseminated intravascular coagulation may be highly suggestive of NBTE. Systemic emboli occur in approximately half of the patients with NBTE. Common sites are the kidneys, spleen, brain, and mesenteric circulations. These findings as well as serial negative blood cultures could be helpful in the antemortem diagnosis of NBTE.[31-32]

Morphologic features. Although all valves may be involved by NBTE, the mitral and aortic valves are the most frequently affected. The characteristic lesions of NBTE are small verrucae, usually less than 3 mm in largest diameter, attached on the atrial surfaces of the mitral and tricuspid valves and the ventricular surfaces of the semilunar valves. Larger vegetations (4 × 2 × 2 cm) have been occasionally described. The lesions are attached to normal valve tissue, are composed of fibrin and platelets, and reveal absence of inflammatory reaction or organization, although older lesions may reendothelialize and have fibroblastic proliferation and fibrosis at their base (Figs. 3-7 and 3-8).[32]

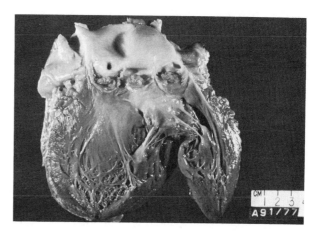

Fig. 3-7. Thrombotic nonbacterial endocarditis involving all three aortic cusps in a patient with sepsis and disseminated intravascular coagulation (DIC).

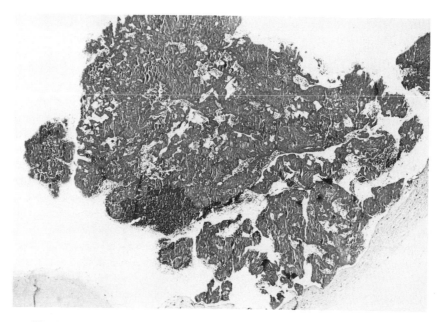

Fig. 3-8. Aortic cusp with attached thrombus composed of fibrin and platelets.

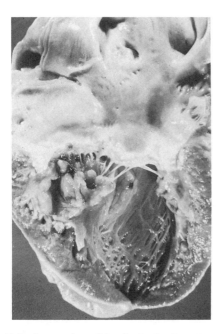

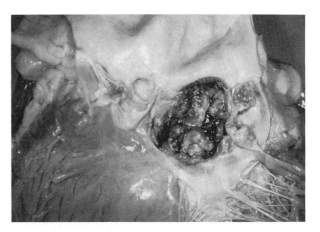

Fig. 3-10. Infectious endocarditis of aortic valve with ring abscess formation. Note extension of vegetations into the undersurface of the anterior mitral leaflet.

Fig. 3-9. Infectious endocarditis of mitral valve. Note extension of vegetations to the chordae.

Pathogenesis. Several hypotheses have been advanced regarding the pathogenesis of NBTE. Although some hypotheses are of rather general nature, such as "nonspecific cardiac stress" or "valvular deformation," most investigators speculate that lesion formation requires a deranged valvular surface, the nature of which may be recent or old.

Immunologic mechanisms have been implicated as immunoglobulin and complement deposition were demonstrated at the base of NBTE lesions. Similar mechanisms may explain the link between malignancy (particularly adenocarcinomas) and NBTE because antibodies are present against mucin-secreting tumors, suggesting the formation of circulating immune complexes. It is also possible that tumor mucin induces a hypercoagulable state resulting in NBTE. Moreover, malignant cells are known to produce a procoagulant state that may contribute to pathogenesis of NBTE.[33-35]

Infectious endocarditis. Infectious endocarditis may affect any of the cardiac valves and usually occurs in patients with underlying valvular or congenital heart disease. Infectious endocarditis usually produces acute valvular regurgitation.

In the elderly, infectious endocarditis is often associated with degenerative heart disease, such as mitral annular calcification. Iatrogenic causes of infective endocarditis (e.g., open heart surgery) account for 1% to 2% of all cases of infectious endocarditis. Mechanical prostheses are more often infected in the early postoperative period. The incidence of infectious endocarditis in aortic valve prostheses is higher than in mitral prostheses.

Transient bacteremias secondary to manipulative procedures such as tooth extractions, bladder or ureter catheterizations, and venous catheterizations are often the cause of infective endocarditis. However, in a number of cases, there is no apparent cause for the development of endocarditis. Whereas in the past, Streptococcus viridans was the most common invader in the heart (preantibiotic era), *Staphylococcus* is currently responsible for approximately 33% of all cases of infectious endocarditis, *Streptococcus* for 24%, *Pseudomonas* for 14%, *Klebsiella* for 5%, *Serratia* for 5%, and *Escherichia coli,* Neisseria, and Proteus for 1% each. While gram-negative bacteria are less commonly the offending organisms, they are recognized as frequent causes of infectious endocarditis among intravenous drug users and diabetics. *Candida* and *Aspergillus* are the two most commonly involved fungi causing infectious endocarditis. Both of these fungi may produce significant valvular damage and may result in serious complications because of their bulky friable vegetations, which are prone to embolization. Immunocompromised patients, as well as those receiving chemotherapy and drug addicts are prone to develop fungal endocarditis.[36-46]

Turbulence of jet lesions induced by different causes may damage the ventricular or valvular endocardium, resulting in deposition of fibrin and platelets at those sites. Quite often, this microthrombus will lyse as a result of the fibrolytic mechanisms, or may become infected in the presence of bacteremia. Virulent organisms, however, have the ability to initiate an infectious process in previously normal tissues, including cardiac valves. Infectious vegetations on incompetent valves are localized at the atrial side of the mitral valve.

Both leaflets of the mitral valve may be involved, and although the infection may occur on a previously normal valve, it is most often seen in valves damaged by either rheumatic disease or patients with mitral valve prolapse (floppy valves) (Figs. 3-9 and 3-10). The anterior leaflet

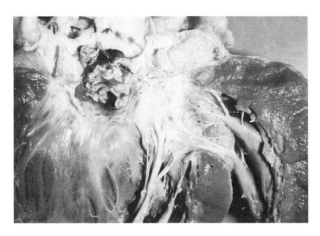

Fig. 3-11. Aortic ring abscess secondary to infectious endocarditis. Note aortotomy from a failed attempt at valve replacement.

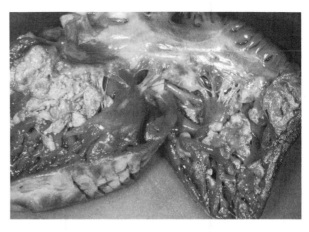

Fig. 3-12. Infectious endocarditis of tricuspid valve with extension into ventricular endocardium in drug addict (pseudomonas).

may be chronically damaged by regurgitant jet lesions such as those produced by aortic incompetence, or may be involved by direct spread from an aortic endocarditis. Similarly, infectious endocarditis high up in the ventricular aspect of the anterior leaflet may spread beneath the aortic cusps and create an infective aneurysm.

The extent of valvular destruction in infectious endocarditis clearly depends on the virulence of the organism involved and the resistance of the host. Flat solid vegetations with more fibrosis and less destruction are seen in less virulent organisms. Vegetations in atrioventricular valves are seen along the line of closure and may extend along the chordae and mural endocardium. These vegetations usually vary in size, are reddish-yellow or gray depending on the stage of organization, are friable and easily embolized (Figs. 3-11 and 3-12). Vegetations are usually made up of platelets, fibrin, polymorphonuclear leukocytes, and colonies of bacteria or fungi. Similar inflammatory phenomena are also seen within the valve substance itself. Healing in endocarditis is manifested by palisading histiocytic mononuclear cells at the base of the vegetation along with foci of lymphocytes. Calcification may be seen in healing infectious endocarditis.

Other causes of valvular heart disease

Several other disease states, such as congenital heart disease, ischemic heart disease and cardiomyopathies, may also result in valvular heart disease. These entities will be described in detail with the valvular abnormalities they produce, in other chapters of the book.

MITRAL VALVE
Anatomy/pathology

Although the two atrioventricular valves are anatomically dissimilar, they have the same modus operandi. Both valves have an annulus on which the base of the leaflets is

attached.[47] The free edges of the leaflets are tethered to the papillary muscles by delicate chordae tendineae. Herniation of the leaflets into the atrium when ventricular pressure rises is prevented by the tense chordae tendineae. However, as the left ventricle is rapidly changing its size, the chordal tension can be maintained only by continuous adjustment of the papillary muscle contraction. Thus the role of the papillary muscles in the functional integrity of the mitral valve is an important one. Chordae of the two mitral leaflets are supplied by both anterolateral and posteromedial papillary muscles. The axes of both papillary muscles runs parallel to the axis of the left ventricular cavity. Ventricular dilatation alters this axis (lateral displacement), and therefore affects the closing of the mitral valve. A prime example of mitral regurgitation secondary to ventricular dilatation is seen in dilated cardiomyopathy.

The floor of the left atrium is made in its greatest portion by the anterior mitral valve leaflet. The valve area of the posterior leaflet is somewhat smaller than that of the anterior, but its attachment to the ring is longer. This arrangement gives the posterior leaflet a crescent shape. There is an important relationship between the anterior mitral leaflet and the outflow tract of the left ventricle. During diastole, the anterior mitral leaflet forms the lateral aspect of the left ventricular outflow tract. This integral association exposes the anterior leaflet to injuries from hemodynamic or morphologic changes in that region. An excellent example of the consequences of this intimate relationship is seen in hypertrophic cardiomyopathy. In this condition the anterior leaflet becomes fibrotic and retracted as a result of systolic anterior motion leading to mitral regurgitation.

The mitral annulus (ring) is one important component of the mitral valve complex. In addition to anchoring the leaflets, it also electrically insulates the atria from the ventricles. The normal mitral valve area in the adult ranges from 4 cm ^{2} to 6 cm^2. In individuals fifty years of age or older, age-related changes in the mitral valve are not uncommon. The leaflets may appear thick and less translucent and reveal lipid deposits on their ventricular surface, particularly in the anterior leaflet. Nodular thickening along the line of closure of both leaflets and/or billowing and hooding of the free edges between chordae insertions is seen in the posterior leaflet in elderly individuals. These morphologic changes are interpreted as wear and tear phenomena, but have no hemodynamic effects.

Calcification of the mitral annulus is another age-related phenomenon. This can occur after the age of 50, but is most common after the age of 70, particularly in women. The calcification occurs at the angle between the ventricular endocardium and the base of the posterior leaflet; when it is nodular it may push the leaflet upwards or it may coalesce with aortic ring calcification. Ulcerated calcified nodules may become the site of endocarditis. Metaplastic bone and/or cartilage may develop at the area of the calcification. Occasionally, giant cells are noted at the periphery of the calcium deposits. Extension of the calcification process into the ventricular septum may create conduction defects. Calcification of the mitral annulus may produce interference with its sphincteric function and mitral regurgitation.[47-49]

MITRAL STENOSIS
Etiology

Mitral stenosis may result from a number of etiologies, such as congenital, infective endocarditis, and metabolic. However, all of these different etiologies account only for a small proportion of mitral stenosis. The etiology is chronic rheumatic valvular disease in the overwhelming number of cases. In certain cases rare conditions may mimic mitral stenosis.[50-51]

Rheumatic mitral stenosis

The chronic sequelae of acute rheumatic fever appear years after the acute episode. The time of the appearance of chronic valvular disease is related to the age of the development of acute rheumatic fever and to the recurrences of the acute episodes. The earlier in life the rheumatic fever attacks, the more frequent the recurrences and the earlier the appearance of the chronic valvular sequelae. What exactly happens in the interim is not absolutely clear. It seems unlikely, however, that a smoldering subclinical valvulitis is present during the latent period. It is more possible that the damage to the valvular apparatus is caused by continuous fibrin deposition on the damaged valve leaflets and chordae tendineae, followed by endothelialization of such deposits, and resulting in thickening and fibrosis. Therefore it is this process that seems to be responsible for the fusion of the commissures, fibrosis, and retraction of the leaflets and chordae. One should keep in mind, however, that the histologic findings in the mitral

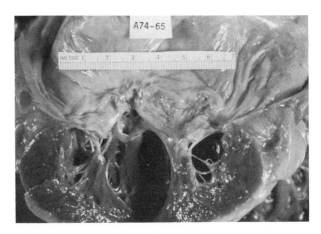

Fig. 3-13. Mitral stenosis of rheumatic etiology. Note fusion of commissures and chordae and atrial dilatation.

valve secondary to past rheumatic disease are not pathognomonic. Vascularization of the valvular leaflets, along with a few chronic inflammatory cells and occasional Anitschkow cells, is often seen in surgically excised valves or at postmortem in conditions other than old rheumatic valvulitis.[50-51]

Morphology and pathology. The morphologic features characterizing mitral stenosis vary from patient to patient; subtypes of morphologic variants of mitral stenosis have been recognized. All valve components may be potentially involved in mitral stenosis, although in a different degree and in a variety of combinations. Therefore, fusion of the commissures (perhaps the most important factor), fibrosis and rigidity of leaflets (particularly when heavy calcification is present) and thickening, retraction and fusion of chordae are all seen in the rheumatic etiology of mitral stenosis. It appears that mitral stenosis in the younger patient is characterized by more prominent commissural fusion and less leaflet fibrosis and calcification. The distribution of calcium varies according to the localization and amount. It may have a linear distribution along the lines of closure of the valve or it may present as nodular masses, particularly at the commissures. The latter arrangement may lead to ulceration of the calcific masses with subsequent thrombosis at that site. Chordae may be thick and retracted (papillary muscles reaching to the edge of leaflet) and when fused may form a fibrous tunnel below the leaflets (Fig. 3-13). Heavy calcification is more common in men than women, in older persons than in young, and is heavier in people in Western countries than in underdeveloped countries.[47,50]

Physical properties. Certain fundamental differences in physical properties exist between the normal mitral valve and the stenotic mitral valve, and between the noncalcific stenotic valve and the calcific stenotic mitral valve. There is a significant and progressive increase in weight from normal mitral valves to stenotic noncalcific valves, and

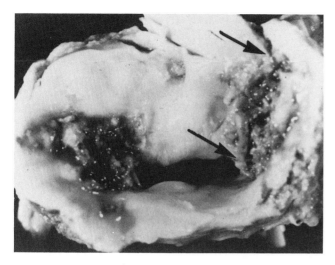

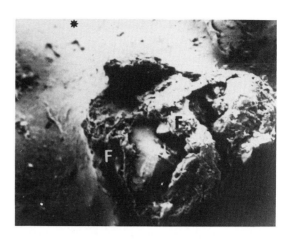

Fig. 3-14. Calcific mitral stenosis, surface morphology. Gross appearance of a calcified and ulcerated mitral valve that has been surgically resected. The anterolateral commissure (on the left) shows a gross thrombus over an ulcer. The posteromedial commissure (on the right) shows an ulcer formed by eruption of a calcific mass through the surface endothelium. This ulcer is free of gross thrombus. Arrows show the extent of calcification and ulceration. ($\times$ 2.5) (From Wooley CF, Sparks EA and Boudoulas H: *Mitral stenosis: The anatomic lesion and the physiologic state.* In Bashore TM, Davidson CJ, eds: *Percutaneous balloon valvuloplasty and related techniques,* Baltimore, 1991, Williams & Wilkins.)

Fig. 3-15. Calcific mitral stenosis, surface morphology. Scanning electron micrograph of an ulcer. Intact nonulcerated endothelial surface appears smooth as marked by asterisk (*). The jagged border of an irregularly shaped surface ulcer is shown. The ulcer base is covered with fibrin (**F**). ($\times$ 30). (From Wooley CF, Sparks EA and Boudoulas H: *Mitral stenosis: The anatomic lesion and the physiologic state.* In Bashore TM, Davidson CJ, eds: *Percutaneous balloon valvuloplasty and related techniques,* Baltimore, 1991, Williams & Wilkins.)

from stenotic noncalcific valves to stenotic valves with advanced calcification. Similarly, there are progressive increases in volume, specific gravity, and weight, from normal to stenotic noncalcific valves and from stenotic noncalcific to calcific valves. The mitral valve area is also decreased from normal to stenotic noncalcific valves, and from stenotic noncalcific valves to stenotic calcific valves.[50]

Thrombotic calcific mitral stenosis. The most striking difference in calcific stenotic mitral valves involves surface morphology (Fig. 3-14). Surface ulceration is due to eruption of underlying calcific focus through the valvular endothelium (Fig. 3-15). Thrombus formation in the area of ulceration may be associated with arterial embolization. Whisker formation (filamentous stalks along the line of valve closure) is also present. The moderately-to-heavily calcified stenotic mitral valve also has a small fixed mitral valve orifice.[50]

The calcific stenotic mitral valves influence clinical expression in various ways. The obvious clinical implications include alterations in valve mobility and mobility-related phenomena such as intensity and presence of the mitral component of the first heart sound and mitral opening snap at auscultation. More severe obstruction with very small fixed orifice size occurs in heavily calcified valves with regional changes in mitral dome dynamics. These changes may be appreciated with imaging techniques.

Pathophysiology (Fig. 3-16). As the affected area of the mitral valve becomes narrow, (valve area < 2 cm^2), obstruction of normal diastolic blood flow begins to occur.[50] The obstruction of blood flow during diastole will result in a pressure gradient across the mitral valve, an increase in pressure in the left atrium, and consequently increase in pressure in the pulmonary veins, capillaries, and arteries. In mild cases of mitral stenosis, the mitral valve gradient is mainly in early diastole and presystole. With increasing severity of stenosis, however, the left atrial pressure rises, and the mitral valve gradient is usually present throughout diastole. Because of the unpredictable behavior of the pulmonary vascular resistance, pulmonary artery pressure is not a direct function of left atrial pressure. In cases of severe mitral stenosis with high pulmonary vascular resistance and/or right ventricular failure, the cardiac output is often markedly reduced. In such settings the cardiac output is not increased with exercise. As the mitral valve area decreases, flow across the valve is maintained by gradually increasing left atrial pressure and the development of a diastolic gradient (Fig. 3-17). The left atrial pressure and gradient across the mitral valve are not only related to mitral valve area but also to cardiac output and to diastolic filling times. Conditions that may increase cardiac output such as exercise, fever, or pregnancy will increase the pressure gradient. An increase in heart rate will shorten the duration of diastole and also will result in an increase in pressure gradient.[50-59]

Left atrial function. A wide spectrum of left atrial size has been observed in patients with mitral stenosis. Normal

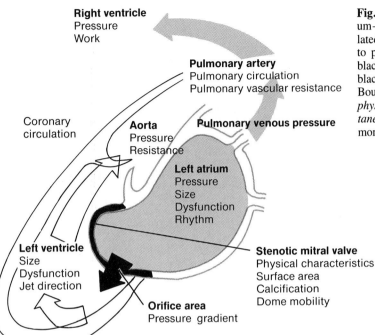

Fig. 3-16. Mitral stenosis: clinical determinants. Left atrium—gray area and arrows indicate hemodynamic changes related to increased left atrial pressure and volume transmitted to pulmonary circulation and right ventricle. Orifice area = black arrows. Stenotic mitral valve labeled and indicated in black. See text for details. (From Wooley CF, Sparks EA and Boudoulas H: *Mitral stenosis: The anatomic lesion and the physiologic state.* In Bashore TM, Davidson CJ, eds: *Percutaneous balloon valvuloplasty and related techniques,* Baltimore, 1991, Williams & Wilkins.)

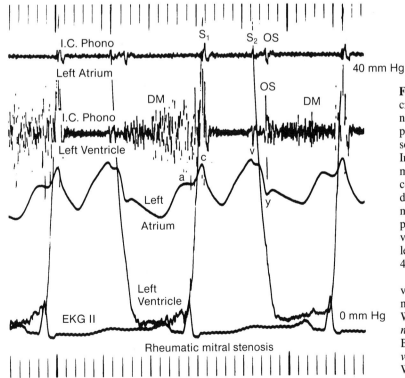

Fig. 3-17. Left atrial and left ventricular pressure pulse crossover relations in severe mitral stenosis. Two-manometer study, first manometer recording sound and pressure in left atrium, second manometer recording sound and pressure in the left ventricle. Top to bottom: Intracardiac sound (IC phono) in left atrium—S_1 = mitral component of the first heart sound: S_2 = aortic component of S_2; OS = mitral opening snap. Intracardiac sound (IC phono) left ventricle—DM = diastolic murmur;)S—mitral opening snap. Left atrial pressure pulse (left atrium)—A, C, V waves and y descent. Left ventricular pressure pulse. Bottom: Electrocardiogram lead II. Scale 1 to 40 mm Hg, right border. Time lines 40 ms.

Note the diastolic murmur was recorded in the left ventricle; in the first two complexes the diastolic murmur continued into a "presystolic" murmur. (From Wooley CF, Sparks EA and Boudoulas H: *Mitral stenosis: The anatomic lesion and the physiologic state.* In Bashore TM, Davidson CJ, eds: *Percutaneous balloon valvuloplasty and related techniques,* Baltimore, 1991, Williams & Wilkins.)

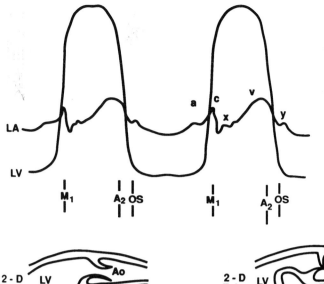

Fig. 3-18. Mitral stenosis—pressure pulse, sound, and echocardiographic correlates. LA = left arterial pressure pulse with A, C, V waves, x and y descents; LV = left ventricular pressure pulse. Heart sounds: M_1 = mitral component of first heart sound; S_2 = aortic component of second heart sound; OS = mitral opening snap. Bottom left: Two-dimensional echo at M_1. Bottom right: Two-dimensional echo at OS. LA = left atrium; LV = left ventricle; Ao = aorta. (From Wooley CF, Sparks EA and Boudoulas H: *Mitral stenosis: The anatomic lesion and the physiologic state.* In Bashore TM, Davidson CJ, eds: *Percutaneous balloon valvuloplasty and related techniques,* Baltimore, 1991, Williams & Wilkins.)

size atria with no mural thrombi, to huge left atria with thrombi of different sizes (most often in the atrial appendage) have been recorded.

As the left atrial pressure increases, there is enlargement of the left atrium along with certain sequelae such as premature atrial contractions, paroxysmal atrial tachycardia, atrial flutter, and atrial fibrillation. Atrial fibrillation may precipitate acute pulmonary edema in severe mitral stenosis and in turn may predispose to thromboembolism. Intramural thrombi may embolize to a number of organs such as the brain, kidneys, and spleen. In some instances, a massive thrombus may be formed within the left atrium, obstructing the emptying of the pulmonary veins. On such an occasion, severe pulmonary edema, syncope, or sudden death may occur.[60]

Atrial dysfunction in mitral stenosis is related to the effects of progressive and chronic left atrial hypertension, with increased left atrial volume, prolonged left atrial systole, interruption of the left atrial contraction-relaxation phase by ventricular systole, increased left atrial work, the gradual development of an atrial myopathic state, and the eventual onset of atrial fibrillation (Fig. 3-18). Large atria reveal very little muscle or no muscle at all in their walls. Whether this is the result of muscle destruction during the acute phase of rheumatic carditis or the result of the dilatation is not clear. A very large left atrium may impinge and shift the left main bronchus and also compress the recurrent laryngeal nerve.

Analysis of left atrial volume dynamics and distribution of atrial emptying fractions provide additional insights into left atrial dysfunction. Blood flow from the left atrium to the left ventricle is normally biphasic. The first phase is passive, begins with mitral valve opening, and ends with the beginning of left atrial systole. The second phase, the active phase, begins with left atrial systole and ends with mitral valve closure. All left atrial volumes—maximal, minimal, and initial atrial systole—are increased in patients with mitral stenosis (Fig. 3-19). When compared with those of normal subjects, left atrial passive emptying volume is not different in patients with mitral stenosis, while the left atrial active emptying volume is larger. The net result is a normal left atrial total emptying volume (maximal minus minimal volume). In contrast, the left atrial emptying fractions (passive, active, and total) are significantly decreased in mitral stenosis. The increased left atrial volumes in patients with mitral stenosis in sinus rhythm compensate for the decreased left atrial emptying fractions and maintain left atrial total emptying volume[60] (Fig. 3-20).

Atrial natriuretic factors (ANF) secretion is regulated by atrial stretch; ANF are increased in patients with mitral stenosis in sinus rhythm without congestive heart failure, depending on left atrial pressure. ANF secretion is also high in patients with mitral stenosis and atrial fibrillation but does not respond appropriately to changes in left atrial pressure. The pathophysiologic role of ANF in mitral stenosis is gradually being defined and may involve regulation of the pulmonary circulatory response to elevated left atrial pressure.[61]

Left ventricular function. The existence of a significant myocardial factor in mitral stenosis as contrasted to the mechanical factors associated with the stenotic valve has been a source of controversy for almost a century. The mitral stenosis left ventricle is small, with greater systolic emptying and inferoposterior systolic wall motion abnormalities. Evidence of systolic dysfunction includes the ab-

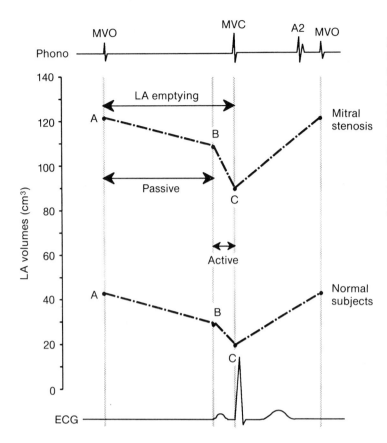

Fig. 3-19. Mitral stenosis: left atrial function. Phonocardiogram (phono), left atrial (LA) volumes, and electrocardiogram (ECG), schematic presentation. **A,** LA maximal volume (mitral valve opening). **B,** LA volume at onset of atrial systole, at ECG P wave. **C,** LA minimal volume (mitral valve closure). Changes of LA volume from **A** to **B** represent the LA passive emptying volume, changes of LA volume from **B** to **C** represent the LA active emptying volume, and changes of LA volume from **A** to **C** represent the LA total emptying volume. A_2 = aortic component of the second heart sound; MVC = mitral valve closure; MVO = mitral valve opening. See text under left atrial function. (Modified from Triposkiadis F, Wooley CF, Boudoulas H: Mitral stenosis: left atrial dynamics reflect altered passive and active emptying, *Am Heart J* 120:124-132, 1990.)

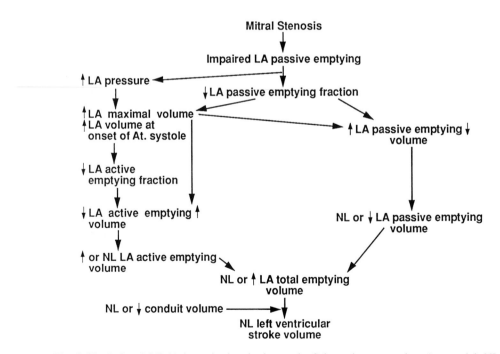

Fig. 3-20. Left atrial (LA) dynamics in mitral stenosis. Schematic presentation; At = atrial, NL = normal.(Modified from Triposkiadis F, Wooley CF, Boudoulas H: Mitral stenosis: left atrial dynamics reflect altered passive and active emptying, *Am Heart J* 120:124-132, 1990.)

normally prolonged left ventricular pressure rise time, the loss of ventricular efficiency related to movement of the mitral dome toward the left atrium in the presence of left atrial hypertension, and alterations in left ventricular function related to disturbances of ventricular filling. Left ventricular isovolumetric contraction time is markedly decreased since ventricular filling continues during early ventricular systole as a result of prolonged atrial systole extending well into early ventricular systole.[50]

Evidence of left ventricular diastolic dysfunction in mitral stenosis is more apparent. The diastolic pressure gradient at the stenotic valve, abnormal patterns of left ventricular dimensional change, absence of the atrial kick in the ventricular pressure pulse, altered diastolic inflow patterns, and the configurations of color flow jets through the mitral orifice from the mitral dome (either as central-apical or eccentric jets) are significant factors affecting or reflecting left ventricular diastolic dysfunction. Diastolic regional left ventricular wall motion abnormalities associated with a significantly reduced peak filling rate have been described. Striking nonuniformity and asynchrony of wall motion are present; regional asynchrony includes abnormal outward wall movement during isovolumic relaxation.[62]

Pulmonary circulation. Pulmonary edema does not occur until the pulmonary venous pressure exceeds 25 mm Hg, which is, of course, higher than the colloid osmotic pressure of the blood. Left atrial pressure reaches approximately 25 mm Hg (mean) when the mitral orifice is reduced to about 1 cm^2; it is after this point that pulmonary arteriolar reactive changes develop. With progressive pulmonary vascular obstruction, pulmonary arterial hypertension develops with eventual right ventricular hypertension, hypertrophy, and dysfunction. In some patients, however, with pulmonary venous pressures higher than 25 mm Hg, pulmonary edema might not occur. This most likely is related to thickening of the alveolar capillary membrane and reactive pulmonary arteriolar constriction in the pulmonary vascular bed. Unfortunately, this protective mechanism occurs at the expense of a decrease in cardiac output. As long as the stenosis occurs gradually, the increased capacity of the pulmonary lymphatics to remove the interstitial fluid may prevent the occurrence of pulmonary edema. However, longstanding elevated pressure in the pulmonary veins ultimately will lead to pulmonary arterial hypertension, the pathogenesis of which is due to both retrograde transmission of elevated left atrial pressure and direct pulmonary arterial constriction. Eventually this chronic vasoconstriction may result in obliterative changes in the walls of small pulmonary arteries. The sequela of a persistent pulmonary hypertension will be tricuspid and pulmonary incompetence, as well as right ventricular failure. As the pulmonary venous pressure increases, collateral connections with the bronchial venous system may increase the pressures in the submucosal bronchial veins, which may result in hemoptysis in patients with mitral stenosis.[50-51]

Mitral stenosis—clinical recognition. Patients with mitral stenosis may present with a progressive symptom complex, with evidence of pulmonary hypertension, or with a complication of mitral stenosis, the evaluation of which leads the clinician back to the underlying diagnosis. The diagnosis may be quite straightforward in a young woman with appropriate symptoms, a history of rheumatic fever, clear-cut physical findings, and confirmatory laboratory studies. The real life questions for the clinician are more complicated. When do you suspect mitral stenosis? When should you think of mitral stenosis? Some representative scenarios include: patients who are short of breath, elderly patients with atrial fibrillation, and patients with hemoptysis. In these cases echocardiography and Doppler echocardiography will establish not only the diagnosis but also the severity of the disease.[50-63]

Mitral stenosis—natural history. Most of the natural history studies of mitral stenosis were written in the 1950s and 1960s and reflected the European and North American experiences from another time in medicine. Are these studies still valid as a benchmark? A more recent natural history study from Greece extended into the diuretic-antibiotic era. There were significant parallels with Wood's earlier study; no striking differences were detected between patients with and without a history of rheumatic fever. One hundred and seventy-six patients with mitral stenosis hospitalized in the AHEPA Hospital Á Medical Clinic of Aristotelian University of Thessaloníki, Greece, from 1963 to 1972 were analyzed.[64] Patients with a history of rheumatic fever (93 patients) were compared to those without a history of rheumatic fever (83 patients). The average age at symptom onset was similar in the two groups (history of rheumatic fever: 36.5 ± 14 years; no history of rheumatic fever: 36.7 ± 13 years). However, there was a wide distribution in the age of the beginning of symptoms in both groups, as the large standard deviation indicates (Fig. 3-21). The frequency of major symptoms was also similar in both groups (Fig. 3-22). The time interval from the beginning of symptoms (functional class II) to total incapacitation (functional class IV) was approximately 10 years in both groups (Fig. 3-21). This time interval varied significantly from patient to patient, as the large standard deviation indicates. Infective endocarditis may alter the natural history, although mitral stenosis seldom becomes involved by infective endocarditis, except when it is combined with mitral regurgitation. The natural history varies from patient to patient. Patients with mitral stenosis should have periodic evaluations when asymptomatic. Periodic evaluation is replaced by more frequent evaluation with the development of symptoms or events. Interventional therapy may indicate different degrees of the disease in symptomatic patients[50,65] (Fig. 3-23).

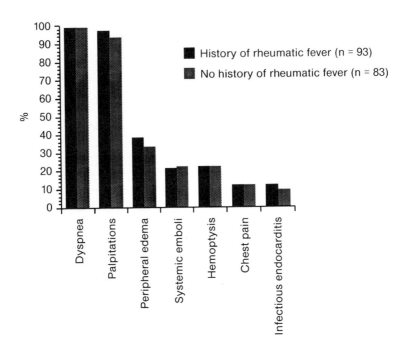

Fig. 3-21. Mitral stenosis: 1963-1972 study in Greece. Frequency of symptoms-events in patients with and without history of rheumatic fever. Note the similarity between the two groups.(Figure constructed with data from Boudoulas H, et al: The natural history of rheumatic valvular heart disease. Comparison of patients with a history of rheumatic fever to those without rheumatic fever, *Helliniki Iatriki* (Greek Medicine) 43:107-115, 1974.)

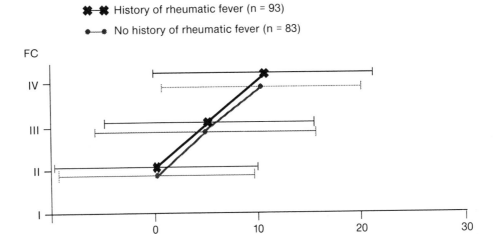

Fig. 3-22. Mitral stenosis: 1963-1972 study in Greece. Time intervals from the beginning of symptoms (functional class, FC II) to total incapacitation (FC IV) in patients with mitral stenosis with and without history of rheumatic fever (mean values = 1 standard deviation). Note the large standard deviation and the similarities between the two groups.(Figure constructed with data from Boudoulas H, et al: The natural history of rheumatic valvular heart disease. Comparison of patients with a history of rheumatic fever to those without rheumatic fever, *Helliniki Iatriki* (Greek Medicine) 43:107-115, 1974.)

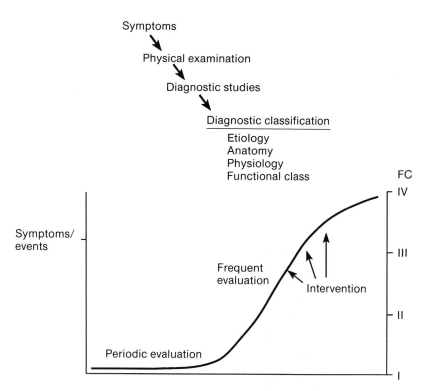

Fig. 3-23. Individual Patient Analysis. Schematic incorporates the diagnostic steps—history, physical examination, diagnostic studies—necessary to develop a diagnostic classification. An individual patient profile plots symptoms, events, time, patient age, and functional classification (FC). Periodic evaluation is replaced by more frequent evaluation with the development of symptoms or events. Intervention (indicated by multiple arrows) may involve medical therapy, or valvuloplasty by surgical procedure or with angioplasty at varying times during the course of the disease.(From Wooley CF, Sparks EA and Boudoulas H: *Mitral stenosis: The anatomic lesion and the physiologic state.* In Bashore TM, Davidson CJ, eds: *Percutaneous balloon valvuloplasty and related techniques,* Baltimore, 1991, Williams & Wilkins.)

Other causes of mitral stenosis

Congenital abnormalities such as a parachute mitral valve may also present as mitral stenosis. Infective endocarditis may produce mitral stenosis when there are large bulky vegetations like those occasionally seen in fungal endocarditis. Mitral stenosis may be secondary to metabolic or enzymatic abnormalities such as seen in gout, deposits of aramide trihexoside as it occurs in Fabry's disease, or large mucopolysaccharide deposits as seen in Hurler-Scheie syndrome. Whipple's disease may involve the mitral valves, resulting in stenosis. Rare examples of massive ring calcification producing mitral stenosis have been seen in elderly women. Therapy with methysergide may also produce mitral stenosis.[50]

Mitral stenosis—mimics. Atrial myxoma is the most common primary neoplasm of the heart. This neoplasm (which will be described in more detail in Chapter 10) is found more commonly in the left atrium and is attached to the limb of the foramen ovale. The atrial myxoma is often pedunculated and falls through the mitral annulus into the left ventricle during diastole, only to be propelled back into the left atrium during ventricular systole.[50]

Cor triatriatum, essentially a third left atrial chamber,

usually produces symptoms similar to mitral stenosis in early life and is rare in adult life. Membranous supravalvular mitral stenosis and other left atrial membranous lesions may mimic certain aspects of mitral stenosis. These lesions have distinctive clinical, hemodynamic, and imaging characteristics that permit discrimination from rheumatic mitral stenosis.

MITRAL REGURGITATION

Normal mitral valve closure is a complex mechanism resulting from a combination of atrial and ventricular events. Effective systolic sealing of the mitral valve depends on proper function, size, position, motion, and integrity of the mitral leaflets, chordae tendineae, papillary muscles, and mitral valve annulus in the presence of a normal left atrium and a normal left ventricle. Abnormal function in any of the structures mentioned above may result in mitral regurgitation.[66-68]

Etiology

Contrary to mitral valve stenosis, in which for all practical purposes there is one etiology (rheumatic disease), mitral regurgitation has several etiologies (box on p. 82).

Common causes of mitral regurgitation

Chronic

- Mitral valve prolapse associated with floppy mitral valve—isolated or a part of recognized connective tissue disorder syndromes (e.g., Marfan syndrome, Ehlers-Danlos syndrome)
- Chronic rheumatic valvulitis
- Mitral annular calcification
- Coronary artery disease
- Kawasaki disease
- Cardiomyopathy
    Dilated
    Hypertrophic
- Congenital
- Therapy with ergotamine

Acute

- Severe papillary muscle ischemia or rupture
- Infectious endocarditis
- Chordae tendineae rupture

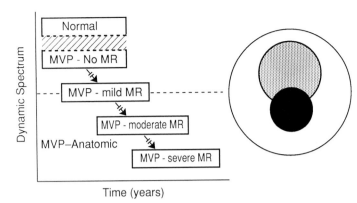

Fig. 3-24. *Left:* The dynamic spectrum and progression of mitral valve prolapse (MVP) are shown. A subtle gradation (cross-hatched area) exists between the normal mitral valve and valves that produce mild MVP without mitral regurgitation (No MR). The condition may remain at the level of *MVP—No MR* or may progress. Most patients with MVP syndrome (MVPS) occupy the area above the dotted line, and patients with progressive mitral valve dysfunction occupy the area below. *Right:* The large circle represents the total number of patients with MVP-symptomatic and asymptomatic. Symptoms may be directly related to mitral valve dysfunction *(black circle)* or to autonomic dysfunction *(dotted area)*. Some patients with symptoms directly related to mitral valve dysfunction may subsequently experience symptoms secondary to autonomic dysfunction. (From Boudoulas H, Wooley CF: *Mitral valve prolapse and the mitral valve prolapse syndrome.* Mount Kisco, New York, 1988, Futura.)

Acute or chronic abnormalities of the mitral valve apparatus may lead to mitral regurgitation. In the past rheumatic heart disease was reported to be the most common cause of chronic mitral regurgitation, but more recently mitral valve prolapse resulting from a floppy mitral valve has become the most frequent cause of chronic mitral regurgitation necessitating surgery in the Western world.[66-68]

Rupture of chordae tendineae is the most common cause of acute mitral regurgitation. Papillary muscle rupture and infective endocarditis may also cause severe acute mitral regurgitation.

One should realize, however, that the above statistics are gathered from operatively excised mitral valves and do not necessarily reflect the overall incidence of the different etiologies of pure mitral regurgitation in the general population. For example, papillary muscle dysfunction is more common than mitral valve prolapse in producing pure mitral regurgitation, although it does not always necessitate surgical intervention. Therefore it appears statistically as a less frequent cause.

Chronic mitral regurgitation
Mitral valve prolapse

Although mitral valve prolapse is a common valvular abnormality, a clinically relevant classification is incomplete and the pathogenesis of symptoms is not completely understood.[66-87] Based on our experience and on the experience of others, we developed a clinical classification in order to better identify subsets of patients with mitral valve prolapse, and develop greater insight into the mechanism of symptoms in these patients. Symptoms or complications may be primarily or directly related to progressive mitral valvular dysfunction (mitral valve prolapse–anatomic), or related to neuroendocrine or autonomic dysfunction rather than valvular dysfunction (Mitral valve prolapse[66,70,80] syndrome, Fig. 3-24).

Recent evidence suggests that mitral valve prolapse is inherited as an autosomal dominant phenotype and that a large proportion of patients with mitral valve prolapse have evidence of the systemic features that occur in patients with heritable disorders of connective tissue. Examples of such features are deformity of the anterior chest, vertebral column, dolichostenomelia, and joint hypermobility. Further, biochemical studies of mitral valves obtained from patients with severe mitral valve prolapse and significant mitral regurgitation demonstrated collagen abnormalities. Mitral valve prolapse has been documented in a number of recognized heritable connective tissue disorders such as Marfan syndrome, Ehlers-Danlos syndrome, Stickler syndrome, and adult polycystic kidney disease. In recognition of this worldwide experience, committee experts classified familial mitral valve prolapse as one of the heritable connective tissue disorders. By virtue of its high frequency in the general population, mitral valve prolapse designates the largest group of patients with a connective tissue abnormality of the heart.

Pathology and histology. Patients with mitral valve prolapse and symptoms directly related to mitral valve dysfunction are classified as mitral valve prolapse–anatomic. Surgical patients usually have large, "floppy" myxomatous mitral valves (Figures 3-25, 3-26, and 3-27). Ruptured chordae tendineae are common in these patients.

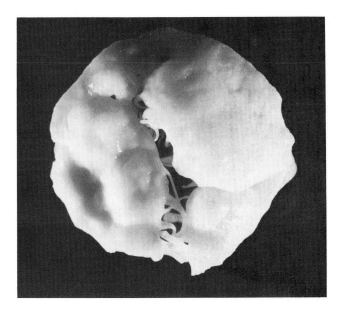

Fig. 3-25. Atrial view of a ballooned, prolapsed mitral valve.

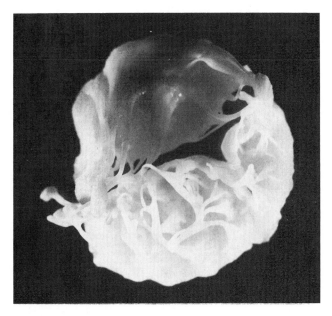

Fig. 3-26. Ventricular view of a prolapsed mitral valve. Note attenuated and elongated chordae tendineae.

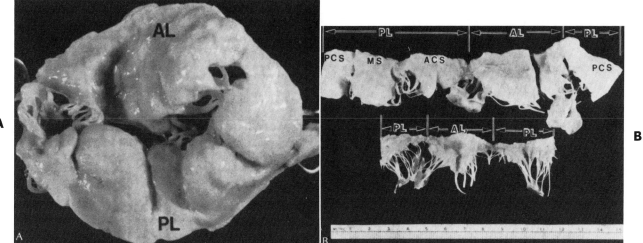

Fig. 3-27. A, Myxomatous mitral valve, atrial view, from a patient with severe mitral regurgitation. The surface area of the valve is increased, with increased folding of the valve surface. The widths of the anterior leaflet (AL) and the posterior leaflet (PL) are almost equal. Individual scallops of the posterior leaflet are enlarged and redundant. **B,** Comparison of an excised myxomatous mitral valve from a patient with severe mitral regurgitation (top) with a normal mitral valve from a patient who died of noncardiac causes (bottom), showing the increased surface area of both anterior leaflets (AL) and posterior leaflets (PL) of the myxomatous valve with enlarged and redundant posterior leaflet scallops, enlarged mitral annulus, and elongated chordae tendineae. *PCS* = posteromedial commissural scallop; *MS* = middle scallop; *ACS* = anterolateral commissural scallop. (From Boudoulas H and Wooley CF: *Mitral valve prolapse and the mitral valve prolapse syndrome.* In Yu P, Goodwin J eds: *Progress in cardiology,* Philadelphia, 1986, Lea & Febiger.)

Extensive gross morphologic and histologic studies in the excised mitral valves show increased surface area, increased annular diameter, elongated chordae tendineae, and collagen dissolution or disruption (Fig. 3-28).

Scanning electron photomicrographs demonstrated surface folds and focal loss of endothelial cells on mitral valve leaflets obtained from patients with severe mitral valve prolapse and significant mitral regurgitation (Fig. 3-29). These abnormalities may be responsible for thromboembolic complications and infectious endocarditis.

Histologic abnormalities and abnormal mechanical properties have been demonstrated in chordae tendineae from "floppy" mitral valves in a recent study conducted in our laboratory. Normal mitral valve chordae tendineae uni-

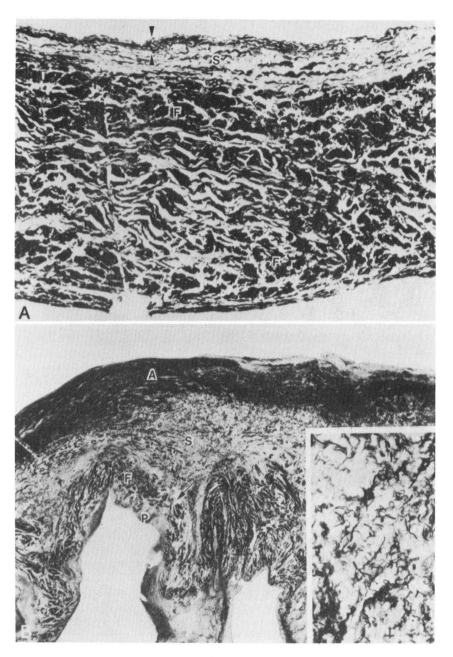

Fig. 3-28. A, A normal mitral valve cusp. The histologic zones are represented in a cross-section. The atrialis is a thin zone of dense collagen immediately below the inflow surface (between arrowheads). The next zone, the spongiosa *(S),* consists of loose connective tissue, and the remainder of the cusp, composed of dense collagen, is the fibrosa *(F).* (Jones' silver stain; original magnification ×25.) **B,** Floppy mitral valve cusp. The cusp has a large expanded central zone of myxomatous connective tissue with focal thinning and disruption of the fibrosa (arrow). The dense layer seen at the top just below the inflow surface is the markedly thickened atrialis (A). Fibrous connective tissue "pads" are seen on the ventricular surface. (Jones' silver stain; original magnification ×4.) The lower right inset is a high magnification view of the myxomatous area showing disoriented, separated collagen bundles. A Mowry's colloidal iron stain demonstrated abundant accumulation of acid mucopolysaccharides in this area. (Jones' silver stain; original magnification ×100.)(From Boudoulas H et al: Mitral valve prolapse and the mitral valve prolapse syndrome: A diagnostic classification and pathogenesis of symptoms, *Am Heart J* 118:796-818, 1989.)

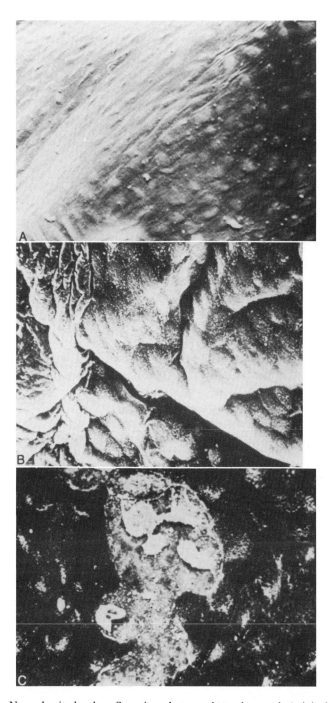

Fig. 3-29. A, Normal mitral valve. Scanning electron photomicrograph (original magnification ×280) shows smooth valve cusp surface covered by endothelial cells. **B,** Floppy mitral valve. Scanning electron photomicrograph (original magnification ×400) shows an irregular surface with deep infolding. **C,** Floppy mitral valve. Scanning electron photomicrograph (original magnification ×600) shows an area of denuded endothelium exposing the underlying collagen. (From Lewis RP: *Cerebral embolism in mitral valve prolapse*. In Boudoulas H, Wooley CF, eds: *Mitral valve prolapse and the mitral valve prolapse syndrome*, Mount Kisco, NY, 1988, Futura.)

formly have a dense central collagenous core surrounded by a thin layer of compact elastic fibers with or without small deposits of acid mucopolysaccharides. Collagen alterations and moderate-to-severe acid mucopolysaccharide accumulation rarely found in normal mitral valve chordae tendineae were frequently present in floppy mitral valve chordae tendineae. The collagen alterations in floppy mitral valve chordae tendineae are illustrated in Figure 3-30. The histology of floppy mitral valve chordae tendineae is not uniform, ranging from a normal histologic appearance to severe collagen fragmentation, attenuation, and separation with associated severe acid mucopolysaccharide accumulation.[66,70,80-81]

Mechanical abnormalities in floppy mitral valve chordae tendineae were demonstrated. Chordae tendineae were tested in a uniaxial tension mode, and load versus elongation curves were obtained for each chorda by increasing the load until the chorda fractured. The fracture stress in floppy mitral valve chordae tendineae was significantly lower compared with that in normal mitral valve chordae tendineae. This indicates a loss of tissue strength that may contribute to chordal elongation and rupture.

Natural history. Symptoms and serious complications related to mitral valve dysfunction associated with anatomic mitral valve prolapse include infectious endocarditis, progressive mitral regurgitation, ruptured chordae tendineae, thromboembolic phenomena, supraventricular or ventricular arrhythmias, atrioventricular conduction defects, congestive heart failure, and death. The natural history of mitral valve prolapse may be accelerated by infectious endocarditis, the development of atrial fibrillation, rupture of chordae tendineae, and left atrial and left ventricular dysfunction. To date, there have been few long-term follow-up studies in adult patients with mitral valve prolapse.[66,80,85,87]

Kolibash et al[88] reported the natural history of 86 patients who had severe mitral regurgitation. Eighty patients had a preexisting heart murmur first detected at an average age of 34 years. An average of 25 years elapsed before the onset of clinical symptoms. After significant symptoms developed, consideration of mitral valve surgery was necessary in most patients within 1 year. This rapid deterioration could generally be attributed to chordal rupture or the development of atrial fibrillation as a late manifestation of left atrial myopathy. Serial evaluations performed in 28 patients demonstrated progressive mitral regurgitation, cardiomegaly, and left atrial enlargement. It is apparent from this study that progressive, severe mitral regurgitation will develop in a subset of patients with mitral valve prolapse.

Duren and colleagues[89] reported the results of a long-term, prospective follow-up study of 300 patients with mitral valve prolapse who ranged form 10 to 87 years of age (mean 42.2 years). The patients were diagnosed by clinical, cineangiographic, and echocardiographic criteria and all had auscultatory findings consistent with mitral valve prolapse. The study encompassed all patients with mitral valve prolapse, irrespective of clinical condition at the onset. The average follow-up period was 6.2 years. The clinical condition in 153 patients remained stable; 27 of these patients experienced supraventricular tachycardia that was controlled with medications. Signs of mitral regurgitation developed in 20 patients, but they remained clinically asymptomatic. Serious complications developed in 100 patients. Sudden death occurred in 3 patients, ventricular fibrillation in 2, ventricular tachycardia in 56, and infective endocarditis in 18. Twenty-eight patients underwent mitral valve surgery because of progressive mitral regurgitation, and an additional 8 patients with severe mitral regurgitation were considered surgical candidates. Eleven patients had cerebrovascular accidents. Although the study population may not be representative of the entire anatomic mitral valve prolapse population, the results strongly support the concept that anatomic mitral valve prolapse may be associated with significant morbidity and mortality.

Nishimura et al[75] determined prognosis in a prospective follow-up study in 237 minimally symptomatic or asymptomatic patients with mitral valve prolapse documented by echocardiography. The patients age ranged from 10 to 69 years (mean 44 years); the mean follow-up period was 6.2 years. Sudden death occurred in six patients. A multivariate analysis of echocardiographic factors identified redundant mitral valve leaflets (present in 97 patients) as the only variable associated with sudden death. Of the 10 patients who sustained a cerebral embolic event, 1 had left ventricular aneurysm with apical thrombus, 1 had infectious endocarditis, 6 had atrial fibrillation with left atrial enlargement, and 2 were in sinus rhythm. Infectious endocarditis occurred in 3 patients, and progressive mitral regurgitation prompted valve replacement in 17 patients. Left ventricular end-diastolic diameter exceeding 60 mm was the best echocardiographic predictor of the subsequent need for mitral valve replacement. Twenty patients had no clinical auscultatory findings of a systolic click or murmur; none of these patients had complications during follow-up. The authors concluded that although most patients with echocardiographic evidence of mitral valve prolapse have a benign course, subsets of patients identified by echocardiography are at high risk for the development of progressive mitral regurgitation, sudden death, cerebral embolic events, or infectious endocarditis.

Marks et al[90] confirmed Nishimura's data in a retrospective study in which they analyzed clinical and two-dimensional echocardiographic data from 456 patients with mitral valve prolapse. Patients with thickening and redundancy of the mitral valve leaflet were compared with those without leaflet thickening. Complications, concurrent or past (i.e., infectious endocarditis, significant mitral regurgitation, the need for mitral valve replacement), were more prevalent in the group with leaflet thickening and redundancy than in those without leaflet thickening. The in-

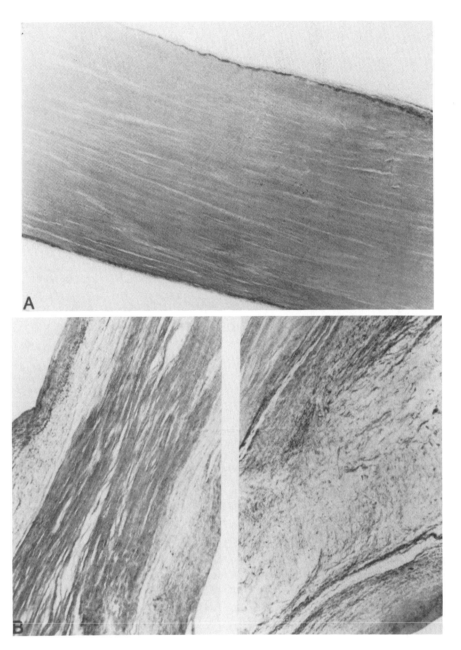

Fig. 3-30. A, Normal mitral valve chordae tendineae. The chorda has a large central core of dense collagen surrounded by a thin dark-staining elastic tissue layer. (Weigert's elastic stain; original magnification ×25.) **B,** Floppy mitral valve chordae tendineae. These chordae show two patterns of histopathologic alterations. The chorda on the left shows myxomatous expansion of the peripheral connective tissue with loss of the distinct elastic layer. The central collagenous core is not extensively involved. The chorda on the right has severe separation and attenuation of collagen in the central core with fragmentation of the elastic layer. Mowry's colloidal iron stain demonstrated abundant acid mucopolysaccharide accumulation in the myxomatous areas of both chordae. (Weigert's elastic stain; original magnification ×25.) (From Boudoulas et al: Mitral valve prolapse and the mitral valve prolapse syndrome: A diagnostic classification and pathogenesis of symptoms, *Am Heart J* 118:796-818, 1989.)

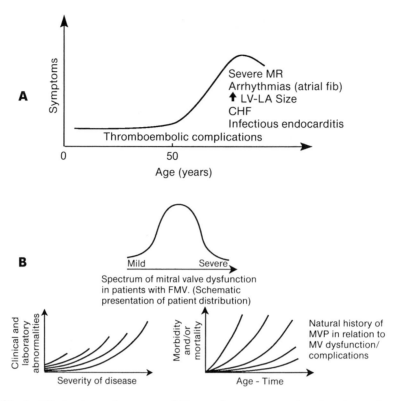

Fig. 3-31. A, Mitral valve prolapse, natural history. Symptoms are plotted against patient age in years. Increased symptoms occur after age 50 and are related to progressive mitral regurgitation (MR), atrial fibrillation (Atrial fib), left atrial (LA), and left ventricular (LV) dysfunction, congestive heart failure (CHF), and infectious endocarditis. Thromboembolic complications have been reported at a wide range of ages. **B,** Floppy mitral valve (FMV), natural history considerations. (Top) The spectrum of mitral valve abnormalities in patient with MVP is compared with the natural history (left lower). Relationship between the number of clinical and laboratory abnormalities and the severity of the disease (schematic presentation). FMV includes a wide spectrum of mild and severe valvular abnormalities and at any particular time the number of abnormal clinical (e.g., click, click plus late systolic murmur, holosystolic murmur, gallop rhythm, and cardiac arrhythmias) and laboratory findings (e.g., late systolic prolapse, thickened mitral leaflets, holosystolic prolapse, left ventricular and left atrial enlargement on echocardiogram, and mitral regurgitation on Doppler) is directly related to the severity of the disease. (Right lower) FMV patients may have a wide spectrum of valvular abnormalities, from mild to severe. The natural history of patients with FMV is directly related to the severity of mitral valve abnormalities. Lines represent morbidity and mortality related to complication such as infective endocarditis, thromboembolic phenomena, cardiac arrhythmias, and mitral regurgitation (schematic presentation).(From Boudoulas H and Wooley CF: *Mitral valve prolapse and the mitral valve prolapse syndrome.* Mount Kisko, NY, 1988, Futura.)

cidence of stroke, however, was similar in the two groups.

These long-term follow-up studies in patients with mitral valve prolapse support several conclusions:

Serious complications do occur in patients with anatomic mitral valve prolapse.

Mitral valve prolapse patients constitute a heterogeneous population: complications relate directly to the specific subset of mitral valve prolapse under consideration[85,87] (Fig. 3-31).

Complications appear to occur primarily in mitral valve prolapse patients with diagnostic auscultatory findings.

Redundant mitral valve leaflets and increased left ventricular size in patients with mitral valve prolapse are associated with a high frequency of serious complications.

The possibility that a patient with mitral valve prolapse will require mitral valve surgery increases with age. Male mitral valve prolapse patients required mitral valve surgery more often than do female patients (Fig. 3-32).

The high-risk patient. Published studies and our experience have identified clinical and laboratory findings that characterize the high-risk patient[87] (see box on p. 90, Fig. 3-33).

Individuals with mitral valve prolapse and thick redundant mitral valve leaflets (i.e., floppy mitral valve) are at high risk of developing complications; men and those more than 50 year of age are at particularly high risk. A

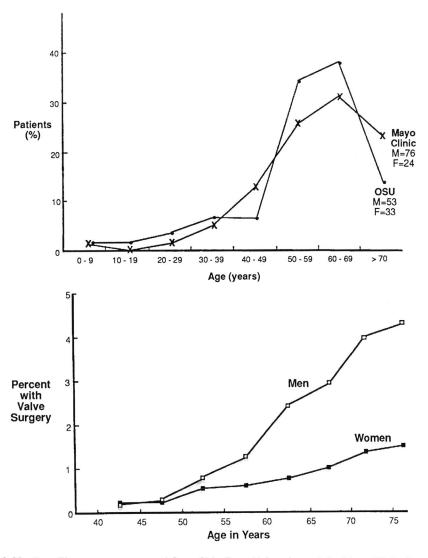

Fig. 3-32. Top: Figure was constructed from Ohio State University and the Mayo Clinic data; it shows the age-related frequency of mitral valve surgery for MR secondary to MVP. Bottom: Estimated lifetime risks of mitral valve surgery by age and sex among cohorts diagnosed as having MVP. (From Wilcken DE, Hickey AJ: Lifetime risk for patients with mitral valve prolapse of developing severe valve regurgitation requiring surgery, *Circulation* 78:10-14, 1988.)

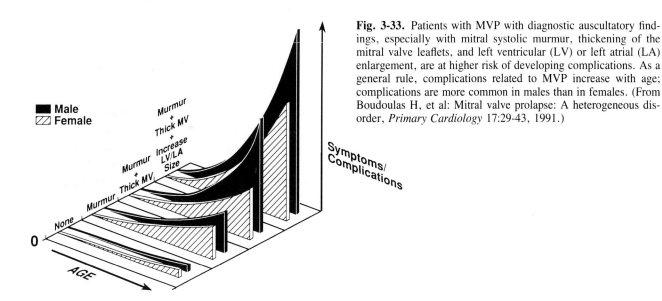

Fig. 3-33. Patients with MVP with diagnostic auscultatory findings, especially with mitral systolic murmur, thickening of the mitral valve leaflets, and left ventricular (LV) or left atrial (LA) enlargement, are at higher risk of developing complications. As a general rule, complications related to MVP increase with age; complications are more common in males than in females. (From Boudoulas H, et al: Mitral valve prolapse: A heterogeneous disorder, *Primary Cardiology* 17:29-43, 1991.)

*From Boudoulas, et al: Mitral valve prolapse: The high risk patient,
Pract Cardiol 17(9):15-31, 1991.

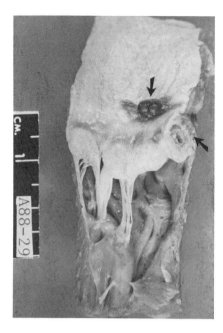

Fig. 3-34. Cross section of left atrial wall, posterior mitral leaflet, and left ventricular wall. Note the calcification of the mitral
ring *(oblique arrow)* and the endocardial ulceration at the lower
atrium with secondary thrombosis *(vertical arrow)*.

mitral systolic murmur detected before the onset of infectious endocarditis has also been shown to be an independent risk factor for complications. Left ventricular enlargement in patients with mitral valve prolapse is a good predictor of the subsequent need for mitral valve surgery.
When two or more of the above abnormalities coexist, the
possibility of complications is increased. The absence of
all three of these features, in contrast, identifies patients
with mitral valve prolapse at exceedingly low risk.

In patients in whom mitral valve prolapse is part of a
recognized heritable disorder of connective tissue or is associated with other cardiovascular abnormalities, the natural history may be more related to coexistence of other abnormalities than to mitral valve prolapse.

Chronic rheumatic valvulitis

Pure mitral valve regurgitation of rheumatic cause is
rather rare and is more often associated with mitral stenosis. In the pure form of mitral regurgitation of rheumatic
cause, one will note that there is no fusion of the commissures, but there is significant loss of actual surface area of
the leaflets because of scarring and retraction, particularly
of the posterior mitral leaflet. Similar scarring and fusion
is seen in the chordae tendineae, which also contribute to
regurgitation of the mitral valve by preventing the leaflets
from coming into apposition. Marked dilatation of the left
atrium secondary to regurgitation will enhance the degree
of the regurgitant stream as the atrium falls posteriorly,
pulling the posterior leaflet backward and downward.
Rheumatic cause of mitral regurgitation should be considered if the patient has both mitral valve stenosis and regurgitation, or in the presence of both mitral and aortic valve
lesions.[67,70,91]

Mitral annular calcification

A rather infrequent cause of mitral valve regurgitation
is calcification of the mitral annulus. Under normal conditions, the portion of the annulus to which the posterior mitral leaflet is attached contracts during systole (Figs. 3-34
and 3-35). Calcification of the mitral annulus, particularly
the portion of the circumference that the posterior leaflet is
attached to, may prevent this contraction. Mitral annular
calcification preferentially involves the posterior leaflet,
but massive mitral annular calcification with involvement
of both mitral leaflets may also occur, which occasionally
may cause mitral stenosis. In a review of 13,043 autopsies
in patients older than 40 years of age, 142 of them had calcification of the mitral annulus. Calcific deposits may ulcerate and embolize to the brain, heart, spleen, or kidneys.
Mitral annular calcification is more common in women
(particularly in the sixth and seventh decades), in patients
with mitral valve prolapse, hypertrophic cardiomyopathy,
arterial hypertension, aortic stenosis, and chronic renal
failure.[49,92-93]

Byrd et al,[93] using echocardiographic techniques studied 114 patients (61 men, 53 women) with end-stage renal
disease, ages 17 to 81 (mean age 48 years). The length of
time of dialysis treatment ranged from 1 to 158 months,
with a mean of 29.4 months. Twenty patients had undergone renal transplantation, although seven of them were
again receiving dialysis. Mitral annular calcification was
present in 40 patients (35%), ages 33 to 84 years, mean

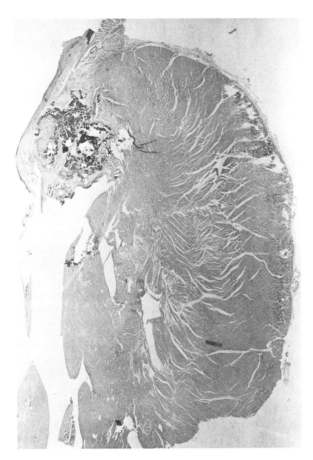

Fig. 3-35. Massive calcification of the mitral valve ring extending into the adjacent ventricular myocardium.

age 54 years. Patients with mitral annular calcification younger than 50 years of age were treated with dialysis for 61 months, versus 26 months for those older than 50 years. Patients with mitral annular calcification usually have higher parathyroid hormone levels compared with patients without mitral annular calcification. Studies have shown that total plasma calcium concentrations are not different in patients with mitral annular calcification compared with those without calcification. However, the ionized plasma calcium level appears to be significantly higher in the patients with mitral annular calcification. Additionally, the plasma phosphorus level and the calcium-phosphorus product are higher in patients with chronic renal failure and mitral annular calcification compared with those without the calcification process. The duration of dialysis may also play some role in the development of mitral annular calcification. As the duration of maintenance dialysis increases, so does the likelihood of mitral annular calcification. The calcification may extend to the aortic valve, which rarely may cause aortic stenosis.

The degree of mitral regurgitation in patients with mitral annular calcification is usually mild unless the calcification is massive and circumferential. In some patients the

calcium deposits are extensive and may extend into the atrioventricular node, producing conduction defects.

Coronary artery disease

Papillary muscle dysfunction due to ischemic heart disease is a very common cause of regurgitation of the mitral valve. Ischemic papillary muscle damage may produce varying degrees of mitral regurgitation at the acute phase of an infarct. This occurs in about 15% of all anterior myocardial infarctions and approximately 40% of all inferior myocardial infarctions. However, most of this dysfunction resolves shortly after the acute myocardial ischemic episode. Valvular dysfunction several months after an ischemic episode is generally due to residual scarring of the papillary muscles and related to asynchronous contraction of the papillary muscles, i.e., contraction of one papillary muscle is not in phase with that of the other.[94-97]

Hickey et al,[97] reported the incidence, the clinical spectrum, and the prognosis in patients with ischemic mitral regurgitation. Over a 6.5 year period, mitral regurgitation was demonstrated ventriculographically in 2343 (19%) of 11,748 patients with angiographically proven coronary artery disease. Moderate or severe mitral regurgitation had a progressively negative impact on survival, regardless of treatment. Acute presentation of congestive heart failure requiring treatment in an intensive care unit, decreased ejection fraction, severity of coronary artery obstruction, and advanced age were associated with a worse prognosis. Reperfusion therapy was highly successful in restoring valve competence in patients with acute mitral regurgitation. In patients requiring mitral valve surgery procedures, valve repair, as opposed to replacement, was associated with improved survival.

Kawasaki disease

Mitral valve regurgitation may be present in children with Kawasaki disease.[98] The mechanisms for it may differ depending on the duration of the disease. When mitral regurgitation develops in the acute phase and improves rapidly, it may be due to pancarditis of Kawasaki disease. Mitral regurgitation that persists for a longer period may be secondary to valve dysfunction (sequela of valvulitis) or dysfunction of the papillary muscles (sequela of the coronary lesions).

Cardiomyopathy

Dilated. Ventricular dilatation may cause functional mitral valve regurgitation, because of stretching of the mitral valve annulus. The severity of this type of regurgitation usually fluctuates, depending on the performance of the left ventricle. Some cardiac pathophysiologists believe that annular dilatation is an infrequent cause of mitral regurgitation, except if it is accompanied by papillary muscle lateral displacement. This mechanism of regurgitation most commonly occurs in patients with the dilated cardiomyopathy. A mitral annulus over 12 cm in circumference probably indicates regurgitation. An annulus which is stretched for a long period of time because of changes in the ventricular geometry may remain permanently stretched.[68,99-100]

Hypertrophic. Mitral regurgitation is often present in patients with hypertrophic cardiomyopathy. Systolic anterior motion of the mitral valve during ventricular systole in patients with hypertrophic cardiomyopathy may result in mitral regurgitation.[101]

Congenital abnormalities

Unusual causes of pure mitral regurgitation are seen in congenital cardiac abnormalities such as common A-V canal and corrected transposition of the great vessels.

Therapy with ergotamine

Mitral regurgitation due to valvular lesions in patients treated with methysergide has been reported. Patients with left-sided valvular lesions requiring valve replacement were recently reported after ergotamine therapy for migraine headaches. These patients revealed histopathologic changes in both aortic and mitral valves, although the alterations in the latter were more pronounced. The leaflets of the mitral valve in patients on ergotamine therapy were diffusely thickened and revealed commissural and chordal fusion without calcification. The thick leaflets were caused primarily by an irregular proliferation of fibroblasts and smooth muscle cells within an avascular collagenous matrix. These morphologic lesions are quite similar to the lesions seen in patients treated with methysergide, and to lesions produced by carcinoid heart disease.[79,102]

Natural history of causes of chronic mitral regurgitation other than mitral valve prolapse

The natural history in these situations depends on the natural history of the underlying disease. The natural course of rheumatic mitral regurgitation associated with mitral stenosis usually is gradual. Certain patients, however, with postinflammatory mitral regurgitation secondary to rheumatic fever develop acute or subacute mitral regurgitation, both of which require early surgical intervention. To date, such reports have come primarily from South Africa and Japan.[14]

Mitral regurgitation is present in approximately 20% of patients with coronary artery disease. Moderate to severe mitral regurgitation, however, is present in only a small percentage of patients with coronary artery disease. Increasing severity of mitral regurgitation has a progressive negative impact on survival regardless of treatment.

Mitral regurgitation is frequent in dilated cardiomyopathy and may contribute to the poor prognosis in this group of patients.

Pathophysiology of chronic mitral regurgitation. Clinical progression in patients with chronic mitral regur-

gitation is usually gradual, permitting adaptive compensatory mechanisms. During ventricular systole, part of left ventricular volume is ejected into the low-pressure left atrium. The left atrium dilates gradually and accommodates this extra volume load; as a result there is only minimal or moderate increase in left atrial pressure during ventricular systole. The left ventricular diastolic volume also increases gradually, since in addition to the blood flow from the pulmonary veins, blood ejected into the left atrium during ventricular systole returns into the left ventricle during diastole. As a result of this gradual dilatation the left ventricle ejects two or more times its normal stroke volume, a portion of which goes into the left atrium (regurgitant volume).[67,100,103-104]

Chronic left ventricular and left atrial dilatation result in increased diastolic compliance of these chambers. Thus the left ventricular diastolic and left atrial systolic and diastolic pressures remain relatively normal despite the large volumes.

Because the left ventricle ejects blood into the low-pressure left atrium in addition to that ejected into the aorta, left ventricular ejection is rapid and brief with a supernormal ejection fraction prior to the development of left atrial and left ventricular muscle dysfunction. Because left ventricular diastolic and left atrial pressures are relatively normal, there is little or no pulmonary congestion; the patient often complains of fatigue rather than dyspnea on exertion (Fig. 3-36).

Timing for surgery in patients with chronic mitral regurgitation

Mitral valve prolapse. The timing of surgery for mitral regurgitation, particularly in the asymptomatic or mildly asymptomatic patient, may be a difficult decision. Preservation of left atrial and left ventricular function are important considerations. If left ventricular dysfunction is mild and contractile reserve still exists, patients will generally experience relief of symptoms or limitations with only a mild fall in left ventricular ejection performance. If left ventricular dysfunction has become severe, surgery may precipitate a severe fall in ejection performance, persistence of symptoms, and even death from congestive heart failure. Thus the ideal timing for mitral valve surgery is at the onset of left ventricular dysfunction, when good surgical results should be expected.[67,105-109]

Proper timing of mitral valve surgery requires recognition of left ventricular dysfunction before it has become severe. Unfortunately, the clinical evaluation of left ventricular function has been difficult in mitral regurgitation because the lesion causes significant alterations in loading conditions. Indeed, in mitral regurgitation, increased preload with decreased afterload results in an augmentation of the ejection performance with a supernormal ejection fraction. After ejection fraction has fallen into the low normal range, a severe postoperative fall in ejection performance

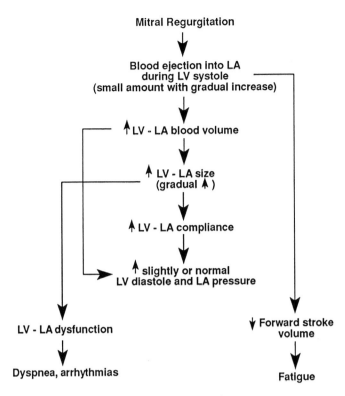

Fig. 3-36. Chronic mitral regurgitation. Pathophysiologic mechanisms. Schematic presentation. LA = left atrium, LV = left ventricle, ↑ = increase, ↓ = decrease. (From Boudoulas H and Wooley CF: *Mitral regurgitation chronic versus acute: Implications for timing of surgery.* In Bowen JM, Mazzaferri EL, eds: *Contemporary internal medicine,* New York and London, 1991, Plenum.)

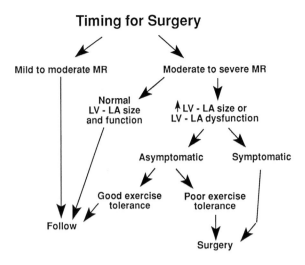

Fig. 3-37. Timing for surgery in patients with chronic MR, based on left ventricular (LV) and left atrial (A) size and function and exercise tolerance. (From Boudoulas H and Wooley CF: *Mitral regurgitation chronic versus acute: Implications for timing of surgery.* In Bowen JM, Mazzaferri EL, eds: *Contemporary internal medicine,* New York and London, 1991, Plenum.)

may occur. Thus preoperative ejection fraction may not be a good predictor of postoperative ejection fraction, but when the ejection fraction is frankly subnormal survival is greatly reduced. This decision must be made with comprehensive knowledge of the individual patient's natural history, individual indicators of left ventricular function, and the evolving state of mitral valve surgery for mitral regurgitation.

Development of symptoms in chronic mitral regurgitation usually coincides with onset of left ventricular dysfunction. As such, even mild symptoms are probably significant. If symptoms are present and ventricular function has begun to decline, surgery should be considered. A question often asked is "how should I manage the asymptomatic patient who is beginning to show signs of left ventricular dysfunction by physical or echocardiographic examination?" It is difficult to recommend surgery for a truly asymptomatic patient. The guidelines for operative intervention, based in part on signs of developing left ventricular dysfunction, are not perfect predictors of outcome. Thus a poor outcome could occur despite favorable preoperative indexes. Some patients who claim to be asymptomatic have in fact limited their activities to avoid symptoms. In most instances, an exercise tolerance test will

help delineate normal or reduced exercise tolerance. The patient who is truly asymptomatic, who has normal exercise tolerance in an objective evaluation, and who is beginning to show signs of left ventricular dysfunction by echocardiography, requires very close follow-up. If symptoms intervene, left ventricular function continues to worsen, or response to medical therapy is limited, mitral valve surgery should be considered (Fig. 3-37).

Timing for surgery for chronic mitral regurgitation other than mitral valve prolapse

Patients with coronary artery disease and mitral regurgitation should undergo cardiac diagnostic studies to delineate coronary anatomy, mitral valve, left atrial and left ventricular function. Myocardial revascularization with or without mitral valve surgery should be considered with hemodynamic deterioration. It is likely, but not proven, that mitral valve repair is preferable to replacement. Surgical mortality in patients with coronary artery disease and mitral regurgitation is high (between 10% and 30%). Surgery before hemodynamic deterioration may improve survival; data are lacking at present, however. Nevertheless, at present the long-term prognosis for patients with associated severe left ventricular dysfunction remains poor.

The indications for mitral valve surgery in patients with rheumatic mitral regurgitation are similar to those outlined for patients with mitral valve prolapse. Reconstructive surgery can be performed in certain patients with rheumatic mitral valve disease and can result in low hospital and late mortality. In certain patients with acute or subacute mitral regurgitation secondary to rheumatic fever, early surgical intervention may be necessary.[105-109]

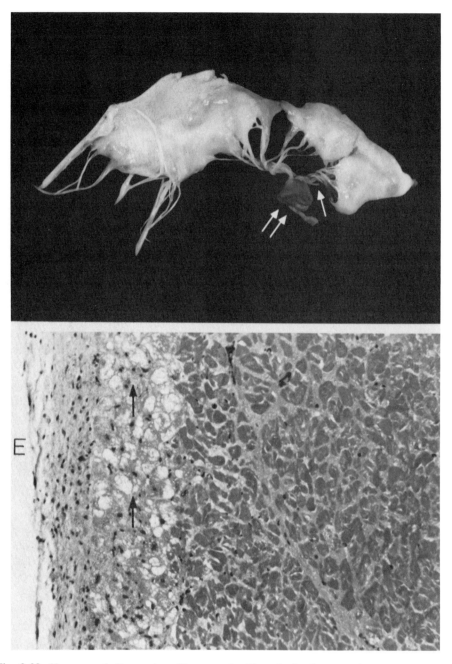

Fig. 3-38. Upper panel: Ruptured papillary muscle. The mitral valve posterior papillary muscle rupture was due to recent infarction *(arrows)*. Anterior papillary muscle is not shown. The ruptured end had been previously excised for histology. The muscle is mottled. Note the twisting of the attached chordae tendineae (arrow) which reflects the free movement of the avulsed papillary muscle tip. Lower panel: Ruptured papillary muscle with recent infarction. This is a histologic section of the papillary muscle seen in the upper panel. Endocardium *(E)* is present at the far left with advanced necrosis of muscle fibers in the center and right portion of the photograph. Between the endocardium and necrotic myocardium is a zone of ischemic myocytes showing cytoplasmic vacuolization or myocytolysis *(arrows)*. Hematoxylin and eosin, × 180. (From Boudoulas H and Wooley CF: *Mitral regurgitation chronic versus acute: Implications for timing of surgery.* In Bowen JM, Mazzaferri EL, eds: *Contemporary Internal Medicine,* New York and London, 1991, Plenum.)

Acute mitral regurgitation

Papillary muscle rupture. This condition occurs in 0.3% to .95% of acute myocardial infarctions, usually within the first week of the acute episode (see also Ischemic Heart Disease). The posterior papillary muscle is affected several times more often than the anterior papillary muscle. The explanation given for this propensity of the posterior papillary muscle to rupture is an anatomic one. The posterior papillary muscle is commonly supplied by branches of both the circumflex and the right coronary arteries. Thus the likelihood of reperfusion is enhanced in the posterior papillary muscle. In a recent autopsy study of 133 cases of acute myocardial infarction, 25 cases of papillary muscle rupture were identified. The anterior papillary muscle was involved in 4 cases, the posterior in 13 cases, and both muscles in 8 cases.[97] Morphologically, one sees the detachment of the head of the papillary muscle because of the formation of hematoma and contraction band necrosis of myocytes (Fig. 3-38).

The usual typical clinical presentation of complete rupture of the papillary muscle is that of abrupt development of acute pulmonary edema. However, the clinical picture is somewhat different, and the survival of the patient is more likely if only one of the apical heads of a papillary muscle is ruptured.[67,110-12]

Infectious endocarditis. Both leaflets of the mitral valve may be involved in infectious endocarditis. Although the infection may occur in a previously normal valve, it is most often seen in valves damaged by either rheumatic disease or mitral valve prolapse. Infectious endocarditis high up in the ventricular aspect of the anterior mitral valve leaflet may spread beneath the aortic cusps and create an infective aneurysm. The extent of the valvular destruction in infectious endocarditis clearly depends on the virulence of the organism involved and the resistance of the host. Flat solid vegetations with more fibrosis and less destruction are seen in less virulent organisms. Vegetations in atrioventricular valves are seen along the line of closure and may extend along the chordae and mural endocarditis. These vegetations usually vary in size, are reddish-yellow or gray depending on the stage of organization, are friable and easy to embolize.[67]

Rupture of chordae tendineae. As it has been stated previously, chordae tendineae may rupture secondary to trauma, infectious endocarditis, rarely due to acute rheumatic fever, during pregnancy, or in cases of mitral valve prolapse. There are, however, cases that are not associated with the above conditions in which the chordae are ruptured, and therefore are classified as idiopathic. A histologic examination of these cases reveals some myxomatous degeneration of the ruptured chordae almost identical to the myxoid changes seen in chordae of mitral valve prolapse. The degree of regurgitation resulting from chordal rupture depends on the number and location of the chordae, as well as the condition of the mitral valve.[67]

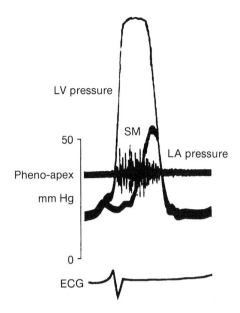

Fig. 3-39. Simultaneous recordings of left ventricular (LV) and left atrial (LA) pressures with external phonocardiogram obtained from the cardiac apex (phono-apex) in a patient with acute mitral regurgitation. Note the large V wave in the LA pressure tracing. As the LA pressure increases during LV systole the systolic pressure gradient diminishes and the intensity of the systolic murmur decreases. (From Boudoulas H and Wooley CF: *Mitral regurgitation chronic versus acute: Implications for timing of surgery.* In Bowen JM, Mazzaferri EL, eds: *Contemporary Internal Medicine,* New York and London, 1991, Plenum.)

Pathophysiology of acute mitral regurgitation. Patients with acute mitral regurgitation have entirely different clinical presentation than patients with chronic mitral regurgitation. This reflects the unique pathophysiology of acute mitral regurgitation.

The immediate direct effects of regurgitant blood flow into the left atrium in patients with acute mitral regurgitation are obvious because there is no time for left atrial adaptation. In severe acute mitral regurgitation, a large regurgitant volume is ejected into the left atrium during ventricular systole. Since there is no time for the left atrium and left ventricle to dilate, the large left atrial volume and consequently the large left ventricular diastolic volume will result in striking elevation of left atrial and left ventricular diastolic pressures. Left atrial V wave pressures of 60 mm Hg or greater are not uncommon (Fig. 3-39). The marked increase in pulmonary venous pressure results in pulmonary congestion and pulmonary edema. The patient complains of severe dyspnea. Since the left ventricle is of normal size and a large amount of blood goes into the left atrium during ventricular systole, the forward left ventricular stroke volume is markedly diminished. The net result is tissue hypoperfusion, low cardiac output, hypotension, and shock[67,113-115] (Fig. 3-40).

Diagnostic evaluation. The etiology of most common causes of acute mitral regurgitation are shown in the box

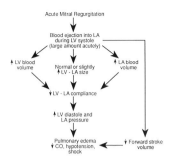

Fig. 3-40. Pathophysiologic mechanisms in acute mitral regurgitation. Schematic presentation. LV = left ventricle, LA = left atrium, CO = cardiac output, ↑ = increase, ↓ = decrease. (From Boudoulas H and Wooley CF: *Mitral regurgitation chronic versus acute: Implications for timing of surgery.* In Bowen JM, Mazzaferri EL, eds: *Contemporary Internal Medicine,* New York and London, 1991, Plenum.)

on p. 82. Clinically distinguishing the three most common types of acute mitral regurgitation (papillary muscle rupture, infectious endocarditis, and chordae tendineae rupture) is reasonably straightforward.

Acute myocardial infarction often results in transient or permanent mild mitral regurgitation. Papillary muscle rupture or significant papillary muscle dysfunction results in severe mitral regurgitation; this usually leads to death in hours or a few days, unless surgical correction is possible.

Patients with infectious endocarditis usually have other systemic manifestations of the disease; mitral regurgitation usually is mild to moderate in severity, but occasionally, especially in patients with preexisting mitral regurgitation, severe mitral regurgitation may occur.

Rupture of chordae tendineae is the most common cause of acute mitral regurgitation in an otherwise healthy person. Thus, rupture of chordae tendineae should be suspected in the absence of other obvious causes.[67,99,110,116-117]

Natural history of acute mitral regurgitation

In cases of severe acute mitral regurgitation, the patient's clinical status deteriorates rapidly despite "good" medical management and usually leads to death without surgical intervention. The natural history of other causes of acute mitral regurgitation (without myocardial infarction) depends on the etiology, the degree of mitral valve dysfunction, the severity of the mitral regurgitation, and the functional status of the left ventricle and left atrium. Patients with less severe mitral regurgitation, especially with mitral regurgitation secondary to infectious endocarditis, may progress less rapidly, respond to medical therapy, and may not require emergency surgical intervention. The same is true in certain patients with chordae tendineae rupture when the mitral regurgitation is not severe and the patient remains in sinus rhythm.[67]

Timing for surgery of acute mitral regurgitation

Patients with acute severe mitral regurgitation, pulmonary congestion and hypotension require emergency surgical intervention. Any delay will result in irreversible clinical deterioration. Mitral valve reconstructive surgery is preferable when feasible, but mitral valve replacement may be necessary in certain circumstances. Patients with less severe acute mitral regurgitation without pulmonary congestion or tissue hypoperfusion may be managed medically without emergency surgical intervention. Decisions about surgical therapy should be based on the patient's symptoms, clinical status, the presence of atrial fibrillation, left ventricular and left atrial size and function as discussed above in patients with chronic mitral regurgitation. Reperfusion therapy with thrombolysis or angioplasty has been successful in restoring valve competence in patients with less severe ischemic acute mitral regurgitation.[67]

Hemodynamically unstable patients with acute mitral regurgitation should be considered for emergency surgery regardless of the etiology. Occasionally, emergency surgery may be necessary in hemodynamically stable patients with infectious endocarditis who have extensive floating mitral valvular vegetations with a threat of embolism; however, data about these patients are limited at present.

Mixed mitral valve disease

As it has been stated earlier, chronic rheumatic valve disease might be presented by fusion of the commissures, as well as scarring and shrinkage of the valvular leaflets. These morphologic changes may produce a combination of mitral valve regurgitation and mitral valve stenosis in patients with rheumatic valvular disease. Patients with mixed mitral valve disease usually have hemodynamic and, therefore, clinical findings of both stenosis and regurgitation, although one of the two conditions usually predominates. Fatigue favors dominant regurgitation, while dyspnea favors dominant stenosis. The size of the left ventricular chamber is a good way to determine the dominant lesion in mixed mitral valve disease. An enlarged left ventricle most often suggests valvular regurgitation; a small left ventricle points to mitral valve stenosis. However, definite recognition of the combination of the two conditions requires noninvasive or invasive diagnostic procedures.

Lupus erythematosus can be the cause of mixed mitral disease, the so-called Libman-Sacks endocarditis, producing bland vegetations, fibrinoid necrosis, and diffuse inflammation of the valve substance and chordae, which may lead to fusion of those structures.

Mitral valve regurgitation associated with prosthetic heart valves

Regurgitation in such valves may be due to paravalvular leaks secondary to dehiscence, or secondary to a thrombus positioned in a manner that interferes with the motion of the poppet or disc. With porcine mitral valve prosthesis

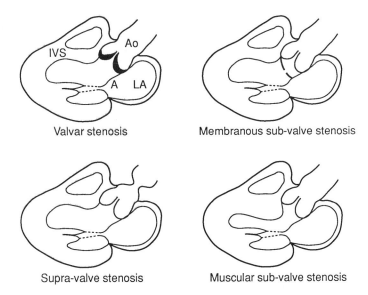

Valvar stenosis   Membranous sub-valve stenosis

Supra-valve stenosis   Muscular sub-valve stenosis

Fig. 3-41. Left ventricular outflow obstruction. The levels at which left ventricular outflow obstruction can occur. The diagrams represent a long-axis echocardiographic plane and highlight the fact that the anterior cusp of the mitral valve *(A)* is one component of the left ventricular outflow at sub valve level. The other component is the interventricular septum (IVS). Obstruction can occur above the valve, at the valve or below the valve. Below the valve, obstruction arises either from muscular hypertrophy of the interventricular septum, or from a membrane. (From Davies MJ: *Color atlas of cardiovascular pathology.* Oxford, UK, 1986, Harvey Miller Publishers, Oxford University Press.)

one may observe degenerative changes of the leaflets, which may become stiff and therefore improperly closed.

AORTIC VALVE
Anatomy and pathology

Although the aortic and pulmonary valves are essentially identical in structure, their function and susceptibility to disease are quite different, because of pressure differences in the two circulations.[47] Both valves contain three cusps which are prevented from prolapsing into the respective ventricles during diastole as the pressure in the two major vessels exceeds that of the ventricles. The semilunar shape of the cusps permits significant overlap and apposition, which during diastole is 40% or more.

In the aortic valve the three cusps are referred to as the right coronary cusp, the left coronary cusp, and the noncoronary cusp. The sinuses of Valsalva, which are located behind the cusps, are saccular dilatations of the proximal aorta. The upper border of the sinuses is defined by an intimal thickening first described by Leonardo da Vinci. This supraaortic ridge, which runs circumferentially at the level of the uppermost point of the commissures, is an important landmark because it represents the functional diameter of the aorta. The tricuspid configuration of the semilunar valves allows them to open completely without impediment of the blood flow. Therefore there is no measurable pressure gradient across a normal semilunar valve.[47]

Age-related changes in the aortic valve are well known and are interpreted as wear and tear phenomena. One of

these changes with age is increased diameter of the aortic annulus. Calcification of the annulus after the age of 65 is not uncommon. Paracommissural fenestrations of cusps are part of the aging process, although those have no hemodynamic significance. Lambl's excrescences at the free, closing edge and nodule of Arantius are common with aging. These early aging changes result from deposits of fibroelastic tissue that cause stiffness of the cusps. Similarly, deposits of lipid in the cusps, as well as calcium deposits are noted in elderly individuals. The more advanced phenomena of wear and tear of the aortic valve are characterized by nodular calcific lesions towards the aortic wall of the cusps, often in continuation with the aortic annulus calcification. The hinge-like motion of the annulus and cusps is often abolished as the result of these calcific deposits. All of the above degenerative changes favor stenosis and only rarely regurgitation, with or without stenosis.

As is the case with mitral valve disease, the type and character of aortic valve diseases have changed considerably in the last 30 years. The most important factors for these changes are the decline of rheumatic heart disease and the increased longevity of the population. As the above changes in recent years have altered the etiologies of mitral valve disease, they have also changed the etiology of aortic stenosis from rheumatic to nonrheumatic.

AORTIC STENOSIS

The outflow tract of the left ventricle may be obstructed at the valvular, supravalvular or subvalvular level (Fig. 3-41). Of these, valvular aortic stenosis is by far the most

A 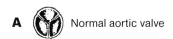 Normal aortic valve

B Bicuspid aortic valve (congenital)

C Rheumatic aortic valve

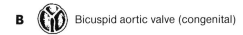

Fig. 3-42. Pathology of aortic stenosis. Normal tricuspid aortic valve, bicuspid aortic valve, and rheumatic aortic stenosis are shown. Note that in rheumatic aortic stenosis the commissures are fused and the valve leaflets are thickened. Calcium deposits are present in senile aortic stenosis. within the cups of the aortic valve without primarily affecting the commissaries. (Modified from Brandenburg RO, Fuster V, Giuliani E: Valvular heart disease. When should the patient be referred? *Pract Cardiol* 5:50, 1979; Fuster V, Brandenburg RO, Giuliani E, [119] et al, with permission *Pract Cardiol;* 3:50, 1979.)

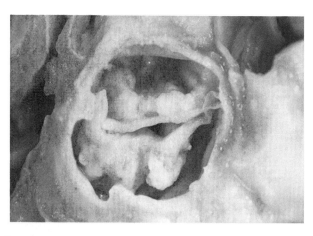

Fig. 3-43. Postinflammatory aortic stenosis (rheumatic). Note fusion of all three commissures.

Valvular aortic stenosis: etiology

Congenital
Postinflammatory
Calcific bicuspid
Calcific senile

---

common.[118] Whatever the level of obstruction, the functional effect on the left ventricular myocardium is the same, i.e., chronic pressure overload. In this chapter only valvular aortic stenosis will be described; the other entities will be discussed in other chapters.

Valvular aortic stenosis

The major etiologies of valvular aortic stenosis are shown in the box below and Fig. 3-42.[118-126]

Congenital malformed valves. In this category, conditions such as bicuspid valve with fused commissures, dome-shaped valves with a central orifice, or unicommissural valves, are associated with stenosis at birth. In all such conditions calcification occurs as early as the teens.

Postinflammatory aortic stenosis. This term was devised to stress that not all cases are postrheumatic. Rheumatoid arthritis, ankylosing spondylitis, systemic lupus erythematosus, and other conditions may give somewhat similar anatomic alterations.

The fibrosis of the cusps in postrheumatic aortic stenosis is fairly uniform and appears like a coating of white candle wax over the cusps (Fig. 3-43). Fusion of one or more commissures results in stenosis of the valve. Calcification of both the ventricular and aortic aspects of the cusps produces rigidity and contributes to stenosis. In some cases with primarily fibrosis and cusp retraction, but no significant commissural fusion, the result may be aortic insufficiency. Certain combinations of anatomic alterations may result in both stenosis and regurgitation. There is no annular dilatation in the post-inflammatory aortic valve disease.

Histologic examination of excised valves from postin-flammatory aortic valve disease offers limited information, particularly when the cusps are heavily calcified. The presence of vascularization of the cusps indicates rheumatic or other inflammatory etiologies. However, any specificity of such histologic findings as to the rheumatic etiology is questionable.

Calcific bicuspid. The most common variety (3/4) of this congenital abnormality is the one that has two cusps, one anterior and one posterior. The two coronary ostia arise from the anterior cusp, which contains a raphe (false commissure) in the anterior cusp. In the right and left cusp variety (1/4) of bicuspid valve, the ostia arise from the two sinuses; the raphe is always in the right cusp.

Identifying an acquired bicuspid valve is not always easy. In the acquired bicuspid valve, the cusp containing the fused commissure is almost twice as long as the remaining cusp. However, in congenital bicuspid valve the cusp with the raphe may be equal with the other cusp or only slightly longer, but never twice the length of the non-conjoined cusp. An interesting identification point for the conjoined cusp is that it is usually notched on the free edge.

Biscuspid aortic valve is seen three to four times more often in men than in women. It occurs in about 1% of the normal population. Therefore, theoretically at least 1% of the population is at risk of developing aortic valve stenosis

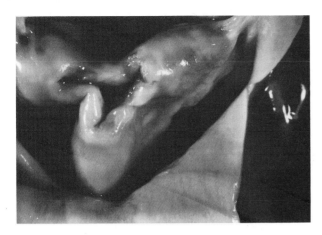

Fig. 3-44. Severely calcified, stenotic bicuspid aortic valve. Note that the commissures are not fused.

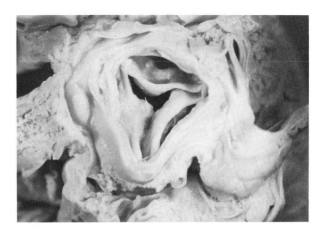

Fig. 3-45. Calcific, senile, (degenerative) aortic stenosis. Note that the commissures are not fused, the calcific deposits are deep in the sinuses and the free edges of the cusps are thick.

by 40 to 50 years of age. Since 1% of the population does not develop aortic valvular stenosis, there must be considerable variation in the susceptibility of individuals to develop cusp calcification, the causes of which are unknown.

The histoarchitecture of distribution of calcific deposits seen in a bicuspid aortic valve are quite different from the ones seen in calcification of tricuspid, senile, stenotic aortic valve. In the bicuspid stenotic valve, the distribution of calcium is throughout the body of the cusp (Fig. 3-44). In the senile form of nodular aortic stenosis, there is a cleavage plane between the calcific nodules and the underlying fibrotic cusp. The reason for the differences in those two histoarchitectural types of aortic stenosis may be related to the duration of the degenerative process. The degenerative process starts earlier in life in the congenital bicuspid valve than in the tricuspid aortic valve. Different types of stress distribution in the two valves may also play a role. Poststenotic dilatation is a common finding in patients with aortic stenosis. Although morphologic changes of the aortic wall have not been described, aortic distensibility has been reported to be abnormal.[126a]

Calcific senile. Primary degenerative calcification of tricuspid aortic valves occurs in the seventh to ninth decades, starts at the base of the cusps and progresses towards the edges (Fig. 3-45). This senile aortic stenosis accounts for approximately 10% to 30% of all cases. Statistics may underestimate the incidence of degenerative calcification of the aortic valve because most of the information available comes from surgically excised valves. Many elderly people with degenerative calcific aortic stenosis may not be candidates for surgery and therefore are not included in the above statistics.

Pathophysiology

In patients with significant aortic stenosis there is a pressure gradient across the aortic valve (Fig. 3-46), which results in increased left ventricular systolic and diastolic

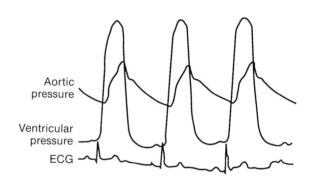

Fig. 3-46. Simultaneous recordings of aortic pressure, left ventricular pressure, and the electrocardiogram (ECG) in a patient with aortic stenosis. Note the pressure difference (gradient) between the left ventricle and the aorta.

pressure, decreased aortic pressure, and prolongation of the left ventricular ejection time (Fig. 3-47). Further, the stenotic valve prevents rapid ejection of blood during ventricular systole. Therefore the left ventricle ejects the blood by a sustained rather than the normal rapid ejection. Normally the blood flow through the aortic valve peaks early in systole. In moderate aortic stenosis, flow is delayed and peak is reached at the midpoint of the systolic period; in severe aortic stenosis, peak flow is reached at the end of the systolic ejection period. Thus in aortic stenosis, maximal wall tension is delayed and mean systolic wall tension is higher than that expected from the increased left ventricular pressure alone.[127-129]

In patients with stenosis, the left ventricular end-diastolic pressure is increased. This is caused by left ventricular hypertrophy and decreased left ventricular compliance while the left ventricular volume is normal (Fig. 3-48).

The most common symptoms in patients with aortic ste-

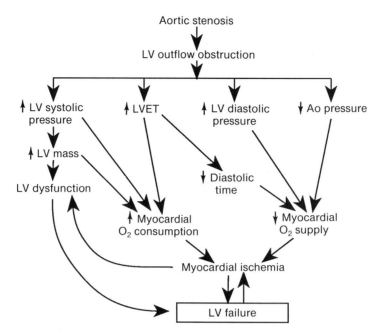

Fig. 3-47. Pathophysiology of aortic stenosis. Left ventricular (LV) outflow obstruction results in an increased LV systolic pressure, increased left ventricular ejection time (LVET), increased left ventricular diastolic pressure and decreased aortic (Ao) pressure. Increased LV systolic pressure with LV volume overload will increase LV mass, which may lead to LV dysfunction and failure. Increased LV systolic pressure, LV mass and LVET will increase myocardial oxygen (O_2) consumption. Increased left ventricular ejection time will result in a decrease of diastolic time (myocardial perfusion time). Increased LV diastolic pressure and decreased Ao diastolic pressure will decrease coronary perfusion pressure. Decreased diastolic time and coronary perfusion pressure will decrease myocardial O_2 supply. Increased myocardial O_2 consumption and decreased myocardial O_2 supply will produce myocardial ischemia, which will further deteriorate LV function. (↑ = increased, ↓ = decreased)

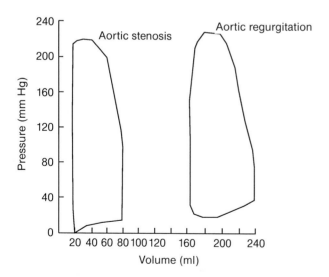

Fig. 3-48. Pressure volume relationship in patients with aortic stenosis and regurgitation. Note that in aortic stenosis the left ventricular volume (ml/m²) remains within normal range while the pressure increases. In aortic regurgitation the left ventricular volume could be markedly increased.

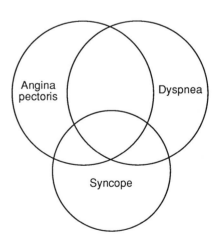

Fig. 3-49. Major symptoms in aortic stenosis. Angina pectoris, dyspnea and syncope may be present as isolated symptoms or in combination.

nosis are congestive heart failure, angina and syncope (Fig. 3-49). The pathophysiologic mechanism of these symptoms is described briefly.

Congestive heart failure. Two major pathophysiologic factors for the pathogenesis of congestive heart failure in patients with aortic stenosis have been identified. The first factor is left ventricular diastolic dysfunction with decreased ventricular compliance. The second factor is systolic dysfunction, secondary to left ventricular pressure work load (see Fig. 3-47). The increased left ventricular work load results in concentric left ventricular hypertrophy. Due to the compensatory concentric left ventricular hypertrophy, end-systolic and end-diastolic left ventricular volumes remain normal until the late stages of the disease. Left ventricular hypertrophy, however, results in decreased compliance and increased ventricular diastolic pressure. High left ventricular diastolic pressure will be transmitted to the left atrium, pulmonary veins, and pulmonary capillaries, resulting in pulmonary edema and dyspnea.[127-130]

In addition to left ventricular hypertrophy there is a left atrial enlargement in patients with aortic stenosis that is directly related to left ventricular mass. The underlying mechanism(s) for the increased left atrial maximal volume are incompletely understood. It is reasonable, however, to assume that the structural and functional changes of the left ventricle lead to an impediment of blood flow during left atrial passive emptying and induce a decrease in left atrial passive emptying fraction, thus increasing left atrial volume at onset of atrial systole. Increased left atrial volume at onset of atrial systole with normal or decreased left atrial active emptying fraction will result in an increased left atrial minimal volume. Assuming the flow from the pulmonary venous return remains within normal limits, the increased left atrial minimal volume will lead to an increased left atrial maximal volume.

There is a rapid deterioration of patients with aortic stenosis with the development of symptoms of congestive heart failure (Fig. 3-50). A vicious cycle is then created, because increased afterload may depress left ventricular function further on. When the compensatory mechanism of myocardial hypertrophy is consumed, the only remaining compensatory mechanism is to increase preload by water and salt retention, elevation of plasma volume, and end-diastolic volume. In a stiff chamber this would lead to further elevation of the diastolic pressure and pulmonary edema. Dyspnea in patients with aortic stenosis indicates increase of left ventricular diastolic pressure, which interferes with the ventricular diastolic filling from the left atrium.

Angina and syncope may develop in the early symptomatic stage of aortic stenosis, even though the left ventricular function is still good.

Angina. Hypoperfusion of the subendocardial layers with anginal pain may develop in patients with aortic stenosis, even in the absence of significant coronary artery

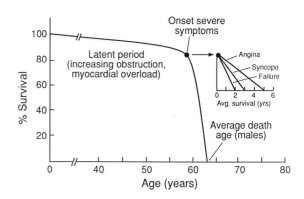

Fig. 3-50. Natural history of aortic stenosis without operative treatment. (From Ross J Jr, Braunwald E: Aortic stenosis, *Circulation* 38 [Suppl V]: 61, 1968.)

disease (See also Ischemic Heart Disease, Chapter 2). In aortic stenosis, reduced coronary artery pressure is due to left ventricular aortic pressure gradient. In addition, increased left ventricular diastolic pressure will result in decreased coronary perfusion pressure and decreased coronary blood flow. The Venturi effect (reduced flow into coronary ostia because of the rapid flow through a constricted valve orifice) is another factor contributing to low coronary flow. Several other factors have also been suggested as playing a role in the angina seen in aortic stenosis. Mechanical compression of the intramural vessels by the contracting hypertrophic myocardium results in increased distance between capillaries because the left ventricular hypertrophy is not accompanied by a parallel increase in capillaries. The increased duration of left ventricular ejection and increased wall tension will increase myocardial oxygen consumption. The net result is increased myocardial oxygen consumption and decreased coronary blood flow. These changes create an imbalance between oxygen demand and supply, resulting in myocardial ischemia and angina pectoris. Coexisting coronary artery disease in aortic stenosis obviously will precipitate myocardial ischemia and chest pain.[121,123,128]

Syncope. Characteristically, syncope occurs during exercise but may also occur immediately after exercise. An abrupt rise in left ventricular pressure during exercise without a corresponding increase in aortic pressure may stimulate left ventricular baroreceptors, resulting in decreased peripheral vascular resistance, hypotension and syncope. Syncope may be mediated by access vagal tone triggered by ventricular stretch receptors that are activated by increased wall stress during exertion. Obviously cardiac arrhythmias and decreased cardiac output are contributory factors. Syncopal attacks may be associated with sudden death.[131-133]

Evaluation of the severity of aortic stenosis

Recommendations for replacement of the stenotic aortic valve are usually based on clinical symptoms, such as angina, syncope and dyspnea, and laboratory data obtained from the echocardiographic and Doppler echocardiographic studies, and cardiac catheterization. To date aortic valve area can be measured with a high degree of accuracy. Coexisting aortic regurgitation, however, decreases the accuracy of the methods, especially of Doppler echocardiography.[58,134-138]

As people of different body size need different size valves, valve area should be corrected for body surface area, to obtain the aortic valve area index (aortic valve area cm^2/m^2).

Natural history of aortic stenosis

It is known that aortic stenosis may have a long asymptomatic stage that may last for decades[139-149] (see Fig. 3-50). It seems that the resistance to flow presented by a transvalvular gradient occurs when the orifice is reduced to about 1 cm^2. Symptoms are rarely developed before moderate or moderately severe aortic stenosis develops, and sometimes patients remain asymptomatic even with severe aortic stenosis. It has been reported though, that symptomatic patients with hemodynamically significant aortic stenosis are at significant risk for serious cardiac events within 2 to 4 years.[141]

In a prospective study of 35 patients with severe aortic stenosis who refused surgery (valve area <.8 cm^2 documented by cardiac catheterization), the average survival after the onset of symptoms was 23 months.[144] The mean survival after occurrence of angina was 45 months, after syncope 27 months, and after onset of heart failure 11 months. The same authors followed 142 patients who had an aortic valve area greater than 1.5 cm^2 as defined by invasive hemodynamic techniques. Eighty-eight percent of those patients after 10 years continue to have mild aortic stenosis. Four percent had the moderate form, and 8% progressed to severe aortic stenosis and required aortic valve replacement.

Progression in severity of stenosis may occur by either the size of the valve orifice becoming smaller (fixed orifice type) or the cusps becoming more rigid (calcific type). Remember, however, that in children with congenital type aortic stenosis, changes in severity of stenosis may reflect growth of the heart with general body growth in relation to possible changes in aortic valve and valve orifice.

It appears that the progression of aortic stenosis in patients with postinflammatory valvular disease is rather slow. Stenosis, however, progresses rapidly in patients with calcific aortic stenosis, particularly in the elderly. This is probably due to increased calcification and reduced valve mobility.

There is a well-known propensity to sudden death in patients with aortic stenosis. This is of particular concern in congenital aortic stenosis in the pediatric population. The risk, however, for cardiac sudden death in aortic stenosis is significantly less than that of either hypertrophic cardiomyopathy or congenital abnormalities of the coronary arteries.

Although data regarding infectious endocarditis in aortic stenosis are insufficient, evidence suggests that the incidence of infectious endocarditis in congenital aortic stenosis is 1.6 in 1000 patient years.

Cardiac arrhythmias are also seen in patients with aortic stenosis. Atrial fibrillation, estimated to be present in about 10% of the patients (particularly older patients), probably reflects the presence of left atrial myopathy. First degree atrioventricular block is relatively common in patients with aortic stenosis but complete atrioventricular block is rare. The incidence of ventricular arrhythmias is also high and reflects the degree of left ventricular hypertrophy, fibrosis, and myocardial ischemia.

Aortic stenosis in the elderly may manifest with gastrointestinal bleeding due to colonic vascular ectasia (angiodysplasia).[143] This is more common in the cecum and ascending colon. Microscopically, dilated mucosal and submucosal vessels are visible.

AORTIC REGURGITATION

In contrast to aortic valvular stenosis, which has a rather limited number of causes, aortic valvular regurgitation may be caused by a multiplicity of conditions (see box

---

Chronic aortic regurgitation: etiology

Congenital

Bicuspid aortic valve
Interventricular septal defect
Sinus of Valsalva aneurysm

Heritable disorders of connective tissue

Marfan syndrome
Ehlers-Danlos syndrome
Adult polycystic kidney disease
Osteogenesis imperfecta
Annuloaortic ectasia
Cystic media necrosis
Prolapse

Rheumatic

Less common disorders associated with aortic regurgitation
Syphilis
Aortitis (Takayasu)
Autoimmune diseases
Ankylosing spondylitis
Reiter's syndrome
Rheumatoid arthritis
Systemic lupus erythematosus

Hypertension (pressure and volume overload)
Regurgitation following aortic valve surgery

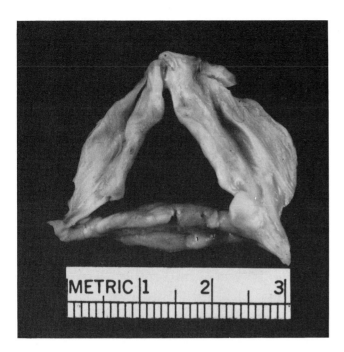

Fig. 3-51. Aortic insufficiency of postinflammatory etiology. Note rolled, reduced height of cusps, and fusion of one commissure (Courtesy of Dr. William D. Edwards, Mayo Clinic).

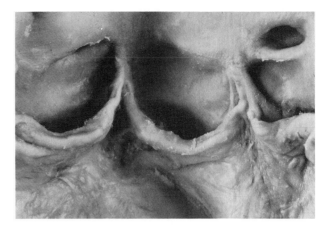

Fig. 3-52. Postinflammatory (rheumatic) chronic aortic regurgitation. Note rolled free cuspal edges, reduced height of cusps with exposure of the coronary ostia, and minimal commissural fusion (Courtesy of Dr. William D. Edwards, Mayo Clinic).

above). Disease processes that directly affect the valve and the proximal aorta may result in aortic regurgitation.[150-154]

Conditions that produce aortic regurgitation by primarily affecting the aortic valve are rheumatic heart disease, bicuspid aortic valve, infectious endocarditis, idiopathic myxomatous degeneration of the aortic valve (aortic valve prolapse), trauma, and aortic regurgitation in prosthetic valves.

Conditions that produce aortic regurgitation by affecting the diameter of the proximal portion of the ascending aorta are heritable disorders of the connective tissue, inflammatory diseases including Takayasu disease, ankylosing spondylitis, and syphilis.

Aortic regurgitation could be acute or chronic. The pathophysiology, hemodynamics and natural history of chronic aortic regurgitation differ considerably from the acute aortic regurgitation. Similarly, the anatomic findings from the heart are quite dissimilar in chronic compared to acute aortic regurgitation.

Chronic aortic regurgitation

Chronic aortic regurgitation subjects the left ventricle to volume overload, resulting in increased left ventricular volume with a globular heart, and increased left ventricular mass. Anatomic findings indicating altered hemodynamics in regurgitant valves may present as jet lesions in the ventricular endocardium at the outflow tract of the left ventricle, apparently induced by the regurgitant stream.[154] Similarly, white fibrous pockets may be found below the

aortic valve, indicative of an impinging regurgitant flow. Fibrosis, thickening, and retraction may be seen in the anterior leaflet of the mitral valve in cases of longstanding chronic aortic regurgitation.

Aortic regurgitation due to congenitally malformed valve. Although in the majority of cases the valve has a bicuspid configuration, a quadricuspid or unicuspid aortic valve may also be incompetent. In rare cases a tricuspid valve may be incompetent because of an inequality of the cusps (most often one cusp is smaller than the other two), resulting in imperfect apposition during diastole. Aortic regurgitation due to a congenital malformation of the aortic valve is usually mild and well tolerated, except when the abnormal valve becomes the site of infectious endocarditis.

A high ventricular septal defect is occasionally associated with aortic regurgitation as one of the cusps (usually the noncoronary cusp) prolapses into the defect below. Secondary phenomena of these prolapsed valves may occur, resulting in fibrosis and retraction of the cusps.

In some cases aortic regurgitation may be secondary to sinus of Valsalva aneurysm.

Rheumatic etiology aortic regurgitation. Rheumatic valvulitis is a disease process that is known to affect primarily the mitral valve or a combination of mitral and aortic valve and rarely the tricuspid valve. Therefore isolated rheumatic aortic regurgitation without mitral disease is considered uncommon. Aortic regurgitation is usually associated with some degree of aortic stenosis secondary to a commissural fusion, which as it was stated before, is the hallmark of chronic rheumatic valvular disease (Figs. 3-51 and 3-52).

Aortic regurgitation due to aortic root dilatation. In cases of aortic root dilatation, aortic regurgitation occurs because the area of the valve leaflets is not sufficient to seal the area of the aortic valve (Fig. 3-53).

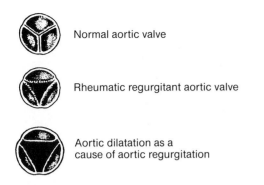

Fig. 3-53. Variations of the aortic valve. Normal aortic valve, shortening of the cusps in rheumatic aortic regurgitation, and dilatation of the aorta as the cause of aortic regurgitation are shown. (Modified from Roberts WC: *Valvular, subvalvular, and supravalvular aortic stenosis: Morphologic features.* In *Clinical pathologic correlations,* Philadelphia, 1973, F.A. Davis.)

Pathophysiology of chronic aortic valve regurgitation. Aortic regurgitation causes an increase of left ventricular stroke volume, and results in left ventricular volume overload (Fig. 3-54). The left ventricular end-diastolic volume is increased proportionally to the quantity of regurgitant blood flow. Over a long period the left ventricular diastolic pressure will increase and will be transmitted to the left atrium, pulmonary veins and pulmonary capillaries, with resulting pulmonary congestion and dyspnea. Large stroke volume will result in increased left ventricular and aortic systolic pressure. Large regurgital flow back to the ventricle will result in decreased aortic diastolic pressure. Early in the course of the disease left ventricular compliance is normal or increased, but later when the contractile function of the left ventricle starts to decline, diastolic function also becomes abnormal and ventricular compliance decreases. Decreased compliance perhaps reflects intramyocardial changes, such as myocyte degeneration and interstitial fibrosis.[154-160]

The wide pulse pressure (high systolic low diastolic pressure) creates marked pulsations in peripheral arteries. The decreased aortic diastolic pressure affects the coronary perfusion and further compromises the marginal supply and demand of a hypertrophic myocardium.

Aortic insufficiency results in significant increase of left ventricular afterload and systolic wall stress. Systolic wall stress in its simplest form is expressed by the Laplace relation, stress $= \dfrac{p \times r}{2h}$ (p = left ventricular pressure, r = radius and h = wall thickness). In aortic insufficiency, both systolic pressure and radius are increased, and wall thickness, even if slightly increased, cannot compensate for the increases of the other two factors (see Fig. 3-48).

Systolic wall stress and oxygen consumption are much greater in patients with aortic regurgitation compared with patients with an equivalent volume of mitral regurgitation. Recovery of ventricular function after valve replacement is better for patients with aortic regurgitation compared with

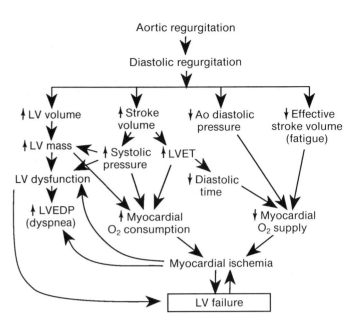

Fig. 3-54. Pathophysiology of aortic regurgitation. Aortic regurgitation will result in an increased left ventricular (LV) volume, increased stroke volume, increased aortic (Ao) systolic pressure, and decreased effective stroke volume. Increased LV volume will result in an increased LV mass, which may lead to LV dysfunction and failure. Increased LV stroke volume will produce an increased systolic pressure and prolongation of left ventricular ejection time (LVET). Increased LV systolic pressure will result in further increase in LV mass. Increased LV systolic pressure and LVET will increase myocardial oxygen (O_2) consumption. Increased LVET will result in a decrease in diastolic time. Decreased diastolic time (myocardial perfusion time), diastolic aortic pressure, and effective stroke volume will decrease myocardial O_2 supply. Increased myocardial O_2 consumption and decreased myocardial O_2 supply will produce myocardial ischemia, which will further deteriorate LV function. (↑ = increased, ↓ = decreased)

patients with mitral regurgitation with the same degree of left ventricular enlargement, because in aortic regurgitation left ventricular afterload will decrease with surgery; in mitral regurgitation the afterload will increase. The degree of aortic regurgitation and effective forward stroke volume are influenced by the diastolic gradient between the aorta and the ventricle, the size of the aortic valve orifice during diastole, the duration of diastole, and the peripheral vascular resistance. Decreased peripheral resistance (e.g., vasodilators) will reduce the regurgital volume and improve forward stroke volume. The ventricular dilatation in aortic regurgitation may produce mitral insufficiency, which is due to stretching of the mitral valve annulus, plus the lateral displacement and malfunction of the papillary muscles.

The coronary flow reserve is decreased in patients with aortic regurgitation and remains low even months after aortic valve replacement. Selection of optimal time for valve surgery is particularly difficult in patients with aortic regurgitation because the deterioration of left ventricular function may be insidious.

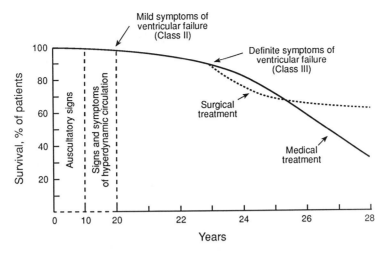

Fig. 3-55. Scheme of clinical presentation and natural history of chronic aortic regurgitation. (From McGoon MD, et al: *Aortic regurgitation.* In Guiliani ER, et al, eds: *Cardiology: Fundamentals and practice,* ed 2, St. Louis, 1991, Mosby Year Book.)

Natural history of chronic aortic regurgitation

The natural course of chronic aortic regurgitation is slow; the patient may be asymptomatic for many years. When symptoms of left ventricular failure occur, the course of the disease is accelerated[154] (Fig. 3-55).

Acute aortic regurgitation

The most common causes of acute aortic regurgitation are shown in the Box at right.

Infectious endocarditis. Data from Mayo Clinic indicated that 79% of the aortic valves with infectious endocarditis had pure aortic regurgitation and 21% combined aortic stenosis and regurgitation. The valve was bicuspid in 45% of the cases, normal in 41%, and postinflammatory (rheumatic) in 10%. The almost equal numbers of bicuspid and normal valves definitely indicates that the risk of infectious endocarditis in the bicuspid valve is much greater compared to normal aortic valve. Infectious endocarditis involving the aortic valve is fatal more often than when the infection is localized to other cardiac valves.[154]

Although vegetations produced by infectious endocarditis are usually seen on the ventricular surface of the semilunar valves, the entire underlying valve substance also reveals inflammatory infiltrations. The vegetations may vary from few millimeters to several centimeters and may be sessile or polypoid. Most of the vegetations are friable, yellowish-brown and hemorrhagic. The core of the vegetation is usually composed of necrotic tissue. The surface contains fibrin, platelets, bacteria and leukocytes. Depending on the virulence of the invading organism, infectious endocarditis may produce significant damage to the cusps, resulting in defects that are often localized in the lunulae or near the annulus. Partial perforation of the cusps may lead to small aneurysms. Calcification, either preexisting or after the inflammation heals, may lead to stenotic and

---

Acute aortic regurgitation: etiology
Infectious endocarditis
Trauma
Acute aortic dissection
Following prosthetic valve surgery

---

regurgitant valves. It seems, however, that previously calcified valves are less prone to develop infectious endocarditis. Less virulent organisms produce more fibrosis and retraction in the cusps, but no perforations.

Aortic valve infectious endocarditis has a propensity to produce ring abscesses that may be difficult to eradicate by antibiotics and may have an adverse affect on any attempt to replace the valve. Extensions from the aortic valve infectious endocarditis may involve the anterior mitral leaflet and the mural endocardium of the left ventricle. An upward spread into the sinus of Valsalva may result in an aneurysm. Such an aneurysm may rupture into either the atria or the ventricles, or may reach the pericardium and produce cardiac tamponade. Ring abscesses may extend into the interventricular septum, produce destruction of the conduction system, or create a ventricular septal defect.

Trauma. Trauma is not a frequent cause of acute aortic valve regurgitation, but it has been encountered with a nonpenetrated steering wheel-type of chest injury. Tearing of the free edge of the cusp may occur, as well as detachment of the cusp from the aortic wall. Such a detachment will create a prolapsed cusp, resulting in regurgitation. The left anterior cusp is more prone to be involved in traumatic injury. Valves that reveal some myxoid change, either as an isolated finding or in association with the Marfan syndrome, are more often predisposed to rupture after thoracic trauma.

Pathophysiology of acute aortic regurgitation. Sudden loss of valvular support is poorly tolerated in cases of acute aortic regurgitation. The left ventricle cannot dilate in the face of sudden diastolic volume overload. Due to the sudden increase of diastolic volume within the stiff pericardium, the diastolic filling pressure will rise markedly. This pressure will transmit to the left atrium, pulmonary veins, and pulmonary capillaries. Such an event will lead to pulmonary congestion and edema. The increased left ventricular end-diastolic pressure (30 to 40 mm Hg) may produce early closure of the mitral valve, an event which may be viewed as protection of the pulmonary vasculature. Unfortunately, this is not a long lasting event; therefore pulmonary edema will eventually develop. Increased left ventricular diastolic pressure will also result in a decreased coronary perfusion pressure and decreased coronary blood flow. Tachycardia, often present in acute aortic regurgitation, will result in a decreased diastolic time that will further compromise coronary blood flow.

High left atrial and pulmonary venous pressure may result in pulmonary artery hypertension and right ventricular dysfunction. Sudden increase in the left ventricular volume inside a tight, normal pericardium with increased left ventricular pressure in diastole will increase right ventricular pressure through the interventricular septum, which will interfere with right ventricular filling and increase right atrial pressure. As a result of these phenomena, one may expect an elevated systemic venous pressure and signs of right ventricular failure.[154]

Natural history of acute aortic regurgitation

Acute aortic regurgitation usually is severe and rapidly leads to left ventricular decompensation and failure. For these reasons valve replacement may be needed early in the course of the disease. In less severe cases, the progress of the disease is usually fast; most of the patients will need valve surgery within 12 months.

TRICUSPID VALVE
Anatomy-pathology

Although the anatomy of the tricuspid valve is quite different from that of the mitral valve, the two valves have, with the exception of minor differences, similar physiology. The circumference of the tricuspid annulus is oriented in a semivertical plane, while the leaflets are thin and delicate and reveal very shallow commissures. Fanlike delicate chordae denote the location of the commissures.[47] The tricuspid valve has three leaflets, the anterior, posterior, and septal. The latter leaflet is small and somewhat rudimentary. The septal leaflet is a significant anatomic landmark, however. Its base is inserted diagonally across the membranous interventricular septum. The anterior leaflet is the largest one and appears to be suspended across the right ventricular outflow tract. The three papillary muscles present in the right ventricle are highly variable. The

anterior, which is the largest, is located inferiorly at the level of the commissure of the posterior septal leaflet. Aging changes are often observed in the tricuspid valve. Expansion and doming are not infrequent. These changes are exacerbated in patients with chronic lung disease and are the sequelae of increased ventricular pressure.

Several factors make morphologic alterations of the tricuspid valve distinctly different from the changes seen in the mitral valve. While some reasons for such differences are anatomic, another equally important factor is the low pressure in which the tricuspid valve operates. However, when the low pressure is changed, such as seen in pulmonary hypertension, even minor anatomic changes affect the tricuspid valve's functional integrity.

The tricuspid valve is the least frequently excised cardiac valve (1.3%). The great majority of these excised tricuspid valves were regurgitant (84%) and only a small minority were stenotic (16%).

Tricuspid stenosis

Etiology. The most common causes of tricuspid stenosis are shown in the Box below. Although causes such as carcinoid syndrome, Whipple disease, Fabry disease, infectious endocarditis or congenital abnormalities have been reported to produce tricuspid stenosis, rheumatic etiology is the overwhelming cause for this condition. Tricuspid stenosis is almost always associated with mitral stenosis of rheumatic etiology.[160-163]

Rheumatic. The morphologic alterations of the tricuspid valve involved by rheumatic heart disease are characterized by fibrous thickening of the leaflets and retraction, but no calcification. Fusion of all three commissures creates a diaphragm with a fixed central opening, but the valve remains mobile. Contrary to the mitral rheumatic involvement, the chordae tendineae in tricuspid stenosis do not usually fuse, although they may become thick and short.

Carcinoid. Carcinoid plaques may appear on either the atrial or ventricular side of the leaflets and are composed of fibrous connective tissue with no elastic fibers (contrary to fibroelastosis) (Fig. 3-56). Those plaques have certain similarities with methysergide lesions, which, however, are usually left-sided. The carcinoid plaques may produce tricuspid stenosis or tricuspid regurgitation. It is estimated that approximately 35% of patients with carcinoid syn-

---

Tricuspid stenosis: etiology

Rheumatic
Carcinoid
Congenital
Right atrial tumor
Pacemaker leads

drome reveal heart involvement. Whether a carcinoid tumor will cause the carcinoid syndrome depends on its ability to release vasoactive and other substances, its site of origin and its ability to metastasize. In more than 50% of cases, when the carcinoid syndrome develops, the primary tumor is in the small intestine.[163] Abnormalities of serotonin metabolism may explain some symptoms and signs. Kinins, prostaglandins, dopamine, and a variety of peptides including gut peptides and particularly the substance P-related peptides, and bradykinins, have been incriminated for the different symptoms seen in carcinoid syndrome, although the exact pathogenetic mechanisms are not well understood.

Congenital. Congenital abnormal tricuspid valve stenosis is diagnosed in infants whose valvular components may all be malformed, reducing the tricuspid orifice. Rarely, Ebstein's anomaly may produce tricuspid stenosis.

Other causes. Infectious endocarditis may be a rare cause of tricuspid stenosis when large, bulky vegetations obstruct the inflow tract. The rare occurrence of a right atrial myxoma may also be the cause of tricuspid stenosis.

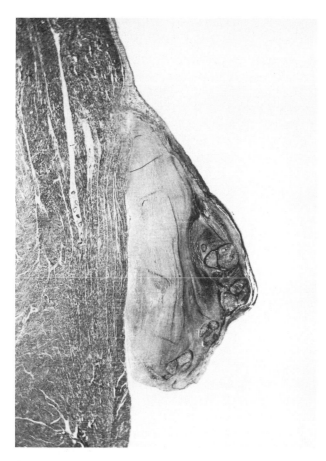

Fig. 3-56. Tricuspid valve with carcinoid plaque completely immobilizing the valvular leaflet. Note absence of elastic tissue within the plaque (ventricular surface of leaflet). Elastic stain.

Pathophysiology

The tricuspid valve orifice is the largest of all cardiac valves, measuring in circumference from 11 cm to 13 cm with an area of 10 cm^2 or more. An orifice of 5 cm^2, which is considered a mild tricuspid stenosis, cannot be detected clinically. At this stage of mild early tricuspid stenosis, there may be no diastolic filling pressure gradient across the tricuspid valve. As the severity of stenosis increases, a diastolic pressure gradient may be measured across the tricuspid valve. Even so, the gradient is usually small compared with the mitral valve stenosis and rarely exceeds 10 mm Hg. A valve area of 1.5 cm^2 or less represents severe tricuspid stenosis.[160-162]

In tricuspid stenosis, a prominent A-wave and a slow Y-descent are present in the right atrial pressure if the patients are in sinus rhythm[164] (Fig. 3-57). When atrial fibrillation develops, the A-wave disappears and the V-wave becomes prominent. In severe tricuspid stenosis increased right atrial pressure will result in systemic venous hypertension, hepatic congestion, and signs of right heart failure such as peripheral edema, hepatomegaly, and ascites.

If tricuspid stenosis is combined with mitral stenosis, pulmonary edema almost never occurs, even though the mitral stenosis might be severe. The tricuspid stenosis reduces the volume of blood in the pulmonary circulation and therefore decreases the capillary pressure in the lungs, preventing the transudation of fluid into the pulmonary interstitium.

Tricuspid regurgitation

Etiology. The most common causes of tricuspid valve regurgitation are shown in the Box on p. 108. Pure tricuspid regurgitation may be due to anatomic alterations or it

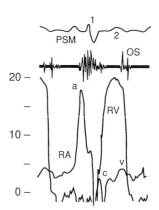

Fig. 3-57. Phonocardiogram and right heart pressure in a patient with tricuspid stenosis. The giant right atrial *a* wave (a) nearly equals right ventricular (RV) systolic pressure and produces a large diastolic gradient (shaded area). A presystolic murmur (PSM), loud first heart sound (1), and early diastolic opening snap (OS) simulate the findings in mitral stenosis. (Time lines = 0.2 sec.) (From Criley JM, et al: *Departures from the expected auscultatory events in mitral stenosis.* In Likoff W, ed: *Valvular heart disease,* Philadelphia, 1973, FA Davis.)

Tricuspid regurgitation: etiology

Chronic

Dilated annulus (elevated right ventricular pressure)
Ebstein's anomaly
AV canal defect
Carcinoid
Prolapse
Connective tissue disorders
Cardiomyopathy
Right ventricular infarction
Radiation therapy

Acute

Infectious endocarditis
Right ventricular infarction
Trauma

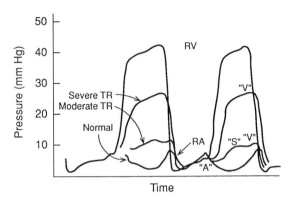

Fig. 3-58. Appearance of right atrial (RA) pressure contour in patients with severe tricuspid regurgitation (TR), moderate TR, and no TR (normal). Note the regurgitant systolic ("S") wave that blends with the normal filling ("V") wave in severe TR. The resultant RA pressure waveform resembles a right ventricular (RV) pressure recording. (From Grossman W, ed: *Cardiac catheterization and angiography,* ed 3, Philadelphia, 1986, Lea & Febiger.)

may be functional. The latter occurs when there is an elevation of right ventricular systolic and/or diastolic pressure.[160-161]

Chronic tricuspid regurgitation. In practical terms, the predominant cause of tricuspid regurgitation is tricuspid annular dilatation. Even with anatomic alterations such as destruction, fibrosis, and retraction of the tricuspid leaflets, significant regurgitation does not occur unless annular dilatation is present.[160-161]

A rule of thumb may be applied in deciding the cause of tricuspid valve regurgitation. If the annular circumference is normal and the leaflets are also normal, the reason for regurgitation may be papillary muscle dysfunction. If the annular size is normal, but the leaflets are abnormal, then rheumatic disease, carcinoid, or infective endocarditis may be the cause of the regurgitation. If the annulus is enlarged (over 13 cm) and the leaflets are normal, then pulmonary hypertension or dilated cardiomyopathy may be the cause. In fact, pulmonary hypertension as the cause of tricuspid regurgitation accounts for at least 50% of all cases. There are several reasons that may explain the frequency of the functional regurgitation of the tricuspid valve. One of those is the weak anatomic support of the tricuspid leaflets, which cannot adequately anchor the tricuspid valve as the right ventricle dilates. Therefore any condition that produces right ventricular failure, such as pulmonary hypertension, myocarditis, left ventricular failure, massive pulmonary emboli, and mitral valve disease, can result in functional tricuspid regurgitation.

Pathophysiology of chronic tricuspid regurgitation

Tricuspid regurgitation develops most commonly as a result of volume or pressure overload of the right ventricle. Compensatory dilatation of the right ventricle, however, can also occur as a result of tricuspid regurgitation, regardless of etiology. The right ventricle dilates and fails more rapidly than the left ventricle when it is subjected to

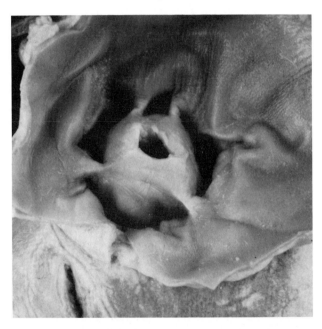

Fig. 3-59. Congenital pulmonary valve stenosis (dome-shaped) with marked post-stenotic pulmonary artery dilatation (Courtesy of Dr. William D. Edwards, Mayo Clinic).

increased pressure work. Reasons for such failure are the thin wall of the right ventricle and the crescentic architecture of that chamber. Because of the anatomic structure of the right ventricle, this chamber can handle increased volume work better than increased pressure work.[160-161,165]

Prominent systolic venous pulsations in the neck (large CV waves) and a large, pulsatile liver are present in patients with tricuspid regurgitation (Fig. 3-58). Chronic tricuspid regurgitation will lead to right ventricular dilatation, right ventricular dysfunction and right ventricular failure.

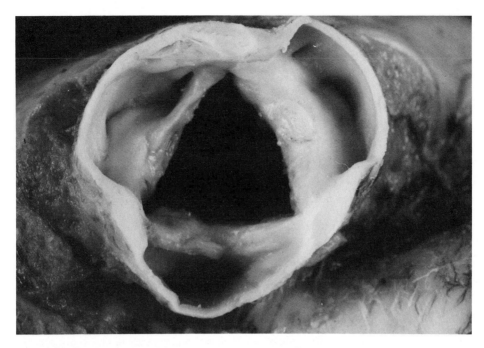

Fig. 3-60. Carcinoid etiology pulmonary stenosis and insufficiency. All three cusps are thick and imobilized. (Courtesy of Dr. William D. Edwards, Mayo Clinic).

Acute tricuspid regurgitation

Acute tricuspid regurgitation usually is secondary to infectious endocarditis, right ventricular myocardial infarction and trauma. Tricuspid valve infectious endocarditis, in the majority of cases is seen in intravenous drug abusers. Acute tricuspid regurgitation most of the time is well tolerated and if the left ventricle is functioning normally, severe tricuspid regurgitation does not produce significant hemodynamic compromise. Tricuspid valve resection without valve replacement has been proposed as initial therapy in intravenous drug abusers and tricuspid valve infectious endocarditis.[160-161]

PULMONIC VALVE

With age, the pulmonic valve may reveal fenestrations of the cusps at the lunulae, which, however, have no hemodynamic effect. In cases of pulmonary hypertension the pulmonic cusps usually appear opaque, thick, and fibrotic.[160]

Pulmonic valve stenosis

Etiology. Congenital malformations are the most common causes for valvular pulmonic valve stenosis (Figure 3-59). It is estimated that it occurs from 1.5 to 6.5 times per 10,000 live births. Bicuspid and quadricuspid pulmonic valves are extremely rare. However, a unicuspid dome-shaped valve is more often the cause of congenital pulmonic stenosis. This type of congenital malformation has an opening of variable size, is like a dome-shaped diaphragm, and its commissural sites are often marked by ridges. Pulmonic valve congenital stenosis may be followed by development of infundibular stenosis as a sec-

ondary phenomenon. In the tetralogy of Fallot, the infundibular stenosis is one of the components of the malformation.

Hypertrophic obstructive cardiomyopathy may produce a right subvalvular outflow tract obstruction. Neoplasms, primary or metastatic, in the outflow tract of the right ventricle may present as pulmonary stenosis. Anomalous hypertrophic muscle bundles crossing the right ventricular cavity may obstruct the outflow tract of the right ventricle.

Pulmonic valve involvement by rheumatic valvulitis is extremely rare. In the few cases that have been reported, the pulmonic valve was involved along with the other three valves.

Pathophysiology. Chronic pulmonic stenosis will produce right ventricular pressure overload, right ventricular hypertrophy and eventually right ventricular failure. Isolated valvular pulmonic stenosis, however, may be well tolerated for many years.[160]

Pulmonic valve regurgitation

Etiology. An isolated cusp abnormality of the pulmonic valve that produces regurgitation is rare. There are no significant changes even with complete destruction of cusps. However, as is the case with the tricuspid valve, dilatation of the main pulmonary artery (high flow pulmonary hypertension) may lead to annular dilation and pulmonic regurgitation. The major cause of pulmonic annular dilatation is either primary or secondary pulmonary hypertension.[160]

Pulmonic incompetence, as well as stenosis, may be caused by carcinoid involvement of the pulmonic valve (Fig. 3-60). The cusps involved by the carcinoid plaques become thick, shrunken, and pearly white. These fibrous plaques do not affect the cusp substance but appear to be sitting on the surface of the valve. A commissural indrawing may result in some degree of stenosis.

The pathophysiology of pulmonic regurgitation due to pulmonary hypertension is totally different from congenital pulmonic insufficiency (see also congenital heart disease).

MULTIVALVULAR DISEASE

Multivalvular involvement is common, particularly in patients with rheumatic heart disease. Development of pulmonic regurgitation and tricuspid regurgitation secondary to dilatation of the annulus of the pulmonic valve and tricuspid valve, as a consequence of pulmonary hypertension secondary to disease (involving the mitral valve or aortic valve or both) may occur. A combination of organic rheumatic tricuspid and mitral valvular disease may also occur. In patients with multivalvular disease, the clinical manifestations depend on the relative severities of each of the lesions. When the valvular abnormalities are of approximately equal severity, as a general rule, the clinical manifestations produced by the more proximal of two valvular lesions, i.e., the mitral valve in patients with combined mitral and aortic valvular disease and the tricuspid valve in patients with combined tricuspid and mitral valvular disease, are more pronounced. In patients with multivalvular disease, the relative severity of each lesion may be difficult to estimate by clinical examination, noninvasive and even invasive techniques, because one lesion may mask the manifestations of the other.[160]

Mitral stenosis and aortic regurgitation

Approximately two thirds of patients with severe mitral stenosis also have aortic regurgitation. In 90% of the cases aortic regurgitation is of little clinical importance, but approximately 10% of patients with mitral stenosis have severe rheumatic aortic regurgitation. Echocardiography and Doppler echocardiography are of decisive value in the detection of both lesions.

Mitral stenosis and aortic stenosis

When severe mitral stenosis and aortic stenosis coexist, the mitral stenosis masks many of the manifestations of the latter condition. Cardiac output tends to be reduced further than in patients with isolated aortic stenosis. Reduction in cardiac output lowers both the transaortic valvular pressure gradient and left ventricular systolic pressure, diminishes the incidence of angina, and retards the development of aortic calcification and left ventricular hypertrophy. On the other hand, clinical manifestations associated with mitral stenosis, such as pulmonary congestion and hemoptysis, atrial fibrillation, and systemic embolization, occur more frequently than in patients with isolated aortic stenosis.

Aortic stenosis and mitral regurgitation

The combination of severe aortic stenosis and mitral regurgitation is a hazardous one, but fortunately it is relatively uncommon. Obstruction to left ventricular outflow augments the volume of mitral regurgitant flow, whereas the presence of mitral regurgitation diminishes the ventricular preload necessary for maintenance of the left ventricular stroke volume in aortic stenosis. The result is a reduced forward cardiac output and marked left atrial and pulmonary venous hypertension.

Aortic regurgitation and mitral regurgitation

This relatively frequent combination of lesions may be caused by rheumatic heart disease or by prolapse of both valves due to myxomatous degeneration, or dilatation of both annuli, as is seen in patients with connective tissue disorders. The clinical features of aortic regurgitation usually predominate. When both valvular leaks are severe, this combination of lesions is poorly tolerated. The normal mitral valve ordinarily serves as a "backup" to the aortic valve, and premature closure of the mitral valve limits the volume of reflux that occurs in patients with acute aortic regurgitation. With combined regurgitant lesions, regardless of the etiology of the mitral lesion, blood may reflux from the aorta through both chambers of the left side of the heart into the pulmonary veins.

MECHANICAL PROSTHETIC AND BIOPROSTHETIC HEART VALVES

Approximately 40,000 valves are replaced yearly in the United States. Examination of removed cardiac valve prostheses serve several purposes and enhance valve selection criteria for other patients. An analysis of those devices may reveal information beyond that obtained by in vitro trials or animal investigations.[166,167]

All prostheses function passively, i.e., they respond to intracardiac pressure and flow changes. Mechanical prostheses include caged-ball, caged-disk, and tilting-disk models (Fig. 3-61). Bioprosthetic valves are trileaflet with a function similar to natural counterparts. Bioprosthetic valves include porcine aortic valves, bovine pericardium, human dura mater valves, fascia lata valves and human aortic homografts.

Mechanical prostheses are prone to thrombosis; therefore patients receiving such devices should be anticoagulated. Bioprostheses need not be anticoagulated, but those valves are more prone to degeneration and calcification.[166-184]

Mechanical heart valves

In the selection of a particular type of prosthesis, several factors should be considered such as age of the patient, lifestyle, previous medical history and access to medical care. The major advantage of the mechanical valves is their durability. In most medical centers, inser-

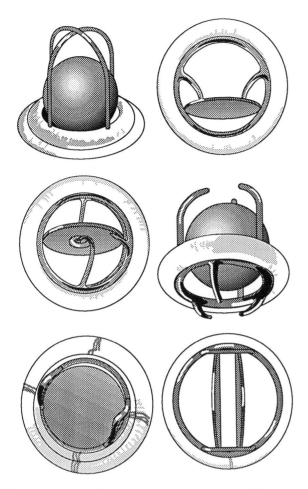

Fig. 3-61. Mechanical valvular prostheses available in the United States. **Upper Panel.** *Left:* Starr-Edwards ball valve, *Right:* Bjork-Shiley convexo-concave tilting disk; **Middle Panel.** *Left:* Medtronic-Hall tilting disk, *Right:* Sutter ball; **Lower Panel.** *Left:* Omniscience tilting disk, *Right:* St. Jude bileaflet valve. (From Edmunds H Jr, et al: *Valvular heart disease: Prosthetic valve replacement.* In Parmley WW, Chatterjeek, eds: *Cardiology,* vol 2, Philadelphia, 1983, JB Lippincott.)

tion of a single valve prosthesis has a 2% to 5% operative mortality.[173-181] Complications in the first 2 postoperative weeks are rarely attributable to the prosthesis itself (see Box above. A prosthetic valve may be placed in a less than ideal position, or it may be disproportional to the orifice. The result will be interference with its function, which may encourage thrombus formation. Less than optimal angle of insertion may create disproportion and subsequent damage to adjacent structures, resulting in obstruction of left ventricular outflow tract or arrhythmias by mitral prosthetic impingement on the septal wall.

Annular injury is seen more often in the aortic than in the mitral location. Such injury of the annulus or the adjacent left ventricular myocardium may result in significant bleeding during surgery or from a false aneurysm in the early postoperative period, which may rupture and produce hemopericardium. The reason for the annular damage may

---

Complications related to prosthetic valves

Early complications

Myocardial injury
Vascular injury
Damage to the conduction system
Paravalvular leaks (dehiscence)
Infectious endocarditis

Late complications

Thromboembolic phenomena
Infectious endocarditis
Hemolysis
Hemorrhage (related to antithrombolitic therapy)
Structural failure

---

be too much calcium debridement or stretching from a large prosthetic device. The most common complications of mechanical prosthetic valves are described briefly.

Early complications

Myocardial injury. The most common of the fatal complications of prosthetic insertion results from myocardial tears. Lesions at the midventricular wall are usually caused by excessive removal of papillary muscle tissue.[183] Other tears may occur in the endocardium in more proximal locations. With improvement in perfusion techniques, contraction band necrosis often seen in the past after prosthesis insertion is rare now.

Vascular injury. The circumflex artery may get caught in the sutures of the prosthesis, particularly if it has an anomalous course. Such an event will lead to myocardial infarction.

Damage to the conduction system. Permanent damage to the atrioventricular node or bundle of His with complete heart block is rather uncommon. It can result from a misplaced suture during insertion of an aortic prosthesis, although more often microhemorrhages are seen within the conduction system. Rarely, remnants of the native valve may interfere with the proper function of the prosthesis.

Paravalvular leaks (dehiscence). Paravalvular leaks are usually early complications. They may have significant hemodynamic effect. The most common cause of dehiscence is infection. A regurgitant murmur may be heard and, on fluoroscopy or echocardiography, one may detect a "dancing" or "rocking" prosthesis. Doppler echocardiography will demonstrate the regurgitant jet(s).

Late complications

Thromboembolic phenomena. Foreign body emboli are estimated to occur in about 10% of hearts examined at autopsy in patients with mechanical valves. Emboli may also be found in organs other than the heart. For example, they may lodge in pulmonary vessels from a tricuspid

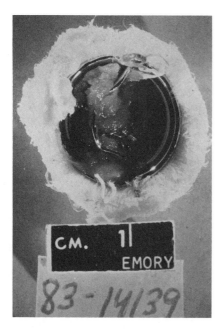

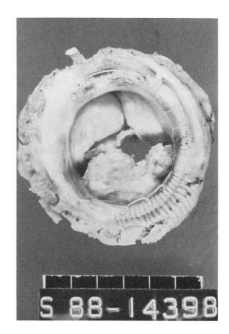

Fig. 3-62. Bjork-Shiley prosthesis with thrombi covering the strut, preventing the proper opening of the disk.

Fig. 3-63. Bioprosthetic valve showing perforations, tears, and calcification of one cusp.

prosthesis. Pieces of cloth from a sewing ring, or calcium may embolize. A granuloma may be formed at the intravascular site or in the adjacent tissues. In time, the cloth surface of a mechanical valve is covered by thrombi that will eventually organize. Thrombi may be formed at several locations on the prosthetic valve, particularly at sites where there is a relative blood stasis (Fig. 3-62).

Patients with atrial fibrillation are more prone to thrombus formation, as are patients in whom the anticoagulant therapy is inadequate. Prosthetic dysfunction enhances the formation of the thrombus. Embolism may occur from those thrombi, some of which may be infected. The brain is one of the common locations for such emboli. Thromboembolism is more common with mitral prosthesis. Infectious endocarditis may also result in thromboembolic phenomena.

Infectious endocarditis. In infectious endocarditis of prosthetic valves, the three most commonly involved pathogens are Staphylococcus epidermitis, *Staphylococcus aureus,* and gram-negative bacilli. Usually, infection in the prosthetic valve starts around the sewing ring and annulus, resulting in ring abscess. Dehiscence of the valve may occur, resulting in paravalvular leaks. A sinus may be formed that communicates with the epicardium or extends into the conduction tissues. Mitral valve prosthesis infectious endocarditis usually produces mitral stenosis, unlike the aortic valve prosthesis, which produces aortic regurgitation. Jet lesions in the mural endocardium may also become infected. Transvalvular gradients exist in all mechanical prosthetic valves, although in some valves this

phenomenon is more pronounced. All prostheses create turbulence, which may induce endocardial thickening.

Hemolysis. Hemolysis with renal hemosiderosis is a common event in prostheses that have been placed for a long period. In about 5% to 15% of cases, the hemolysis may lead to iron deficiency anemia.[183]

Bioprosthetic cardiac valves

Certain abnormalities are best detected by inspection of the prosthetic valve in situ. Perivalvular leaks often are caused by placement of sutures through infected tissues, extensive calcification, or by abnormal connective tissue (e.g., in patients with Marfan syndrome). Necrosis of the valve annulus may also be caused by the toxic effect of residual glutaraldehyde on the cusps if not adequately washed. Abnormal angulation of the axis may occur when a valve annulus is distorted by calcification, infection or scarring.[172,175-183]

A certain hemodynamic obstruction of forward flow and minimal regurgitation occurs in almost all bioprosthetic valves. Obstruction of the coronary ostium may result from a malpositioning of the stent of a bioprosthetic valve implanted in the aortic position.[180] Ventricular rupture may occur either at the atrioventricular groove, the site of excision of the papillary muscle, or midway between the mitral annulus and the papillary muscles.[182]

Porcine valves are asymmetric because the right coronary cusp is larger. This larger cusp, at its basal portion, has a strip of ventricular muscle that has the propensity to calcify after implantation. Some postimplantation changes

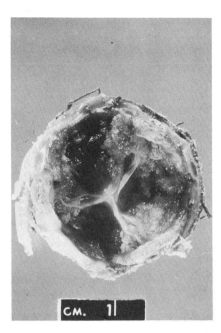

Fig. 3-64. Bioprosthetic valve with diffuse thrombotic deposits in all three cusps.

in bioprosthetic valves are common to all types and include tears, perforations and calcification of collagen (Fig. 3-63). These changes may lead to either stenosis or regurgitation of the bioprosthetic valve. As time goes on after implantation, the cusps will endothelialize, particularly at their basal region, and may even be covered by a fibrous sheath of host origin.[178] Formation of thrombi is less common but may also occur in bioprosthetic valves, (Fig. 3-64). Infection is a problem similar to that seen in mechanical valves.

Ishihara et al[179] proposed a system of classification of cuspal lesions in bioprosthetic valves. Type I lesions (flail cusps) are tears of the cusp near the stent post. This is more common in pericardial and dura mater valves, but it has also been recorded in porcine valves. Type II lesions are linear defects along the base of the cusp and are thought to be the result of "hinging" motion of the cusps. Type III lesions are the result of infection and can present as destruction of the cusps at the edges or as a hole in the middle of the cusp. Type IV lesions are small fenestrations occurring in the vicinity of calcifications. Shearing mechanical forces at the edges of calcification may be responsible for these types of lesions. As it has been already stated, bioprosthetic valves gradually become covered by fibrous sheath of host origin. This sheath usually covers both surfaces of the cusp. Although the sheath may have a somewhat reinforcing effect, it may also cause extensive stiffening of the cusps and even commissural fusion. Bioprosthetic valve at the tricuspid location is more prone to excessive sheathing.

Calcification occurs after 3 years or longer. It can cause both stenosis and regurgitation, the latter because of concomitant perforations. Calcium may be deposited intrinsically or on the surface of microthrombi. Several factors predispose to calcification, such as young age, chronic renal failure, infection and hyperparathyroidism, but the exact pathogenesis of calcification is not clear. Calcium deposits are made of hydroxyapatite. Studies show that the initial nuclei of calcification may occur in cuspal surface debris and membrane fragments. Intracuspal hematomas leading to stiffness are probably produced by penetration of blood from the sewing ring down to the cusp substance.

Progressive inward bending of the polypropylene struts ("stent creep") may result in stenosis of bioprosthetic valves. Infiltration by plasma-derived lipids of the bioprosthetic cusps has been reported.[167]

Amyloid deposits have also been found in bioprosthetic valves. Usually, this is observed after the third posttransplantation year.

While hemolytic anemia is a relatively common complication after insertion of mechanical valve prosthesis, it is rare after porcine valve implantation.[175] A recent report stresses that although hemolysis in patients with porcine valves is uncommon, it may be the initial manifestation of valve malfunction even without a detectable regurgitation murmur.[176]

Sudden death of patients with prosthetic valves

A multiplicity of events may cause death. Obstruction of poppet movement by either entrapment by thrombus or disproportion may occur. Emboli that may occlude coronary arteries or cerebral arteries are some of the autopsy findings in these patients.

REFERENCES

1. Gordis L: The virtual disappearance of rheumatic fever in the United States; Lessons in the rise and fall of disease, *Circulation* 72:1155, 1985.
2. Markowitz M: The decline of rheumatic fever: Role of medical intervention, *J Pediatr* 106:545-50, 1985.
3. Congeni B, Rizzo C, Congeni J, et al: Outbreak of acute rheumatic fever in North Eastern Ohio, *J Pediatr* 111:176-9, 1987.
4. Wald ER, Dashefsky B, Feidt C, et al: Acute rheumatic fever in Western Pennsylvania and the tri-state area, *Pediatrics* 80:371-4, 1987.
5. Bisno AL, Shulman ST, Dajni AS: The rise and fall (rise?) of rheumatic fevers, JAMA 259:728-9, 1988.
6. Guilherme L, Weidebach W, Kiss MH, et al: Association of human leukocyte class II antigens with rheumatic fever or rheumatic heart disease in a Brazilian population, *Circulation* 83: 1995-8, 1991.
7. Ayoub EM, Barrett DJ, Maclaren NK, et al: Association of class II human histocompatibility leukocyte antigens with rheumatic fever, *J Clin Invest* 77:2019-26, 1986.
8. Chopra B, Narula J, Tandon R: Aschoff nodule revisited, *Jpn Heart J* 30:479-85, 1989.
9. Barnert AL, Terry EE, Persellin HR: Acute rheumatic fever in adults, *JAMA* 232:925, 1975.

10. Schwartz B, Facklam RR, Breiman RF: Changing epidemiology of group A streptococcal infection in the USA, *Lancet* 336:1167-71, 1990.

11. Bland EF, Jones TD: Rheumatic fever and rheumatic heart disease; A twenty-year report of 1,000 patients followed since childhood, *Circulation* 4:836-843, 1951.

12. Bisno AL: Group A streptococcal infections and acute rheumatic fever, *N Engl J Med* 325:783-93, 1991.

12a. Cunningham MW, Hall NK, Krisher KK et al: A study of anti-group A streptococcal monoclonal antibodies cross-reactive with myosin, *J Immunol* 136:293, 1986.

13. Zabriskie JB: Rheumatic fever: The interplay between host, genetics, and microbe, *Circulation* 71:1077, 1985.

14. Marcus RH, Sarels P, Pocock WA, et al: Functional anatomy of severe mitral regurgitation in acute rheumatic carditis, *Am J Cardiol* 63:577-84, 1989.

15. Archer JR, Winrow VR: HLA-B27 and the course of arthritis: Does molecular biology help?, *Ann Rheum Dis* 46:713, 1987.

16. Brewerton DA, Gibson DG, Goddard DH, et al: The myocardium in ankylosing spondylitis, *Lancet* 1:995-9, 1987.

17. Roberts WC, Hollingsworth JF, Balkley BH, et al: Combined mitral and aortic regurgitation in ankylosing spondylitis. Angiographic and anatomic features, *Am J Med* 56:237-43, 1974.

18. Albes MG, Espirito-Snato J, Queirez MV, et al: Cardiac alterations in ankylosing spondylitis, *Angiology* 567-71, 1988.

19. Bowen J, Boudoulas H, Wooley CF: Cardiovascular disease of connective tissue origin, *Am J Med* 82:481, 1987.

20. Pyeritz RE: *Heritable disorders of connective tissue.* In Boudoulas H, Wooley CF, eds: *Mitral valve prolapse and the mitral valve prolapse syndrome,* Mount Kisco, NY, 1988, Futura.

21. Hollister DW, Godfrey M, Sakai LY, et al: Immunohistologic abnormalities of the microfibrillar-fiber system in the Marfan syndrome, *N Engl J Med* 323:515, 1990.

22. Dietz HC, Cutting GR, Pyeritz RE, et al: Marfan syndrome caused by a recurrent de novo missense mutation in the fibrillin gene, *Nature* 352:337, 1991.

23. Lima SD, Lima JAC, Pyeritz, et al: Relation of mitral valve prolapse to ventricular size in Marfan's syndrome, *Am J Cardiol* 55:739-43, 1985.

24. Leier CV, Call TD, Fulkerson PK, et al: The spectrum of cardiac defects in the Ehlers-Danlos syndrome, types I and II, *Ann Int Med* 92:171-78, 1980.

25. Leier CV, Baker PB, Kilman JW, et al: Cardiovascular abnormalities associated with adult polycystic kidney disease. *Ann Intern Med* 100:683-88, 1984.

26. Sohval AR: Gumma of the heart, *Arch Pathol Lab Med* 20:429-44, 1935.

27. Johns DR, Tierney M, Sclsenstein D: Alteration in the natural history of neurosyphilis by concurrent infection with the human immunodeficiency virus, *N Engl J Med* 316:1569-72, 1987.

28. Dickens P, Chan ACL: Nonbacterial thrombotic endocarditis in Hong Kong Chinese, *Arch Pathol Lab Med* 115:359, 1991.

29. Cammarosano C, Lewis W: Cardiac lesions in acquired immune deficiency syndrome (AIDS), *J Am Coll Cardiol* 5:703, 1985.

30. Patchell RA, White CL, Clark AW, et al: Nonbacterial thrombotic endocarditis in bone marrow transplant patients, *Cancer* 55:631, 1985.

31. Lopez JA, Ross RS, Fishbein MC, et al: Nonbacterial thrombotic endocarditis: A review, *Am Heart J* 113:773, 1987.

32. Habbab MA, Al-Zaibag AM, Al-Hilali AM, et al: Unusual presentation and echocardiographic features of surgically proven nonbacterial thrombotic endocarditis, *Am Heart J* 119:404, 1990.

33. Lehto VP, Stenman S, Somer T: Immunohistochemical studies on valvular vegetations in nonbacterial thrombotic endocarditis (NBTE), *Acta Pathol Microbiol Immunol Scand* (A) 90:207, 1982.

34. Cook DJ, Tanser PH: Nonbacterial thrombotic endocarditis complicating mitral valve prolapse presenting as Parinaud's syndrome. A case report, *Angiology-J* 5:494, 1989.

35. Gordon SG, Cross BA: A factor x-activating cysteine protease from malignant tissue, *J Clin Invest* 67:1665, 1981.

36. Applefeld MM, Woodward TE: *Infective endocarditis: A clinical overview.* In Harvey PW, ed: *Current Problems in Cardiology,* Chicago, 1977, Year Book.

37. Hayward GW: Infective endocarditis: a change in disease, *Br Med J* 2:706, 1973.

38. Walshe TJ, Hutchins JM, Bulkley BH, et al: Fungal infections of the heart: Analysis of fifty-one autopsy cases, *Am J Cardiol* 45:357, 1980.

39. Middlemost S, Wisenbaugh T, Meyerowitz C, et al: A case for early surgery in native left-sided endocarditis complicated by heart failure: Results in 203 patients, *J Am Coll Cardiol* 18:663-7, 1991.

40. Child JS: Infective endocarditis: Risks and prophylaxis, *J Am Coll Cardiol* 18:311-42, 1991.

41. Steckelberg JM, Murphy JG, Ballard D, et al: Emboli in infective endocarditis: The prognostic value of echocardiography, *Ann Intern Med* 114:635-40, 1991.

42. Vegetations, valves, and echocardiography, *Lancet* 2:1118-9, 1988 (editorial).

43. Dresler FA, Roberts WC. Infective endocarditis in opiate addicts. Analysis of eighty cases studied at necropsy, *Am J Cardiol* 63:1240-57, 1989.

44. Silverman NA, Levitsky S: Acute infective endocarditis: When is surgical treatment warranted? *Primary Cardiology* 40-52, 1989.

45. Boudoulas H: *Involvement of other structures of the heart and other disease processes induced by renal failure.* In Leier CV, Boudoulas H, eds: *Cardiorenal Disorders and Diseases,* Mount Kisco, New York, 1986, Futura.

46. Boudoulas H: *Pericardial disease: Clinical presentation, diagnostic evaluation and management.* In Leier CV, Boudoulas H, eds: *Cardiorenal Disorders and Diseases,* Mount Kisco, New York, 1986, Futura.

47. Davis MJ: *Pathology on cardiac valves.* London, 1980, Butterworths.

48. Boudoulas H, Wooley CF: Mitral valve disorders, *Current Opinion in Cardiology* 5:162-70, 1990.

49. Fulkerson PK, Beaver BM, Auseon JC, et al: Calcification of the mitral annulus. Etiology, clinical associations, complications and therapy, *Am J Med* 66:967-77, 1979.

50. Wooley CF, Sparks EA, Boudoulas H: *Mitral stenosis: The anatomic lesion and the physiologic state.* In Bashore TM, Davidson CJ, eds: *Percutaneous Balloon Valvuloplasty and Related Techniques,* Baltimore, 1991, Williams and Wilkins.

51. Wood P: An appreciation of mitral stenosis, *Br Med J* 1:1051-63; 1113-24, 1954.

52. Barlow JB, Lakier JB, Pocock JA: *Mitral stenosis.* Barlow JB, ed: In: *Perspectives on the Mitral Valve,* Philadelphia, 1987, FA Davis.

53. Wooley CF, Baba N, Kilman JW, et al: Thrombotic calcific mitral stenosis: Morphology of the calcific mitral valve, *Circulation* 49:1167-74, 1974.

54. Wooley CF, Klassen KP, Leighton RF, et al: Left atrial and left ventricular sound and pressure in mitral stenosis, *Circulation* 38:295-307, 1968.

55. Barrington WW, Boudoulas H, Bashore T, et al: Mitral stenosis: Mitral dome excursion at M^1 an the mitral opening snap. The concept of reciprocal heart sounds, *Am Heart J* 115:1280-90, 1988.

56. Wooley CF, Klassen KP, Leighton RF, et al: The left atrial pressure pulse of mitral stenosis in sinus rhythm, *Am J Cardiol* 25:395-400, 1970.

57. Criley JM, Herner AJ: Crescendo presystolic murmur of mitral stenosis with atrial fibrillation, *N Engl J Med* 285:1284, 1971.

58. Gorlin R, Gorlin SG: Hydraulic formula for calculation of the area of the stenotic mitral valve, other cardiac valves and central circulatory shunts, *Am Heart J* 41:1-29, 1981.

59. Cheitlin MD, Byrd RC: *Mitral valve disease.* In Greenberg BH, Murphy E, eds: *Valvular Heart Disease,* Littleton, 1987, PSB.

60. Triposkiadis F, Wooley CF, Boudoulas H: Mitral stenosis: Left atrial dynamics reflect altered passive and active emptying, *Am Heart J* 120:124-132, 1990.

61. Dussaule JC, Vahanian A, Michel PL, et al: Plasma atrial natriuretic factor and cyclic GMP in mitral stenosis treated by balloon valvulotomy, *Circulation* 78:276-85, 1988.

62. Hui WKK, Lee PK, Chow JSF, et al: Analysis of regional left ventricular wall motion during diastole in mitral stenosis, *Br Heart J* 50:231-9, 1983.

63. Naito M, Morganroth J, Mardelli TJ, et al: Rheumatic mitral stenosis: Crossectional echocardiographic analysis, *Am Heart J* 100:34-40, 1980.

64. Boudoulas H, Kontopoulos A, Parcharidis G, et al: The natural history of rheumatic valvular heart disease. Comparison of patients with a history of rheumatic fever to those without history of rheumatic fever, *Helliniki Latriki* (Greek Medicine) 43:107-115, 1974.

65. Lock JE, Khallilullah M, Shrivastava S, et al: Percutaneous catheter commissurotomy in rheumatic mitral stenosis, *N Engl J Med* 313:1515-8, 1985.

66. Boudoulas H, Wooley CF: *Mitral valve prolapse and the mitral valve prolapse syndrome.* Mount Kisko, NY, 1988, Futura.

67. Boudoulas H, Wooley CF: *Mitral regurgitation chronic versus acute: Implications for timing of surgery.* In Bowen JM, Mazzaferri EL, eds: *Contemporary Internal Medicine,* New York, 1991, Plenum.

68. Perloff JK, Roberts WC: The mitral apparatus: Functional anatomy of mitral regurgitation, *Circulation* 46:227-39, 1972.

69. Barlow JB, Bockock WA: The mitral valve prolapse enigma—two decades later, *Mod Conc Cardiovasc Dis* 53:13-17, 1984.

70. Boudoulas H, Wooley CF: *Mitral valve prolapse and the mitral valve prolapse syndrome.* In Yu P, Goodwin J, eds: *Progress in Cardiology,* Philadelphia, 1986, Lea & Fibiger.

71. Barlow JB: Aspects of mitral and tricuspid regurgitation, *J Cardiol* 21(suppl XXV):3-33, 1991.

72. Gravanis MB, Campbell WG Jr: The syndrome of prolapsed mitral valve; its etiologic and pathogenic enigma, *Arch Pathol Lab Med* 106:369, 1982.

73. Bel-Kahn JVD, Duren DR, Bocker AE: Isolated mitral valve prolapse; chordal architecture as an anatomic basis in older patients, *J Am Coll Cardiol* 5:335, 1985.

74. Virmani R, Atkinson JB, Forman MB, et al: *Mitral valve prolapse, Hum Pathol* 18:596-602, 1987.

75. Nishimura RA, McGoon MD, Shub C, et al: Echocardiographically documented mitral valve prolapse. Long-term follow-up of 237 patients, *N Engl J Med* 313:1305, 1985.

76. Davies MJ, Moore PB, Brainbridge MV: The floppy mitral valve: Study of incidence, pathology and forensic material, *Br Heart J* 40:468, 1978.

77. Hanson TP, Edwards BS, Edwards JE: Pathology of surgical excised mitral valves. One-hundred consecutive cases, *Arch Pathol Lab Med* 109:823, 1985.

78. Pickering NJ, Brody JL, Barrett MJ: Von Willebrands' syndrome and mitral valve prolapse linked mesenchymal dysplasias. *N Engl J Med* 305:131, 1981.

79. Waller BF, Morrow AG, Maro BJ, et al: Etiology of clinically isolated, severe, chronic, pure, mitral regurgitation: Analysis of ninety-seven patients over thirty years of age having mitral valve replacement, *Am Heart J* 4:288, 1982.

80. Boudoulas H, Kolibash AJ, Baker P, et al: Mitral valve prolapse and the mitral valve prolapse syndrome: A diagnostic classification and pathogenesis of symptoms, *Am Heart J* 118:796-818, 1989.

81. Wooley CF, Baker PB, Kolibash AJ, et al: The floppy, myxomatous mitral valve, mitral valve prolapse, and mitral regurgitation, *Prog Cardiovasc Dis* 33:397-433, 1991.

82. Fontana ME, Sparks EA, Boudoulas H, et al: Mitral valve prolapse and the mitral valve prolapse syndrome, *Curr Prob Cardiol* 16, 1991.

83. Perloff JK, Child JS: Mitral valve prolapse. Evolution and refinement of diagnostic techniques, *Circulation* 80:710-1, 1989.

84. Levine RA, Handschumacher MD, Sanfilippo AJ, et al: Three-dimensional echocardiographic reconstruction of the mitral valve, with implications for the diagnosis of mitral valve prolapse, *Circulation* 80:589-98, 1989.

85. Boudoulas H, Kolibash AJ, Wooley CF: Mitral valve prolapse: A heterogeneous disorder, *Primary Cardiology* 17:29-43, 1991.

86. Akasaka T, Yoshikawa J, Yoshida K, et al: Temporal resolution of mitral regurgitation in patients with mitral valve prolapse: A phonocardiographic and Doppler echocardiographic study, *J Am Coll Cardiol* 13:1053-61, 1989.

87. Boudoulas H, Kolibash AJ, Wooley CF: Mitral valve prolapse: The high risk patients, *Pract Cardiol* 17(9):15-31, 1991.

88. Kolibash AJ, Kilman JW, Bush CA, et al: Evidence for progression from mild to severe mitral regurgitation in mitral valve prolapse, *Am J Cardiol* 58:762-67, 1986.

89. Duren DR, Baker AE, Dunning AJ: Long-term follow-up of idiopathic mitral valve prolapse in 300 patients. A prospective study, *J Am Coll Cardiol* 11:42-47, 1988.

90. Marks AR, Choong CY, Sanfilippo AJ, et al: Identification of high-risk and low-risk subgroups of patients with mitral valve prolapse, *N Engl J Med* 320:1031-36, 1989.

91. Duran CMG, Gometza B, De Vol EB: Valve repair in rheumatic mitral disease, *Circulation* 84[suppl III]:III-125-III-132, 1991.

92. Shiraki M, Miyagawa A, Akiguchi I, et al: Evidence of hypovitaminosis D in patients with mitral ring calcification, *Jpn Heart J* 29:801-8, 1988.

93. Byrd RJ, Gordon PB, Digdal SD: Doppler-detected tricuspid, mitral or aortic regurgitation in end-stage renal disease, *Am J Cardiol* 63:750, 1989.

94. Kaul S, Spotnitz WD, Glasheen WP, et al: Mechanism of ischemic mitral regurgitation. An experimental evaluation, *Circulation* 84:2167-80, 1991.

95. Rankin JS, Hickey MSJ, Smith LR, et al: Ischemic mitral regurgitation, *Circulation* 79(suppl I):I-116-I-121, 1989.

96. Jackman JD, Tcheng JE, Califf RM, et al: Current concepts in the management of ischemic mitral regurgitation, *Cardiology* 4:76-83, 1991.

97. Hickey M, Smith RL, Muhlbeuer LH, et al: Current prognosis of ischemic mitral regurgitation: Implications for future management, *Circulation* 78(Suppl I):51-59, 1988.

98. Akagi T, Kato H, Inoue O, et al: Valvular heart disease in Kawasaki's syndrome: Incidence and natural history, *Am Heart J* 120:366-372, 1990.

99. Cosby RS, Giddings JA, See JR, et al: The echocardiogram in nonrheumatic mitral insufficiency, *Chest* 66:642-646, 1974.

100. Carabello BA: Mitral regurgitation, part 1: Basic pathophysiological principles, *Mod Conc Cardiovasc Dis* 57:53-64, 1988.

101. Boudoulas H, Mantzouratos D, Geleris P, et al: Hypertrophic cardiomyopathy: Noninvasive identification of patients with significant pressure gradient, *Am J Noninvas Cardiol* 1:24-29, 1987.

102. Hauck AJ, Edwards WD, Danielson GK, et al: Mitral and aortic valve disease associated with ergotamine therapy for migraine, *Arch Pathol Lab Med* 114:62-4, 1990.

103. Urabe Y, Mann DL, Kent RL, et al: Cellular and ventricular contractile dysfunction in experimental canine mitral regurgitation, *Circ Res* 70:131-47, 1992.

104. Vokonas PS, Gorlin R, Cohn PF, et al: Dynamic geometry of the left ventricle in mitral regurgitation, *Circulation* 48:786-95, 1973.

105. Galloway AC, Colvin SB, Baumann FG, et al: Long-term results of mitral valve reconstruction with Carpentier techniques in 148 patients with mitral insufficiency, *Circulation* 78(suppl I):I-97-I-105, 1988.

106. Assey ME, Usher BW, Hendrix GH: Valvular heart disease: Use of invasive and noninvasive techniques in clinical decision-making. Part 2: Mitral valve disease, *Mod Conc Cardiovasc Dis* 58:61-66, 1989.

107. Shah PM: Quantitative assessment of mitral regurgitation, *J Am Coll Cardiol* 13:591-3, 1989.

108. Spain MG, Smith MD, Grayburn PA, et al: Quantitative assessment of mitral regurgitation by Doppler color flow imaging: Angiographic and hemodynamic correlations, *J Am Coll Cardiol* 13:585-90, 1989.

109. Sasayama S, Takahashi M, Osakada G, et al: Dynamic geometry of the left atrium and left ventricle in aortic and mitral regurgitation, *Circulation* 60:177, 1979.

110. Sutton GC, Chatterjee K, Caves PK. Diagnosis of severe mitral regurgitation due to non-rheumatic chordal abnormalities. *Br Heart J* 35:877-86, 1973.

111. Koma-Canella I, Gamallo C, Onsurbe PM, et al: Anatomic findings in acute papillary muscle necrosis, *Am Heart J* 118:1188-92, 1989.

112. Sanders CA, Armstrong PW, Willerson JT, et al: Etiology and differential diagnosis of acute mitral regurgitation, *Prog Cardiovasc Dis* 14:129, 1971.

113. Yoran C, Yellin EL, Becker RM, et al: Dynamic aspects of acute mitral regurgitation; effects of ventricular volume pressure and contractility on the effective regurgitant orifice area, *Circulation* 60:170, 1979.

114. Boudoulas H, Lewis RP, Dervenagas S, et al: Abbreviation of systolic time intervals in acute mitral regurgitation with observations on the effect of mitral valve replacement, *Am J Cardiol* 44:595, 1979.

115. Boudoulas H, Weinstein PB, Shaver JA, et al: Atrial septal defect: Attenuation of respiratory variation in systolic and diastolic time intervals, *J Am Coll Cardiol* 9:53, 1987.

116. Lie JT, Wright KE, Titus JL: Sudden appearance of systolic murmur in acute infarction, *Am Heart J* 90:507, 1975.

117. Cohn LH: Surgery for mitral regurgitation, *JAMA* 260:2883-87, 1988.

118. Davies MJ: *Color atlas of cardiovascular pathology.* Harvey Miller Publishers, Oxford, UK, 1986, Oxford University Press.

119. Brandenbkurg RO, Fuster V, Giuliani E: Valvular heart disease. When should the patient be referred? *Pract Cardiol* 3:50, 1979.

120. Isner JM, Khokshi SK, DeFranco A, et al: Contrasting histoarchitecture of calcified leaflets from stenotic bicuspid vs. stenotic tricuspid aortic valves, *J Am Coll Cardiol* 15:1104-8, 1990.

121. Lerer PK, Edwards WD: Coronary arterial anatomy in bicuspid aortic valve: Necropsy study of 100 hearts, *Br Heart J* 45:142, 1981.

122. Edwards JE: Calcific aortic stenosis: Pathologic features. proceedings staff meet, *Mayo Clin Proc* 36:444-51, 1961.

123. Lombard JT, Selzer A: Valvular aortic stenosis. A clinical and hemodynamic profile of patients, *Ann Intern Med* 106:292-8, 1987.

124. Letac B, Cribier A, Koning R, et al: Aortic stenosis in elderly patients aged 80 or older. Treatment by percutaneous balloon valvuloplasty in a series of 92 cases, *Circulation* 80:1514-20, 1989.

125. Levinson JR, Akins CW, Buckley MJ, et al: Octogenarians with aortic stenosis. Outcome after aortic valve replacement, *Circulation* 80(suppl I):I-49-I-56, 1989.

126. Pellikka PA, Tajik AJ: Adults with asymptomatic severe aortic stenosis, *Cardiol* 10:43-48, 1990.

126a. Stefanadis C, Wooley CF, Bush CA et al: Aortic distensibility in post stenotic aortic dilatation: the effect of co-existing coronary artery disease, *J Cardiol* 18:189-195, 1988.

127. Danielsen R, Nordrehaug JE, Vik-Mo H: Clinical and haemodynamic features in relation to severity of aortic stenosis in adults, *Eur Heart J* 12:791-5, 1989.

128. Marcus ML, Doty DB, Hiratzka LF, et al: Decreased coronary reserve. A mechanism for angina pectoris in patients with aortic stenosis and normal coronary arteries, *N Engl J Med* 307:1362-7, 1982.

129. Sprigings DC, Chambers JB, Cochrane T, et al: Ventricular stroke work loss: Validation of a method of qualifying the severity of aortic stenosis and elevation of an orifice formula, *Am J Cardiol* 16:1608-14, 1990.

130. Brent BN: Aortic valve stenosis: Comparison of patients with and those without congestive heart failure, *Am J Cardiol* 57:419-22, 1986.

131. Johnson AM: Aortic stenosis, sudden death, and left ventricular baroreceptors, *Br Heart J* 33:1-5, 1971.

132. Schwartz LS, Goldfischer J, Sprague GJ, et al: Syncope and sudden death in aortic stenosis, *Am J Cardiol* 23:647-58, 1969.

133. Boudoulas H, Weissler AM, Lewis RP, et al: The clinical diagnosis of syncope, *Curr Prob Cardiol* 7:7-40, 1982.

134. Jawad IA, Boudoulas H, Stark C, et al: A noninvasive index of severity of valvular aortic stenosis, *Am J Noninvas Cardiol* 1:102-108, 1987.

135. Dunn M: Evaluating severity of aortic stenosis: New validation of an old method, *J Am Coll Cardiol* 16:1615-6, 1990.

136. Conway MA, Allis J, Ouwerkerk R, et al: Detection of low phosphocreatine to ATP ratio in failing hypertrophied human myocardium by ^{31}P magnetic resonance spectroscopy, *Lancet* 338:973-6, 1991.

137. Assey ME, Usher BW, Hendrix GH: Valvular heart disease: Use of invasive and noninvasive techniques in clinical decision-making. Part 1: Aortic valve disease, *Mod Concep Cardiovasc Dis* 58:55-60, 1991.

138. Krayenbuehl HP, Hess OM, Monrad ES, et al: Left ventricular myocardial structure in aortic valve disease before, intermediate, and late after aortic valve replacement, *Circulation* 79:744-55, 1989.

139. Ross J Jr, Braunwald E: Aortic stenosis, *Circulation* 38(Suppl V):61, 1968.

140. Wagner S, Selzer A: Patterns of progression of aortic stenosis. A longitudinal hemodynamic study, *Circulation* 65:709-12, 1982.

141. Pillikka PA, Nishimura RA, Bailey et al: The natural history of adults with asymptomatic hemodynamically significant aortic stenosis, *J Am Coll Cardiol* 15:1012-1017, 1990.

142. Cheitlin MD: Severe aortic stenosis in the sick octogenarian. A clear indicator for balloon valvuloplasty as the initial procedure, *Circulation* 80:1906-8, 1989.

143. Weaver GA: Gastrointestinal bleeding in the patient with aortic stenosis, *Med Interne* 3:42-55, 1982.

144. Horstkotte D, Loogen F: The natural history of aortic valve stenosis, *Eur Heart J* 9(suppl E):57-64, 1988.

145. Davies SW, Gershlick AH, Balcon R: Progression of valvular aortic stenosis: a long-term retrospective study, *Eur Heart J* 12:10-14, 1991.

146. Deleted in galleys.

147. Kontusaari S, Tromp G, Kuivaniemi H, et al: A mutation in the gene for type III procollagen (COL3A1) in a family with aortic aneurysms, *J Clin Invest* 86:1465-73, 1990.

148. Gaasch WH: Management of aortic valve disease, *Hosp Prac* September:133-8, 1982.

149. When to operate in aortic valve disease, *Lancet*, 2:981-2, 1991 (Editorial).

150. Arvan S: Aortic valve prolapse in congenital and acquired systemic disease, *Arch Intern Med* 145:1601-3, 1985.

151. Woldow AB, Parameswaran R, Hartman J, et al: Aortic regurgitation due to aortic valve prolapse, *Am J Cardiol* 55:1435-8, 1985.

152. Greenberg B: Selecting high-risk patients with chronic aortic insufficiency, *Primary Cardiology* 17:47-59, 1991.

153. Michel PL, Acar J, Chomette G, et al: Degenerative aortic regurgitation, *Eur Heart J* 12:875-82, 1991.

154. McGoon MD, Fuster V, Shub C, et al: *Aortic regurgitation.* In Giuliani ER et al, eds: *Cardiology: Fundamentals and Practice,* ed 2, St. Louis, 1991, Mosby Year Book.

155. Henry WL, Bonow RO, Borer JS, et al: Observations on the optimum time for operative intervention for aortic regurgitation. I. Evaluation of the results of aortic valve replacement in symptomatic patients, *Circulation* 61:471-95, 1980.

156. Siemienczuk D, Greenberg B, Morris C, et al: Chronic aortic insufficiency: Factors associated with progression to aortic valve replacement, *Ann Intern Med* 110:587-92, 1989.

157. Lewis RP, Bristow JD, Griswold HE: Exercise hemodynamics in aortic regurgitation, *Am Heart J* 80:171-6, 1970.

158. Eberli FR, Ritter M, Schwitter J, et al: Coronary reserve in patients with aortic valve disease before and after successful aortic valve replacement, *Eur Heart J* 12:127-38, 1991.

159. Bonow RO: Left ventricular structure and function in aortic valve disease, *Circulation* 79:966-9, 1989.

160. Braunwald E: *Valvular heart disease.* In Braunwald E, ed: *Heart Diseases,* ed 4, Philadelphia, 1992, WB Saunders.

161. Wooley CF: *Rediscovery of the tricuspid valve.* In Harvey PW, ed: *Current Problems in Cardiology,* Chicago, 1981, Year Book.

162. Wooley CF, Fontana ME, Kilman JW, et al: Tricuspid Stenosis. Atrial systolic murmur, tricuspid opening snap, and right atrial pressure pulse, *Am J Med* 78:375-84, 1985.

163. Maton PN: The carcinoid syndrome, *JAMA* 260:1602-5, 1988.

164. Criley M, et al: *Departures from the expected auscultatory events in mitral stenosis.* In Likoff W, ed: *Valvular Heart Disease,* Philadelphia, 1973, FA Davis.

165. Grossman W: *Cardiac catheterization and angiography,* ed 3, Philadelphia, 1986, Lea & Febiger.

166. Edmunds H Jr, Addonizio P Jr, Tepe NA: *Valvular heart disease: Prosthetic valve replacement.* In Parmley WW, Chatterjeek, eds: *Cardiology,* Philadelphia, 1987, JB Lippincott.

167. Ferrans VJ, McManus B, Roberts WC: Cholesterol ester crystals in porcine aortic valvular bioprosthesis implanted for eight years, *Chest* 83:698, 1983.

168. Olesen KH, Rygg IH, Wennevold A, et al: Aortic valve replacement with the Lillehei-Kaster prosthesis in 262 patients: An assessment after 9 to 17 years, *Eur Heart J* 12:680-9, 1991.

169. Schoen FJ: Surgical pathology of removed natural and prosthetic heart valves, *Hum Pathol* 18:558-67, 1987.

170. Collins JJ: The evolution of artificial heart valves, *N Engl J Med* 324:624-6, 1991.

171. Bloomfield P, Wheatley DJ, Prescott RJ, et al: Twelve-year comparison of a Bjork-Shiley mechanical heart valve with porcine bioprostheses, *N Engl J Med* 324:573-9, 1991.

172. Moxley JH, Beljan JR, Bertozzi S, et al: Xenografts, *JAMA* 254:3353-7, 1985.

173. Lund O, Pilegaard H, Nielsen TT, et al: Thirty-day mortality after valve replacement for aortic stenosis over the last 22 years. A multivariate risk stratification, *Eur Heart J* 12:322-331, 1991.

174. Hosking MP, Warner MA, Lobdell CM, et al: Outcomes of surgery in patients 90 years of age and older, *JAMA* 261:1909-15, 1989.

175. Schaer DH, Cheng TO, Aaron BL: Hemolytic anemia in acute mitral regurgitation caused by a torn cusp of a porcine mitral prosthetic valve seven years after its implantation, *Am Heart J* 113:404-6, 1987.

176. Enzenauer RJ, Berenberg JL, Cassell PF: Microangiopathic hemolytic anemia as the initial manifestation of porcine valve failure, *South Med J* 83:912-7, 1990.

177. Ishihara T, Ferrans VJ, Barnhart GR, et al: Intracuspal hematomas in implanted porcine aortic valvular bioprosthesis, *J Thorac Cardiovasc Surg* 83:399, 1982.

178. Ishihara T, Ferrans J, Jones M, et al: Occurrence and significance of endothelial cells in the implanted porcine bioprosthetic valves, *Am J Cardiol* 48:443, 1981.

179. Ishihara T, Ferrans VJ, Boyce SW, et al: Structure and classification and cuspal tears and perforation in porcine bioprosthetic cardiac valves implanted in patients, *Am J Cardiol* 48:665, 1981.

180. Roberts WC, Ferrans VJ: *Complications of replacement of either the mitral or aortic valve or both by either mechanical or bioprosthetic valves.* In Cohn LH, Gallucci V, eds: *Cardiac Bioprosthesis,* New York, 1982, Worke.

181. Nellessen U, Masuyama T, Appleton CP: Mitral prosthesis malfunction. Comparative Doppler echocardiographic studies of mitral prostheses before and after replacement, *Circulation* 79:330-6, 1989.

182. Ferrans VJ, Tomita Y, Hilbert SL, et al: Pathology of bioprosthetic cardiac valves, *Hum Pathol* 18:586-95, 1987.

183. Silver MD, Butany J: Mechanical heart valves: Methods of examination, complications, and modes of failure, *Hum Pathol* 18:577-85, 1987.

Chapter 4

CARDIAC HYPERTROPHY AND HYPERTENSIVE HEART DISEASE

W. Dallas Hall Jr.
Michael B. Gravanis

CARDIAC HYPERTROPHY

During fetal and early postnatal life (3 to 6 months), demand for increased cardiac mass is provided by an increase in the number of myocytes (hyperplasia). Later in life, similar demands are fulfilled by an increase in the size of a fixed number of preexisting myocytes (hypertrophy). The heart is an efficient protein-synthesizing organ when challenged by an increased hemodynamic load.

The failure of myocytes to resume mitotic activity does not mean that they have lost their capacity to synthesize DNA by the nuclei. In fact, a fraction of the nuclei endoreplicate their DNA complement.[1] Furthermore, induced cardiac growth activates biosynthetic pathways and results in rapid changes in RNA. The end result is an increase in all species of RNA (ribosomal, transfer and messenger) at a proportional level.[1] As biosynthesis is activated, organelles accumulate so that cellular symmetry is properly maintained. In the acute stage of hypertrophy, however, a modest degree of disproportionate growth of mitochondria is observed, but the relation between plasma membrane volume and cell volume remains unchanged.[1] The ratio of sarcotubular membranes to myofibrillar volume is also maintained.

The early preferential proliferation of mitochondria changes as the hypertrophic process advances; eventually, myofibrils accumulate more rapidly than mitochondria. These ultrastructural changes in cellular components differ between pressure and volume overload hypertrophy, and between gradual and abrupt increases in the hemodynamic demand.

Pressure and volume overload hypertrophy

Pressure overload myocyte hypertrophy is characterized by an accumulation and/or alteration of myofibrils, mitochondria, and sarcoplasmic reticulum. Microtubules and intermediate filaments are apparently involved in the assembly of sarcomeres during postnatal development of cardiac muscle.[2] During the development of hypertrophy, intermediate desmin filaments are mainly involved in the process of myofibril registration, whereas microtubules increase in number and change in their distribution. Microtubules have a dynamic role in sarcomerogenesis.[3]

Hypertrophy entails the addition of new contractile proteins and mitochondria. However, this adaptive process is not merely an addition of identical units; it is accompanied by reorganization at the cellular and subcellular level. Furthermore, besides the quantitative response of the myocardium, there is a qualitative change in the composition of contractile proteins in hypertrophic myocytes. Induction of fetal isogenes occurs in adult hearts during pressure overload hypertrophy. However, reexpression of the fetal program is not an obligatory process; similar degrees of hypertrophy in hyperthyroidism reveal no induction of fetal isogenes.[4] The reexpression of fetal isogenes is viewed as a beneficial adaptation to the hemodynamic overload, resulting in the production of sarcomeres with useful functional properties. The myosin heavy chain (MHC) transition from the normal adult type (a-MHC) to the fetal (b-MHC) isoform is interpreted as an adaptation to a bioenergetically more efficient type of myosin. A similar fetal shift can also occur in other enzymes that regulate intermediary metabolism and muscle contraction, resulting in a greater percentage of fetal isoenzymes of creatine kinase (CK) and lactate dehydrogenase (LDH).[5] Such changes reflect the heart's ability to adapt to stress by synthesis of fetal isoenzymes, a favorable adaptation that ensures that the resynthesis of ATP via the CK reaction remains high.

Various isoforms of both myosin light and heavy chains are known. In cardiac muscle the two types of myosin heavy chains are alpha and beta. These form myosin molecules composed of an alpha-alpha homodimer, an alpha-beta heterodimer, and a beta-beta homodimer, known respectively as the V1, V2, and V3 isoforms. Both pressure and volume-induced hypertrophy are accompanied by a shift from the V1 toward the V2 and V3 isomyosins. The V3 isoform is characterized by low speed muscle shortening, calcium activated ATPase activity, and oxygen consumption, resulting in an improved economy of force generation.[6] V1 has opposite effects and V2 is intermediate. Thus the pressure and volume overload–related shift toward the V3 isoform is a beneficial adaptational process. Humans do not have the same adaptational capacity as small mammals; poor adaptation can result in decreased contractility in the hypertrophied myocardium.[7] One possible beneficial adaptive mechanism in humans may involve myosin light chains, which influence myofibrillar ATPase activity.[8]

The molecular mechanism by which pressure overload induces myosin isoform switching remains unknown. Knowledge is also limited regarding the biochemical signal that regulates myosin gene expression in the pressure overloaded condition. The specific signals that initiate myocyte hypertrophy and the intracellular mechanisms that transduce these signals have not been completely elucidated.

Another change observed in pressure overload hypertrophy is that of the atrial natriuretic factor (ANF) mRNA, expressed primarily in the atria in normal hearts. High levels of ANF occur in pressure-overloaded adult ventricles. The induction of ANF mRNA in the left ventricle in pressure overload hypertrophy is an adaptational response that reduces the hemodynamic load imposed on the ventricle.[9]

Other conditions that can induce myocardial hypertrophy include hypoxia, anemia, exercise, loss of myocardial mass, and excess of thyroid hormone or catecholamines. Although many investigators hope that a single mediator for all those types of hypertrophy will be found, such a discovery has not materialized.

Molecular biology of cardiac hypertrophy

Role of protooncogenes. Mechanical stimuli (stretching) on myocytes can directly induce specific gene expression and protein synthesis without the participation of humoral factors.[10] Hemodynamic overload, such as stretching of myocytes, will induce expression of specific genes such as protooncogenes and a major heat shock protein gene (hsp 70).[4]

Protooncogenes (cellular oncogenes) are normal cellular genes encoding critical regulatory proteins. The importance of protooncogenes in growth regulation was confirmed by the discovery of homology of protooncogenes with known growth factors and growth factor receptors.[11] Functional groups of protooncogenes include growth factors and growth factor receptors, protein kinases, guanosine nucleotide binding proteins, and RNA transcription factors. Such grouping advances the concept that any gene encoding a growth factor, a receptor, an intracellular signaling molecule, or a protein that regulates transcription, can be considered a protooncogene.[12] However, not all protooncogenes have a role in growth regulation. More than 20 peptide growth factors have been defined, some with broader than physiologic effects on growth.[13] Growth factors that originate from the target cell are referred to as autocrine; those from neighboring cells are called paracrine; and those from remote tissues are designated as endocrine. Furthermore, growth factors may modulate cell growth, differentiation, or function (e.g., contraction or secretion) in a positive or negative way.[14,15,16] These diverse cellular effects may not be mutually exclusive, and may depend on the total growth factor environment of a cell and its phase of development.[11]

The bulk of information about growth factors and myocyte hypertrophy is derived from studies in experimental animals. Within 1 hour following pressure overload in rats, c-fos and c-myc protooncogenes and a major head shock protein gene (hsp 70) are induced in the ventricular myocardium. The physiologic significance of such induction is not clear, but the extremely rapid response to pressure overload mimics the early mitogenic response to growth factors by a variety of cells.[17,18] There is adequate evidence, however, that c-fos and c-myc are transcription factors[19] and that both can rapidly be induced in response to a wide variety of stimuli. However, induction of c-fos and c-myc in response to pressure overload is transient and returns to baseline within 24 to 48 hours.[4] For the development of hypertrophy, a continuous hemodynamic overload is necessary, which indicates that expression of genes per se may not be enough to trigger the hypertrophic response. A permissive role in mediating the hypertrophic response has been suggested for c-fos and c-myc proteins because they are localized in the nucleus.[18] Hemodynamic overload is one of the main factors that stimulates expression of the c-fos gene in the heart. The protein that it encodes, fos, is localized in the nucleus and is believed to play an important role in regulating the subsequent expression of other genes.[20] Fos appears to be regulated by multiple factors in myocytes. For example, fos mRNA in the myocardium is increased by high coronary flow or pressure,[21] contractility induced by α or β-adrenergic stimulation, and by histamine H1 and prostaglandin E1 (PGE1).[22]

Another protooncogene that may be associated with cardiac hypertrophy is c-Ha-ras. Ha-ras genes encode 21-KDa proteins that appear to be involved in control of cellular growth and differentiation.[23]

Additional growth factors or receptors in the myocardium include c-sis mRNA (PDGF B chain) and the PDGF receptor, which may constitute an autocrine or paracrine heart cell growth factor system.[24] The alpha-1-adrenergic receptor was the first well-documented growth factor receptor for cardiac myocytes.[11] Stimulation of this receptor on cultured neonatal rat myocytes increased cell size, total and myofibrillar protein synthesis, total RNA content, and c-myc mRNA content.[25,26]

The biologic effects of protooncogenes seem to depend on the cell type, although the biochemical function of the proteins (growth factor, receptor, transducer, or transcription factor) may be the same in all cells.[11] Different types of hypertrophy may denote the actions of various combinations of growth factors on myocyte-specific genes.[11] The current emphasis on growth factors should not overshadow the acknowledgment that physical stimuli (such as stretch) activate cell transduction stimuli with synthesis of total and specific cardiac proteins.[11]

Pressure overload also induces myocardial hypertrophy by expanding the myocyte capacity for protein synthesis, a reaction not dependent on an increase in myocardial work.

Protein synthesis increases as perfusion pressure is raised, even after removing ventricular preload.[27]

Accepting the premise that protooncogenes orchestrate the important early changes in contractile protein synthesis requires identification of a biochemical signal linking the increase in aortic pressure to activation of the protooncogenes. Possible receptors for mechanical stimuli may include ion channels[28] and receptors for extracellular matrix proteins, such as integrins.[29] Search for the crucial link between the initial stimulus for pressure overload hypertrophy and the secondary increase in gene expression has led to the hypothesis that an increase in cytosolic free Ca^{2+} concentration may trigger the expression of protooncogenes with subsequent protein synthesis.[30]

In perfused, isovolumically contracting ferret hearts, both diastolic and peak systolic intracellular Ca^{2+} increased when perfusion pressure was raised from 80 mm Hg to 120 mm Hg.[31] The exact mechanism by which intracellular Ca^{2+} increases in response to perfusion pressure is not known. However, increases in Ca^{2+} and protein kinase C induce protooncogenes such as c-fos and c-myc.[32,33]

Thyroid hormone hypertrophy

The hypertrophic response to some stimuli does not require new protooncogene expression. It can occur with hypertrophy induced by thyroxine where triiodothyronine permeates the cell membrane and interacts directly with a nuclear protein to modulate transcription without activation of protooncogenes.[34] Administration of thyroid hormone in rats (10 weeks) increases the myocyte volume in both ventricles, most noticeably in the right ventricle. In the left ventricle, subepicardial myocytes reveal more hypertrophy than do myocytes in the middle myocardium and subendocardium.[35] After cessation of hormonal treatment a precipitous drop in right ventricular and subepicardial myocyte cell volume occurs within 4 days.

During thyroid treatment, animals reveal a moderate increase in systemic blood pressure and a marked increase in heart rate. The concept that heart rate might play a prominent role in myocyte hypertrophy was dispelled by normalizing the heart rate with propranolol in hyperthyroid rats, which did not decrease the amount of hypertrophy.[36] The hypertrophy is characterized by increase of both cross-sectional area and length of the myocytes. The mechanism proposed for thyroid hormone-induced cardiac hypertrophy is as follows: after binding to its membrane receptor, the hormone is internalized, binds to sites on sensitive DNA, and mediates or modulates transcriptional processes that result in the regulation of specific genes.[37]

Renin-angiotensin-aldosterone system in cardiac hypertrophy

Recent attention has been directed to the renin-angiotensin system and its relation to left ventricular hypertrophy. Available data indicate that an inverse relation exists between renin-angiotensin system activity and LV performance in human hypertension.[38] Furthermore, patients with primary or secondary low renin hypertension appear to develop concentric LVH proportional to the blood pressure elevation, whereas patients with high renin hypertension are more likely to develop eccentric LVH with lesser and inadequate wall thickening to offset the increased pressure load.[38]

A local renin-angiotensin system in the heart has been isolated and characterized biochemically.[39] In rhesus monkeys, angiotensin-II levels were higher in the atria (especially the right atrium) than in the ventricles.[40] Components of the renin-angiotensin system required for local angiotensin production have also been identified in the vascular wall.[41] Locally generated vascular angiotensin II may be involved in various hemodynamic functions (e.g., spasm) and might modulate the vascular angiotensin receptors and their response to circulating angiotensin.[42]

Angiotensin II can be a direct stimulus for myocyte growth, independent of its effects on raising vascular resistance and cardiac afterload.[43] Angiotensinogen mRNA is present in the left ventricle in pressure overload hypertrophy and is upregulated in both atria and ventricles. It remains unclear, however, whether the presence of angiotensinogen mRNA is the result of pressure overload, or a mere accompaniment of left ventricular hypertrophy. Whether the contribution of the renin-angiotensin system in pressure-overload hypertrophy derives from circulating or cardiac-produced angiotensin II is also uncertain, but current information suggests that a localized cardiac renin-angiotensin system has a paracrine or autocrine function for inducing and perpetuating cell growth.[44]

Myotrophin and other mitogenic peptides

Recent experimental work has demonstrated a factor, "myotrophin," that exists in the hypertrophic myocardium of spontaneous hypertensive rats (SHR) and stimulates protein synthesis in cultured adult rat myocytes in vitro.[45] Myotrophin is a protein of 12KDa capable of enlarging cell surface area and enhancing maturation of myocardial cells; it has no mitogenic properties.

A high molecular-weight (135 KDa) polypeptide has also been found in the sera of experimental animals with pressure overload.[46] This phosphoprotein persists until a certain stage of hypertrophy is reached and then disappears. The protein, probably present in repressed levels in the normal animal, may not be obligatory for a rapid increase in myocardial mass, as is the case in thyroxine-induced hypertrophy.[46] Data indicate that this polypeptide is synthesized in cardiac cells, is present in nuclei, and could traverse cardiac cells and extracellular fluid, suggesting an autocrine/paracrine role during the development of cardiac hypertrophy.

Normal human atrial and ventricular myocardium also contain mitogens for fibroblasts and endothelial cells. These mitogens resemble aFGF and bFGF in their molecular weight and affinity to heparin.[47] Suggested possible functions for cardiac FGF peptides include development of myocyte hypertrophy, healing of myocardial infarction, development of coronary collaterals, and proliferation of vascular smooth muscle. The precise role of these peptides has not been clarified.

Although several factors modulate the rate and degree of myocardial hypertrophy, increased hemodynamic loading per se appears to be an important factor for the compensatory hypertrophy of the pressure or volume-overloaded heart in the adult.[48] Furthermore, there are only quantitative differences between the anabolic effects of diastolic and systolic loading of the myocardium.[49] Adult myocardium exhibits a remarkable plasticity in response to either increased or decreased loading in terms of rapid and reversible changes in composition, structure, and function. The germane question is how the cardiocyte translates changes in physical properties into intracellular signals that regulate protein synthesis. Whether higher organisms can transduce mechanical stimuli into electrical responses (such as is described in protozoa) is unknown.[50] Other cells, such as hair cells of the auditory, vestibular cells, or even embryonic chick skeletal myocytes, have stretch-activated ion channels that, when activated by deformation, allow the gated entry of one or more cations. Similar principles may apply to stress-induced cardiac deformation through hemodynamic loading. Such transduction of load into growth may be accomplished by activation of ion channels that constitute the most important routes by which environmental information reaches the interior of the cell.[51]

TYPES OF CARDIAC HYPERTROPHY
Normal postnatal cardiac growth

Postnatal physiologic growth of the heart is characterized by a well-balanced expansion of parenchymal cells, subcellular components, extracellular matrix, and capillary microvasculature, all of which grow in proportion to the increase in cardiac mass. Transition from the fetal to the adult form of circulation is accompanied by a progressive increase in volume load affecting both sides of the heart, and significant increase in pressure load affecting the left ventricle.[52] Pressure overload on the myocardium of the left ventricle results in a relatively greater LV muscle mass in the adult heart (Fig. 4-1).

In rats, myocytes continue to proliferate (hyperplasia) up to approximately 3 weeks, although the major increase in cell numbers occurs within the first few days after birth.[53] When myocyte enlargement (hypertrophy) becomes the main growth mechanism, an increased cross-sectional diameter of the myocytes is responsible for the increases in wall thickness with age. With maturation, the myocyte undergoes a significant increase in length and di-

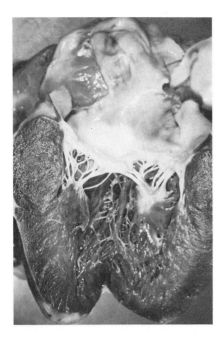

Fig. 4-1. Severe left ventricular hypertrophy in a patient with long-standing systemic hypertension.

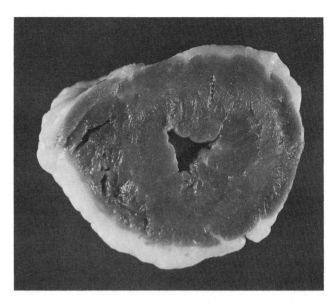

Fig. 4-2. Cross heart section, midventricular level, showing marked concentric left ventricular hypertrophy. Note small left ventricular chamber.

ameter. The maturation process also changes the composition of the myocyte at the cellular level, with increases in the volume fractions of mitochondria and myofibrils.

In the first month of postnatal life in the rat, capillary growth exceeds myocyte growth. In the adult heart, capillary luminal volume and surface per unit volume of myocytes remain nearly constant.[52]

Concentric hypertrophy

Increased pressure load in the adult heart induces *concentric hypertrophy* of the left ventricle without chamber enlargement (Fig. 4-2). The resulting hypertrophy is not uniform in the various layers of the free wall of the left ventricle, interventricular septum, and papillary muscles.[52] Although cardiac hypertrophy secondary to chronic systemic hypertension has been described as concentric with symmetric involvement of all segments of the left ventricular wall, some hypertensive patients exhibit an asymmetric distribution of hypertrophy and can even simulate the asymmetric hypertrophy of primary hypertrophic cardiomyopathy. Studies using two dimensional (2-D) echocardiography have shown that the distribution of LV hypertrophy was asymmetric in as many as one third of hypertensive patients.[54] Some patients also exhibit a circumscribed hypertrophy confined to the anterior basal ventricular septum under the aortic valve, similar to that seen in hypertrophic cardiomyopathy. The severity and duration of hypertension may be the major determinants of the extent and form of left ventricular hypertrophy.

The increased cross-sectional diameter of myocytes reflects an adaptive response that tends to minimize the ef-

fects of an increased pressure load. The increased myocyte diameter and wall thickness help offset the higher peak systolic wall stress, according to LaPlace's law.[55] Mitochondrial growth exceeds myofibril growth early in the hypertrophic process (pressure overload), but later there is a reduction of the mitochondrial to myofibrillar volume ratio that can lead to impaired cardiac muscle function.[56]

Some reports have also demonstrated hypertrophy of the right ventricle in essential hypertension, with average anterior right ventricular wall thickness of 6 mm to 7 mm in hypertensive patients with echocardiographic left ventricular hypertrophy, compared with 3 mm to 4 mm in normotensive controls.[57,58]

Angiogenesis and capillary proliferation in cardiac hypertrophy

Although capillary length is not significantly altered in pressure overload hypertrophy, indicating lack of capillary proliferation, the average size of capillaries does increase. The larger capillary size compensates for the inadequate lengthening of the capillary microvasculature and maintains a somewhat constant capillary luminal volume and surface in the hypertrophic ventricle.[56] A number of studies have suggested that coronary vascular growth lags behind that of cardiac muscle growth during the development of left ventricular hypertrophy. However, other data in experimental studies provide evidence that angiogenesis of major resistance vessels can parallel the ventricular hypertrophy associated with chronic hypertension.[59] Contrary to experimental animal studies, however, there is no evidence for significant angiogenesis in humans with left ventricular hypertrophy. Therefore a number of problems can occur in the coronary circulation of the hypertrophic heart.

In humans, hypertrophic hearts reveal a relative decrease in capillary density (increased intercapillary distance), and greater intramyocardial compressive forces (high cavitary pressures) that can compromise coronary perfusion. These anatomic and physiologic factors contribute to the hypertrophic heart's susceptibility to ischemia.

Hypertension is an established risk factor for myocardial infarction and its complications, including heart failure, arrhythmias, cardiac rupture, or sudden death.[60] In hypertension with left ventricular hypertrophy, coronary autoregulation is shifted toward higher pressures, likely due to impaired vasodilator reserve.[61]

Until lately, the prevailing concept was that hypertensive patients were predisposed to earlier and more severe coronary atherosclerosis. In recent years more attention has focused on the reserve and autoregulation of small intramyocardial vessels. If myocardial hypertrophy is present, coronary flow is increased and a higher autoregulatory line is established. The upward shift of the lower range of autoregulation would make it possible that coronary flow declines even when the aortic pressure is returned to levels that are within the normal range.[62]

Endothelial factors in cardiac hypertrophy

Studies in humans have confirmed older observations that the endothelium modulates the activity of vascular smooth muscle and resistance vessels.[63] Vascular relaxation is related to endothelium-derived relaxing factor (EDRF), which may be nitric oxide. Several studies in experimental animals and humans indicate that endothelial-mediated vasodilatation is reduced in atherosclerotic arteries.[64] A defective vasodilator response to acetylcholine, possibly caused by decreased release of EDRF by endothelial cells,[65] led to the discovery of altered endothelium-mediated vascular relaxation in patients with essential hypertension. Whether endothelial dysfunction in such patients is primary or secondary has not been determined. However, even if it is secondary, it could still exacerbate the primary vascular wall abnormality and further raise peripheral resistance.

A reduction in coronary artery reserve in hypertrophic hearts may also reflect altered vasodilating capacity. Additional factors (e.g., medial hypertrophy) may also contribute to the reduction of coronary reserve in hypertrophic hearts. Intramyocardial small artery disease has been considered as a possible mechanism for myocardial ischemia in patients with hypertensive heart disease. Indeed, autopsy studies have revealed that the mean percentage luminal diameter of intramyocardial small arteries was lower in hypertensive hearts than in normal hearts, and correlated inversely with the area of fibrosis.[66]

Biochemical studies of impaired contractility of the hypertrophied myocardium have not clarified why this normally efficient system fails. Moreover, it is not clear whether any given biochemical abnormality is primary or secondary. A search for a structural basis for left ventricular dysfunction in the hypertrophied myocardium has considered both myocyte and nonmyocyte compartments (e.g., connective tissue matrix, vasculature). We have already discussed the cellular and molecular myocyte alterations in cardiac hypertrophy; thus the following discussion will concentrate on the role of the nonmyocyte compartments in the pathologic remodeling of the myocardium.

Connective tissue components of cardiac hypertrophy

The cardiac connective tissue, or endoskeleton, is primarily composed of collagen (types I, III and IV), but it also includes fibronectin, laminin, elastin, and microfibrils, along with glycoproteins that serve as intercellular lubricants. Collagen fibrils extending from lateral myocyte to myocyte, and from myocyte to blood vessel connections, are called struts.[67] Meshes of connective tissue that surround individual and groups of myocytes are called weaves, and interstitial and thick spring-like structures are called coils.[68] It is suggested that weaves and struts maintain myocyte alignment, permitting reversible interdigitation of contracting myocytes while restricting slippage between myocytes and limiting the dissipation of generated tension.[69]

In essence, collagen may control the extent to which myocytes stretch and contract. In that respect, collagen contributes to the mechanical (viscoelastic) behavior of the myocardium, although it composes only 2% to 3% of the heart.[69]

The majority of cardiac collagen is type I, which comprises approximately 85% of the total collagen; lesser amounts of type III (11%) and type V (perivascular space) are (4%) present. Fibroblasts produce type I, III, and IV types of collagen; myocytes (within the basement membrane) and endothelial cells produce type IV collagen. Intracellular procollagen synthesis is rapid, but extracellular collagen turnover is slow.[70]

The collagen network of the heart consists of three components: epimysium, perimysium, and endomysium. On the epicardial surface, the epimysium is found below the visceral pericardium. On the endocardial side, the epimysium is located under the endothelium and basement membrane. Arborizations of the epimysium become the perimysium, which surrounds muscle bundles. Attachments between muscle bundles are provided by perimysial fibers that have a wavy, tendinous, or cable-like configuration. The endomysium gives rise to fibers that surround individual muscle fibers and connect adjacent ones.[71]

At birth, the collagen concentration in the left and right ventricles is equal. In the adult heart, collagen concentration of the right ventricle is 30% greater than that of the left ventricle, probably due to reduction in the size of right ventricular myocytes after birth.[72]

Collagen is important for the support and alignment of

myocytes and is a major determinant of myocardial stiffness. Other mechanical functions of the cardiac extracellular matrix are transduction of myocyte-generated force to the ventricular chamber, protection of sarcomeres from excessive stretching, and the active relengthening of myocytes that help diastolic filling.[72] Thus a connective tissue matrix maintains cardiac integrity, transmits and possibly amplifies contractile forces, buffers abnormal increases in intracavitary pressure, and stores energy during systole, which aids the relengthening of myocytes during relaxation.

Increases in extracellular matrix, seen in various pathologic conditions (including myocardial hypertrophy), can decrease chamber compliance and adversely affect myocardial contractility and LV filling. Reduction of extracellular matrix can lead to ineffective contraction, increased chamber compliance, and myocyte slippage, resulting in myocardial wall thinning. Such loss of matrix can be regional or global. Although definitive correlations with clinical evidence of cardiac failure are often lacking, the importance of extracellular connective tissue matrix and the status of the intramyocardial coronary arteries is gaining recognition.

The structural remodeling of nonmyocyte compartments in cardiac hypertrophy is not the same in all disease states because hypertrophy is a heterogenous process. Perhaps this heterogeneity exists either because the compartments, namely the myocyte and nonmyocyte, are under the influence of different regulatory mechanisms, or because they respond in a different way to the same signals.[73] It has been suggested that myocyte and nonmyocyte cells grow independently of each other, as seen in radiation-induced myocardial fibrosis, where there is growth and remodeling of nonmyocyte cells without myocyte growth.[74]

In contrast, cardiac hypertrophy associated with exercise training, arteriovenous fistulas, chronic anemia, or thyroxine or growth hormone excess reveals myocyte growth without increase in collagen concentration. Conditions in which both myocyte hypertrophy and disproportionate non-myocyte cell growth occur include various forms of hypertension, aortic stenosis, and coarctation of the aorta.[74]

In morphologic terms the remodeling of the myocardium in hypertrophy can be either homogenous or heterogenous, depending on the degree of growth of nonmyocyte cells.[75] In instances in which the proportionality of muscular, vascular, and interstitial compartments is maintained, the hypertrophy is physiologic. In instances where there is a disproportionate nonmyocyte cell growth and a heterogeneity in myocardial structure, the hypertrophy is pathologic.

In both human and nonhuman primate hypertension, the morphologic features consist of interstitial fibrosis with thick fibrillar collagen, perivascular fibrosis, replacement fibrosis (reparative), and a plexiform fibrosis of collagen fibers associated with myocyte disarray.[74]

In the nonhuman primate, the sequence of events after induction of renovascular hypertension includes interstitial edema followed by accumulation of fibrillar collagen in the perivascular space and interstitium surrounding muscle bundles. In this model, the functional effect of the increased collagen is characterized by an early (8 to 12 weeks) increase in diastolic stiffness, but systolic function (ejection fraction) is preserved. The later stages (32 weeks) are characterized by systolic dysfunction with chamber dilatation and reduced ejection fraction.

Collagen components in cardiac hypertrophy related to pressure or volume overload

Although there is ample evidence from studies in humans and in experimental animals that myocardial collagen is increased with the hypertrophic process, the degree of collagen growth relative to muscle appears to be a function of several factors, including age, species, rapidity of induction of pressure overload, nature of the initiating lesion, and the severity and duration of the overload. Whether the collagen-forming capacity of the myocardium is increased because of greater synthesis by existing fibroblasts or a greater number of fibroblasts is not entirely clear.[75]

Furthermore, the interrelation between the structural features of the two major types of the collagen matrix (i.e., type I and III), their biochemical characteristics and biophysical properties, and the function they serve in the myocardium have not been defined.[76] This information is of considerable importance because myocardial stiffness does not correlate directly with total collagen content, and changes in collagen phenotypes could be responsible for compromised function in hypertensive heart disease. The possibility that the myocardial collagen phenotype could be more important than the total amount of collagen present in the myocardium has prompted several investigations. For example, in spontaneously hypertensive rats a marked increase in the type I:III ratio has been noted in the established phase of hypertensive hypertrophy.[77] Increased deposition of collagen type III was associated with a transition from compensated hypertrophy to decompensation with myocardial dysfunction. In humans, during the compensated phase of concentric hypertrophy with normal or reduced LV chamber size, increased deposition of thick bundles of type I collagen occurs.[77] With the onset of decompensation and a dilated left ventricle, there is an increase in the deposition of Type III collagen fibers.[78]

Similar to other cardiac proteins, myocardial collagen gene expression is altered in experimental hypertension. In animal experiments, collagen type IV mRNA levels increase rapidly after induction of pressure overload. Changes in mRNA levels of type-I collagen also occur

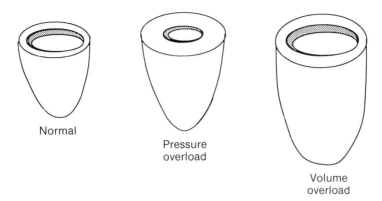

Fig. 4-3. Schematic presentation of pressure vs volume overload left ventricular hypertrophy.

early, but discernible fibrosis occurs only at later stages. The reason for this delay in deposition of mature collagen is that posttranslational modifications, such as intermolecular and intramolecular covalent cross-linking of the secreted collagen molecules, are necessary for the formation of mature collagen.[79]

Similar to myocytes, myocardial fibroblasts participate actively in the hypertrophic process of pressure overload. However, the precise signal and transducer of fibroblast collagen synthesis secondary to increased chamber pressure is not known. From a limited number of reports it appears that myocyte necrosis is not the stimulus for this reactive fibrosis, and that the interstitial and muscular compartments may be under separate controls.[80] Perhaps release of stored mitogens in the interstitium (e.g., norepinephrine) may stimulate collagen synthesis and fibroblast proliferation. This view is supported by the observation that enhanced collagen formation is not found in the pressure overloaded heart following denervation.[81]

Although there are adequate data to suggest that mechanical factors (e.g., stretch) can induce myocyte hypertrophy, it is uncertain whether they can promote the growth of cardiac fibroblasts or enhance their synthesis of collagen. As was stated earlier, collagen concentration remains normal in myocardial hypertrophy secondary to arteriovenous fistulas, chronic anemia, or thyroxine administration, but increases in the hypertensive heart or with aortic stenosis. Thus comparable elevations in wall stress resulting from ventricular pressure or volume overload can result in disproportionate accumulation of collagen in myocardial hypertrophy. These findings support the view that ventricular loading is the critical determinant of myocyte growth. However, nonmyocyte growth can occur in the absence of myocyte growth, and can be induced by nonhemodynamic factors such as circulating hormones that act as growth stimuli to cardiac fibroblasts.[74]

Recent evidence suggests that the remodeling of the collagen network and intramyocardial coronary arteries is related to the concentration of circulating hormones such as angiotensin II or aldosterone. Circulating aldosterone may bind to a cell surface receptor of the fibroblast, or its action may be mediated through a cytosolic receptor. The interaction of circulating aldosterone with the corticoid receptor of fibroblasts (and its possible stimulation of collagen synthesis) is probably accomplished through DNA binding and collagen gene synthesis.[74]

Several studies have indicated different effects of various antihypertensive drugs on total collagen content.[82] The exact mechanism of action of those drugs on cardiac collagen metabolism has not been elucidated.

In patients with aortic stenosis, collagen volume fraction (determined by endomyocardial biopsies) and the degree of fibrosis was unchanged in the majority of patients before and after valve replacement.[72] Similar to aortic stenosis, reversal of hypertensive hypertrophy with most antihypertensive drugs may shift the relation between contractile and noncontractile proteins in favor of the noncontractile components.[83] However, antihypertensive therapy with calcium blockers in spontaneously hypertensive rats was associated with regression of the myocardial collagen in parallel with cardiac muscle mass, leaving myocardial distensibility unchanged.[83]

The studies and observations mentioned above clearly indicate that the pathophysiology of myocardial dysfunction in hypertensive heart disease is multifactorial, with altered collagen matrix having an important role.[76] The myocardial responses to pressure overload are complicated, and hemodynamic factors alone do not account for the hypertrophic response of the ventricle in hypertension.

Increased volume load induces enlargement of the left ventricular chamber of the heart without, or only mild, increase in its wall thickness. This is *eccentric hypertrophy* (Fig. 4-3). Adaptive mechanisms in dynamic exercise and endurance training are accompanied by an elevated preload, a condition that progresses to eccentric hypertrophy.[52] In the physiologic LV hypertrophy of endurance athletes, diastolic function is normal.[84] Moreover, unlike hypertrophic or hypertensive cardiomyopathy, reactive antimitochondrial antibodies are not found.[85]

In strenuous exercise, however, the adaptive hypertrophy is greater in the right ventricle, which begins with a thinner wall, less mass, and a smaller total number of myocytes.[86] Volume overload hypertrophy in exercise produces chamber enlargement through lengthening of myocytes by replication of sarcomeres in series.[87] The volume fractions of mitochondria and myofibrils remain nearly constant in volume overload exercise-induced hypertrophy.[86] Moderate exercise hypertrophy is associated with increases in total capillary volume, surface, and length. In cases of strenuous exercise and/or pathologic conditions (e.g., aortocaval fistula), capillary luminal volume remains nearly constant, but the absolute increases in capillary surface and length are less by one third of the overall growth of the ventricle.[52] Therefore excessive volume overload hypertrophy can lead to a state that leaves the myocardium more susceptible to ischemia, and may contribute to the transition from cardiac hypertrophy to cardiac failure. Different data have been reported, however, by others using an infrarenal aortocaval shunt in dogs. Transition from cardiac hypertrophy to cardiac failure occurred in the absence of significant changes in the geometry of the capillary network.[88]

In experimental volume overload hypertrophy (arteriovenous shunt) there is an increased diastolic stiffness of the left ventricle. This is thought to be associated with either a quantitative or qualitative (structural) change in the collagen content.[89] It also has been suggested that the collagen concentration does not increase in volume overload hypertrophy, and often the ratio of type I to type III collagen remains unaltered.[90] Recent evidence, however, indicates that there is a greater degree of collagen cross-linking associated with increase in passive compliance in volume overload hypertrophy.[91]

Postinfarction reactive nypertrophy

Reactive hypertrophy. This condition can result from focal or diffuse loss of myocytes such as occurs in ischemic heart disease. Postinfarction alterations in ventricular geometry include areas of thinning and bulging, which may obscure the overall morphology. However, on a cellular basis, postinfarction hypertrophy includes both an increase in myocyte diameter and length; the hypertrophic cell maintains a constant mitochrondrial to myofibrillar volume ratio.[92,93] Thus the anatomy of postinfarction reactive hypertrophy is like that of a combination of pressure and volume overload hypertrophy. This reactive hypertrophy lags in the adaptive growth of the microvasculature with respect to myocytes. Therefore the hypertrophic infarcted ventricle is more vulnerable to subsequent ischemic episodes.[93]

Hypertrophy of blood vessels

Morphologic changes, such as hypertrophy or thickening of the walls of large arteries as the result of increased systemic blood pressure, are well known. Elastin and collagen, the two major connective tissue components of blood vessels, compose about three-fourths of the dry weight of the vessel wall, with elastin more abundant in the thoracic aorta and collagen predominating in the abdominal aorta. These proteins are major contributors and account in large part for the physical properties of the walls of large arteries, such as distensibility, elastic recoil, and tensile strength. Elastin is rapidly synthesized and accumulates in the aorta during the perinatal period. Once it reaches adult levels, the synthesis of the protein rapidly decreases, and its turnover is very slow.[94]

Regardless of the specific model of hypertension used, there are increases in both total aortic segment weight and content of insoluble elastin early in the development of hypertension. The increased synthesis of aortic elastin in hypertension is rapid but transient, reaching a maximum and then returning to normal levels of synthesis.[95] It is believed that the stimulus for increased connective tissue production is an increase in hydraulic stress in the vascular wall. Therefore the transient nature of this response could be explained by Laplace's law: as wall thickness increases (elastic, collagen), wall stress decreases, reducing the drive for connective tissue production.[95]

FUNCTIONAL CHANGES IN THE HYPERTROPHIED LEFT VENTRICLE
Left ventricular diastolic dysfunction in hypertension

A variety of noninvasive methods are used currently to assess diastolic function in hypertensive patients.[96] Radionuclide angiography uses R-wave gated scintigraphy to detect chamber filling rates of erythrocytes labeled with technetium-99m pertechnetate.[97] Other techniques include digitized M-mode echocardiography[98,99] and the diastolic mitral inflow velocity profile obtained by Doppler echocardiography.[100] Most methods assess diastolic filling during rest and again following a stimulus designed to increase the rate of diastolic filling, such as exercise,[97] volume loading, or 45° leg elevation for 5 minutes.[101]

Ventricular relaxation is an energy-dependent process that requires ATP for removal of Ca^{2+} from the cytoplasm and contractile proteins of myocardial cells, allowing lengthening and ventricular filling without an increase in filling pressure.[102,103] The majority of diastolic filling (up to 80%) occurs during the first one-third of diastole. This is referred to as the rapid or "early" ventricular filling phase; derived indices during this phase include the peak filling rate, the time to peak filling rate, and the first-third filling fraction.[104] Early diastolic filling is followed by a slow and passive filling period where less than 5% of diastolic filling occurs. The final "late" phase of diastolic filling represents atrial contraction when 15% to 20% of filling occurs normally.

Diastolic dysfunction may be the earliest indicator of the effects of hypertension on the heart.[96,97,105] It is detectable in up to 84% of hypertensive patients[97] and, although often associated with evidence of left ventricular hypertrophy, can precede it.[106] The diastolic dysfunction associated with hypertension is characterized by a decreased early peak filling rate, prolongation of the time to peak filling rate, and often, a greater than usual contribution of atrial contraction to late diastolic filling.

When inadequate filling of the left ventricle occurs during diastole, the increased left ventricular filling pressure can be transmitted to the left atrium and lungs, leading to dyspnea and pulmonary congestion despite a normal contractility and ejection fraction.[107]

In the conscious dog made hypertensive by bilateral renal artery constriction, accentuation of the diastolic filling rate was noted early in the course to return to normal at the time of the appearance of LV hypertrophy. Such findings are highly suggestive that intracardiac structural changes may be responsible for the alteration in LV diastolic function rather than the presence of hypertension.[108] Furthermore, comparative studies of hypertensive patients and normotensive individuals have shown that left ventricular diastolic dysfunction in hypertension may be associated with an impairment in cardiopulmonary reflexes, and therefore may influence peripheral vascular regulation.[109]

Left ventricular systolic dysfunction in hypertension

Prolonged periods of hypertension in the spontaneous hypertensive rat are often associated with abnormal myocardial performance due to progressive impairment of intrinsic muscle function as the rat develops heart failure.[110] Proposed mechanisms for depressed myocardial contractility include, (1) alteration in intracellular Ca^{2+} availability, (2) alterations of myofilament Ca^{2+} responsiveness, or (3) a combination of these two mechanisms.[111] Recent data indicate that with the development of hypertrophy, calcium sensitivity of the left ventricular muscle remains unaffected, but maximal calcium-activated force declines with the development of left ventricular failure, despite the continued presence of significant hypertrophy. These changes are thought to represent important physiologic adaptive mechanisms.[112]

In eccentric hypertrophy an increased end-diastolic volume and increased systolic wall stress become important factors for left ventricular performance. In this form of hypertrophy, the afterload is increased while cardiac index and ejection fraction are depressed and myocardial oxygen consumption is increased.[113] Coronary reserve is significantly reduced in eccentric hypertrophy.

Mechanisms that may lead to decrease in myocardial function and congestive heart failure in hypertension include left ventricular pressure overload with myocardial ischemia and focal myocyte necrosis, impairment of oxygen diffusion capacity (increased distance between capillary and myocyte), reduction in protein synthesis, increased myocardial extracellular matrix, and decreased myosin-ATPase activity.[113]

Left ventricular hypertrophy and cardiovascular risks

Left ventricular hypertrophy (LVH) is associated with an increased risk of cardiovascular mortality and sudden death. Both simple and complex ventricular arrhythmias occur more often in hypertensive patients with LVH than in those without it.[114] However, the relationship between ventricular arrhythmias in hypertensive LVH and other variables (e.g., coexistent coronary artery disease or left ventricular dysfunction) that influence arrhythmia frequency is not clear. A recent study of hypertensive patients evaluated coronary arteriography, echocardiographic left ventricular mass, left ventricular function, and left endomyocardial biopsy in relation to ventricular arrhythmias.[115] The findings suggest that the increased frequency of ventricular arrhythmias among hypertensive patients with LVH could not have resulted solely from coexistent coronary artery disease or left ventricular dysfunction. Furthermore, patients with ventricular arrhythmias had significantly more endomyocardial fibrosis than those without it, and also tended to have higher left ventricular mass.

Left ventricular hypertrophy, coronary vascular reserve, and myocardial ischemia

Pressure overload hypertrophy as seen in essential hypertension is associated with a higher coronary blood flow and myocardial oxygen consumption, despite a significant increase in coronary vascular resistance.[113]

The coronary vascular reserve of the left ventricle in compensated hypertensive patients without coronary artery disease remains at about ⅔ of normal values, but is reduced below 50% in compensated hypertensive patients with coronary disease.[113] It appears, however, that there is no relationship between the decrease in coronary reserve and the end-diastolic pressure, nor between the end-diastolic volume and wall stress. Coronary reserve decreases with increasing peak systolic wall stress.[113] On a quantitative basis, the impairment of the coronary reserve (left ventricle) in essential hypertension with coronary stenosis greater than 75% is comparable to that in normotensive coronary disease with similar degree of stenosis.[113]

However, the risk for myocardial ischemia in the hypertensive patient with coronary disease is higher because of the higher systolic left ventricular pressure load (Fig. 4-4). Patients with essential hypertension, even with normal coronary angiograms, can experience angina or silent ischemia similar to those with coronary artery disease, indicating that the ischemia may be due to a functional coronary microangiopathy.

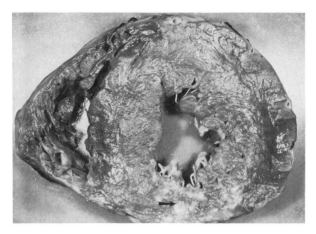

Fig. 4-4. Concentric left ventricular hypertrophy in a patient with systemic hypertension. Note transmural posterior wall scars of ischemic etiology *(arrow).*

Cardiopulmonary reflexes

Observations in both animals and humans indicate that reflex control of the circulation depends to a significant degree on cardiopulmonary receptors that reduce sympathetic vasoconstrictor tone to several regional circulations (such as splanchnic, or skeletal muscle).[116] In addition, these receptors can inhibit renin secretion from the kidney and contribute to regulation of blood pressure and blood volume.[117]

Changes in forearm vascular resistance induced by fluctuations in central venous pressure (at a constant blood pressure and heart rate) are reduced in patients with mild or moderate essential hypertension, as compared with those of normotensive patients. A further reduction of these vasomotor responses occurs in hypertensive patients with left ventricular hypertrophy.[118] The pathophysiologic implication of the impairment of the cardiopulmonary receptor may be reflected in the inability of hypertensive patients with hypertrophic heart to regulate blood volume adequately. Similarly, the impairment of the cardiopulmonary reflex means less tonic restraint on neural and humoral influences that tend to elevate blood pressure.[118]

Impairment of the cardiopulmonary reflex in hypertension with cardiac hypertrophy may result from cardiac receptors being reset in cardiac hypertrophy, and from the thick, less compliant ventricle becoming less sensitive to physiologic stimuli.[119] This proposed mechanism suggests that the derangement of the cardiopulmonary reflex has an afferent origin, akin to the resetting in cardiac transplantation patients who depend mainly on intracardiac receptors.[120]

Regression of left ventricular hypertrophy in experimental animals

Regression of left ventricular hypertrophy improves the cardiopulmonary reflex and restores its normal role in reflex cardiovascular homeostasis. Regression of cardiac hypertrophy also improves the baroreceptor-heart rate reflex.[118]

Investigations with different experimental models have yielded a wide range of morphologic findings in hearts after reversal of the increased pressure load. Removal of aortic banding in one set of animals led to complete normalization of the heart weight without any qualitative or quantitative changes of the myocardium. In another set of animals, degeneration of mitochondria and disintegration of myofibers was observed even after release of the aortic constriction.

Cardiac hypertrophy induced by physical training in rats regresses completely as a result of diminished protein synthesis within 14 days after termination of conditioning. However, regression of cardiac hypertrophy in this model is not synchronous; there is a delay in regression of capillary hypertrophy relative to that of the myocyte hypertrophy.[121]

Regression of left ventricular hypertrophy in hypertensive humans

Multiple studies in hypertensive patients treated with a variety of antihypertensive drugs have not conclusively established whether complete normalization occurs after regression of cardiac hypertrophy. Furthermore, it has not been clarified whether regression of cardiovascular structural changes in hypertensive patients significantly improves prognosis independent of the blood pressure reduction. There is, however, considerable agreement among investigators that many factors other than the level of blood pressure are involved in the regression of LVH by antihypertensive therapy.[122] Factors that interfere with the reduction of LV mass include activation of sympathetic nervous system or the renin-angiotensin system, older age, male gender, genetic factors, duration of treatment, and effectiveness of blood pressure control.[123] In humans, systolic cardiac performance, assessed by ejection fraction or fractional shortening at rest, was maintained by reduction in LV mass after hypertensive therapy.[124] Regression of left ventricular hypertrophy has variable effects on diastolic function.

Regression of arteriolar hypertrophy

The issue of regression of medial hypertrophy in arteries and arterioles of hypertensive patients after therapy is somewhat cloudy because the results of effective antihypertensive therapy in different vascular beds are nonuniform. Present studies indicate, however, that antihypertensive drugs that induce vasodilation without stimulating an adrenergic response appear to be effective in reducing structural vascular changes.[123]

Epidemiology of hypertension

Demographics of left ventricular hypertrophy associated with essential hypertension

The prevalence of LVH is consistently higher among men than among women with hypertension.[125] Also, a significant increase in relative wall thickness, which is an index of concentric LVH, was found in black patients compared with white patients of similar age, duration of hypertension, and prior treatment status.[126,127]

It has also been reported that several groups of patients with uncomplicated essential hypertension have only a weak relationship between office measurements of systolic blood pressure and echocardiographically determined LV mass.[128] However, in men with uncomplicated essential hypertension, detection of LVH by echocardiogram identified patients at high risk for morbid events independent of age, blood pressure, or resting left ventricular performance.[129]

Prevalence and incidence. The overall prevalence of hypertension, defined as a systolic level of $\geq$ 160 mm Hg or a diastolic level of $\geq$ 95 mm Hg, is 21.7% of the U.S. population between the ages of 25 to 74 years.[130] The use of lower criteria, $\geq$ 140 mm Hg systolic or $\geq$ 90 mm Hg diastolic, indicates a prevalence of 29% in whites and 38% in blacks.

In the Hypertension Detection and Follow-up Program (HDFP), initially normotensive individuals (age 30 years to 69 years) were rescreened after 3 years.[131] The 3-year incidence of hypertension was 11.8% and related directly to the level of the initial blood pressure. The incidence was markedly higher in black men (28.6%) than in white men (8.2%), and higher in black women (23.3%) than in white women (9.6%). The National Health and Nutrition Examination Survey Epidemiologic Follow-up Study provided data on a 10-year follow-up of 7073 normotensive individuals between the ages of 25 to 74 years.[132] Body mass index was positively related to the subsequent development of hypertension in all race and gender groups. These data emphasize the importance of body weight as a strong predictor for the risk of developing hypertension.[133,134]

Sociodemographic features. The prevalence of hypertension is inversely related to socioeconomic status and educational level. It is higher in urban than rural areas, and higher in the Southeastern region than in other regions of the United States. Hypertension is associated with obesity, and the prevalence of being overweight is higher in black women (63%) than in white women (35%), and higher in black men (36%) than in white men (32%).[135]

Diet. A higher prevalence of hypertension, and a greater rise in blood pressure with age, is found in populations whose diet contains excess sodium and inadequate potassium. The relation between blood pressure and dietary salt intake was again confirmed by results of the recent INTERSALT study, in which a significant association was found between sodium excretion and median systolic blood pressure, the prevalence of hypertension, and the rise in blood pressure with age.[136]

There is also an association between hypertension and low dietary intake of calcium, although the data are confounded by lower calcium intakes in blacks and individuals of lower socioeconomic status.[137]

Etiology of hypertension

Secondary causes

Renovascular disease. The most common secondary correctable cause of hypertension, renovascular disease, occurs in up to 5% of all hypertensive individuals.[138,139] The two pathologic varieties are fibromuscular dysplasia and atherosclerosis of the renal artery. Fibromuscular dysplasia occurs primarily in young women and is often unilateral at the time of diagnosis. The histology is typically noninflammatory hyperplasia of the media with multiple small mural aneurysms[140] (Fig. 4-5). Less often, the hyperplasia is localized to the fibroblasts of the intima. Overgrowth of these layers of the arterial wall can also occur in other arteries, commonly the carotids, but also sometimes in the superior mesenteric and iliac arteries; coronary artery involvement is rare. Approximately 10% of cases have a hereditary component with autosomal dominant transmission.[141] No one has yet investigated what factors lead to stimulation of growth in these different segments of the arterial wall, or why the renal artery is particularly susceptible.

The clinical occurrence of atherosclerotic renovascular hypertension is increasing as the population ages. When present, the lesions are bilateral in 35% or more of cases and also are sometimes associated with atherosclerotic abdominal aneurysms in the region of the renal arteries. The areas of stenosis are often at the ostium of the renal artery, typical of the localization of atherosclerotic plaques in other systemic arteries. An excellent review of the pathophysiology of renovascular hypertension and the hyperreninemic state has been published recently by Martinez-Maldonado.[142]

Renoparenchymal disease. This condition occurs with a frequency similar to that of renovascular disease as a

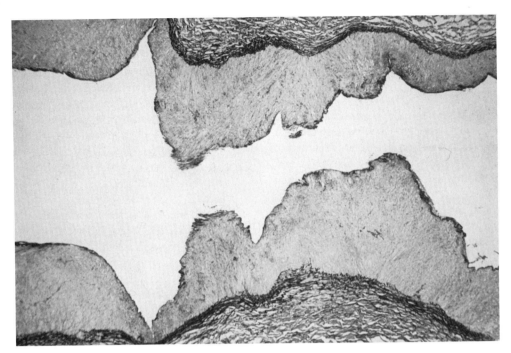

Fig. 4-5. Longitudinal section of a renal artery showing fibromuscular ridges protruding into the arterial lumen, alternating with areas of medial thinning. (Courtesy of Dr. William D. Edwards– Mayo Clinic).

secondary cause of hypertension. Unlike renovascular disease, however, the hypertension is not usually correctable. In general, the glomerular diseases are more strongly associated with hypertension than are the tubular and interstitial diseases.[143] By far, the two most common forms are diabetic nephropathy and chronic glomerulonephritis. Renin levels tend to be somewhat higher in hypertensive patients with underlying primary renoparenchymal disease (compared with patients with essential hypertension and normal glomerular filtration rates),[144] but the major mechanism of hypertension in this setting is renal retention of sodium and water, leading to a volume-dependent variety of hypertension.

Aldosteronism. An uncommon but correctable form of hypertension, aldosteronism, is suspected clinically because of hypokalemia. The two major forms are adrenal cortical adenoma and adrenal cortical hyperplasia, both of which lead to excessive production of aldosterone. Other types of aldosteronism have now been identified, including congenital and acquired enzymatic defects.[145] Awaiting clarification, however, is the reason for hyperplasia in the idiopathic form of bilateral adrenocortical hyperplasia. The three major known stimuli for aldosterone production are renin, potassium, and ACTH, but with bilateral hyperplasia the renin and potassium levels are low, and the ACTH level is not elevated. An aldosterone stimulating factor (ASF) of pituitary origin has been described.[146]

Cushing disease. Another uncommon secondary cause of hypertension, this condition is suspected clinically in hypertensive patients who present with an appearance of excess glucocorticoids (truncal obesity, moon facies, striae, bruising). In the past decade, a progressively larger number of cases have been found to be of pituitary rather than adrenal origin. Magnetic resonance imaging (MRI) has revolutionized the diagnosis of Cushing disease because it is so much more sensitive than the CT scan for detection of pituitary microadenomas. Even with MRI, however, many patients have biochemical evidence of a pituitary lesion when the MRI is negative. Oldfield et al[147] found a 48% difference of ACTH levels between the two petrosal veins to be predictive for localization of a pituitary microadenoma with an accuracy of about 70%.

Pheochromocytoma. This condition is a rare (about 1 in every 5000 hypertensive patients) but reversible cause of hypertension, suspected clinically by labile blood pressures in a patient with episodes of tachycardia, headaches, palpitations, and sweating.[148] Approximately 90% of tumors arise from the adrenal gland, and 97% occur within the abdomen. Bilateral and extraabdominal pheochromocytomas occur primarily in the familial form of the disease associated with medullary thyroid carcinoma and hyperparathyroidism (multiple endocrine neoplasia, MEN-type II, Sipple's syndrome). Like essential hypertension, the primary hemodynamic abnormality is an increased total peripheral resistance.[149] The preferred diagnostic screening tests include urinary excretion of metanephrine, and measurement of plasma catecholamines before and after administration of clonidine.[148,150]

Primary essential hypertension. Much has been learned about the anatomy, physiology, hemodynamics, endocrinology, and molecular biology of essential hypertension. The current level of understanding can be gleaned from a *hypothetic* construct of the pathophysiology.[151-153]

Heredity explains much of the variance in the level of blood pressure and it may be that predisposed individuals are born with a genetic defect in membrane ion transport. This might result from deficiency of a specific enzyme or receptor, or from a direct biochemical abnormality of the cell membrane, either of which could impair the transport of ions such as Na^+, Ca^{2+}, H^+, or Cl^-. The defect could be generalized in the vascular walls, or involve only ion transport in specific organs such as the kidney. Such a renal defect might limit the capacity to excrete salt, resulting in early expansion of the blood volume with increased venous return to the heart. Hyperinsulinemia also occurs early in the course of essential hypertension, and directly increases proximal tubular reabsorption of sodium. The resultant increased venous return and expanded cardiopulmonary blood volume distend the atria and cause release of atrial natriuretic peptide (ANP) to evoke natriuresis and help restore sodium homeostasis, provided that renal ANP receptors are intact.

The increased venous return would further stretch the fibers of the left ventricle, which would respond according to Frank-Starling law with an increase in cardiac output. Alternatively, the cardiac output could be driven by increased sympathetic outflow from the central nervous system (CNS), leading to a high turnover rate of norepinephrine at sympathetic nerve terminals. The norepinephrine would stimulate postsynaptic alpha receptors to cause venular and arteriolar constriction, and cardiac beta receptors to increase myocardial contractility and heart rate. Increased CNS sympathetic outflow would also cause the renal sympathetic nerves to release renin. Renin then cleaves angiotensin I (extrarenally and intrarenally) to the vasoconstrictor angiotensin II. Angiotensin II then stimulates adrenal secretion of aldosterone, which further increases sodium retention and vascular reactivity. A high cardiac output could also result from more vigorous myocardial contractility induced by an increase in the amount, availability, or binding kinetics of intracellular calcium.

The net result from any of these proposed mechanisms is an early increase in cardiac output, often associated with a modest increase in heart rate; total peripheral resistance (TPR) remains normal or low at this stage. The increase in cardiac output causes a mild and labile increase in blood pressure that serves to enhance natriuresis ("pressure natriuresis") in an effort to restore sodium balance. The higher arterial pressure also stimulates carotid sinus baroreceptors to reduce CNS sympathetic outflow, heart rate and blood pressure. In this compensated but tenuous state, hypertension can become fixed and progressive if any component of the system goes awry. This is the first, or labile, phase of essential hypertension.

Renal sodium retention leads to an increase in intracellular sodium, including in the blood vessel walls. The accumulation of intracellular sodium is especially prominent if the intracellular sodium pump is defective or inhibited. Digitalis-like substances emerge to assist in the membrane exchange of Na^+ for K^+, but they have vasoconstrictive effects per se. Calcium exchanges for extruded sodium by way of the Na-Ca and other exchange mechanisms, and the gain in intracellular calcium causes further constriction of the vascular smooth muscle wall.

Hence, arteriolar vasoconstriction is mediated by increased vascular wall sodium and calcium, as well as stimulation by catecholamines and angiotensin II. The arteries and veins attempt to relax by endothelial secretion of prostacyclin (PGI2) and endothelium-derived relaxing factor (EDRF), but their capacity to vasodilate is impaired. Increased vasoconstriction narrows the radius (r) of the arteriolar wall, markedly increasing the resistance (R) to flow, according to Poiseuille's law ($R = 8v1/\pi r^4$). The mean arterial blood pressure (i.e., cardiac output × total peripheral resistance) now increases primarily because of a high TPR. This is the second, or fixed, stage of essential hypertension.

Fixed elevation of blood pressure causes structural changes in the vascular wall. Endothelial damage accelerates atherosclerosis and causes release of endothelin, a potent vasoconstrictor. Stimulation of smooth muscle growth with medial hypertrophy of the vascular wall causes more encroachment on the radius of the vessel lumen, with a further increase in TPR. Chronic elevation of TPR creates a significant work load ("afterload") on the left ventricle, which responds by augmenting its protein synthesis to increase myofibril size and the thickness of its posterior and septal walls. The hypertrophy of muscle and collagen tis-

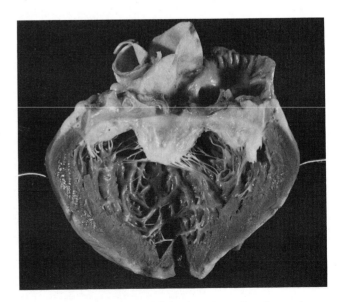

Fig. 4-6. Left ventricular wall hypertrophy and moderate chamber dilatation in a patient with long-standing systemic hypertension.

sue stiffens the left ventricle so much that left ventricular filling and diastolic function are impaired. The newly formed compensatory myosin and collagen fibrils may result in a suboptimal blend of isoforms that impairs contractility. Systolic dysfunction eventually occurs with a decrease in ejection fraction and cardiac output. Incomplete ejection of blood then leads to residual left ventricular diastolic volume that can no longer be pumped out. The hypertrophied left ventricle now begins to dilate with the appearance of clinical signs of left ventricular dysfunction and failure (Fig. 4-6). This is the third, or final, stage of hypertensive heart disease.

Malignant hypertension

The renal lesion that accompanies chronic essential hypertension is arteriolar nephrosclerosis. The primary changes affect the afferent arteriole, beginning with multifocal areas of smooth muscle hypertrophy and ending with diffuse replacement of the smooth muscle by fibrous tissue, leading to elongated and tortuous vessels.[154] Arteriolar wall thickness eventually exceeds luminal diameter. The ratio between the wall and lumen increases progressively with increasing severity and duration of the hypertension.

More acute deterioration of renal function occurs with malignant hypertension, in which the severity of the blood pressure elevation produces fibrinoid necrosis of the renal arteriolar walls (Fig. 4-7), often with thrombi that can extend into the glomerular tuft.[155] The acute renal ischemia leads to marked hyperreninemia and a vicious cycle of vasoconstriction as angiotensin II constricts the renal efferent arterioles and, along with the primary glomerular lesions,

promotes proteinuria. The high levels of angiotensin II also stimulate aldosterone and cause secondary aldosteronism, often with hypokalemia despite impaired renal function.[156] The marked elevation of blood pressure creates such an afterload that even a hypertrophied left ventricle fails, with resultant acute pulmonary edema. Small retinal arterioles burst and result in retinal hemorrhages. Intense cerebral vasospasm alters vascular permeability and leads to cerebral edema, increased intracranial pressure, papilledema, and hypertensive encephalopathy.

Fortunately, all of these acute changes are reversible with adequate control of blood pressure. The prognosis of this condition has improved from a 6 to 12 month mortality of 80% in the era prior to antihypertensive drugs (hence, the term *malignant*)[157] to a more recent 1-year survival as good as 80% to 90%.[158]

Target organ damage due to hypertension

Left ventricular hypertrophy and left ventricular dysfunction. Both conditions are prominent sequelae of chronic hypertension and have been reviewed in the preceding sections on left ventricular hypertrophy and function.

Atherosclerotic complications of hypertension. Coronary artery disease and cerebrovascular accidents are the two most common causes of death in hypertensive individuals.[159,160] Smooth muscle proliferation is a prominent component of both the atherosclerotic lesion and the resistance vessels of hypertensive persons; as such, hypertension and atherosclerosis might be regarded as two independent expressions of a common cellular defect.[161-164]

Other factors inherent in the atherosclerotic process are

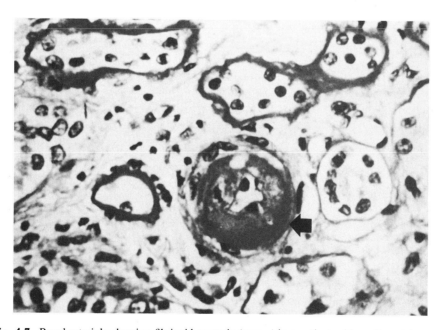

Fig. 4-7. Renal arteriole showing fibrinoid necrosis *(arrow)* in a patient with malignant hypertension.

lipids and platelets. Cholesterol levels of 240 mg/dl or more are present in approximately 40% of hypertensive patients and contribute to the accelerated risk of atherosclerosis.[165] In addition to the altered risk imposed by systemic and regional hemodynamic changes in hypertension, other factors shared by both hypertension and atherosclerosis include the added risks of increased blood viscosity, increased fibrinogen, and the high renin state. For example, Alderman and coworkers[166] have recently reported a direct and independent association between a high renin profile and the 8-year risk of myocardial infarction in 1717 hypertensive patients.

Previous studies have shown that excessive angiotensin II had a direct pathologic effect on vascular and myocardial tissue. Recent data demonstrate that angiotensin II also stimulates vascular smooth muscle cell migration and growth and promotes intimal hyperplasia after vascular injury.[167,168] Hence, factors central to the pathogenesis of hypertension may also be involved directly in the consequence of atherosclerosis.

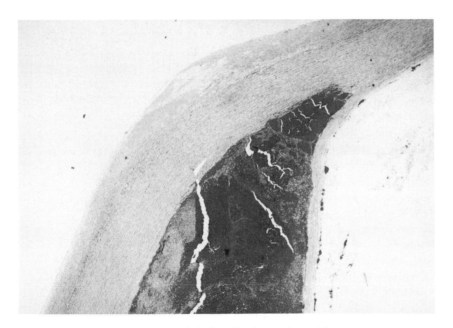

Fig. 4-8. Aortic dissection (outer third of media) in a patient with systemic hypertension.

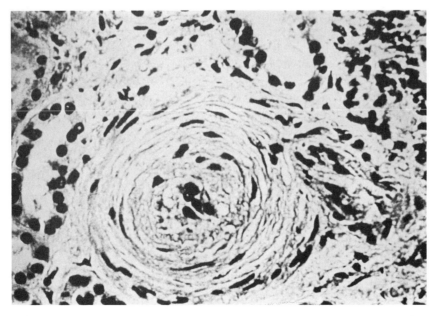

Fig. 4-9. Myxoid, laminated intimal thickening in a small renal artery from a black patient with malignant hypertension.

The well-known association between systemic hypertension and aortic dissection is shown in Fig. 4-8.

Chronic renal failure. This condition is a serious consequence of mild, moderate, severe, accelerated and malignant hypertension.[169] Hypertensive nephrosclerosis is the second leading cause of end-stage renal disease (ESRD) in the United States, surpassed only by diabetes.[170] The risk is staggering in hypertensive black individuals,[169-171] but the reasons for this are unclear, particularly in context of the low renin profile typical of hypertension in blacks.

Some physiologic, anatomic, and histologic differences have been reported in hypertensive blacks compared with whites with similar levels of blood pressure. For example, Frohlich, et al[172] reported a lower renal blood flow (and higher renal resistance) in blacks compared with whites with similar levels of creatinine clearance. Levy, et al[173] noted more tortuosity of the renal arcuate arteries when arteriograms were compared in blacks and whites with similar levels of blood pressure. Pitcock, et al[174] reported a striking absence of fibrinoid necrosis, but did find a prominent myxoid thickening of the small arteries in the renal biopsies of black patients with malignant hypertension (Fig. 4-9).

The pathophysiology of nephrosclerosis is not well defined, especially because it occurs in some patients but not others with similar levels of blood pressure. Like the model for diabetic nephropathy, there is some evidence to suggest that hyperfiltration may occur early and lead to subsequent glomerulosclerosis.[175] For example, Schmieder and associates[176] reported that a creatinine clearance above 130 mL/min/1.73m^2 was associated with increased echocardiographic left ventricular mass in patients with essential hypertension. Another early marker of renal damage is microalbuminuria, detectable in approximately 25% of patients with essential hypertension whose routine urinalysis and serum creatinine levels are normal.[177] Thus hyperfiltration and microalbuminuria may be early indicators of hypertensive nephrosclerosis.

REFERENCES

1. Umeda PK, Darling DS, Kennedy JM, et al: Control of myosin heavy chain expression in cardiac hypertrophy, *Am J Cardiol* 59:49A, 1987.
2. Cartwright J Jr, Goldstein MA: Microtubules in the heart muscle of the postnatal and adult rat, *J Mol Cell Cardiol* 17:1, 1985.
3. Watkins SC, Samuel JL, Marotte B, et al: Microtubules and desmin filaments during onset of heart hypertrophy in rat: a double immunoelectron microscope study, *Circ Res* 60:317, 1987.
4. Izumo S, Nadal-Ginard B, Mahvadi V: Protooncogene induction and reprogramming of cardiac gene expression produced by pressure overload, *Proc Natl Acad Sci USA* 85:339, 1988.
5. Smith SH, Kramer MF, Reis I, et al: Regional changes in creatine kinase and myocyte size in hypertensive and nonhypertensive cardiac hypertrophy, *Circ Res* 67:1334, 1990.
6. Alpert NR, Mulieri LA: Increased myothermal economy of isometric force generation in compensated cardiac hypertrophy induced by pulmonary artery constriction in the rabbit: a characterization of heat liberation in normal and hypertrophied right ventricular papillary muscle, *Circ Res* 77:225, 1982.
7. Swynghedauw B, Schwartz K, Apstein CS: Decreased contractility after myocardial hypertrophy: cardiac failure or successful adaption? *Am J Cardiol* 54:437, 1984.
8. Pauletto P, Piccolo D, Scannapieco G, et al: Left ventricular hypertrophy in hypertension: changes in isomyosins and creatine-kinase isoenzymes, *Am J Med* 84:122, 1988.
9. de Bold AJ: Atrial natriuretic factor: a hormone produced by the heart, *Science* 230:767, 1985.
10. Komuro I, Kurabayashi M, Shibazaki Y, et al: Molecular mechanism of cardiac hypertrophy, *Jpn Circ J* 54:526, 1990.
11. Simpson PC: Proto-oncogenes and cardiac hypertrophy, *Annu Rev Physiol* 51:189, 1988.
12. Kahn P, Graf T: *Oncogenes and growth control.* Berlin, 1986, Springer-Verlag.
13. Carpenter G: Receptors for epidermal growth factor and other polypeptide mitogens, *Annu Rev Biochem* 56:881, 1987.
14. Berk BC, Alexander RW, Brock TA, et al: Vasoconstriction: a new activity for platelet-derived growth factor, *Science* 232:87, 1986.
15. Massague J: The TGF-b family of growth and differentiation factors, *Cell* 49:437, 1987.
16. Sparn MB, Roberts AB: Peptide growth factors are multi-functional, *Nature* 332:217, 1988.
17. Wu BJ, Morimoto RI: Transcription of the human hsp70 gene is induced by serum stimulation, *Proc Natl Acad Sci USA*, 82:6070, 1985.
18. Weinberg RA: The action of oncogenes in the cytoplasm and nucleus, *Science* 230:770, 1985.
19. Varmus HE: Oncogenes and transcriptional control, *Science* 238:1337, 1987.
20. Marx JL: Searching land and sea for the dinosaur killer, *Science* 237:856, 1987.
21. Bauters C, Moalic JM, Bercovici J, et al: Coronary flow as a determinant of a c-myc and c-fos proto-oncogenes expression in an isolated adult rat heart, *J Mol Cell Cardiol* 20:97, 1988.
22. Barka T, van der Noen H, Shaw PA: Proto-oncogene fos (c-fos) expression in the heart, *Oncogene* 1:439, 1987.
23. Mulcahy LS, Smith MR, Stacey DW: Requirement for ras proto-oncogene function during serum-stimulated growth of NIT 3T3 cells, *Nature* 313:241, 1985.
24. Claycomb WC, Lanson NA Jr: Proto-oncogene expression in proliferating and differentiating cardiac and skeletal muscle, *Biochem J* 247:701, 1987.
25. Meidell RS, Sen A, Henderson S, et al: a1-adrenergic stimulation of rat myocardial cells increases protein synthesis, *Am J Physiol* 251:H1076, 1986.
26. Starksen NE, Simpson PC, Bishopric N, et al: Cardiac myocyte hypertrophy is associated with c-myc proto-oncogene expression, *Proc Natl Acad Sci* USA 83:8348, 1986.
27. Gordon EE, Kira Y, Morgan HE: Aortic pressure, protein synthesis, and protein degradation, *Circulation* 75 (suppl I):I78, 1987.
28. Sachs F: Biophysics of mechanoreception, *Membr Biochem* 6:175, 1986.
29. Hynes RO: Integrins: a family of cell surface receptors, *Cell* 48:549, 1987.
30. Marban E, Koretsume Y: Cell calcium, oncogenes, and hypertrophy, *Hypertension* 15:652, 1990.
31. Marban E, Kitakaze M, Chacko VP, et al: Ca^{2+} transients in perfused hearts revealed by gated FNMR spectroscopy, *Circ Res* 63:673, 1988.
32. Morgan JT, Curran T: Role of ion influx in the control of c-fos expression, *Nature* 322:552, 1986.
33. Kaibuchi K, Tsuda T, Kikuchi A, et al: Possible involvement of protein kinase C and calcium ion in growth factor-induced expression of c-myc oncogene in Swiss 3T3 fibroblast, *J Biol Chem* 261:1187, 1986.

34. Simpson PC: Role of proto-oncogenes in myocardial hypertrophy, *Am J Cardiol* 63:13G, 1988.

35. Campbell SE, Gerdes AM: Regional changes in myocyte size during the reversal of thyroid-induced cardiac hypertrophy, *J Mol Cell Cardiol* 20:379, 1988.

36. Gerdes AM, Moore JA, Hines JM: Regional changes in myocyte size and number in propranolol-treated hyperthyroid rats, *Lab Invest* 57:708, 1987.

37. Carter WJ, van der Weijden Benjamin WS, Faas FH: Effect of thyroid hormone on protein turnover in cultured cardiac myocytes, *J Mol Cell Cardiol* 17:897, 1985.

38. Devereux RB, Pickering TG, Cody RJ, et al: Relation of renin-angiotensin system activity to left ventricular hypertrophy and function in experimental and human hypertension, *J Clin Hypertens* 3:87, 1987.

39. Campbell DJ: Tissue renin-angiotensin system: sites of angiotensin formation, *J Cardiovasc Pharmacol* 10 (suppl 7):S1, 1987.

40. Ganten D, Balz W, Hense HW, et al: Characterization and regulation of angiotensin (ANG) peptides in tissue of rabbits and primates (abstr), *Hypertension* 3 (suppl 3):S552, 1985.

41. Dzau VJ: Vascular angiotensin pathways: a new therapeutic target, *J Cardiovasc Pharmacol* 10 (suppl 7):S9, 1987.

42. Unger T, Gohlke P: Tissue renin-angiotensin systems in the heart and vasculature: possible involvement in the cardiovascular actions of converting enzyme inhibitors, *Am J Cardiol* 65:3I, 1990.

43. Khairallah PA, Robertson AL, Davila D: *Effects of angiotensin II on DNA, RNA and protein synthesis.* In Genest J, Koiw R, eds: *Hypertension,* New York, 1972, Springer-Verlag.

44. Baker KM, Chernin MI, Wixson SK, et al: Renin-angiotensin system involvement in pressure-overload cardiac hypertrophy in rats, *Am J Physiol* 259:H324, 1990.

45. Sen S, Kundu G, Mekhail N, et al: Myotrophin: purification of a novel peptide from spontaneously hypertensive rat heart that influences myocardial growth, *J Biol Chem* 265:16635, 1990.

46. Mariappan M, Selvamurugan N, Rajamanickam C: Purification and characterization of a high-molecular-weight protein induced in rat serum during development of cardiac hypertrophy, *Arch Biochem Biophys* 281:297, 1990.

47. Casscells W, Speir E, Sasse J, et al: Isolation, characterization, and localization of heparin-binding growth factors in the heart, *J Clin Invest* 85:433, 1990.

48. Cooper G: Cardiocyte adaptation to chronically altered load, *Annu Rev Physiol* 49:501, 1987.

49. Kent RL, Hoover K, Cooper G IV: Load responsiveness of protein synthesis in adult mammalian myocardium: role of cardiac deformation linked to sodium influx, *Circ Res* 64:74, 1989.

50. Naitoh Y: *Mechanosensory transduction in protozoa.* In Colombetti G, Lenci F, eds: *Membranes and sensory transduction,* New York, 1984, Plenum.

51. Barnes O: How cells respond to signals, *Science* 234:286, 1986.

52. Anversa P, Ricci R, Olivetti G: Quantitative structural analysis of the myocardium during growth and induced cardiac hypertrophy: a review, *J Am Coll Cardiol* 7:1140, 1986.

53. Anversa P, Olivetti G, Loud AV: Morphometric study of early postnatal development in the left and right myocardium of the rat, I: hypertrophy, hyperplasia, and binucleation of myocytes, *Circ Res* 46:495, 1980.

54. Lewis JF, Moran BJ: Diversity of patterns of hypertrophy in patients with systemic hypertension and marked left ventricular wall thickening, *Am J Cardiol* 65:874, 1990.

55. Grossman W, Jones D, McLaurin LP: Wall stress and patterns of hypertrophy in the human left ventricle, *J Clin Invest* 56:56, 1975.

56. Anversa P, Olivetti G, Loud AV: *Morphometric studies of left ventricular hypertrophy.* In Tarazi RC, Dunbar JB, eds: *Cardiac hypertrophy in hypertension,* New York, 1983, Raven.

57. Nunez BD, Shmieder R, Garavaglia E, et al: Right ventricular involvement in hypertensive patients with isolated septal and concentric left ventricular hypertrophy, *J Hypertens* 4 (suppl 5):S300, 1986.

58. Cuspidi C, Sampieri L, Angioni L, et al: Right ventricular wall thickness and function in hypertensive patients with and without left ventricular hypertrophy: echo-Doppler study, *J Hypertens* 7 (suppl 6):S108, 1989.

59. Tomanek RJ, Schalk KA, Marcus ML, et al: Coronary angiogenesis during long-term hypertension and left ventricular hypertrophy in dogs, *Circ Res* 65:352, 1989.

60. Levy D, Garrison RJ, Savage DD, et al: Prognostic implications of echocardiographically determined left ventricular mass in the Framingham study, *N Engl J Med* 322:1561, 1990.

61. Harrison DG, Florentine MS, Brooks LA, et al: The effect of hypertension and left ventricular hypertrophy on the lower range of coronary autoregulation, *Circulation* 77:1108, 1988.

62. Polese A, DeCesare N, Montorsi P, et al: Upward shift of the lower range of coronary flow autoregulation in hypertensive patients with hypertrophy of the left ventricle, *Circulation* 83:845, 1991.

63. Vallance P, Collier J, Moncada S: Effects of endothelium-derived nitric oxide on peripheral arteriolar tone in man, *Lancet* 2:997, 1989.

64. Forstermann V, Mugge A, Alheid V, et al: Selective attenuation of endothelium-mediated vasodilatation in atherosclerotic human coronary arteries, *Circ Res* 62:185, 1988.

65. Panza JA, Quyyumi AA, Brush JE, et al: Abnormal endothelium-dependent vascular relaxation in patients with essential hypertension, *N Engl J Med* 323:22, 1990.

66. Tanaka M, Fujiwara H, Onodera T, et al: Quantitative analysis of narrowings of intramyocardial small arteries in normal hearts, hypertensive hearts, and hearts with hypertrophic cardiomyopathy, *Circulation* 75:1130, 1987.

67. Factor SM, Robinson TF: Comparative connective tissue structure-function relationships in biologic pumps, *Lab Invest* 58:150, 1988.

68. Weber KT: Cardiac interstitium in health and disease: the fibrillar collagen network, *J Am Coll Cardiol* 13:1637, 1989.

69. Weber KT, Janicki JS, Pick R, et al: Collagen in the hypertrophied, pressure-overloaded myocardium, *Circulation* 75 (suppl I):I40, 1987.

70. Karim MA, Ferguson AG, Wakim BT, et al: In vivo collagen turnover during development of thyroxine-induced left ventricular hypertrophy, *Am J Physiol* 260:C316, 1991.

71. Pick R, Janicki JS, Weber KT: Myocardial fibrosis in nonhuman primate with pressure overload hypertrophy, *Am J Pathol* 135:771, 1989.

72. Eghbali M, Weber KT: Collagen and the myocardium: fibrillar structure, biosynthesis and degradation in relation to hypertrophy and its regression, *Mol Cell Biochem* 96:1, 1990.

73. Silver MA, Weber KT: *Structural basis of left ventricular dysfunction: role of collagen network remodeling and potential therapeutic interventions.* In Brachmann J, Dietz R, Kubler W, eds: *Heart failure and arrhythmias,* Berlin, 1990, Springer-Verlag.

74. Weber KT, Brilla CG: Pathological hypertrophy and cardiac interstitium: fibrosis and renin-angiotensin-aldosterone system, *Circulation* 83:1849, 1991.

75. Weber KT, Clark WA, Janicki JS, et al: Physiologic versus pathologic hypertrophy and the pressure-overload myocardium, *J Cardiovasc Pharmacol* 10:S37, 1987.

76. Mukherjee D, Sen S: Collagen phenotypes during development and regression of myocardial hypertrophy in spontaneous hypertensive rats, *Circ Res* 67:1474, 1990.

77. Thiedmann KV, Hollubarsch CH, Medugorac I, et al: Connective tissue content and myocardial stiffness in pressure overload hypertrophy, *Basic Res Cardiol* 78:140, 1983.

78. Robbins SL, Cotran RS, Kumar V: *Pathological basis of disease,* ed 3, Philadelphia, 1984, WB Saunders.

79. Chapman D, Weber KT, Eghbali M: Regulation of fibrillar collagen

types I and III and basement membrane type IV collagen expression in pressure-overloaded rat myocardium, *Circ Res* 67:787, 1990.

80. Doering CN, Jalil JE, Janicki JS, et al: Collagen network remodeling and diastolic stiffness of the rat left ventricle with pressure overload hypertrophy, *Cardiovasc Res* 22:686, 1988.

81. Cooper G, Kent RL, Uboch CE, et al: Hemodynamic versus adrenergic control of rat right ventricular hypertrophy, *J Clin Invest* 75:1403, 1985.

82. Ruskoaho HJ, Savolainen ER: Effect of long term verapamil treatment on blood pressure, cardiac hypertrophy, and collagen metabolism in spontaneously hypertensive rats, *Cardiovasc Res* 19:355, 1985.

83. Motz W, Strauer BE: Left ventricular function and collagen content after regression of hypertensive hypertrophy, *Hypertension* 13:43, 1989.

84. Colan SD, Sanders SP, MacPherson D, et al: Left ventricular diastolic function in elite athletes with physiologic cardiac hypertrophy, *J Am Coll Cardiol* 6:545, 1985.

85. Autore C, Fiorito E, Pelliccia A, et al: Antimitochondrial autoantibodies in myocardial hypertrophy: comparison between hypertrophic cardiomyopathy, hypertensive heart disease, and athlete's heart, *Am Heart J* 116:496, 1988.

86. Loud AV, Beghi C, Olivetti G, et al: Morphometry of right and left ventricular myocardium after strenuous exercise in preconditioned rats, *Lab Invest* 51:104, 1984.

87. Grossman W, Jones D, McLaurin LP: Wall stress and patterns of hypertrophy in the human left ventricle, *J Clin Invest* 56:56, 1975.

88. Legault F, Rouleau JL, Juneau C, et al: Functional and morphologic characteristics of compensated and decompensated cardiac hypertrophy in dogs with chronic infrarenal aorto-caval fistulas, *Circ Res* 66:846, 1990.

89. Thiedemann KV, Houbarsch CH, Medugorac I, et al: Connective tissue content and myocardial stiffness in pressure overload hypertrophy: a combined study of morphologic, morphometric, biochemical, and mechanical parameters, *Basic Res Cardiol* 78:140, 1983.

90. Medugorac I: Myocardial collagen in different forms of heart hypertrophy in the rat, *Res Exp Med* (Berlin) 177:201, 1988.

91. Iimoto DS, Covell JW, Harper E: Increase in cross-linking of type I and type III collagens associated with volume-overload hypertrophy, *Circ Res* 63:399, 1988.

92. Anversa P, Loud AV, Levicky V, et al: Left ventricular failure induced by myocardial infarction, I, Myocyte hypertrophy, *Am J Physiol* 248:H876, 1985.

93. Anversa P, Loud AV, Levicky V, et al: Left ventricular failure induced by myocardial infarction, II, Tissue morphometry, *Am J Physiol* 248:H883, 1985.

94. Dubick MA, Rucker RB, Cross CE, et al: Elastin metabolism in rodent lung, *Biochim Biophys Acta* 672:303, 1981.

95. Keeley FW, Alatawi A: Response of aortic elastin synthesis and accumulation to developing hypertension and the inhibitory effect of colchicine on this response, *Lab Invest* 64:499, 1991.

96. Harizi RC, Bianco JA, Alpert JS: Diastolic function of the heart in clinical cardiology, *Arch Intern Med* 148:99, 1988.

97. Inouye I, Massie B, Loge D, et al: Abnormal left ventricular filling: an early finding in mild to moderate systemic hypertension, *Am J Cardiol* 53:120, 1984.

98. Shapiro LM, McKenna WJ: Left ventricular hypertrophy: relation of structure to diastolic function in hypertension, *Br Heart J* 51:637, 1984.

99. Papademetriou V, Gottdiener JS, Fletcher RD, et al: Echocardiographic assessment by computer-assisted analysis of diastolic left ventricular function and hypertrophy in borderline or mild systemic hypertension, *Am J Cardiol* 56:546, 1985.

100. Spirito P, Maron BJ, Bonow RO: Noninvasive assessment of left ventricular diastolic function: comparative analysis of Doppler echocardiographic and radionuclide angiographic techniques, *J Am Coll Cardiol* 7:518, 1986.

101. Marmor AT, Blondheim DS, Frankel A, et al: Early detection of diastolic impairment in longstanding hypertension by a noninvasive volume challenge method, *Clin Cardiol* 8:154, 1985.

102. Smith V-E, Weisfeldt ML, Katz AM: *Relaxation and diastolic properties of the heart.* In Fozzard HA, Haber E, Jennings RB, et al, eds: *The heart and cardiovascular system,* vol 2, New York, 1986, Raven.

103. Grossman W: Diastolic dysfunction in congestive heart failure, *N Engl J Med* 325:1557, 1991.

104. Shephard RJF, Zachariah PK, Shub C: Hypertension and left ventricular diastolic function, *Mayo Clin Proc* 64:1521, 1989.

105. Fouad FM, Slominski JM, Tarazi RC: Left ventricular diastolic function in hypertension: relation to left ventricular mass and systolic function, *J Am Coll Cardiol* 3:1500, 1984.

106. Smith V-E, Schulman P, Karimeddini MK, et al: Rapid ventricular filling left ventricular hypertrophy: II, Pathologic hypertrophy, *J Am Coll Cardiol* 5:869, 1985.

107. Topol EJ, Traill TA, Fortuin NJ: Hypertensive hypertrophic cardiomyopathy of the elderly, *N Engl J Med* 312:277, 1985.

108. Fouad-Tarazi FM: Ventricular diastolic function of the heart in systemic hypertension, *Am J Cardiol* 65:85G, 1990.

109. Madkour MA, Fouad-Tarazi FM: Alterations in cardiopulmonary receptors in hypertensive patients with impaired left ventricular filling, *J Hypertens* 7 (suppl 6):S106, 1989.

110. Conrad GH, Brooks WW, Robinson KG, et al: Impaired myocardial function in the spontaneously hypertensive rat with heart failure (abstr), *J Mol Cell Cardiol* 19 (suppl 4):565, 1987.

111. Endoh M, Blinks JR: Actions of sympathomimetic amines on Ca transients and contractions of rabbit myocardium: reciprocal changes in myofibrillar responsiveness to Ca mediated through a- and b-adrenoreceptors, *Circ Res* 62:247, 1988.

112. Perreault CL, Bing OHL, Brooks WW, et al: Differential effects of cardiac hypertrophy and failure on right versus left ventricular calcium activation, *Circ Res* 67:707, 1990.

113. Strauer BE: Regression of myocardial and coronary vascular hypertrophy in hypertensive heart disease, *J Cardiovasc Pharmacol* 12 (suppl 4):545, 1988.

114. McLenachan JM, Henderson E, Morris KI, et al: Ventricular arrhythmias in patients with hypertensive left ventricular hypertrophy, *N Engl J Med* 317:787, 1987.

115. McLenachan JM, Dargie HJ: Ventricular arrhythmias in hypertensive left ventricular hypertrophy: relationship to coronary artery disease, left ventricular dysfunction, and myocardial fibrosis, *Am J Hypertens* 3:735, 1990.

116. Mancia G, Lorenz RR, Shepherd JT: Reflex control of circulation by heart and lungs, *Int Rev Physiol* 9:111, 1976.

117. Stella A, Zanchetti A: Neural control of renin secretion, *J Hypertens* 2 (suppl 2):83, 1984.

118. Grassi G, Giannattasio C, Cleroux J, et al: Cardiopulmonary reflex before and after regression of left ventricular hypertrophy in essential hypertension, *Hypertension* 12:227, 1988.

119. Thoren P, Noresson E, Ricksten E: Resetting of cardiac C-fiber endings in the spontaneously hypertensive rat, *Acta Physiol Scand* 107:13, 1979.

120. Mohanty PK, Thames MD, Arrowd JA, et al: Impairment of cardiopulmonary baroflex after cardiac transplantation in humans, *Circulation* 75:914, 1987.

121. Frenzel H, Schwartzkopff B, Holtermann W, et al: Regression of cardiac hypertrophy: morphometric and biochemical studies in rat heart after swimming training, *J Mol Cell Cardiol* 20:737, 1988.

122. Tarazi RC, Fouad FM: Reversal of cardiac hypertrophy in man, *Hypertension* 6 (suppl II):140, 1984.

123. Agabiti-Rosei E, Muiesan ML, Nuiesan G: Regression of structural alterations in hypertension, *Am J Hypertens* 2:705, 1989.

124. Fouad-Tarazi FM, Liebson P: Echocardiographic studies of regression of left ventricular hypertrophy in hypertension, *Hypertension* 9 (suppl II):65, 1987.

125. Devereux PB, Pickering TG, Alderman MH, et al: Left ventricular hypertrophy in hypertension: prevalence and relation to pathophysiologic variables, *Hypertension* 9 (suppl II):53, 1987.

126. Devereux RB: Cardiac involvement in essential hypertension: prevalence, pathophysiology, and prognostic implications, *Med Clin North Am* 71:813, 1987.

127. Dunn FE, Oigman W, Sundgaard-Riise K, et al: Racial differences in cardiac adaptation to essential hypertension determined by echocardiographic indexes, *J Am Coll Cardiol* 1:1348, 1983.

128. Hammond JW, Devereux RB, Alderman MH, et al: The prevalence and correlates of echocardiographic left ventricular hypertrophy among employed patients with uncomplicated hypertension, *J Am Coll Cardiol* 7:639, 1986.

129. Devereux RB: Echocardiographic insights into the pathophysiology and prognostic significance of hypertensive cardiac hypertrophy, *Am J Hypertens* 2:186S, 1989.

130. Kaplan NM: *Clinical hypertension,* ed 5, Baltimore, 1990, Williams & Wilkins.

131. Apostolides AY, Cutter G, Daugherty SA, et al: Three-year incidence of hypertension in thirteen U.S. communities, *Prev Med* 11:487, 1982.

132. Ford ES, Cooper RS: Risk factors for hypertension in a National Cohort Study, *Hypertension* 18:598, 1991.

133. Kotchen TA, Kotchen JM, Boegehold MA: Nutrition and hypertension prevention, *Hypertension* 18 (suppl I):I-115, 1991.

134. Stamler J: Blood pressure and high blood pressure: aspects of risk, *Hypertension* 18 (suppl I):I-95, 1991.

135. Saunders E: *Cardiovascular diseases in blacks.* Philadelphia, 1991, FA Davis.

136. Stamler J, Rose G, Stamler R, et al: INTERSALT study findings: public health and medical care implications, *Hypertension* 14:570, 1989.

137. McCarron DA, Morris CD: The calcium deficiency hypothesis of hypertension, *Ann Intern Med* 107:919, 1987.

138. Wollam GL, Hall WD: *Hypertension management. Clinical practice and therapeutic dilemmas.* Chicago, 1988, *Year Book.*

139. Barnes R, Berson A, Dean R, et al: NHLBI workshop on renovascular disease, summary report and recommendations, *Hypertension* 7:452, 1985.

140. Harrison EG, Hunt JC, Bernatz PE: Morphology of fibromuscular dysplasia of the renal artery in renovascular hypertension, *Am J Med* 43:97, 1967.

141. Rushton AR: The genetics of fibromuscular dysplasia, *Arch Intern Med* 140:233, 1980.

142. Martinez-Maldonado M: Pathophysiology of renovascular hypertension, *Hypertension* 17:707, 1991.

143. Hall WD: *Renoparenchymal hypertension.* In Hurst JW, ed: *Medicine for the practicing physician,* ed 3, Boston, 1992, Butterworth.

144. Del Greco F, Simon NM, Goodman S, et al: Plasma renin activity in primary and secondary hypertension, *Medicine* 46:475, 1967.

145. Biglieri EG: Spectrum of mineralcorticoid hypertension, *Hypertension* 17:251, 1991.

146. Saito I, Saruta T: Regulation of aldosterone secretion by a new aldosterone stimulating factor, *Jpn Circ J* 46:523, 1982.

147. Oldfield EH, Doppman JL, Nieman LK, et al: Petrosal sinus sampling with and without corticotropin-releasing hormone for the differential diagnosis of Cushing's syndrome, *N Engl J Med* 325:897, 1991.

148. Manger WM, Gifford RW Jr: *Pheochromocytoma.* In Laragh JH, Brenner BM, eds: *Hypertension. Pathophysiology, diagnosis and management,* New York, 1990, Raven.

149. Bravo E, Fouad-Tarazi F, Rossi G, et al: A reevaluation of the hemodynamics of pheochromocytoma, *Hypertension* 15 (suppl I):I-128, 1990.

150. Bravo EL: Diagnosis of pheochromocytoma. Reflections on a controversy, *Hypertension* 17:742, 1991.

151. Dustan HP: *Pathophysiology of systemic hypertension.* In Hurst JW, Schlant RC, eds: *The heart. Arteries and Veins,* New York, 1990, McGraw-Hill.

152. Hall WD: Pathophysiology of hypertension in blacks, *Am J Hypertens* 3 (suppl):366S, 1990.

153. Reaven GM: Insulin resistance, hyperinsulinemia, hypertriglyceridemia, and hypertension, *Diabetes Care* 14:195, 1991.

154. Sommers SC, Melamed J: Renal pathology of essential hypertension, *Am J Hypertension* 3:583, 1990.

155. Jespersen B, Eiskjaer H, Christiansen NO, et al: Malignant arterial hypertension, relationship between blood pressure control and renal function during long-term observation of patients with malignant nephrosclerosis, *J Clin Hypertens* 3:409, 1987.

156. Laragh JA, Ulich S, Januszewicz V, et al: Electrolyte metabolism and aldosterone secretion in benign and malignant hypertension, *Ann Intern Med* 53:259, 1960.

157. Keith NM, Wagener HP, Barker NW: Some different types of essential hypertension: their course and prognosis, *Am J Med Sci* 197:332, 1939.

158. Labeeuw M, Zech P, Pozet N, et al: Renal failure in essential hypertension, *Contrib Nephrol* 71:90, 1989.

159. Curry CL: Coronary artery disease in African-Americans, *Circulation* 83:1474, 1991.

160. Caplan LR: Strokes in African-Americans, *Circulation* 83:1469, 1991.

161. Chobanian A: Overview: hypertension and atherosclerosis, *Am Heart J* 116:319, 1988.

162. Bondjers G, Glukhova M, Hansson GK, et al: Hypertension and atherosclerosis. Cause and effect, or two effects with one unknown cause? *Circulation* 84 (suppl VI):VI-2, 1991.

163. Hadrava V, Kruppa U, Russo RC, et al: Vascular smooth muscle cell proliferation and its therapeutic modulation in hypertension, *Am Heart J* 122:1198, 1991.

164. Frohlich ED, Apstein C, Armstrong ML, et al: Target organ consequences in hypertension: pathogenesis and prevention, *Hypertension* 18 (suppl I):I-143, 1991.

165. Working Group on Management of Patients with Hypertension and High Blood Cholesterol: National Educations Programs Working Group Report on the Management of Patients with Hypertension and High Blood Cholesterol, *Ann Intern Med* 114:224, 1991.

166. Alderman MH, Madhavan S, Ooi WL, et al: Association of the renin-sodium profile with the risk of myocardial infarction in patients with hypertension, *N Engl J Med* 324:1098, 1991.

167. Griffin SA, Brown WCB, MacPherson F, et al: Angiotensin II causes vascular hypertrophy in part by a non-professor mechanism, *Hypertension* 17:626, 1991.

168. Daemen MJAP, Lombardi DM, Bosman FT, et al: Angiotensin II induces smooth muscle cell proliferation in the normal and injured rat arterial wall, *Circ Res* 68:450, 1991.

169. Whelton PK, Klag MJ: Hypertension as a risk factor for renal disease. Review of clinical and epidemiological evidence, *Hypertension* 13 (suppl I):I-19, 1991.

170. National High Blood Pressure Education Program: National High Blood Pressure Education Program Working Group Report on hypertension and chronic renal failure, *Arch Intern Med* 151:1280, 1991.

171. Shulman NB, Hall WD: Renal vascular disease in African-Americans and other racial minorities, *Circulation* 83:1477, 1991.

172. Frohlich ED, Messerli FH, Dunn FG, et al: Greater renal vascular involvement in the black patient with essential hypertension: a comparison of systemic and renal hemodynamics in black and white patients, *Miner Electrolyte Metab* 10:173, 1984.

173. Levy SB, Talner LB, Coel MN, et al: Renal vasculature in essential hypertension: racial differences, *Ann Intern Med* 88:12, 1978.

174. Pitcock JA, Johnson JG, Hatch FE, et al: Malignant hypertension in blacks: malignant intrarenal arterial disease as observed by light and electron microscopy, *Hum Pathol* 7:333, 1976.

175. Anderson S, Brenner BM: Intraglomerular hypertension: implications and drug treatment, *Annu Rev Med* 39:243, 1988.

176. Schmieder RE, Messerli FH, Garavaglia G, et al: Glomerular hyperfiltration indicates early target organ damage in essential hypertension, *JAMA* 264:2775, 1990.

177. Cerasola G, Cottone S, D'lgnoto G, et al: Micro-albuminuria as a predictor of cardiovascular damage in essential hypertension, *J Hypertens* 7 (suppl 6):S332, 1989.

Chapter 5

PULMONARY HYPERTENSION AND COR PULMONALE

Robert H. Franch
Michael B. Gravanis

MORPHOLOGY OF PULMONARY ARTERIES

The morphology of the pulmonary artery tree continues to undergo scrutiny and reclassification with efforts made toward more quantitative descriptions. In pioneering work done on uninjected lungs, Brenner[1] classified the pulmonary arteries into (1) elastic arteries, (2) muscular arteries 100 to 1000 μm external diameter, and (3) arterioles (less than 100 μm external diameter). Elliott and Reid in work quoted by Lamb[2] subsequently believed that the anatomy of the medial layer could not be predicted by the outside diameter of the artery. In their classification of smaller arteries they discarded the term *arteriole*. They defined a muscular artery as (1) having internal and external elastic lamina whose media have continuous muscle coats and fragmented elastic laminae (2) a partially muscular artery as one which has muscle in a noncontinuous strip-like pat-

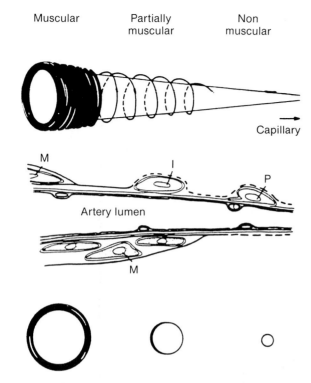

Muscular   Partially muscular   Non muscular

Capillary

Artery lumen

Fig. 5-1. By light microscopy (top and bottom, longitudinal and cross section), the muscle layer of the normal pulmonary artery gradually disappears as the alveolar capillary is approached. By electron microscopy (middle) two precursor smooth muscle cells are shown distally: the intermediate cell (I) and the pericyte (P), and two mature muscle cells, (M) are shown proximally. (From Reid LM:[3] Structure and function in pulmonary hypertension, *Chest* 89:279-288, 1986.)

tern, and (3) the nonmuscular artery as one which has no media and only a single elastic lamina that histologically resembles a vein (Fig. 5-1).[3]

The authors mentioned above regarded the presence of muscle in an artery distal to the terminal bronchiole as abnormal and considered it to be a sign of pulmonary artery hypertension. Continuous intimal thickening was related to cellular proliferation and to an increase in collagen, whereas organization of a thrombus produced an eccentric or cushion pattern of intimal thickening. Dilatation lesions, including plexiform, angiomatoid and vein-like branches, are associated with thickened, usually totally obstructed pulmonary arteries and are an indication of advanced pulmonary vascular disease.

Morphometric assessment of pulmonary arteries at lung biopsy

Morphometric classification attempts to grade the vascular changes in a lung biopsy specimen obtained from patients with pulmonary hypertension secondary to a potentially correctable shunt. The purpose of the biopsy is to predict whether the pulmonary hypertension will regress postsurgically.[4] The open lung biopsy should avoid the dependence segments of the right middle lobe and lingula, as well as small subpleural samples. The procedure should include pulmonary arteries that accompany respiratory bronchioles, alveolar ducts, and alveolar walls.

In Grade A changes, the smooth muscle extends into the nonmuscular arteries. An increase in medial wall thickness of up to 1.5 times may be present. In Grade B, the medial wall thickness of 1.5 to 2 times normal is rated mild; an increase to greater than 2 times normal is considered severe. In Grade C, the presence of more than half the usual number of small pulmonary arteries and arterioles per unit area judged by the number of alveoli is rated mild; less than half the usual number is rated severe. The pulmonary vascular resistance in severe Grade C is significantly elevated (greater than 6 Wood units).

Two thirds of the complete number of acinar arteries are present at age 1½ years, and nearly all are present by 5 years of age. Because some lung growth continues, acinar growth is complete by 8 years to 10 years of age. In the neonate, the normal alveolar-arterial ratio is 20:1; in the 2-year-old it is 12:1, and in the adult it is 6:1. The ratio was 25:1 in a 2-year-old child with a large ventricular septal defect and a high pulmonary vascular resistance.

PULMONARY VASCULAR RESISTANCE

Developed in 1842, the Poiseuilles formula described the factors controlling steady state laminar nonturbulent flow of a homogenous fluid through a long cylindrical glass tube.

$$Q = \frac{nr4 \, (p1 - p2)}{8 \, nl} \qquad R = \frac{8 \, nl}{\pi \, r \, 4} = \frac{P1 - P2}{Q}$$

Q = volume flow per unit
P1 = upstream pressure
P2 = pressure at a downstream point
n = viscosity of fluid
l = length of tube

Volume flow is affected most by luminal size because the radius is raised to the fourth power; thus volume flow increases 16 times if the radius is doubled. The formula applies only to rigid tubes or vessels with a circular cross-sectional area. In the chest, the shape of the pulmonary vessel, (e.g., elliptical or circular) may be related to the transmural pressure. Inside the thorax, the pressure around the artery or vein may be lower than atmospheric pressure. Thus the true lateral pressure in the vessel is equal to the pressure difference between intravascular and extra-vascular or intrathoracic pressure. This is called the transmural pressure. There is a reciprocal relation between flow and the vessel length and/or blood viscosity.

The resistance to blood flow in the pulmonary vascular bed is estimated by analogy to Ohm's law: resistance =

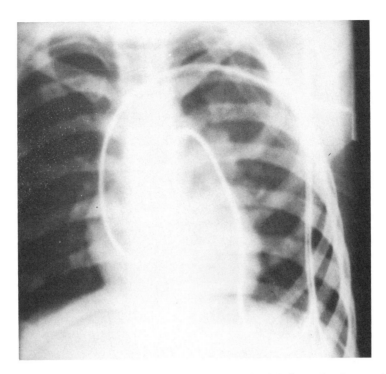

Fig. 5-2. The catheter is passed from the left arm through the right heart chambers so that its tip wedges in a 2 mm (in diameter) pulmonary artery in the lower lobe of the left lung. The pressure recorded is equal to the pulmonary venous pressure and thus left atrial pressure.

the mean pressure drop across the vascular bed (volts) ÷ by flow (amperes).[5] By the Poiseuilles formula,

$$R = \frac{8 \, nl}{\pi \, r \, 4} = \frac{p1 - P2}{Q}$$

Thus pulmonary vascular resistance (R) is the ratio of mean alveolar pressure (PA) minus mean left atrial pressure divided by the pulmonary blood flow. The latter is equal to the cardiac output in the absence of a left-to-right shunt. The resistance should be normalized for body size by indexing the flow to body surface area. The left atrial pressure is obtained by wedging the catheter tip into a branch pulmonary artery (Fig. 5-2) or by inflating a balloon tip catheter in a PA branch. Flow is interrupted and a static column of blood extends via pulmonary vein branches to the left atrium, reflecting its pressure and wave form. Theoretically, wedging is best done in the lung base to avoid collapse of the column by increased alveolar pressure, but this is usually not a problem because most studies are done in the supine position. Factors other than flow and axial pressure difference that alter resistance include changes in the velocity profile, bifurcations, flow pulsation, the nature of blood changes in vessel geometry, and recruitment of previously closed or partially closed vessels.[6,7]

RIGHT VENTRICULAR VOLUME AND WEIGHT

The angiographic estimation of right ventricular volume by biplane right ventriculography can use one of three mathematical models[8] (Fig. 5-3). The first model, the prolate ellipsoid form, uses an area length method. The second model involves an assumed triangular shaped cylinder form of the right ventricle, using Simpson's rule and adding up the volume of each slice. BB and AA, the height and base of the triangle, are gotten from the frontal and lateral views of the right ventricular angiogram. Slices are perpendicular to a long axis common to the two views. The final model involves assumed elliptic slices of the RV model using Simpson's rule. The latter is favored mathematically because of the right ventricle's unconventional form, although volume results agree well for clinical purposes with all three models. The RV ejection fraction equals $0.51 \pm .08$ whereas the left ventricular ejection fraction equals $0.67 \pm .16$. Thus the right ventricle has a somewhat greater end diastolic volume (81 ± 12 ml/m^2 vs. 70 ± 20 ml/m^2) and a lower ejection fraction than the left ventricle[9] (Fig. 5-4).

Isolated right ventricular weight (without the septum) of more than 80 grams represents right ventricular hypertrophy. Each ventricle should be weighed separately because total heart weight is not a useful way to assess right hyper-

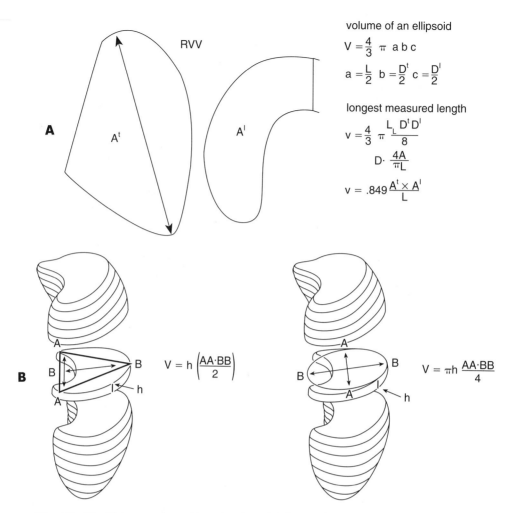

volume of an ellipsoid

$$V = \frac{4}{3} \pi \, a \, b \, c$$

$$a = \frac{L}{2} \quad b = \frac{D^t}{2} \quad c = \frac{D^l}{2}$$

longest measured length

$$v = \frac{4}{3} \pi \frac{L \, D^t D^l}{8}$$

$$D \cdot \frac{4A}{\pi L}$$

$$v = .849 \frac{A^t \times A^l}{L}$$

$$V = h \left(\frac{AA \cdot BB}{2} \right)$$

$$V = \pi h \frac{AA \cdot BB}{4}$$

Fig. 5-3. The biplane angiographic estimation of right ventricular volume may use one of three mathematical models. **A,** Prolate ellipsoid form. a, b, c = 3 hemi-axes of the ellipsoid; L = the long axis of the ventricle; D1 = two mutually perpendicular short axes at the midpoint of L, Af Ab = planimetered area in the frontal and lateral projections. **B,** Triangular cylinder form using Simpson's rule. **C,** Elliptical cylinder form using Simpson's rule. (From Horn V, Mullins CB, Soffer SI et al: A comparison of mathematical models for estimating right ventricular volumes in animals and man, *Clin Cardiol* 2:341-47, 1979.)

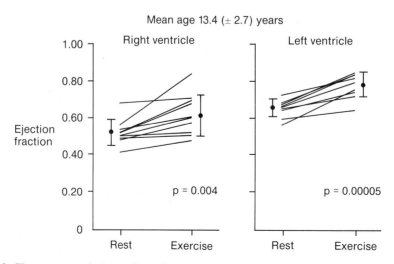

Fig. 5-4. First pass quantitative radionuclide angiocardiography was done at rest and with upright bicycle exercise in 10 normal children. Note that both RV and LV ejection fractions (EF) rise significantly with exercise and that the LVEF is greater than the RVEF.

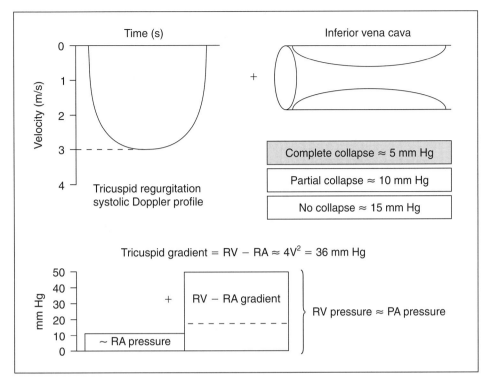

Fig. 5-5. The echocardiographic Doppler technique can provide an accurate noninvasive estimate of peak PA pressure (see text). (From Liebson PR: What role for echocardiography in primary pulmonary artery hypertension? *J Crit Illness* 6:882-88, 1991.)

trophy. An RV to LV ratio of less than 2.2 with a normal weight left ventricle is indicative of RVH.[10]

NONINVASIVE ESTIMATION OF PA PRESSURE

Continuous wave Doppler echocardiography allows us to measure PA systolic pressure with excellent accuracy in noninvasive fashion.[11,12] The peak tricuspid valve regurgitant velocity is measured by Doppler echocardiography; this value, substituted into the modified Bernoulli equation (velocity^2 × 4), is equal to the systolic pressure gradient between the RV and the RA (Fig. 5-5). Thus if the tricuspid regurgitant velocity jet is 5 meters per second, then the peak RV systolic pressure exceeds right atrial pressure by 100 mm Hg. The peak PA systolic pressure is equal to the RV RA systolic gradient plus the right atrial pressure. An arbitrary value of 10 mm Hg may be used for the right atrial pressure, or the right atrial pressure may be estimated to be as much as 20 mm Hg if there is no inspiratory collapse of the inferior vena cava.

Other echocardiographic techniques have estimated pulmonary artery systolic pressure by using a nomogram and measuring the isovolumic pulmonary closure to tricuspid valve opening time, i.e., the duration of right ventricular isovolumic relaxation, which increases as pulmonary hypertension increases. The acceleration time from the onset to peak velocity progressively shortens as pulmonary artery pressure increases, but this measurement does not give as exact an estimation of pulmonary artery pressure as other techniques.

Diastolic pulmonary valve regurgitant velocity is measured at end diastole in the main pulmonary artery (MPA) and reflects RV pressure difference at the time RV diastolic pressure is lowest. The measurement of end diastolic pulmonary valve regurgitant velocity estimates the diastolic gradient between the RV and MPA by the simplified Bernoulli equation, yielding the pulmonary artery diastolic pressure.

DISTRIBUTION OF PULMONARY BLOOD FLOW IN THE LUNG

West and Dollery[13] have shown that pulmonary blood flow in the erect position is highest at the lung base and decreases moving toward the apex of the lung, where flow is the lowest. The distribution of blood flow and the presence of three hydrostatic zones in the upright lung is determined by the value of the pulmonary artery (Pa) and the pulmonary venous (PV) pressure in each zone and the alveolar pressure (PA), which tends to be constant from apex to base[14] (Fig. 5-6).

At the apical lung zone (zone 1), alveolar pressure is greater than pulmonary artery pressure; consequently, alveolar capillaries collapse or are severely compressed, and apical flow is very low.

In the midlung (zone 2), pulmonary artery pressure is

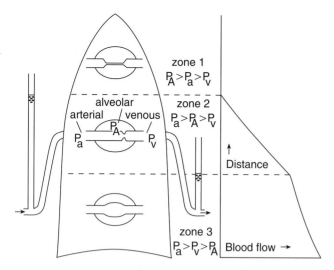

Fig. 5-6. The classic model West used to explain the zones of increasing blood flow passing from apex to base of the lung in the upright position in relation to vascular and alveolar pressures. Pa = pulmonary artery pressure; PA = alveolar pressure; PV = pulmonary venous pressure. (From West JB, Dollery CT, Narmack A: Distribution of blood flow in isolated lung relation to vascular and alveolar pressure, *J Appl Physiol* 19:713-24, 1964.)

1. Physical expansion of the lungs and increased alveolar PO2 produces a marked decrease in pulmonary artery vasoconstriction and a dramatic fall in pulmonary vascular resistance.
2. Elimination of the low-resistance placental circulation is followed by a significant rise in systemic vascular resistance.
3. Abolition of the umbilical venous return results in decreased blood flow to the right atrium.
4. The abrupt rise (tenfold) in pulmonary blood flow is promptly translated into a rise in the left atrial volume and pressure.
5. The rise in left atrial pressure and the concomitant fall in right atrial pressure results in functional closure of the foramen ovale.
6. Largely in response to an increase in systemic arterial PO2 constriction and closure of the ductus arteriosus occurs at about 12 hours.

Postnatal pulmonary arterial remodeling has been studied by electron microscopy.[16,17] Such studies have revealed that at birth the media of the pulmonary artery at the level of the terminal bronchiole is comprised of overlapping smooth muscle cells that are rectangular in shape, closely packed and surrounded by only a small amount of connective tissue.

The reduction in wall thickness in these arteries, observed about a month after birth, appears to result from thinning of endothelial and smooth muscle cells. The latter exhibit less overlap at this stage of remodeling, plus reduction in the mean diameter and more spindle-shaped configuration.[18] Thus the postnatal adaptation of the pulmonary arteries is manifested by thinning of the wall and increase in luminal diameter probably achieved by changes in smooth muscle cell shape that spread the cells within the arterial wall. Therefore this adaptation is accomplished without a reduction in the amount of pulmonary vascular smooth muscle.[19] Both the media and adventitia at birth contain predominantly collagen type III. Lesser amounts of collagen type I, which has a high tensile strength, enhance the plasticity of the vessel walls at birth. Unlike the small peripheral pulmonary arteries, the proximal elastic conducting pulmonary arteries retain the shape of the endothelial and smooth muscle cells from birth to adulthood, although some increase in the connective tissue between muscle cells occurs more than 6 months after birth. Although at birth the morphologic features of the smooth muscle cells in the intrapulmonary arteries suggest an abundance of secretory rather than contractile organelles, the volume density of myofilaments appears to increase with age.

At birth a reduction in vasoconstrictor tone could be caused by increased PO2, reduction of the effects of vasoconstrictor leukotrienes (LIC4 and LTD4), and release of prostacyclin (PGI2) with the onset of respiration.[20,21,22]

Although debatable currently, it appears that the ana-

greater than alveolar pressure. However, PA pressure rises and pulmonary venous pressure is persistently greater than alveolar pressure as one moves down within zone 2, where flow increases and is proportional to the Pa − PV difference, or pressure drop.

In the base of the lung (zone 3), pulmonary artery and venous pressures constantly exceed alveolar pressure. Thus the alveolar capillary bed is opened widely by the increased venous pressure, permitting the highest flow. The geometry of the alveolar vessels, and the resistance to flow within them (pulmonary capillaries) changes in response to the hydrostatic column extending from the apex to the base of the lung.[15] The role of active tension in alveolar vessels is not well defined.

Zonal flow in the lung secondary to the erect posture is primarily a resting phenomenon that disappears even with mild exercise. The previously unopened apical lung vessels serve to accommodate the increase in pulmonary blood flow with exercise with only a slight increase in pulmonary artery pressure; thus the basal vessels distend with increased pulmonary blood flow as pulmonary artery pressure and pulmonary venous pressure exceed alveolar pressure. In the supine position at rest, pulmonary blood flow is nearly uniform from apex to base of the lung. The flow is somewhat increased in the posterior dependent portion of the supine lung.

POSTNATAL CHANGES IN THE PULMONARY CIRCULATION

Several events that occur immediately after birth alter the pulmonary blood flow and pressure. These are:

tomic innervation of the lungs is relatively sparse. Thus the combination of less smooth muscle in the pulmonary arteries and arterioles and fewer adrenergic nerve endings provides the structural basis for the comparatively modest intrinsic vasomotor activity of the adult pulmonary circulation and the relative greater importance of passive effects.

Local regulatory mechanisms intrinsic to the lung appear to determine its ventilation and perfusion. For example, when a segment of the lung is not ventilated because of a bronchial obstruction, a local rise of CO_2 and fall of PO_2 and pH in the alveoli will occur. These changes will induce vasoconstriction in an attempt to shunt blood away from this lung segment and match the local perfusion and ventilation.

PULMONARY HYPERTENSION SECONDARY TO CONGENITAL HEART DISEASE

In infants born with large communications between the two circulations, four developmental patterns may occur in the pulmonary arteries: (1) normal regression of the media of the fetal pulmonary arteries, with a proportionate fall in pulmonary vascular resistance, permitting a large left-to-right shunt at 3 weeks to 6 weeks of age; (2) delayed or incomplete regression, resulting in a moderate left-to-right shunt; (3) recurrence of an elevated pulmonary vascular resistance months or years after partial or complete regression, resulting in gradual decrease of a large left-to-right shunt; or (4) persistence of the high pulmonary vascular resistance of the newborn, resulting in no significant left-to-right shunt or a small bidirectional shunt.[23]

Atrial septal defect with pulmonary hypertension usually occurs beyond age 20 and is rare in infancy and childhood (Fig. 5-7). Early adult onset pulmonary hypertension in large atrial septal defect (ASD) occurs in 5% to 15% of cases and is likely multifactorial.[24] Pulmonary hypertension with ASD predominates in females, a predominance that is unrelated to the already increased prevalence of ASD in women. Genetic predisposition toward hyperreactivity of the pulmonary arterioles to the increased pulmonary flow may be a factor.

In the infant with increased pulmonary blood flow and a high pressure drop across the pulmonary vascular bed, arteriolar obstructive disease and abnormalities in pulmonary artery remodeling occur in the first 1 to 2 years. The defects most commonly responsible for the large left-to-right shunt include ventricular septal defect, patent ductus arteriosus, or aortopulmonary window, common AV canal, and truncus arteriosus. Pulmonary vascular obstructive dis-

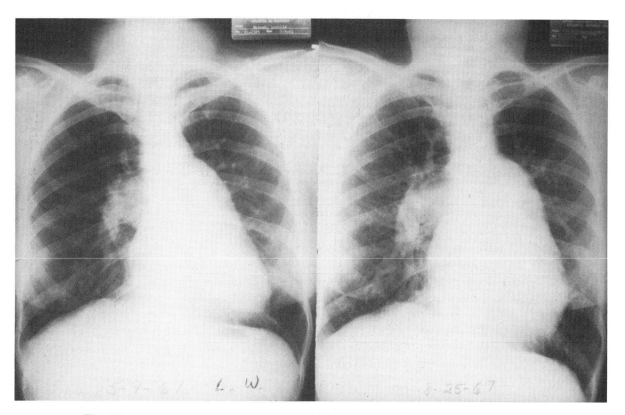

Fig. 5-7. Frontal chest films of a 41-year-old housewife taken 6 years apart show progressive RV, and PA enlargement as the mean PA pressure (MPAP) rose from 32 mm Hg to 64 mm Hg and the pulmonary vascular resistance (PVR) from 4 units to 9 units. A large atrial septal defect was closed at age 29; the preoperative MPAP was 62 with a PVR of 10 units. Despite initial palliation, the PVR has returned to near systemic levels.

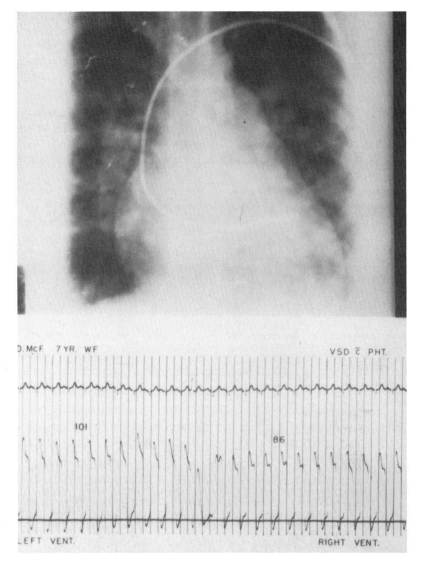

Fig. 5-8. Frontal chest film of a 7-year-old girl. The catheter tip lies in the LV after crossing a large VSD. A pull back pressure tracing shows the RV systolic pressure to be 85% of LVSP. A significant left-to-right shunt is still present.

ease is especially accelerated in the infant, with transposition of the great arteries and ventricular septal defect occurring as early as 6 months after birth. In general, to prevent irreversible pulmonary vascular changes, repair of shunt defects with significant pulmonary hypertension should be optimally done before 1 year of age[25] (Fig. 5-8).

Damage to the endothelial cells may occur from the increase in shear stress secondary to the large pressure drop (ΔP) across the long axis of the pulmonary vascular bed, i.e., shear stress (dynes/cm^2) = ΔP · r. "R" is the distance from the center of the artery to the point of shear measurement; thus shear stress is 0 at the center of the artery and maximal along the wall (Fig. 5-9). "L" is the length of the artery. Endothelial cell alterations may change circulating catecholamines, arachidonate metabolites, and endothelial

derived relaxing factor. The function of von Willebrand's factor is shear rate-dependent. It is the largest protein known in mammalian plasma, acting as "mortar" for platelet aggregation.

Increased flow to a normal pulmonary vascular bed or normal flow to a restrictive vascular bed results in the extension of mature smooth muscle into the pulmonary arteries normally non-muscular of 20 to 30 microns in diameter. In the larger proximal pulmonary arteries, the smooth muscle cells of the medial layer increase in number while there is a concomitant increase in collagen in both the medial and adventitial connective tissue. In addition, a constellation of cellular factors alters the endothelial cells and breaks down the internal elastic lamina so that endothelium and smooth muscle come in close proximity. Elastase

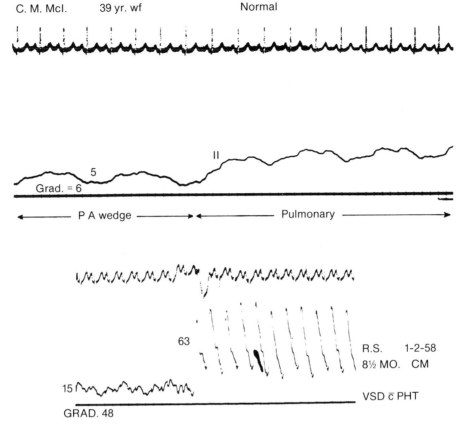

Fig. 5-9. The PA mean minus PA wedge pressure difference in a normal adult is 6 mm Hg; it is 48 mm Hg in an infant with a VSD. PA hypertension and pulmonary blood flow is 2.5 times normal, leading to increased shear stress and progressive pulmonary vascular damage.

degrades elastin in the nonmuscular and muscular pulmonary arteries. Growth factors in the basement membrane encourage migration of smooth muscle cells from the media to the intima.

As the pulmonary vascular resistance and pulmonary artery pressure rise to or beyond systemic levels, a significant right-to-left-shunt occurs across a preexisting septal defect or aorto-pulmonary communication, resulting in desaturation of systemic arterial blood (Fig. 5-10). This hemodynamic state is called Eisenmenger's physiology (EP). In the discussion below, patients with EP will be considered as a group independent of the underlying congenital shunt defect, unless otherwise specified.

Progression of pulmonary vascular disease in those surviving infancy results in dyspnea, fatigue, and increasing cyanosis peaking in the second to fourth decade of life. Activity is limited by exertional syncope and RV angina in some patients. Increasing cyanosis, especially with exercise, occurs due to the right-to-left shunting of mixed venous blood of low oxygen saturation. A fall in peripheral vascular resistance caused by postural or vasovagal hypotension is catastrophic, permitting massive right-to-left shunting through the defect. Sitting with the legs pulled up is a learned comfortable position to avoid dependent ve-

nous pooling. In cases with balanced vascular resistances, the shunting across the defect at rest is small, and no murmur is audible.

Overt right ventricular failure is not common in EP. The right ventricle adapts early to facing pressure at systemic levels and is bolstered by continued myocyte hypertrophy in early life. In non-ASD EP, right ventricular systolic pressure is dependent on both the pulmonary and the systemic vascular resistance. RA pressure is within normal limits, and RV function remains good unless systemic vascular resistance rises. Isometric exercise causes a rise in systemic vascular resistance and thus an increase in right ventricular afterload, but it causes little or no increase in pulmonary blood flow. Isotonic exercise causes a decrease in systemic vascular resistance, an increase in the right-to-left shunt, a decrease in arterial oxygen saturation, and an increase in systemic flow. In contrast, in EP with an atrial septal defect, RV afterload can be greater than LV afterload. Thus isotonic exercise may increase the RV end diastolic pressure, yielding an increased right-to-left shunt but no satisfactory increase in systemic flow. Therefore blood pressure may fall, resulting in syncope.[26] Visible cyanosis occurs when 5 grams of reduced hemoglobin per 100 ml of blood is present. The degree of arterial blood

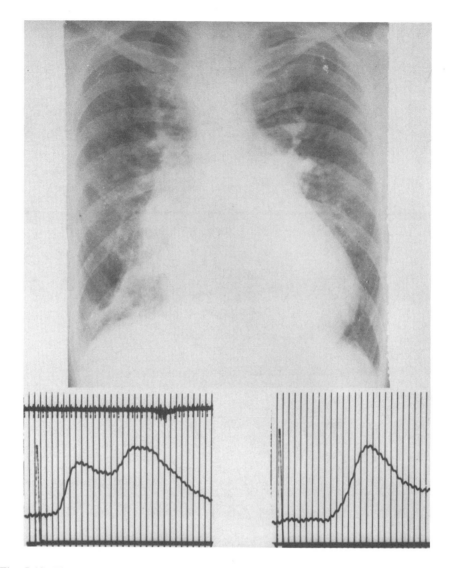

Fig. 5-10. The chest film of a 44-year-old cyanotic man with atrial septal defect shows cardiomegaly secondary to enlargement of the right atrium (RA), right ventricle (RV), and main and right descending pulmonary artery. The pulmonary artery pressure is 124/53 mm Hg. RA dye injection is followed by early appearance at the earpiece densitometer recording site. RV injection shows a normal appearance time. A right-to-left shunt at the atrial level equals 34% of systemic flow. The interval between the vertical time lines is 1 sec. (From Franch RH: *Cyanotic congenital heart disease.* In Fowler NO, ed: *Cardiac diagnosis and treatment,* Hagerstown, 1980, Harper & Row.)

unsaturation depends not only on the size of the right-to-left shunt but also on the oxygen saturation of the systemic venous blood shunted. Thus even if the percentage of right-to-left shunt is not increased, the fall in systemic venous blood saturation occurring with exercise causes a fall in arterial oxygen saturation. Of course, pulmonary venous blood remains normally saturated.

Brain abscess is the result of a chronic, frequently anaerobic infection in the sinuses, middle ear, or respiratory tract. Localization in the brain may occur at an area of low oxygen tension, which is either an area of previous infarction or softening, or at a junction of the gray and white matter, where vascularization may be poor.

Hemoptysis is usually mild, self-limited and may not recur for years. If the pulmonary vascular resistance has remained persistently high from infancy, the heart may be only slightly enlarged, and the pulmonary arteries of normal size. If the pulmonary vascular resistance has increased progressively and the pulmonary flow decreased, stepwise the heart and pulmonary arteries are large. The calculated pulmonary vascular resistance is equal to or greater than the systemic vascular resistance in cases of EP, and pulmonary blood flow is equal to or less than systemic flow. The only surgical form of treatment is heart-lung or lung transplant[27] (see Table 5-1).

Table 5-1. Hemodynamics in recipients (n=8) with primary pulmonary hypertension and Eisenmenger syndrome, before and after transplantation[27]

Parameter*	Before Transplantation	After Transplantation
Time period, days	367 ± 618	235 ± 116
Pulmonary artery pressures, mm Hg		
Systolic	93 ± 18	27 ± 6†
Diastolic	40 ± 5	13 ± 4†
Mean	58 ± 6	19 ± 5†
Cardiac index, L/min/m²	2.15 ± 0.37	2.75 ± 0.50†
Pulmonary vascular resistance (Wood units)	14.4 ± 4.5	2.3 ± 1.3†

*All values shown as mean ± standard deviation (SD).
†P < .01 before vs. after transplantation.

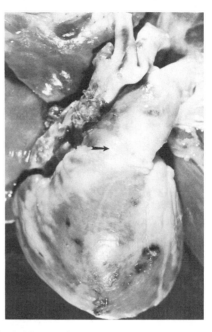

Fig. 5-11. A 27-year-old woman was diagnosed with anomalous right pulmonary venous return and a small atrial septal defect. Two years before her demise, she developed primary pulmonary hypertension (plexogenic). Note the marked dilatation of the pulmonary trunk (3.2 cm in diameter) *(arrow)*. The aortic diameter was 1.6 cm *(curved arrow)*.

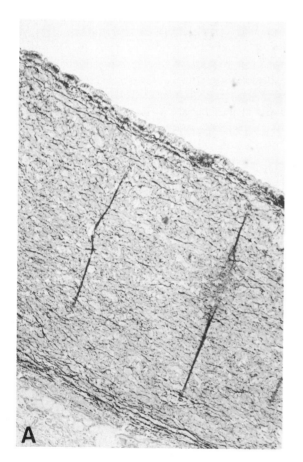

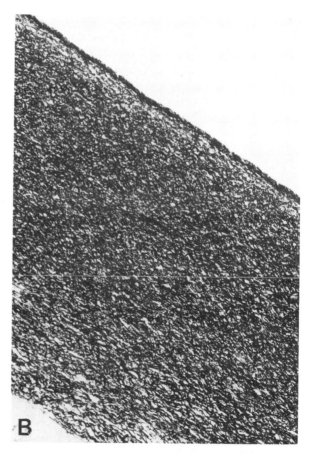

Fig. 5-12. Main pulmonary artery from a 27-year-old female patient with primary pulmonary arterial hypertension of 2 years duration. Note the marked paucity and fragmentation of elastic fibers in the media **(A)** (Elastic stain of the same case depicted in Fig. 5-11). Normal pulmonary artery **(B)**.

PATHOLOGY OF PULMONARY ARTERIES IN CONGENITAL HEART DISEASE

A multiplicity of histoarchitectural alterations is seen in the pulmonary vasculature in patients with pulmonary hypertension secondary to cardiac shunts. The large elastic arteries are dilated and exhibit increased medial thickening. In time these arteries may develop atherosclerotic lesions that are modest in extent and do not ulcerate. In cases in which the hypertension has been present from birth, the elastic fibers of these arteries are continuous, as they are in the fetus. When hypertension develops after the third year of life, the elastic fibers are fragmented (Figs. 5-11; 5-12).

The preacinar and terminal bronchiolar pulmonary arteries reveal increased medial thickness. In the majority of cases the intraacinar arteries also show medial hypertrophy, and muscle is seen in more peripheral arteries than normal (extension). The medial hypertrophy is considered a secondary phenomenon resulting from stretching of the small arteries and arterioles, which is caused by increased pulmonary pressure. Intimal proliferation and fibrosis is seen only in small preacinar and terminal bronchiolar pulmonary arteries (Fig. 5-13). This intimal thickening may be noted as early as 1.4 years of age and occurs with increasing frequency after 2.4 years. Intimal proliferation and fibrosis increase with age, producing luminal narrowing, whereas medial hypertrophy is less marked, at least in the intraacinar arteries.[28]

Plexiform lesions have been observed as early as 2.4 years of age and increase in frequency in older children and young adults (Fig. 5-14). The alveolar: arterial ratio is increased in approximately one-fourth of the cases, indicating a reduction in number of peripheral arteries. Complete cellular occlusion tends to occur in the younger patient (3 months to 2.4 years); fibrotic occlusion occurs in the older patient (2.4 years to 10.8 years). In the majority of the cases, the preacinar veins show an increase in wall thickness, whereas the intraacinar veins develop external elastic laminae similar to those of arteries.[28]

The mechanism(s) by which the abnormal pulmonary hemodynamics cause the vascular alterations enumerated above is still unknown. Similarly, our understanding about the rate of progression of different vascular lesions among different individuals is rather incomplete.

Lacking such fundamental information about the pathogenesis of the vascular reactivity in pulmonary hypertension makes prognostication about which patients will favorably respond to corrective surgery very difficult.

PULMONARY ENDOTHELIUM AND PULMONARY ARTERY HYPERTENSION IN CONGENITAL CARDIAC DEFECTS

The possible interactions of the pulmonary endothelium with blood elements in patients with congenital cardiac defects, before and after corrective surgery, have been studied by light, scanning, and transmission electron microscopy. The main goal of Rabinovitch's[29] study was to demonstrate endothelial cell surface alterations and changes in intracytoplasmic composition that may reflect functional abnormalities in these cells. Alterations in endothelial surface characteristics, such as deep infolding and twisting of endothelial ridges, may result from either an increase in thickness of the arterial wall or altered pulmonary hemodynamics (increased PA pressure and flow). Pulmonary ar-

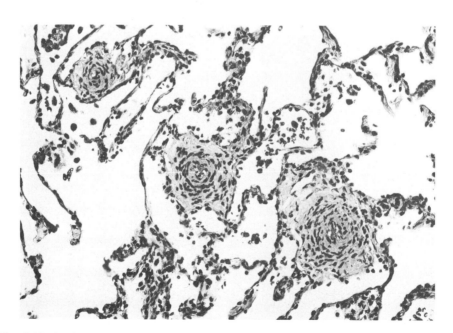

Fig. 5-13. Small pulmonary arteries and arterioles showing marked intimal proliferation in a patient with congenital heart disease (common AV canal).

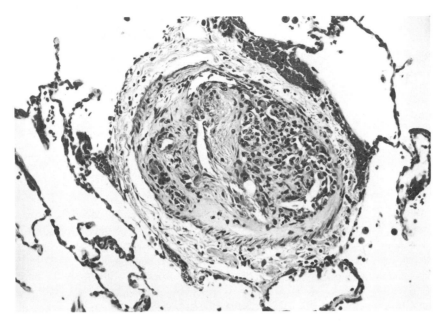

Fig. 5-14. Early stage of a plexiform lesion in a patient with congenital heart disease (VSD).

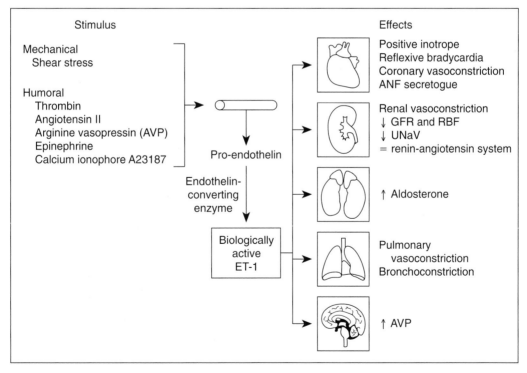

Fig. 5-15. A chart by Underwood depicts the stimuli for the secretion of proendothelin and its transformation, and the physiologic effects of endothelin. (From Underwood RD, Chan DP, Burnett JC: Endothelin: an endothelin-derived vasoconstrictor peptide and its role in congestive heart failure, *Heart Failure* 7:50-58, 1991.)

teries with medial hypertrophy or medial hypertrophy plus intimal hyperplasia reveal increased areal proportion of microvilli or cytoplasmic surface projections. However, it remains unknown whether the increase of microvilli is instrumental in reducing the speed of the plasma flow at the cell surface and therefore enhance the exchange of metabolites between the plasma and the endothelium. It has also been suggested, but not proved, that an increase in microvilli may enhance the adherence of platelets and leukocytes, and facilitate their degranulation and release of vasoconstrictive substances (thromboxane or leukotrines).[30]

Von Willebrand's factor (vWF), a large multimeric plasma glycoprotein produced by endothelial cells, may also alter platelet adherence and increase the release of vasoactive substances and smooth muscle mitogens. Quantitative and qualitative abnormalities in vWF have been noted in patients with congenital heart defects and pulmonary hypertension. The majority of these patients reveal increased levels of vWF:Ag (increase antigenic activity).[31]

The peptide endothelin has potent vasoconstricting activity and induces smooth muscle proliferation[32,33] (Fig. 5-15). Plasma endothelin-like immunoreactivity (ET-LI) was measured in patients with congenital heart defects and pulmonary hypertension age 6 months to 12 years and was compared with age-matched controls. Patients with pulmonary hypertension revealed elevated concentration of plasma ET-LI.[34]

Measurement of endothelin levels at different sites in the circulation showed that substantial amounts of the peptide are produced in the endothelium of pulmonary arteries, capillaries, and veins. Whether the increased endothelin production in pulmonary hypertension reflects an increased metabolic activity of pulmonary endothelial cells remains unknown.

SYSTEMIC-PULMONARY ARTERY COLLATERAL CIRCULATION IN THE LUNG

The systemic-to-pulmonary artery collateral circulation (SPAC) is made up of arteries that supply the bronchi, and arteries that supply other intrathoracic structures. The bronchial arteries vary highly in number and site of origin. They usually originate in the proximal descending thoracic aorta from level T3 to T8, with most arising at T6. The right bronchial artery may arise jointly with an intercostal artery. Bronchial arteries anastomose with the subclavian, internal mammary, superior intercostal, and pericardiophrenic arteries, as well as with direct pericardial, esophageal and pleural, and transpleural and transdiaphragmatic rami. There are also direct primitive aortopulmonary collaterals that join with the true pulmonary arteries at the hila of the lungs, especially in patients with cyanotic congenital heart disease who have decreased pulmonary blood flow due to pulmonary valve atresia.

The oxygen demand of the normal lung is small, representing 1% to 2% of the cardiac output. However, the systemic arterial network supplying the lung can expand dramatically in the presence of parenchymal lung disease,[35] pulmonary artery obstruction, and cyanotic congenital heart disease. For example, 3 months after ligation of the pulmonary artery in a dog, collateral flow can supply ⅔ of the original pulmonary artery flow.[36]

In cases of pulmonary atresia, the greatly expanded SPAC supplies desaturated blood to multiple prealveolar PA branches providing the sole blood flow for the entire gas exchange of the lungs.[37] Occasionally the collateral flow may be so large and effective that the LV enlarges secondary to the voluminous left-to-right-shunt, and the O₂ saturation may approach 90%.

In acquired pulmonary lesions, severe bronchiectasis, fibrothorax, post-resection of emphysematous bullae, tuberculosis, cancer of the lung, and chronic pulmonary artery thromboembolism, SPAC may be so marked that at pulmonary angiography the collateral circulation causes a phasic reversal of pulmonary blood flow in the pulmonary arteries supplying the involved lung. In these cases a continuous murmur is present. In a housewife (Fig. 5-16) the

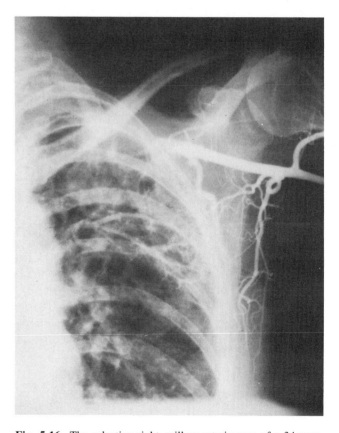

Fig. 5-16. The selective right axillary arteriogram of a 34-year-old housewife opacifies the lateral thoracic artery, the transpleural systemic to pulmonary artery collateral and retrogradely, the right upper lobe (RUL) pulmonary artery. One year previously she had undergone resection of RUL bullae with removal of chest wall pleura. A right infraclavicular continuous murmur was subsequently found.

murmur was audible over the thoracotomy scar at the site of removal of an emphysematous bulla. At the site of the surgical intervention a communication between the arterial branches of the chest wall occurred with the pulmonary artery transpleurally. On selective pulmonary artery angiography there was a negative washout of contrast media from the SPAC.

A 5-year old girl with a contracted fibrotic right lung supplied by SPAC had a marked increase in the oxygen content of the blood obtained in the RPA but not in the LPA. The pulmonary-to-systemic flow ratio was 1.5. The pneumonectomy specimen revealed thick pleura containing arteries leading to the underlying lung. The source of hemoptysis is most often from the SPAC rather than from the pulmonary arteries themselves. Identification of the culprit collateral artery by selective arteriography and its occlusion by percutaneous catheter embolization has proved to be a therapeutic modality.[38]

CAVOPULMONARY ARTERY ANASTOMOSIS AND NONPULSATILE BLOOD FLOW TO THE LUNGS

In patients with tricuspid atresia or single ventricle, if the pulmonary vascular resistance is normal and systemic ventricular function adequate, caval blood can be surgically shunted directly to the lungs. This results in low pulsatile or nonpulsatile blood flow through the pulmonary vascular bed.

If the superior vena cava is anastomosed end-to-end to the right pulmonary artery (the classic Glenn shunt), pulmonary arterial venous fistulae develop in the right lower lobe of up to 25% of patients.[39,40]

If the superior vena cava is anastomosed end to side into the right pulmonary artery (bidirectional cavopulmonary anastomosis or modified Glenn shunt), the lung perfusion pattern is normal in ⅓ of patients (i.e., one lung receives at least 45% of the total pulmonary blood flow). However, in ⅓ of the cases moderate to severe abnormalities in the distribution of pulmonary blood flow are noted.[41] The bidirectional cavopulmonary anastamosis can be used to palliate a high-risk patient because effective pulmonary blood flow is increased, whereas total pulmonary flow and ventricular volume load is decreased.[42]

If the inferior vena cava is connected to the right pulmonary artery at the time of the superior vena cava anastomosis (modified Fontan procedure) or at a subsequent operation, then these patients are no longer cyanotic because the systemic venous return no longer enters the right atrium and the obligatory right-to-left shunt ceases. Long-term follow-up will determine whether the post-Fontan patient is at risk for development of pulmonary AV fistulae and whether this is related to altered lung perfusion patterns.[43]

If the right atrium is joined directly to the pulmonary artery, the RA mean pressure comes to equal or be slightly greater than the PA pressure. Total caval to pulmonary artery end-to-side anastomosis tends to raise the RA pressure less than the direct right atrial PA communication. The onset of atrial fibrillation does not alter PA filling in cases of RA to PA anastomosis, but the loss of left atrial kick may decrease systemic ventricular output and result in an increase in LA pressure, thus increasing resistance to pulmonary blood flow.

Patients who have the Fontan procedure are improved subjectively and are no longer cyanotic. In 16 patients with RA to PA anastomoses, upright bicycle exercise was carried out for 7 minutes. The heart rate increased from 92 to 155 beats per minute, and the cardiac index rose by a factor of 1.8. The rise in systemic output tends to occur by an increase in heart rate rather than an increase in stroke volume.[44] However, oxygen consumption at peak exercise is significantly decreased compared with that of normal patients.

THE ANATOMIC RIGHT VENTRICLE SERVING AS THE FUNCTIONAL LEFT VENTRICLE

The right ventricle contracts in sequence starting from the sinus, or inflow portion, and ending in the infundibulum, or outflow channel, of the right ventricle. When the contraction pattern of the right ventricle is studied in normal patients by cine x-ray CT scanner, no change in the area of the interventricular septum is noted during systole.[45] This lack of change suggests that the systolic reduction in area of the right ventricular free wall is primarily responsible for right ventricular ejection. The right ventricle is designed to eject a relatively large amount of blood with minimal myocardial shortening. It has a high diastolic compliance and tolerates the large diastolic overload from an atrial septal defect for a lifetime if the pulmonary artery pressure remains in the normal range.

When the right ventricle must function as the systemic ventricle (e.g., in patients with transposition of the great arteries after an interatrial baffle repair, or in patients who have congenitally corrected transposition of the great arteries), then the ejection fraction of the right ventricle is decreased, and the end diastolic volume is increased.[46,47] With exercise the right ventricular ejection fraction fails to rise or may decrease[48] (Fig. 5-17). Concern about the long-term function of the right ventricle as the systemic ventricle has led to surgically switching the great vessels and reimplanting the coronary arteries in patients with transposition. One of our 20-year-old patients who had an interatrial baffle procedure early in life developed a right (systemic) ventricular end diastolic pressure of 32 mm Hg and a PA mean of 54 mm Hg.

Many patients with isolated congenitally corrected transposition of the great arteries (ICCTGA) will show clinical evidence of systemic or anatomic (RV) dysfunction by age 50. However, one of our elderly patients, (82 years old) an active asymptomatic man with ICCTGA, has

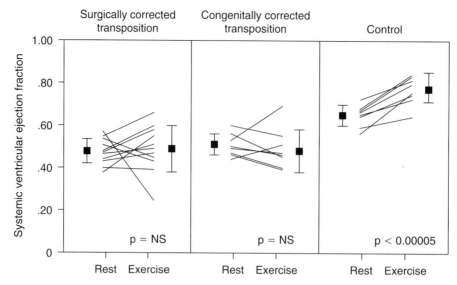

Fig. 5-17. The systemic ventricular (i.e., anatomic right ventricle) ejection fraction from rest to exercise for surgically corrected (intraatrial baffle) transposition of the great arteries (N=11), congenitally corrected transposition of the great arteries without other defects (N=8), and control (N=10). When the anatomic RV functions as the systemic ventricle for the EF with exercise does not change significantly. (From Peterson RJ et al: Comparison of cardiac function in surgically corrected and congenitally corrected transposition of the great arteries, *J Thorac Cardiovasc Surg* 96:223-36, 1988.)

a mean PA pressure of 24, an RV (systemic) end diastolic pressure of 20, and an RV ejection fraction of 32. In his case the anatomic right ventricle continues to function as the systemic ventricle at an adequate level for the eighty-second year.

PULMONARY HYPERTENSION SECONDARY TO ELEVATION OF PULMONARY VENOUS PRESSURE

An elevation in left ventricular end diastolic pressure caused by systolic or diastolic dysfunction of the left ventricle (Fig. 5-18), or a rise in left atrial pressure caused by mitral stenosis, results in moderate and occasionally severe pulmonary venous and pulmonary artery pressure elevation.[49] A patient with hypertrophic cardiomyopathy without mitral regurgitation had a PA systolic pressure of 80 mm Hg. Congenital or, less commonly, acquired stenosis or obstruction of the pulmonary veins at or near their junction with the left atrium, total anomalous pulmonary venous return with obstruction, cor triatriatum, congenital mitral stenosis, or mitral or aortic atresia, and hypoplastic left ventricle are all associated with severe pulmonary artery hypertension requiring surgical intervention (Fig. 5-19). Fibrosing mediastinitis also may obstruct pulmonary veins.[50,51]

The patient with mitral stenosis may have mild, moderate, or severe chronic pulmonary venous pressure (PVP) elevation at rest, depending on the mitral valve area. Acute rises in PVP with exercise, which occur secondary to the increased cardiac output, and the decreased left ven-

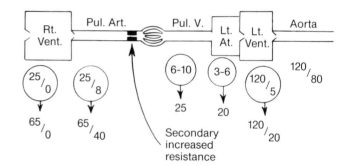

Fig. 5-18. In PA hypertension secondary to LV systolic or diastolic dysfunction the PA pressure rises disproportionately to the elevation in pulmonary venous pressure, indicating a "reflex" increase in pulmonary arteriolar resistance.

tricular filling time resulting from tachycardia can double the resting PA pressure. Chronic PVP elevation results in muscularization of arteries and medial thickening of the arteries in the lung bases. The lung becomes stiffer because of chronic interstitial fluid sequestration, which may also compress the alveolar vessels. Blood flow tends to be redistributed toward the apices of the lungs. Decreased vital capacity and diffusing capacity, increased alveolar-arterial gradients for oxygen, and increased airway resistance correlate well with the increased PVP.

In patients with mitral stenosis, the PA pressure rises passively and mildly in keeping with the mild rise in PVP. A PVP of 20 mm Hg to 25 mm Hg, may trigger reactive pulmonary hypertension, i.e., PA pressure rises dispropor-

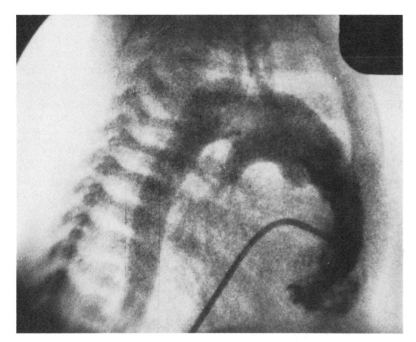

Fig. 5-19. Selective RV angiography in the lateral view shows filling of the descending thoracic aorta via reversed flow through a patent ductus arteriosus (PDA). This 7-week-old boy with aortic atresia had equal aortic and pulmonary artery pressures. The hypoplastic ascending aorta also filled from the PDA.

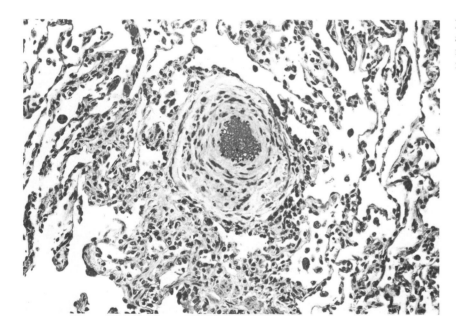

Fig. 5-20. Nonocclusive medial hypertrophy and intimal proliferation within a small pulmonary artery in a patient with long-standing mitral stenosis.

tionately to the rise in PVP. Pulmonary artery hypertension at systemic levels or above may be associated with a PVP of 30 mm Hg to 35 mm Hg. The response of the pulmonary arterioles to chronic PVP elevation varies from patient to patient, suggesting individual susceptibility to neural or hypoxic vasoconstrictor stimuli. Because bronchial veins drain primarily into the pulmonary veins, PVP elevation may result in slowing of bronchial venous return or even reversing of flow toward collateral veins.[52] Distended bronchial veins and varices are the presumed sources of hemoptysis.

In longstanding mitral stenosis the morphologic alter-ations in the pulmonary vasculature include interstitial fibrosis and destruction of alveolar capillaries. Changes in the veins and venules consist of medial thickening and arterialization of veins (separate internal and external elastica). Medial hypertrophy of the muscular pulmonary arteries and arterioles, and intimal proliferation with fibrosis are also observed. The latter may be concentric or eccentric, or mild to moderate, but does not become occlusive (Fig. 5-20). The pulmonary vascular changes in mitral stenosis tend to be more pronounced in the lower lobes. As a rule, pulmonary hypertension secondary to mitral stenosis is reversible after complete surgical correction regardless of the preoperative level of pulmonary hypertension or vascular resistance.

In patients who have pulmonary hypertension secondary to advanced cardiomyopathy, if the pulmonary vascular resistance can be acutely reduced to less than 2.5 Wood units with a nitroprusside infusion, the 3-month mortality after heart transplantation is reduced.[53]

COR PULMONALE IN ACUTE THROMBOEMBOLISM

Acute cor pulmonale secondary to pulmonary artery embolization occurs as a complication of several clinical conditions, such as malignancy, trauma, post-surgery events (especially after orthopedic procedures), immobilization, or prolonged bed rest. Patients with dilated left ventricular cardiomyopathy may die of acute cor pulmonale from either massive or recurrent pulmonary emboli. Mural throbmi may occur in the right atrium and right ventricle without clinical evidence of venous thrombosis. Deep femoral, iliac, ovarian, and testicular veins are sites of venous thromboses.[54] A normal thin-walled right ventricle after a large or massive pulmonary embolus is suddenly confronted with a significant rise in PA pressure and develops a high wall stress.[55] (Table 5-2) The right atrial pressure increases; irreversible right ventricular failure ensues, and death may occur in less than an hour. If there is right ventricular hypertrophy from previous heart or lung disease, a higher PA pressure can be generated without RV failure.[56] During the acute rise in RV pressure, the LV may undergo changes in systolic geometry, especially in the septal-free wall minor axis, resulting in reduced systolic function. Hypoxemia results from venous admixture, decreased diffusion, and ventilation perfusion imbalance.[57] Dyspnea, pleurisy, and hemoptysis occur in less than a third of the patients, therefore confirmatory tests are needed. Small emboli are particularly hard to detect.[58] If labeled human albumin particles of 30 μm are injected, the particles will lodge in the precapillary arterioles. A normal perfusion scan will thus exclude a pulmonary embolus. Unfortunately, a false positive scan may result from lung disease, infection, or heart failure. Pulmonary angiography can detect thrombi as small as 3 mm and is one of the best studies for pulmonary embolism because it is less subjective and has the least interobserver variation in interpretation. A ventilation scan using xenon in combination with a perfusion scan may not be conclusive because other causes of abnormal ventilation may coexist. If single or multiple pulmonary defects occur without associated defects on the chest radiogram, a positive scan is thought to be 80% predictive.

Although sudden obstruction is the principal cause of pulmonary hypertension in acute pulmonary embolus, individual reactivity of the pulmonary vascular bed to hypoxemia from ventilation-perfusion mismatch or from thrombin-induced bronchoconstriction may be a factor. Release of thromboxane, endogenous catecholamines, histamine, and serotonin may be contributory.[59] Acute pulmonary emboli most often lodge in the muscular arteries at the lobular level; resolution when it occurs, is often apparent after the seventh day. Spontaneous resolution explains why less than 2% of patients develop chronic pulmonary hypertension.[60]

Sustained elevation in pulmonary artery pressure and vascular resistance was induced by the continuous infusion of air emboli for 1 to 12 days into the pulmonary arterial bed of chronically instrumented awake sheep.[61] Arteriograms revealed marked dilation of the large pulmonary arteries and tapering of the peripheral ones.[62] A sequence of structural changes was identified. Interstitial lung granulocyte sequestration and interstitial edema was noted on day 1. The concentration of elastin peptides in lung lymph was evident by day 2, reflecting the increased elastin deposition required in arterial remodeling. Medial thickness increased and smooth muscle appeared in small arteries by day 4, progressing up to day 8. Both the media and adventitia showed increased proteoglycans; eccentric intimal hyperplasia was present. Transforming growth factor-b (TGF-b) was increased in lung lymph, suggesting its potential role in stimulating smooth muscle proliferation and enhancing endothelin release.[63,64,65]

COR PULMONALE IN CHRONIC PULMONARY THROMBOEMBOLISM

The natural history of chronic pulmonary hypertension secondary to persistent thromboembolic obstruction of the lobar vessels begins with a deep venous thrombosis fol-

Table 5-2. Spectrum of hemodynamic sequelae of pulmonary embolism

SYNDROMES	% PA OBSTR	$\overline{PA}$	PAWP	PAVR	$R\overline{AP}$	CO	BP
Unexplained dyspnea or	< 50%	$\overline{25}$	−N	N	N	SL	N
pulmonary infarction syndrome	50-75%	25-40	N or SL ↓	↑ 2-4u	<8	N or SL ↓	N or SL ↓
Acute cor pulmonale	75% or >	$\overline{45}$	N or SL ↓	4-6u	≥10	↓	SL ↓
Cardiogenic shock	> 75%	35-45	N or ↓	↑ 6u	>10	↓ ↓	↓
Chronic unresolved pulmonary emboli	60-80%	> 25*	N	4u	N or ↑	SL ↓	N

$\overline{PA}$ = Pulmonary artery mean pressure, mm HG Hg (normal 14-18); PAWP = Pulmonary artery wedge pressure, mm Hg; PAVR = Pulmonary artery vascular resistance, units (normal 1-2); $R\overline{AP}$ = Right atrial mean pressure, mm Hg; CO = Cardiac output; BP = Systemic arterial pressure.

lowed by extensive pulmonary embolization.[66] Morphologic findings in large pulmonary arteries and their branches at the site of the thromboembolism are characterized by variable stages of organization of the thromboembolus and/or recanalization. The latter appears as a web-like structure within the lumen of the occluded artery (Fig. 5-21). In smaller arteries, however, organization of the thrombus creates a patchy, cushion-like lesion of intimal fibrosis (Fig. 5-22). Recovery seems to occur, but slight dyspnea on exertion may persist because the emboli inex-

plicably do not dissolve but organize, recanalize, and endothelialize, thus remaining chronically obstructive.[67] Retrograde propagation of the initial embolus with in situ thrombosis proximally has been postulated.[68] The stimulus for a procoagulant condition in chronic pulmonary thromboembolism is hypothesized to be persistent pulmonary endothelial disruption secondary to the acute embolism. Findings of increased levels of fibrinopeptide A, a small peptide released by the action of thrombin from fibrinogen, in patients with pulmonary hypertension associated

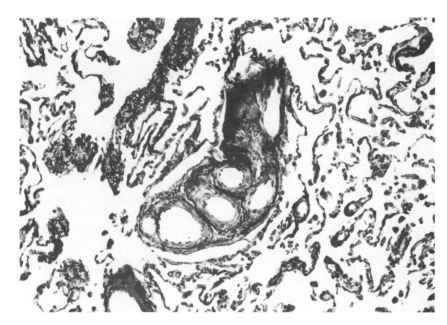

Fig. 5-21. Recanalized (luminal web) medium-sized pulmonary artery in a patient with thromboembolic pulmonary arterial hypertension.

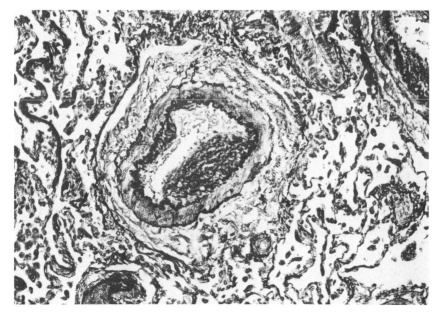

Fig. 5-22. Cushion-like lesion in a small pulmonary artery. Thromboembolic pulmonary arterial hypertension in a middle-aged man.

with thromboembolism support this hypothesis.[69] This finding provides in vivo evidence that active intravascular thrombosis is occurring in these patients. Vigorous search for abnormalities in clotting or lytic mechanisms in patients with chronic proximal pulmonary thromboembolism has not been rewarding. Special coagulation studies of most patients yield normal results. Deterioration in the functional capacity of the patient occurs over several years as pulmonary vascular changes occur in the nonobstructed areas of the lung. These changes are in part secondary to increased blood flow and occur as progressive pulmonary hypertension ensues. An erroneous diagnosis of primary pulmonary hypertension or psychogenic dyspnea may be made. The lung scan in chronic thromboembolism shows several or multiple segments of V/Q mismatch, whereas primary pulmonary hypertension has diffuse mottling on the scan. Nearly all patients have a decreased arterial pO_2 and a widened alveolar-arterial O_2 tension. Hypoxemia is related to a moderate VA/Q abnormality that is accentuated by low mixed venous oxygen saturation secondary to the low cardiac output. Right heart catheterization with

measurement of moderate to severe PA pressure elevation at rest confirms the presence of significant pulmonary artery hypertension. The pulmonary vascular resistance is usually greater than 6 Wood units. Selective pulmonary angiography is the diagnostic technique of choice and shows a variable pattern of lobar artery total or partial occlusion. The upper left lobe and lingula are frequently spared. While acute emboli are red and gelatinous, these chronic emboli are pale, show fibrous ingrowth, and adhere to the pulmonary artery wall. Surgical removal requires endarterectomy, yielding a cast-like specimen of the peripheral hilar and lobar arterial tree.[70] Because of marked enlargement of the systemic and bronchial collateral artery circulation to the lung, the pleural approach should be avoided by surgeons; embolectomy attempts must involve a sternal approach. After the main pulmonary artery is opened, the dissection plane progresses distally to both the right and left main branches. The patent foramen ovale is closed to prevent the inevitable right-to-left shunting. Acute respiratory distress syndrome is a postoperative complication presumably related in some way to reperfusion of the lung. The appearance of lung edema may be immediate or occur within 3 days. Both hypoxemia and low output failure may result from a combination of inadequate right ventricular myocardial perfusion during surgery, and persistent pulmonary hypertension caused by pulmonary arteriolar vasoconstriction and reduced cross sectional area of the pulmonary vascular bed. A successful operation results in a decrease in pulmonary vascular resistance of greater than 50% and a return to improved physical function capacity.

COR PULMONALE SECONDARY TO PARENCHYMAL LUNG DISEASE
Pathogenesis of pulmonary artery hypertension in parenchymal lung disease

Chronic bronchitis in the advanced stage is the most common chronic lung disease associated with cor pulmonale; less often cystic fibrosis,[71] late stages of emphysema, or chronic suppurative or granulomatous lung disease are the causes (Fig. 5-23).[72] In the past bronchitic patients with advanced cor pulmonale caused by obstructive airways disease and mismatched alveolar ventilation and perfusion were called polycythemic obstructive emphysema patients or black cardiacs (cardiacos negroes) in order to differentiate them from the dyspneic but noncyanotic emphysematous patients (pink puffers). Fishman[73] describes the hemodynamic state of one of these cyanotic and edematous patients: The PA pressure, 70/40; hematocrit, 65%; blood volume, 50% greater than normal; elevated cardiac output; arterial saturation 60%; and pCO_2 65 mm Hg. The majority of deaths in patients with cystic fibrosis are caused by cor pulmonale secondary to pulmonary artery hypertension associated with parenchymal lung disease and hypoxia secondary to maldistribution of air and blood in the lungs.

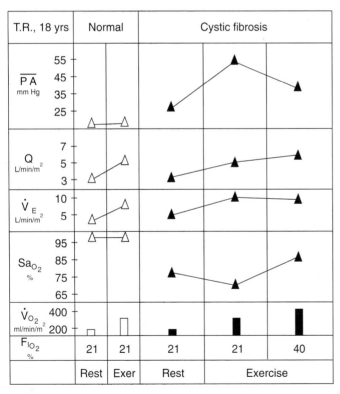

Fig. 5-23. A patient with cystic fibrosis shows a reduction in PA hypertension during exercise on a 40% oxygen mixture compared to exercise on room air. Relief or reduction of hypoxia is mandatory in this group of patients. PA = PA mean pressure; Q = cardiac index; VE = minute ventilation; Sa_{O_2}, arterial oxygen saturation; VO_2, oxygen consumption; FI_{O_2}, fraction of oxygen in inspired air. (From Goldring RM, Fishman AF, Turino GM et al: Pulmonary hypertension and cor pulmonale in cystic fibrosis of the pancreas, *J Pediatr* 65:501-524, 1969.)

The increased pulmonary vascular resistance in COPD is made up of two components. The first, a fixed anatomic component, results from a reduction in the total area of the pulmonary vascular tree, as well as to mild structural changes in the arteries themselves, including slight thickening of the pulmonary arterioles caused by muscularization.[73,74] There is no intimal disease of significance, and the media of the large and pulmonary arteries is within normal limits or only minimally thickened. The second and most important factor is a dynamic component that is related to widespread alveolar hypoxia. Hypoxia is a potent constrictor of pulmonary arterioles whose media are increasingly muscularized, although their intima shows no occlusive disease.

The mechanism by which hypoxia acts on the smooth muscle cells to cause vasoconstriction remains unclear.[75] Whether it is via the action of a mediator or through direct action of the low oxygen tension on the muscle cell, especially in the presence of acidosis, which acts to enhance the hypoxic vasoconstriction, is not known.[76,77,78] It is unlikely, however, that intermittent episodes of hypoxia independent of severe persistent pulmonary artery hypertension can cause permanent intimal pulmonary vascular changes.

Rings of the pulmonary artery, measuring 1.2 mm to 3.4 mm in diameter, were harvested from patients undergoing heart/lung transplant who had COPD with hypoxic respiratory failure. Similar rings of pulmonary artery were also obtained from control patients having lobectomy for cancer of the lung. It was noted that acetylcholine and adenosine, which act through endothelium-derived relaxing factor (EDRF), caused significantly less relaxation in the pulmonary arteries of the COPD group than in those of the control group.[79] On the other hand, nitroprusside, which acts independently of EDRF, relaxed COPD and control group rings of PA to a similar degree. Less relaxation occurred in the COPD patients whose arterial Po_2 was decreased, whose pulmonary artery intima was thickened, or whose Pco_2 was elevated. Thus COPD patients with pulmonary artery hypertension and hypoxia may not have endothelial-dependent pulmonary artery relaxation; therefore they may be predisposed to worsening of the pulmonary artery hypertension.

Calcium channel blockers inhibit hypoxic pulmonary vasoconstriction in the isolated rat lung preparation and in the in situ pig lung. Thus calcium channel blockers have been used in humans to counteract hypoxia-induced pulmonary vasoconstriction and to decrease pulmonary vascular resistance. Other calcium-dependent processes triggered by alveolar hypoxia may release a mediator from perivascular mast cells, and initiate the enzymatic steps in the leukotriene synthesis.

Polycythemia is not a major factor in causing an increase in pulmonary vascular resistance. Hypercapnia affects the central nervous system but has no major affect on the pulmonary vascular bed.

Right and left ventricular function in cor pulmonale

Normally the right ventricle (RV) is a high-volume, low-pressure pump. RV dysfunction is usually related to increased RV afterload. Adaptive right ventricular hypertrophy increases the systolic pressure development and helps reduce ventricular wall tension. The right ventricle of a patient who has acquired pulmonary artery hypertension gradually develops an intact contractile state that responds normally to changes of preload or afterload. As pulmonary vascular resistance increases, pulmonary artery hypertension develops, and there is decreased compliance in the pulmonary artery tree (Fig. 5-24). As pulmonary vascular resistance increases significantly, there is a decrease in resting stroke volume and in the right ventricular ejection fraction.[80] Cardiac output may decrease because an increase in heart rate cannot fully compensate for the decrease in stroke volume. In advanced pulmonary artery hypertension the stiffer walls of the main and branch pulmonary arteries result in a widened PA pulse pressure. Although peak pulmonary artery velocity in pulmonary hypertension peaks early, PA systolic pressure peaks later. Thus late elevated peak systolic pressure results in an increased late systolic load on the right ventricle.[81] With exercise the rise in cardiac output in the patient with pulmonary hypertension is blunted. If pulmonary artery hypertension is severe, right ventricular filling does not increase despite elevation of the right atrial pressure. The coronary blood flow to the right ventricle that normally occurs in both systole and diastole, occurs only in diastole in the presence of severe pulmonary artery hypertension. The electrocardiogram shows right atrial abnormality reflected

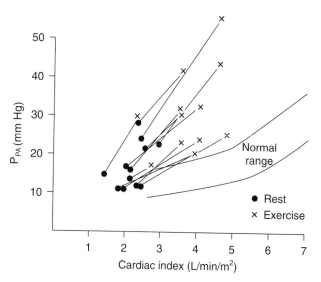

Fig. 5-24. Twelve patients with COPD show an abnormal rise in mean PA pressure (P_{PA}) with exercise when compared to the normal range of P_{PA} rise with exercise in 75 normal subjects. (From Mahler PA, Brent BN, Lake J et al: Right ventricular performance and central circulatory hemodynamics during upright exercise in patients with chronic obstructive pulmonary disease, *Am Rev Respir Dis* 130:722-729, 1984.)

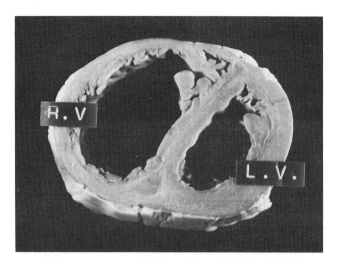

Fig. 5-25. Cross-heart section, midventricular level, showing hypertrophy and dilatation of the right ventricle. Note the straight ventricular septum.

by tall pointed P waves in leads 2, 3 and AVF. The heart has a vertical electrical position with clockwise rotation and right axis deviation. The ECG criteria for right ventricular hypertrophy are relatively weak. Much more useful is the echocardiographic Doppler technique, which gives an estimate of right ventricular peak systolic pressure and the ratio of RV to LV volume.[12] In the patient with cor pulmonale, the effect of loading one ventricle on the function of its partner ventricle is intriguing. This so-called ventricular interdependence is related to sharing a common ventricular septum, sharing encircling muscle fibers, and experiencing a common pericardial and intrathoracic pressure. Animal and physical models have been used to attempt to predict the effect of changes in compliance, ventricular volume, and pressure on ventricular interdependence.[82,83] The straightening of the interventricular septum from its usual curved form is well documented in patients with right ventricular hypertrophy (Fig. 5-25). Left ventricular hypertrophy of unexplained cause has been found at autopsy in some patients with cor pulmonale. Diastolic dysfunction of the left ventricle secondary to right heart failure may result from elevation of the coronary venous pressure, increased myocardial blood volume, and decreased left ventricular distensibility.[84] Whether clinically significant changes in left ventricular function occur in patients with cor pulmonale remains to be documented.

Pathogenesis of right ventricular failure in parenchymal lung disease

The pulmonary circulation has the ability to recruit additional pulmonary vessels or to expand those already recruited (Fig. 5-26). Pulmonary blood flow of three to four times normal can be tolerated without a PA pressure rise during exercise in normal individuals,[85] or in the patient

with an atrial septal defect. After pneumonectomy, the pulmonary artery pressure in the normal sole lung remains at the upper limits of normal at rest, and can tolerate a twofold increase in flow with only mild increases in pulmonary artery pressure. Thus in mild or moderately advanced parenchymal lung disease with an anatomically restricted vascular bed, the resting pulmonary artery pressure is only mildly elevated. The right ventricle generally adapts nicely by hypertrophy without significant right ventricular fibrosis and without significant dysfunction. Thus one may be justified in stating that patients with chronic lung disease develop acute right ventricular dysfunction when additional triggering mechanisms occur. Commonly a superimposed pulmonary infection results in progressive ventilation perfusion mismatch, decreased alveolar ventilation, increased work of breathing through airways obstruction and abnormal respiratory mechanisms, and an alveolar diffusion defect. Global hypoxemia and local alveolar hypoxia develops, leading to intense pulmonary arteriolar constriction, increased pulmonary vascular resistance, and acute increase in right ventricular afterload. As the PA pressure rises a patent foramen ovale may stretch open, resulting in right-to-left shunting at the atrial level. Hypoxemia may also aggravate existing LV dysfunction caused by coronary disease or by systemic hypertension with left ventricular hypertrophy and diastolic dysfunction. Superimposed multifocal atrial tachycardias, or atrial flutter or fibrillation may result in loss of the atrial kick. The tricuspid valve ring may dilate; the resultant tricuspid regurgitation may add a significant volume load to the right ventricle.[86] Respiratory acidosis compounds the vasoconstrictive properties of hypoxemia. There may be increased plasma renin and aldosterone with sodium and water retention and increased blood volume. Superimposed pulmonary emboli in the presence of acute respiratory failure is catastrophic, as is the rupture of a subpleural bleb with pneumothorax.

Relief of the hypoxemia by administered oxygen and prompt treatment of the respiratory infection has been shown to decrease pulmonary hypertension and improve RV function. Pulmonary artery hypertension is significantly improved by administering oxygen in the absence of any consistent change in pulmonary blood flow or pulmonary artery wedge pressure (Fig. 5-27). The reduction of PA pressure with oxygen strongly suggests pulmonary artery vasodilation by the latter. The use of chronic oxygen for patients with COPD with a P_{O_2} of 55mm Hg or lower has been shown to increase survival.[87] One should strive for a P_{O_2} of 60mm Hg without inducing hypercapnia (Fig. 5-28). Single lung transplant for bilateral pulmonary fibrosis is a limited option.[88]

MYOCARDIAL INFARCTION OF THE RIGHT VENTRICLE

Coronary blood flow to the right ventricle normally occurs throughout the cardiac cycle because right ventricular systolic and diastolic pressure is lower than aortic systolic

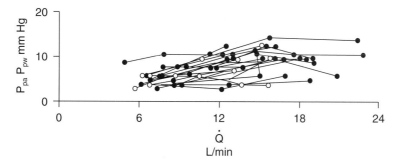

Fig. 5-26. The pressure difference between the pulmonary artery (Ppa) and the pulmonary veins (Ppw) remains unchanged in normal subjects as pulmonary blood flow increases significantly with exercise, indicating significant decrease in calculated pulmonary vascular resistance. (From Linehan JH, Dawson CA: *Pulmonary vascular resistance (P:Q relations)*. In Fishman A, ed: *The pulmonary circulation: normal and abnormal,* Philadelphia, 1990, University of Pennsylvania Press.)

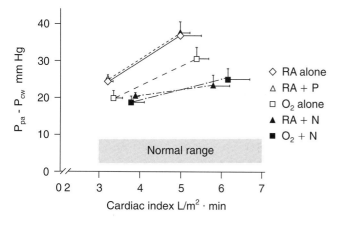

Fig. 5-27. In exercising patients with stable COPD, oxygen alone lowers the PA-pulmonary venous pressure difference; if nifedipine is added the difference decreases further, especially at higher pulmonary flows, but this response is no different than that of nifedipine without supplemental oxygen. *RA* = room air, *P* = placebo, *N* = nifedipine. (From Kennedy TP, Michael JR, Huang CK et al: Nifedipine inhibits hypoxic pulmonary vasoconstriction during rest and exercise in patients with COPD, *Am Rev Respir Dis* 129:544, 1984.)

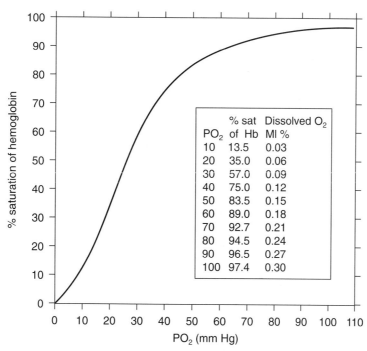

Fig. 5-28. Hypoxia is mild at a pO$_2$ of 65 mm Hg to 70 mm Hg, moderate at a pO$_2$ between 50 mm Hg and 60 mm Hg, and severe below a pO$_2$ of 50 mm Hg. Chronic oxygen administration should strive for pO$_2$ between 60 mm Hg to 65 mm Hg. (From Miller WC: The ABCs of blood gases, *Emerg Med* 2:37-58, 1984.)

and diastolic pressure. In 90% of cases, the right coronary artery supplies the posterior right ventricular wall and the posterior interventricular septum. In 10% of cases, the left coronary artery supplies these areas; the right coronary artery supplies most of the anterior and all the lateral wall of the right ventricle. The left anterior descending branch of the left coronary artery may encircle the apex, supplying the distal septal portion and the apical area of the right ventricle. Because coronary disease may occur in the patient with cor pulmonale, it is comforting to know that isolated right ventricular infarcts occur in perhaps only 2% to 3% of patients with coronary artery disease. However, combined right ventricular and left ventricular infarctions are much more common with the posterior right ventricular wall being predominantly involved. If this occurs despite relatively good left ventricular function, the cardiac output may be low. The jugular venous pressure is elevated with a decrease in blood pressure or with shock-like symptoms caused by severe right ventricular dysfunction. If left ventricular function is good, there is an excellent prognosis after the acute phase of RV dysfunction is treated. Left ventricular stroke volume is reduced by decreased left ventricular preload secondary to decreased right ventricular systolic function.[89] Increased intrapericardial pressure associated with right ventricular myocardial infarction occurs, restricting LV filling. The IV septum is noted to shift leftward. It is imperative to increase right ventricular preload with fluids and albumin (especially if the right atrial pressure is low or normal) in order to use residual Starling function in the right ventricle to maintain pulmonary blood flow and filling of the left ventricle. Inotropic stimulation of the right ventricle with dobutamine and maintenance of good arterial oxygenation to decrease the pulmonary vascular resistance is also important. Prompt reperfusion treatment is desirable in this setting. Vasodilator infusion with nitroprusside or nitroglycerin may be helpful.

ALVEOLAR HYPOVENTILATION

Alveolar hypoventilation is related to dysfunction in the mechanics of breathing or to dysfunction in the regulatory mechanism of respiration in the respiratory center.[90] Alveolar hypoventilation from primary muscle disease, neurologic disorders, or bilateral diaphragmatic dysfunction may

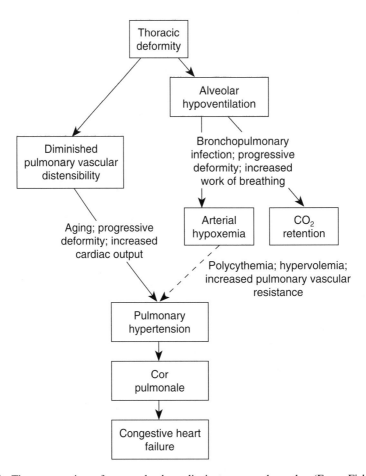

Fig. 5-29. The progression of severe kyphoscoliosis to cor pulmonale. (From Fishman AP, Turino GM, Bergofsky EH: Disorders of the respiration and circulation in subjects with deformities of the thorax. *Mod Conc Cardiovasc Dis 27:449-453, 1958.*)

require ventilatory support to avoid acute episodes of respiratory failure, or chronic support to prevent cor pulmonale.

The known potential respiratory plight of the kyphotic dates back to Hippocrates and includes the case of Richard III. Only in severe posterolateral spine angulation that occurs in advanced kyphoscoliosis does generalized alveolar hypoventilation occur through inadequate respiratory muscle leverage and lung compression (Fig. 5-29).[91] In addition, disparity and inhomogeneity of ventilation and perfusion lead to hypoxemia. One of our patients, a 13-year-old girl with severe right kyphoscoliosis whose left chest could be pinched between one's thumb and index finger, had a resting arterial O_2 saturation of 90% that decreased to 76% after walking up and down 9″ steps for 3 minutes. The P_{CO_2} was 54mm Hg at rest. Pectus excavatum (funnel chest) is a congenital hereditary posterior displacement of the sternal body toward the vertebra. In severe cases of this condition the heart is displaced to the left. Although dramatic in appearance, pectus excavatum rarely produces objective cardiopulmonary dysfunction and is usually not associated with cor pulmonale.

Alveolar hypoventilation may occur in some obese people but not in others equally obese, a fact that suggests some predisposing factor in the ventilatory response of the respiratory center to abnormal blood gases in cases of pickwickian syndrome. The latter patients are somnolent, plethoric, and edematous with hypoxemia, increased P_{CO_2}, and cor pulmonale, and are at major risk for pulmonary embolism. Weight reduction is required to improve alveolar hypoventilation.

Apneic breathing disorders during sleep may be central, obstructive, or of mixed origin.[92] Nocturnal periodic sleep apnea can result in phasic hypoxemia (half normal oxygen saturation of the blood) marked hypercapnia, cardiac bradyarrhythmias, tachy-arrhythmias, episodic sinus arrest, and asystole.[93] Pharyngeal airway narrowing is related to decreased activity of the upper airway muscles during inspiration. For example, poor genioglossus contraction allows for tongue relaxation. A short neck and obesity seem to be additive factors. Hypertrophied tonsils and adenoids may cause chronic upper airway obstruction particularly in childhood, resulting in alveolar hypoventilation.[94] It is especially important to detect this problem in children with pulmonary hypertension and to differentiate from that caused by a large left-to-right shunt. One of our patients, a 6-year-old girl with a large ventricular septal defect, was noted to snore heavily, have fitful sleep patterns, and to kneel at the side of her bed in order to sleep in a semierect prone position. Her P_{CO_2} was 56 mm Hg. While she was supine during catheterization, wide swings in her intrathoracic pressure were noted with respiration. The patient's pulmonary artery pressure was 100/59 with a mean of 78 mm Hg before removal of her tonsils, and 79/54 with a mean of 65 mm Hg afterwards. The pulmonary flow index

rose from 3.6 liters/min/M^2 to 10.9 liters/min/M^2, and total pulmonary resistance index fell from 21 units × M^2 to 6 units × M^2 after her tonsillectomy. As a result of relief of upper airway obstruction and the subsequent fall in calculated pulmonary vascular resistance accompanied by an increase in the pulmonary/systemic flow ratio, she became a candidate for closure of the ventricular septal defect.

Alveolar hypoventilation and decreased sensitivity of the respiratory center is an acquired condition caused by a past occurrence of central nervous system disease. Rarely the disorder is idiopathic or congenital in origin, occurring in infancy and early childhood (Ondine's curse). Such patients have an elevation of arterial P_{CO_2} and fail to increase ventilation normally with exercise, i.e., ventilation barely doubles with exercise although the arterial P_{CO_2} increases. At rest a decreased ventilatory response to the administration of inspired CO_2 is noted (Fig. 5-30).

HIGH ALTITUDE AND THE RESPONSE OF THE PULMONARY CIRCULATION

Skiing, trekking in the Himalayas, and visits to tourist attractions in the Andes bring low altitude dwellers abruptly to high altitudes. The swiftness of air travel allows little time for acclimatization.[95] Headache, nausea, dizziness, vomiting, and ataxia may reflect acute mountain sickness. The skier or the mountaineer may develop high altitude pulmonary edema (HAPE) in association with the rapid arrival of altitudes of 2500 to 3000 meters. Dyspnea

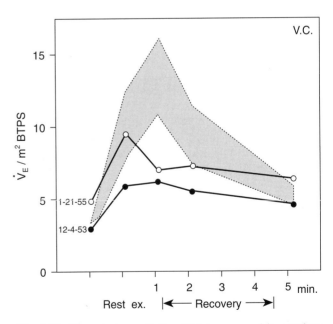

Fig. 5-30. The minute ventilation (V_E) is measured in a patient with diminished sensitivity of the respiratory center on 2 dates. An abnormally low ventilatory response to exercise is noted, compared to the range of normal response *(dotted area)*. (From Richter T, West JR, Fishman AP: The syndrome of alveolar hypoventilation and diminished sensitivity of the respiratory center, *N Engl J Med* 256:1165-70, 1957.)

and cough are prominent, frequently associated with rales and pinkish sputum. Right-to-left shunting across a patent foramen ovale may add to the hypoxemia.[96] The chest x-ray film shows diffuse pulmonary infiltrates.

The prevalence of HAPE is said to be 1% of the general climbing population; it increases to 10% if arrival at 4500 meters is within a time period of 24 hours. If a previous history of HAPE exists (and thus implied susceptibility), then estimates are that 60% of this group will develop HAPE. In the presence of hypoxia and pulmonary hypertension of high altitude, a calcium-mediated inflammatory response may occur, liberating thromboxane B2 or leukotriene B, and resulting in increased permeability of the pulmonary vascular endothelium. Similar increases in permeability may occur in the vessels of the brain, resulting in high altitude cerebral edema (HACE), and in the vessels of the subcutaneous tissues, resulting in facial or peripheral edema. The high pulmonary artery pressures (especially with exercise) accentuate the fluid leak. Nonhomogeneous pulmonary vasoconstriction may result in high flow to some areas (regional over perfusion), which is accelerated by exercise or sleep hypoxia. Individuals who lack one pulmonary artery are particularly susceptible to HAPE. These individuals have overperfusion of one lung with increased sheer stress. Four such skiers with absence of the right pulmonary artery developed life-threatening HAPE, and one of them died.[97] One of these skiers was studied 2 years later at age 58 and had a pulmonary artery pressure of 44/17 with a mean of 28, rising to 75/37 after 2 minutes of exercise in the supine position. These values were obtained at sea level 2 years after the original episode of HAPE.

Venous and cerebral artery thrombosis are also noted at high altitude accentuated by dehydration. At altitudes greater than 17,000 feet, 50% of individuals may develop retinal hemorrhages, most of which are asymptomatic. Nearly all people with HAPE or HACE have retinal hemorrhages. Early descent to restore the partial pressure of arterial oxygen to that of persons living close to sea level is mandatory to avoid the greater than 50% chance of fatality that may occur in HAPE. Bartsch[98] found that giving the calcium antagonist nifedipine 3 days before and on the day of the rapid ascent to those with a previous history of the disease prevented HAPE in 9 of 10 climbers at 4559 meters. In the placebo group, 7 of 11 developed HAPE. Doppler-determined systolic pulmonary artery pressure and alveolar-arterial O_2 pressure differences were significantly lower in the treated group; oxygen saturation was higher.

Acclimatization to high altitude

On the summit of Mt. Everest the inspired Po_2 is 42 mm Hg, but increasing the alveolar ventilation by fivefold or sixfold results in an alveolar Po_2 of 35 mm Hg, an alveolar Pco_2 of 7.5 mm Hg, and an arterial Po_2 of 28 mm Hg. The arterial PH is 7.75. If alveolar ventilation were that of sea level, the arterial Po_2 would be 0.[99]

Following 6 weeks at high altitude the hemoglobin was 20.5 with a hematocrit of 60% to 62%. There was increased myoglobin in the skeletal muscles. The number of capillaries remained the same but capillary density was increased by a decrease in the size of muscle fibers. Physical training in humans increases mitochondrial volume density, but climbing at high altitudes decreases muscle mass, fiber diameter and mitochondrial volume density.[99] Cattle born and raised at high altitude have an increased number of mitochondria.

Living at high altitude

Native residents at high altitude tend to have delayed pulmonary vascular maturation, muscular pulmonary arterioles and mild pulmonary artery hypertension directly related in severity to altitude and duration of altitude exposure. Peruvian residents at 17,500 feet have an inspired oxygen partial pressure of 74 mm Hg at a barometric pressure of 401 mm Hg. The PAo_2 is 42 and the hemoglobin saturation is 79%.

Cattle may develop pulmonary artery hypertension at high altitudes.[100] Sheep and Peruvian llamas are much less reactive. Cattle grazing at high altitude with free access to salt develop edema of the anterior torso-brisket area. The edema and the pulmonary hypertension in cattle is reversible on transport to low altitude. In newborn calves at 4300 meters, elastin synthesis increased by a factor of four compared with controls.[101] Elastin, a highly cross-linked protein, is primarily localized in the media, but in the presence of pulmonary artery hypertension it increases significantly in the adventitia, probably caused by a phenotypic transition of adventitial fibroblasts to elastogenic cells.[102]

Human pulmonary artery pressure varies in response to living at high altitude. Those native to high altitude or well adapted have functionally normal abilities and muscularization of the pulmonary arterioles, but no intimal thickening or thrombotic occlusion. In cases of chronic mountain sickness, or Monge's disease, there is usually chronic pulmonary vascular obstruction.

Catheterization of 28 Colorado high school students by Grover[103] at 10,200 feet, where they lived and attended school, revealed an average resting mean PA pressure of 25 mm Hg (normal = 12 mm Hg) and as a group, during exercise a mean of 54 mm Hg. All but three developed a mean pulmonary artery pressure of greater than 35 mm Hg; one fourth of the students had a mean PA pressure greater than 65 mm Hg. A 15-year-old girl who was a champion skier had a PA pressure of 165/95 with exercise.

A decrease in oxygen concentration causes pulmonary vascular beds to constrict. Regulation or mediation may occur by the endothelium through an endothelium-derived relaxing factor. In the laboratory nitric oxide, which may be identical to this factor, reverses the increased pulmonary artery pressure and vascular resistance in dogs made hypoxic by breathing a low oxygen mixture ($FIO_2 = .11$).

Hypoxemia during air travel

At 22,500 feet pressurization provides a cabin altitude at sea level; at 35,000 feet compromise is necessary, and cabin altitude is equivalent to 5000 to 8000 feet.[104] Arterial saturation is 87% at the latter in the normal individual, or a reduction of 9%. If a patient with COPD begins the trip at a Po_2 of 60 at sea level, he or she may have a Po_2 of 40 at the cabin equivalent of 8000 feet. As a rule supplemental oxygen should be given during flight if the patient with COPD has a very recent blood gas measuring a Po_2 of less than 55 mm Hg, or if one suspects that the PAO_2 may fall below 50 during the flight.[105] If in doubt, giving the patient a 15% oxygen test mixture to breathe in the office would adequately check the PAO_2 response of traveling at 8000 feet.

PRIMARY PULMONARY HYPERTENSION (PPH) IN CIRRHOSIS

Cirrhosis may be associated with mild cyanosis, clubbing, and hypoxemia. Intrapulmonary arteriovenous channels have been defined by postmortem injection and by angiography. Isotope and inert gas techniques have shown mild to moderate intrapulmonary right-to-left shunting. Ventilation perfusion mismatch associated with pulmonary hypertension may also contribute to the hypoxemia. Some centers will not perform liver transplantation if the PAO_2 on ambient air is less than 50 mm Hg, because it is not clear whether the transplant will reverse the hypoxemia.

Unexplained pulmonary hypertension occurs in about 0.5% of all cases of established cirrhosis of the liver with portal hypertension. Roughly one third of these patients have surgical portosystemic shunts.[106] There is no female predilection; mean survival is 15 months, and the average age at diagnosis is 41 years. Portal hypertension results in right-to-left shunting from esophageal and mediastinal venous collaterals to the pulmonary veins. In patients with portosystemic anastomosis there is a potential for pulmonary emboli from the splanchnic venous circulation, but this is not considered to be a cause of the pulmonary hypertension. Cirrhosis is associated with a decrease in peripheral vascular resistance, increased plasma volume, and a high cardiac output. Thus increased pulmonary blood flow results in increased shear stress on pulmonary artery endothelial cells. Furthermore, the presence of abnormal humoral agents caused by metabolic or detoxification failure of the liver cell may play a role in the susceptible patient, inducing pulmonary vasoconstriction. Pathologic findings in the small pulmonary arteries are similar to those of PPH.

COEXISTENT PULMONARY AND PORTAL HYPERTENSION

Although such coexistence is rare, it is statistically significant. The association is most commonly reported in patients with hepatic cirrhosis, but it seems that portal hypertension, not cirrhosis, is the necessary prerequisite.[107,108]

Nodular regenerative hyperplasia of the liver (NRH) has also been reported to be associated with pulmonary hypertension.[109,110] The morphologic vascular features in the pulmonary tree in this syndrome have been reported to be most often of the plexogenic variety, occasionally of the thrombotic type, or a combination of the two.

Although the histologic changes in the pulmonary vasculature in patients with coexistent pulmonary and portal hypertension are well delineated, the pathogenesis and etiology for this association remains unclear. Several hypotheses has been proposed in an attempt to explain the exact pathogenetic mechanism involved in this puzzling syndrome.

One hypothesis suggests that in patients with portal hypertension and portosystemic shunts substances normally metabolized by the liver may reach the pulmonary vasculature and induce vasoconstriction. Stated another way, failure of hepatic synthetic or metabolic functions may effect the pulmonary vasculature. Factors suspected for such action, although not confirmed, include serotonin, neuropeptide Y, thromboxane, or a deficiency of vasodilatory prostaglandins.[111] However, in cirrhotic patients, increased blood volume and generalized vasodilatation are almost universal.

The role of small thromboemboli reaching the lung through collaterals has also been considered as a possible cause for the pulmonary hypertension in patients with increased portal pressures. An example often cited in this regard is that of the *Schistosoma mansoni* eggs, which cause pulmonary hypertension in patients with hepatic Schistosomiasis.[112] Whether there is a hypercoagulable state in these patients that may enhance in situ thrombosis is not clear.

Liver-associated hypoxemia (cyanosis accompanying cirrhosis) was described long ago, but of all proposed causes the concept of intrapulmonary shunts through arteriovenous channels has attracted the most attention. Evidence of intrapulmonary arteriovenous channels in liver-associated hypoxemia was obtained from angiographic and physiologic studies.[113]

However, certain questions about liver-associated hypoxemia and arteriovenous communications remain unanswered. Two of the most important concerns involve the pathogenesis of these intrapulmonary arteriovenous channels, and whether the hypoxemia accompanying liver disease is reversible (liver transplantation).

PULMONARY VASCULITIS

Pulmonary vasculitis may occur predominantly in the lung or it may be associated with a systemic vasculitis or systemic disease that also involves the lung (Fig. 5-31) (see Box on p. 167).[114,115]

The patient with Wegener's necrotizing granulomatosis vasculitis, if untreated, usually dies of renal insufficiency. There is also involvement of the upper and lower respiratory tract and the CNS. One fourth of patients may have

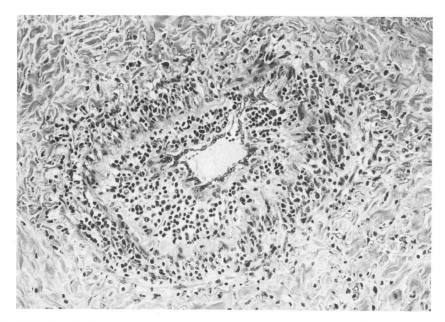

Fig. 5-31. Small pulmonary artery in a patient with Wegener's granulomatosis. Note transmural lymphocytic infiltrate of the arterial wall, loose intimal proliferation, and luminal narrowing.

pericarditis or occasionally pancarditis and coronary artery vasculitis. One third of patients have pulmonary symptoms at the time of the diagnosis. The lung in Wegener's granulomatosis has bilateral nodular densities, some of which are cavitated; old lesions may regress and new crops of pulmonary lesions occur. Severe pulmonary bleeding and/or respiratory insufficiency is noted in a minority of patients.

The CREST syndrome (calcinosis, Raynaud's phenomenon, esophageal dysmotility, sclerodactyly, telangiectasias) is a variant of systemic sclerosis (scleroderma). Pulmonary hypertension occurs in about 9% of systemic sclerosis patients, but develops after years in over half of patients with CREST syndrome; it is considered one of the leading causes of mortality among such patients.[116] Vascular changes observed consist of medial hyperplasia, intimal proliferation and fibrosis, reduplication of the internal elastic membrane, and adventitial fibrosis. There is a lack of correlation between the presence and severity of pulmonary hypertension and the presence of interstitial fibrosis, suggesting that obstructive pulmonary vascular disease is the major factor. Oral nifedipine causes a decrease in pulmonary vascular resistance, (in short-term and long-term) in some patients with diffuse systemic sclerosis, the CREST syndrome, and mixed connective tissue disease, especially in those who have mild to moderate pulmonary hypertension.

The diffuse interstitial pneumonitis and fibrosis of rheumatoid pulmonary disease is usually associated with active arthritis, circulating immune complexes, and cryoglobulinemia. Chest radiographs show progression from fine nodularity to coarse reticulation, and honeycombing of the lung. A rare but serious complication of rheumatoid arthritis is pulmonary hypertension secondary to vasculitis without dilatation or plexiform lesions.[117]

PULMONARY HYPERTENSION SECONDARY TO ORAL INGESTION OF SUBSTANCE

The ingestion of several oral compounds has been associated with pulmonary artery hypertension in mammals. Powdered crotalaria seeds (*C. spectabilis,* a legume) produce pulmonary hypertension in the rat, beagle, and macaque monkey, causing endothelial cell swelling, medial thickening, and decreased angiotensin-converting enzyme activity. The medicinal bush tea from *C. fulva* causes hepatic venoocclusive disease in humans, and tea made from *C. luburnoides* caused pulmonary artery hypertension in a 9-year-old child.

In an animal model, monocrotaline injected into rats produces immediate swelling of the endothelial cells in the distal small pulmonary arteries.[118] Subsequently, migration of muscle cells distally in the pulmonary tree, and hypertrophy of smooth muscle in the media of muscular pulmonary arteries result in progressive pulmonary hypertension and right ventricular hypertrophy. If the small peripheral arteries are assayed there is increased elastolytic activity per milligram (and per cell) of pulmonary artery. The administration of an elastase inhibitor drug results in decreased muscularization of peripheral arteries, decreased differentiation of smooth muscle, decreased elastolytic activity, and blunting of the pulmonary hypertension response.

The use of aminorex fumarate (menocil), an alpha sympathomimetic anorexiant in Europe, was associated with a twentyfold rise in the prevalence of idiopathic pulmonary artery hypertension, presumably in hyperreactors. Pulmonary vascular disease could not be reproduced predictably in an animal model. The anorexigenic agents chlorphentermine and fenfluramine have been suspect; so has phenformin, used to treat noninsulin dependent diabetics who are obese. The rapeseed oil epidemic (later named the toxic oil syndrome [TOS] by the World Health Organization) appeared in Spain in 1981.[119]

Rapeseed oil containing aniline and acetanilid dyes (oleoanilid) was ingested by the populace, resulting in acute interstitial pneumonitis with residual pulmonary artery hypertension and right ventricular failure in approximately 12% of cases. Pulmonary vasculitis, intimal hyperplasia, and in situ thrombosis were noted. Approximately 369 deaths have been attributed to TOS, with about 32 of those caused by pulmonary hypertension. No definite caus-

ative agent has yet been identified in TOS. The pathologic changes in the pulmonary vasculature consisted of medial hypertrophy, concentric myointimal proliferation with fibrosis, and frequent plexiform lesions. Some cases revealed organized and recanalized thrombi. Changes in the veins were manifested by intimal fibrosis and intraluminal septa. Early lesions, however, were characterized by endothelial injury and perivascular inflammatory infiltrates. The endothelial injury may result from the release of free peroxide radicals induced by oleoanilids contained in rapeseed oil acting on cell membranes. The incidence of severe pulmonary artery hypertension in TOS is 1.6 per 1000.[120]

PRIMARY PULMONARY HYPERTENSION (PPH)
Clinical findings and pathophysiology

PPH is a clinical syndrome associated with unexplained severe pulmonary hypertension with a relentless fatal course. The diagnosis is one of exclusion.[121] It is common in females of child-bearing age. The female/male ratio is 1.7:1. Most patients are in the mid 30s.[122] Symptoms are present for approximately 2 years, and the median survival following diagnosis is 2.8 years. Generally less than one fourth of people are alive 5 years after the diagnosis. Right ventricular hypertrophy and right ventricular dysfunction is followed by sudden death. Symptoms include breathlessness, increased fatigue, dizziness, palpitations, and chest pain.[123] Near syncope or syncope especially associated with exertion occurs in 55% of patients and is caused by a rapid decrease in cardiac output secondary to a sudden increase in right ventricular afterload and subsequent decreased LV preload. Hemoptysis is noted in 15% of such patients. Occasionally PPH is noted during or after pregnancy but causality is not clear.[124,125] Amniotic and trophoblastic embolism must be excluded.[126] The detection of right ventricular hypertension is possible by such noninvasive techniques as Doppler echocardiography,[127] but PPH is uncommon and insidious in onset; therefore early screening is difficult.

At the onset and in the midcourse of PPH, the cardiac output is normal, as is the right atrial pressure, even though pulmonary artery pressure is gradually rising. At the end stage cardiac output begins to fall and right atrial pressure rises as RV dysfunction increases and gas exchange becomes impaired.[128] A rise in right atrial pressure greater than 11 mm Hg and a fall in cardiac index to below 2.1 liters/min $\times$ m^2 means a short survival time. As the right ventricular ejection fraction decreases, there is decreased systolic RV ejection velocity and main pulmonary artery blood velocity. The IV septum may move paradoxically as tricuspid regurgitation and pulmonary regurgitation occur. Arterial hypoxemia is common, caused by ventilation perfusion abnormalities or shunting through a patent foramen ovale. Lung perfusion scans may be normal or show diffuse, patchy defects. There is mild altered lung compliance and a reduction in diffusing capacity. In a

10-year-old girl the heart, primarily because of RV hypertrophy, weighed 340 grams, more than twice the normal weight for her age.

Finding the disease early so that an attempt may be made to therapeutically modify its course is desirable but difficult.[129] When the patient is first seen, the increased pulmonary vascular resistance may be fixed in most of the lung. Usually the PA mean pressure is 60mm Hg or above, although pulmonary artery wedge pressure is normal. Although no prospective controlled trial has been performed, chronic anticoagulation with warfarin is sometimes used but it does not seem to alter the natural history.

Although the potential for improvement seems small, nearly every known vasodilator drug has been tried.[130] Potential candidates in studies are selected by acute testing after defining criteria for a favorable response. Palevsky[131] used a decrease in calculated pulmonary vascular resistance of greater than 30% accompanied by a decrease in PA mean pressure of 10% to define vasodilatation. Four of 19 patients with PPH responded by these criteria. Qualitative histology of the lung was not a predictor of response, but quantitative morphologic study of the initial open lung biopsy was helpful in predicting vasodilatation; the procedure had an 85% predicted value in identifying patients who did poorly in a 3-year follow-up. It is of interest to note that the greater the decrease in pulmonary vascular resistance with testing, the better the long-term survival and clinical relief of symptoms. However, survival is identical whether treatment with vasodilators is or is not given. The two main vasodilators used include the calcium antagonist nifedipine in high dose,[132] and prostacyclin, which has a half-life of only 2 to 3 minutes.[133] If refractoriness to oral vasodilators occurs, continuous IV prostacyclin (or epoprostenol sodium) is given via a Hickman catheter connected to a portable infusion pump. Such treatment has been carried on for up to a year; dosage must be increased over time. If a patient is desaturated, supplemental oxygen may be used for an additive vasodilator effect on the pulmonary bed. The anticoagulant heparin is also thought to inhibit smooth muscle and endothelial proliferation. The question of whether to use chronic vasodilator drug treatment even though there is no decrease in resistance during acute testing has not been answered.

Because a patent foramen ovale may result in a better prognosis in PPH by unloading the right ventricle and maintaining LV filling, creation of an atrial septal defect with a blade catheter with subsequent ballooning has been performed to vent the right atrium and increase systemic output. Despite the creation of a right-to-left shunt with a possibility of fatal hypoxemia, overall oxygen transport to the periphery can be improved in some patients.[134]

Heart lung transplant in patients with PPH show a 65% survival in the first year. One third of patients develop obliterative bronchiolitis; one-half of these require retransplantation. The internal mammary artery has been anasto-mosed to the bronchial arteries to increase the blood supply in order to facilitate healing of the airway anastomosis. Transplantation achieves excellent hemodynamic results with pulmonary pressure, pulmonary vascular resistance, and cardiac output returning to normal values. By echocardiography the IV septum, which formerly bulged into the left ventricle, returns to a more normal position.

Pathology of primary pulmonary hypertension (PPH)

The World Health Organization (WHO) defined PPH as pulmonary arterial hypertension associated with normal pulmonary capillary wedge pressure and right ventricular hypertrophy that was not caused by a cardiac, macroembolic, or pulmonary parenchymal disorder. WHO has proposed three histopathologic categories for clinically apparent PPH: (1) plexogenic pulmonary arteriopathy, (2) pulmonary venoocclusive disease, and (3) recurrent microthromboembolic arteriopathy.[135]

Thromboembolic arteriopathy, the most common of the three pathologic entities, often afflicts adults. Venoocclusive disease, the least common of the three, is more common in infants and children.[136] The plexogenic variety, the second most common type of primary pulmonary hypertension, afflicts children and young adults. Correlation between each of the three histologic subtypes of PPH and presenting symptoms showed no significant statistical differences.

However, patients with plexogenic arteriopathy had higher mean pulmonary vascular resistance (44.5 ± 12.4 units) and mean pulmonary pressure (76.4 ± 22.2 mm Hg) at the initial baseline catheterization than patients with either the thrombotic variety or venoocclusive disease.[137] Patients with thrombotic lesions had the best survival. Since the clinical presentation of all three categories is comparable at the initial diagnosis, differences in survival apparently reflect the rate of progression of the underlying processes. Patients with plexogenic arteriopathy are more often young and female (M/F ratio is 1:3).

Regarding reversibility of different histopathologic vascular lesions, most authors agree that hypertrophy and cellular hyperplasia are capable of regressing. If intimal fibrosis is significant, regardless of the status of other structures, the vessel is functionally fixed, and likely unresponsive to vasodilator agents.

Plexogenic pulmonary arteriopathy

The histologic features of the pulmonary arteries in the early stages of plexogenic pulmonary arteriopathy do not include lesions such as fibrinoid necrosis, onionskin intimal proliferation, or plexiform lesions. In the early stages important alterations involve the small muscular pulmonary arteries, arterioles, and precapillaries.

Medial hypertrophy in the muscular arteries is made up of circumferentially oriented smooth muscle cells. In the

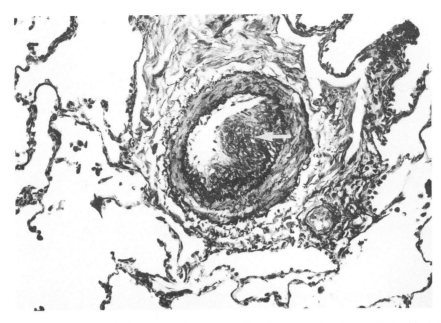

Fig. 5-32. Cushion-like lesions *(arrow)* on the small pulmonary artery in a patient with thromboembolic variety of primary pulmonary arterial hypertension.

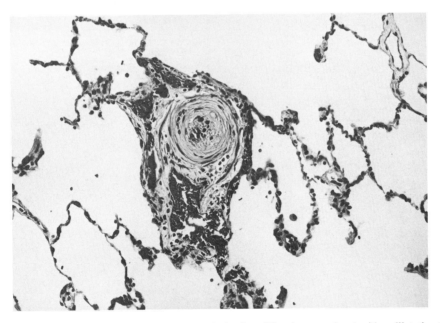

Fig. 5-33. Severe, onion skin-like concentric intimal proliferation associated with a dilatation lesion in a patient with primary pulmonary arterial hypertension.

zone adjacent to the internal elastic lamina these cells have a radial orientation, as if preparing for migration towards the intima.[138] Proliferating cells inside the interna elastica with ultrastructural features, such as myofilaments, disclose their muscular origin. Fine fibrillary ground substance, collagen fibers, and small deposits of elastin occupy the intercellular spaces. The internal elastic lamina reveals fragmentation.

Proliferation of myofibroblasts is seen in the intima of pulmonary arterioles, although the intercellular ground substance and collagen are less than in muscular arteries. Myofibroblasts seen in terminal arterioles do not form a continuous intimal layer, but instead produce small cushions projecting into the lumen (Fig. 5-32). Medial hypertrophy with or without intimal thickening is seen in both primary and secondary pulmonary hypertension.

Although the early intimal proliferation is primarily cellular, in the later stages the intimal lesions are characterized by fibrosis, often called intimal fibroelastosis or concentric laminar fibrosis (Fig. 5-33). With development of laminar fibrosis, there is a detectable secondary medial di-

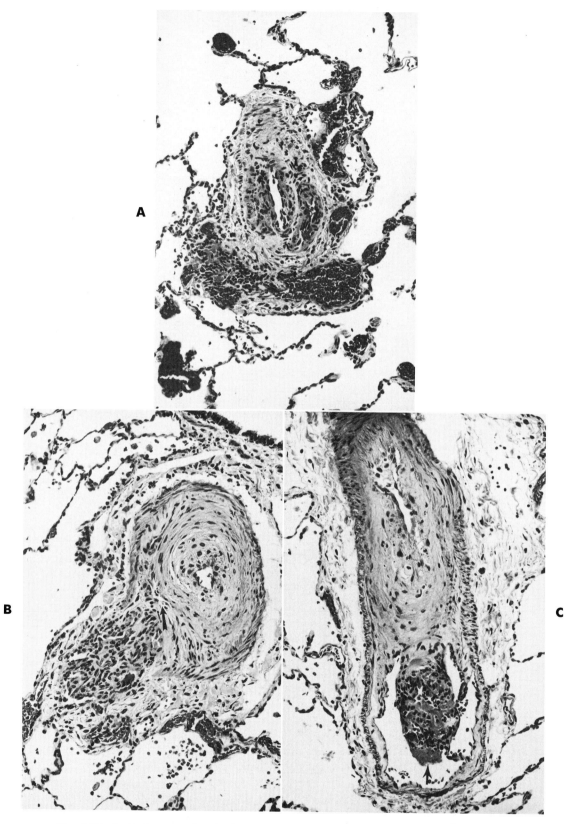

Fig. 5-34. A, Early stage of a plexiform lesion in primary pulmonary arterial hypertension, in small-sized artery. **B,** A developing plexiform lesion in primary pulmonary arterial hypertension. Note gap *(arrow)* in the muscular coat of the artery in continuity with the plexiform lesion. **C,** Plexogenic primary pulmonary arterial hypertension. A medium-sized pulmonary artery shows a well-established plexiform lesion. Note proliferating cells in the plexiform lesion glued together with fibrin *(arrow)*.

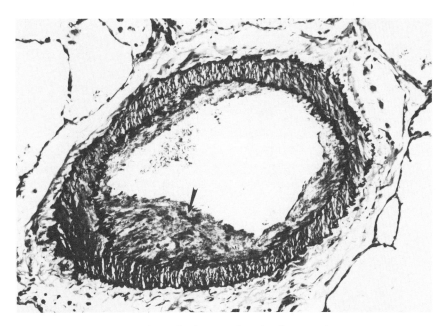

Fig. 5-35. Thromboembolic variety of primary pulmonary hypertension. Note cushion-like intimal lesion *(arrow)*.

latation. The intimal fibrosis may not be concentric with onionskin-like proliferation of intimal cells and elastic tissue, but eccentric, with cushion-like thickening of the intima.

A late-stage finding in the so-called vasoconstrictive form of primary pulmonary hypertension is the plexiform lesion, which is by no means pathognomonic for PPH; it is also seen in the pulmonary hypertension secondary to cardiac shunts. It is widely believed that plexiform lesions do not have a unique hemodynamic etiology because besides the two conditions mentioned above, they are also seen in pulmonary hypertension associated with portal hypertension, ingestion of the appetite depressant aminorex, or menocil, and schistosomiasis.[139]

Plexiform lesions appear as dilated branches of small muscular pulmonary arteries in which a proliferation of myofibroblasts and primitive vasoformative reserve cells form a plexiform tuft. (Fig. 5-34).

Fibrinoid necrosis within the wall of these arteries with plexiform lesions is not always present. It has been suggested that the intraluminal cells of the plexiform lesion are muscular in origin and migrate from the arterial media.

At the stage of mature plexiform lesions, ultrastructural studies show muscular pulmonary arteries of all dimensions to contain extensive intimal fibrosis arranged in a circumferential manner. The intimal layer close to the endothelium appears more cellular than the deeper part, and the cells within the fibrosis appear to be identical to medial smooth muscle.[140] These intimal cells are able to form a wide variety of connective tissue components, including collagen, elastin, and proteoglycans.

Recurrent microthromboembolic arteriopathy

The second major pathologic subdivision of PPH is called the thrombotic type, although the term thromboembolic variety is still used. In this subcategory, plexiform lesions are not present, whereas thrombi in arteries and arterioles are the main histologic findings (Fig. 5-35). If these arterial thrombi are embolic in nature, clinical evidence of the site of origin is lacking. In all likelihood, these arterial thrombi represent in situ thrombosis, which may be fresh, organized, or recanalized, reflecting the time of formation and the subsequent fibrinolytic action. Recanalized thrombi may reveal intraluminal septa, fibroelastic intimal pads, or eccentric intimal fibrosis.[141]

Pathogenetic mechanisms responsible for this in situ thrombosis in the pulmonary vasculature are not entirely clear, although they may result from procoagulant stimuli, impaired inhibition of procoagulant activity, or reduced fibrinolytic response. If indeed this clinicopathologic entity is the result of impaired coagulation mechanisms, then anticoagulation may reduce morbidity and mortality in these patients.[142] Unfortunately, such a favorable outcome has been reported in only a limited number of patients.

Increased plasma concentrations of fibrinopeptide A were found in patients with thrombotic primary pulmonary hypertension, indicating the presence of a procoagulant stimulus that results in thrombin activity and fibrin formation. Perhaps inadequate fibrinolytic activity is the cause of the thrombosis observed in primary pulmonary hypertension. Increased plasminogen activator inhibitor-1 (PAI-1) activity, in spite of normal t-PA concentration, may be insufficient to induce thrombolysis in patients with PPH.[143]

Pulmonary venoocclusive disease

The third morphologic variety of PPH is pulmonary venoocclusive disease, which is quite distinct from the other two forms because it involves veins and venules. In this entity intraluminal thrombi in various stages of organization and recanalization are seen in veins and venules, and there is thickening of the adventitia. The more proximal venules may reveal arterialization with medial hypertrophy, perhaps as the result of increased luminal pressure. Because the obstruction is postcapillary, hemosiderosis and septal edema are more prominent in this entity.[144] The luminal obstruction of pulmonary veins and venules consists of loose, myxoid paucicellular connective tissue.

Recanalization with the formation of intravascular septa is another feature of venoocclusive disease. It is assumed that the luminal obliteration of veins and venules is the result of thrombosis, although disturbances in the clotting mechanism have not been demonstrated. In addition to the changes in veins, the muscular pulmonary arteries reveal medial hypertrophy and intimal fibrosis of similar nature with the veins, and recanalization with formation of intravascular fibrous septa. However, fibrinoid necrosis, arteritis, or plexiform lesions are absent.[145] Contrary to the plexogenic arteriopathy, venoocclusive disease affects more adult males than females, although there is no sex predominance in children.

There is no known etiology for venoocclusive disease. However, proposed etiologies include viral infections, immunologic mechanisms, genetic influence, or hormonal factors. Some writers like to consider venoocclusive disease a morphologic rather than an etiologic entity with perhaps a common pathogenesis, such as intraluminal thrombosis.

Although there are several distinguishing morphologic features among the three entities of PPH described above, there are also some overlapping features. For example, thrombotic lesions are seen to some extent in all three conditions. Furthermore, absence of plexiform lesions in some of the three entities may be a sampling error.

Invasive pulmonary capillary hemangiomatosis

According to some authors, a fourth histopathologic entity described recently under the name invasive pulmonary capillary hemangiomatosis, associated with pulmonary hypertension, should be added to the list of causes of PPH.[146] About 14 cases of this morphologic entity have been reported since the original description in 1978. Pulmonary capillary hemangiomatosis is characterized by proliferating capillary channels within the lung interstitium, which may also invade the walls of airways, veins, and arteries. The cause for the hypertension in these patients is unexplained, and its clinical and histologic distinction from other causes of pulmonary hypertension, particularly the pulmonary venoocclusive disease, is difficult to ascertain.

The morphologic features of this condition consist of capillary proliferation with widening of the pulmonary interstitium. The proliferation is more intense around veins and venules, with occasional extension into the venous walls, resulting in intimal fibrosis and venoocclusion.[147] Infiltration of the wall of small pulmonary arteries, although to a lesser degree than in veins, is also noted. Reticulin stains delineate the proliferating capillaries growing on both sides of the alveolar walls in a back-to-back fashion (Fig. 5-36).

Plexiform lesions were not observed in any of the reported cases, although venoocclusion, marked muscular hypertrophy of pulmonary arteries, and intimal thickening were present in all cases.

Hemoptysis was one of the presenting clinical symptoms in some patients with capillary hemangiomatosis.

The exact nature of this condition is unclear. The suggested neoplastic nature seems unlikely because almost all cases revealed no endothelial atypia, and the proliferating vessels varied from capillaries to venules.

Whether pulmonary capillary hemangiomatosis constitutes a separate morphologic cause of PPH remains to be elucidated. In almost all reported cases, the capillary proliferation was accompanied with significant changes in veins (venoocclusive) as well as arteries.

The question, therefore, arises whether the hemangiomatosis is the result of the vascular alterations in both arteries and veins rather than the cause. Furthermore, we have seen in our material (unpublished data) plexiform lesions in association with capillary hemangiomatosis and pulmonary hypertension.

Morphologic alterations associated with the intimal lesions

The migration and proliferation of smooth muscle cells from the media in PPH indicates that some trophic or mitogenic substance is exerting an effect on those cells. Similar phenomena have been repeatedly described in systemic arteries in relation to the atherogenesis, or after damage of the endothelium by a balloon catheter. Perhaps a certain zoning of the intimal proliferation indicates that intimal fibrosis develops in a series of episodes, and that the most cellular lesions with little or no collagen represent early changes. EM studies have shown that smooth muscle cells that arrive in the intima lose most of their myofilaments, become somewhat irregular in shape, and interdigitate with their peers. Although they contain few synthetic organelles, they still secrete mucopolysaccharides. The next step for the smooth muscle cells is to transform into myofibroblasts by acquiring rough endoplasmic reticulum, free ribosomes, and a peripheral layer of myofilaments.

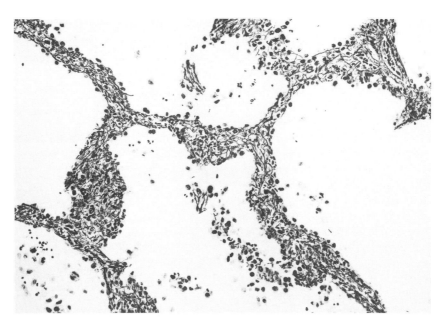

Fig. 5-36. Primary pulmonary arterial hypertension. Note the back-to-back arrangement of pulmonary capillaries in a case of capillary hemangiomatosis.

At this stage of their development, they secrete large amounts of ground substance along with fine collagen fibrils. After the myofibroblasts are embedded in extracellular matrix, they lose their endoplasmic reticulum, gain myofilaments, and revert fully to their muscular origin. During this evolution, the myofibroblasts also lose their cytoplasmic extensions, become elongated, and arrange in an organized circumferential fashion. The final result is a concentric laminar intimal fibrosis, the so-called onionskin proliferation that is a characteristic lesion of plexogenic arteriopathy. With maturation of the intimal fibrosis, migration of smooth muscle cells from the media stops. This endstage lesion somewhat resembles advanced vascular lesions of systemic hypertension.

It has been assumed that the stimulus that causes smooth muscle to migrate to the intima involves a chemical attractant. Light and electron microscopy studies of the bronchial epithelium in patients with PPH have revealed increased number of neuroendocrine cells that are immunoreactive for bombasin and to a lesser degree, calcitonin.[148] As the result of these studies, it was suggested that bombasin plays a role in the migration of the smooth muscle cells either directly or indirectly through an intermediary, such as the endothelium.

Pathogenesis of PPH

Theories regarding the pathogenesis of PPH are many, but few are supported by hard data because no good animal model is available. Many initiating factors have been considered: hormonal, autoimmune, neurohumoral, toxic metabolic, abnormal pulmonary vascular reactivity, and genetic predisposition. For many years, it has been as-

sumed that the initial event in plexogenic arteriopathy is vasoconstriction followed by medial hypertrophy of muscular pulmonary arteries and arterioles. Such a vascular spasm was thought to arise from imbalances of vasoactive substances, catecholamine-induced injury, or from neurogenic mechanisms. After the aminorex epidemic and a few cases of primary pulmonary hypertension related to catecholamine-like drugs, another unproven hypothesis was advanced, that of PPH being the result of susceptibility of the vasculature to catecholamine agents. The vasoconstrictive hypothesis gained some strength by studies showing hemodynamic improvement of some patients with calcium channel blockers.[149] Moreover, approximately 10% of female patients with PPH have Raynaud's syndrome. Animal studies indicate that the humoral regulation of pulmonary vascular tone is likely more complex than previously imagined. Vasoconstriction may result from a variety of stimuli, such as enzymes and oxidants from activated leukocytes, arachidonic acid metabolites (e.g., leukotrienes), components of the coagulation system, and thromboxane, a prostaglandin released from activated platelets. Whether the autonomic and central nervous systems play a role in pulmonary hypertensive disorders remains unclear. The traditional thinking that pulmonary vascular reactivity is predominantly regulated by local influences may need revision.

The involvement of an immunologic mechanism in PPH has been suggested, although experimental evidence is lacking.[150] Clinically, about 40% of patients with PPH have positive antinuclear antibody titers greater than or equal to 1:80 dilution, compared with positive titers in 6% of patients with a secondary type of pulmonary hypertension. Childhood PPH may be associated with major histocompatibility complex alleles. ANA and HLA typing was done in patients with PPH and in those with shunt lesions and pulmonary artery hypertension. Positive ANA and increased frequency of HLA-DR were found in the PPH group.[151]

Support for an immunologic mechanism comes also from the association of pulmonary hypertension with plexogenic arteriopathy in patients with systemic lupus erythematosus, mixed connective tissue disease, diffuse systemic sclerosis, CREST syndrome, and polymyositis, all of which are regarded as autoimmune disorders.

A genetic predisposition to PPH has been suggested as familial occurrences were reported. Familial PPH is an autosomal dominant disease indistinguishable from the sporadic one. A recent study of 12 families with 23 affected members revealed that plexiform and thrombotic lesions often coexist in familial PPH, with great heterogeneity of lesions among members in each family.[152]

Data about possible pathogenetic mechanisms involved in secondary forms of plexogenic arteriopathy (e.g., congenital heart disease, aminorex, portal hypertension) point towards an important role of the endothelium in the development of the vascular lesions. The hypothesis advanced states that functional abnormalities of the endothelium may lead to pulmonary vasoconstriction.[153] In a system of low resistance, such as the pulmonary vascular bed, the endothelium (through its relaxing factors) maintains a state of chronic smooth muscle relaxation. Therefore a state of increased pulmonary vascular tone may be the result of abnormal endothelial cell mediation.

Study of the endothelium and its interaction with the humoral and cellular blood elements is likely to yield important information about the pathogenesis of PPH.

It is also entirely possible that diffuse eccentric intimal proliferation seen in the thrombotic variety of PPH is probably the result of endothelial damage rather than the cause. Endothelial damage and in situ thrombosis seem the most logical explanation for this form of pulmonary hypertension. Perhaps models used to study proliferative vascular lesions in systemic arteries may be applied to the pulmonary circulation. Factors such as platelet-derived growth factor and macrophage-derived factors and other platelet-endothelial interactions may initiate the proliferative response in PPH.

Similar to the systemic arteries, abnormal cell adhesion may also be an important problem in PPH; smooth muscle cells migrating into the intima may have altered adhesiveness to the underlying basement membrane or in cell interactions.[154]

Adhesive proteins or integrins present in the extracellular matrix and blood include thrombospondin, fibronectin, fibrinogen, and von Willebrand's factor. Preliminary studies have shown that interactions of cells with integrins may influence vascular cell behavior, such as anchorage and

polarity of cells, and traction for cell migration across cells.[155] One may hypothesize that abnormalities of the receptor sites of vascular wall cells to integrins also occur in PPH.

REFERENCES

1. Brenner O: Pathology of the vessels of the pulmonary circulation, *Arch Intern Med* 56:211,457,724,976,1139, 1936.
2. Lamb D: *Cor pulmonale and pulmonary hypertension.* In Pomerance A, Davies MJ, eds: *The pathology of the heart*, London, 1975, Blackwell.
3. Reid LM: Structure and function in pulmonary hypertension, *Chest* 89:279-288, 1986.
4. Rabinovitch M, Keane JF, Norwood WI, et al: Vascular structure in lung tissue obtained at biopsy correlated with pulmonary hemodynamic findings after repair of congenital heart defects, *Circulation* 69:655, 1984.
5. Linehan JH, Dawson CA: *Pulmonary vascular resistance* (P:Q Relations). In Fishman AP, ed: *The pulmonary circulation: normal and abnormal*, Philadelphia 1990, University of Pennsylvania Press.
6. Mitzner W, Chang HK: *Hemodynamics of the pulmonary circulation*. In Reeves JT, Weir EK, eds: *Lung biology in health and disease*, New York, 1989, Marcell-Dekker.
7. Grant BJB: *Functional aspects of pulmonary vascular anatomy. In Dantzler DR, ed: Cardiopulmonary critcal care*, ed 2, Philadelphia, 1991, WB Saunders.
8. Horn V, Mullins CB, Saffer SI, et al: A comparison of mathematical models for estimating right ventricular volumes in animals and man, *Clin Cardiol* 2:341-47, 1979.
9. Gentzler RD, Briselli MF, Gault JH: Angiographic estimation of right ventricular volume in man, *Circulation* 50:324-330, 1974.
10. Lamb D: *Cor pulmonale and pulmonary hypertension.* In Pomerance A, Davis MJ, eds: *The pathology of the heart*, London, 1975, Blackwell.
11. Liebson PR: What role for echocardiography in primary pulmonary artery hypertension, *J of Crit Illness* 6:882-88, 1991.
12. Himelman R, Stulbarg M, Kucher B, et al: Noninvasive evaluation of pulmonary artery pressure during exercise by saline enhanced Doppler echocardiography in chronic pulmonary disease. *Circulation* 79:863-871, 1989.
13. West JB, Dollery CT, Narmack A: Distribution of blood flow in isolated lung relation to vascular and alveolar pressure. *J Appl Physiol* 19:713-24, 1964.
14. West JB, ed: *Regional difference in the lung*. New York, 1977, Academic Press.
15. Staub NC: *Pulmonary and bronchial circulations*. In Staub NC, ed: *Basic respiratory physiology*, New York, 1991, Churchill-Livingstone.
16. Allen KA, Haworth SG: Cytoskeletal features of immature pulmonary vascular smooth muscle cells: the influence of pulmonary hypertension on normal development, *J Pathol* 158:311-317, 1989.
17. Hall S, Haworth SG: Conducting pulmonary arteries: structural adaptation to extra-uterine life, *Cardiovasc Res* 21:208-216, 1986.
18. Allen K, Haworth SG: Human postnatal pulmonary arterial remodeling. Ultrastructural studies of smooth muscle cell and connective tissue maturation, *Lab Invest* 59:702-709, 1988.
19. Haworth SG, Hall SM, Chew M, et al: Thinning of fetal pulmonary arterial wall and postnatal remodeling. Ultrastructural studies on the respiratory unit arteries of the pig, *Virchows Arch A Pathol Anat Histopathol* 411:161, 1987.
20. Piper PJ, Levene S: Generation of leukotrienes from fetal and neonatal porcine blood vessels, *Biol Neonate* 49:109, 1986.
21. Leff CW, Hessler JR, Green RS: The onset of breathing at birth stimulates pulmonary vascular prostacyclin synthesis, *Pediatr Res* 18:938, 1984.

22. Rudolph AM: *Perinatal pulmonary circulation.* In Bongpanich B, Sueblinoong V, Vongprateep C, eds: *Pediatric cardiology,* Amsterdam, 1990, Excerpta Medica Amsterdam.

23. Burnell RH, Joseph MC, Lees MH: Progressive hypertension in newborn infants, *Am J Dis Child* 123:167, 1972.

24. Steele PM, Fuster V, Cohen M, et al: Isolated atrial septal defect with pulmonary vascular obstructive disease - long-term follow-up and prediction of outcome after surgical correction, *Circulation* 76:1037-1042, 1987.

25. Hoffman JIE, Rudolph AM, Heymann MA: Pulmonary vascular disease with congenital heart lesions: pathologic features and causes, *Circulation* 64:873-877, 1981.

26. Perloff JK, Sietsema KE: *Response to exercise in cyanotic congenital heart disease: intracardiac and extracardiac venoarterial shunts.* In Weir EK, Reeves JT, eds *Lung biology in health and disease,* New York, 1989, Marcell-Dekker.

27. Trulock EP, Cooper JD, Kaiser LR, et al: The Washington University-Barnes Hospital experience with lung transplantation, *JAMA* 266:1943-46, 1991.

28. Haworth SG: Pulmonary vascular disease in ventricular septal defect: structural and functional correlations in lung biopsies from 85 patients with outcome of intracardiac repair, *J Pathol* 152:157-168, 1987.

29. Rabinovitch M, Bothwell T, Hayakawa BN, et al: Pulmonary artery endothelial abnormalities in patients with congenital heart defects and pulmonary hypertension. A correlation of light with scanning electron microscopy and transmission electron microscopy, *Lab Invest* 55:632-553, 1986.

30. Yokochi K, Olley PM, Sideris E, et al: *Leukotriene D4: A potent vasoconstrictor of the pulmonary and systemic circulations in the newborn lamb.* In Samuelson B, *Leukotrines and other lipoxygenase products,* New York, 1982, Raven.

31. Rabinovitch M, Andrew M, Thom H, et al: Abnormal endothelial factor VIII associated with pulmonary hypertension and congenital heart defects, *Circulation* 76:1043-1052, 1987.

32. Stewart DJ, Levy RD, Cernacek P: Increased plasma endothelin-1 in pulmonary hypertension: marker or mediator of disease? *Ann Intern Med* 114:464-469, 1991.

33. Miller WL, Redfield MM, Burnett JC Jr: Integrated cardiac, renal, and endocrine actions of endothelin, *J Clin Invest* 83:317, 1989.

34. Yoshibayashi M, Nishioka K, Nakao K, et al: Plasma endothelin concentrations in patients with pulmonary hypertension associated with congenital heart defects. Evidence for increased production of endothelin in pulmonary circulation, *Circulation* 84:2280, 1991.

35. Hutchin P, Terzi RG, Peters RM: Bronchial-pulmonary artery reverse flow: angiographic demonstration in bronchiectasis, *Ann Thorac Surg* 4:391-398, 1967.

36. Bloomer WE, Harrison W, Liebow AA: Respiratory function and blood flow in the bronchial artery after ligation of the pulmonary artery, *Am J Physiol* 157:317, 1949.

37. Benson LN, Laks H, Lois J, et al: Surgical correction of pulmonary atresia and ventricular septal defect with large systemic-pulmonary collaterals, *Ann Thorac Surg* 38:522, 1984.

38. Lois JF, Gomes AS, Smith DC, et al: Systemic-to-pulmonary collateral vessels and shunts: treatment with embolization, *Circulation* 64:1234, 1981.

39. Clauther A, Ash JM, Smallhorn JF, et al: Abnormal distribution of pulmonary blood flow after the Glenn shunt or Fontan procedure: risk of development of arteriovenous fistulae, *Circulation* 72:471-479, 1985.

40. Trusler G, Williams WG, Cohen AJ, et al: The Cavopulmonary shunt: evolution of a concept, *Circulation* (Suppl IV) 82:131-138, 1990.

41. Seliem M, Murphy J, Heyman S, et al: Lung perfusion patterns following bidirectional cavopulmonary anastamosis: a reflection of the pulmonary vascular bed status, *J Am Coll Cardiol* 17:257A, 1991.

42. Bridges ND, Jonas RA, Mayer JE, et al: Bidirectional cavopulmonary anastomosis as interim palliation for high risk Fontan candidates, *Circulation* (Suppl IV) 82:170-176, 1990.

43. Mair DD, Hagler DJ, Julsrud PR, et al: Early and late results of the modified Fontain Procedure for double-inlet LV, *J Am Coll Cardiol* 18:1727-32, 1991.

44. Peterson RJ, Franch RH, Fajman WA, et al: Noninvasive determination of exercise cardiac function following Fontan operation, *J Thorac Cardiovasc Surg* 88:263-272, 1984.

45. Santamore EA, Hoffman EA, Santamore WP: Contraction pattern of the right ventricle, *Clin Res* 39:681A, 1991.

46. Peterson RJ, Franch RH, Fajman WA, et al: Comparison of cardiac function in surgically corrected and congenitally corrected transposition of the great arteries, *J Thorac Cardiovasc Surg* 96:227-36, 1988.

47. Graham TP: Ventricular performance in congenital heart disease, *Circulation* 84:2259-74, 1991.

48. Benson LN, Bonet J, McLaughlin P, et al: Assessment of right ventricular function during supine bicycle exercise after Mustard's operation, *Circulation* 65:1052-1059, 1982.

49. Niederman MS, Matthay RA: Cardiovascular function in secondary pulmonary hypertension, *Heart Lung* 15:341-351, 1986.

50. Berry DF, Buccigrossi D, Peabody J, et al: Pulmonary vascular occlusion and fibrosing mediastinitis, *Chest* 89:296-301, 1986.

51. Cordasco EM, Ahmad M, Mehta A, et al: The effects of steroid therapy on pulmonary hypertension secondary to fibrosing mediastinitis, *Cleve Clin J Med* 57:647-652, 1990.

52. Agostoni PG, Deffebach ME, Kirk W, et al: Upstream pressure for systemic to pulmonary flow for the bronchial circulation in dogs, *J Appl Physiol* 63:485-91, 1987.

53. Castard-Jackle A, Fowler MB: Influence of preoperative pulmonary artery pressure on mortality after heart transplantation: testing of potential reversibility of pulmonary hypertension with nitroprusside is useful in defining a high risk group. *J Am Coll Cardiol* 19:48-54, 1992.

54. Lensing AWA, Levi MM, Büller HR, et al: Diagnosis of deep-vein thrombosis using an objective Doppler method, *Ann Intern Med* 113:9-13, 1990.

55. Sharma GV, McIntyre KM, Sharma S, et al: Clinical and hemodynamic correlates in pulmonary embolism, *Clin Chest Med* 5:421-37, 1984.

56. Benotti JR, Ockene IS, Alpert JS, et al: The clinical profile of unresolved pulmonary embolism, *Chest* 84:669-78, 1983.

57. Sasahara AA, Sidd JJ, Tremblay G, et al: Cardiopulmonary consequences of acute pulmonary embolism, *Prog Cardiovasc Dis* 9:259-274, 1966.

58. Schriner RW, Ryu JH, Edwards WD: Microscopic pulmonary tumor embolism causing subacute cor pulmonale: a difficult antemortem diagnosis, *Mayo Clin Proc* 66:143-148, 1991.

59. Stein M, Levy SE: Reflex and humoral responses to pulmonary embolism, *Prog Cardiovasc Dis* 17:167-174, 1974.

60. Paraskos JA, Adelstein SJ, Smith RE, et al: Late prognosis of acute pulmonary embolism, *N Engl J Med* 289:55-8, 1973.

61. Perkett EA, Davidson JM, Meyrick B: Sequence of structural changes and elastin peptide release during vascular remodelling in sheep with chronic pulmonary hypertension induced by air embolization, *Am J Pathol* 139:1319-1332, 1991.

62. Perkett EA, Brigham KL, Meyrick B: Continuous air embolization into sheep causes sustained pulmonary hypertension and increased pulmonary vasoreactivity, *Am J Pathol* 132:444-454, 1988.

63. Perkett EA, Lyons RM, Moses HL, et al: Transforming growth factor-b activity in sheep lung lymph during the development of pulmonary hypertension, *J Clin Invest* 86:1459-1464, 1990.

64. Assoian RK, Sporn MB: Type b transforming growth factor in human platelets, release during platelet degranulation and action on vascular smooth muscle cells, *J Cell Biol* 102:1217-23, 1986.

65. Kurihara HM, Yoshizumi T, Suriyama F, et al: Transforming

growth factor-b stimulates the expression of endothelium mRNA by vascular endothelial cells, *Biochem Biophys Res Commun* 159:1435-1440, 1989.

66. Moser KM, Auger WR, Fedullo PF: Chronic major-vessel thromboembolic pulmonary hypertension, *Circulation* 81:1735-43, 1990.

67. Palevsky HI, Weiss DW: Pulmonary hypertension secondary to chronic thromboembolism, *J Nucl Med* 31:1-9, 1990.

68. Rich S, Levitsky S, Brundage BH: Pulmonary hypertension from Chronic Pulmonary thromboembolism. Ann Inter Med, 108:425-434; 1988.

69. Eisenberg PR, Rich S, Kaufmann L, et al: Evidence for increased thrombin activity in patients with primary pulmonary hypertension, *Circulation* 76:1246, 1987.

70. Moser KM, Spragg RG, Utley J, et al: Chronic thrombotic obstruction of major pulmonary arteries: results of thromboendarterectomy in 15 patients, *Ann Intern Med* 99:299-305, 1983.

71. Goldring RM, Fishman AF, Turino GM, et al: Pulmonary hypertension and cor pulmonale in cystic fibrosis of the pancreas, *J Pediatr* 65:501-524, 1964.

72. Palevsky HI, Fishman AP: Chronic cor pulmonale. Etiology and management, *JAMA* 263:2347-53, 1990.

73. Fishman AP: *Pulmonary hypertension and cor pulmonale*. In: Fishman AP, ed: *Pulmonary diseases and disorders*, ed 2, New York, 1988, McGraw-Hill.

74. Dunnill MS: An assessment of the anatomical factor in cor pulmonale in emphysema, *J Clin Pathol* 14:246, 1961.

75. Fishman AP: Hypoxia on the pulmonary circulation: how and where it acts, *Circ Res* 38:721, 1976.

76. Archer SL, McMartry IF, Weir EK: *Mechanisms of acute hypoxic and hyperoxic changes in pulmonary vascular reactivity*. In Weir EK, Reeves JT, eds: *Pulmonary vascular physiology and pathophysiology*, New York, 1989, Marcel Dekker.

77. Weitzenblum E, Schrijen F, Mohan-Kumar T, et al: Variability of the pulmonary vascular response to acute hypoxemia in chronic bronchitis, *Chest* 94:772-78, 1988.

78. Matthay RA, Niederman MS, Wiederman HP: Cardiovascular-pulmonary interaction in chronic obstructive pulmonary disease with special reference to the pathogenesis and management of cor pulmonale, *Med Clin North Am* 74:571-618, 1990.

79. Dinh-Xuan AT, Higenbottam TW, Clelland CA: Impairment of endothelium-dependent pulmonary-artery relaxation in chronic obstructive lung disease, *New Engl J Med* 324:1539-1547, 1991.

80. Berger HJ, Matthay RA, Lake J, et al: Assessment of cardiac performance with quantitative radionuclide angiocardiography: right ventricular ejection fraction with reference to findings in chronic obstructive pulmonary disease, *Am J Cardiol* 41:897-905, 1978.

81. Reeves JT, Graves BM, Turkevich D, et al: *Right ventricular function in pulmonary hypertension*. In Reeves JT, Weir EK, eds: *Lung biology in health and disease,* New York, 1989, Marcell-Dekker.

82. Santamore WP, Shaffer T, Papa L: Theoretical model of ventricular interdependence: pericardial effects, *Am J Physiol* 259 (Heart Circ Physiol 28) H181-H189, 1990.

83. Santamore WP, Shaffer T, Hughes D: A theoretical and experimental model of ventricular interdependence, *Basic Res Cardiol* 81:529-537, 1986.

84. Grossman W: Diastolic dysfunction in congestive heart failure, *New Engl J Med* 325:1557-1564.

85. Brower R, Permutt: *Exercise and the pulmonary circulation*. In Reeves JT, Weir EK, eds: *Lung biology in health and disease,* New York, 1989, Marcell-Dekker.

86. Morrison DA, Ovitt T, Hammermeister KE, et al: Functional tricuspid regurgitation and right ventricular dysfunction in pulmonary hypertension, *Am J Cardiol* 62:108-112, 1988.

87. Nocturnal oxygen therapy trial group. Continuous or nocturnal oxygen therapy in hypoxemic chronic obstructive lung disease, *Ann Intern Med* 93:391-398, 1980.

88. Grossman RF, Frost A, Zamel N, et al: Results of single-lung transplantation for bilateral pulmonary fibrosis, *N Engl J Med* 322:727-33, 1990.

89. Isner JM: Right ventricular myocardial infarction, *JAMA* 259:712-718, 1988.

90. Millman RP, Fishman AP: *Disorders of alveolar ventilation. In* Fishman AP, ed: *Pulmonary diseases and disorders,* ed 2 New York, 1988, McGraw-Hill.

91. Fishman AP, Turino GM, Bergofsky EH: Disorders of the respiration and circulation in subjects with deformities of the thorax, *Mod Conc Cardiovasc Dis* 27:449-453, 1958.

92. Cherniack NS: Sleep apnea and its causes, *J Clin Invest* 73:1501, 1984.

93. Fletcher EC, Schoof JW, Miller J: Long-term cardiopulmonary sequelae in patients with sleep apnea and chronic lung disease, *Am Rev Respir Dis* 135:525-533, 1987.

94. Levy AM, Tabakin BS, Hanson JS, et al: hypertrophied adenoids causing pulmonary hypertension and severe congestive heart failure, *N Engl J Med* 277:506-510, 1967.

95. Sutton JR: Helping your patients avoid high-altitude sickness, *J Respir Dis* 12(2):125-134, 1991.

96. Levine BD, Grayburn PA, Voyles WF, et al: Intracardiac shunting across a patent foramen ovale may exacerbate hypoxemia in high-altitude pulmonary edema, *Ann Intern Med* 114:569-570, 1991.

97. Hackett PH, Creagh CE, Grover RF, et al: High-altitude pulmonary edema in persons without the right pulmonary artery, *N Engl J Med* 302:1070-73, 1980.

98. Bärtsch P, Maggiorini M, Ritter M, et al: Prevention of high-altitude pulmonary edema by Nifedipine, *N Engl J Med* 325:1284-89, 1991.

99. West JB: *Acclimatization and adaptation: organ to cell*. In Lahisi S, Cherniak NS, Fitzgerald RS, eds: *Response and adaptation to hypoxia: organ to organelle*, New York, 1991, Oxford University Press.

100. Grover RF, Reeves JT, Will DH, et al: Pulmonary vasoconstriction in steers at high altitude, *J Appl Physiol* 18:567-574, 1963.

101. Mecham RP, Whitehouse LA, Wrenn DS, et al: Smooth muscle-mediated connective tissue remodeling in pulmonary hypertension. *Science* 237:423-426, 1987.

102. Stenmark KR, Fasules J, Voelkel NF, et al: Severe pulmonary hypertension and arterial adventitial changes in new born calves at 4300 M, *J Appl Physiol* 62 (2):821-830, 1987.

103. Vogel JH, Blount SC, Grover RF: *Pulmonary hypertension on exertion in normal man living at 10,150 feet (Leadville, Colorado)*. In Grover RF, ed: *Normal and abnormal pulmonary circulation*, Basle, Switzerland, 1963, Karger.

104. Gong H: Advising pulmonary patients about commercial air travel, *J Respir Dis* 11(5):484-499, 1990.

105. Dillard TA, Beninati WA, Berg BW: Air travel in patients with chronic obstructive pulmonary disease, *Arch Intern Med* 151:1793-95, 1991.

106. Moodie DS: Association between primary pulmonary hypertension and portal hypertension, *J Am Coll Cardiol* 17:492-498, 1991.

107. Edwards BS, Weir EK, Edwards WD, et al: Coexistent pulmonary and portal hypertension: morphologic and clinical features, *J Am Coll Cardiol* 10:1233-8, 1987.

108. Sherlock S: The liver-lung interface, *Semin Respir Infect* 9:247-53, 1988.

109. Yutani C, Imakita M, Ishibashi-Ueda H, et al: Nodular regenerative hyperplasia of the liver associated with primary pulmonary hypertension, *Hum Pathol* 19:726-731, 1988.

110. Morrison EB, Gaffney FA, Eigenbrodt EH, et al: Severe pulmonary hypertension associated with macronodular (postnecrotic) cirrhosis and autoimmune phenomena, *Am J Med* 69:513-519, 1980.

111. Vanhoutte PM: Serotonin and the vascular wall, *Int J Cardiol* 14:189-203, 1987.

112. Wanless IR: Coexistent pulmonary and portal hypertension: yin and yang, *Hepatology* 10:255-257, 1989.

113. Bank ER, Thrall JH, Dantzker DR: Radionuclide demonstration of intra-pulmonary shunting in cirrhosis, *Am J Roentgenol* 140:967-69, 1983.

114. Fauci AS, Haynes BF, Katz P: The spectrum of vasculitis: clinical, pathologic, immunologic, and therapeutic consideration, *Ann Intern Med* 89:660-676, 1978.

115. Foster G, Kvale PA: Differentiating and managing the primary pulmonary vasculitides, *J Respir Dis* 11:1052-60, 1990.

116. Stupi AM, Steen VD, Owens GR, et al: Pulmonary hypertension in the CREST syndrome variant of systemic sclerosis, *Arthritis Rheum* 29:515-524, 1986.

117. Young ID, Ford SE, Ford PM: The association of pulmonary hypertension with rheumatoid arthritis, *J Rheumatol* 16:1266-9, 1989.

118. Todd L, Mullen M, Rabinovitch M, et al: Pulmonary toxicity of monocrotaline differs at critical periods of lung development, *Pediatr Res* 19:731-737, 1985.

119. Gomez-Sanchez MA, Mestre de Juan MJ, Gomez-Pajuelo C, et al: Pulmonary hypertension due to toxic oil syndrome. A clinicopathologic study, *Chest* 95:325-31, 1989.

120. Gomez-Sanches MA, Saeny De La Calzada C, Gomez-Pajuelo, et al: Clinical and pathologic manifestations of pulmonary vascular disease in the toxic oil syndrome, *J Am Coll Cardiol* 18:1539-45, 1991.

121. Johnson WJ, Lie JT: Pulmonary hypertension and familial mediterranean fever: a previously unrecognized association, *Mayo Clin Proc* 66:919-925, 1991.

122. Braman SS, Eby E, Kuhn C, et al: Primary pulmonary hypertension in the elderly, *Arch Intern Med* 151:2433-2438, 1991.

123. Hawkins JW, Dunn MI: Primary pulmonary hypertension in adults, *Clin Cardiol* 13:382-87, 1990.

124. Fuster V, Giuliani ER, Brandenburg RO: The natural history of idiopathic pulmonary hypertension, *Am J Cardiol* 47:422, 1981.

125. Dawkins KD, Burke CM, Billingham ME, et al: Primary pulmonary hypertension and pregnancy, *Chest* 89:383-88, 1986.

126. Carlson JA, Day TG, Kuhns JG, et al: Endoarterial pulmonary metastasis of malignant trophoblast associated with a term intrauterine pregnancy, *Gynecol Oncol* 17:241-248, 1984.

127. Nishimura RA, Miller FA, Callahan MJ et al: Doppler echocardiography: theory, instrumentation, technique and application, *Mayo Clin Proc* 60:321-43, 1985.

128. Rhodes J, Barst RJ, Garofano RP, et al: Hemodynamic correlates of exercise function in patients with primary pulmonary artery hypertension, *J Am Coll Cardiol* 18:1738-44, 1991.

129. Rich S, Dantzker DR, Ayres SM, et al: Primary pulmonary hypertension: a national prospective study, *Ann Intern Med* 107:216-223, 1987.

130. Morgan JM, McCormack DG, Griffiths MJD, et al: Adenosine as a vasodilator in primary pulmonary hypertension, *Circulation* 84:1145-1149, 1991.

131. Palevsky HI, Schloo BL, Pietra GG, et al: Primary pulmonary hypertension. Vascular structure, morphometry, and responsiveness to vasodilator agents, *Circulation* 80:1207-1221, 1989.

132. Rich S, Kaufmann: High dose titration of calcium channel blocking agents for primary pulmonary hypertension: guidelines for short term drug testing, *J Am Coll Cardiol* 18:1323-27, 1991.

133. Rubin LJ, Mendoza J, Hood M, et al: Treatment of primary pulmonary hypertension with continuous intravenous prostacyclin (epoprostenol), *Ann Intern Med* 112:485-491, 1990.

134. Nihill MR, O'Laughlin MP, Mallins CF: Effects of atrial septostomy in patients with terminal cor pulmonale due to pulmonary vascular disease, *Cathet Cardiovasc Diagn* 24:166-72, 1991.

135. Hatano S, Strasser T: Primary pulmonary hypertension, Geneva, 1975, World Health Organization.

136. Bjornsson J, Edwards WD: Primary pulmonary hypertension: a histopathologic study of 80 cases *Mayo Clin Proc* 60:16-25, 1985.

137. Pietra GG, Edwards WD, Kay JM, et al: Histopathology of primary pulmonary hypertension. A quantitative and qualitative study of pulmonary blood vessels from 58 patients in the National Heart, Lung and Blood Institute, primary pulmonary hypertension registry, *Circulation* 80:1198-1206, 1989.

138. Heath D, Smith P, Gosney J, et al: The pathology of the early and late stages of primary pulmonary hypertension, *Br Heart J* 58:204-13, 1987.

139. Pietra GG, Rutther JR: Specificity of pulmonary vascular lesions in primary pulmonary hypertension. A reappraisal, *Respiration* 52:81-85, 1987.

140. Smith P, Heath D, Yacoub M, et al: The ultrastructure of plexogenic pulmonary arteriopathy, *J Pathol* 160:111-121, 1990.

141. Fein SA, Frishman WH: The pathophysiology and management of primary pulmonary hypertension, *Cardiol Clin* 5:563-576, 1987.

142. Fuster V, Steele PM, Edwards WD, et al: Primary pulmonary hypertension: natural history and the importance of thrombosis, *Circulation* 70:560-587, 1984.

143. Fuchs J, Mlczoch J, Niessner H: Abnormal fibrinolysis in primary pulmonary hypertension (abstract), *Eur Heart J* 2:A168, 1981.

144. Burke AP, Farb A, Virmani R: The pathology of primary pulmonary hypertension, *Mod Pathol* 4:269, 1991.

145. Wagenvoort CA, Wagenvoort N, Takahashi T: Pulmonary venoocclusive disease: involvement of pulmonary arteries and review of the literature, *Hum Pathol* 16:1033-41, 1985.

146. Wagenvoort CA, Beetstra A, Spijker J: Capillary haemangiomatosis of the lungs, *Histopathology* 2:401-6, 1978.

147. Tron V, Magee F, Wright JL: Pulmonary capillary hemangiomatosis, *Hum Pathol* 17:1144-1150, 1986.

148. Gosney J, Heath D, Smith P, et al: Pulmonary endocrine cells in pulmonary arterial disease, *Arch Pathol Lab Med* 113:337-341, 1989.

149. Rich S, Brundage BH: High dose calcium channel-blocking therapy for primary pulmonary hypertension: evidence for long-term reduction in pulmonary arterial pressure and regression of right ventricular hypertrophy, *Circulation* 76:135-41, 1987.

150. Hughes JD, Rubin LJ: Primary pulmonary hypertension: an analysis of 28 cases and a review of the literature, *Medicine* 65:56-72, 1986.

151. Barst RJ, Flaster ER, Menon A: Evidence for the association of unexplained pulmonary hypertension in children with the major histocompatibility complex, *Circulation* 85:249-258, 1992.

152. Loyd JE, Atkinson JB, Pietra GG, et al: Heterogeneity of pathologic lesions in familial primary pulmonary hypertension, *Am Rev Respir Dis* 138:952-957, 1988.

153. Vanhoutte PM: The endothelium-modulator of vascular smooth-muscle tone, *N Engl J Med* 319:512-3, 1988.

154. Newman JH, Ross JC: Primary pulmonary hypertension: a look at the future, *J Am Coll Cardiol* 14:551-55, 1989.

155. Ruoslahti E, Pierschbacher MD: New perspectives in cell adhesion: RGD and integrins, *Science* 238:491-7, 1987.

Chapter 6

MYOCARDITIS

Ahvie Herskowitz
Kenneth L. Baughman

Myocarditis has come under increasing investigation by clinicians, virologists, molecular biologists, and immunologists. Recent key advances include (1) the acceptance of a histologic definition of myocarditis, (2) the affirmation of the hypothesis that cardiotropic viruses play a role in the pathogenesis of myocarditis and cardiomyopathy by nucleic acid hybridization molecular techniques and (3) further documentation of the importance of the host's genetic predisposition to the development and severity of myocarditis. Despite these critical advances, myocarditis remains one of the most daunting challenges in modern cardiology. The diagnosis of myocarditis remains problematic due to the lack of a distinctive clinical syndrome, the lack of noninvasive mechanisms to diagnose the condition, the focal histologic nature of the disease, and the difficulties inherent to the interpretation of endomyocardial biopsies. These barriers have prevented an accurate assessment of the true incidence and prevalence of myocarditis and therefore blunted its potential public health significance. Nevertheless, as increasing numbers of human and animal studies identify immune and genetically based links between myocarditis and idiopathic dilated cardiomyopathy, the possibility that studies of myocarditis will yield fundamental insights into the pathogenesis and treatment of cardiomyopathy broadens the scope of this enigmatic disorder. The purpose of this chapter is to review the current criteria and methods for diagnosis of human myocarditis and weigh the evidence for and against the concept that myocarditis is an immunopathic consequence of an initiating viral infection.

The current definition of myocarditis is a histologic one, frequently based on the examination of an endomyocardial biopsy performed during the evaluation of a patient with new onset of unexplained congestive heart failure or arrythmias. The criteria for the diagnosis of myocarditis were established by a group of cardiac pathologists known as the Dallas panel and are as follows: **Myocarditis is a process characterized by an inflammatory infiltrate of the myocardium with necrosis and/or degeneration of** adjacent myocytes not typical of the ischemic damage associated with ischemic heart disease.[1-2] This definition has established uniformity in the diagnosis of myocarditis, the lack of which previously prevented investigators from determining that the entity they were evaluating was indeed myocarditis. It is clear that myocarditis can be caused by almost all forms of infectious diseases including bacteria, viruses, fungi, protozoa, spirochetes and Rickettsiae (Table 6-1). In many of these infections, an associated acute cardiomyopathy has also been described. The development of long-standing dilated cardiomyopathy associated with myocarditis has been largely limited to either viral infections (Coxsackieviruses, influenza, cytomegalovirus, echoviruses, and human immunodeficiency virus) or Chagas' disease (South American trypanosomiasis). In Chagasic myocarditis and cardiomyopathy, more than any other form of postinfectious cardiomyopathy, serologic and epidemiologic studies in endemic areas of Central and South America have clearly documented the role of *Trypanosoma cruzi* as the initiator of a persistent myocarditis leading to dilated cardiomyopathy.[3-7]

Primary, or idiopathic, myocarditis must be distinguished from myocarditis found in association with known etiologies (Table 6-1). Patients presenting with a clinical suspicion of myocarditis therefore should be fully evaluated to exclude secondary or known etiologies. A recent drug history including those that are known to provoke hypersensitivity myocarditis, as well as cardiotoxic drugs such as vasopressors and immunosuppressive agents, should be sought. Blood work should be obtained to rule out collagen vascular disease. In addition, other causes of dilated cardiomyopathy should also be evaluated. This evaluation should include obtaining a negative history for coronary disease, excessive alcohol ingestion, or illicit drug abuse. Thyroid disease, and 24-hour urinary metanephrine excretion should be obtained to rule out pheochromocytoma. A family history of cardiomyopathy should be sought. It should be emphasized that in the appropriate clinical setting, coronary angiography may be necessary to rule out ischemic disease as the etiology of suspected myocarditis. Coronary angiography should be considered in patients over 35 years of age when no other etiology is found and in patients with a suggestion of ischemic heart disease by history, electrocardiographic changes or coronary artery disease risk factors such as hyperlipidemia, family history of premature vascular disease, history of cigarette smoking, or diabetes mellitus.

CLINICAL PRESENTATION

The classical clinical presentation of myocarditis is characterized by the rapid onset of congestive heart failure, syncope, or unexplained tachyarrythmias with a recent history of a viral-type illness. Symptoms typically include malaise, fever and chills, upper respiratory and/or gastrointestinal symptoms, myalgias, and chest pain.[8] In

Table 6-1. Etiologies of human myocarditis

Infectious	Noninfectious
Viral	
Coxsackievirus (A & B)	**Cardiotoxic drugs**
Echovirus	Cocaine
Influenza	Catecholamines
Cytomegalovirus	Doxorubicin
Hepatitis	
Mumps	**Hypersensitivity drug reactions**
herpes simplex	Antibiotics
EBV	Amphotericin B
HIV	Ampicillin
	Chloramphenicol
Rickettsial	Penicillin
Q fever	Tetracycline
Rocky mountain spotted fever	Streptomycin
Scrub typhus	Sulfisoxazole
	Diuretics
Fungal	Chlorthalidone
Cryptococcus	Acetazolamide
Candidiasis	Hydrochlorothiazide
Histoplasmosis	Spironolactone
Aspergillus	Others
	Isoniazid
Protozoal and metazoal	Nucleoside analogues
Trypanosomiasis	Lithium
Toxoplasmosis	Methyldopa
Malaria	Tetanus toxoid
Schistosomiasis	Indomethacin
Trichinosis	
	Systemic illness
Bacterial	SLE
Diptheria	Other autoimmune diseases
Tuberculosis	Sarcoidosis
Legionella	Kawasaki disease
Brucella	
Clostridium	
Salmonella	
Meningococcus	
Spirochetal	
Borrelia (lyme)	

cases with congestive heart failure, global left ventricular hypokinesis, often with a nondilated LV cavity and associated increased left ventricular wall thickness, is found by noninvasive testing. Mild to moderate pericardial effusions are not uncommon. In patients presenting with syncope or unexplained tachyarrythmias, left ventricular function may be only mildly impaired or entirely normal. Electrocardiographic findings are frequently nonspecifically abnormal with diffuse ST-T wave abnormalities, interventricular conduction delays, low QRS voltage, poor R wave progression, and premature atrial and ventricular beats. Occasionally, Q waves and ST-T changes mimicking myocardial infarction are present. Before the availability of endomyocardial biopsy, a presumptive diagnosis of myocarditis was based on this type of clinical information alone and could only be confirmed by postmortem examination.

None of the clinical features of myocarditis described above define myocarditis as a unique entity. It is important to note that a wide range of frequencies (0% to 63%) of myocarditis have been reported upon histologic examination of cardiac biopsies of patients diagnosed as having dilated cardiomyopathy.[9-14] Perhaps the most important reason for this wide discrepancy in reporting myocarditis prevalences is the imprecise clinical relationship of subacute or chronic presentations of congestive heart failure and tachyarrythmias to myocarditis. It is now evident from endomyocardial biopsy studies that many patients who were clinically diagnosed with myocarditis, particularly those with subacute presentations, did not indeed have myocarditis. Before the Dallas criteria were formulated in 1986, reported studies on myocarditis were plagued by variability in histologic criteria. They were also hampered by geographic differences, which likely reflect exposures to different types and strains of cardiotropic viruses, as well as genetic differences in host populations, both of which are capable of manifesting a wide variety of clinical presentations. Active myocarditis cases in Japan appear more likely to present in direct association with a viral-type illness than those in the United States, where patients frequently cannot clearly recall a preceding viral illness before congestive heart failure or arrythmias appear.[15-16] Viral cultures of blood or endomyocardial biopsy specimens, or rising serum viral titers have not been commonly utilized in adults. Therefore the linking of virus as an etiologic basis for myocarditis in patients with subacute or chronic presentations of cardiac disease remains a subject for debate.

EPIDEMIOLOGY

Virus-associated myocarditis was recognized in the 1800s during epidemics of mumps and pleurodynia, which are now known to be due to coxsackievirus and echovirus.[17] Although human myocarditis is found after infection with a wide range of viruses (Table 6-1), RNA viruses predominate, with picornaviruses being the most commonly identified agents. Coxsackieviruses are members of the *Enterovirus* genus within the *Picornavirus* family and were distinguished from polioviruses and other enteroviruses by their pathogenicity for suckling mice.[18] Group A coxsackieviruses typically produce severe, generalized skeletal myositis in neonatal mice. Group B coxsackieviruses produce more severe damage to the nervous system, brown fat, pancreas, and heart. Although these general distinctions remain helpful, considerable clinical overlap, particularly with syndromes of myositis and upper respiratory infection, occur among echoviruses, enteroviruses, and coxsackieviruses. The members of the EV genus are most prevalent in warm climates and during the warm seasons in temperate countries and are more commonly isolated from children and young adults and from patients living in low socioeconomic conditions. Infection can spread both by the fecal-oral route or via the respiratory route. Reinfections can occur, and certain types of enterovirus tend to be endemic in most years, whereas others appear in outbreaks or epidemics at longer intervals. Therefore the types of EV prevalent in any given community will vary from year to year.

Of the list in Table 6-1, only a small number of viruses have been either cultured or identified using nucleic acid hybridization techniques from the hearts of infected patients: coxsackieviruses A and B, polio, echovirus, vaccinia, rabies, influenza, HIV, and hepatitis. Most often the association of a particular viral infection and heart disease has been based either on serologic studies, the isolation or identification of the virus in tissues or fluids outside the heart, or recognition of a characteristic clinical picture associated with a viral infection. Serologic evidence of viral infections require the demonstration of at least a fourfold rise in specific antibody in paired acute (less than 1 week) and convalescent (2 weeks or longer) serum specimens. Initially, IgM antibody is present, reaching peak titers by 2 to 3 weeks and declining to undetectable levels thereafter. IgG antibody production is the predominant immunoglobulin class after the first month of disease.

Incidence of myocarditis

The true prevalence and incidence of viral myocarditis and cardiomyopathy in the general population is unknown. Evidence indicates that approximately 5% of a virus-infected population may experience some form of cardiac involvement associated with the acute illness. Studies of cardiac tissues from two series of unselected autopsy cases involving 40,000[19] and 12,474[20] patients showed a prevalence of myocarditis of 3.5% and 1.06%, respectively (the latter used the currently accepted Dallas criteria). In 417 young adult and middle-aged male victims of sudden accidental death[21] and 214 children who died a sudden violent death,[22] the overall prevalence of myocarditis was also <5%. In cases of unexpected sudden death, however, the prevalence is higher and ranges from 17 to 21%.[17-23] There is also evidence that during epidemics of coxsackievirus B, poliomyelitis and influenza, approximately 5% to 10%[22] of those affected experience cardiac symptoms. Unlike adults, lethal myocarditis may occur in up to 50% of infected infants[24] during outbreaks of coxsackie B viral disease. These agents are known to produce a high prevalence of myocarditis in infected babies in the first year of life, particularly during the neonatal period. These cases of myocarditis are characterized by a fulminant course with short incubation times, frequently less than 1 week. Myocarditis becomes less common in early childhood and increases again in adolescence and adulthood.[17] In contrast to the often fatal disease in the neonatal period, viral myocarditis in adolescents and adults usually has a delayed onset (1 to 4 weeks) and is rarely fatal.

Idiopathic myocarditis characterized by a progressive

downhill course over a period of months to years, ending in death from heart failure or intractable arrythmias, has been recognized for decades.[11,15,17,25] Although the true incidence of this pattern of chronic disease is not yet known, studies utilizing the Dallas criteria suggest that the prevalence of myocarditis in patients with recent onset (<12 months) of congestive heart failure is approximately 5% to 15%. At our institution 60 of 348 (17%) patients undergoing endomyocardial biopsy for recent onset heart dysfunction were found to have either active or borderline myocarditis.[16] Of these 60 patients, idiopathic or primary myocarditis was diagnosed histologically in 35 patients (10%). The additional 25 patients (7%) were diagnosed with myocarditis associated with an underlying condition such as postpartum cardiomyopathy (n = 15), SLE (n = 3), AIDS (n = 3), hepatitis A (n = 1). The preliminary data from the Myocarditis Treatment Trial (MTT) have demonstrated a 9% prevalence of active myocarditis in 2242 adult patients.[26] Other studies include Vasiljevic, et al,[27] who found a 12% prevalence of active myocarditis in 85 patients thought to have idiopathic dilated cardiomyopathy, in 2 of 6 patients with alcoholic cardiomyopathy, and 12 of 16 patients with clinical myocarditis. The criteria used for clinical myocarditis in this study was a fourfold increase in antiviral titers. Latham, et al,[28] studied 52 patients with idiopathic dilated cardiomyopathy with a mean duration of symptoms of < 2 months and found active myocarditis in 7 patients (13%). Although the Dallas criteria were not specifically employed, in a prospective trial of prednisone for dilated cardiomyopathy, Parillo, et al,[29] diagnosed lymphocytic myocarditis in 2 of 102 patients with idiopathic dilated cardiomyopathy who were symptomatic for a median of 8 months before entering the study. These findings may reflect a low prevalence of myocarditis in patients with chronic dilated cardiomyopathy, whereas a prevalence of 40% to 60% has been suggested in patients with acute onset of symptoms of less than 4 weeks duration.[16,30-31]

A male predominance of myocarditis was seen both in the MTT study (62%) and in our own series of 546 patients (60%).[32] This male predominance is consistent with the epidemiology of coxsackieviruses group A and B, which show a male/female infectivity predominance of approximately 2.5:1.[17,33] This indirect correlation for coxsackieviruses as the cause of myocarditis is now being confirmed by recent studies that utilize molecular techniques such as in situ hybridization and polymerase chain reaction on endomyocardial biopsy samples. These studies, which will be discussed in detail in the following sections, are now providing concrete evidence that point to enteroviruses as possible primary initiators in the more common cases of myocarditis with subacute or chronic presentations of dilated cardiomyopathy.[34-39] These major advances in technology will continue to elaborate on the relationship between these and other viruses to myocarditis and idiopathic dilated cardiomyopathy.

ENDOMYOCARDIAL BIOPSY
The Dallas criteria

In 1986-1987 Aretz[1-2] and colleagues, in an attempt to establish a uniform histologic classification for the diagnosis of myocarditis on endomyocardial biopsy, published a classification that was proposed by eight cardiac pathologist (the Dallas panel).

Two separate classifications were described for the first and subsequent biopsies. On the first biopsy, *active myocarditis* required the presence of myocardial inflammation associated with adjacent myocyte damage. Myocyte damage could either take the form of necrosis, which by definition would require the presence of neutrophils engulfing the myocyte (Fig. 6-1, *A-D*), or may consist of myocyte vacuolization, irregular cellular outlines, or cellular disruption associated with lymphocytes that appear adjacent to the sarcolemma; these latter degenerative changes presumably reflect irreversible myocyte injury. *Borderline myocarditis* is diagnosed when an unequivocal diagnosis of myocarditis cannot be made, either because the inflammatory infiltrate is too sparse or because the damage to myocytes is not clearly demonstrable (Figure 6-1, *E*). *No myocarditis* is diagnosed when the myocardium is entirely normal, shows nonspecific changes such as mild myocyte hypertrophy and mild interstitial fibrosis, or shows more advanced features of idiopathic dilated cardiomyopathy (Fig. 6-1, *F*). Since advanced cases of idiopathic dilated cardiomyopathy frequently contain scattered collections of interstitial infiltrates not associated with myocyte necrosis,[40-41] care must be used not to diagnose borderline myocarditis in cases with extensive interstitial fibrosis and myocyte hypertrophy.

The inflammatory infiltrate in idiopathic myocarditis is frequently composed exclusively of mononuclear cells, although in cases with a more acute presentation, the presence of polymorphonuclear cell infiltration is common. This type of infiltrate is in contrast to the prominent interstitial eosinophilic infiltrate seen in hypersensitivity myocarditis (Figure 6-1, *G*) and the prominent polymorphonuclear infiltrates in toxic and pressor-induced myocarditis. The Dallas criteria specifically mention that myocarditis must be distinguished from the histologic pattern of injury seen with ischemic heart disease. This type of histologic injury can also be seen in patients experiencing prolonged hypotensive episodes prior to endomyocardial biopsy. The histologic features of these ischemic lesions demonstrate that they typically spare the subendocardial myocardium, frequently involve larger clusters of myocytes and contain granulation tissue with mixed infiltrates that include plasma cells and pigment laden macrophages, and may contain dense scarring, termed *replacement fibrosis*.

The terminology used for subsequent biopsies is *ongoing, resolving* and *resolved* myocarditis, and is reserved only for patients with previous biopsies. Ongoing (persistent) myocarditis is used if myocardial inflammation associated with myocyte damage persists. Resolving (healing)

Text continued on p. 186.

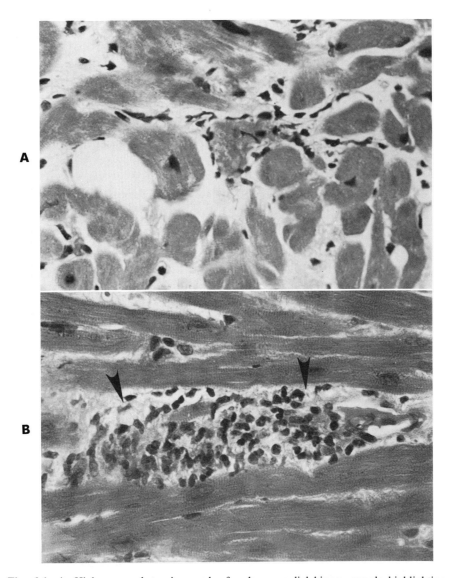

Fig. 6-1. A, High power photomicrograph of endomyocardial biopsy sample highlighting one isolated myocyte undergoing myocyte necrosis. The presence of myocyte degeneration associated with an adjacent inflammatory infiltrate is characteristic of active myocarditis. **B,** A small cluster of longitudinally oriented myocytes engulfed in a dense infiltrate composed primarily of mononuclear cells. Outside the focus of active myocarditis, the adjacent myocardium appears relatively normal.

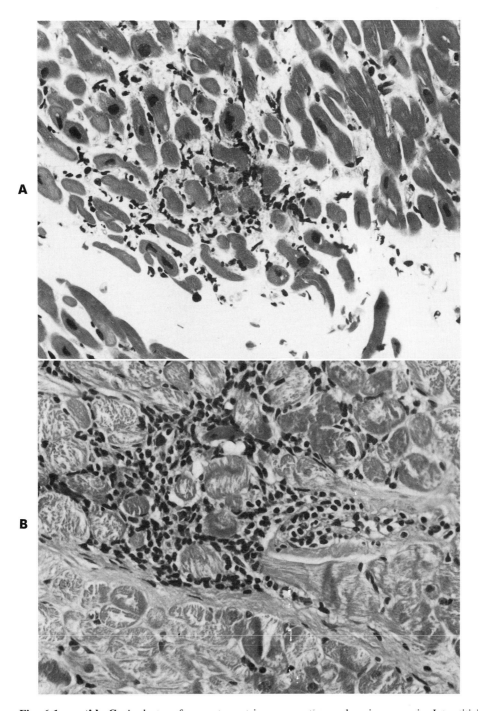

Fig. 6-1, cont'd. C, A cluster of myocytes cut in cross-section undergoing necrosis. Interstitial mononuclear cells surround the cluster of myocytes, which no longer have crisp cellular outlines. The interstitial space between affected myocytes contains granular basophilic material, which likely is fibrin. The inflammatory cells appear to extend from the central core of necrotic myocytes into the adjacent myocardium. **D,** A high power photomicrograph of tangentially sectioned myocytes engulfed by a dense cluster of mononuclear cells. This example of active myocarditis highlights the pattern of myocyte vacuolization associated with irregular myocyte surface outlines caused by lymphocytes adjacent to the sarcolemmal surfaces of individual myocytes.

continued.

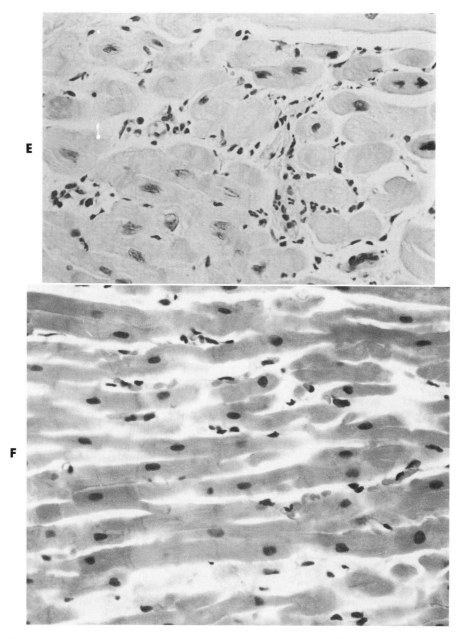

Fig. 6-1, cont'd.   E, A focus of interstitial inflammatory cell infiltration without associated myocyte necrosis. This histologic pattern is characteristic of borderline myocarditis. **F,** Normal-appearing myocardium characteristic of no myocarditis. In this example there is no appreciable interstitial fibrosis or myocyte hypertrophy.

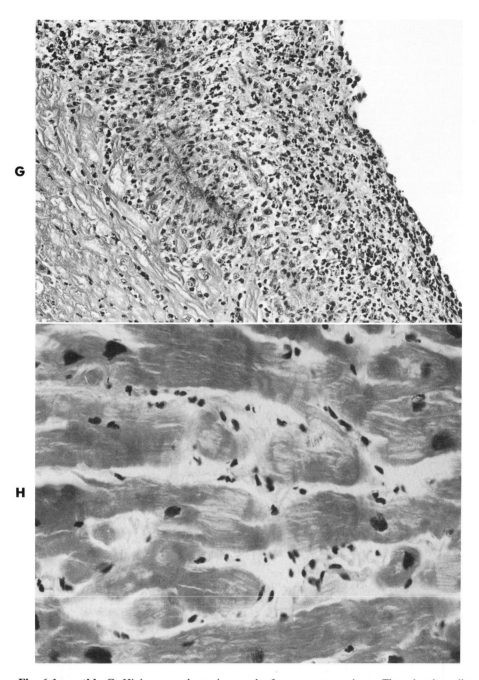

Fig. 6-1, cont'd. G, High power photomicrograph of an autopsy specimen. The subendocardium contains dense collections of polymorphonuclear eosinophils as well as large mononuclear histiocytes, characteristic of hypersensitivity myocarditis. **H,** Repeat endomyocardial biopsy in a patient previously with active myocarditis. Only a sparse interstitial mononuclear cell infiltrate is seen, which is consistent with resolving myocarditis.

myocarditis can be identical to borderline myocarditis, although reparative fibrosis may be also seen (Figure 6-1 *H*). Resolved (healed) myocarditis is diagnosed if no inflammatory infiltrate is present. The precise role of repeat endomyocardial biopsies in the routine follow-up of patients with myocarditis has not yet been systematically studied. A recent published study has suggested that there may be no relationship between histologic findings of myocarditis on repeat, serial biopsies and hemodynamic improvement.[42] Our own experience confirm these observations. In many cases of myocarditis, serial biopsies with resolving or resolved myocarditis have been associated with continued or deteriorating contractile function; likewise, ongoing myocarditis has been occasionally seen, despite complete resolution of cardiac symptoms. The Myocarditis Treatment Trial (MTT) protocol of four serial biopsies over a 12-month period will likely be able to systematically address the role of the follow-up endomyocardial biopsy in patients with myocarditis.

The role of electron microscopy in the evaluation of endomyocardial biopsies appears to be limited. This technique does not appear to offer any added specificity for the diagnosis of myocarditis, although it may provide some clinically useful information regarding prognosis. In a recent study involving 79 patients with suspected myocarditis, those patients with significant myocyte myofilament loss had a 37% 18-month mortality, compared with 10% in patients without such loss.[43]

Other studies conducted before the Dallas criteria were developed have proposed quantitative criteria for the diagnosis of lymphocytic myocarditis using light microscopy.[44-45] They suggested that more than five lymphocytes per high power field ($\times 400$) (30 cells/mm^2) is indicative of myocarditis. To utilize these criteria effectively, one would have to overcome considerable interobserver discordance in identifying lymphocytes on hematoxylin-eosin stained sections.[46] This is at least partially due to the difficulty in distinguishing myocardial lymphocytes from endothelial cells, fibroblasts, pericytes, and mast cells.[41] Immunohistochemical quantitative studies using common leukocyte antigen to specifically mark inflammatory cells[45,47-49] are likely to yield more specific criteria that could determine whether quantitative methods will be useful in the future for diagnosis and follow-up of patients with myocarditis.

Pitfalls of endomyocardial biopsy interpretation

Interobserver variability: In an early study performed in 1987 by Shanes, et al,[50] 16 specimens from patients with idiopathic dilated cardiomyopathy were sent to 7 cardiac pathologists. The prevalence of abnormal lymphocyte counts ranged from 0% to 30%. One or more pathologists diagnosed definite or possible myocarditis in 11 of 16 patients, although of these 11 cases, the highest concordance rate was when 3 of the pathologists agreed on 3 cases. This study highlights the need for special training in interpreting endomyocardial biopsies in a reproducible fashion. The Pathology Panel associated with the Myocarditis Treatment Trial (MTT) has developed extensive experience in interpreting endomyocardial biopsies and has a concordance rate of > 90% (personal communication).

Sensitivity

Several studies have now clearly demonstrated that diagnostic histologic features of myocarditis are focal; the small sampling size of endomyocardial biopsies produce a potentially insensitive diagnostic procedure. Hauck, et al,[51] took 10 biopsies from each ventricle from 38 autopsy hearts of patients with lymphocytic myocarditis. Right ventricular endomyocardial biopsies were positive in only 63% of the 38 cases and in only 17% of the individual biopsy specimens. Left ventricular endomyocardial biopsies were positive in only 55% of the cases and in 20% of the individual specimens. Chow, et al,[52] sampled 14 autopsy hearts from patients with myocarditis using both Stanford and Cordis bioptomes from apical and nonapical locations on the right side of the septum. Of the samples examined, 43% to 57% were diagnostic for myocarditis for each bioptome in each region. By analyzing all available samples, 11 of 14 cases could be diagnosed, requiring a mean of 17.2 samples/patient, a clinically unrealistic number. It is difficult to judge precisely how these autopsy studies can be related to studies of living patients undergoing endomyocardial biopsy. It is unlikely that the subendocardium in an autopsy heart specimen accurately represents the subendocardium that is biopsied in a living patient. Nonetheless, these studies suggest that the endomyocardial biopsy may be an insensitive diagnostic tool in a disease characterized by its focal histologic changes. In support of this, Dec, et al,[53] performed repeat endomyocardial biopsies on 28 patients with strong clinical evidence of myocarditis despite nondiagnostic initial biopsies. Of the six patients initially diagnosed with borderline myocarditis, four were found to have active myocarditis on repeat biopsy. None of the remaining patients with the initial diagnosis of no myocarditis had active myocarditis on repeat biopsy. These results are consistent with the histologic observation that in many cases of active myocarditis, focal zones of borderline myocarditis can also be seen throughout the biopsy. These observations suggest that when borderline myocarditis is diagnosed, an effort must be made to cut through the whole paraffin block to maximize the possibility of finding a diagnostic focus of active myocarditis. If no definite diagnosis is made, then a repeat right ventricular endomyocardial biopsy could be considered.

DETECTION OF MYOCARDITIS USING NONINVASIVE IMAGING TECHNIQUES
Radionuclide imaging

The first radionuclide scanning technique to be actively used in the diagnosis of myocarditis was gallium-67 citrate. This imaging technique has been used clinically for its affinity for inflammatory reactions such as localization of occult abscesses. Latham, et al,[28] found positive gallium scans in 4/52 patients with IDCM, only 1 of which had myocarditis on biopsy. In contrast, O'Connell, et al,[13] studied 39 patients with IDCM and found 19 patients with positive gallium scans (49%). More recently, indium-111 antimyosin antibody imaging has been studied as a diagnostic tool in myocarditis. This imaging technique has been well characterized in imaging acute myocardial infarction and cardiac transplant rejection, and may be ideally suited to identify small foci of myocyte necrosis in a sensitive fashion. In a study by Dec, et al,[54] indium-111 antimyosin imaging was evaluated in 82 patients undergoing endomyocardial biopsy for suspected myocarditis. Seventy-four patients had dilated cardiomyopathy of less than one year's duration, and eight patients had normal left ventricular function. Symptoms at presentation included congestive heart failure (92%), chest pain mimicking myocardial infarction (6%) and life-threatening ventricular tachyarrhythmias (2%). On the basis of the right ventricular histologic examination, the sensitivity of antimyosin imaging was 83%, its specificity was 53% and the predictive value of a normal scan was 92%. The clinical importance of a positive scan was highlighted by the finding that improvement in left ventricular function occurred within 6 months of treatment in 54% of patients with an abnormal antimyosin scan, compared with 18% of those with a normal scan (p < 0.01). In addition, a normal antimyosin scan was associated with a very low rate (8%) of detecting myocarditis on endomyocardial biopsy. Similarly, Yasuda, et al,[55] studied 28 patients clinically suspected of having myocarditis, 25 of whom had left ventricular ejection fractions of less than 45%. Antimyosin scans were positive in 9 patients who had evidence of myocarditis, and negative in 11 who had no evidence of myocarditis by biopsy. The remaining eight had positive antimyosin scans but showed no evidence of myocarditis on right ventricular biopsy. On the basis of a right ventricular biopsy standard, the sensitivity of this method was 100%, its specificity 58%. These studies are consistent with the hypothesis that the sensitivity of antimyosin scanning to diagnose myocarditis is higher than that of endomyocardial biopsy. In addition to its diagnostic role, the role of this noninvasive scan in directing which patients require initial, repeat or serial biopsies requires further evaluation.

The role of antimyosin scanning in patients with chronic idiopathic dilated cardiomyopathy is less clear. In a study by Obrador, et al,[56] 12 of 17 patients (71%) with chronic idiopathic dilated cardiomyopathy (> 12 months duration), had abnormal antimyosin uptake. This result is in stark contrast to the typically low prevalence of myocarditis in this population on endomyocardial biopsy. A possible explanation for this discrepancy is that with a chronic presentation of myocarditis, inflammatory foci with myocyte necrosis become increasingly more sparse

and are therefore more apt not to be identified by the endomyocardial biopsy technique. This explanation would suggest an important role for antimyosin scanning in patients with long-standing idiopathic dilated cardiomyopathy. On the other hand, end-stage dilated cardiomyopathy associated with elevated end-diastolic pressures is frequently associated with foci of endocardial myocytolysis, which most likely reflect chronic ischemia rather than immune-mediated myocyte necrosis.[4] Therefore the role for antimyosin scanning in patients with idiopathic dilated cardiomyopathy also requires further evaluation.

Echocardiography

The echocardiographic features of myocarditis are nonspecific and can simulate a variety of other conditions. The study by Pinamonti, et al,[57] analyzed 41 patients with histologically proven myocarditis and variable clinical presentations: congestive heart failure (63%), atrioventricular block (17%), chest pain (15%) and supraventricular arrhythmias (5%). Left ventricular dysfunction was particularly common in patients with congestive heart failure (88%), often without or with only minor cavity dilatation. Patients with atrioventricular block or chest pain alone usually had preserved ventricular function. Right ventricular dysfunction was present in only 23% of the patients. Additional findings included asynergic ventricular areas (64%), sometimes reversible left ventricular "hypertrophy" (20%), and ventricular thrombi (15%). In addition, transient concentric[58] and asymmetric[59] increases in left ventricular wall thickness have also been observed by others and is consistent with our own experience. These changes may represent compensatory hypertrophy, although in patients with a fulminant presentation and multifocal zones of inflammation and necrosis, ventricular thickening may represent interstitial edema. Transient akinetic or dyskinetic ventricular segments may also be seen[60-61] and can mimic acute myocardial infarction.

Echocardiographic features that may be associated with a better overall prognosis are regional wall motion abnormalities[62] and the presence of preserved right ventricular function.[28] The latter finding was associated with a 95% 24-month survival versus 47% for patients with right ventricular end-diastolic pressures >11 mm Hg. In our experience with 30 consecutive patients with myocarditis, the echocardiographic predictor of hemodynamic improvement after immunosuppressive therapy was the ratio of wall thickness to left ventricular cavity dimension. The combination of a normal or modestly dilated left ventricular cavity and left ventricular hypertrophy either at presentation or developing early in the course of therapy, was a strong predictor of improvement in contractile function.

IMMUNOPATHOGENESIS
Experimental animal studies

Most of our understanding of the immunopathogenetic mechanisms of viral myocarditis in humans come from experimental studies in mice. Coxsackievirus-induced myocardial disease in mice was developed by Lerner, et al.[63-64] They demonstrated that after intraperitoneal inoculation of coxsackievirus B3 (CVB3), 14 day-old mice developed severe myocarditis after 5 to 7 days. Woodruff, et al,[65-66] confirmed these results using different strains of mice. From these studies, the earliest damage in myocarditis did not appear to be due to host responses, but rather to direct virally-mediated injury. This finding was consistent with our own observations that the earliest histologic abnormality in myocarditis was a contraction band necrosis of small clusters of myocytes that could be seen before any inflammatory cell reaction was present.[67] Contraction band necrosis characteristically seen in reperfusion injury and in patients given high doses of catecholamines, is believed to represent a histologic pattern reflecting calcium overload of myocardial cells. The mechanism(s) by which direct viral infection of myocytes may produce irreversible calcium overload are not known. In addition, since small clusters of myocytes with contraction band injury are seen, a form of reperfusion injury could be playing a role; direct viral injury of arteriolar endothelium and/or smooth muscle cells could predispose to arteriolar spasm with secondary myocyte injury. Irrespective of the precise mechanism of injury, necrosis of small clusters of myocytes appears to be the histologic hallmark of early myocarditis, before an inflammatory cell reaction can be identified.

Susceptibility to acute myocarditis. Susceptibility to the acute phase of myocarditis appears to be subject to a number of factors including: the age and sex of the host,[68] the myocarditic nature of the virus strain,[69] and the genetic background of the host.[67,70] The genetically determined viral neutralizing antibody response appears to be determined by non-MHC genes, and a delayed antibody response is associated with more severe acute myocarditis.[70] In contrast, an adequate natural killer cell response in the earliest stages of disease, protects a host from severe viral myocarditis.[71] Enhancing factors which, in conjunction with a cardiotropic viral illness, potentiate the manifestations of myocarditis include hypoxia, pregnancy, nutritional deficiencies of B vitamins, prolonged ingestion of ethanol, forced exercise and increased afterload.[6-7] In addition, in acute myocarditis in animal models, drug therapy, particularly cyclophosphamide, cyclosporine, cortisone, levamisole and nonsteroidal antiinflammatory drugs[72-73] likely increases viral replication and has been repeatedly shown to increase the severity of myocarditis. In further support of the direct role of virus and viral replication in early injury in myocarditis, studies involving the antiviral agent ribavirin[74] and interferon[75] have shown that an inhibition of myocardial virus replication reduces the early inflammatory response in virus-induced myocarditis.

Susceptibility to chronic myocarditis. The genetic background of the host has also been shown to determine

which immunologic effector mechanisms are elicited after CVB3 infection. Huber, et al,[76] have shown that in CVB3-infected BALB/c mice, cytotoxic T cells (CD8[+]) were primarily responsible for a primary cell-mediated cardiac injury. In other strains of mice (DBA/2), humoral immunity plays a more dominant role with production of heart-specific autoantibodies and a pathogenic population of CD4[+] helper-T cells. Huber, et al,[76-77] have shown that 3 distinct T lymphocyte subpopulations were produced in CVB3 infected BALB/c mice. These populations include virus-specific cytotoxic T lymphocytes (CTLs) that probably recognize viral peptides in association with MHC-Class I or Class II molecules, CTLs that nonspecifically lyse normal myocytes, and a population of T cells that express the gamma-delta T cell receptor (TcR) and presumably recognize heat shock proteins. These observations suggest that the epitope recognized by the autoreactive CTL population is present on normal myocytes that are not manipulated by virus infection. The specificity of this autoreactive CTL population was demonstrated by showing that CTLs generated from mice infected with a nonmyocarditic strain of CVB3 could only lyse virus-infected myocytes, whereas CTLs generated from mice infected with a myocarditic CVB3 variant were cytotoxic to both infected and uninfected normal myocytes. One population of T cells is therefore viral specific and one reacts to nonviral epitopes, which were later characterized by Gauntt, et al, as glycoproteins of cellular rather than viral origin.[78-79] Recent studies by Traystman, et al, have mapped the susceptibility to CVB3-chronic myocarditis near the murine T cell receptor (Tcr-alpha) and myosin heavy chain (Myhc-alpha) loci on chromosome 14.[80] Their observations suggest that genetic predisposition to myocarditis may reflect the genetic predisposition of a host's T cell receptor to recognize specific antigenic epitopes of cardiac proteins, such as myosin heavy chain.

Humoral autoimmunity is another pathogenic mechanism in those mouse strains susceptible to chronic myocarditis. Studies in our laboratory[81-82] have shown that CVB3-infected mice with ongoing myocarditis frequently produced circulating heart-reactive IgG autoantibodies reactive with cardiac myosin heavy chain. If these heart autoantibodies were important in the pathogenesis of myocarditis, then immunization of mice with myosin should elicit a potent antibody response and myocarditis. Indeed, immunization of susceptible mice with cardiac myosin by several laboratories has induced severe myocarditis associated with high titers of antimyosin antibodies.[83-84] The antigenic specificity of cardiac myosin has also been demonstrated; immunization with skeletal or brain myosin does not produce myocarditis. These results affirmed the importance of cardiac myosin in the induction of autoimmune myocarditis in mice.

To link the appearance of these antibodies to myocardial injury it was first important to determine whether they bind to heart tissue in vivo. Neumann, et al,[85-86] showed that IgG immunoglobulin could be eluted from CVB3 myocarditic hearts, even from those with mild interstitial inflammation. The eluate was primarily reactive to cardiac myosin heavy chain; specific B cells reactive to cardiac myosin could also be isolated from those hearts. When CVB3-infected and myosin-immunized mice with myocarditis were tested for in vivo immunoglobulin G (IgG) deposition, diffuse IgG deposition could be demonstrated within the myocardium even in areas remote to myocyte necrosis or inflammation. These results indicated that some of the reactivity was directed against the surface of intact myocytes. When the eluates themselves were tested for their reactivity to normal mouse heart tissue, a diffuse reactivity both within the myocyte fibrils as well as the myocyte surface could be demonstrated, once again supporting the view that these antibodies react with the normal myocyte sarcolemma.

In CVB3-induced myocarditis an antigenic cross-reactivity between myosin and coxsackievirus has not yet been clearly demonstrated,[87] although recently a homology between viral neutralizing antibody to CVB4 and cardiac myosin has been suggested.[88] This form of molecular mimicry would be analogous to that described both with rheumatic carditis and Chagasic myocarditis. In rheumatic heart disease, the streptococcal M protein shares epitopes with cardiac myosin,[89-90] as well as the alpha-helical coiled-coil proteins such as tropomyosin.[91] The concept of molecular mimicry as a pathogenic mechanism directly involved in valvular injury in rheumatic heart disease also has been supported in more recent observations that human heart valves have numerous sites of immunoreactivity with antistreptococcal antibodies and acute rheumatic fever sera.[92] Similarly, in Chagasic myocarditis and cardiomyopathy, antisera directed against the *Trypanosoma cruzi* organism cross-react with sarcolemmal proteins, which may have a direct pathogenic role in cardiac contractile dysfunction.[93]

The simplest explanation for the induction of autoimmunity in experimental postviral myocarditis is virus-mediated myocyte damage promoting the accessibility of myosin to immunoreactive cells. This can occur from leakage of myosin from virally damaged myocytes with subsequent uptake, processing and presentation of the myosin epitopes by resident dendritic cells, or infiltrating macrophages (antigen presenting cells, APCs). Alternatively, IFN-gamma or other cytokine-induced expression of MHC-Class II antigens on myocytes may allow the presentation of processed forms of myosin by myocytes directly.[94] Either an intracellular protein such as myosin can be transported to the myocyte sarcolemma, or myosin and/or a cross-reactive epitope of myosin is a normal resident of the sarcolemma. By either of these mechanisms, the presence of autoimmunity to heart proteins in CVB3 myocarditis has been firmly established.

However, the presence of autoimmunity in heart proteins does not demonstrate that the myocardial injury is due to heart-reactive autoantibodies. Similar autoantibodies to cardiac myosin are produced after cytomegalovirus (CMV)-induced myocarditis in mice.[95] This fact demonstrates that the antigenic stimulus arises from the host's own myocardial cells rather than from the virus itself. Autoimmunity may be elicited in a final common pathway after myocardial damage takes place. Huber, et al,[96] have recently reported that heart-reactive T cells from CVB3-infected mice also recognize cardiac myocytes treated with the cardiotoxic drug adriamycin, suggesting that both virally-induced and drug-induced changes may induce the expression and/or presentation of similar antigens.

Physiologic effects of cytokines and antibodies on cardiac function

Several studies have characterized the inflammatory infiltrates in murine myocarditis using immunohistochemical techniques.[48,79,97] A mixed inflammatory cell infiltrate similar to that seen in human myocarditis[47] is composed of T cells, macrophages and natural killer (NK) cells, and peaks 5 to 10 days after infection. T cells may produce injury either by direct cytotoxic effects or by production of cytokines. In-vitro studies of CTL cytotoxicity reveal that after contact with the target cell, lymphocyte granules distributed adjacent to the target fuse with the cell membrane and are released into the extracellular microenvironment. One of the effector molecules contained within cytoplasmic granules of CTLs (CD8+) and asialo-GM1 positive cells (natural killer or NK type) is a pore-forming protein or perforin. This protein has recently been demonstrated in cardiac tissues of CVB3-infected mice during the acute phase of myocarditis.[98] Since NK cells are known to be protective during the earliest phases of acute viral myocarditis (day 3), it is likely that virally infected cells have altered sarcolemmal surfaces that act as targets for perforin-containing CTLs for eradication of the virus. The role of such CTLs in the late, chronic autoimmune phase of myocarditis is not known, although recent studies in our laboratory[99] have shown that a mouse strain genetically resistant to CVB3 myocarditis will develop myocarditis when treated with tumor necrosis factor (TNF) or interleukin-1 along with the viral inoculum. Mononuclear cells secreting TNF and IL-1 have also been recently identified in CVB3 myocarditis. These recent findings suggest that local cytokine production may play a significant direct role in myocyte injury. Studies by Leiros et al,[100] have demonstrated that the addition of IFN-gamma to beating rat atria decreased contractile function in a dose-dependent manner. Studies by Hassein[101] et al, have recently demonstrated that cultured rat cardiocytes infected with mengovirus and incubated with lymphocytes sensitized to the virus produce irreversible depolarization. Treatment with verapamil and early washout of lymphocytes reversed these abnormalities. Leiros[102] et al, induced autoimmune myocarditis in mice and found that splenic T lymphocytes induced a negative inotropic response in normal atrial tissue from allogeneic mice.

As noted earlier, in addition to a mixed inflammatory infiltrate, murine myocarditis is characterized by diffuse IgG deposition, which has been shown to react with cardiac myosin.[85-86] The direct role for antimyosin antibodies in the pathogenesis of cardiac dysfunction has not yet been fully characterized, but recent studies by Leiros et al,[102-103] have demonstrated that circulating autoantibodies in animals immunized with whole heart extracts (A) bind to myocardial muscarinic cholinergic receptors and reduce contractility, and (B) inhibit the binding of [(3)H]-dihydroalprenolol to a beta-adrenergic receptor of purified myocardial membranes, behaving as a beta-adrenergic antagonist. These findings support the potential pathogenic role of myosin autoantibodies in murine myocarditis.

We and others have searched for circulating autoantibodies to other putative human autoantigens, such as the adenine nucleotide translocator (ANT) and the branched chain ketoacid dehydrogenase (BCKD). Antibodies to these 2 mitochondrial proteins have been widely described in human myocarditis and idiopathic dilated cardiomyopathy.[104-106] Of interest was the observation that sera from CVB3 infected mice, in addition to antimyosin antibodies, also develop antibodies to the ANT and BCKD proteins (Neumann, personal communication). This finding has potential physiologic consequences since Schultheiss, et al,[107] and Schultz, et al,[108-109] have demonstrated that (1) rabbit anti-ANT cross-reacts with a normal Ca^{++} channel plasma membrane protein of cardiac myocytes, (2) anti-ANT antibodies enhance intracellular calcium transport when added to isolated beating cardiac myocyte,[110] and (3) immunization of guinea pigs with purified ANT induces abnormal ANT carrier function in vivo[108] and causes marked impairment in cardiac function in vivo.[109] These studies suggest that in virus-induced myocyte injury a variety of myocyte proteins are accessible to antigen-presenting cells that initiate an antigen-specific immune response. For intracellular molecules to become targets for specific immune effectors, it would seem that myocyte surface expression would be required. While it is widely accepted that myosin is not expressed on the myocyte surface, certain nonmuscle myosin isoforms are membrane-associated and may extend into the extracellular milieu. To determine whether myosin was the major antigen recognized by tissue-bound immunoglobulin in CVB3-infected mice, Neumann, et al,[85] eluted cardiac-bound IgG and demonstrated that it reacted primarily with myosin, which suggests that it was indeed the major protein eliciting an antibody response. In terms of human disease, myosin, ANT and BCKD have been demonstrated on the surface membrane of isolated cardiac myocytes from acute myocarditis patients,[106] supporting the hypothesis that the myocardial microenvironment in myocarditis may promote surface expression of nominally intracellular proteins. These studies as a whole strongly suggest that humoral autoimmune mechanisms may play a significant primary or enhancing role in the pathogenesis of cardiac dysfunction in human myocarditis.

Murine myocarditis and cardiomyopathy

CMV and CVB3 infection in mice do not usually produce a dilated cardiomyopathy with congestive heart failure acutely, although both can produce a chronic cardiomyopathy over 5 to 12 months.[111-113] In contrast, encephalomyocarditis (EMC) infection of DBA/2 mice frequently produces a severe myocarditis with cardiomegaly, clinical congestive heart failure and death within 2 weeks of inoculation.[114] Modification of viral dose can produce a milder form of myocarditis similar histologically to borderline myocarditis in humans.[115]

The potential use of serologic studies for autoantibodies as diagnostic tools in chronic myocarditis leading to cardiomyopathy is supported by the recent identification of circulating autoantibodies to cardiac myosin demonstrated in mice with chronic CMV myocarditis until 100 days postinfection.[113] These findings are consistent with in situ hybridization techniques that demonstrate persistent viral genome within infected hearts as late as 2 to 3 months postinoculation.[34-35] Similarly, the potential use for antimyosin antibody scanning in myocarditis and cardiomyopathy is also supported by studies performed by Kishimoto et al,[116] who have demonstrated that mice infected with EMC have intensely abnormal antimyosin antibody scans on day 10 during the acute phase of myocarditis. Abnormal scans persisted in 30% to 40% of the animals through day 150, at which point mice were found to have persistent left ventricular dysfunction (ejection fractions of 30%) by technetium-99m radionuclide ventriculography.

In conclusion, although the histologic features of murine myocarditis may appear more similar to the most severe cases of myocarditis in humans, the entire histologic spectrum of human myocarditis can be reproduced by using genetically inbred strains of mice,[67] by altering the host conditions such as the age and sex of the animal, exposure to exercise and toxins, pregnancy or secondary viral infection,[117] or by altering the virus conditions (such as the use of less virulent strains of virus).[118] Strong evidence exists for viral persistence in infected mice long after viral cultures and viral neutralizing antibody assays are negative. The development of a chronic myocarditis associated with aberrant MHC expression within the myocardium in genetically susceptible strains, as well as the persistence of cardiac-specific circulating autoantibodies as late as 5 months after infection, suggest a role for both cellular and humoral autoimmune responses. The potential role of cytokines and circulating autoantibodies in direct modulation of cardiac function are now becoming elucidated. **These** findings lead to the hypothesis that genetic susceptibility, the presence of enhancing environmental factors, and the immunogenicity of the virus itself are all likely to play a significant role in human disease and are the basis for understanding the wide spectrum of clinical presentations of myocarditis.

Potential effects of viruses on endothelial cells, smooth muscle cells and the extracellular matrix

In addition to myocytes, CVB3 is known to infect fibroblasts, endothelial cells and smooth muscle cells.[78,119-120] Direct or indirect virus-mediated injury to the interstitial connective tissue matrix and to the microcirculation are significant potential causes of cardiac dysfunction in myocarditis and postmyocarditis cardiomyopathy. Extensive abnormalities within the collagen matrix have been demonstrated in murine myocarditis[115,121] and in murine Chagas' disease.[122] Of particular importance, the pattern of collagen deposition and reduplication characteristic of reactive interstitial fibrosis in human cardiomyopathy is closely associated with persistent interstitial inflammation. This suggests that cytokines may play a significant role in the modulation of the cardiac interstitium during chronic myocarditis. In addition, cytokines have been demonstrated to modulate endothelial and smooth muscle cell function, and may therefore play a critical role in affecting the microcirculation during an episode of myocarditis. The hypothesis that microcirculatory spasm plays an important role in dilated cardiomyopathy is well described.[123-124] An important role for microvascular spasm in the pathogenesis of Chagasic cardiomyopathy, a clear example of a postinflammatory cardiomyopathy, has been elucidated.[125] In addition, as mentioned previously, the earliest histologic pattern of myocyte injury in CVB3 myocarditis is contraction band necrosis of small clusters of myocytes. This finding is consistent with an injury pattern caused by microcirculatory spasm of small and medium sized arterioles, with subsequent ischemia and reperfusion of small regions of myocardium. Future studies using in situ hybridization techniques will be needed to precisely locate viral proteins or genes within the myocardium in both early and late phases of myocarditis, and thus characterize the role of direct viral infection of vascular and interstitial elements in myocarditis.

Human studies

Human myocarditis is characterized by microscopic, discrete areas of myocyte necrosis with focal interstitial infiltrates. The inability to relate the severity of myocardial damage to the severity of cardiac contractile function suggests a role for tissue-bound autoantibodies and locally produced cytokines in the pathogenesis of cardiac dysfunction in myocarditis. The prevailing dogma states that a triggering event such as a cardiotropic virus induces initial cardiac tissue damage, which leads to infiltration by mononuclear cells. The majority of patients that recover quickly without lasting sequelae likely have the immune response genes that produce a rapid viral neutralizing antibody response, an adequate natural killer cell response, and adequate removal of virally infected myocardial cells expressing MHC Class I by cytotoxic T lymphocytes. The mechanisms responsible for the induction and perpetuation of mononuclear cell infiltrates (which recognize self-proteins by an undefined pathway), leading to the local production of cytokines and circulating heart-reactive autoantibodies, are not yet known. It is likely though, that chronic, episodic effervescence of latent virus (such as enteroviruses and cytomegalovirus) or a secondary viral infection may trigger ongoing cardiac tissue damage over longer periods of time, eventually leading to dilated cardiomyopathy.[117]

Role of enteroviruses. Isolation of enteroviruses from cardiac tissue of patients with myocarditis is rarely successful. Coxsackieviruses B4 and B5 have been isolated as well as echovirus 22.[126] Because viral recovery has not been clinically useful, the evidence implicating enteroviruses in the etiology of human myocarditis has come largely from observations of increased enteroviral antibody titers among patients with myocarditis. Because enteroviruses are very common human pathogens and the actual temporal relationship between an acute viral infection and clinical heart disease is frequently unclear, these results do not firmly establish an enteroviral etiology to myocarditis. Conclusive evidence that viruses play a role in human myocarditis requires the identification of virus within the myocardium of patients with myocarditis in contract to patients with other specific heart muscle diseases in whom no virus is identified. Recently, in situ nucleic acid hybridization techniques have been successfully applied to the detection of virus-specific nucleotide sequences in endomyocardial biopsy samples.

Easton and Eglin[127] detected enteroviral RNA in 5 (42%) of 12 biopsy samples from cardiac tissues of patients with clinical symptoms of myocarditis. Tracy, et al,[126,128] detected enteroviral RNA foci in 3 of 17 (18%) frozen biopsy samples, 2 of which showed myocarditis by histologic criteria. Studies by Kandolf, et al,[34,35] have demonstrated enteroviral RNA in 19 of 81 (23%) patients with a clinical suspicion of myocarditis, including 8 of 27 (29%) patients with idiopathic dilated cardiomyopathy. His studies utilized 30 control patients with other specific cardiac disorders, all of which were negative for enteroviral RNA. Archard, et al,[37,129] found 17 of 44 (39%) patients with either "acute or healing myocarditis" to be positive, and 22 of 54 (41%) of patients with "healed myocarditis/dilated cardiomyopathy." None of 36 control patients were found to be positive.

In addition to nucleic acid hybridization techniques, which can usually localize the site of nucleic acid hybridization within tissue slices, the polymerase chain reaction (PCR) amplification technique allows rapid and substantive amplification of specific nucleic acid sequences in extracts prepared from tissue samples. Jin, et al,[39] applied the PCR technique to cardiac biopsies taken from 48 patients with clinically suspected myocarditis or dilated cardiomyopathy, and found 5 of 48 (10%) demonstrating a positive enteroviral signal by PCR. In another study, Weiss, et al,[38] using PCR amplification for the detection of coxsackievirus B3 RNA, found that 1 of 5 myocarditis specimens and none of 11 idiopathic cardiomyopathy samples were positive.

These studies provide the first compelling evidence that enteroviral genomic material is present in some human hearts with myocarditis and cardiomyopathy. Great care must now be exercised in the performance of future studies.[126,128] Enteroviral probes that share homology with all or many enteroviruses (group specific) must be distinguished from strain specific probes (e.g., CVB3 specific). Greater experience with the use of these probes regarding standardization of assays, reproducibility of results and the further documentation of the specificity of these assays by continued studies with control tissues will be most helpful. Utilization of these probes on tissues derived from the Myocarditis Treatment Trial would, as an initial step, document the prevalence of enteroviral genomic material in a well-characterized group of patients.

Evidence of genetic factors. Numerous studies have described multiple immunologic defects in patients with idiopathic dilated cardiomyopathy, including defects in natural killer cells,[130] suppressor lymphocyte activity,[131] myocyte specific cytotoxic T cell responses,[132] and the production of a number of cardiac-specific autoantibodies. Because of the immune hypothesis of idiopathic dilated cardiomyopathy (IDCM) and the association between autoimmune disease and HLA molecules, in 1984, Anderson, et al,[133] published a retrospective HLA-typing study in IDCM patients that revealed an increased frequency of HLA-DR4 and a decreased frequency of HLA-DRw6 in idiopathic dilated cardiomyopathy patients. These findings were corroborated by studies performed by Limas et al,[134] who demonstrated an increased prevalence of HLA-DR4 in idiopathic dilated cardiomyopathy patients. Furthermore, a genetic predisposition towards cardiac autoantibody production was also demonstrated by the fact that 72% of HLA-DR4–positive patients had anti-B-receptor antibodies, versus 21% of HLA-DR4–negative patients. In the largest study to date, Carlquist et al,[135] has reconfirmed these findings and also found that the DR4-DQw4 haplotype bears an indeterminantly high risk of disease. In a metaanalysis of five studies he confirmed that the DR4 association could be replicated in several different patient populations. His study concluded that there were predisposing genetic factors linked to immunoregulatory loci in idiopathic dilated cardiomyopathy. Similar studies involving large numbers of patients with myocarditis have not yet been performed.

Evidence of autoimmunity. Autoantibodies have been identified in human myocarditis and cardiomyopathy in two ways. Organ-specific autoantibodies have been identified using an indirect immunofluorescence testing[132,136-138] in approximately 40% to 60% of patients with myocarditis, and in 20% to 26% of patients with IDCM (Fig. 6-2). Patterns of reactivity are noted, such as antifibrillary or antisarcolemmal (Fig. 6-2). These assays are nonquantitative screening methods which are now commercially available. Specific autoantibodies have been identified using Western immunoblotting and ELISA techniques. These include two intracellular mitochondrial proteins, the adenine nucleotide translocator (ANT) protein and the branched chain alpha-ketoacid dehydrogenase (BCKD) protein,[106] as well as the cell membrane B-adrenoreceptor[134,139] protein. These assays are quantitative and may represent future methods of assessing both diagnosis, therapy and prognosis in myocarditis. The direct pathogenic significance of these autoantibodies are not established, although a number of recent studies described earlier highlight their pathogenic significance in experimental myocarditis.

Although antibodies to these putative antigens have clearly been demonstrated in patients with myocarditis and cardiomyopathy, cross-reactivity against some other protein that shares epitopes with these putative autoantigens remains a possibility. Antigenic mimicry has been considered as a possible mode for the pathogenic mechanisms in a variety of autoimmune diseases, similar to the relationship between streptococcal M protein and myosin.[90] Preliminary findings in our laboratory suggest that IgG antibodies to CVB3 do cross-react with as yet undetermined cardiac proteins are consistent with this view, although previous studies in CVB3 murine myocarditis have failed to identify cross-reactivity between myosin antibodies and CVB3.[87]

Evidence of immune targeting of the myocardium. Products of the major histocompatibility complex (MHC) genes have been shown to present processed forms of antigens such as viruses to the immune system. T lymphocytes can recognize antigens only in the context of self-MHC molecules. MHC Class I molecules in the presence of viral antigens appear to be the target of sensitized, predominantly CD8[+] cytotoxic T lymphocytes. MHC Class II molecules on the other hand, in the presence of processed antigen predominantly activate CD4+ helper-T lymphocytes. Normal human fetal and adult cardiac myocytes express low levels of (MHC) Class I antigens (HLA A, B and C regions) and do not express detectable levels of MHC Class II antigens[140] (HLA DP, DQ and DR regions) (Fig. 6-3, A). Increased expression of these MHC antigens have been demonstrated in a number of tissues undergoing autoimmune injury, allograft rejection and viral illnesses. In a recent series of studies we have demonstrated the induction of aberrant MHC Class I and MHC Class II antigens on myocytes from endomyocardial biopsy samples

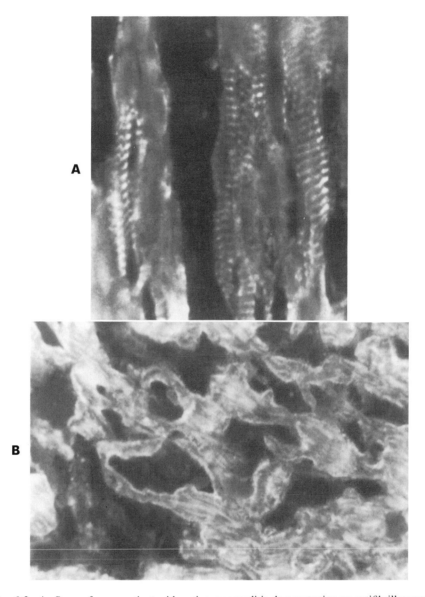

Fig. 6-2. A, Serum from a patient with active myocarditis demonstrating an antifibrillary reactivity pattern using an indirect immunofluorescence assay. The tissue used was normal rat myocardium. **B,** Similarly, another patient with active myocarditis whose serum demonstrates an antisarcolemmal reactivity pattern.

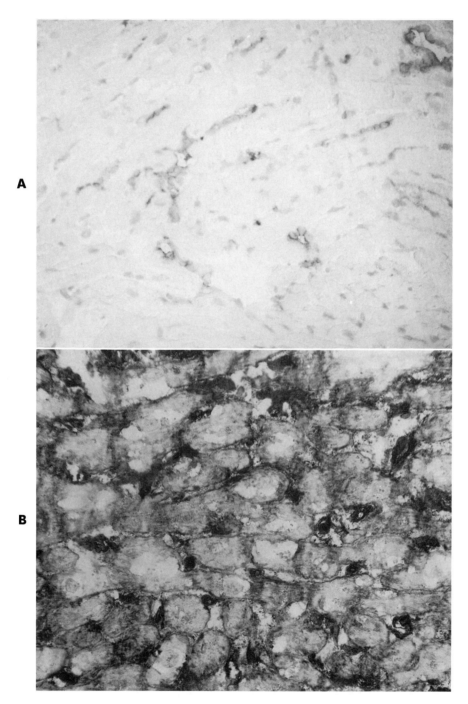

Fig. 6-3. A, Immunoperoxidase staining for MHC Class I antigen expression of a frozen section taken from an endomyocardial biopsy sample from a patient with ischemic cardiomyopathy. Note the sparse staining of microvascular endothelium with no appreciable staining of myocytes. **B,** Similar immunoperoxidase staining for MHC Class I antigen expression of a frozen section taken from an endomyocardial biopsy sample from a patient with active myocarditis. Note the intense staining of the microvascular capillary bed, as well as the discrete staining of sarcolemmal surfaces of myocytes.

from 11/13 myocarditis patients and 5/15 patients with idiopathic dilated cardiomyopathy[140-141] (Fig. 6-3, *B*). In addition, Ansari, et al, have recently shown that small discrete foci of cardiac tissue in DCM and myocarditis patients express quantitatively high levels of ANT and BCKD.[106] These findings were most clearly defined in several pediatric cases of fulminant myocarditis, in which flow cytometry revealed that ANT and BCKD were aberrantly expressed on the surface membrane of cardiac myocytes. These findings were not seen in tissue from patients with a variety of other forms of cardiomyopathy and normal tissue. Thus the identification of putative myocyte autoantigens being presented to the immune system in the context of abnormal expression of MHC antigens, provides the first clear immunohistochemical evidence that both myocarditis and idiopathic dilated cardiomyopathy may represent a spectrum of immune-mediated myocardial injury.

CLINICAL CLASSIFICATION

Although the Dallas criteria provide diagnostic guidelines for the histologic diagnosis, thereby aiding in patient identification, the varied clinical presentations of myocarditis also require some form of uniform description and classification. Recent efforts at our institution[16] has led to a classification of myocarditis based on both clinical and pathologic information, analogous to the accepted classification of viral hepatitis (Table 6-2). Four categories are described: fulminant, acute, chronic persistent and chronic active myocarditis.

Fulminant myocarditis is heralded by a nonspecific flu-like illness and distinct onset of cardiac involvement. The patient's condition rapidly deteriorates and frequently results in profound hemodynamic compromise. Endomyo-

cardial biopsies from such patients demonstrate unequivocal active myocarditis, and are particularly notable for very extensive inflammatory infiltrates and numerous foci of myocyte necrosis (Fig. 6-4). Finally, within 1 month, the patients either completely recover left ventricular function or they succumb to their disease.[142]

Acute myocarditis represents the clinical spectrum of the largest group of patients with active or borderline myocarditis. These patients have minimally dilated, hypokinetic left ventricles on presentation. The onset of their cardiac symptoms is frequently indistinct and some patients provide a vague history consistent with but not diagnostic of an antecedent viral illness. Active or borderline myocarditis is present on initial but not subsequent endomyocardial biopsies. In our experience, some patients appear to respond to immunosuppressive therapy[143] and experience a partial recovery in ventricular function. Others within this group continue to show deterioration to end-stage dilated cardiomyopathy.

Similarly, *chronic active myocarditis* has an indistinct clinical presentation. These patients pursue a slowly progressive, inevitably deteriorating course which may be punctuated by brief, often dramatic but unsustained responses to immunosuppressive therapy. Serial endomyocardial biopsies demonstrate ongoing myocarditis, the development of extensive interstitial fibrosis and frequently, giant cells (Fig. 6-5).

Chronic persistent myocarditis patients come to medical attention with atypical chest pain, palpitations or other noncongestive heart failure symptoms. They display no signs or symptoms of left ventricular dysfunction and all invasive and noninvasive studies of ventricular function are normal despite unequivocal histologic evidence of ongoing myocardial inflammation. In our experience, the

Table 6-2. Clinical classification of myocarditis

	Fulminant	Acute	Chronic active	Chronic persistent
Onset of clinical symptoms	Distinct	Indistinct	Indistinct	Indistinct
Initial presentation	Cardiogenic shock; severe LV dysfunction	CHF; LV dysfunction	CHF; LV dysfunction	No CHF; normal LV function
Initial endomyocardial biopsy	Multiple foci of active myocarditis	Active or borderline myo.	Active or borderline myo.	Active or borderline myo.
Clinical natural history	Complete recovery or death	Incomplete recovery or DCM	DCM	Non-CHF symptoms normal LV function
Histologic natural history	Complete resolution of active myocarditis	Complete resolution	Ongoing or resolving myo., fibrosis and giant cells	Ongoing or resolving myo.
Immunosuppressive therapy	No benefit	Sometimes beneficial	No benefit	No benefit
Estimated percentage of myocarditis population	20%	65%	10%	5%

CHF = congestive heart failure; DCM = dilated cardiomyopathy; LV = left ventricular; myo = myocarditis.

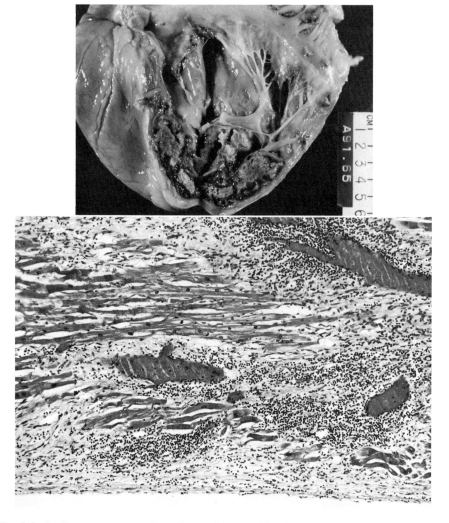

Fig. 6-4. A, Gross autopsy specimen from a 31-year-old male with fulminant myocarditis. The right ventricle is cut along its long axis to demonstrate an apical mural thrombus. **B,** Microscopic examination of the myocardium revealed extensive mononuclear inflammation, replacing large clusters of myocytes which have undergone necrosis.

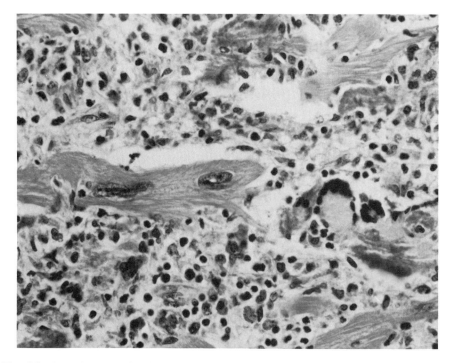

Fig. 6-5. An endomyocardial biopsy specimen from a 37-year-old female with chronic active myocarditis. There is an extensive mononuclear infiltrate associated with dense interstitial fibrosis. A large, multinucleated giant cell can be seen within the interstitial infiltrate.

myocardial infiltrate does not appear to be improved with immunosuppressive therapy.

Controversies regarding efficacy of immunosuppression in myocarditis

In the early 1900s the only treatment for myocarditis was absolute bedrest. The potential role for immunosuppressive therapy in myocarditis should be great, if patients with immune-mediated cardiac injury could be identified in a sensitive and specific fashion. Numerous centers have treated small numbers of patients during the last 20 years, and in the mid-1980s the need for a multicenter study became evident. The Myocarditis Treatment Trial is the recently completed National Institutes of Health sponsored study designed to assess the efficacy of immunosuppressive therapy in patients with active myocarditis. Patients with biopsy-proven active myocarditis and left ventricular dysfunction (ejection fractions < 45%) were randomly assigned to receive either conventional therapy alone for congestive heart failure, or conventional therapy plus immunosuppression (prednisone and cyclosporine) for a total of 6 months. Noninvasive measures of LV function were assessed for 1 year. A total of 206 patients of 2236 that underwent endomyocardial biopsy were diagnosed with active myocarditis (9%). The strict biopsy criteria for entry into the Myocarditis Treatment Trial ensured the histologic homogeneity of the population. Pending the results of this trial, the benefits of immunosuppressive therapy for patients with myocarditis are not yet established with certainty. The benefits of immunosuppressive therapy for patients with borderline myocarditis, as well as positive gallium and antimyosin antibody scans were not endpoints of the MTT.

Another landmark placebo controlled study was performed by Parrillo, et al,[29] who studied a heterogeneous group of patients with idiopathic dilated cardiomyopathy. Most of these patients had long-standing idiopathic dilated cardiomyopathy. Patients were randomly assigned to receive prednisone or placebo, and randomization was stratified according to the presence or absence of self-described "indicators" of myocardial inflammation (e.g., elevated erythrocyte sedimentation rate, positive gallium scan or biopsy specimen positive for immunoglobulin or complement deposition). It is not known whether any of these "indicators" are reflective of immune-mediated cardiac injury. The patients were treated with prednisone for 3 months; then steroid therapy was altered or discontinued until the completion of follow-up. The study demonstrated that unselected patients with dilated cardiomyopathy do not benefit substantially from immunosuppressive therapy. A small, significant short-term benefit in ventricular function was demonstrated in patients who had evidence of inflammation as defined by the investigators. Becuase only 2 of 102 patients had histologic evidence of myocarditis by our current criteria, these results suggest that other nonhis-

tologic "indicators" may be clinically useful markers of immune-mediated injury and that the population of patients with immune-mediated cardiac injury may be substantially larger than the patients with diagnostic biopsy changes.

Other nonrandomized studies appear to corroborate the potential role for immunosuppressive therapy in myocarditis as defined by scintigraphic studies. O'Connell, et al,[14] demonstrated that in 15 patients with positive gallium scans (all treated with immunosuppressive drugs), those with unchanged scans (n = 9) did not improve hemodynamically, while those with improved scans (n = 6) clinically improved. In a study by Dec, et al,[54] where indium-111 antimyosin imaging was performed in 82 patients, improvement in left ventricular function occurred within 6 months of immunosuppressive treatment in 54% of patients with an abnormal antimyosin scan, compared with 18% of those with a normal scan (p < 0.01).

In a preliminary study at our institution involving 20 patients with either active (n = 9) or borderline (n = 11) myocarditis, Jones, et al,[143] found that short-term immunosuppressive therapy (6 to 8 weeks with prednisone 1.0 mg/kg/d and azathioprine, 1.5 mg/kg/d) improved LV contractile function and was associated with regression of ventricular dilatation in patients with borderline myocarditis to a greater extent than patients with active myocarditis. Although these findings require further study, they suggest that patients with borderline myocarditis should be considered for inclusion in subsequent trials of immunosuppressive therapy in myocarditis. The possibility that borderline myocarditis may also represent immune-mediated cardiac injury is also supported by studies by Dec, et al,[53] that have shown that on repeat biopsy, many of these patients indeed have active myocarditis, reflecting problems with sampling error rather than a different disease. In addition, in our own experience, the prevalence of anti-heart antibodies and aberrant MHC expression by immunohistochemistry are no different in patients with active or borderline myocarditis.[136,140]

SPECIFIC ENTITIES
HIV-associated myocarditis and cardiomyopathy

Early in the AIDS epidemic, autopsy series described a variety of cardiac abnormalities in patients infected with the human immunodeficiency virus (HIV). Marantic endocarditis, metastatic Kaposi's sarcoma and opportunistic infection of the myocardium and pericardium were noted. Later studies confirmed that clinically significant and life-threatening cardiomyopathy was also part of the spectrum of HIV-related cardiac disease.[144] Echocardiographic studies have further documented common abnormalities that are clinically silent, e.g., pericardial effusions and marantic endocarditis, as well as clinically significant dilated cardiomyopathy, in 11% to 22% of adults with HIV infection.[145]

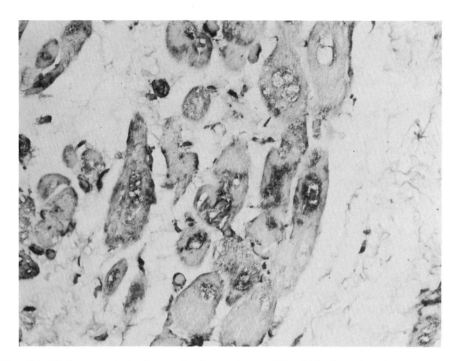

Fig. 6-6. High power photomicrograph of the antisense CMV IE-2 riboprobe taken from an endomyocardial biopsy of a patient with HIV-associated myocarditis. Note the intense staining within clusters of myocytes, which are predominantly within nuclear and perinuclear regions.

A direct HIV myocardial cell cytotoxicity has yet to be demonstrated, although HIV has been cultured from one endomyocardial biopsy specimen and HIV viral genome has been identified within myocardial autopsy tissue in AIDS patients with no known cardiac dysfunction during life.[146] In addition, a recent study by Rodriguez et al, using a polymerase chain reaction, found both cardiac myocytes and dendritic cells to harbor HIV-1 sequences in patients with and without cardiac dysfunction.[147] Lymphocytic myocarditis has been frequently found in autopsies of HIV-infected patients with and without known cardiac disease during life. In addition, a high prevalence of myocarditis has recently been described in endomyocardial biopsies from HIV-infected patients with cardiomyopathy.[47,148] Current hypotheses concerning the etiology of cardiomyopathy related to HIV infection include coinfection with other cardiotropic viruses, postviral cardiac autoimmunity, selenium deficiency, autonomic dysfunction and cardiotoxicity from illicit drugs such as cocaine and heroin, as well as commonly used antiretroviral drugs. One commonly used drug in HIV-infected patients, pentamidine, is known to exhibit cardiotoxicity in the form of recurrent ventricular tachycardia.

The role of cardiotropic viruses. Recently we undertook a study using nucleic acid hybridization techniques to determine the prevalence of HIV and cytomegalovirus genomic material in 20 HIV-infected patients with left ventricular dysfunction, 13 with congestive heart failure and 7 without congestive heart failure. A positive HIV signal

was found in 5 endomyocardial biopsy samples (20%) and showed clear myocyte localization in 4 of 5 cases. The remaining case showed positive HIV signal within interstitial mononuclear cells. Cytomegalovirus genomic probes for immediate early (IE-2) gene products (consistent with "latent" or nonpermissive viral infection) were demonstrated in 9 patients (45%), and showed clear hybridization signal within myocyte nuclei, nucleoli and perinuclear regions (Fig. 6-6). CMV hybridization, utilizing probes for delayed early gene products (consistent with lytic or permissive CMV viral infection), was present in only one case. In none of the cases were classic intranuclear inclusions revealed by histologic examination. All 5 patients with HIV genomic material within the myocardium had concurrent CMV involvement, indicating some possible interaction between the two viruses. All patients with abnormal hybridization signals clinically presented with congestive heart failure with either active or borderline myocarditis on biopsy, and aberrant myocardial expression of MHC Class I on immunohistochemical stains.[47] At this point, the role of enteroviruses in HIV-related myocarditis and cardiomyopathy is not known.

Myocarditis in immunosuppressed patients (Fig. 6-7, *A-D*)

Immunosuppressed patients appear to be at increased risk of myocarditis secondary to opportunistic infection of the myocardium. Patients post-organ transplantation, undergoing chemotherapy for tumor eradication, and patients

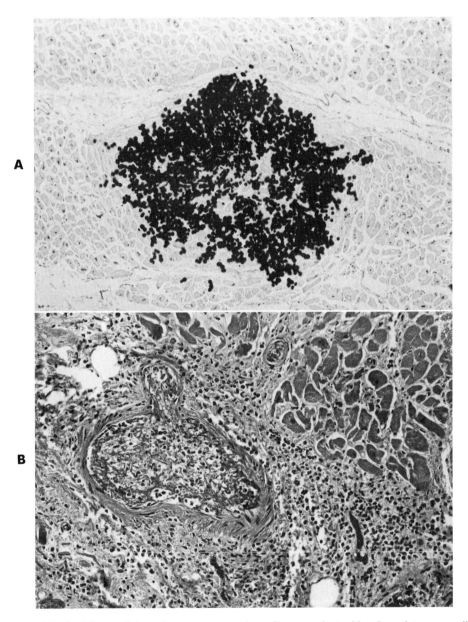

Fig. 6-7. A, Silver staining of an autopsy specimen from a patient with a large intramyocardial abscess secondary to *Candida*. **B,** An autopsy case of *Aspergillus* myocarditis associated with a mycotic mural coronary thrombus and vasculitis.   *continued*.

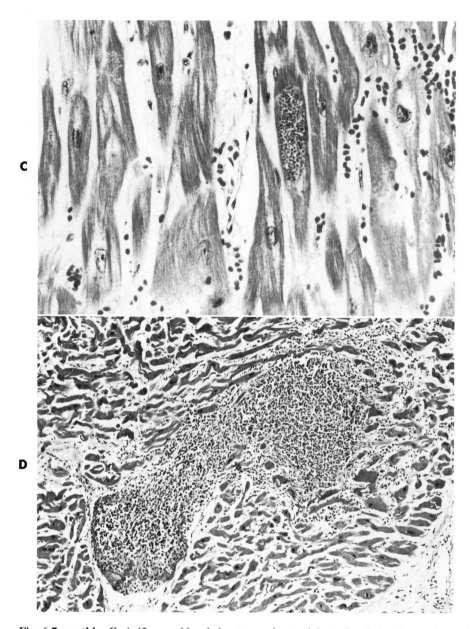

Fig. 6-7, cont'd. **C,** A 42-year-old male heart transplant recipient who died with toxoplasmosis. Typical organisms can be easily identified in one myocyte. There is an increased number of interstitial mononuclear cells, and a few noninfected myocytes appear to be undergoing necrosis. **D,** A case of acute suppurative myocarditis with a characteristic myocardial abscess.

with acquired immunodeficiency syndrome are commonly found to have evidence of myocarditis at autopsy. The most common cardiotropic fungal organisms are *Candida, Aspergillus* and *Cryptococcus*,[149-150] all of which may produce myocarditis, endocarditis, pericarditis or pancarditis. Patients may be asymptomatic from a cardiovascular perspective, or may present with regional or global cardiac contractile dysfunction, conduction system abnormalities such as heart block, or mycotic embolic events secondary to endocarditis. In addition to fungal organisms, opportunistic protozoal infection with *Toxoplasma gondii* has been similarly reported in immunosuppressed patients.[151] Myocarditis associated with *Toxoplasma gondii* has been more commonly associated with severe left ventricular dysfunction than with fungal myocarditis, and clinical congestive heart failure is not uncommon. Bacterial myocarditis is probably diminishing in frequency because of prompt antibiotic treatment of systemic bacterial infections. In most cases, cardiac symptoms and signs are overshadowed by the systemic illness, but its contribution to mortality can still be appreciated during autopsy examination. Viral myocarditis, particularly with cytomegalovirus (CMV), has been recognized with increasing frequency in patients post-cardiac transplantation. Classic intranuclear inclusion bodies within myocytes indicate active, replicating viral infection requiring antiviral therapy.

Chagas disease

Trypanasoma cruzi is a protozoan that causes Chagas disease, the most important cause of heart disease in Latin America.[152] It is estimated that approximately 50,000 deaths annually can be linked to this infection. Most individuals who are naturally infected lack evidence of clinical disease. However, children, and less frequently adults, may develop acute symptoms after a short incubation period. In the acute phase, severe active myocarditis is present, and parasitism of individual myocytes may be evident, although the severity of myocarditis does not predict the subsequent development of chronic cardiomyopathy. The appearance of arrythmias, heart block or progressive congestive heart failure during the acute phase of illness are poor prognostic indicators. The majority of acutely infected patients recover within 3 to 4 months and remain asymptomatic. Approximately 5% to 10% of patients die of cardiac or CNS complications.

During acute disease, pathologic damage probably follows as a consequence of direct parasite-associated cytolysis, or via interference with myocyte metabolism.[152] Infection of endothelial cells may also contribute to myocardial injury secondary to focal coronary microvascular spasm reported in acute murine infection.[125] It has also been recently reported that trypanasomes contain a variety of degradative enzymes such as collagenases and proteases capable of degrading collagen.[122] These enzymes may play an important role in the degradation of the extracellular matrix, which may result in chronic pathology such as aneurysmal thinning of the apex, a characteristic gross feature of Chagas disease.[153]

Dilated cardiomyopathy usually occurs years or decades after acute infection and may present with arrythmias, thromboembolic events or congestive heart failure, which is often associated with four-chamber cardiac dilation. The number of parasites appear to bear little relationship to chronic myocardial pathology supporting the hypothesis that the pathogenesis of chronic chagasic cardiomyopathy has an autoimmune basis. Spleen cells from *T. cruzi*-infected mice have been found to be cytotoxic to normal syngeneic neonatal myocytes.[154] More recent studies have shown that CD4 T cells from chronically infected mice proliferate in response to myosin,[155] and serum from patients with chagasic heart disease contains antibodies directed against a 25kDα *T. cruzi* polypeptide.[3] In addition, Mesri, et al,[156] demonstrated that a major antigenic determinant of *T. cruzi* shares homology with the systemic lupus erythemmatosus ribosomal P protein, and that anti-P autoantibodies are present in patients with chronic Chagas heart disease. The link between the variety of these autoantibodies and the pathogenesis of chagasic heart disease is still unresolved.

Myocarditis and drugs

Drugs can induce myocarditis and/or cardiomyopathy in a number of ways. Anthracycline analogues are the best characterized compounds that cause drug-induced cardiomyopathy.[157] This condition may be idiosyncratic but is usually characterized by being dose-dependent, with its effects sometimes progressing despite the discontinuation of the causative agent. Acute idiosyncratic doxorubicin cardiotoxicity can also be associated with myocarditis on endomyocardial biopsy, which may reflect a component of immune-mediated injury in a certain subpopulation of patients receiving such compounds. Experimental studies in mice receiving adriamycin support the concept that myocytes treated with adriamycin may be immunogenic in genetically susceptible strains.[96] In our own experience, in a small number of adriamycin-treated patients with cardiomyopathy out of proportion to the cumulative dose of adriamycin, active myocarditis associated with circulating anti-heart antibodies has been found. In addition, we have recently described a myocarditis leading to severe LV dysfunction in HIV-infected patients receiving nucleoside analogues such as zidovudine, DDI or DDC.[158]

Drug-induced hypersensitivity or allergic hypersensitivity is not dose-dependent and may arise at any time during treatment.[159-160] Patients are usually not critically ill with respect to their cardiovascular status and usually respond within days to withdrawal of the medication, if it is recognized in a timely fashion. The patient may have classic allergic symptoms with rash, fever, sinus tachycardia and peripheral eosinophilia. A high index of suspicion for this entity should be considered whenever new electrocardiographic changes appear in association with unexpected tachycardia, mildly elevated cardiac enzymes and cardiomegaly in a patient with an allergic drug reaction and eosinophilia. A list of the best known drugs associated with hypersensitivity myocarditis are found in Table 6-1, although the main offenders appear to be sulfonamides, methyldopa, and penicillin and its derivatives. The histologic features of hypersensitivity myocarditis clearly distinguish this entity from the histologic features of active myocarditis described previously. There is usually a mixed infiltrate including plasma cells, lymphocytes and eosinophils, often with concomitant vasculitis. Minimal or no myocyte necrosis is typical. This histologic pattern is distinct from acute necrotizing eosinophilic myocarditis,[161] which is characterized by extensive myocyte necrosis and no notable systemic symptoms of drug allergy. This latter disorder may represent a severe form of hypersensitivity myocarditis and likely highlights an aberrant immunologic reaction, possibly stimulated by drugs in a patient predisposed to myocarditis.

Cocaine. It is estimated that as many as 5 million Americans use cocaine regularly and until recently, there was little information about the cardiovascular effects of cocaine. The most common cardiovascular complications of cocaine are angina, myocardial infarction and arrythmias,[162] although dilated cardiomyopathy and myocarditis are being seen more frequently now.[163-164] Regarding myocarditis, Virmani and colleagues studied 40 medical examiner cases of cocaine-associated deaths and found histologic evidence of myocarditis in 8 patients (20%).[163] Similarly, Turnicky, et al,[165] studied 15 HIV negative intravenous drug abusers with sudden traumatic death and found active myocarditis in 5 (33%), and borderline myocarditis in 5 (33%). Myocarditis in intravenous drug users, particularly cocaine users, is prevalent, and this must be taken into account in the interpretation of endomyocardial biopsy samples from patients with a history of intravenous drug use. In addition, with a high prevalence of contraction band necrosis in intravenous drug abusers secondary to a catecholamine-like microvascular spasm, the presence of ischemic injury on biopsy could also be another histologic pitfall. The possibility that cocaine is a direct myocardial cell toxin has been highlighted by recent studies demonstrating deleterious effects of cocaine on cardiac contractile function in animals. Although the incidence of cardiomyopathy associated with myocarditis in intravenous drug users is uncertain, it has been considered to be rare in the past. Considering the recent coexistence of HIV infection in many intravenous drug users, the possibility exists for a growing number of cases with multiple cardiotoxic factors simultaneously involved in the pathogenesis of cardiomyopathy. In our own experience during the last 2 years, of 35 patients with HIV-associated cardiomyopathy, 19 (54%) were intravenous drug users. While over 70% of the patients presenting with congestive heart failure had

active or borderline myocarditis, the immunohistochemical features of the biopsies (aberrant MHC expression within the myocardium) distinguished these cases from cases with incidental myocarditis. In our study,[165] incidental myocarditis with intravenous cocaine use was not associated with aberrant expression of MHC within the myocardium.

Lyme carditis

Lyme borreliosis, or Lyme disease, is a systemic disorder caused by the spirochete Borrelia burgdorferi, a recently discovered species of borrelia. The organism is endemic to most of the United States, all of Europe, China, Japan, and both the European and Asian parts of Russia. Symptoms usually begin in the summer with a characteristic skin lesion, erythema chronicum migrans, which first appears at the site of the bite. Some patients, particularly those with the B-cell alloantigen HLA-DRw2, develop an abnormal immune response associated with neurologic, cardiac, or joint involvement, days to months after the initial exposure. Although the most common form of cardiac involvement is AV block, often associated with myocarditis and normal LV contractile function, cardiomyopathy has also been described.[166] In a study by Steere, et al,[162] 20 patients with cardiac involvement of Lyme disease were recognized over a 4-year period. Nineteen of them had the onset of erythema chronicum migrans within 3 weeks before the onset of cardiac involvement, and most still had multiple skin lesions when heart disease was present. Some patients also had migratory polyarthritis, oligoarticular arthritis, meningoencephalitis or facial palsy, findings typical of nervous system or joint involvement of Lyme disease. Eighteen of 20 patients had AV block. Ten of them had intermittent high-degree AV block and for those requiring temporary pacemakers, all were removed within 1 week. In addition to AV block, 13 of the 20 patients also had diffuse nonspecific ST and T wave changes on electrocardiograms. Although not performed in this study, endomyocardial biopsies taken from patients with AV block secondary to Lyme disease frequently show nonspecific active or borderline myocarditis. Rare spirochetes can be seen by using modified silver stains.[166] Patients with high degree AV block may also develop cardiac symptoms such as syncope, dizziness, shortness of breath or substernal chest pain. A minority of patients experience transient, mild left ventricular dysfunction, but severe cardiomyopathy has only been rarely observed.[166] The true prevalence of myocarditis and cardiomyopathy associated with Lyme disease is not known but epidemiologically, cardiac involvement of any kind was found in 8% of patients.[167] The study by Steere et al, would suggest that for most patients with Lyme cardiac disease, symptoms are transient and reverse either spontaneously or with treatment with antibiotics or corticosteroids. The role for these therapeutic strategies in Lyme cardiac disease has not yet been systematically studied.

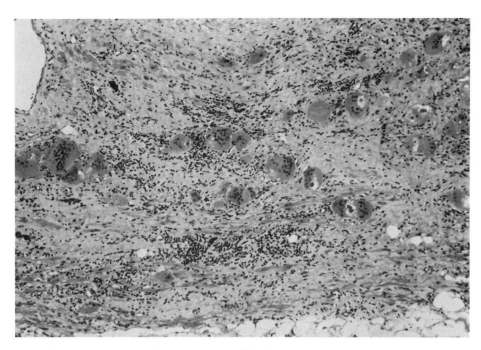

Fig. 6-8. An autopsy case of giant cell myocarditis characterized by multifocal mononuclear cell infiltrates within extensive areas of replacement fibrosis. Multiple multinucleated giant cells are scattered throughout the field (courtesy of Dr. Henry D. Tazelaar, Mayo Clinic).

Peripartum myocarditis

The onset of unexplained dilated cardiomyopathy occurring for the first time during the last month of pregnancy or within 5 months after delivery has been termed *peripartum* or *postpartum cardiomyopathy*. It has been described more commonly in patients older than 30 years of age, in multiparous and eclamptic patients, and in twin gestation. Although viral infections, nutritional deficiencies, small vessel coronary disease, and immunologic responses to fetal and myometrial antigens have all been postulated as possible causes, the etiology of peripartum cardiomyopathy remains unknown. In a study by O'Connell, et al,[168] 14 patients with peripartum cardiomyopathy were studied. Eight of them (57%) were multiparous, 6 (43%) required cesarean section and 2 (14%) had twin gestations. The initial presentation of cardiac disease occurred before delivery in 8 (57%) patients and in the first week postpartum in 3 (21%). The remaining 3 patients first developed symptoms of heart failure between the second and eighth week postpartum. Of the 14 patients, 7 died during the follow-up period. All patients who improved did so within 6 weeks of presentation. The prevalence of myocarditis was 29%. Midei, et al,[31] studied 18 patients with an average time from delivery to the onset of symptoms of 34 days. Eleven of eighteen (59%) were multiparous, and myocarditis was found in 14 (78%) of the biopsy samples. All patients improving spontaneously presented with congestive heart failure within 1 month of delivery and others improved dramatically within days of presentation. Of 10 patients with myocarditis treated with

immunosuppressive therapy, 9 showed improvement in cardiac function. The patient failing to respond presented for biopsy and treatment more than 5 months postpartum. Of the four patients without myocarditis, none were treated with immunosuppressive therapy and two deteriorated and required transplantation. These studies suggest that peripartum cardiomyopathy may be a distinct entity from idiopathic dilated cardiomyopathy. Pregnant women may have an enhanced susceptibility to viral myocarditis when infected with a cardiotropic virus, as has been demonstrated in mouse models of myocarditis.[169] In addition, the third trimester of pregnancy may be associated with an augmentation of suppressor cell function, and elevated levels of cytokines such as tumor necrosis factor are associated with labor and eclampsia.[170] With recent observations in mouse models that cytokines modulate susceptibility to viral myocarditis, patients during the peripartum period are at particular risk of enhancing a preexisting cardiotropic viral infection. A postviral etiology is also suggested by our finding that anti-heart antibodies and aberrant MHC expression within the myocardium, both reliable markers in myocarditis patients, are seen with equal frequency in patients with peripartum myocarditis.

Giant cell myocarditis

The term *giant cell myocarditis* is used to describe a rare form of myocarditis of unknown etiology characterized by widespread degeneration, necrosis and replacement of myocardial fibers, and formation of multinucleated giant cells (Fig. 6-8). The natural history of giant cell myocarditis is largely unknown, although it has been associated with a rapidly downhill course resulting in death with 1 to 3 months of presentation. Systemic illnesses associated with giant cell myocarditis include sarcoidosis, rheumatoid arthritis and other autoimmune diseases, Whipple disease, Wegner granulomatosis, tuberculosis, fungal infections, syphilis, and drug hypersensitivity.[171-172] Its existence as a separate entity from myocardial sarcoidosis continues to be debated. Its differentiation may be difficult in cases where myocarditis is the only manifestation of cardiac sarcoidosis during life and when pulmonary involvement is absent. Davidoff et al,[173] recently described their experience with 10 patients with giant cell myocarditis and found a high prevalence of ventricular tachycardia (90%) and AV block requiring pacemaker insertion (60%). Seven of the ten patients either died or required transplantation. At autopsy, four patients had histologic evidence consistent with cardiac sarcoidosis and one had evidence for widespread Whipple disease. At our institution we have observed a small number of patients with chronic active myocarditis progressing to giant cell myocarditis.[16] These patients were characterized by progressive deterioration of cardiac contractile function leading to transplantation, or death within 6 months of the biopsy diagnosis.

CONCLUSIONS

The advent of new technology has spurred renewed interest in the field of myocarditis research. As an inflammatory disorder, the direct relationship of viral injury to myocytes, as well as the indirect triggering of persistent humoral and cell-mediated autoimmunity, are now beginning to be understood. It is now clear that enteroviral infection of the myocardium plays a role in a substantial group of patients with myocarditis. The recent findings of CMV immediate early (IE-2) gene products within myocytes of patients with HIV-related myocarditis suggests that other cardiotropic viruses are also likely to be associated with myocarditis. It appears unlikely, though, that virus-mediated myocytolysis directly produces the cardiac contractile dysfunction in the majority of cases of adult human myocarditis. In some neonatal cases, the direct viral insult may be severe and result in irreversible cardiac damage. The lack of extensive myocyte necrosis and inflammatory infiltrate in most adult cases of myocarditis makes it attractive to hypothesize that the primary insult(s) in myocarditis are secondary to a response to virally altered myocytes.

Putative intracellular autoantigens ANT, BCKD, and myosin have been demonstrated on the surface membrane of isolated cardiac myocytes from acute CVB3 myocarditis patients.[106] Circulating autoimmune antibodies to these three autoantigens suggest that in the setting of myocarditis, multiple proteins may be aberrantly transported to the plasma membrane of myocytes. Other putative autoantigens, such as the beta-adrenergic receptor, already reside

within the plasma membrane. Myocardial proteins are likely to be either processed intracellularly within myocytes, or extracellularly by interstitial mononuclear cells. The resulting peptides are complexed to self-MHC antigens and presented to T cells, thus initiating an autoimmune process. The abnormal expression of autoantigens induced by cryptic cardiotropic viruses may also indirectly result in cardiac dysfunction. The literature is now replete with demonstrations of pathophysiologic effects of immune mediators such as antibodies to ANT and the beta-adrenergic receptor in idiopathic myocarditis, and of a cross-reacting antigen (SRA) in Chagas' disease. Pathogenic properties of these antibodies may be manifested physiologically rather than histologically, which is consistent with clinical findings in myocarditis where severe functional impairment may be associated with only sparse inflammation and rare myocyte necrosis. In addition to humoral-mediated autoimmune injury, local production of cytokines by infiltrating inflammatory cells may also have a role in altering myocardial metabolism. It has been reasoned for some time that abnormal expression of MHC antigens on cardiac myocytes is most likely secondary to the release of gamma interferon from infiltrating mononuclear cells. The role of cytokines such as tumor necrosis factor (TNF) and IL-1 in modulating myocyte function are currently being investigated.

Cardiotropic viruses may therefore initiate some cardiac tissue damage that results in clones of immune cells, which are activated against intracytoplasmic and sarcolemmal proteins, producing a delayed and often prolonged humoral and cell-mediated injury in a genetically predisposed host.

The identification of enteroviral gene products in a proportion of patients with IDCM suggests that in a group of patients where the acute phase of myocarditis is only partially controlled by a protective immune response, offending viruses may become sequestered (latent) and undergo periodic activation. This latency may be associated with excessive accumulation of the same intracytoplasmic proteins that subsequently activate the immune cells and result in focal tissue injury. The long-term effects of such focal tissue injury may result in the development of dilated cardiomyopathy with only a limited inflammatory reaction.

The ultimate goal of all the investigations of myocarditis is the prevention of ongoing myocardial injury leading to cardiomyopathy. From a preventive cardiology perspective, high-risk viruses and high-risk patients must be identified if there is to be a significant role for antiviral therapy in this disorder. Noninvasive and invasive markers of immune-mediated cardiac injury need to be further characterized in order to sensitively identify cardiomyopathy patients with potentially reversible cardiac dysfunction. With patients accurately identified, the elucidation of the pathogenic mechanisms of injury induced by autoantibodies and cytokines will likely lead to new therapeutic strategies involving more specific immunosuppression and drug therapy tailored to defend the myocardium.

REFERENCES

1. Aretz HT: Myocarditis: the Dallas criteria, *Hum Pathol* 18:619-624, 1987.

2. Aretz HT, Billingham ME, Edwards WD, et al: Myocarditis. A histopathologic definition and classification, *Am J Cardiovasc Pathol* 1(1):3-14, 1986.

3. Santos-Buch CA, Acosta AM, Zweerink HJ, et al: Primary muscle disease: definition of a 25-kDa polypeptide myopathic specific Chagas antigen, *Clin Immunol Immunopathol* 37:334-350, 1985.

4. Factor SM, Sonnenblick EH: The pathogenesis of clinical and experimental congestive cardiomyopathies: recent concepts, *Prog Cardiovasc Dis* 27:395-420, 1985.

5. de Paola AAV, Horowitz LN, Miyamoto MH, et al: Angiographic and electrophysiologic substrates of ventricular tachycardia in chronic Chagasic myocarditis, *Am J Cardiol* 65:360-363, 1990.

6. Abelmann WH, Lorell BH: The challenge of cardiomyopathy, *J Am Coll Cardiol* 13(6):1219-1239, 1989.

7. Abelmann WH: *The etiology, pathogenesis and pathophysiology of dilated cardiomyopathies.* In Schultheiss HP, ed: *New Concepts in Viral Heart Disease,* New York, 1988, Springer-Verlag.

8. Sekiguchi M, Hiroe M, Hiramitsu S, et al: *Natural history of acute viral or idiopathic myocarditis: a clinical and endomyocardial biopsy follow-up.* In Schultheiss HP, ed: *New Concepts in Viral Heart Disease,* New York, 1988, Springer-Verlag.

9. McManus BM, Gauntt CJ, Cassling RS: Immunopathologic basis of myocardial injury, *Cardiovasc Clin* 18:163-184, 1988.

10. Nippoldt TB, Edwards WD, Holmes DR Jr, et al: Right ventricular endomyocardial biopsy: clinicopathologic correlates in 100 patients, *Mayo Clin Proc* 57:407-418, 1982.

11. Strain JE, Grose RM, Factor SM, et al: Results of endomyocardial biopsy in patients with spontaneous ventricular tachycardia but without apparent structural heart disease, *Circulation* 68:1171-1181, 1983.

12. Fenoglio JJ Jr, Ursell PC, Kellogg CF: Diagnosis and classification of myocarditis by endomyocardial biopsy, *N Engl J Med* 308:12-18, 1983.

13. O'Connell JB, Robinson JA, Henkin RE, et al: Immunosuppressive therapy in patients with congestive cardiomyopathy and myocardial uptake of gallium-67, *Circulation* 64(4):780-786, 1981.

14. O'Connell JB, Henkin RE, Robinson JA, et al: Gallium-67 imaging in patients with dilated cardiomyopathy and biopsy-proven myocarditis, *Circulation* 70:58-62, 1984.

15. Kitaura Y, Morita H: Secondary myocardial disease: virus myocarditis and cardiomyopathy, *Jpn Circ J* 43:1017, 1979.

16. Lieberman EB, Hutchins GM, Herskowitz A, et al: A clinicopathologic description of myocarditis, *J Am Coll Cardiol* 18(7):1617-1626, 1991.

17. Woodruff JF: Viral myocarditis. A review, *Am J Pathol* 101:427-479, 1980.

18. Grist NR: *Epidemiology and pathogenicity of coxsackieviruses.* In Schultheiss HP, ed: *New Concepts in Viral Heart Disease,* New York, 1988, Springer-Verlag.

19. Gore I, Saphir O: Myocarditis: a classification of 1402 cases, *Am Heart J* 34:827-830, 1947.

20. Gravanis MB, Sternby NH: Incidence of myocarditis: a 10-year autopsy study from Malmo, Sweden, *Arch Pathol Lab Med* 115:390-392, 1991.

21. Stevens PJ, Underwood-Ground KE: Occurrence and significance of myocarditis in trauma, *Aerospace Medicine* 47:776-780, 1970.

22. Bandt CM, Staley NA, Noren GR: Acute viral myocarditis: clinical and histologic changes, *Minn Med* 62:234-237, 1979.

23. Ito M, Baba M, Mori S, et al: Tumor necrosis factor antagonizes inhibitory effect of azidothymidine (AZT) on human immunodeficiency virus (HIV) replication in vitro, *Biochem Biophys Res Commun* 166(3):1095-1101, 1990.

24. Gear JHS, Measroch V: Coxsackievirus infections of the newborn, *Prog Med Virol* 15:42-62, 1973.

25. Smith WG: Coxsackie B myopericarditis in adults, *Am Heart J* 80:34, 1980.

26. Mason JW, Herskowitz A: Incidence and clinical characteristics of myocarditis, *Circulation* 84(4 Suppl 2):2, 1991.

27. Vasiljevic JD, Kanjuh V, Seferovic P, et al: The incidence of myocarditis in endomyocardial biopsy samples from patients with congestive heart failure, *Am Heart J* 120:1370-1377, 1990.

28. Latham RD, Mulrow JP, Virmani R, et al: Recently diagnosed idiopathic dilated cardiomyopathy: Incidence of myocarditis and efficacy of prednisone therapy, *Am Heart J* 117(4):876-882, 1989.

29. Parrillo JE, Cunnion RE, Epstein SE: A prospective, randomized, controlled trial of prednisone for dilated cardiomyopathy, *N Engl J Med* 321(16):1061-1068, 1989.

30. Dec GW Jr, Palacios IF, Fallon JT, et al: Active myocarditis in the spectrum of acute dilated cardiomyopathies: Clinical features, histologic correlates, and clinical outcome, *N Engl J Med* 312:885-890, 1985.

31. Midei MG, DeMent SH, Feldman AM, et al: Peripartum myocarditis and cardiomyopathy, *Circulation* 81:922-928, 1990.

32. Deckers JW, Hare JM, Baughman KL: Complications of transvenous right ventricular endomyocardial biopsy in adult cardiomyopathy patients: a seven year survey of 546 consecutive diagnostic procedures in a tertiary referral center, *Circulation* (in press):1992.

33. Sainani GS, Kromptogic E, Slodki SJ: Adult heart disease due to coxsackievirus B infection, *Medicine* 47:133-147, 1968.

34. Kandolf R, Ameis D, Kirschner P, et al: In situ detection of enteroviral genomes in myocardial cells by nucleic acid hybridization: an approach to the diagnosis of viral heart disease, *Pro Natl Acad Sci USA* 84:6272-6276, 1987.

35. Kandolf R, Kirschner P, Ameis D, et al: *Enteroviral heart disease: diagnosis by in situ hybridization.* In Schultheiss HP, ed: *New Concepts in Viral Heart Disease.* Berlin, 1988, Springer-Verlag.

36. Foulis AK, Farquharson MA, Cameron SO, et al: A search for the presence of the enteroviral capsid protein VP1 in pancreases of patients with type 1 (insulin-dependent) diabetes and pancreases and hearts of infants who died of coxsackieviral myocarditis, *Diabetologia* 33:290-298, 1990.

37. Bowles NE, Richardson PJ, Olsen EGJ, et al: Detection of coxsackie-B-virus-specific RNA sequences in myocardial biopsy samples from patients with myocarditis and dilated cardiomyopathy, *Lancet* I(May 17):1120-1123, 1986.

38. Weiss LM, Movahed LA, Billingham ME, et al: Detection of Coxsackievirus B3 RNA in myocardial tissues by the polymerase chain reaction, *Am J Pathol* 138:497-503, 1991.

39. Jin O, Sole MJ, Butany JW, et al: Detection of enterovirus RNA in myocardial biopsies from patients with myocarditis and cardiomyopathy using gene amplification by polymerase chain reaction, *Circulation* 82:8-16, 1990.

40. Tazelaar HD, Billingham ME: Leukocytic infiltrates in idiopathic dilated cardiomyopathy. A source of confusion with active myocarditis. *Am J Surg Pathol* 10:405-412, 1986.

41. Tazelaar HD, Billingham ME: Myocardial lymphocytes. Fact, fancy, or myocarditis? *Am J Cardiovasc Pathol* 1:47-50, 1987.

42. Dec GW Jr, Fallon JT, Southern JF, et al: Relation between histological findings on early repeat right ventricular biopsy and ventricular function in patients with myocarditis, *Br Heart J* 60(4):332-337, 1988.

43. Hammond EH, Menlove RL, Anderson JL: Predictive value of immunofluorescence and electron microscopic evaluation of endomyocardial biopsies in the diagnosis and prognosis of myocarditis and idiopathic dilated cardiomyopathy, *Am Heart J* 114:1055-1065, 1987.

44. Edwards WD, Holmes DR Jr, Reeder GS: Diagnosis of active lymphocytic myocarditis by endomyocardial biopsy: quantitative criteria for light microscopy, *Mayo Clin Proc* 57:419-425, 1982.

45. Linder J, Cassling RS, Rogler WC, et al: Immunohistochemical characterization of lymphocytes in uninflamed ventricular myocardium. Implications for myocarditis, *Arch Pathol Lab Med* 109:917-920, 1985.

46. Schnitt SJ, Ciano PS, Schoen FJ: Quantitation of lymphocytes in endomyocardial biopsies: use and limitations of antibodies to leukocyte common antigen, *Hum Pathol* 18:796-800, 1987.

47. Beschorner WE, Baughman K, Turnicky RP, et al: HIV associated myocarditis: pathology and immunopathology, *Am J Pathol* 137:1365-1371, 1990.

48. McManus BM, Kandolf R: Evolving concepts of cause, consequence and control in myocarditis, *Curr Opin Cardiol* 6:418-427, 1991.

49. Kinney EL, Brafman D, Wright RJ II: Echocardiographic findings in patients with acquired immunodeficiency syndrome (AIDS) and AIDS-related complex (ARC), *Cathet Cardiovasc Diagn* 16:182-185, 1989.

50. Shanes JG, Ghali J, Billingham ME, et al: Interobserver variability in the pathologic interpretation of endomyocardial biopsy results, *Circulation* 75:401-405, 1987.

51. Hauck AJ, Kearney DL, Edwards WD: Evaluation of postmortem endomyocardial biopsy specimens from 38 patients with lymphocytic myocarditis: implications for role of sampling error, *Mayo Clin Proc* 64:1235-1245, 1989.

52. Chow LH, Radio SJ, Sears TD, et al: Insensitivity of right ventricular endomyocardial biopsy in the diagnosis of myocarditis, *J Am Coll Cardiol* 14(4):915-920, 1988.

53. Dec GW, Fallon JT, Southern JF, et al: "Borderline" myocarditis: an indication for repeat endomyocardial biopsy, *J Am Coll Cardiol* 15(2):283-289, 1990.

54. Dec GW, Palacios I, Yasuda T, et al: Antimyosin antibody cardiac imaging: its role in the diagnosis of myocarditis, *J Am Coll Cardiol* 16(1):97-104, 1990.

55. Yasuda T, Palacios IF, Dec GW, et al: Indium 111-monoclonal antimyosin antibody imaging in the diagnosis of acute myocarditis, *Circulation* 76:306-311, 1987.

56. Obrador D, Ballester M, Carrio I, et al: High prevalence of myocardial monoclonal antimyosin antibody uptake in patients with chronic idiopathic dilated cardiomyopathy, *J Am Coll Cardiol* 13:1289-1293, 1989.

57. Pinamonti B, Alberti E, Cigalotto A: Role of echocardiography in myocarditis, *Cardio Board Rev* 6(9):70-81, 1989.

58. Arvan S, Manalo E: Sudden increase in left ventricular mass secondary to acute myocarditis, *Am Heart J* 116(1 Pt 1):200-202, 1988.

59. Kondo M, Takahashi M, Shimono Y, et al: Reversible asymmetric septal hypertrophy in acute myocarditis -serial findings of two-dimensional echocardiogram and thallium-201 scintigram, *Jpn Circ J* 49:589-593, 1985.

60. Pasquini JA, Gottdiener JS, Cutler DJ: Myocarditis with transient left ventricular apical dyskinesis, *Am Heart J* 109(2):371-373, 1985.

61. Nieminen MS, Heikkila J, Karjalainen J: Echocardiography in acute infectious myocarditis: relation to clinical and electrocardiographic findings, *Am J Cardiol* 53:1331-1337, 1984.

62. Wallis DE, O'Connell JB, Henkin RE, et al: Segmental wall motion abnormalities in dilated cardiomyopathy: a common finding and good prognostic sign, *J Am Coll Cardiol* 4(4):674-679, 1984.

63. Khatib R, Chason JL, Silberberg BK, et al: Age-dependent pathogenicity of group B coxsackieviruses in Swiss- Webster mice: infectivity for myocardium and pancreas, *J Infect Dis* 141:394-403, 1980.

64. Reyes MP, Lerner AM: Coxsackievirus myocarditis—with special reference to acute and chronic effects, *Prog Cardiovasc Dis* 27:373-394, 1985.

65. Huber SA, Job LP, Woodruff JF: Lysis of infected myofibers by coxsackievirus B-3-immune T lymphocytes, *Am J Pathol* 98:681-694, 1980.

66. Wong CY, Woodruff JJ, Woodruff JF: Generation of cytotoxic T lymphocytes during coxsackievirus B-3 infection: II. Characterization of effector cells and demonstration of cytotoxicity against viral-infected myofibers, *J Immunol* 118(4):1165-1169, 1977.

67. Herskowitz A, Wolfgram LJ, Rose NR, et al: Coxsackievirus B3 murine myocarditis: a pathologic spectrum of myocarditis in genetically defined inbred strains, *J Am Coll Cardiol* 9:1311-1319, 1987.

68. Huber SA, Job LP, Woodruff JF: Sex-related differences in the pattern of coxsackievirus B-3-induced immune spleen cell cytotoxicity against virus-infected myofibers, *Infect Immun* 32:68-73, 1981.

69. Gauntt CJ, Trousdale MD, LaBadie DR, et al: Properties of coxsackievirus B3 variants which are amyocarditic or myocarditic for mice, *J Med Virol* 3:207-220, 1979.

70. Wolfgram LJ, Beisel KW, Herskowitz A, et al: R. Variations in the susceptibility to Coxsackievirus B3-induced myocarditis among different strains of mice, *J Immunol* 136:1846-1852, 1986.

71. Godeny EK, Gauntt CJ: Murine natural killer cells limit coxsackievirus B3 replication, *J Immunol* 139:913-918, 1987.

72. O'Connell JB, Reap EA, Robinson JA: The effects of cyclosporine on acute murine Coxsackievirus B3 myocarditis, *Lab Invest* 73(2):353-359, 1986.

73. Rezkalla S, Khatib G, Khatib R: Coxsackievirus B3 murine myocarditis: deleterious effects of nonsteroidal anti-inflammatory agents, *J Lab Clin Med* 107:393-395, 1986.

74. Matsumori A, Wang H, Abelmann WH, et al: Treatment of viral myocarditis with ribavirin in an animal preparation, *Circulation* 71:834-839, 1985.

75. Matsumori A, Crumpacker CS, Abelmann WH: Prevention of viral myocarditis with recombinant human leukocyte interferon alpha A/D in a murine model, *J Am Coll Cardiol* 9:1320-1325, 1987.

76. Huber SA, Lodge PA: Coxsackievirus B-3 myocarditis. Identification of different pathogenic mechanisms in DBA/2 and Balb/c mice, *Am J Pathol* 122:284-291, 1986.

77. Lodge PA, Herzum M, Olszewski J, et al: Coxsackievirus B-3 myocarditis. Acute and chronic forms of the disease caused by different immunopathogenic mechanisms, *Am J Pathol* 128:455-463, 1987.

78. Lutton CW, Gauntt CJ: Coxsackievirus B3 infection alters plasma membrane of neonatal skin fibroblasts, *J Virol* 60:294-296, 1986.

79. Godeny EK, Gauntt CJ: In situ immune autoradiographic identification of cells in heart tissues of mice with coxsackievirus B3-induced myocarditis, *Am J Pathol* 129:267-276, 1987.

80. Traystman MD, Chow LH, McManus BM, et al: Susceptibility to coxsackievirus B3-induced chronic myocarditis maps near the murine Tcr-alpha and Myhc-alpha loci on chromosome 14, *Am J Pathol* 138(3):721-726, 1991.

81. Neu N, Beisel KW, Traystman MD, et al: Autoantibodies specific for the cardiac myosin isoform are found in mice susceptible to Coxsackievirus B3-induced myocarditis, *J Immunol* 138(8):2488-2492, 1987.

82. Alvarez FL, Neu N, Rose NR, et al: Heart-specific autoantibodies induced by Coxsackievirus B3: identification of heart autoantigens, *Clin Immunol Immunopathol* 43:129-139, 1987.

83. Neu N, Rose NR, Beisel KW, et al: Cardiac myosin induces myocarditis in genetically predisposed mice, *J Immunol* 139(11):3630-3636, 1987.

84. Smith SC, Allen PM: Myosin-induced acute myocarditis is a T cell mediated disease, *J Immunol* 147(7):2141-2147, 1991.

85. Neumann DA, Lane JR, Lafond-Walker A, et al: Elution of autoan-

tibodies from the hearts of Coxsackievirus-infected mice, *Eur Heart J* 12(Suppl D):113-116, 1991.

86. Neumann DA, Lane JR, Lafond-Walker A, et al: Heart-specific autoantibodies can be eluted from the hearts of Coxsackievirus B3-infected mice, *Clin Exp Immunol* 86:405-12, 1991.

87. Neu N, Craig SW, Rose NR, et al: Coxsackievirus induced myocarditis in mice: cardiac myosin autoantibodies do not cross-react with the virus, *Clin Exp Immunol* 69:566-574, 1987.

88. Beisel KW, Srinivasappa J, Olsen MR, et al: A neutralizing monoclonal antibody against coxsackievirus B4 cross-reacts with contractile muscle proteins, *Microb Pathog* 8(2):151-156, 1990.

89. Krisher K, Cunningham MW: Myosin: a link between streptococci and heart, *Science* 227(4685):413-415, 1985.

90. Cunningham MW, McCormack JM, Talaber LR, et al: Human monoclonal antibodies reactive with antigens of the group A Streptococcus and human heart, *J Immunol* 141:2760-2766, 1988.

91. Fenderson PG, Fischetti VA, Cunningham MW: Tropomyosin shares immunologic epitopes with group A streptococcal M proteins, *J Immunol* 142(7):2475-2481, 1989.

92. Gulizia JM, Cunningham MW, McManus BM: Immunoreactivity of anti-streptococcal monoclonal antibodies to human heart valves. Evidence for multiple cross-reactive epitopes, *Am J Pathol* 138(2):285-301, 1991.

93. Borda ES, Pascual J, Cossio P, et al: A circulating IgG in Chagas' disease which binds to beta-adrenoceptors of myocardium and modulates their activity, *Clin Exp Immunol* 57:679-686, 1984.

94. Wang YC, Kanter K, Lattouf O, et al: Characterization of human cardiac infiltrating cells posttransplantation: II. CD4+ cloned T-cell lines with "anti-idiotype:-like reactivity, *Hum Immunol* 28:141-152, 1990.

95. Bartholomaeus WN, O'Donoghue H, Foti D, et al: Multiple autoantibodies following cytomegalovirus infection: virus distribution and specificity of autoantibodies, *Immunology* 64:397-405, 1988.

96. Huber SA, Heintz N, Tracy R: Coxsackievirus B-3-induced myocarditis. Virus and actinomycin D treatment of myocytes induces novel antigens recognized by cytolytic T lymphocytes, *J Immunol* 141:3214-3219, 1988.

97. Chow LH, Gauntt CJ, McManus BM: *Early cellular infiltrates in coxsackievirus B3 myocarditis.* In Schultheiss HP, ed: *New Concepts in Viral Heart Disease,* New York, 1988, Springer-Verlag.

98. Seko Y, Shinkai Y, Kawasaki A, et al: Expression of perforin in infiltrating cells in murine hearts with acute myocarditis caused by coxsackievirus B-3, *Circulation* 84:788-795, 1991.

99. Lane JR, Neumann DA, Lafond-Walker A, et al: LPS promotes CB3-induced myocarditis in resistant B10.A mice, *Cell Immunol* 136:219-223, 1991.

100. Borda E, Perez-Leiros C, Sterin-Borda L, et al: Cholinergic response of isolated rat atria to recombinant rat interferon-gamma, *J Neuroimmunol* 32(1):53-59, 1991.

101. Hassin D, Fixler R, Shimoni Y, et al: Physiological changes induced in cardiac myocytes by cytotoxic T lymphocytes, *Am J Physiol* 252:C10-C16, 1987.

102. Perez-Leiros C, Sterin-Borda L, Borda E: Beta-adrenergic cardiac antibody in autoimmune myocarditis, *Autoimmun* 2(3):223-234, 1989.

103. Leiros CP, Sterin-Borda L, Cossio P, et al: Muscarinic cholinergic antibody in experimental autoimmune myocarditis regulates cardiac function, *Proc Soc Exp Biol Med* 195(3):356-363, 1990.

104. Schultheiss HP, Bolte HD: Immunological analysis of auto-antibodies against the adenine nucleotide translocator in dilated cardiomyopathy, *J Mol Cell Cardiol* 17:603-617, 1985.

105. Schultheiss HP: The significance of autoantibodies against the ADP/ATP carrier for the pathogenesis of myocarditis and dilated cardiomyopathy—clinical and experimental data, *Springer Semin Immunopathol* 11:15-30, 1989.

106. Ansari AA, Wang YC, Danner DJ, et al: Abnormal expression of histocompatibility and mitochondrial antigens by cardiac tissue from patients with myocarditis and dilated cardiomyopathy, *Am J Pathol* 139(2):337-354, 1991.

107. Schultheiss HP, Kuhl U, Janda I, et al: Antibody-mediated enhancement of calcium permeability in cardiac myocytes, *J Exp Med* 168(6):2105-2119, 1988.

108. Schulze K, Becker BF, Schultheiss HP: Antibodies to the ADP/ATP carrier, an autoantigen in myocarditis and dilated cardiomyopathy, penetrate into myocardial cells and disturb energy metabolism in vivo, *Circ Res* 64(2):179-192, 1989.

109. Schulze K, Becker BF, Schauer R, et al: Antibodies to ADP-ATP carrier, an autoantigen in myocarditis and dilated cardiomyopathy—impair cardiac function, *Circulation* 81:959-969, 1990.

110. Morad M, Davies NW, Ulrich G, et al: Antibodies against ADP-ATP carrier enhance Ca2+ current in isolated cardiac myocytes, *Am J Physiol* 255(4 Pt 2):H960-H964, 1988.

111. Reyes MP, Ho KL, Smith F, et al: A mouse model of dilated-type cardiomyopathy due to coxsackievirus B3, *J Infect Dis* 144:232-236, 1981.

112. Khatib R, Chason JL, Lerner AM: A mouse model of transmural myocardial necrosis due to coxsackievirus B4: observations over 12 months, *Intervirology,* 18:197-202, 1982.

113. O'Donoghue HL, Lawson CM, Reed WD: Autoantibodies to cardiac myosin in mouse cytomegalovirus myocarditis, *Immunology* 71:20-28, 1990.

114. Matsumori A, Kawai C: An animal model of congestive (dilated) cardiomyopathy: dilatation and hypertrophy of the heart in the chronic stage in DBA/2 mice with myocarditis caused by encephalomyocarditis virus, *Circulation* 66:355-360, 1982.

115. Neumann DA, Wulff SM, Leppo MK, et al: Pathologic changes in the cardiac interstitium of mice infected with encephalomyocarditis virus, *Cardivasc Pathol* (in press):1992.

116. Kishimoto C, Hung G-L, Ishibashi M, et al: Natural evolution of cardiac function, cardiac pathology and antimyosin scan in a murine myocarditis model, *J Am Coll Cardiol* 17(3):821-827, 1991.

117. Beck MA, Chapman NM, McManus BM, et al: Secondary enterovirus infection in the murine model of myocarditis: pathologic and immunologic aspects, *Am J Pathol* 136(3):669-681, 1990.

118. Chow LH, Gauntt CJ, McManus BM: Differential effects of myocarditic variants of coxsackievirus B-3 in inbred mice: a pathologic characterization of heart tissue damage, *Lab Invest* 64(1):55-64, 1991.

119. Godeny EK, Sprague EA, Schwartz CJ, et al: Coxsackievirus group B replication in cultured fetal baboon aortic smooth muscle cells, *J Med Virol* 20:135-149, 1986.

120. Huber SA, Job LP, Woodruff JF: In vitro culture of coxsackievirus group B, type 3 immune spleen cells on infected endothelial cells and biological activity of the cultured cells in vivo, *Infect Immun* 43:567-573, 1984.

121. Leslie KO, Schwarz J, Simpson K, et al: Progressive interstitial collagen deposition in coxsackievirus B3-induced myocarditis, *Am J Pathol* 136(3):683-693, 1990.

122. Factor SM, Wittner M, Tanowitz H, et al: Collagen matrix damage and trypanosome induced collagenolysis in murine Chagas' disease, *Circulation* 82:Abstract #1155, 1990.

123. Factor SM, Cho SH, Scheuer J, et al: Prevention of hereditary cardiomyopathy in the Syrian hamster with chronic verapamil therapy, *J Am Coll Cardiol* 12:1599-1604, 1988.

124. Sonnenblick EH, Fein F, Capasso JM, et al: Microvascular spasm as a cause of cardiomyopathies and the calcium- blocking agent verapamil as potential primary therapy, *Am J Cardiol* 55:179B-184B, 1985.

125. Factor SM, Cho S, Wittner M, et al: Abnormalities of the coronary microcirculation in acute murine Chagas' disease, *Am J Trop Med Hyg* 34(2):246-253, 1985.

126. Tracy SM, Wiegand V, McManus BM, et al: Molecular approaches

to enteroviral diagnosis in idiopathic cardiomyopathy and myocarditis, *J Am Coll Cardiol* 15:1688-1694, 1990.

127. Easton A, Eglin R: The detection of coxsackievirus RNA in cardiac tissue by in situ hybridization, *J Gen Virol* 69:285-291, 1988.

128. Tracy SM, Chapman NM, McManus BM, et al: A molecular and serologic evaluation of enteroviral involvement in human myocarditis, *J Mol Cell Cardiol* 22:403-414, 1990.

129. Archard L, Freeke C, Richardson P, et al: *Persistence of enterovirus RNA in dilated cardiomyopathy: a progression from myocarditis.* In Schultheiss HP, ed: *New Concepts in Viral Heart Disease,* New York, 1988, Springer-Verlag.

130. Anderson JL, Carlquist JF, Hammond EH: Deficient natural killer cell activity in patients with idiopathic dilated cardiomyopathy, *Lancet* 2:1124-1127, 1982.

131. Eckstein R, Mempel W, Bolte HD: Reduced suppressor cell activity in congestive cardiomyopathy and in myocarditis, *Circulation* 65(6):1224-1229, 1982.

132. Maisch B, Deeg P, Liebau G, et al: Diagnostic relevance of humoral and cytotoxic immune reactions in primary and secondary dilated cardiomyopathy, *Am J Cardiol* 52:1072-1078, 1983.

133. Anderson JL, Carlquist JF, Lutz JR, et al: HLA A, B and DR typing in idiopathic dilated cardiomyopathy: a search for immune response factors, *Am J Cardiol* 53(9):1326-1330, 1984.

134. Limas CJ, Limas C, Kubo SH, et al: Anti-beta-receptor antibodies in human dilated cardiomyopathy and correlation with HLA-DR antigens, *Am J Cardiol* 65:483-487, 1990.

135. Carlquist JF, Menlove RL, Murray MB, et al: HLA class II (DR and DQ) antigen associations in idiopathic dilated cardiomyopathy, *Circulation* 83:515-522, 1991.

136. Neumann DA, Burek CL, Baughman KL, et al: Circulating heart-reactive antibodies in patients with myocarditis or cardiomyopathy, *J Am Coll Cardiol* 16(4):839-846, 1990.

137. Caforio ALP, Bonifacio E, Stewart JT, et al: Novel organ-specific circulating cardiac autoantibodies in dilated cardiomyopathy, *J Am Coll Cardiol* 15:1527-1534, 1990.

138. Maisch B, Berg PA, Kochsiek K: Clinical significance of immunopathological findings in patients with post-pericardiotomy syndrome. I. Relevance of antibody pattern, *Clin Exp Immunol* 38:189-197, 1979.

139. Limas CJ, Goldenberg IF, Limas C: Autoantibodies against beta-adrenoceptors in human idiopathic dilated cardiomyopathy, *Circ Res* 64:97-103, 1989.

140. Herskowitz A, Ansari AA, Neumann DA, et al: Induction of major histocompatibility complex (MHC) antigens within the myocardium of patients with active myocarditis: a nonhistologic marker of myocarditis, *J Am Coll Cardiol* 15(3):624-632, 1990.

141. Herskowitz A, Baughman KL, Rose NR, et al: Induction of major histocompatibility antigens on myocardial cells in patients with active myocarditis and idiopathic cardiomyopathy. In Schultheiss HP, ed: *New Concepts in Viral Heart Disease,* Berlin 1988, Springer-Verlag.

142. Rockman HA, Adamson RM, Dembitsky WP, et al: Acute fulminant myocarditis: Long-term follow-up after circulatory support with left ventricular assist device, *Am Heart J* 121 (3 Part 1):922-926, 1991.

143. Jones SR, Herskowitz A, Hutchins GM, et al: Effects of immunosuppressive therapy in biopsy-proved myocarditis and borderline myocarditis on left ventricular function, *Am J Cardiol* 68:370-376, 1991.

144. Cohen IS, Anderson DW, Virmani R, et al: Congestive cardiomyopathy in association with the acquired immunodeficiency syndrome, *N Engl J Med* 315(10):628-630, 1986.

145. Himelman RB, Chung WS, Chernoff DN, et al: Cardiac manifestations of human immunodeficiency virus infection: a two-dimensional echocardiographic study, *J Am Coll Cardiol* 13(5):1030-1036, 1989.

146. Grody WW, Cheng L, Lewis W: Infection of the heart by the human immunodeficiency virus, *Am J Cardiol* 66:203-206, 1990.

147. Rodriguez ER, Nasim S, Hsia J, et al: Cardiac myocytes and dendritic cells harbor human immunodeficiency virus (HIV) in infected patients with and without cardiac dysfunction : detection by multiplex, nested, polymerase chain reaction in individually microdissected cells from right ventricular endomyocardial biopsy tissue, *Am J Cardiol* 68:1511-1520, 1991.

148. Baroldi G, Corallo S, Moroni M, et al: Focal lymphocytic myocarditis in acquired immunodeficiency syndrome (AIDS): a correlative morphologic and clinical study in 26 consecutive fatal cases, *J Am Coll Cardiol* 12:463-469, 1988.

149. Cox JN, di Dio F, Pizzolato GP, et al: Aspergillus endocarditis and myocarditis in a patient with the acquired immunodeficiency syndrome (AIDS). A review of the literature, *Virchows Arch* 417:255-259, 1990.

150. Rogers JG, Windle JR, McManus BM, et al: Aspergillus myocarditis presenting as myocardial infarction with complete heart block, *Am Heart J* 120(2):430-432, 1990.

151. Hoffman P, Bernard E, Michiels JF, et al: Myocardite aigue toxoplasmique, *Arch Mal Coeur* 83:1735-1738, 1990.

152. Tanowitz HB, Morris SA, Factor SM, et al: Parasitic diseases of the heart. I. Acute and chronic Chagas' disease, *Cardiovasc Pathol* 1(1):7-15, 1992.

153. Oliveira JSM, De Oliveira JAM, Frederigue U, et al: Apical aneurysm of Chagas' heart disease, *Br Heart J* 46:432-437, 1981.

154. Acosta AM, Santos-Buch CA: Autoimmune myocarditis induced by Trypanosoma cruzi, *Circulation* 71(6):1255-1261, 1985.

155. Rizzo LV, Cunha-Neto E, Teixeira AR: Autoimmunity in Chagas' disease: specific inhibition of reactivity of CD4: p1 T cells against myosin in mice chronically infected with Trypanosoma cruzi, *Infect Immun* 57:2640-2644, 1989.

156. Mesri EA, Levitus G, Hontebeyrie-Joskowicz M, et al: Major Trypanosoma cruzi antigenic determinant in Chagas' heart disease shares homology with the systemic lupus erythematosis ribosomal P protein epitope, *J Clin Microbiol* 28:1219-1224, 1990.

157. Rowan RA, Masek MA, Billingham ME: Ultrastructural morphometric analysis of endomyocardial biopsies. Idiopathic dilated cardiomyopathy, anthracycline cardiotoxicity, and normal myocardium. *Am J Cardiovasc Pathol* 2:137-144, 1988.

158. Herskowitz A, Willoughby SB, Baughman KL, et al: Cardiomyopathy associated with anti-retroviral therapy in patients with human immunodeficiency virus infection: a report of six cases, *Ann Intern Med* (In press): 1991.

159. Gravanis MB, Hertzler GL, Franch RH, et al: Hypersensitivity myocarditis in heart transplant candidates, *J Heart Lung Transplant* 10:688-697, 1991.

160. Kounis NG, Zavras GM, Soufras GD, et al: Hypersensitivity myocarditis, *Ann Allergy* 62(2):71-74, 1989.

161. Getz MA, Subramanian R, Logemann T, et al: Acute necrotizing eosinophilic myocarditis as manifestation of severe hypersensitivity myocarditis, *Ann Intern Med* 115(3):201-202, 1991.

162. Isner JM, Estes NAM III, Thompson PD, et al: Acute cardiac events temporally related to cocaine abuse, *N Engl J Med* 315:1438-1443, 1986.

163. Virmani R, Robinowitz M, Smialek JE, et al: Cardiovascular effects of cocaine: an autopsy study of 40 patients, *Am Heart J* 115(5):1068-1076, 1988.

164. Tazelaar HD, Karch SB, Stephens BG, et al: Cocaine and the heart, *Hum Pathol* 18:195-199, 1987.

165. Turnicky RP, Goodin J, Smialek JE, et al: Incidental myocarditis with intravenous drug abuse: the pathology, immunopathology, and potential implications for HIV associated myocarditis, *Hum Pathol* (In press): 1991.

166. Stanek G, Klein J, Bittner R, et al: Isolation of Borrelia Burgdorferi from the myocardium of a patient with longstanding cardiomyopathy, *N Engl J Med* 322:249-252, 1990.

167. Steere AC, Batsford WP, Weinberg M: Lyme carditis: cardiac abnormalities of Lyme disease, *Ann Intern Med* 93:8-16, 1980.

168. O'Connell JB, Costanzo-Nordin MR, Subramanian R, et al: Peripartum cardiomyopathy: clinical, hemodynamic, histologic and prognostic characteristics, *J Am Coll Cardiol* 8(1):52-56, 1986.

169. Lyden DC, Huber SA: Aggravation of coxsackievirus, group B, type 3-induced myocarditis and increase in cellular immunity to myocyte antigens in pregnant Balb/c mice and animals treated with progesterone, *Cell Immunol* 87:462-472, 1984.

170. Beutler B, Cerami A: Cachectin: more than a tumor necrosis factor, *N Engl J Med* 316(7):379-385, 1987.

171. Lemery R, McGoon MD, Edwards WD: Cardiac sarcoidosis: a potentially treatable form of myocarditis, *Mayo Clin Proc* 60(8):549-554, 1985.

172. Ferrans VJ, Rodriguez ER, McAllister HA Jr: Granulomatous inflammation of the heart, *Heart Vessels Suppl* I:262-270, 1985.

173. Davidoff R, Palacios I, Southern J, et al: Giant cell versus lymphocytic myocarditis: a comparison of their clinical features and long-term outcomes, *Circulation* 83:953-961, 1991.

Chapter 7
====

THE CARDIOMYOPATHIES

Celia M. Oakley
Michael B. Gravanis
Aftab A. Ansari

PART I DILATED CARDIOMYOPATHY

Cardiomyopathy is the term given to myocardial dysfunction of unknown cause. The definition excludes structural heart disease with failure resulting from coronary artery disease, hypertension, cor pulmonale, or valvular or congenital heart disease. Even after such exclusions, cardiomyopathy still encompasses a broad category of diseases.

The WHO classification of cardiomyopathies into dilated, hypertrophic, and restrictive forms is currently based on clinical presentation, pathophysiologic alterations refined by echocardiography, and morphologic findings from endomyocardial biopsy or necropsy.

Although these categories are helpful for clinical definition, they do not provide a basis from which to conduct research or question specific pathogenetic mechanisms because of significant heterogeneity[1] and overlap.

Although the cardiomyopathic process involves the entire heart, it is primarily reflected in the left ventricle, which shows dilatation and hypertrophy. Dilated cardiomyopathy is undoubtedly multifactorial in causation, i.e., not a single disease but the final common path of an insult to the ventricular myocardium. This insult may have been a virus or other infection; the effect of toxins such as cobalt, nickel, lithium, and antracyclines; or associated with alcohol abuse, pregnancy, systemic hypertension, and genetic predisposition based on inheritance of HLA-linked genes. All of these may be considered as risk factors. It is possible that a combination of these is responsible for triggering an immune-mediated myocarditis in genetically predisposed individuals.

Morphologic features

The globular shape of the heart in dilated cardiomyopathy is caused by dilatation of all chambers, particularly of the left ventricle (Fig. 7-1). The weight of the heart is increased by 25% to 50%, indicating hypertrophy, but the walls of the ventricles appear only mildly thickened or normal as a result of stretching (Fig. 7-2). Grossly visible left or right ventricular subendocardial and occasionally, transmural scars are found in approximately one tenth of hearts examined in the absence of identifiable occlusive coronary disease.[2] Endocardial fibrosis is commonly present particularly in children. It is patchy and irregular and may be caused by organization of mural thrombi (Fig. 7-3), or secondary to the stretching of the dilated ventricle (Fig. 7-4). Mural thrombi at different stages of organization are present in all four chambers unless anticoagulant therapy has been given (Fig. 7-5).

Significant variability of histologic findings in different cases of dilated cardiomyopathy depend on the stage of the process and the severity of the disease. The myocardial cells are hypertrophied, as shown by the enlarged hyperchromatic nuclei, but the individual fibers may be of normal diameter because they are attenuated as a result of chamber dilatation. Rare small clusters of lymphocytes may be present in areas of ongoing myocyte degeneration. Another morphologic finding in the myocardium is the significant increase in interstitial fibrous connective tissue along with evidence of individual myocyte degeneration

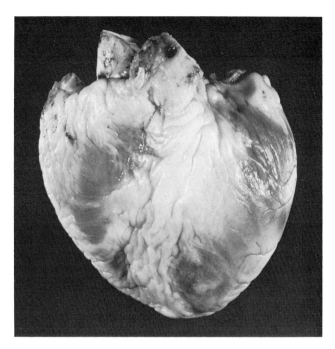

Fig. 7-1. Explanted idiopathic dilated cardiomyopathy. Note the globular shape of the heart caused by biventricular dilatation.

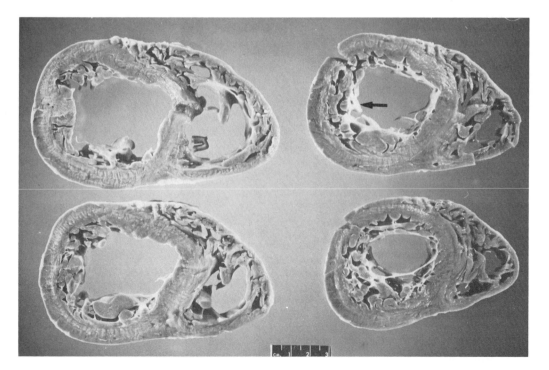

Fig. 7-2. Multiple biventricular cross-sections from a case of idiopathic dilated cardiomyopathy. The left ventricular wall thickness appears normal, the ventricular cavity is markedly increased, and the endocardium is thick and fibrotic *(arrow)*.

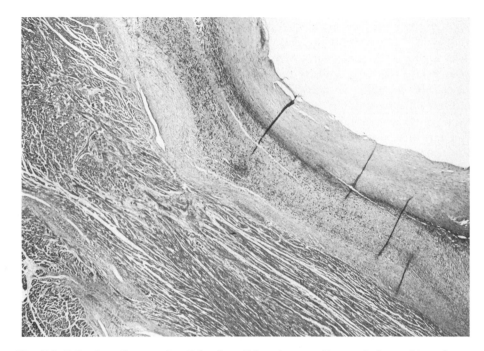

Fig. 7-3. Dilated cardiomyopathy. Subendocardial region revealing marked stretching of myocytes and endocardial thickening secondary to an organized mural thrombus.

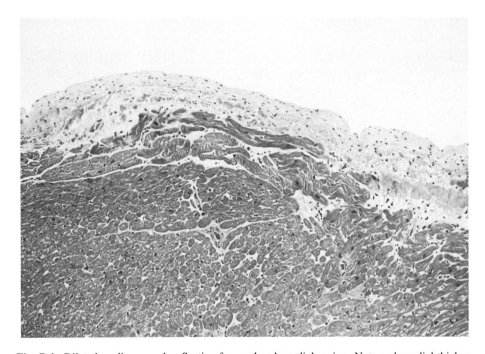

Fig. 7-4. Dilated cardiomyopathy. Section from subendocardial region. Note endocardial thickening containing an increased number of smooth muscle cells, and stretched myocytes with hypertrophic nuclei.

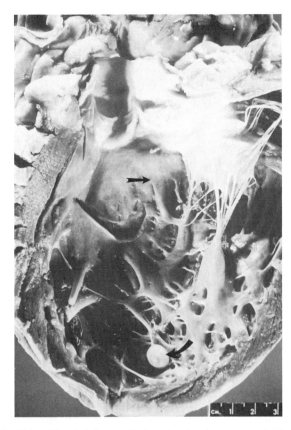

Fig. 7-5. Dilated left ventricular chamber in a case of dilated cardiomyopathy. Note normal left ventricular wall thickness, patchy endocardial fibrosis *(arrow),* and organized mural thrombus *(curved arrow).*

(empty sarcolemmal membranes), which may account for the focal replacement fibrosis (Fig. 7-6). The endocardium reveals a patchy thickening that on microscopy reveals young connective tissue cells and reactive smooth muscle cells. This proliferation of smooth muscle cells is attributed to long-standing dilatation of the ventricular chambers[3] and is therefore not specific.

As with light microscopic findings, ultrastructural changes are also nonspecific. Therefore a clear distinction between dilated cardiomyopathy and other cardiac conditions cannot always be made on morphologic grounds. In some cases ultrastructural studies have shown decreased nuclear chromatin aggregation, which has been interpreted to mean either heightened metabolic activity or an alteration in DNA concentration caused by increased nuclear size (edema) without corresponding increase in DNA.[4]

A recent study using monoclonal antibodies has reported a slightly reduced myosin and actin content of the left ventricular myocardium. However, no evidence of a primary derangement of myosin myofibrils to explain the reduced myocardial contractility was detected.[5]

According to some reports, ultrastructural abnormalities in myocardial cells from patients with end-stage dilated cardiomyopathy reveal alterations in the cytoskeleton that may contribute to the deterioration of contractile function of the myocardium in this disorder.[6] The cytoskeleton proper consists of microtubules actin filaments, and intermediate filaments such as desmin for muscle cells and vimentin for interstitial cells, although other proteins such as vinculin and laminin are closely linked to these structures.[7]

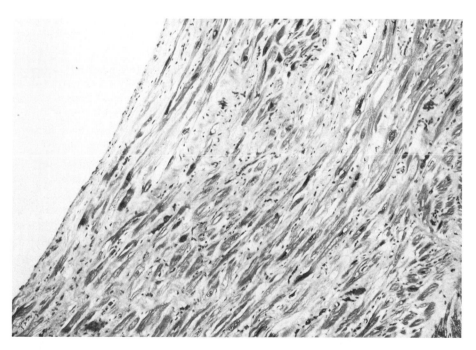

Fig. 7-6. Subendocardial section from an end-stage dilated cardiomyopathy. Note stretching of myocytes, marked nuclear hypertrophy, and significant interstitial and replacement fibrosis.

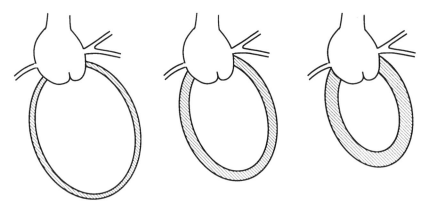

Fig. 7-7. Diagrammatic representation of the left ventricle in dilated cardiomyopathy with varying degrees of dilatation. The crosshatched area can be regarded either as the wall thickness or as the difference between the end-diastolic and end-systolic cavity size. This is the stroke volume, which could be the same in the greatly dilated, poorly contracting left ventricle shown on the left as it is in the more nearly normally contracting left ventricle on the right. This similarity may occur even though the ejection fraction may be below 10% in the heart on the left, compared with 50% on the right. The left ventricular filling pressure might be near normal in the heart on the left and the patient free from symptoms, whereas the patient whose less dilated heart is shown on the right may have a restrictive cardiomyopathy and be in pulmonary edema. The heart in the middle has intermediate characteristics. The diagram illustrates the observed fact that symptomatic class cannot be guessed from the echocardiographic or angiographic degree of dilatation, or from the calculated ejection fraction.

The study by Schaper et al revealed loss of myofibrils in many areas in both the center and the periphery of a myocyte, prominent dilated parts of the T-tubular system, fat droplets, myelin figures, and vacuoles. Furthermore, it showed disproportionate increases of cytoskeletal proteins such as desmin, tubulin, and vinculin. These ultra-structural changes in the myocytes were thought to be the morphologic correlates of the reduced function in end-stage dilated cardiomyopathy and, perhaps more accurately, in chronic cardiac failure.[6]

Preliminary data from studies on the structural characteristics of the extracellular matrix and in particular its collagen matrix, suggest a pathologic remodeling of the extracellular matrix in dilated cardiomyopathy.[8] Weber et al observed an increase in proportion of thin collagen fibers (type III collagen), which are known to have considerably less tensile strength than type I collagen; thus it may not adequately resist deformation or provide adequate support. An additional finding was a reduction in the number of thick collagen fibers that represent lateral connections between muscle bundles (collagen tethers). Such reduction may favor muscle slippage, muscle fiber rearrangement, and wall thinning. These abnormalities of the collagen matrix may represent the anatomic milieu for thinning, dilatation, and general compromise of the mechanical properties of the myocardium all of which leads to dilated cardiomyopathy.

If indeed the changes in the extracellular matrix are consistent and reproducible, Weber's suggestion of calling this cardiac disorder "cardiopathy" instead of cardiomyopathy may have some justification.

A broad spectrum of electromyographic or histologic abnormalities or both in skeletal muscle of patients with dilated cardiomyopathy have been reported.[9] A reduction of single motor unit potential duration was found in about 40% of patients with dilated cardiomyopathy who had no evidence of overt clinical skeletal myopathy.[10] These patients reveal selective involvement of type I fibers which have predominant oxidative metabolism. It was suggested that the myopathy is not secondary to heart failure because it was similar among patients with symptoms varying from mild to severe. However, although cardiac and skeletal myopathy occasionally coexist, the changes in skeletal muscle are usually secondary to reduction in blood flow during exercise coupled with the detraining effects of inactivity.

Mitral and tricuspid regurgitation are frequent occurrences in dilated cardiomyopathy and are related to the increased end-systolic volumes resulting from impaired myocardial contraction. Annular dilatation, lack of sphincteric contraction of the valve ring, and lateral malalignment of papillary muscles have all been considered to contribute. Recent studies have concluded that although mitral annular size is greater in patients with dilated cardiomyopathy, neither the presence nor the degree of mitral or tricuspid regurgitation correlate with the observed size of the annulus.[11] In general, regurgitation diminishes as failure is treated. It occurs least in mild cases, is greatest in severe failure, and is clearly related to the impaired contractile efficiency.

Symptomatic class is dependent upon maintenance of cardiac output on exercise together with a sufficiently low diastolic filling pressure. These basic functions cannot be assessed from measurement of left ventricular size. Increasing dilatation provides automatic compensation for systolic failure (Fig 7-7), but after distention ceases and diastolic pressure rises, clinical symptoms and failure occur. This provides some support for Weber's concepts concerning the extracellular matrix and explains a clinical continuum between typical dilated cardiomyopathy and restrictive cardiomyopathy with a mainly or exclusively diastolic failure.

Morphologic evidence of hypoperfusion of the subendocardial myocardium in dilated cardiomyopathy has been attributed to raised end-diastolic pressure combined with low aortic systolic pressure, plus compression caused by dilatation. Anginal chest pain occurs in at least 10% of patients with dilated cardiomyopathy, even in the absence of detectable coronary artery disease. Recent studies have suggested an abnormality of the microvasculature and that patients with dilated cardiomyopathy and chest pain have true myocardial ischemia resulting from dynamic abnormality of coronary resistance vessels, which is characterized by an abnormal vasodilator response to metabolic and pharmacologic stimuli.[12] In view of the absence of organic alteration in the microvasculature, the defect in dilatation must be functional or result from a combination of increased vasoconstrictor and reduced vasodilator tone coupled with abnormal response or production of regulatory endothelial peptides. Thus an impaired relaxation of the microvasculature in patients with dilated cardiomyopathy in response to the endothelium-dependent vasodilator acetylcholine has been demonstrated. This impairment is out of proportion to the mildly impaired response to adenosine, a dilator of vascular smooth muscle.[13] Triggered by impaired endothelium-dependent vasodilatation, microvascular spasm could impair myocardial metabolism, interfere with its contractile function and possibly induce focal myocardial necrosis. The cause of the endothelial impairment is not known. If it is secondary to heart failure it does not shed light on the cause of the failure.

Myocardial alterations (hypertrophy, nuclear changes, myofibrillar lysis, and interstitial fibrosis) are considered nonspecific and are poorly correlated with systolic functional variables. Others, however, have suggested that structural alterations of the myocardium with increased amounts of fibrous tissue are probably responsible for the observed changes in passive elastic properties of the myocardium in patients with dilated cardiomyopathy.[14] Still others have found good correlations between the ejection fraction and either the volume fraction of myofibrils, interstitial fibrosis, or muscle fiber diameter.[15]

Reduced myofibril volume fraction may have an adverse prognostic significance, whereas myocellular hypertrophy seems to have a compensatory role in idiopathic dilated cardiomyopathy.[16]

It is evident that comparison of clinical and hemody-namic parameters or comparison of prognosis with morphometric data has yielded conflicting results. Different case mixes and interpretations may account for the differences.

Pathogenesis and etiology of dilated cardiomyopathy

A variety of agents have been implicated in the pathogenesis of human dilated cardiomyopathy (DCM).[17] Picornaviruses,[18] parasites,[19] and cardiotoxic drugs are among the agents that have received the greatest attention.[20] In addition, several recent studies have documented the association of major histocompatibility gene products (MHC) as factors that play a role in genetic predisposition of a select group of patients with idiopathic dilated cardiomyopathy.[21,22] It is becoming increasingly clear that cardiac tissue injury induced by the insulting agents results in an immune response of the host against cardiac tissue self-antigens. The initial acute cardiac tissue injury leads to infiltration of host inflammatory cells that accumulate around areas of tissue injury. It is reasonable to assume that whereas the infiltrating host polymorphonuclear phagocytes perform their normal function, as is common in most acute inflammations, the infiltration of host mononuclear cells in the area of cardiac tissue injury results in the activation of non–antigen-specific (natural killer, or NK, cells) and antigen-specific (T cells, B cells, and macrophages) immune responses. Such activation thus results in the recognition not only of the foreign insulting agents, but also a variety of structural and nonstructural physiologically important cardiac tissue self-proteins, a number of which have been described in the literature.[23-26] In some cases, such acute cardiac tissue injury results in global myocarditis that leads to death, as seen in cases of acute myocarditis. In most cases it is reasonable to assume that such acute episodes of cardiac tissue injury and subsequent immune responses result in removal of the insulting agents, local necrosis followed by replacement fibrosis, dampening of the immune responses, and return to normal physiology and health of the patient. However, there appears to be increasing evidence that in select cases following such acute cardiac tissue injury, a chronic form of auto-immune–based pathology ensues. It is hypothesized that episodic effervescence of cryptic and persistent viruses and/or chronic exposure to cardiotoxic drugs results in metabolic perturbation of the affected cells. Such alterations lead to chronic exposure of the host immune system not only to the foreign proteins, but also to either altered forms of self-proteins, or self-proteins that have not been previously exposed to the host immune system during ontogeny. Such inaccessibility of these proteins to the immune system during early development (whereby positive and negative selection of antigen-specific T-cell clones occurs in the thymus) results in the recognition of these proteins that share sequences with host proteins. Thus, immune responses against these shared sequences result in an autoimmune immunologic response, a phenomenon known as "immunologic mimicry".[27] These autoimmune-based injuries, although secondary, may during a prolonged period of time induce cardiac tissue dysfunction, resulting in human dilated cardiomyopathy (DCM). It is clear, however, that such autoimmune-based pathology is very focal and localized. Therefore, examination of cardiac biopsies and/or cardiac tissue of DCM patients at autopsy rarely shows fulminant pathologic manifestations. Histopathologic studies of cardiac tissue specimens from autopsy cases of human DCM support this concept.[17] Thus it is a common finding that in most cases only nonspecific patchy areas of fibrosis are noted in cardiac tissues of DCM patients.[17] Patchy areas of replacement fibrosis, however, may represent the tombstones of myocytes that at one time either harbored cardiotropic enteroviruses in a latent form or were metabolically altered by exposure to cardiotoxic drugs or other agents. Based on the above concepts, this chapter is designed to provide a review of (1) our current evidence for a link between acute myocarditis and dilated cardiomyopathy; (2) the descriptive studies on the immunologic status of patients with DCM and the role of genetic factors; (3) the various autoimmune antibodies characterized in the sera of DCM patients, with the identification of the putative autoantigens; (4) a description of the cellular infiltrates, their phenotype and function; and (5) immunopathologic studies of cardiac tissue from DCM patients. It is important to note that there are several animal models of myocarditis that have provided insights on the pathogenesis of human DCM, and in vitro models have been described that may be useful in understanding the basic interactions between the host's immune system and cardiac tissue. However, these issues are discussed in Chapter 6 of this textbook.

Evidence for a link between myocarditis and human DCM

The finding of mononuclear cell infiltrates and necrosis in cardiac tissues has been used to define human myocarditis. As described above, many infectious disease agents and cardiotoxic drugs induce such cardiac tissue injury. Of the agents incriminated, picornaviruses have gained the largest attention. This is based largely on results from three general areas of investigation. First, in one study approximately 15% of patients who recovered from clinically diagnosed acute viral myocarditis developed chronic cardiac disease with clinical manifestations that were indistinguishable from those of human DCM.[28]

Second, a high frequency of DCM patients report a flu-like syndrome 4 to 8 weeks before the onset of clinical symptoms. About 36% to 53% of patients diagnosed with myocarditis have quantitatively high circulating antibody titers against coxsackie virus group B.[29] Such antibody titers were not seen in the sera of patients with other forms of heart disease.[29] The increased titers of coxsackie virus B were more pronounced in patients with congestive cardi-

omyopathy disease of less than 1 year's duration.[30] Sera from 90% of patients with myocarditis and DCM associated with coxsackie B influenza and mumps contain high titers of heart-reactive antibodies (HRAs). Such HRAs induce lysis of cultured cardiac tissue cells in vitro either in the presence of complement or by antibody-dependent cell-mediated cytotoxicity (ADCC) assays in the absence of complement, denoting their potential to induce cardiac tissue injury in vivo. Although similar HRAs were also seen in sera from otherwise healthy normal individuals and in sera from patients with other forms of cardiac diseases, the incidence and titers were much lower.[31] In this regard, it is interesting to note that a recent study showed that diffuse cytoplasmic staining of both atrial and ventricular myocytes was seen in sera from 26% of 65 DCM patients examined. The same sera did not stain skeletal muscle. Of importance was the finding that similar organ-specific tissue staining was seen in only 3.5% of the 200 normal sera screened; in only 1% of the sera from 205 patients with other forms of heart disease (coronary, hypertrophic cardiomyopathy, rheumatic, right ventricular dysplasia, and congenital); and in 0% of the sera from 41 patients with heart failure following myocardial infarction. It was suggested that this finding provides a new diagnostic criterion for human DCM.[32]

Third, several laboratories utilizing molecular tools have recently described the presence of enteroviral sequences in cardiac tissue specimens of a high frequency of myocarditis and DCM patients.[33-36] Finally, our laboratory results (described in detail below) strongly suggest that sera from patients with acute viral myocarditis, as compared with sera from DCM patients, contain similar autoantibodies against several putative cardiac tissue autoantigens that selectively react with cardiac tissues but not skeletal tissues.[37]

Consequently, the circumstantial epidemiologic data that document the progression from myocarditis to dilated cardiomyopathy, clinically and hemodynamically, together with results of cardiac tissue organ-specific autoimmune antibodies and the recent data (using molecular tools) on the presence of viral RNA sequences in cardiac tissue of a high frequency of patients with myocarditis and DCM, provide compelling evidence for a link between myocarditis and human DCM. It is important to note that such evidence does not account for the pathogenic mechanisms of all cases of DCM. As noted above, DCM is a multifaceted disease that results in insult to ventricular myocardium, and as such, other mechanisms are most likely involved. It is clear that further studies are required to refine our clinical and laboratory criteria for the classification of human cardiomyopathies.

Studies on the immunologic status of patients with DCM and the role of genetic factors

The concept that autoimmunity is involved in the pathogenesis of human DCM prompted investigations on the immunologic profile of patients, similar to the phenomenologic studies of patients with a variety of other autoimmune diseases. These investigations included assays for natural killer cell activity and nonspecific suppressor cell activity, analysis of responses to a battery of recall antigens by skin testing, and a study of levels of immune complexes in the sera of DCM patients. In addition, studies on the frequency of HLA types in patients with DCM were prompted by the knowledge that a variety of autoimmune diseases may be related to inheritance of major histocompatibility complex (MHC) genes. The findings of these studies are summarized below.

Studies of natural killer cell activity have shown varying results, depending on the target cells used in the assay. Some laboratories showed no difference in peripheral blood NK cell activity of patients with DCM as compared with controls using the K-562 as the target cell, whereas others have shown decreased NK cell activity in patients with DCM.[38,39] Maisch et al,[40] similar to Jacobs et al,[41] using myocytes as target cells from presumably HLA incompatible donors (thus presumably measuring NK cell activity against myocytes), demonstrated that peripheral blood lymphocytes from 30% of the patients with primary myocardial disease had detectable cytotoxic activity. It is interesting to note that 24% of patients with other cardiac diseases also showed significant cytotoxicity against cardiomyocytes,[41] indicating that such cytotoxic activity was present in one third of all patients with cardiac diseases in this study. Of interest was the finding that such NK-type activity was not seen against Chang liver cells, denoting an element of cell lineage specificity for this type of NK cell function. The addition of autologous serum in these cytotoxicity assays revealed interesting data. Only autologous sera from patients with secondary (alcoholic) myocardial disease significantly abrogated such cell-mediated cytotoxicity. Sera from patients with primary myocardial disease or postmyocarditic disease failed to show significant blocking activity, denoting perhaps a method for differential diagnosis of myocardial disease.

In addition, studies of Cambridge et al,[42] showed a reduced ability of mononuclear cells to respond to the induction of NK cell activity by interferon in patients with primary myocardial disease as compared with control subjects.

In a study conducted by Lowry et al,[43] no major abnormality of the normal cellular immune response was noted in patients with dilated cardiomyopathy. The tests included a variety of in vivo skin test antigens, such as tuberculin (PPD), SK-SD, candida albicans, and BCG. They also included a variety of in vitro tests, such as the blastogenic response of the peripheral blood mononuclear cells to nonspecific mitogens PHA and con-A, and the ability to produce migration inhibition factor in response to the skin test antigens described above. In addition, the frequency of total T cells, helper and suppressor T cells, NK cells and Ia+ cells in the recirculating pool of peripheral blood lymphocytes was also measured using mononuclear reagents and flow microfluorometry. All of these tests failed to reveal major differences between patients and control subjects.[44] These data on cell-mediated immunity are in contrast to those published by Das et al,[45] who observed that more than 40% of patients with congestive cardiomyopathy showed decreased levels of cell-mediated immunity. The data on the frequency of cell subpopulations determined by Das et al[45] are in agreement with those obtained by Anderson et al,[44] who, in addition to examining the frequency of helper, suppressor, and total T cells, examined the frequency of NK cells (using Leu-7 and Leu 11) and macrophages (OKM-1) and failed to show any marked difference. However, reduced NK cell function in the peripheral blood of patients with DCM was seen in this study. In contrast, Kipshidze et al[46] demonstrated a decrease in the frequency of suppressor T cells in 22 patients with DCM. Analysis of the frequency of lymphoid cell subsets in the PBMC (Peripheral blood mononuclear cells) of patients with acute myocarditis revealed elevated frequencies of B cells and activated T lymphocytes (HLA-DR+). However, no significant differences in the level of suppressor cell function or frequency of CD8+ T cells were noted.

Suppressor cell function has been examined in patients with cardiomyopathies. Fowles et al[47] demonstrated a marked impairment of suppressor cell induction in peripheral blood mononuclear cells of patients with idiopathic congestive cardiomyopathy, but not in patients with end-stage coronary artery disease (using con-A as an inducing agent and alloreactivity in mixed lymphocyte cultures as an assay system). These data were supported by studies of Eckstein et al,[48] who further demonstrated that such lack of suppressor cell induction in PBMC from DCM patients was also seen in patients with myocarditis. Nonspecific suppressor factors in the sera of patients with dilated cardiomyopathy have also been reported,[49] and it has been suggested that these inhibitors play a role in the pathogenesis of this disease.

As far as immune complexes are concerned, it is interesting to note that about 10% of patients with primary or secondary (alcoholic) cardiomyopathy demonstrate circulating levels of immune complexes, as compared with about 5% seen in healthy control subjects.[40] However, 30% of the patients with postmyocarditic disease demonstrated up to 64 μg/ml of IgG immune complexes. Sera from a significant number of patients with coxsackie virus infections have also been shown to contain significant levels of immune complexes. These complexes were shown to contain coxsackie virus-specific antigens.[50]

Although the above studies are to a large extent phenomenologic, they are consistent with the hypothesis that the phenomenologic findings in DCM patients, at least in a significant number of them appear to resemble findings seen in a variety of other autoimmune diseases. In addition to the above analyses, the finding of disorders of immune regulation in human DCM has prompted studies of the genes that regulate immune response. It has been established that gene products of the major histocompatibility complex (MHC) in both humans and a variety of animal species play a major role in the regulation of immune responses at the cellular and molecular level. There are three major classes of MHC gene products: MHC class I, MHC class II, and MHC class III. The MHC class I gene products are glycoproteins expressed on nearly all nucleated cells; the MHC class II gene products are glycoproteins that have a more restricted tissue distribution being expressed on B cells, macrophages, dendritic cells, and activated T cells; and the MHC class III gene products code for tumor necrosis factor and complement proteins. Our recent knowledge of the nature of these gene products shows that endogenously derived peptides, such as those coded by viruses intracellularly, appear to associate predominantly with MHC class I gene products and are then expressed on the cell surface, whereas exogenously added proteins appear to be processed intracellularly, then associated with MHC class II gene products, and subsequently expressed on the cell surface. The MHC class I and class II gene products expressed on the cell surface thus contain endogenously and exogenously derived peptides, respectively, which they present to the cells of the immune system. The CD4$^+$ T cells appear to predominantly recognize exogenously derived peptides in association with MHC class II molecules, whereas the CD8$^+$ T cells appear to predominantly recognize endogenously derived peptides in association with MHC class I molecules. However, notable exceptions of CD4$^+$/MHC class II and CD8$^+$/MHC class I interactions do exist. Such specific interactions of CD4$^+$ and CD8$^+$ T cells with self-MHC molecules define the concepts of MHC restricted immune reactions. Antigen-specific CD4$^+$ T cells thus become activated only subsequent to recognition of the appropriate peptide in context of self-MHC class II molecules. These self–MHC-restricted activated CD4$^+$ T cells have been shown to be functionally heterogeneous. Some provide helper function for the activation and synthesis of Ig by B cells, whereas others have been shown to provide signals for the activation of CD8$^+$ suppressor T cells; yet, other populations appear to help in the induction of CD8$^+$ cytotoxic T cells. These T cells and their subpopulations recognize the peptide-MHC ligand by virtue of clonally distributed T-cell receptors. Antigen (peptide)-specific recognition thus requires the availability of appropriate clones of T cells with TcR specific for peptide self-MHC complex. This repertoire of T-cell clones develops in the thymus through a process known as negative and positive selection whereby clones of T cells, upon exposure to self peptides in the context of self-MHC molecules, lead to activation and specific clonal elimination by way of a process referred to as *apoptosis* (negative selection).

The precise molecular events leading to positive as compared with negative selection are still poorly under-

stood. It is however, readily apparent that our ability to recognize self vs. nonself is governed to a large extent by the emergence and/or deletion of T-cell clones that recognize self-proteins and subsequent peptides in the context of MHC molecules. The knowledge that immunologic dysfunction occurs in patients with a variety of autoimmune diseases has prompted the study of the association of MHC (particularly class II gene products) and the autoimmune diseases. As examples, rheumatoid arthritis has been shown to be associated with HLA-DR4 and DR1; myasthenia gravis with HLA-DR3 and DR7; systemic lupus erythematosus with HLA-DR2 and DR3; multiple sclerosis with HLA-DR2, and insulin-dependent diabetes mellitus with HLA-DR3 and DR4.

Regarding cardiomyopathies, whereas there is considerable knowledge about the familial genetic transmission of hypertrophic cardiomyopathy, very few studies have been conducted on genetic factors that may be associated with human DCM. Results of these are summarized here. A recent prospective study revealed that 7% of DCM cases had at least one other member of the family affected.[51] This figure may underestimate the real incidence of familial occurrences because the disorder may be latent in some relatives within the family. The mode of inheritance of familial dilated cardiomyopathy was originally thought to be autosomal dominant, but recently a recessive autosomal allele has been identified. Therefore both modes of inheritance may be involved.[52] Furthermore, an x-linked genetic transmission has also been observed.[53]

Of the more definitive studies on the genetic association of DCM, the studies by Carlquist et al[21] have been the most extensive. These investigators have recently confirmed their previous findings and shown an increase of DR4 (49% in DCM patients, compared with 21% in normal controls) frequency and a trend toward decreased association with DRW6 (10% in DCM patients, compared with 23% in control subjects). In addition, the combined DR4-DQW4 haplotype was seen in 5 of 41 white DCM patients, compared with 0 of 53 control subjects. The increased association of DR4 with DCM was seen by these investigators in a series of five studies conducted over time in several different patient populations. Arbustini et al[22] have basically confirmed the increased frequency of DR4 in DCM patients. In addition, they have performed histologic studies on biopsy specimens of these patients and observed that a group of DCM patients showed large abnormal nuclei in hypertrophic myocytes. Based on such morphologic parameters and myocyte diameter, the nuclear size and nuclear/cytoplasmic ratio allowed them to subgroup DCM patients. Whereas an increased DR4 association was seen with the entire group of DCM patients, the group with bizarre nuclei appeared to be more strongly associated with DR5. There was also a decreased frequency of DR3 in DCM patients as compared with the HLA type of 400 normal individuals. The association of DCM with

HLA-DR4 has also been reported by Limas et al,[54] who have shown that 40% of DCM patients were HLA-DR4 positive, compared with 24% in control groups. Also of considerable interest is their finding that there is no correlation between presence of HLA-DR4 and the severity of duration of the disease, which indicates that this genetic marker does not influence the progression of the disease.

These data, in general, appear to show that careful characterization of DCM patients, in addition to more refined studies of endomyocardial biopsies, may provide further insights regarding the association of DR4 and, more importantly, both the positive and the negative association with certain MHC class II alleles. The aspects of negative association of MHC types with autoimmune diseases are gaining increased importance as our knowledge about putative autoimmune peptide binding with MHC class II molecules increases. Thus (as in the case with RA), it appears that lack of inheritance of a certain class II molecule may allow the preferential competitive association with another class II molecule that may result in disease. The former may thus be regarded as a "protective" class II molecule, whereas lack thereof may result in a "nonprotective" disease-inducing MHC class II molecule. Studies of the molecular analysis of MHC class II genes, coupled with identification of the precise autoepitopes in DCM, may provide exciting future directions for the diagnosis and mechanisms of this confounding disease.

Presence of autoantibodies in the sera of DCM patients

Historically, the presence of autoantibodies against myocardial tissue was most widely recognized in patients following myocardial infarction, or cardiac surgery. It was reasoned that tissue injury led to the release of cardiac tissue proteins that were recognized as neoantigens, thus resulting in immune responses. Dressler[55] was among the first to describe autoantibodies against heart tissue in patients with rheumatic carditis, postmyocardial infarction, and postpericardiotomy syndromes. Subsequently, heart-reactive antibodies (HRAs) were characterized in the sera of patients with a number of disease conditions involving cardiac tissue injury, such as post-infectious (presumably viral) myocarditis, Chagas disease, postadriamycin cardiotoxicity, and dilated cardiomyopathy. In collaboration with the laboratories of Herskowitz et al (The Johns Hopkins University, Baltimore, MD), our laboratory screened sera from patients with various forms of cardiomyopathy and showed that a high frequency of sera from patients with clinical myocarditis, idiopathic DCM, postpartum cardiomyopathy and postadriamycin cardiomyopathy contained high titers of HRAs as compared with sera from patients with hypertrophic cardiomyopathy, the so-called ischemic cardiomyopathy, alcoholic cardiomyopathy, and sera from normal control individuals (see Table 7-1). Maisch et al[40] were the first to study the subcellular pattern of HRAs in patients with cardiomyopathies. Using clinical criteria, they compared patients who had primary cardiomyopathies with those who had secondary cardiomyopathies and showed that sera from 89% of the patients with postmyocarditic cardiomyopathy stained the sarcolemma and intracellular cardiac proteins, whereas only 9% of individual sera from patients with primary cardiomyopathy showed such a staining pattern. The titers of the reactive sera correlated with the degree of myocytolysis induced by

Table 7-1. Human heart-reactive antibody titers in the sera of DCM patients and patients with other forms of cardiomyopathies* as determined by an indirect fluorescent antibody (IFA) technique[†]

Source of sera	No. of sera tested	No. of sera positive/Total no. tested			
		<1:10	1:40	1:80	>1:160
DCM	46	2/46	6/46	10/46	28/46
Myocarditis	12	—	—	—	12/12
Postpartum cardiomyopathy	4	—	—	1/4	3/4
Adriamycin cardiomyopathy	3	—	—	—	3/3
Hypertrophic cardiomyopathy	12	9/12	3/12	—	—
Alcoholic cardiomyopathy	26	10/12	2/12	—	—
Coronary artery disease	32	26/32	4/32	2/32	—
Normal	24	24/24	—	—	—

*Sera were obtained from patients with dilated cardiomyopathy (DCM), patients following acute myocarditis (presumably viral), pediatric cases, patients with other forms of cardiomyopathies, and normal adult healthy laboratory volunteers. Patients with coronary artery disease comprised those with myocardial infarction infraction (N = 14) and without myocardial infarction (N = 18).

[†]The IFA technique utilized serial sections of fresh frozen human cardiac tissue (obtained at autopsy from a patient who died of other than cardiac disease). The tissue section was incubated with 0.1 ml of normal rabbit serum (to block nonspecific binding) for 30 min. After decanting, twofold dilutions of the sera to be tested were added, and following incubation for 30 min at 4° C, the sections were washed with PBS pH 7.4. This was followed by the addition of 0.1 ml of a fluorescein-conjugated F(ab′)₂ fraction of rabbit anti-human IgG diluted 1/100. The sections were washed and then immediately scored for reactivity, using a fluorescence microscope.

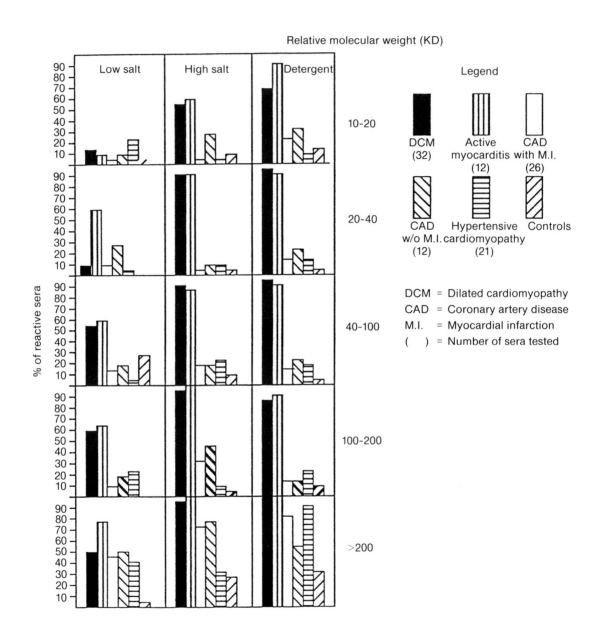

Relative molecular weight (KD)

Table 7-2. Autoantibodies in the sera of patients against structural proteins detected by ELISA

	Frequency (% positive)*				
	Sera from				
Structural proteins†	DCM‡ (N = 57)	Alcoholic CM (N = 28)	CAD (N = 41)	RA (N = 48)	SLE (N = 44)
Myosin	92.5	73.4	81.6	64.7	41.3
Actin	68.4	77.3	78.2	71.4	81.3
Alpha-actinin	24.3	34.6	43.1	23.7	28.6
Tropomyosin	48.6	27.3	26.9	28.4	37.2
Vinculin	21.2	10.2	9.2	10.8	10.4
Desmin	37.4	18.2	26.8	34.1	32.6
Keratin	84.4	87.4	91.6	92.4	94.0
Collagen type I	72.1	82.1	92.4	88.4	92.6
Collagen type II	75.1	72.6	88.6	81.2	88.4
Collagen type III	72.1	83.2	92.8	91.4	86.8
Laminin	53.4	38.9	48.8	43.4	49.6

*Sera was considered positive if reactivity was greater than 2 S.D. above background control. Sera was diluted 1/40 for this assay.
†Structural proteins were purchased commercially, and positive controls consisted of monoclonal and/or heterologous commercially available antisera.
‡DCM = dilated cardiomyopathy, alcoholic CM = alcoholic cardiomyopathy, CAD = coronary artery disease with myocardial infarction (N=26) and without myocardial infarction (N=15), RA = rheumatoid arthritis, and SLE = systemic lupus erythematosus.

such sera. In contrast, antiinterfibrillary antibodies were found in the sera from 49% of the patients with primary dilated cardiomyopathy and 61% of the patients with alcoholic cardiomyopathy. These data were interpreted to indicate that different proteins and epitopes were being recognized in the sera of patients with cardiomyopathies, based on the etiology of the disease. Subsequently, various other laboratories, including ours, have shown that these HRAs occur in the sera of a high frequency of DCM patients. The pathologic significance of such HRAs was strengthened by the finding that cardiac biopsy tissue from patients with primary congestive cardiomyopathy contained significant levels of tissue-bound Ig.[56] In studies of cardiac biopsies, there also appeared to be a correlation between the ejection fraction of the patient and the presence of such cardiac tissue-bound Ig. Cardiac biopsies of 77% of these patients with ejection fractions of less than 35% had tissue-bound Ig, as compared with 45% of the patients with ejection fraction less than 35%. Elution of tissue bound Ig from cardiac tissue of DCM patients revealed that such Ig contained high titers of myosin-reactive antibodies (Dr. Ahvie Herskowitz, personal communications). Studies by other laboratories showed that high titers of HRAs were seen when cardiac tissue from DCM patients, rather than rat heart tissue, was used as a substrate. Biochemical studies were initiated in efforts to identify the targets of such HRAs in the sera of DCM patients. One study reported that sera from about 25% of DCM patients contained antibodies that reacted with submitochondrial particles from beef heart but not pig kidney or rat liver.[57] The predominant reactivity, characterized to be an antigen between 67 kDa and 72 kDa, was termed *M-7*, based on the classical scheme of Berg et al for the identification of mitochondrial

proteins of various molecular weights that react with sera from patients with autoimmune-involved liver disease.[57] The reactivity of DCM sera against M-7 was shown to be specific because sera from a variety of patients with other diseases and from control subjects failed to react.[57] Furthermore, a link between the acute stages of myocarditis and chronic DCM was implied by the finding that sera from the myocarditis cases contained IgM-specific anti–M-7 antibody, whereas IgG-Specific–M-7 antibody was detected in the sera from DCM patients. As an initial attempt to identify the spectrum of proteins that are recognized by sera from DCM patients, our laboratory prepared sequential extracts of low salt, high salt, and detergent-solubilized proteins from human cardiac tissue. These extracts were then subjected to electrophoretic separation, and Western blot analysis was used to screen sera from patients with DCM (N = 32), postacute presumed viral myocarditis (N = 12), cardiomyopathy associated with coronary artery disease with myocardial infarction (N = 26) and without myocardial infarction (N = 12), hypertensive cardiomyopathy (N = 21), and sera from normal adult healthy laboratory volunteers (N = 24). As summarized in Table 7-1 Fig. 7-A, studies showed that a high frequency of sera from DCM patients and postmyocarditis patients reacted with bands of various molecular weights. Of interest was the finding that the majority of the reactivity appeared to be directed against detergent-solubilized and high salt extracts of human heart tissue. It was also interesting that a high frequency of sera from patients with various forms of cardiomyopathies, including DCM, reacted with antigens of high molecular weight (>200 kDa), denoting an element of nonspecific reactivity against these normal cardiac tissue proteins. These findings are supported by previous reports that sera from DCM patients react with a number of structural proteins such as myosin, actin, alpha-actinin, tropomyosin, vinculin, desmin, keratin, and collagen. Unfortunately, such reactivity against structural proteins is also found in sera from patients with other forms of cardiac disease and with other autoimmune diseases, such as rheumatoid arthritis (RA) and systemic lupus erythematosus (SLE). Table 7-2 presents a comparison of the frequency of sera that react with such structural proteins. These sera were from patients with DCM, other forms of cardiomyopathies, and autoimmune diseases such as RA and SLE. The reactivity of these sera against these structural proteins makes it difficult to ascertain the pathogenic significance of these autoantibodies. Based on the high index of suspicion that DCM is a chronic autoimmune disease that results from infectious viral autoimmune disease that occurs following infectious viral myocarditis, sera from post-coxsackie virus B myocarditis patients have been studied for reactivity against cardiac tissue antigens. In one such study, it was shown that sera from 40% to 50% of such patients reacted with cardiac tissue proteins of 34 kDa, 48 kDa, and 110 kDa, and sera from 15% reacted with proteins of 28 kDa, 31 kDa, and 220 kDa. As expected, such sera also had high titers of antibodies against coxsackie virus antigens. It was suggested that antibodies against coxsackie virus antigens cross-react with normal cardiac myocyte antigens, supporting the concept that "molecular mimicry," as proposed by the laboratory of Oldstone et al,[27] is involved in the pathogenic mechanisms of myocarditis-induced disease. Such cross-reacting antibodies between coxsackie antigens and self-tissue proteins were reasoned to be the underlying mechanisms that, in a select group of patients following acute infections, lead to the development of DCM. In this regard, it is important to note that a monoclonal antibody against the VP-1 capsid protein of coxsackie virus B4 was shown to cross-react with the contractile muscle proteins,[57a] one of which may be the v-1 isoform of cardiac myosin.

Identification of the major autoantigens

The laboratories of Schulteiss in association with Klingenberg[58-60] were the first to report the identification of the putative autoantigens that react with sera from DCM patients. The protein was identified as the adenine nucleotide translocator (ANT) inner mitochondrial membrane protein of 31-32 kDa. The functional significance of such antibody reactivity was strengthened by the finding that a rabbit antibody raised against ANT was shown to induce irreversible contractile dysfunction in cultures of cardiac myocytes in vitro.[61] In addition, immunization of guinea pigs with the ANT protein not only induced a decrease in the cytosolic mitochondrial difference in the phosphorylation potential of adenosine triphosphate,[59,61] but also appeared to induce diminished cardiac performance in these animals.[59] The ANT is the predominant protein found in cardiac mitochondria. In humans, there are at least three isoforms

(ANT1, ANT2 and ANT3)[62-64]; of these, only ANT1 and ANT2 are expressed in cardiac tissue. The genes encoding these three isoforms have been cloned and their full-length sequence established.[62-64] Recent studies by the laboratory of Schultheiss et al[65] have identified two peptide sequences of the ANT that react with DCM sera. Our laboratory has confirmed the observation that sera from DCM patients react with a mitochondrial protein of 31-32 kDa, biochemically purified as described by Schultheiss et al.,[65a] and therefore presumably native ANT.[66] However, in vitro translation and transcription of the full-length human skeletal muscle ANT, using a rabbit reticulocyte lysate assay, failed to show reactivity against sera from DCM patients. In addition, fusion proteins generated by cloning the translated region of the ANT, cDNA[62] into the bacterial expression vector pGEX2T failed to show reactivity with not only sera from DCM patients, but also the rabbit anti-ANT sera. The reason for this failure is not clear at present. It is also important to know that the rabbit anti-ANT sera has been shown to cross-react with the Ca^{++} channel plasma membrane protein[24] of guinea pig myocytes and to cause increased Ca^{++} uptake and myocyte injury. Previously, it was difficult to ascertain the pathogenic significance of antibodies against an intracellular protein. However, the cross-reactivity of the rabbit anti-ANT sera against a plasma membrane Ca^{++} channel protein makes it reasonable to visualize its pathogenic role.*

In addition to ANT, sera from DCM patients have also been shown to react with cardiac myosin. The pathogenic significance of such antibodies was strengthened by the finding that mice immunized with myosin develop myocarditis that is indistinguishable from that induced by experimental infection of these mice with coxsackie virus B3. A prominent role for cytokines in the inflammatory process of coxsackie virus-induced myocarditis in the murine model has recently been documented.[66b] The precise mechanism by which these antimyosin antibodies induce cardiac damage in human DCM patients remains to be determined. Recent data seem to suggest that the α and β cardiac myosin heavy chain isoforms may be the major autoantigens in DCM.[66c] In this regard, the murine model (described in detail in another chapter) of myosin-induced myocarditis provides an excellent model for studying the potential mechanisms of this autoimmune-based disease. In addition to ANT and myosin, two other proteins have been shown to react with sera from DCM patients. These include the branched chain alpha ketoacid dehydrogenase (BCKD-E2) mitochondrial protein[23,37] and the cardiac B-adrenoceptor proteins.[25] Sera from about 70% of DCM patients were shown to react with BCKD-E2,[66] and 30%-40% of them with cardiac B-adrenoceptor. Once again, it is not presently clear how an antibody against the intracellular BCKD-E2 protein induces cardiac damage. However, sera from DCM patients have been shown to induce internalization of the B-adrenoceptors, which are subsequently degraded intracellularly. Antireceptor anti-

---

*It should be noted that a high degree of correlation exists between the presence of ANT-reactive antibodies and DCM. In particular, the disease association is highest when such ANT-reactive sera are shown to inhibit the biologic activity of ANT in vitro (Schultheiss et al., personal communication). It is also important to note that recent evidence suggests that the mitochondrial benzodiazepine receptor appears to be a trimolecular

complex of 18 kDa, 30 kDa, and 32 kDa. The 30 kDa and 32 kDa proteins have been identified as the voltage-dependent anion channel and the adenine nucleotide translocator proteins.[66a] It is thus possible that the 32 kDa reactivity may indeed be directed against the VDAC rather than ANT, which may help explain the lack of reactivity of sera from DCM patients with in vitro translated and transcribed ANT.

bodies have been shown to selectively inhibit the activity of isoproterenol-sensitive adenylate cyclase, using a membrane preparation in vitro. The presence of such anti–beta-receptor antibodies in DCM patients was shown to be linked to the HLA-DR4 MHC allele. In this study, sera from 77% of the HLA-DR4$^+$ DCM patients contained such antibodies, as compared with the presence of such antibodies in only 22% of the DCM patients that were HLA-DR4.[67] Current efforts have resulted in the mapping of the putative epitopes of the β-adrenoreceptor proteins (Hoebeke J, personal communication) that are the target of the autoimmune response against this protein.

In summary, there are currently several identified autoantigens for human DCM. These include the intracellular mitochondrial proteins ANT and BCKD, cardiac myosin, and the B-adrenoceptor protein. In addition, the possibility that the Ca^{++} channel protein also reacts with a rabbit anti-ANT sera provides another potential target auto-antigen. These proteins still need to be considered as putative autoantigens until the full pathogenic significance of such autoantibodies is identified.

Immunopathologic studies of cardiac tissue from DCM patients

Endomyocardial biopsies, cardiac tissue sections prepared from recipient explanted hearts during transplantation, and cardiac tissue sections prepared from recipient explanted hearts during transplantation, and cardiac tissue sections prepared from autopsy tissues of DCM patients have been utilized for a variety of studies designed to elucidate the mechanisms of pathogenesis of this disease. Several laboratories have conducted studies to quantitate the frequency of mononuclear cell infiltrates in such cardiac tissue. Results from these studies have been variable, primarily because of differences in criteria used for diagnosis of the patients who were the source of the tissue and/or the definition of the constitution of mononuclear cell infiltrates (i.e., 2 to 5 vs. 5 to 10 or 10 to 20 leukocytes per high power field). It is nonetheless the consensus opinion that, whereas massive leukocyte infiltrates are readily observed in cardiac biopsies and tissues from patients during episodes of acute myocarditis, it is relatively rare to observe infiltrates in tissue specimens from DCM patients. In general, small isolated foci of mononuclear cells have been reported in select cases of human DCM, accompanied by patchy areas of necrosis and replacement fibrosis. Phenotypic analysis of these mononuclear cell infiltrates has shown them to consist primarily of CD4$^+$ T cells, NK cells, and sIg$^+$ B cells in relative order of predominance. Of interest have been studies dealing with the expression of MHC antigens in cardiac tissues. Normal human cardiac myocytes do not constitutively express MHC class I or class II antigens.[68,69] In contrast, cardiac myocytes from patients with acute myocarditis and select cases of DCM demonstrate a marked increase in the expression of MHC class I antigens and, to a smaller extent, MHC class II antigens.[37] This has been documented by both immunoperoxidase techniques and by a radioimmunoassay developed to more specifically quantitate the lev-

els of MHC class I and class II antigens expressed by cardiac tissues. At face value, these data are consistent with the hypothesis that chronic autoimmune responses must be occurring in cardiac tissues of DCM patients, mediated by the infiltrating mononuclear cells upon recognition of cardiac tissue proteins in the context of expressed MHC antigens. This concept of recognition of cardiac tissue proteins is difficult to reconcile with recent data on the function of such MHC-expressing myocytes.[66] Thus in vitro coculture of isolated single cell cultures of human cardiac myocytes, even after induction of MHC antigens on such cells prior to coculture (by incubation with gamma interferon) with allogeneic PBMC, failed to induce proliferation, interleukin-2 generation, or the development of cytotoxic cells.[66] Such failure to induce allogeneic T-cell activation was not secondary to the absence of IL-1 or IL-2. Preincubation of MHC-expressing cardiac myocytes with highly enriched monocytes for 3 hours to overnight, followed by coculture with T cells, led to marked proliferative responses that appeared to be restricted by the MHC type of the monocytes utilized.[66] These data appeared to suggest that host T-cell sensitization to cardiac myocyte antigens most likely occur via processing and presentation of these antigens by resident dendritic cells or infiltrating antigen-presenting cells (APCs) rather than directly by MHC-expressing cardiac myocytes. It is conceivable, however, that such initial sensitization may lead to secondary responses against MHC-expressing myocytes presenting the same peptide if such myocytes have the potential for processing self-proteins. Such investigations have important implications for our understanding of the mechanisms of cardiac myocyte injury, and the molecular basis for such interactions is currently being analyzed by our laboratory.

The identification of the autoantigens that may be involved in the pathogenesis of human DCM prompted the study of expression of these autoantigens in cardiac tissues from DCM patients. The results of these studies showed that cardiac myocytes in focal areas of the myocardium expressed quantitatively high levels of ANT and BCKD, using immunoperoxidase techniques.[37] This increased expression was selectively seen in cardiac tissue specimens from DCM patients and not in similar cardiac tissue specimens of patients with other forms of cardiomyopathies; nor was it seen in normal control cardiac tissue specimens.[37] The increased expression was also cardiac organ tissue-specific because skeletal muscle tissues or sections from renal, pancreas, or liver tissues of DCM patients failed to show increased expression. It should be emphasized that such increased expression of these putative autoantigens was in *small focal areas* of cardiac tissue sections from DCM patients; it was difficult to distinguish cardiac membrane expression from cytoplasmic expression. Such increased expression of these putative autoantigens was not only detected by using heterologous antisera against ANT and BCKD, but also by using ANT and BCKD affinity-purified sera from human DCM patients. In addition, such staining was not secondary to Fc binding of the antibody (because (F[ab′]$_2$) fractions of the antisera were utilized) and was not secondary to nonspecific staining of necrotic areas of the tissue specimens. Of interest was the observation that isolated myocytes from a few pediatric cases of acute (presumably viral) myocarditis, when analyzed by flow microfluorometric (FMF) techniques, demonstrated increased expression of ANT, BCKD, MHC class I, and (to a lesser extent) MHC class II antigens. Such FMF studies were not possible with tissues from adult DCM patients because of our inability to prepare viable single cell myocyte preparations from such tissues. Examination of cardiac tissue specimens or isolated cardiac myocytes for the expression of myosin were not fruitful because these tissues normally express high levels of this protein. These data, in concert, suggest that (1) there is increased expression of MHC class I and, to a lesser extent, MHC class II antigens by a high frequency of cardiac myocytes from patients with acute myocarditis and by small foci of cardiac myocytes in DCM patients; (2) there is similarly increased expression of ANT, BCKD, and probably myosin in a high frequency of myocytes from patients with acute myocarditis and in small discrete foci of the myocardium in cardiac tissues of DCM patients; (3) the increased expression of these MHC antigens and the putative autoantigens is unique to DCM patients and patients during episodes of acute myocarditis; and (4) the increased expression of the MHC antigens and the putative autoantigens is organ-specific. The recent findings of enteroviral sequences in cardiac tissue specimens from patients with myocarditis and select patients with DCM,[33,36] coupled with the above findings, provide compelling evidence that autoimmune mechanisms may play a role in the pathogenesis of this disease. Within this context, it should be kept in mind that such abnormal expression of MHC antigens is most likely induced by cytokines generated by cellular infiltrates. These cytokines are known to have pleiotropic effects, and it is conceivable that such cytokines may alter normal myocyte physiology and thus result in cytolysis of these cells. Certainly, additional studies need to be performed to delineate more precisely the pathways and mechanisms that lead to myocyte cytolysis.

PATHOPHYSIOLOGY

Dilated cardiomyopathy is characterized by impaired systolic function with dilatation of one or both ventricles. Although preceding myocarditis caused by virus infection or other infective or noninfective agent is favored, such causation is hard to prove by the time a patient is seen, and etiology may be multifactorial. Previous hypertension, often undiagnosed, undoubtedly has a role in some patients, particularly in Africa and the Caribbean. Alcohol is the most common toxin to depress myocardial contractile force. Although the contribution of alcohol to the heart failure may not be obvious from the clinical history or investigations, disclosure is important because abstention may be followed by great improvement in cardiac function. Peripartum cardiomyopathy is a distinct condition with an immunologic basis for the myocarditis that has

been sometimes found on biopsy. When not rapidly lethal, this also may improve markedly, even to apparently total recovery in some patients.

Dilated cardiomyopathy is usually regarded as sporadic, particularly if an infective agent is suspected, but immunologic factors are probably important in causing an inflammatory response and perpetuating myocardial damage and deterioration. An inherited tendency may therefore determine whether a common virus infection of the myocardium is followed by rapid recovery or the development of heart failure. Affected families have been reported and are being found increasingly when a family history is taken carefully and physical examination, electrocardiography and echocardiography examination carried out on as many relatives as possible. In this way 18 relatives from 12 families of 59 index patients with dilated cardiomyopathy were found to be affected out of 315 relatives who had been examined. In addition, 22 of 240 healthy relatives with normal ejection fractions had increased left ventricular diameters during either systole or diastole or both, compared with only 2 of 112 healthy control subjects. In this study from the Mayo Clinic dilated cardiomyopathy was found to be familial in 20% of the patients, a much higher proportion than had previously been reported.[70]

Although reduced systolic function with dilation of one or both ventricles without other explanation are the criteria for recognition, there is a wide spectrum of disease. Most cases first seek help on account of the development of left ventricular failure, but milder cases are seen because of embolism, arrhythmia, or abnormal electrocardiogram or are asymptomatic. They may be detected on echocardiographic screening of relatives when physical examination, the electrocardiogram, and chest x-ray may all be normal. Although previously regarded as a relentlessly progressive and fatal condition, dilated cardiomyopathy, when recognized in these milder forms, may remain stable for many years or for as long as the patients are followed.[71,72] At the other end of the spectrum, patients with a short history and in severe heart failure with greatly dilated hearts when first seen usually do badly and require transplantation.[73,74]

A combination of adequate stroke volume and heart rate at low filling pressure plus trained skeletal muscles is needed for efficient exercise performance. Such efficiency may be achieved despite a dilated left ventricle with a low ejection fraction, or it may fail to be achieved by an undilated left ventricle with a preserved ejection fraction (Fig. 7-1). If the filling pressures rise with normal or near-normal parameters of systolic function, the condition is termed *restrictive cardiomyopathy*.

It has long been recognized that it is impossible to assess a patient's clinical state from the appearance of the left ventricle on angiography or echocardiographic imaging.[75] A substantially dilated ventricle looks worse and has a lower calculated ejection fraction, but such a ventricle needs to contract less in order to eject a normal stroke volume (Fig. 7-7). Provided the stroke volume remains close to normal and exercise-induced tachycardia is associated with continued ability of the left atrium to empty at near normal pressure, symptoms will be absent. The amount of left ventricular dilatation compatible with these characteristics is widely variable, and there is a continuum between "dilated" and "restrictive" cardiomyopathy.

Recent studies have emphasized these differences in diastolic function between left ventricles with varying degrees of dilatation and ejection fraction because functional class depends not upon the degree of left ventricular dilatation, but upon this preservation of output and filling pressure. Severely symptomatic patients in Classes III and IV have higher left ventricular filling pressures than asymptomatic or mildly symptomatic (Class I and II) patients although ejection fraction and left ventricular size may be similar.[76,77]

The development of mitral or tricuspid regurgitation curtails ventricular filling and forward stroke and raises filling pressures. By its onset before the semilunar valves open and its continuation after they have closed, atrioventricular valve regurgitation reduces the time available for diastolic filling. Reversed flow in the pulmonary veins may be seen via Doppler technique when left atrial pressure is high, even when mitral regurgitation is quantitatively not severe. Left atrial contraction may fail to augment left ventricular filling, and regurgitation occurs if the P-R-interval is long. The left atrium then dilates, and atrial fibrillation soon supervenes, with further increase in both tricuspid and mitral reflux. These developments are indicators of poor prognosis in dilated cardiomyopathy.[78]

Patients with dilated cardiomyopathy are helped by modern therapy to reduce left ventricular afterload, left ventricular size, and left atrial pressure.[79,80] The presence of ventricular ectopy found on Holter ECG recording is associated with poor prognosis and the risk of sudden death not preceded by observed deterioration in symptoms, which occurs in about half of the patients. Treatment with antiarrhythmic drugs has so far not been shown to improve prognosis. A proarrhythmic effect together with depression of myocardial function caused by these drugs may be deleterious, whereas improvement in function by the use of angiotensin-converting enzyme (ACE) inhibitors, though in themselves not antiarrhythmic agents, may reduce the incidence of ectopy and improve prognosis.[81]

Although the treatment of heart failure has been revolutionized by the ACE inhibitors, improvement in exercise performance has been disappointing. Skeletal muscles show loss of fast oxidative fibers, reduction of mitochondria, and shrinkage of the capillary network. The resistance vessels show loss of vasodilator capacity in heart failure.[82] They are stiff, perhaps because of increased sodium content, and vasoconstricted through neurohormonal activation. The latter is intensified by diuretic therapy and in addition, there may be abnormal endothelial function

with failure of dilatation to accompany increased flow.[83] Maximal vasodilation seems to be reduced. These changes with reduction of blood flow to exercising muscle caused by the heart failure, together with detraining secondary to inactivity, can be partly reversed by daily exercise training, which improves exercise performance in patients with chronic stable treated failure.[84,85] This explains the delay between clinical control of failure and objective improvement in performance. Exercise is part of the treatment.[86]

RIGHT VENTRICULAR DILATED CARDIOMYOPATHY

Right ventricular cardiomyopathy and arrhythmogenic right ventricular dysplasia are separate conditions in which the right ventricular abnormality is not shared by the left ventricle, whose function remains normal or near normal.

Dilated cardiomyopathy is recognized by ventricular dilatation and a low ejection fraction. In rare cases the right ventricle is predominantly or seemingly solely involved, appearing globally dilated, hypokinetic, and thin-walled.[87] The condition has been termed *partial Uhl's syndrome,* but these patients may present at any age, usually with congestive failure,[88] the right ventricular myocardium, though thinned, is not absent. The natural history of the disorder is unknown because most patients are not seen until the right ventricle is already greatly dilated. The condition may then clinically simulate pericardial effusion or rheumatic heart disease with tricuspid regurgitation, although echocardiography will reveal normal left-sided valves, failure of contraction of the dilated thin-walled right ventricle, and usually no pericardial effusion.

Arrhythmogenic right ventricular dysplasia is a primary disorder of the right ventricular myocardium.[89] It is characterized by gradual replacement of the right ventricular free wall by fibroadipose tissue.[90] The condition should be suspected in patients with ventricular tachycardia of right ventricular origin, or even in young people with ventricular ectopic beats of left bundle branch block configuration. Symptoms may be absent or related to arrhythmia, and sudden death may occur at any stage.[91] Right ventricular enlargement may not be detectable clinically, but the electrocardiogram may reveal T-wave inversion in right ventricular leads or a partial right bundle branch block pattern.[92] Careful echocardiographic examination of the right ventricle may show typical early changes.[93] The condition is progressive; cases with massive replacement of the right ventricular myocardium may show severe right ventricular failure.

In 1961 Della Volta described some bizarrely severe cases of right ventricular cardiomyopathy in a report titled "Auricularization of the right ventricular pressure curve."[94] These patients showed massive cardiomegaly, their right ventricles were dilated and functionally extinct, and their pulmonary arteries were filled as a result of right atrial drive. Replacement of the right ventricular myocardium with fibroadipose tissue was mentioned in these grossly severe patients. The term *right ventricular dysplasia* was initiated in 1982 by Marcus, Fontaine, and Guiraudon, who described 26 adult cases.[89]

Gradually two separate conditions have become recognized, right ventricular cardiomyopathy, the etiology of which is probably diverse and similar to dilated cardiomyopathy involving predominantly the left ventricle, and arrhythmogenic right ventricular dysplasia, which is frequently familial and shows a wide spectrum of severity.

ARRHYTHMOGENIC RIGHT VENTRICULAR DYSPLASIA

This disorder is most common in young adult males. In a study that included 72 members of 9 families, the sex ratio was 1.5:1, the mean age at death was 24 years, and the age range of detected cases was 8 years to 77 years, including 3 generations in 2 families.[95] In Marcus' study of 26 adult cases, the age range was 17 to 65 with a male predominance of 2.7:1.[89] It is of interest that the disorder has not so far been recognized in neonates or infants. This is in sharp contrast to Uhl's syndrome.

The pathologic abnormality consists of transformation of the right ventricular myocardium into fibrotic or adipose tissue. This starts in specific areas of the right ventricle with a triangle of dysplasia in the free wall distal to the tricuspid valve, at the apex and below the pulmonary valve. The ventricular septum is unaffected, thus biopsies taken from there will not show diagnostic changes. Thiene[96] observed inflammatory changes with monocytic infiltration around necrotic myocytes in a quarter of the cases, but no infective cause has been documented.

The left ventricle is usually normal but may develop focal wall motion abnormalities in advanced cases, although it does not dilate and some of the apparent abnormality may be consequent upon the right ventricular dilatation, as has been described in other disorders of the right heart.[97]

As is usual, the first descriptions were of the most florid cases. The condition is now recognized not to be nearly as rare as had been thought. An autosomal dominant mode of inheritance has been shown. Affected families have shown a broad spectrum of severity varying from asymptomatic cases with only very localized adipose transformation, to massive replacement of right ventricular myocardium with gross cardiomegaly and heart failure. The natural history of the disease is unknown, as is its true incidence. Many cases have been described from Italy since the original descriptions, although there is no real evidence that it is regional or ethnic. Sporadic cases are also described, but the definition of sporadic is often arguable because it is dependent on how many family members had been examined and found normal before a case was so regarded.

Waynberger[98] described familial ventricular tachycardia with left bundle branch block pattern in 1974. Such cases showed both a normal electrocardiogram when in sinus rhythm, and a normal echocardiogram. It is not known whether they showed progression to an overt right ventricular cardiomyopathy.

Arrhythmogenic right ventricular dysplasia is thus a cause of sudden death in asymptomatic young people. Ventricular arrhythmias may be induced by exercise. Fragmented conduction times revealed on the signal averaged ECG by late QRS potentials are the substrate for a reentry tachycardia that is usually readily inducible on electrophysiologic study.[99]

Echocardiography may reveal focal right ventricular abnormality with bulging on the inferobasal wall, apex, or outflow tract with bizarre vermiform trabeculation and dilatation. Typical parallel deep fissuring of the anterior wall of the right ventricle resembles a "pile of plates." This resemblance is typically seen in diastole, with a multisaccular bulging visible both on echocardiography and on angiography. In systole the inferior and anterior walls of the right ventricle are seen to be hypokinetic.[100]

The dysplastic changes appear to be progressive but the main concern centers on the risk of fatal ventricular arrhythmia at a stage when there may be little or no hemodynamic impairment and only subtle abnormalities on investigation.

Endomyocardial biopsy taken from the free wall of the right ventricle may reveal the typical fibroadipose changes with some occasional cellular infiltration. Magnetic resonance imaging (MRI) may make biopsy redundant by allowing tissue recognition of the adipose replacement, a specific finding.

PERIPARTUM CARDIOMYOPATHY

Peripartum cardiomyopathy (PPCM) is defined as heart muscle disorder presenting with the onset of heart failure in the last month of pregnancy or the first 5 months postpartum.[101]

The incidence is said to range from approximately 0.005% of white deliveries to as high as 1% of the Hausa tribe deliveries in Zambia, Northern Nigeria.[102] However, the heart failure among the Hausa tribe mothers is completely different, with a high output failure related to local custom involving excessive heat and sodium intake for parturient women. In the United States the condition has been observed to occur most often in older multiparous black women, with an incidence of 0.1%, and in cases of twin gestation, toxemia or pregnancy, hypertension, and women with poor nutritional status. Although earlier reports had indicated a higher prevalence of PPCM in the lower socioeconomic strata, recent studies have revealed similar prevalence in a middle-class population.[103] It is likely that the overall incidence of PPCM is higher than appears from the statistics; for every recognized case numerous others of milder severity and benign course remain undiscovered.

The criteria used in recognizing PPCM are absence of

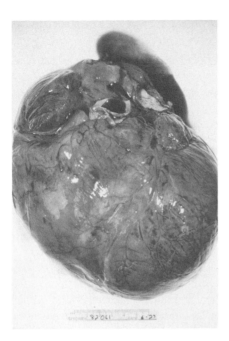

Fig. 7-8. Peripartum cardiomyopathy. Note the globular shape of the enlarged heart caused by biventricular dilatation.

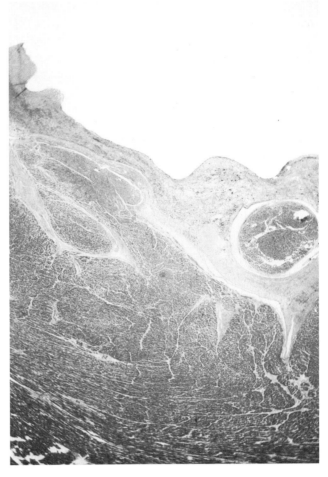

Fig. 7-9. Subendocardial region from a peripartum cardiomyopathy. Note the marked endocardial fibrosis secondary to an organized thrombus.

previously known heart disease or of other detectable causes for heart failure.

On gross examination the heart appears flabby, with enlargement of all four chambers and mural thrombi (Figs. 7-8 and 7-9). Histopathologic findings are characterized by degeneration and hypertrophy of myocytes, edema, and fibrosis. Scattered foci of mononuclear cell infiltrates are occasionally noticed. The latter finding may have an etiologic implication, although reports about the possible inflammatory nature of PPCM are still controversial. There is, however, agreement that both gross and microscopic findings in PPCM are similar to the ones seen in idiopathic dilated cardiomyopathy.

A high incidence of myocarditis in PPCM has been reported (29% to 100%).[103] Differences in the histologic criteria for myocarditis are likely to be responsible for such a wide range, although recent studies have followed the Dallas criteria.[104] An equally important factor in detecting an inflammatory infiltrate in cases of PPCM is the timing of endomyocardial biopsy with respect to the onset of symptoms. A recent study of 18 cases showed evidence of myocarditis in 78% of the patients.[105] The authors suggested that the condition may be caused by viruses, drugs, or toxins, or possibly be of immune origin. They cited alterations in autoreactive T-cell expression by progesterone (occurring at the end of the first trimester) that may predispose peripartum patients to myocarditis.[106] An alternative explanation may be that although these women have normal immune function, viral infection may be responsible for inducing a defect in the immunoregulatory circuits that are involved in maintaining homeostasis.[107] Other re-

searchers have suggested that maternal antibodies against myometrial proteins, or placental or fetal antigens may induce an immune-mediated myocarditis with subsequent cardiomyopathy.[108]

An older hypothesis for the etiology of PPCM included the increased cardiac workload imposed by the demands of pregnancy. Such demands involve an increase in blood volume and stroke output of up to 50% with even greater increases required by multiple pregnancies. Immediately postpartum, an additional increase (up to 30%) in blood volume and cardiac output occur as the uterus contracts and forces a large volume of blood back into circulation.[109]

The urinary excretion of free catecholamines increases by approximately 50% during pregnancy and may rise even higher with exercise.[110] An exaggerated or prolonged adrenergic physiologic response secondary to prolonged stress may play an additional role in the development of cardiac dysfunction in pregnancy and the puerperium.[111] The most common type of presentation occurs in the first week of the puerperium.

Peripartum cardiomyopathy may have a fatal outcome soon after presentation, but survivors usually start to improve. It is alleged that prognosis may be predicted by the rapidity with which the heart returns to its normal size.[112] Patients whose hearts return to normal within 6 months (approximately 50%) do well, whereas approximately 85% of the remainder will eventually die from congestive heart failure. However, recovery may be delayed for a year or more and still appear to be complete, whereas other patients stabilize with impaired left ventricular function.

TOXIC AND DRUG-INDUCED HEART MUSCLE DISEASE

A classification of toxic secondary heart muscle disease includes a variety of agents such as venoms, heavy metals, alcohol, hydrocarbons, tricyclic antidepressants, corticosteroids and several chemotherapeutic agents. Such a diverse group apparently causes a great variety of cardiologic symptoms and a multiplicity of pathologic alterations.

Cyclophosphamide

This alkylating agent used for hematologic malignancies either alone or in combination with other anticancer agents and for immunosuppression may cause fatal heart failure.

The features include ECG voltage loss, pericardial effusion, and elevations in CK, SGOT, and LDH. It is believed that neither the identification of patients at risk for development of cardiac toxicity nor its treatment is feasible.

The characteristic lesions in the heart induced by cyclophosphamide are usually subepicardial ecchymoses associated with hemorrhagic myocardial necrosis.[113] The postulated mechanism of the myocardial lesions is direct damage to the vascular endothelium, capillary rupture, and extravasation of the drug with resultant myocyte damage.

The response of patients to cyclophosphamide is quite variable, perhaps because of differences in the production of various metabolites, differential binding or excretion of these metabolites, and possibly differences in susceptibility to cytoxic effects among individuals.

Adriamycin-induced cardiotoxicity

Adriamycin and its related anthracycline drugs such as doxorubicin and daunorubicin are well known for their effective anticancer action. An important limiting factor is their cardiotoxic effects. Adriamycin-induced myocardial damage often results in a refractory congestive heart failure, has an insidious onset, and may appear weeks or even months after termination of the drug therapy.[113]

The cardiotoxic effect of adriamycin develops as a result of the accumulative effect of successive treatment. A typical treatment utilizes doses of 20 mg/m^2 to 65 mg/m^2/month. For a cumulative dose of less than 550 mg/m^2

there is a 1% incidence of congestive heart failure. However, with a cumulative dose between 550 mg/m^2 and 600 mg/m,^{2} the incidence of heart failure is between 14% and 20%.[117]

Endomyocardial biopsy has had the best rate of success from among a number of invasive and noninvasive techniques in the identification and staging of cardiotoxicity. A scale of 0 to 3 has been devised for scoring the morphologic alterations in the biopsy samples.[115] Zero score indicates normal myocyte appearance, whereas a score of 1 is characterized by rare cells, revealing partial myofibril loss and/or distention of the sarcoplasmic reticulum and T-tubular system. A score of 2 shows more widespread changes of cells with marked or total loss of myofibrils and/or coalescing cytoplasmic vacuoles. Score 3 reveals frank necrosis with loss of cytoplasmic organelles, including mitochondria and nuclear degeneration. Although myofibrillar degeneration is characteristic of adriamycin toxicity, the earliest ultrastructural changes involve the sarcoplasmic reticulum and mitochondria (Figs. 7-10A and B). The former is distended and displaces both contractile elements and mitochondria; the latter reveals positive calcium staining. Finding progressive increase in myocardial fibrosis in hearts after adriamycin treatment at varying periods from cessation of therapy to examination has prompted more detailed studies of the extracellular matrix in an effort to clarify whether altered collagen metabolism is also involved. Such studies have shown that adriamycin administered in rats (single dose of 4.5 mg/kg or 6 mg/kg) elicits marked loss of the myocardial collagen matrix.[116] The mechanism for such loss is not known, but it is suggested that it may account for alterations in form as well as manifestation of poor contractility in adriamycin cardiotoxicity.

There is good correlation between cell damage and cumulative dose of adriamycin. Chest radiation, previous or concurrent, appears independently to accelerate the onset of anthracycline-related cardiomyopathy.[114] Although adriamycin-induced cardiotoxicity has been recognized for several years, the controversy exists regarding what specific agent mediates the toxicity and the pathogenetic mechanism. Unanswered questions remain concerning whether the adriamycin or a specific metabolite are responsible for the myocyte damage. Perhaps endogenous substances such as histamine, arachidonic acid metabolites, platelet activating factor, or high concentrations of calcium are released (directly or indirectly) by the action of anthracyclines. Several other hypotheses still remain unanswered, such as whether the cardiotoxicity results from anthracycline free radicals that generate superoxide anion, lipid peroxides, and oxygen-centerd free radicals that may damage membranes.[117]

Isolated cardiac preparations have been utilized to find answers about the pathogenetic mechanisms involved. How these preparations relate to clinical cardiotoxicity of

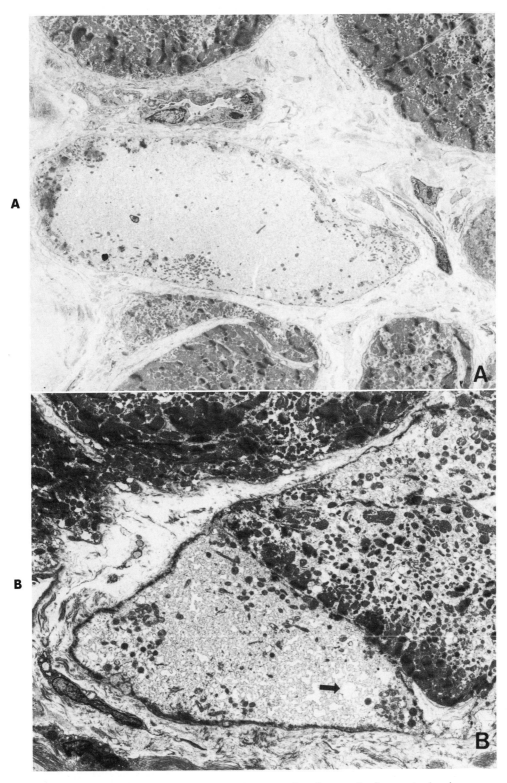

Fig. 7-10. A, Adriamycin cardiotoxicity. Electron microphotograph of myocyte showing severe myofibrillary loss. **B,** Higher magnification of a myocyte with myofibrillary loss and distension of the endoplasmic reticulum *(arrow)* (Courtesy Dr. Henry Tazelaar, Mayo Clinic).

intact organisms remains unclear. In the intact organisms systolic and diastolic cardiac dysfunction occur either acutely or after chronic exposure to anthracyclines. Diastolic dysfunction is an earlier manifestation of toxicity than systolic dysfunction but may be reversible. Furthermore, it has been shown that low cumulative doses of doxorubicin decreased diastolic function without decreasing contractile function in patients.[118] Early cardiac toxicity may be reversible, whereas later changes in cardiac function are irreversible.

Mitochondrial function in doxorubicin toxicity is altered with loss of ability to sequester calcium and therefore inability to offer cytoplasmic calcium.[117] Doxorubicin is known to open calcium release channels of terminal cisternae; thus the cardiac dysfunction induced by this drug may be related to release and subsequent depletion of sarcoplasmic (SR) reticulum calcium.[117] Both low and high concentrations of doxorubicin can cause sarcoplasmic calcium accumulation and may increase cytoplasmic calcium by inhibiting Na/Ca exchange or Ca-ATPase of sarcolemma.[119]

Various proposed hypotheses of anthracycline cardiac toxicity will be discussed briefly, including their strong and weak points. The free radical hypothesis of adriamycin cardiotoxicity has been popular since the mid 1970s. There are several reasons for this, one of which is that it could conceivably account for the time-related nature of anthracycline cardiotoxicity. Free radicals could acutely damage nucleic acids without inducing overt cardiac dysfunction until myocardial cells fail to repair or replace critical enzymes and proteins.[117] The heart is known to be highly susceptible to free radical injury because it contains less free radical detoxifying substances than other organs.[120]

Quinone-containing anthracyclines (doxorubicin, daunorubicin) are potent free radical formers. The quinone moiety can be reduced to a semiquinone by single electron donors. Semiquinone, as it cycles back to quinone, transfers an electron to a molecular oxygen–generating superoxide anion. The latter may initiate lipid peroxidation, damage membranes or macromolecules, and cause myocardial injury.[117] Free radicals may promote extensive calcium release and depletion of SR calcium stores, leading to impaired contractility and relaxation.[121] Free radical formation has been demonstrated by direct spin-trapping techniques in the adriamycin perfused isolated rat heart.[122]

There are, however, several limitations to the free radical hypothesis. Vitamin E, a free radical scavenger, failed to attenuate histologic lesions caused by multiple injection of doxorubicin in dogs. Furthermore, the heart is a relatively poor free radical generator. Thus at doses of doxorubicin that cause cardiac injury, often there is no evidence of oxidative stress or free radical production.[122]

According to the calcium overload hypothesis, anthracyclines may cause excessive levels of intracellular calcium that result in mitochondrial dysfunction, depletion of high energy phosphates, increased muscle stiffness, contractile dysfunction, and cell death.[123] However, recent evidence suggests that calcium accumulation may be a manifestation rather than a cause of anthracycline cardiotoxicity.[124]

The prostaglandins and platelet activating factor (PAF) hypothesis lacks experimental support, except perhaps in regard to PAF, because some preliminary data indicate that it may contribute, in an unclear way, to anthracycline toxicity.[125] Regarding the histamine hypothesis, there is little or no data to suggest that acute or chronic exposure to histamine or histamine-releasing agents causes cardiotoxic effects similar to anthracyclines.[117] The hypothesis that anthracycline metabolites induce cardiotoxicity offers an explanation for the time-related nature of the drug's toxicity. Data indicate that the time-delayed cardiotoxicity of doxorubicin is unrelated to plasma or cardiac levels of doxorubicin and that doxorubicinol, a metabolite of doxorubicin, has been observed to accumulate in cardiac tissue. In addition, doxorubicinol appears much more toxic than doxorubicin in isolated cardiac preparations.[126] Tissue levels of doxorubicinol also correlate with the development of cardiotoxicity.[127] Doxorubicinol is also a potent inhibitor of Na/Ca exchange of sarcolemma.[128] Thus doxorubicinol is a potent inhibitor of several key cationic pumps that directly or indirectly regulate cell calcium and inhibit relaxation.

Current evidence indicates that the heart can convert doxorubicin to doxorubicinol. When the cellular levels of the latter reach toxic limits, inhibition of ion pumps would cause cardiac dysfunction. Such a hypothesis could explain the chronic cumulative nature of doxorubicin cardiotoxicity.[126]

Recent studies have examined adriamycin-induced changes in cardiac mRNA in vivo. Results suggest a selective effect of adriamycin in depressing actin mRNA in the rat heart.[129] This decrease in actin is not related to altered mitochondrial transcription.

Some data indicate that adriamycin has an immuno-enhancing capacity that probably contributes to its antitumor activity. Adriamycin may also produce an antigenic alteration in susceptible cells, which raises the possibility that immunologic mechanisms might contribute to tissue injury.[130]

In summary, one may state that present available data indicate that the most possible pathogenetic mechanism for anthracycline cardiotoxicity is through their metabolites.

Alcoholic heart disease

Although an alcohol-related heart disease has been known for more than a hundred years, debate still continues over whether such an entity actually exists or whether alcohol is simply a myocardial depressant drug that precipitates heart failure in susceptible individuals.

The patient with alcoholic heart disease is usually less

than 50 years old and has a history of alcohol intake, usually daily and often in substantial quantity. Malnutrition and thiamine deficiency (beriberi) must be ruled out and are rarely found. Malnutrition potentiates the adverse effects of ethanol, but most alcoholics seen in the west are not otherwise malnourished.

Chronic alcoholism is also associated with changes in skeletal muscle that are characterized by acute and chronic myopathy.[131] Chronic alcoholic myopathy is characterized by proximal muscle weakness and atrophy with minimal pain. Reports indicate that chronic alcoholism is associated with cardiac dysfunction in as many as one-third of chronic alcoholics and with abnormalities of skeletal muscle in almost half. The injurious effects of ethanol are to some extent dose-related. There is a correlation between damage to the heart and injury to skeletal muscle, but the development of heart failure seems to be idiosyncratic.[132] It is perhaps related to genetically determined differences in isoenzymes such as alcohol dehydrogenase, which also determine the proclivity to alcohol dependence or addiction.

Many of the hemodynamic and morphologic characteristics of alcoholic heart disease are similar to those of dilated cardiomyopathy. Cardiomegaly with ventricular and atrial dilation are observed, and microscopic studies reveal changes in the endocardium, myocytes, and interstitium. The most common findings are an increase in endocardial thickness, focal or diffuse interstitial fibrosis, myocyte hypertrophy, myocytolysis, and fatty infiltration of cardiomyocytes and the interstitium. Electron microscopy shows an increase in myocyte glycogen, loss of myofibrils, enlarged mitochondria with disorganized cristae and myelin bodies, and an increase in the number of lysosomes and dilated sarcoplasmic reticulum. Contrary to idiopathic dilated cardiomyopathy, in which the changes in the sarcoplasmic reticulum are focal, they appear to be generalized in alcoholic cardiomyopathy. However, these changes are not sufficiently different from those in idiopathic dilated cardiomyopathy for it to be possible to diagnose alcoholic heart disease from the morphologic changes found.

The level of enzyme activity in the metabolism of alcohol appears to be of great importance. Histochemical studies of the myocardium in patients with alcoholic heart disease have shown the activity of succinate dehydrogenase, lactate dehydrogenase, alpha-glycerophosphate dehydrogenase and beta-hydroxybutyrate dehydrogenase to be decreased from 15% to 34%.[133] The activity of glucose-6-phosphate dehydrogenase was found to be increased by 23%.

The fact that alcoholic cardiomyopathy does not develop in all cases of chronic alcoholism supports the hypothesis that alcohol alone is not sufficient for the development of the disease.

In rats, heart disease developed only when there was simultaneous alcohol administration and inhibition of catalase activity.[134] The reported increase in catalase activity in rats fed ethanol suggests that cardiac catalase serves a protective function in the pathogenesis of alcoholic cardiomyopathy in that animal.[135] However, no significant increase in catalase activity was detected in human myocardium after alcohol administration.

Catalase represents one of the main metabolic pathways for ethanol in muscle tissue. Catalase is an enzyme of lipid peroxidation and takes part in ethanol oxidation. Some investigations have advanced the hypothesis that lipid peroxidation is responsible for the damage in cardiac muscle in chronic alcoholics. Both the mitochondria and sarcoplasmic reticulum contain the highest amounts of polyunsaturated fatty acids and are particularly vulnerable to damage by peroxidation.[133] The morphologic findings of organelle damage and increased lysosome and lipofuscin granules in the myocyte are also in support of the lipid peroxidation hypothesis regarding the pathogenesis of alcoholic cardiomyopathy.

Several dehydrogenases in the myocardium of chronic alcoholics are decreased, and differing inheritance of isoenzymes may explain differing susceptibility. A reduction of lactate dehydrogenase may cause acidosis, whereas a decrease in alpha-glycerophosphate dehydrogenase activity increases alpha-glycerophosphate, an intermediate product of glycolysis. The latter may stimulate the synthesis of triglycerides, resulting in lipid droplets in cardiomyocytes.[133]

The question regarding whether the toxic effect of acetaldehyde is greater than that of alcohol has not been answered satisfactorily. While acetaldehyde damages protein synthesis and the pump function of the sarcoplasmic reticulum and mitochondria, neither acetaldehyde nor ethanol have a necrotic effect on an isolated heart preparation. This finding may indicate that their actions are not direct ones.[136] Acetaldehyde, the product of alcohol dehydrogenase activity, reacts with many proteins to form acetaldehyde-protein derivatives, which may either be directly harmful or cause pathologic change by provoking an immune response.[137]

Changes in cellular membranes have been observed after long-term exposure to ethanol, whereas short-term effects of ethanol are characterized by adaptive mechanisms that compensate for ethanol-induced changes in function.[138] Such adaptive responses involve ion channels and membrane receptors. For example, it has been shown that cells adapt to long-term ethanol exposure by increasing the concentration and activity of voltage-dependent calcium channels.[139]

A major target of ethanol (short-term and long-term) is the signal transduction system that regulates levels of intracellular cyclic AMP after the activation of receptors. Ethanol increases the production of receptor-dependent cyclic AMP in the short-term and decreases it in the long-term.[138] Such data suggest that ethanol-induced heterologous desensitization of cyclic AMP production could be of widespread pathophysiologic importance in chronic alcoholism.[140]

Cocaine-induced cardiotoxicity

Several studies have presented data documenting the association of cocaine use with angina, myocardial infarction, coronary artery spasm, arrhythmia, and sudden death. Whether cocaine use may induce the development of heart muscle dysfunction remains unclear, and the half dozen cases reported to date have not conclusively put this issue to rest. Cocaine has two primary effects: (1) it inhibits neuronal reuptake of monoamines and (2) it acts as a local anesthetic.[141]

Cocaine affects the cardiovascular system via the central nervous system and also by direct actions on the heart. The latter are dose-related after acute cocaine administration. At low plasma concentrations cocaine is a local anaesthetic with membrane potential stabilizing effects, whereas at higher concentrations cocaine prevents reuptake of norepinephrine by preganglionic sympathetic nerve endings, resulting in a local excess of norepinephrine at the synaptic cleft.[142] However, the relative roles of the central nervous system and the peripheral sympathetic nervous system regarding this involvement in cocaine-induced cardiovascular complications are not fully understood because most earlier studies have been performed in sedated animals.[143]

Circumstantial evidence suggests that cocaine-related life-threatening cardiac events may not be dependent on the amount of drug taken; therefore there may be a subgroup of the population that may be more sensitive to the cardiotoxic effects. Furthermore, cocaine does not follow the usual dose-dependent or first-order elimination kinetics; unexpected marked increases in plasma levels may occur in cocaine abusers after binges.[143]

The most well-known clinical cardiovascular effects of cocaine are ischemic chest pain and myocardial infarction occurring within minutes to hours after cocaine use.[144] Proposed mechanisms for the ischemic episodes include focal vasospasm in a large epicardial coronary artery or a diffuse increase in tone in the resistance vessels, leading to a decrease in coronary blood flow in conjunction with marked cocaine-induced increases in cardiac oxygen consumption.[143]

Two large autopsy studies of cocaine-associated deaths have revealed quite different cardiac morphologic findings. In one of the studies, the most notable abnormality found was the presence of myocardial contraction bands in 93% of the cases (30). According to the authors, the contraction band myocardial damage provided the anatomic pathways for potentially lethal reentrant arrhythmias, whereas the anatomic contraction bands represented a catecholamine-induced disruption of intracellular calcium homeostasis.[145] The second large autopsy study was based on cocaine-as-

sociated deaths and homicide deaths with detectable cocaine. In this study, myocarditis was noted in 20% of the cases. However, the foci of myocarditis described, although small, were associated with myocyte necrosis; as such they may have induced ventricular fibrillation and sudden death.[146] According to these investigators, the cause of myocarditis was not apparent because bacterial, viral, and fungal studies were negative. However, cocaine itself may cause myocardial necrosis and inflammation by one or more mechanisms. Individual myocyte necrosis with accompanying inflammatory infiltrates may be secondary to increased myocardial concentration of norepinephrine, small vessel spasm, or increase of natural killer cell activity.[147]

There are less than six cases reported in which global myocardial dysfunction and/or dilatation occurred after chronic cocaine use. Catechol excess and patchy myocardial infarction have been proposed as mechanisms for the myocardial dysfunction, although neither was morphologically proven. Preliminary experimental data indicate depression of left ventricular function and left ventricular dilatation in dogs after cocaine administration.[148]

Four cases of so-called cocaine cardiomyopathy and four cases of global ventricular dysfunction have been reported.[149-152] However, there is no information available regarding whether any of the four cases of cardiomyopathy reported was caused by cocaine or some other agent or simply by cocaine-induced ischemia. Until a cause-and-effect relationship can be established in a laboratory animal or a large series of cases is studied, the evidence for entity "cocaine cardiomyopathy" will remain weak.

REFERENCES

1. Gravanis MB, Ansari AA: Idiopathic cardiomyopathies: a review of pathogenic mechanisms of pathogenesis, *Arch Pathol Lab Med* 111:915, 1987.
2. Isner JM, Virmani R, Itscoitz SB et al: Left and right ventricular myocardial infarction in idiopathic dilated cardiomyopathy, *Am Heart J* 99:235, 1980.
3. Gravanis MB: (ed) *Cardiovascular Pathophysiology,* New York, 1987, McGraw-Hill.
4. Unverferth BJ, Leir CV, Magorien RD et al: Differentiating characteristics of myocardial nuclei in cardiomyopathy, *Hum Pathol* 14:974, 1983.
5. Wiegand V, Ebecke M, Figulla H et al: Structure and function of contractile proteins in human dilated cardiomyopathy, *Clin Cardiol* 12:656, 1989.
6. Schaper J, Froede R, St. Hein TA et al: Impairment of the myocardial ultrastructure and changes of the cytoskeleton in dilated cardiomyopathy, *Circulation* 83:504, 1991.
7. Steinert PM, Jones JCR, Goldman RD: Intermediate filaments, *J Cell Biol* 99: 22, 1984.
8. Weber KT, Pick Ro, Janicki JS et al: Inadequate collagen tethers in dilated cardiomyopathy, *Am Heart J* 116:1641, 1988.
9. Dunnigan A, Staley NA, Smith SA et al: Cardiac skeletal muscle abnormalities in cardiomyopathy: comparison of patients with ventricular tachycardia or congestive heart failure, *J Am Coll Cardiol* 10:608, 1987.
10. Carofio ALP, Rossi B, Risaliti R et al: Type 1 fiber abnormalities in skeletal muscle of patients with hypertrophic and dilated cardi-

omyopathy: evidence of subclinical myogenic myopathy, *J Am Coll Cardiol* 14:1464, 1989.

11. Dickerman SA, Rubler S: Mitral and tricuspid valve regurgitation in dilated cardiomyopathy, *Am J Cardiol* 63:629, 1989.

12. Cannon RO, Cunnion RE, Parillo JE et al: Dynamic limitation of coronary vasodilator reserve in patients with dilated cardiomyopathy and chest pain, *J Am Coll Cardiol* 10:1190, 1987.

13. Treasure CB, Vita JA, Cox DA et al: Endothelium-dependent dilatation of the coronary microvasculature is impaired in dilated cardiomyopathy, *Circulation* 81:772, 1991.

14. Bortone AS, Hess OM, Chiddo A et al: Functional and structural abnormalities in patients with dilated cardiomyopathy, *J Am Coll Cardiol* 14:613, 1989.

15. Schwarz F, Gerhard M, Zebe H et al: Quantitative morphologic findings of the myocardium in idiopathic dilated cardiomyopathy, *Am J Cardiol* 51:501, 1983.

16. Goodwin JF: The frontiers of cardiomyopathy, *Br Heart J* 48:1, 1982.

17. Gravanis MB, Ansari AA: Idiopathic cardiomyopathies. A review of pathologic studies and mechanisms of pathogenesis, *Arch Pathol Lab Med* 111:915, 1987.

18. Huber SA, Herzum M, Craighead JE: Myocarditis and dilated cardiomyopathy: clinical and experimental evidence implicating autoimmunity in tissue injury, Clin Immunol Newsletter 9:69, 1988.

19. Acosta AM, Santos-Buch CA: Autoimmune myocarditis induced by *Trypanasoma cruzi, Lab Invest* 71:1255, 1985.

20. Billingham ME: *Morphologic changes in drug-induced heart disease.* In Bristow MR, ed: *Drug-induced heart disease,* Amsterdam, 1980, Elsevier.

21. Carlquist JF, Menlove RL, Murray MB et al: HLA class II (DR and DQ) antigen associations in idiopathic dilated cardiomyopathy: validation study and meta-analysis of published HLA association studies, *Circulation* 83:515, 1991.

22. Arbustini E, Gavazzi A, Pozzi R et al: The morphologic spectrum of dilated cardiomyopathy and its relation to immune response genes, *Am J Cardiol* 64:991, 1989.

23. Ahmed-Ansari A, Herskowitz A, Danner DJ et al: Identification of mitochondrial proteins that serve as targets for autoimmunity in human dilated cardiomyopathy, *Circulation* 78:457, 1988.

24. Schultheiss HP, Kuhl U, Janda I et al: Antibody mediated enhancement of calcium permeability in cardiac myocytes, *J Exp Med* 168:2105, 1988.

25. Limas CJ, Goldenberg IF, Limas C: Autoantibodies against beta-adrenoceptors in human idiopathic dilated cardiomyopathy, *Circ Res* 64:97, 1989.

26. Alvarez FL, Neu N, Rose NR et al: Heart-specific autoantibodies induced by coxsackievirus B3: identification of heart antoantigens, *Clin Immunol Immunopathol* 43:129, 1987.

27. Oldstone MBA, Notkins AL: *Molecular mimicry.* In Notkins AL, Oldstone MBA, eds: *Concepts in viral pathogenesis II,* New York, 1986, Springer-Verlag.

28. Edwards WD, Holmes DR, Reeder GS: Diagnosis of active lymphocytic myocarditis by endomyocardial biopsies quantitative 'criteria' by light microscopy, *Mayo Clin Proc* 57:419, 1982.

29. Morgan-Capner P, Richardson PJ, McSorley C: *Virus investigations in heart muscle disease.* In Bolkte HD, ed: *Viral heart disease,* Berlin, 1984, Springer-Verlag.

30. Cambridge G, MacArthur CGC, Waterson AP: Antibodies to coxsackie B viruses in congestive cardiomyopathy, *Br Heart J* 41:692, 1979.

31. Maisch B: *Immunologic regulation and effector mechanisms in myocarditis and perimyocarditis.* In Sekiguchi M, Olsen EGJ, Goodwin E, eds: *Myocardial and related disorders, proc of the Int Symp on Cardiomyopathy and Myocarditis,* Berlin, 1985, Springer-Verlag.

32. Caforio AL, Bonafacio E, Stewart JT et al: Novel organ-specific circulating cardiac autoantibodies in dilated cardiomyopathy, *J Am Coll Cardiol* 15:1527, 1990.

33. Bowles NE, Richardson PJ, Olsen EGJ et al: Detection of coxsackie B virus-specific RNA sequences in myocardial biopsy samples from patients with myocarditis and dilated cardiomyopathy, *Lancet* 1:1120, 1986.

34. Archard L, Freeke C, Richardson P et al: *Persistence of enterovirus RNA in dilated cardiomyopathy: a progression from myocarditis.* In Schultheiss PH, ed: *New concepts in viral heart disease,* Berlin, 1988, Springer-Verlag. 1988.

35. Jin O, Sole MJ, Butany JW: Detection of enterovirus RNA in myocardial biopsies from patients with myocarditis and cardiomyopathy using gene amplification by polymerase chain reaction, *Circulation* 82(1):8, 1990.

36. Kandolf R, Ameis D, Kirschner P et al: In situ detection of enteroviral genomes in myocardial cells by nuclei and hybridization: an approach to the diagnosis of viral heart disease, *Proc Natl Acad Sci USA* 84:6272, 1987.

37. Ansari AA, Wang YC, Danner DJ et al: Abnormal expression of histocompatibility and mitochondrial antigens by cardiac tissue from patients with myocarditis and dilated cardiomyopathy, *Am J Pathol* 139:337, 1991.

38. Carlquist JF, Hammond EH: Cell may lose killer instinct, *JAMA* 249:1126, 1983.

39. Anderson JL, Carlquist JF, Hammond EH: Deficient natural killer cell activity in patients with idiopathic dilated cardiomyopathy, *Lancet* 2:1124, 1982.

40. Maisch B, Deeg P, Liebau G et al: Diagnostic relevance of humoral and cytotoxic immune reactions in primary and secondary dilated cardiomyopathy, *Am J Cardiol* 52:1072, 1983.

41. Jacobs B, Matsuda Y, Deodhar S et al: Cell mediated cytotoxicity to cardiac cells by lymphocytes from patients with primary myocardial disease, *Am J Pathol* 72:1, 1979.

42. Cambridge G, Campbell-Blair L, Wilinshurst P et al: Deficient "natural" cytotoxicity in patients with congestive cardiomyopathy, *Br Heart J* 49:623, 1983.

43. Lowry PJ, Thompson RA, Littler WA: Cellular immunity in congestive cardiomyopathy - the normal cellular response, *Br Heart J* 53:394, 1985.

44. Anderson JL, Carlquist JF, Higashikubo R: Quantitation of lymphocyte subsets by immunofluorescence flow cytometry in idiopathic dilated cardiomyopathy, *Am J Cardiol* 55:1550, 1985.

45. Das SK, Stein LD, Reynolds RT et al: *Immunological studies in cardiomyopathy and pathophysiological implications.* In Goodwin JF, Hjalmarson A, Olsen EGJ, eds: *Congestive cardiomyopathy,* Kiruna, Sweden, 1981, AB Hassle.

46. Kipshidze NN, Chumbunidze VB, Dzidsigmi LM et al: Characteristics of immunoregulatory lymphocyte subpopulations in patients with congestive cardiomyopathy and non-rheumatic myocarditis studied by monoclonal antibodies, *Ter Arkh* 56:56, 1984.

47. Fowles RE, Bieber CP, Stinson EB: Defective in vitro suppressor cell function in idiopathic congestive cardiomyopathy, *Circulation* 59:483, 1979.

48. Eckstein E, Mempel W, Bolte HD: Reduced suppressor cell activity in congestive cardiomyopathy and in myocarditis, *Circulation* 65:1224, 1982.

49. Francescheri R, Peltilo A, Corazzo M et al: Depression of lymphocyte reactivity by serum from patients with dilated cardiomyopathy, *In J Cardiol* 6:431, 1984.

50. Kadiry WA, Gold RG, Behan PO et al: Analysis of antigens in the circulating immune complexes of patients with coxsackie virus infections, *Prog Brain Res* 59:61, 1983.

51. Mestroni L, Miani D, LiLenarda A: Clinical and pathologic study of familial dilated cardiomyopathy, *Am J Cardiol* 65:1449, 1990.

52. Maclennan BA, Tsoi EV, MacGuire C: Familial idiopathic congestive cardiomyopathy in three generations: a family study with eight affected members, *O J Med* 63:335, 1987.

53. Berko BA, Swift M: X-linked dilated cardiomyopathy, *N Engl J Med* 316:1186, 1987.

54. Limas CJ, Limas C: HLA antigens in idiopathic dilated cardiomyopathy, *Br Heart J* 62:379, 1989.

55. Dressler W: The post myocardial infarction syndrome: a report on forty-four cases, *Arch Intern Med* 103:28, 1959.

56. Bolte HD, Schultheiss HP, Cyran J et al: *Binding of immunoglobulins in the myocardium (biopsies)*. In Bolte HD, ed: *Cardiomyopathies,* Berlin, 1980, Springer-Verlag.

57. Klein R, Maisch B, Kochsiek K, et al: Demonstration of organ specific antibodies against heart mitochondria (anti-M7) in sera from patients with some forms of heart diseases, *Clin Exp Immunol* 58:283, 1984.

57a. Beisel KW, Srinivasappa J, Olsen MR, et al. A neutralizing monoclonal antibody against Coxsackievirus B4 cross-reacts with contractile proteins. *Microb Pathog* 8:151; 1990.

58. Schultheiss HP, Bolte HD: Immunochemical characterization of the adenine nucleotide translocator as an organ-specific autoantigen in dilated cardiomyopathy, *J Mol Cell Cardiol* 17:603; 1985.

59. Schulze K, Becker BF, Schauer R et al: Antibodies to ADP-ATP carrier—an autoantigen in myocarditis and dilated cardiomyopathy—impair cardiac function, *Circulation* 81:959, 1990.

60. Maisch B, Bauer E, Cirse M: Cytolytic cross-reactive antibodies directed against the cardiac membrane of adult human myocytes in coxsackie B myocarditis: analysis by Western blot, immunofluorescence test, and antibody-mediated cytolysis of cardiocytes, *Int Symp Inflammatory Heart Disease,* Wurzburg, Germany, 51, 1986(abstract).

61. Schulze K, Becker BF, Schultheiss HP: Antibodies to the ADP/ATP carrier, an autoantigen in myocarditis and dilated cardiomyopathy, penetrate into myocardial cells and disturb energy metabolism in vivo. *Circ Res* 64(2):191, 1989.

62. Neckelmann N, Li K, Wade RP et al: cDNA sequence of a human skeletal muscle ADP/ATP translocator: lack of a leader peptide divergence from a fibroblast translocator cDNA, and coevolution with mitochondrial DNA genes, *Proc Natl Acad Sci USA* 84:7580, 1987.

63. Battini R, Ferrari S, Kaczmarek L et al: Molecular cloning of a cDNA for a human ADP/ATP carrier which is growth-regulated, *J Biol Chem* 262:4355, 1987.

64. Houldsworth J, Attardi G: Two distinct genes for ADP/ATP translocase are expressed at the mRNA level in adult human liver, *Proc Natl Acad Sci USA* 85:377, 1988.

65. Schwimmbeck PL, Schultheiss HP, Strauer BE: Mapping of antigenic determinants of the adenine-nucleotide translocator and coxsackie-B3-virus with synthetic peptides: use for the diagnosis of viral heart disease, Second Int Symp Myocarditis, Airlie House, VA 1991 (abstract).

65a. Schultheiss HP, Klingenberg M. Immunochemical characterization of the adenine nucleotide translocator: Organ and conformational specificity, *Eur J Biochem* 143:599; 1984.

66. Ansari AA, Neckelmann N, Wang YC et al: Immunologic dialogue between cardiac myocytes, endothelial cells and mononuclear cells, Second Int Symp on Myocarditis, Airlie House, VA, 1991 (abstract).

66a. McEnery MW, Snowman AM, Trifiletti RR, Snyder SH. Isolation of the mitochondrial benzodiazepine receptor: Association with the voltage-dependent anion channel and the adenine nucleotide carrier, *Proc Natl Acad Sci (USA)* 89:3170; 1992.

66b. Lane JR, Neumann DA, Lafond-Walker A, Herskowitz A, Rose NR. Interleukin 1 or tumor necrosis factor can promote Coxsackie B3-induced myocarditis in resistant B10.A mice, *J Exp Med* 175:1123; 1992.

66c. Caforio ALP, Grazzini M, Mann JM, et al. Identification of α- and β-cardiac myosin heavy chain isoforms as major autoantigens in dilated cardiomyopathy, *Circulation* 85:1734, 1992.

67. Limas CJ, Limas C, Kubo SH et al: Anti beta-receptor antibodies in human dilated cardiomyopathy and correlation with HLA-DR antigens, *Am J Cardiol* 65:483, 1990.

68. Rose ML, Coles MI, Griffin RJ et al: Expression of Class I and Class II major histocompatibility antigens in normal and transplanted human heart, *Transplantation* 41(6):776, 1986.

69. Ahmed-Ansari, Tadros TS, Knopf WD et al: Major histocompatibility complex Class I and Class II expression by myocytes in cardiac biopsies post transplantation, *Transplantation* 45:972, 1988.

70. Michels VV, Moll PP, Miller FA: The frequency of dilated cardiomyopathy in a series of patients with idiopathic dilated cardiomyopathy, *New Engl J Med* 326:77-82, 1992.

71. Diaz RA, Obasohan A, Oakley CM: Prediction of outcome in dilated cardiomyopathy, *Br Heart J* 58:393 1987.

72. Stewart RAH, McKenna WJ, Oakley CM: Good prognosis for dilated cardiomyopathy without severe heart failure or arrhythmia, *Q J Med* 74:309, 1990.

73. Fuster V, Gersh BJ, Giuliani ER et al: The natural history of idiopathic dilated cardiomyopathy, *Am J Cardiol* 47:525, 1981.

74. Wiles HB, McArthur PD, Taylor AB et al: Prognostic features of children with idiopathic dilated cardiomyopathy, *Am J Cardiol* 68:1372-1376, 1991.

75. Franciosa JA, Park M, Levine TB: Lack of correlation between exercise capacity and indexes of resting left ventricular performance in heart failure, *Am J Cardiol* 47:33, 1986.

76. Dubiel JS, Petkow-Dimitrow P, Reichhart J et al: Comparative studies of systolic and diastolic function of the left ventricle in patients with dilated cardiomyopathy, *Cor Vasa* 33:227-234, 1991.

77. Clements IP, Brown ML, Zinsmeister AR et al: Influence of left ventricular diastolic filling on symptoms and survival in patients with increased left ventricular systolic function, *Am J Cardiol* 67:1245-1250, 1991.

78. Blondheim DS, Jacobs LE, Kotler MN et al: Dilated cardiomyopathy with mitral regurgitation: decreased survival despite a low frequency of left ventricular thrombus, *Am Heart J* 122:763-771, 1991.

79. The SOLVD Investigators: Effect of enalopril on survival in patients with reduced left ventricular ejection fraction and congestive heart failure, *N Engl J Med* 325:293, 1991.

80. Cohn JN et al: A comparison of enalopril with hydralazine - isosorbide dinitrate in the treatment of chronic congestive heart failure, *New Engl J Med* 325:303, 1991.

81. Cleland JGF, Dargie HJ, Hodsman et al: Captopril in heart failure. A double blind controlled trial, *Br Heart J* 52:530, 1984.

82. Zelis R, Mason DJ, Braunwald E: A comparison of the effects of vasodilator stimuli on peripheral resistance vessels in normal subjects and in patients with CHF, *J Clin Invest* 47:960, 1968.

83. Griffith TM, Lewis MJ, Newby AC, et al: Endothelium derived relaxing factor, *J Am Coll Cardiol* 12:797, 1988.

84. Sullivan MJ, Higginbotham MB, Cobb FR: Exercise training in patients with severe left ventricular dysfunction in haemodynamic and metabolic effects, *Circulation* 78:506, 1988.

85. Coats AJ, Adamopoulos S, Meyer TC et al: Effects of physical training in chronic heart failure, *Lancet* 335:63, 1990.

86. Mancini DM, Davis L, Wexler J, et al: Dependence of enhanced maximal exercise performance on increased peak skeletal muscle perfusion during long term captopril therapy in heart failure, *J Am Coll Cardiol* 10:845, 1987.

87. Fitchett DH, Sugrue DD, McArthur CG, et al: Right ventricular dilated cardiomyopathy, *Br Heart J* 51:25-29, 1984.

88. Ribeiro PA, Shapiro IM, Foale RA, et al: Echocardiographic features of right ventricular dilated cardiomyopathy and Uhl's anomaly, *Eur Heart J* 8:65-71; 1987.

89. Marcus FI, Fontaine GH, Guiraudon G et al: Right ventricular dysplasia: a report of 26 adult cases, *Circulation* 65:384-98, 1982.

90. Dalla Volta S: Arrhythmogenic cardiomyopathy of the right ventricle: thoughts on aetiology, *Eur Heart J* 10(Suppl D):2-6, 1989.

91. Maron BJ: Right ventricular cardiomyopathy: another cause of sudden death in the young, *N Engl J Med* 318:178-180, 1988.

92. Scognamiglio R, Fasoli G, Nava A et al: Relevance of subtle echocardiographic findings in the early diagnosis of the concealed form of right ventricular dysplasia, *Eur Heart J* 10(Suppl D):27-28, 1989.

93. Robertson JH, Bardy GH, German LD et al: Comparison of two-dimensional echocardiographic and angiographic findings in arrhythmogenic right ventricular dysplasia, *Am J Cardiol* 55:1506-8, 1985.

94. Dalla Volta S, Battaglia G, Zerbini E: Auricularization of right ventricular pressure curve, *Am Heart J* 61:25-33, 1961.

95. Nava A, Thiene G, Canciani B et al: Familial occurrence of right ventricular dysplasia: a study involving nine families, *J Am Coll Cardiol* 12:1228, 1988.

96. Thiene G, Nava A, Carrado D et al: Right ventricular cardiomyopathy and sudden death in young people, *N Engl J Med* 138:129, 1988.

97. Webb JG, Kerr CR, Huckell VF et al: Left ventricular abnormalities in arrhythmogenic right ventricular dysplasia, *Am J Cardiol* 58:568-70, 1986.

98. Waynberger M, Gourtadon M, Peltier JM et al: Tachycardies ventriculaires familiales: a propos de 7 observations, *Nouv Presse Med* 30:1857-60, 1974.

99. Blomstrom-Lundqvist C, Hirsch I, Olsson SB, et al: Quantitative analysis of the signal-average QRS in patients with arrhythmogenic right ventricular dysplasia, *Eur Heart J* 9:301-312, 1988.

100. Chiddo A, Locuratolo N, Gaglione A, et al: Right ventricular dysplasia in angiographic study, *Eur Heart J* 10 (Suppl D):42-45, 1989.

101. Homans DC: Peripartum cardiomyopathy, *N Engl J Med* 312:1432, 1985.

102. Davidson N, Parry FH: The etiology of peripartum cardiac failure, *Am J Cardiol* 97:535, 1979.

103. O'Connell JB, Costanzo-Nordin MR, Subramanian R et al: Peripartum cardiomyopathy: clinical, hemodynamic, histologic and prognostic characteristics, *J Am Coll Cardiol* 8:52, 1986.

104. Aretz HT, Billingham ME, Edwards WD et al: Myocarditis: a histopathologic definition and classification, *Am J Cardiovasc Pathol* 1:3, 1987.

105. Midei MG, DeMent SH, Feldman AM, et al: Peripartum myocarditis and cardiomyopathy, *Circulation* 81:922, 1990.

106. Lyden DC, Huber SA: Aggravation of coxsackievirus, group B, antigen in pregnant Balb/c mice and animals treated with progesterone, *Cell Immunol* 87:462, 1984.

107. Gravanis MB, Ansari AA: Idiopathic cardiomyopathies. A review of pathological studies and mechanisms of pathogenesis, *Arch Pathol Lab Med* 111:915, 1987.

108. Boleslaw K, Melamud E, Kishon V: Peripartum cardiomyopathy, *Is J Med Sci* 20:1061, 1984.

109. Quilligan EJ: *Maternal physiology.* In *Danforth's obstetrics and gynecology,* Philadelphia, 1982, Harper and Row.

110. Oesterling MJ, Tse RL, Holmes HM: Spectrophotometric determination of catecholamine excretion in the free and conjugated forms, *Fed Proc* 21:192, 1982.

111. Stamler J, Horowitz SF, Goldman ME et al: Peripartum cardiomyopathy. A role for cardiac stress determinants other than during pregnancy? *Mt Sinai J Med* 56:285, 1989.

112. Aroney C, Khafagi F, Boyle C et al: Peripartum cardiomyopathy: echocardiographic features in five cases, *Am J Obstet Gynecol* 155:103, 1986.

113. Barry MA, Roberts RW: Cyclophosphamide-induced cardiomyopathy, *Cancer* 43:2223, 1979.

114. Praga C et al: Adriamycin cardiotoxicity. A survey of 1273 patients, *Cancer Treat Res* 53: 827; 1979.

115. Billingham ME: Some recent advances in cardiac pathology, *Hum Pathol* 10:367, 1979.

116. Caulfield JB, Bittner V: Cardiac matrix alterations induced by adriamycin, *Am J Pathol* 133:298, 1988.

117. Olson RD, Mushlin PS: Doxorubicin cardiotoxicity: analysis of prevailing hypotheses, *FASEB J* 4:3076, 1990.

118. Lee BH, Goodenday LS, Muswick GJ et al: Alterations in left ventricular diastolic function with doxorubicin therapy, *J Am Coll Cardiol* 9:184, 1987.

119. Harada H, Cusack BJ, Olson RD et al: Taurine deficiency and doxorubicin: interaction with the cardiac sarcolemmal calcium pump, *Biochem Pharmacol* 39: 745, 1990.

120. Olson RD, Mushlin PS: *Mechanisms of anthracycline cardiotoxicity: are metabolites involved?* In Acosta D, ed: In *Focus on molecular cellular and In vitro toxiocology,* Boca Raton, 1990, CRC Press.

121. Abramson JJ, Salama G: Sulfhydryl oxidation and calcium release from sarcoplasmic reticulum, *Mol Cell Biochem* 82:81, 1988.

122. Rajogopalan S, Politi PM, Sinha BK et al: Adriamycin-induced free radical formation in the perfused rat heart. Implications for cardiotoxicity, *Cancer Res* 48:4766, 1988.

123. Van Vleet JF, Ferrans VJ, Weirich WE: Cardiac disease induced by chronic adriamycin administration in dogs and an evaluation of vitamin E and selenium as cardioprotectans, *Am J Pathol* 99:13, 1980.

124. Jensen RA: Doxorubicin cardiotoxicity: contractile changes after longterm treatment in the rat, *J Pharmacol Exp Ther* 236:197, 1986.

125. Bristoe MR, Kantrowitz NE, Harrison WD et al: Mediation of subacute anthracycline cardiotoxicity in rabbits by cardiac histamine release, *J Cardiovasc Pharmacol* 5:913, 1983.

126. Olson RD, Mushlin PS, Brenner DE et al: Doxorubicin cardiotoxicity may be due to its metabolite, doxorubicinol, *Proc Natl Acad Sci USA* 85:3585, 1988.

127. Boucek RJ Jr, Olson RD, Brenner DE et al: The major metabolite of doxorubicin is a potent inhibitor of membrane-associated ion pumps, *J Biochem Chem* 262:15851, 1987.

128. Boucek RJ Jr, Kunkel EM, Graham TP Jr et al: Doxorubicinol, the metabolite of doxorubicin, is more cardiotoxic than doxorubicin, *Pediatr Res* 21:1871, 1987.

129. Papoian T, Lewis W: Adriamycin cardiotoxicity in vivo. Selective alterations in rat cardiac mRNAs, *Am J Pathol* 136:1201, 1990.

130. Huber SA, Moraska A: Cytolytic T Lymphocytes and antibodies to myocytes in adriamycin-treated BALB/c mice, *Am J Pathol* 140:233, 1992.

131. Haller RG, Knochell JP: Skeletal muscle disease in alcoholism, *Med Clin North Am* 68:91, 1984.

132. Urbano-Marquez A, Estruch R, Navaro-Lopez F et al: The effects of alcoholism on skeletal and cardiac muscle, *N Engl J Med* 320:409, 1989.

133. Tsiplenkova VG, Vikhert AM, Cherpachenko NM: Ultrastructural and histochemical observations in human and experimental alcoholic cardiomyopathy, *J Am Coll Cardiol* 8:22A, 1986.

134. Kino M: Chronic effects of ethanol under partial inhibition of catalase activity in the rat heart: light and electron microscopic observations, *J Mol Cell Cardiol* 13:5, 1981.

135. Fahimi KD, Kino M, Hicks L, et al: Increased myocardial catalase in rats fed ethanol. *Am J Pathol* 96:373, 1979.

136. Zabirova IG: On the cardionecrotic effect of ethanol, acetaldehyde and teturam in acute rat experiments, *Cardiology* 9:90, 1983.

137. Israel Y, Hurwitz E, Niemela O et al: Monoclonal and polyclonal antibodies against acetaldehyde-containing epitopes in acetaldehyde-protein adducts, *Proc Natl Acad Sci USA* 83:7913, 1986.

138. Diamond I: Alcoholic myopathy and cardiomyopathy, *N Engl J Med* 320:458, 1989.

139. Messing RO, Carpenter CL, Diamond I et al: Ethanol regulates calcium channels in clonal neural cells, *Proc Natl Acad Sci USA* 83:6213, 1986.

140. Moohly-Rosen D, Chang FH, Cheever L et al: Chronic ethanol

causes heterologous desensitization of receptors by reducing as messenger RNA, *Nature* 333:848; 1988.

141. Ritchie JM, Greene NM: *Local anesthetics* I Gilman AG, Goodman LS, Rall TW et al, eds: *The pharmacological basis of therapeutics*, ed 7, New York, 1985, MacMillian.

142. Dart AM, Dietz R, Kubler W et al: Effects of cocaine and desipramine on the neurally evoked overflow of endogenous noradrenaline from the rat heart, *Br J Pharmacol* 79:71, 1983.

143. Thadani PV: Cardiovascular-toxicity of cocaine: underlying mechanisms, *J Appl Cardiol* 5:317, 1990.

144. Smith HWB III, Liberman HA, Brody SL et al: Acute myocardial infarction temporarily related to cocaine use, *Ann Intern Med* 107:13, 1987.

145. Tazelaar HD, Karch SB, Stephens BG et al: Cocaine and the heart, *Hum Pathol* 18:195, 1987.

146. Virmani R, Rabinowitz M, Smialek JE et al: Cardiovascular effects of cocaine: an autopsy study of 40 patients, *Am Heart J* 115:1068, 1988.

147. VanDyke C, Stesin, Jones R et al: Cocaine increases natural killer cell activity, *J Clin Invest* 77:1387, 1986.

148. Rongione AJ, Isner JM: Cocaine-induced contraction of vascular smooth muscle is inhibited by calcium channel blockade, *J Am Coll Cardiol* 13:78A, 1989 (abstract).

149. Wiener RS, Lockhart JT, Schwartz RG: Dilated cardiomyopathy and cocaine abuse, *Am J Med* 81:699, 1986.

150. Duell PB: Chronic cocaine abuse and dilated cardiomyopathy, *Am J Med* 81:601, 1986. (letter).

151. Chokshi SK, Moore R, Pandian NG et al: Reversible cardiomyopathy associated with cocaine intoxication, *Ann Intern Med* 111:1039, 1989.

152. Bertolet BD, Freund G, Martin CA et al: Unrecognized left ventricular dysfunction in an apparently healthy cocaine abuse population, *Clin Cardiol* 13:323, 1990.

PART II RESTRICTIVE CARDIOMYOPATHY

Endomyocardial fibrosis and Loffler's parietal endocarditis were listed in the WHO classification of restrictive cardiomyopathy, although their association with eosinophilia should really place them among the specific heart muscle diseases. Endomyocardial fibrosis occurs predominantly in the tropics,[1] including South India, South and Central America, and Asia. Loffler's endocarditis is seen in temperate zones. It is currently believed that Loffler's parietal endocarditis and endomyocardial fibrosis represent a continuum of the same disease entity caused by hypereosinophilia.[2] They both are now regarded as specific heart muscle diseases.

Primary restrictive cardiomyopathy is rather rare, shows myocyte hypertrophy, interstitial fibrosis, and sometimes disarray. It is characterized by a diastolic fault with increased filling pressures despite maintained systolic function.[3,4]

MORPHOLOGIC FEATURES

The heart in endomyocardial fibrosis is hypertrophied. The ventricular cavities are of varying sizes depending mostly on the extent and severity of the endocardial process, which prevents dilatation and may cause apical oblit-

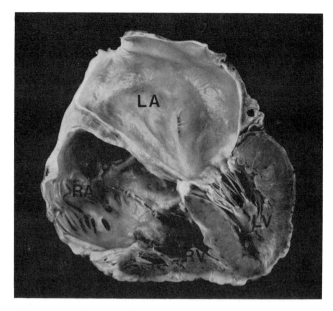

Fig. 7-11. Noneosinophilic restrictive cardiomyopathy. Note fixation of the mitral leaflets and marked left atrial dilatation (Courtesy Dr. William D. Edwards, Mayo Clinic).

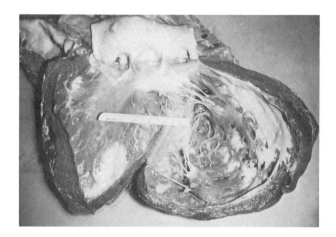

Fig. 7-12. Idiopathic restrictive cardiomyopathy (noneosinophilic). The left ventricle reveals large areas of endocardial thickening localized primarily in the inflow tract and the apex.

eration. The uninvolved parts of the ventricles (particularly the outflow tract) may show dilatation and hypertrophy. Atrial dilatation is always present (Fig. 7-11). The most significant alterations are seen in the endocardium (often in both ventricles) in the form of collagen-rich fibrotic plaques of various sizes and thickness (several millimeters). Their gross characteristics are rolled edges and an abrupt termination. The plaques are commonly located in the inflow tract and apex and only rarely in the outflow tract (Fig. 7-12). A fibrotic plaque in the left ventricle may trap the posterior leaflet, posterior chordae, and papillary muscle of the mitral valve. Mitral and tricuspid insufficiency are common occurrences in endomyocardial fibrosis

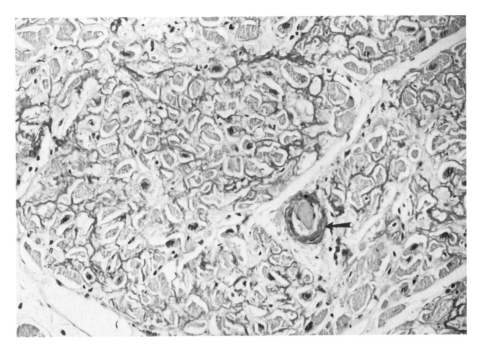

Fig. 7-13. Congo red stain of myocardium from a case of restrictive cardiomyopathy. Linear amyloid deposits are present on almost every myocardial fiber. Note also amyloid deposits in the wall of a small coronary artery *(arrow).*

and contribute greatly to morbidity because of the relatively small size of the abnormal ventricles. Histologically the fibrotic plaque reveals a characteristic layering and, in more than half the cases, a thrombus is superimposed on the plaque. The thrombus is usually attached to a layer of relatively acellular collagen, beneath which there is a collagenous layer containing multiple thin-walled sinusoidal vessels and occasional mononuclear cells. Connective tissue septa extend from this granular layer, into the underlying myocardium. Calcific deposits may be seen in the plaques.[5,6]

In the noneosinophilic forms of restrictive cardiomyopathy, myocardial hypertrophy and/or fibrosis may account for the restrictive pathophysiology. In one type a fine interstitial myocardial fibrosis is found that apparently affects ventricular compliance, other types show myocardial disarray without increase in wall thickness. Cardiac amyloidosis is not an uncommon cause for restrictive heart muscle disease (Fig. 7-13), whereas rare cases of myocardial hemochromatosis may present with restrictive pathophysiology. Constrictive pericarditis has to be considered in the differential diagnosis.[3,4]

A noneosinophilic familial restrictive cardiomyopathy with skeletal myopathy has been reported in five generations of an Italian family. The mode of transmission was autosomal dominant, and the morphologic findings were those of myocardial and epicardial fibrosis, absence of endocardial fibrosis, and fibrosis in the conduction system.[2] Such cases are rare, but seemingly sporadic cases are recurrent. The condition appears to be a specific entity.[7]

THE HYPEREOSINOPHILIC SYNDROME

Although dysfunction of many organs (e.g., lung, nervous system, skin, liver, GI tract) may occur, the primary cause of morbidity and mortality is cardiac.[5] The presence of an elevated number of activated eosinophils in the blood and tissues plays a direct part in cardiac dysfunction.

IMMUNOBIOLOGY

Eosinophilia, characterized by increased bone marrow production, is observed in helminthic parasitic infections, allergic diseases, and conditions with less defined causes that may be designated as idiopathic. Eosinophils, which are predominantly tissue-dwelling cells, are plentiful at epithelial interface with the environment (e.g., in the respiratory, gastrointestinal, or lower genitourinary tracts).

Intracytoplasmic specific granules are the eosinophils' distinguishing morphologic feature. Specific granules contain lysosomal hydrolases, as well as most of the cationic proteins unique to these cells. The granule has a crystalloid core that is composed of major basic protein, whereas the noncore matrix contains eosinophil cationic protein, eosinophil-derived neurotoxin, and eosinophil peroxidase.[8]

Major basic protein (14,000-dalton protein) has no enzymatic activity but is toxic to helminthic parasites, tumor cells, and host cells.[9] Eosinophil cationic protein (18,000 to 21,000 daltons) has bactericidal and helminthotoxic activities[10] but is also toxic to host cells. Eosinophil-derived neurotoxin (18,600 daltons protein) induces cerebrocerebellar dysfunction when injected intracerebrally into rabbits.[11] Another protein associated with eosinophil granules and cell membranes is the protein that forms Charcot-Leyden crystals. This hydrophobic protein (17,000 dalton) has a lysophospholipase activity.[11] Eosinophils express receptors for IgG,IgE, and IgA for complement components (Clq, C3b/C4b, iC3b, C5a) and for three cytokines interleukin-3, interleukin-5, and granulocyte-macrophage colony-stimulating factor.[12]

Eosinophils have receptors for two lipid mediators: platelet-activating factor and leukotriene B4, both of which are chemoattractants for eosinophils[13] and can stimulate their degranulation and the formation of superoxide anion and other oxidant derivatives.[14] Eosinophils also express cell-surface proteins involved in cell-to-cell interactions (integrins) that enable them to emigrate from blood to normal and inflamed tissues.[11]

Other chemoattractants of eosinophils are lymphocyte chemoattractant factor and interleukin-2.[15] Interleukin-5 appears to be the principal cytokine responsible for increased eosinophil production and has been found in the blood of patients with idiopathic hypereosinophilia and parasitic infections.[16]

Eosinophils from patients with eosinophilia who show cardiac involvement are morphologically distinct in that they have cytoplasmic vacuoles, alterations in the size and number of granules, and loss of granule cores containing major basic protein. However, activation reflects stimulation; (not immaturity) the same cytokines that stimulate bone marrow production of eosinophils also stimulate mature cells and activate their effector functions.[11]

Several functions have been attributed to eosinophils. As effector cells, eosinophils can have roles that are both beneficial and detrimental to the host. Eosinophils are particularly toxic to helminths by depositing, after binding to the surface of the parasite, major basic protein and eosinophilic cationic protein.[11] Eosinophils can collaborate with lymphocytes and other immunologic and mesenchymal cells in various ways that are pertinent to health and disease. For example, by elaborating, transforming growth factor-a may stimulate the function of endothelial cells and fibroblasts.[17]

Activation of platelets by eosinophil granule proteins may play a role in the pathogenesis of several diseases, such as asthma or hypereosinophilic syndrome. Major basic protein deposited on the endocardium and intima of blood vessels results in thrombus formation.[18] Eosinophil granule proteins are known to be involved in cardiac injury, producing myocyte damage and vascular alterations that lead to the development of endomyocardial fibrosis. In vitro studies with isolated rat heart cells have revealed that eosinophilic secretion products damaged the plasma membranes of heart cells and inhibited mitochondrial 2-oxoglutarate dehydrogenase.[19]

Recent studies have demonstrated activated eosinophils and eosinophil granule proteins within the endocardium, adjacent thrombus, and myocardium of patients with eosinophilic endomyocardial disease.[20] The intensity of deposits was more marked at early stages of the disease, although they were detected even at the late fibrotic stage. Major basic protein (MBP) was localized on the surface of myocytes and persisted longer than eosinophilic cationic protein (ECP), possibly through formation of disulfide bonds between MBP and the target tissue.[20] It is likely that the eosinophil granule proteins, in association with reactive oxygen products, are involved in the pathogenesis of the endomyocardial damage. The presence of large numbers of activated eosinophils and their products in thrombi and in the walls of the ventricles suggests a causal association.

In Löffler endomyocardial disease three major histopathologic forms may be recognized depending on the length of time between onset of the disease and death of the patient.[21] The *necrotic stage* (weeks between onset to death) is characterized by an eosinophilic myocarditis, myocyte necrosis (mostly in the subendocardial myocardium), and arteritis of small intramural vessels. The *thrombotic stage* (months from onset to death) is indicated by prominent fibrous endocardial thickening, a superimposed thrombus, subendocardial myocardial scars, and focal arteritis. The *fibrotic stage* (years between onset and death) reveals a thick fibrous endocardium with superimposed thrombus and zonal layering of the endocardial plaques similar to that described in cases of tropic endomyocardial fibrosis. The hallmark of endomyocardial fibrosis is the thick, fibrous tissue covering the endocardium of either one or both ventricles. It has been suggested that the fibrous plaques begin at the apex and progress toward the inflow tract, encompassing the papillary muscles on their way up (Figs. 7-14, 7-15).[22]

Survival in endomyocardial fibrosis is influenced by functional class, type of ventricular involvement, degree of right and left ventricular fibrosis, and mitral or tricuspid regurgitation or both.

In the noneosinophilic forms of restrictive cardiomyopathy, myocardial hypertrophy and/or fibrosis may account for the restrictive pathophysiology.

Tropic endomyocardial fibrosis is usually associated with an eosinophil level that is no different from that of the rest of the indigent population, but children in these endemic areas hospitalized with parasitic infections associated with eosinophilia have been shown to exhibit cardiac abnormalities that had earlier gone unobserved.[23] It appears that the difference between endomyocardial fibrosis as it is seen in the West and as it occurs in the tropics is in the severity, acuteness, and duration of the eosinophilic insult. In the tropics this is low grade, chronic, and often absent by the time of presentation with heart failure. The patient is often in the teens or 20s, and the eosinophilic insult is not seen or detected unless or until the cardiac failure is severe. Typically the venous pressure is exceedingly high even with proptosis and facial edema as well as tense ascites, but often there is no peripheral edema. Milder cases

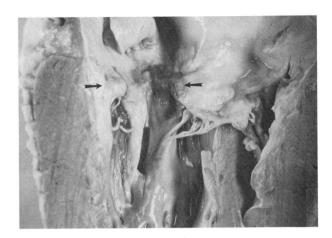

Fig. 7-14. Eosinophilic restrictive cardiomyopathy. Note immobilization of both mitral valve leaflets *(arrow)* by endocardial fibrous plaques in the inflow tract.

are now being recognized in patients from the tropics who may simply show cardiomegaly with mild failure, which is found to be associated with ventricular distortion on echocardiographic readings, a trait typical of endomyocardial fibrosis. Usually, residual myocardial function is well preserved but this varies because extensive fibrosis may eventually splint the muscle, which then becomes hypocontractile. The condition then can be exceedingly chronic with the cause long gone and the condition essentially nonprogressive over the years.

Löffler endocarditis, seen in the West, is usually associated with a hyper-eosinophilic syndrome, idiopathic, or less often, associated with carcinoma, secondary aspergillus infection in chronic atopic asthma, or Churg-Strauss syndrome. In Löffler endocarditis, cardiac involvement may not even be suspected while the ventricles are filling up with thrombus in the necrotic-thrombotic phase until embolism or sudden death occurs. With survival and less acute cardiac damage, necrosis heals with fibrosis which, starting at the apices of the ventricles, may give rise to no abnormal symptoms or signs. Embolism may still occur. As the posterior mitral leaflet becomes immobilized in the fibrotic process, mitral regurgitation develops. Even if mild, this may give rise to symptoms because of the reduced capacity of the left ventricle. Its apex has been obliterated in the scarring process; thus the regurgitant volume cannot be accommodated except at a raised filling pressure. The true nature of the process is readily recognized on echocardiographic or angiographic examination. The appearance on angiography is of an amputated apex resembling a fist in a boxing glove, with obliteration of the internal architecture. On the right side, obliteration of the sinus or cavity of the right ventricle can proceed even further before giving rise to a high venous pressure, hepatomegaly, and edema. During this process the infundibulum tends to dilate and become hypercontractile, compensating in part for the loss of volume. The tricuspid valve becomes

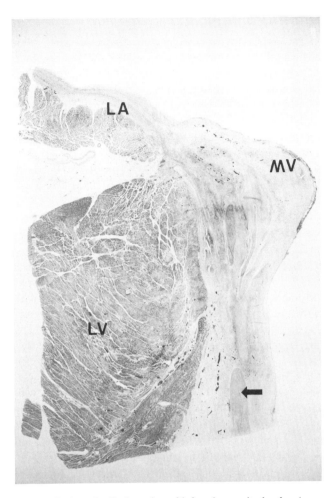

Fig. 7-15. Longitudinal section of left atrium, mitral valve (posterior leaflet), and left ventricular wall from an eosinophilic restrictive cardiomyopathy. Note complete incorporation and immobilization of the valvular leaflet by a fibrous plaque in which the chordae tendineae are also trapped *(arrow)* LA - left atrium, MV = mitral valve, LV = left ventricle.

regurgitant. Eventually the pressures in the pulmonary artery and the right ventricle through to the right atrium become identical, with the right side of the heart becoming simply a conduit.[20,21]

In Löffler endocarditis the condition may also be subacute. When its onset has been observed in patients whose hypereosinophilic syndrome had been discovered but the heart had appeared to be normal, the appearance of degranulation of the eosinophils may be associated temporally with the onset of cardiac abnormality. This may be the development of nonspecific myocardial failure, which subsequently resolves but precedes development of the typical focal changes. Progression of the cardiac damage will be arrested only if the eosinophil activation can be reversed. Unfortunately, efforts to reduce the eosinophilia are often unsuccessful because of an essential failure to understand the cause of the condition despite an abundance of theories. The hypereosinophilic syndrome usually pursues a fatal course.

PRIMARY RESTRICTIVE CARDIOMYOPATHY

Primary restrictive cardiomyopathy unassociated with eosinophilia, amyloid infiltration, or storage diseases such as hemochromatosis or Fabry's disease, is a heterogeneous and relatively rare condition with raised ventricular filling pressures without ventricular dilatation. There also is normal or near normal systolic function in the absence of an increase in wall thickness, as would be found in hypertrophic cardiomyopathy or amyloidosis.[1,2,23,24]

Endomyocardial biopsy or autopsy may show increase in the intracellular matrix with fine interstitial fibrosis in some patients. This is often most marked in the subendocardial regions and accounts for the frequent development of conduction defects that eventually require pacemaker implantation.[7] In other cases, the finding is of generalized myocardial disarray with hypertrophied myocytes and patchy fibrosis in the absence of an increase in wall thickness. Some of these cases are familial; in those with disarray, other members of the family may show typical hypertrophic cardiomyopathy. Thus overlap is shown to be inevitable with the arbitrary (though useful) simple classification that we use. A hereditary pattern may also be seen in the restrictive cardiomyopathy associated with progressive sinoatrial and atrioventricular conduction failure with raised ventricular filling pressures, normal size and activity of the ventricles, and progressive atriomegaly. Association with a slowly progressive proximal limb girdle skeletal myopathy is noted in a few families.[7]

Distinction from amyloidosis is not difficult because of the usually younger age, absence of extra cardiac amyloid, lack of increased ventricular wall thickness, and absence of amyloid fibrils on endomyocardial biopsy.[25] Distinction from constrictive pericarditis can occasionally be difficult. However, the much greater atriomegaly, the common presence of tricuspid regurgitation, the usually much higher left-sided filling pressures (compared with those on the right side), the presence of conduction defects, and the ability to show a pericardial space on echocardiography should differentiate. In the absence of tricuspid regurgitation the left ventricular diastolic pressure and left atrial pressure is usually much higher than the diastolic pressures on the right side. The development of tricuspid regurgitation, however, may result in a rise in right-sided filling pressures to equalize those on the left. The two pressures can be separated by respiration or by fluid challenge at catheterization. The demonstration of tricuspid regurgitation, together with the increased right atrial size resulting from it, distinguish restrictive cardiomyopathy from constrictive pericarditis, in which the heart is usually of normal size. In constrictive pericarditis the interdependence of the two ventricles caused by the restricted total cardiac volume can be demonstrated by Doppler echocardiography, in which inspiration is associated with an increase in right sided E-wave at the expense of the left sided E-wave in those constrictive pericarditis patients who may also show pulsus paradoxus clinically. In restrictive cardiomyopathy atrioventricular inflow does not vary in this way.

The time course of primary restrictive cardiomyopathy is usually long and chronic, but sudden death may occur. Eventually transplantation may be justified for the relief of severe congestive symptoms.

REFERENCES

1. Gravanis MB, Ansari AA: Idiopathic cardiomyopathies: a review of pathologic studies and mechanisms of pathogenesis, *Arch Pathol Lab Med* 111:915, 1987.
2. Isner JM, Virmani R, Itscoitz SB et al: Left and right ventricular myocardial infarction in idiopathic dilated cardiomyopathy, *Am Heart J* 99:235, 1980.
3. Chew CYC, Ziady GM, Raphael MJ et al: Primary restrictive cardiomyopathy. Non-tropical endomyocardial fibrosis and hypereosinophilic heart disease, *Br Heart J* 39:399, 1977.
4. Katritsis D, Wilmshurst PT, Wendon JA et al: Primary restrictive cardiomyopathy: clinical and pathologic characteristics, *J Am Coll Cardiol* 18:1230-5, 1991.
5. Parillo JE: Heart disease and the eosinophil, *N Engl J Med* 323: 1560, 1990.
6. Brockington IF, Olsen EGJ: Loffler's endocarditis and Davies' endomyocardial fibrosis, *Am Heart J* 85:308, 1973.
7. Fitzpatrick AP, Shapiro LM, Richards AF et al: Familial restrictive cardiomyopathy with atrioventricular block and skeletal myopathy, *Br Heart J* 63:114, 1990.
8. Egesten A, Aumets J, von Mecklenburg C et al: Localization of eosinophil cationic protein, major basic protein, and eosinophil peroxidase in human eosinophils by immunoelectron microscopic technique, *J Histochem Cytochem* 34:1399, 1986.8
9. Gleish GJ, Adolphson CR: The eosinophilic leukocyte: structure and function. *Adv. Immunol* 39:177, 1986.
10. Lehrer RI, Szklarek D, Barton A et al: Antibacterial properties of eosinophil major basic protein and eosinophil cationic protein, *J Immunol* 142:4428, 1989.
11. Weeler PF, Bach D, Austen KF: Human eosinophil lysophospholipase: the sole protein component of Charcot-Leyden crystals, *J Immunol* 128:1346, 1982.
12. Chihara J, Plumas J, Gruart V et al: Characterization of a receptor for interleukin-5 on human eosinophils: variable expression and induction by granulocyte/macrophage colony-stimulating factor, *J Exp Med* 172:1347, 1990.
13. Wardlaw AJ, Moqbel R, Cromwell O et al: Platelet-activating factor: a potent chemotactic and chemokinetic factor for human eosinophils, *J Clin Invest* 78:1701, 1986.
14. Kroegel C, Yukawa T, Dent G et al: Stimulation of degranulation from human eosinophils by platelet-activating factor, *J Immunol* 142:3518, 1989.
15. Rand TH, Silberstein DS, Weller PF: Human eosinophils express functional interleukin-2 receptors, *Blood* 76(Suppl 1):191a; 1990 (abstract).
16. Owen WF, Rothenberg ME, Petersen J et al: Interleukin-5 and phenotypically altered eosinophils in the blood of patients with the idiopathic hypereosinophilic syndrome, *J Exp Med* 170:343, 1989.
17. Wong DTW, Weller PF, Galli SJ et al: Human eosinophils express transforming growth factor alpha, *J Exp Med* 172:673, 1990.
18. Tai PC, Stickerman SJ, Spry CJF et al: Deposits of eosinophil granule proteins in cardiac tissues of patients with eosinophilic endomyocardial disease, *Lancet* 1:643, 1987.
19. Tai PC, Hayes DJ, Clark JB et al: Toxic effects of human eosinophil products on isolated rat heart cells in vitro, *Biochem J* 204:75, 1982.
20. Tai PC, Spry CJF, Olsen EGJ et al: Deposits of eosinophil granule proteins in cardiac tissues of patients with eosinophilic endomyocardial disease, *Lancet* 1:643, 1987.
21. Olsen EGJ: Pathological aspects of endomyocardial fibrosis, *Postgrad Med J* 59:135, 1983.

22. Barretto ACP, Lemos da Luz P, de Oliverra SA et al: Determinants of survival in endomyocardial fibrosis, *Circulation* 80(Suppl I):I-177, 1989.

23. Andy JJ, Bishara FF, Soyinka OD: Relation of severe eosinophilia and microfilariasis to chronic African endomyocardial fibrosis, *Br Heart J* 45:672, 1981.

24. Katritsis D, Wilmshurst PT, Wendon JA et al: Primary restrictive cardiomyopathy: clinical and pathologic characteristics, *J Am Coll Cardiol* 18:1230, 1991.

25. Weston LT, Raybuck BD, Robinowitz M et al: Primary amyloid heart disease presenting as hypertrophic obstructive cardiomyopathy, *Cathet Cardiovasc Diagn* 12:176-81, 1986.

PART III HYPERTROPHIC CARDIOMYOPATHY

Hallopeau, a French pathologist, is credited with the first description of the gross anatomic features of hypertrophic cardiomyopathy in 1869.[1] The condition was also recognized by other cardiac pathologists such as Schmincke[2] and Bernheim,[3] and by clinicians such as Osler. This fascinating clinicopathologic entity was then largely ignored for almost half a century, recapturing attention in the late 1950s.[4,5]

Hypertrophic cardiomyopathy (HC) is now defined simply as left ventricular hypertrophy of unknown cause; it may be concentric or asymmetric. The right ventricle also is usually involved.

The disorder is clinically very heterogeneous. The pathogenesis and etiology remain speculative, although significant advances have recently been made in unraveling its genetic inheritance. These advances have shown that hypertrophic cardiomyopathy is also genetically heterogeneous.

Ventricular hypertrophy is described as hypertrophic cardiomyopathy only after excluding systemic hypertension (prominent in Brock's first case in 1957),[5] valvular aortic stenosis, or other identifiable causes of ventricular hypertrophy. Although the left ventricle is predominantly involved, right ventricular hypertrophy may be marked, especially in severe cases.[5] The ventricular cavities are either normally sized or smaller, in contrast to the thick, robust ventricular myocardium. There are considerable changes over the course of the disease; thus survivors to middle and old age may show ventricular wall thinning, although usually no more than slight cavity dilatation.[6]

Anatomic descriptions from echocardiographic or autopsy studies have stressed considerable variability in the site and extent of the hypertrophic process. It has been recognized that the distribution of hypertrophy is asymmetric in the majority of cases. The hypertrophy most commonly involves the septum, with a septal-to-posterior wall thickness ratio equal to or greater than 1.5:1 (Fig. 7-16).[7] Data from Toronto, where interest has centered on surgical relief of outflow obstruction, indicate that one quarter of the cases have localized subaortic hypertrophy. In another quarter the hypertrophy extends down to the papillary

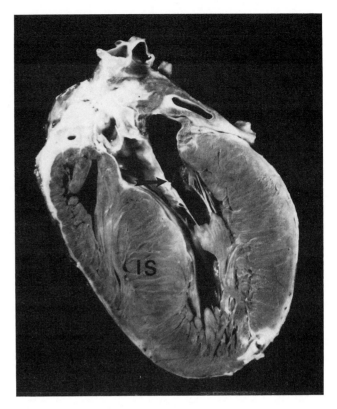

Fig. 7-16. Hypertrophic cardiomyopathy, asymmetric type. The massive hypertrophy of the proximal interventricular septum appears to obstruct the outflow tract of the left ventricle. Note the opposition of the anterior leaflet of the mitral valve *(arrow)* IS = interventricular septum (Courtesy Dr. William D. Edwards, Mayo Clinic).

muscles, whereas in about half of cases the hypertrophy involves the whole length of the ventricular septum. In the last two subgroups the hypertrophy may also extend into the anterolateral wall.[8] Variation in description reflects the highly selected case mix of institutions that specialize in HC.

Although outflow tract gradients on the left side of the heart have generated most interest, dynamic obstruction of the right ventricular outflow may result from hypertrophy of the crista supraventricularis (septal and parietal bands), or at the midright ventricular level from bulging of the hypertrophied septum. Impairment of diastolic filling of the left and often also of the right ventricle provides the major hemodynamic fault, which becomes progressively more severe over the years.

A rare form of hypertrophic cardiomyopathy shows midventricular obstruction as the hypertrophied walls and papillary muscles come into systolic apposition at midventricular level. This functional midventricular obstruction is easily visible on echocardiography and creates two ventricular chambers: a basal hyperkinetic chamber and a partially dyskinetic apical chamber.[9] This rare apical near-aneurysm formation may result from persistently high left ventricular apical pressures in patients with midventricular obstruction.[9]

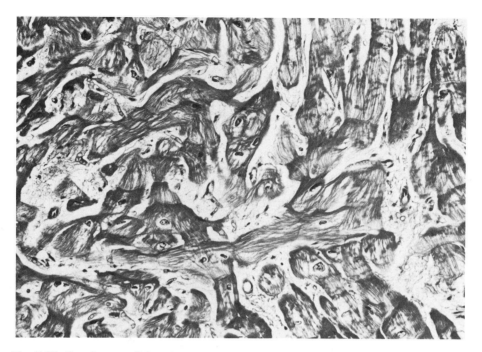

Fig. 7-17. Septal myocardial section from a case of hypertrophic cardiomyopathy. Note myocyte hypertrophy, perinuclear halo, disarray of myocardial fibers, and increased interstitial connective tissue.

Apical hypertrophy is a variant of HC first described in Japan and characterized by giant negative T-waves in a spade-shaped left ventricular cavity in middle-aged, Japanese men with angina.[10] Although this type of HC has been regarded as more common in Japan than elsewhere, sporadic cases are seen in Western countries. Asymmetric apical hypertrophy seems to develop with increasing age.[11] It is clinically benign, has no demonstrable genetic transmission and is not infrequently associated with systemic hypertension. It only rarely results in severe cardiac symptoms or death.[12] A "pure" Japanese type of asymmetric apical hypertrophy is rather rare in non-Asians and is not invariably associated with giant T-wave inversion.[13] It may coexist with asymmetric septal hypertrophy.

This morphologic and clinical diversity of HC was recently emphasized in a report of a subset of 17 patients described because of their atypicality.[14] In contrast to the majority of patients with HC, these patients showed marked thickening of the posterior left ventricular free wall and normal or only modestly increased septal thickness. The majority of these patients (65%) with this pattern of "inverted" asymmetry of the posterior wall relative to the septum were severely symptomatic and had symptoms early in life.[14] This unusual pattern of left ventricular hypertrophy underscores the known limitations of using the ratio of septal-to-posterior free wall thickness as the echocardiographic marker of HC.

The histopathologic features of HC are characterized by myocyte hypertrophy, nuclear polyploidy, and myocardial fiber disarray (Fig. 7-17). Short runs of myocytes are often interrupted by loose intercellular connective tissue with fibrosis and abnormal intramural coronary arteries. The myocardial fiber disarray is not specific to HC because similar disarray may occur in certain locations in normal, developing hearts, and especially in diseased hearts with hypertrophy caused by congenital or acquired disorders.[15]

Although extensive myocardial fiber disarray is typically seen in HC, neither its presence nor its absence is definitively diagnostic; the entire spectrum of histologic features (short fat fibers, myocyte hypertrophy, hyperchromatic nuclei, and loose connective tissue) should be considered in reaching the histologic diagnosis of HC. One should also be aware that when disarray is present it is always in the deepest (innermost) portions of the myocardium. Such a precise histologic search can only be conducted at postmortem because septectomy specimens or endomyocardial biopsies are too superficial to reach the location where the disarray is most likely to be.[16] Disarray is usually most apparent in the ventricular septum.

Widespread myocardial disarray may rarely occur in the absence of increased cardiac mass or wall thickness and be associated with sudden death.[17] Myocyte disarray, when widespread, almost certainly contributes to abnormalities of left ventricular diastolic function and is probably the substrate for reentry ventricular tachycardia and sudden death, although sustained ventricular tachycardia is uncommon in HC.[18]

Another characteristic histopathologic feature of HC is myocardial fibrosis with a variable distribution. Fibrosis is most striking in the ventricular septum, apparently contributing to its thickness, but it is also present in the free wall of the left and right chambers. The cause of myocardial fibrosis is still debated. It may represent myocyte fallout in the course of the myopathy, although ischemia secondary to the hypertrophy or caused by small intramyocardial vessel disease may be important.

Quantitative studies of stainable collagen have revealed a 72% higher level of fibrosis in HC than in hypertrophied control hearts.[19] Fibrosis may be interstitial, perivascular, or replacement type and appears more prevalent in the subendocardium than in the deeper layers. This suggests that ischemia from raised left ventricular end-diastolic pressure is important in its genesis. Silver impregnation techniques have also shown marked increases in all components of the extracellular matrix (struts, weaves, and coils), as well as evidence of matrix disorganization. Marked increase of pericellular weave fibers encasing individual myocytes has been observed, as well as coils of increased thickness and branching.[19]

The alterations in the extracellular matrix, particularly the thick pericellular weaves, may limit lateral and longitudinal excursion of the myocytes, especially when tissue has to stretch during diastolic relaxation.[19] The hypotheses about the contribution of intracellular connective tissue matrix, myocyte disarray, and fibrosis to the increased ventricular chamber stiffness are based on strictly morphologic observations, but the relative contributions of these different abnormalities to the diastolic dysfunction existing in individual patients has not been established for obvious reasons.

Morphologic abnormalities in the intramyocardial small coronary arteries[20] may be responsible for the myocardial fibrosis or vice versa. Vascular intramyocardial changes are rather common in HC and are characterized by medial thickening secondary to smooth muscle proliferation and increased collagen, intimal myofibroblastic proliferation, and luminal narrowing.[20]

These structural changes vary in magnitude in individual patients and cannot be considered unique to HC because they are also present in other cardiac disorders characterized by left ventricular hypertrophy. However, the frequency and severity of the small coronary artery alterations are more marked in HC, although they reveal no clear correlation with the clinical history of chest pain in these patients. It has been suggested that the pressure load on the left ventricular myocardium is insufficient to produce these abnormal intramural arteries, and that this histologic finding may therefore constitute an independent marker of HC and a component of the cardiomyopathic process that may be present at birth. An alternative explanation is that the vascular changes are secondary to transmural fibrous tissue formation, a form of neovascularization.[20]

Patients with HC often have atypical chest pain. Several mechanisms of ischemia have been suggested, including small coronary artery disease, septal perforator artery compression, coronary artery spasm, and inadequate capillary density in relation to increased myocardial mass.[21] Recent reports suggest the presence of a generalized arteriolar dysfunction in HC patients, which may be a contributing factor in the clinical picture.[22] However, diminished vasodilator reserve is also found in secondary hypertrophy, therefore this also is not specific to HC.

Others have suggested different pathogenetic mechanisms, such as transient severe regional ischemia accompanied by reversible systolic wall motion abnormalities, a form of "myocardial stunning."[23] The susceptibility of patients with HC to myocardial ischemia has been shown to result from reduced myocardial perfusion per unit of left ventricular mass and increased coronary resistance at rest with inadequate coronary reserve during pacing stress.[24] Thus hypoperfusion of the subendocardial areas may lead to progressive impairment of ventricular function, focal myocyte necrosis, and fibrosis.

Although the mechanism for transient ischemic episodes in HC remains unclear, recently demonstrated abnormalities of calcium fluxes and calcium antagonist receptors, as well as possible genetic factors affecting vascular smooth muscle, may explain the pathophysiology of ischemia in HC.[25]

The hemodynamic outflow gradients observed in about a quarter of patients with HC have fascinated clinicians. The thick protruding septum narrows the outflow tract, producing a high velocity jet that can be measured by Doppler ultrasound and may pull the anterior mitral leaflet, bending it almost to right angles.[26] Diminished systolic shortening of the left ventricle and its bent shape, with the mitral valve apparatus on the convexity, may also contribute.[27] The contact of the anterior mitral leaflet with the asymmetrically hypertrophied septum during systole (systolic anterior movement, or SAM), creates an endocardial thickening (imprint) at the site of contact (Fig. 7-18).

A synergistic combination of lesions contributing to the development of outflow tract obstruction in older subjects has been observed in recent years. Anterior displacement of the mitral apparatus created by heavy calcification of the annulus narrows the outflow tract, contributing to the development of a pressure gradient and septal-mitral contact.[28] These patients are elderly and have less septal thickness, but they have greater contribution of septal contraction and bowing to the narrowing of the outflow tract than in classic HC.

A higher incidence of mitral annular calcification in HC has been suggested and attributed to minimal, but long-term hemodynamic stresses on the mitral leaflet.[29] Recent data reported from a large autopsy series in patients with HC revealed that patients of less than 40 years of age had no mitral calcification (100 patients), whereas 30% of patients more than 40 years of age had mitral annular calcification (100 patients). The majority of the latter group with mitral annular calcification were women.[30] The frequency of mitral regurgitation was similar in the patients with and without mitral annular calcification, although it is thought that the severity of mitral regurgitation in the individual cases of HC bears a direct relationship to the presence and severity of SAM of the anterior mitral leaflet and therefore to the severity of obstruction.[26]

It was recently suggested that the disease process in HC is not confined to the left ventricular myocardium and that a congenital abnormality of the mitral valve may be present. Increased leaflet length and an increased mitral valve area was found; the abnormality was present in both the obstructive and nonobstructive types of HC and largely independent of other clinical morphologic components of the disease process.[31] However, this abnormality, could well be an acquired secondary change rather than congenital.

An additional congenital abnormality of the mitral valve apparatus in a subset of patients (approximately 14%) with HC was also described recently. The abnormality consisted of an anomalous insertion of papillary muscle directly onto the ventricular surface of the anterior mitral leaflet with total absence of chordae tendineae.[32] In the majority of these patients (approximately 50%), the anomaly was thought to be responsible for systolic contact with the septum and outflow obstruction. The authors of the study emphasize that failure to recognize this congenital anomaly may be responsible for the persistence of a pressure gradient even after adequate myomectomy.

PATHOGENESIS, NATURAL HISTORY, AND PROGNOSIS

The degree and extent of left ventricular hypertrophy may increase significantly during childhood in patients with HC.[33] Whether similar progression may occur in adults after mature body size has been achieved is not clear. Never-the-less, short follow-up of cases of HC has shown that if progression of the hypertrophic process occurs in adults it is probably rare.[34] In contrast, in a minority of adult cases there is progressive thinning of the left ventricular wall and relative cavity enlargement often accompanied by marked clinical deterioration.[6,35] It is estimated that this left ventricular wall thinning occurs in approximately 10% of surviving patients with advanced HC as they approach a stage of terminal myocardial failure.

The prognostic significance of the left ventricular outflow tract gradient in HC remains controversial. Some studies have indicated that a gradient had no adverse prognostic significance,[36] although ejection fraction, mean pulmonary artery pressure, dyspnea, left ventricular end-diastolic pressure, ventricular arrhythmias, and severe mitral regurgitation were all associated with a poor prognosis.[36]

A study of the morphologic, functional, and clinical features of outpatients with HC has revealed that these patients had a substantially more benign and more favorable clinical course than is usually inferred from the litera-

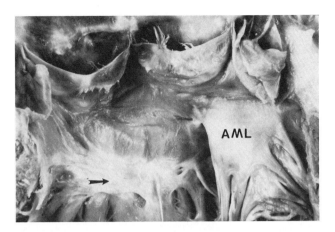

Fig. 7-18. Outflow tract of a hypertrophic cardiomyopathy, asymmetric type. Note the septal endocardial thickening secondary to the anterior mitral leaflet imprint, *(arrow)* AML = anterior mitral leaflet (Courtesy Dr. William D. Edwards, Mayo Clinic).

ture.[37] This is true also of unselected populations with HC from the cardiac departments of community hospitals, partly perhaps because of echocardiographic overdiagnosis, but also because specialist centers are referred the worst cases. There is evidence to suggest that right ventricular hypertrophy is associated with more severe disease. Right ventricular hypertrophy is not related to the occurrence of pulmonary hypertension, although it is not clear whether the increased right ventricular wall thickness is primary and idiopathic, or secondary to other causes such as left ventricular hypertrophy.[38,39]

The risk of syncope in HC is high in young patients who present with low left ventricular filling volume but who do not show ventricular ectopy on electrocardiographic monitoring. This mechanism of syncope indicates a low input-low output failure induced by sudden increase in heart rate and associated with a fall in venous return.[40] Autopsy studies have shown that almost half of competitive athletes under age 35 who died suddenly had HC.[41]

Maximum left ventricular wall thickness (equal to or greater than 30mm) was eight times more common in patients with HC and sudden death than in the control patients with HC of similar age and functional status.[42]

Atrial fibrillation in HC has been called "an ominous milestone" associated with marked clinical and hemodynamic deterioration and a poor prognosis.[43]

In most patients with HC ventricular wall motion is either normal or hyperkinetic. Except for the hypertrophied septum, which is notably akinetic in "classical" HC, segmental or global wall motion abnormality or chamber dilatation in HC are unusual. Hypertrophic cardiomyopathy evolving into a hypokinetic and dilated left ventricle has been estimated to occur in approximately 4% to 7% of cases.[6] This rare evolution is to be distinguished from the progressive failure of systolic function without notable dilatation described by Spirito.[34] The pathophysiologic reasons for such an outcome in HC have not been elucidated. Proposed pathogenetic mechanisms for the hypokinesia and dilatation have often implicated vascular episodes, although these patients characteristically reveal absence of fixed epicardial coronary artery disease (this is quite often seen in older patients with hypertrophy and good systolic function). Infarction in the absence of epicardial coronary disease has been described but is rare.[9]

Mechanisms proposed for the development of hypokinesia and dilatation include (1) myocardial infarction from embolization, coronary spasm, small coronary artery disease, myocardial bridging, or an oxygen supply demand mismatch; (2) intraventricular obliteration; and (3) prior septal myotomy or myomectomy, which is followed by the development of heart failure in about 25% of cases. A further possibility is that this is the evolution of the myopathy in patients who escape earlier sudden death.

Ventricular hypokinesia and dilation in HC can occur if the heart is subjected to an additional injury of surgical or perhaps vascular nature. Ischemic episodes may be initiated by embolization of a large coronary artery or multiple small intramyocardial arteries. However, histopathologic demonstrations of such embolic phenomena is not always feasible.[35]

Genetic studies have shown that HC is often familial (55%) and transmitted in a pattern consistent with autosomal dominant trait. The remaining 45% of cases appear to be sporadic,[38] but the number of "sporadic" cases diminishes with increasing numbers of relatives screened. The definition of "sporadic" needs to be based on a stated number of first-degree relatives who have been examined and found to be normal. It is possible that sporadic cases represent either new mutations or an autosomal recessive inheritance with reduced penetrance. There is little doubt that HC represents a group of related but etiologically distinct diseases rather than a single entity.[39] The type of HC may vary within individual families and patterns of distribution; severity and extent of hypertrophy may be different in various members of an affected family.[44] Genetic heterogeneity has already been shown.

Association of HC with Friedreich's ataxia has long been known,[45] although the hypertrophy in the latter tends to be symmetrical without outflow gradient. An association between familial neurofibromatosis and HC supports the suggestion that both diseases are manifestations of a common hereditary defect of neural crest tissue,[46] as does the association of HC with lentiginosis, another disorder of abnormal neural crest tissue migration. Although immunogenetic factors might be involved in the pathogenesis of HC, data on the frequency of certain HLA antigens are conflicting, partly because of the almost certain inclusion of a very heterogeneous population. HLA-DR3 antigen was found in 50% of European patients with HC but only in 17% of control group patients.[47]

A search for molecular abnormality in hypertrophic cardiomyopathy has directed investigators towards the study of calcium antagonist receptors.[48] Experiments have shown a substantial increase of such receptors in the myocardium in HC. This probably reflects an increased density of voltage-sensitive calcium channels. In contrast, no abnormality in the number of voltage-sensitive sodium channels or beta-adrenoceptors was found, which suggests that the increase in calcium channels does not reflect a generalized membrane defect.[48] However, recent work (unpublished) suggests a decrease in the number of beta-adrenoceptors in HC. Whether the increased number of calcium antagonist receptors is primary or a response to hypertrophy is not known. It may be related to an enhanced calcium flux across the sarcolemma membrane and be responsible for some of the pathophysiologic abnormalities in HC.[48] The rationale discussed above may have been strengthened by a favorable response to therapy with calcium channel-blocking drugs in a few patients with HC, most of whom were young.

Additional studies in myocardial calcium kinetics in HC have demonstrated abnormal prolongation of the ventricular action potential, the calcium transient, and the duration of isometric contraction and relaxation. These abnormalities were exacerbated by interventions that increased the intracellular calcium concentration and were ameliorated by manipulations that reduced it.[49,50]

The first presentation of HC may be with sudden death, and children who are at highest risk may not manifest the typical cardiac morphology until their teens. This fact, along with the tremendous clinical heterogeneity of "idiopathic hypertrophy," makes a genetic marker highly desirable. The first study to identify by linkage analysis the chromosomes responsible in families affected by HC was reported from Boston in 1989.[51] The authors demonstrated that locus D14s26 was genetically linked to the locus responsible for familial hypertrophic cardiomyopathy (FHC) in a large French-Canadian family. Locus D14s26 had been previously mapped to chromosome 14 close to band q11, a chromosome in which a number of genes thought to play a role in cardiac hypertrophy have also been mapped (cardiac myosin heavy chains).[52] However, two other possible links have been revealed, on chromosome 18 in 78 members of 16 families studied in Japan,[53] and on chromosome 16 in one Italian family.[54] These disparities suggested that HC may not be a single gene defect[55]; it may be a final common pathway of different gene defects.

Several different mutations on the myosin heavy chain gene in exons 9, 13, 14, 16, 17, and 23 have since been described by the Boston group.[52,56] The myosin heavy chain (MHC) genes are expressed at high levels in the myocardium and encode a major contractile component of myofibrils, the organization of which is distorted in hypertrophic cardiomyopathy. Recent genetic linkage analyses have raised the possibility that defects in the cardiac myosin heavy chain genes may be responsible for FHC.[52] This intriguing hypothesis was suggested because of close linkage of the cardiac MHC genes and the FHC locus. In this large kindred a unique mutation in the cardiac MHC genes of individuals with FHC was demonstrated. A missense mutation present in exon 13 of the beta-cardiac MHC gene of affected members in the family converts an arginine residue to a glutamine residue.[56]

The gene for heat shock protein (HSP70) and protooncogene c-phos also maps to chromosome 14.[57] The former may be important in the development of myocardial hypertrophy and therefore etiologically implicated.[58] Myosin heavy chain mutations account for the disease in only half of the affected families so far tested. The mutations have been different even in the families that show β-MHC mutations. All of the mutations so far identified have been clustered in the head rod junction of the molecule. It is fascinating that the mutations alter highly conserved amino acid residues, perhaps resulting in poison polypeptides that cause the formation of defective myofibrils. It is likely that particular mutations will be identified with survival; such recognition of a particular genotype will give important prognostic information. Sporadic cases of HC have not yet been found to have mutations, but genetic mutations have been found in clinically unaffected members of large pedigrees with an MHC mutation. This has revealed clinically "skipped" generations and again suggests the need for interaction with other genetic or environmental forces that may determine when and whether the disorder develops.

In families with identified mutations in the β-MHC gene, peripheral blood mononuclear cells have been shown to express the mutant gene. Amplification of B-cardiac MHC transcripts from peripheral blood can be carried out to detect or unequivocally exclude the disorder in as yet unaffected members of families with identified mutations.[59] This can enable preclinical diagnosis in young children who may still be clinically, electrocardiographically, and echocardiographically normal. It is noteworthy that the electrocardiogram may precede the echocardiogram in showing abnormality in young children, although the electrocardiographic abnormalities may be subtle. This is important because an electrocardiogram is inexpensive and more readily available than echocardiography. In the future, genetic analysis will shed light on the nature of left ventricular hypertrophy associated with athletic training or hypertension. Early detection of HC in as yet unaffected children will eventually lead to understanding of the development of the functional disorder, thus enabling early intervention to prevent the development or progression of the disease.

Since its clinical emergence following Teare's autopsy description,[4] hypertrophic cardiomyopathy (HC) has provided material for an ever increasing literature. Much of this material is conflicting. Apart from the undoubted fascination inspired by the disorder, one reason for the extensive literature has been the absence of any absolute criterion for the diagnosis apart from unexplained hypertrophy. Although the family described by Teare lacked outflow tract obstruction in the clinically studied members of the original sibship, left ventricular outflow tract obstruction and "pseudoaortic stenosis" were the striking clinical features that were noted and incorporated into the nomenclature of the time.[60,61,62] Subsequently, the existence of the obstruction came into question.[63,64] Even when this became accepted, its hemodynamic importance was argued. There is still no consensus regarding its only incidental occurrence and lack of prognostic significance.[36] Credit for the first "modern" description should probably go to Davies, who in 1952 reported a family with systolic murmurs, sudden deaths, and pathologic features of HC in one member who died after an injection for asthma.[65]

In 1961 Menges[7] had suggested from a pathologic study that the diagnosis should be considered if the ratio of the thickness of the septum to that of the free wall of the left ventricle exceeded 1.3. However, the disorder became a clinical entity before echocardiography was available, and increased ventricular wall thickness is not well assessed on angiography. With the advent of M-mode echocardiography, asymmetric septal hypertrophy (ASH) was reborn in 1973,[66] only to die[67] when it was recognized that hypertrophy could be symmetrical or preferentially involve the posterior wall rather than the septum.[14] Technical errors abounded when using only M-mode technology. It was common for measurement of the septum to be increased by erroneous inclusion of the papillary muscle of the tricuspid valve or the moderator band. The advent of cross-sectional imaging allowed the thickness of all parts of the left and right ventricle to be evaluated and for the M-mode beam to be directed with precision to obtain accurate and repeatable mensuration.

Natural history studies of the time course of the development (and regression) of hypertrophy cover at most 20 years of the disease, and only then in individual cases in centers concentrating on HC studies. Published studies are usually much shorter.[33,34,68] Sequential studies have enabled appreciation of the acquisition of hypertrophy in the children of familial cases (FHC) during the end of their first decade or beginning of their second decade,[33] but we know nothing of the antecedents of newly diagnosed middle-aged and older patients.[69,70] The literature is swollen with accounts of "HC" in the elderly,[69-78] sometimes in association with mitral annular calcification,[73] sometimes with systolic hypertension,[4,71] and sometimes in extreme old age.[77] These older patients have displayed their good prognosis by their survival, give no past history of known or suspected heart disease, have no family history, and almost certainly do not have the same "HC" as younger and familial cases. The simplified definition has resulted in great clinical heterogeneity caused by the inclusion of a diversity of disorders that have in common unexplained left ventricular hypertrophy. This is represented in Fig. 7-19,

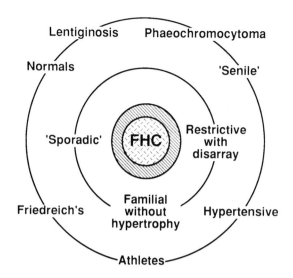

Familial hypertrophic cardiomyopathy with known mutation

Familial hypertrophic cardiomyopathy without determined genetic fault

Fig. 7-19. Hypertrophic cardiomyopathy–umbra and penumbra. The classical condition is depicted in the center (FHC). FHC is surrounded by conditions with left ventricular hypertrophy that are probably different in origin, natural history, and prognosis but that are included under the general descriptive umbrella.

which shows classic FHC in the center. This is the familial disorder inherited as an autosomal dominant. Surrounding the central disorder is sporadic HC, disarray without increased LV mass, restrictive cardiomyopathy with disarray, senile HC, hypertensive HC, athletes with sudden death, and the hypertrophic cardiomyopathies occurring in association with a number of inherited disorders. This latter group includes Friedreich's ataxia, the genetic defect of which is known to be on chromosome 9 and thus far apart from the recently found mutations in FHC.

It is still unknown how the genetic defect and postulated defective myofibrils account for a disorder characterized by myocyte hypertrophy and disarray that is focal rather than generalized. It is quite unclear how or why parts of the myocardium in HC may show no abnormality either in myocyte size or arrangement even when the defective gene is present in every cell. It is also unknown how the myofibril defects affects cell biology in terms of possibly increased density of voltage-sensitive calcium channels and an increased duration of isometric contraction and relaxation. It is possible that expression of the genetic mutation may have need of other enabling genes or be concealed by lack of these or by protective ones. Such expression may indeed require the hormonal changes occurring around puberty, athletic training, or the development of hypertension.

It is certain that we are dealing with many more genetic abnormalities than have yet been identified. It also is clear

that the diagnostic label of hypertrophic cardiomyopathy covers far too broad a canvas. The shape of the left ventricle differs from individual to individual, and with age the amount and site of hypertrophy that occurs in response to stimuli may vary for many different reasons. The myocardium is not very versatile. The echocardiographic appearance of the heart changes with increasing age in a recognizable way.[73,74] The septum becomes more bent with protrusion just below the aortic valve. This curvature, particularly when coupled with hypertrophy caused by hypertension or with anterior displacement of the mitral valve associated with annular calcification, may result in sufficient outflow tract narrowing to generate high blood flow velocity and turbulence. The resulting systolic anterior movement of the mitral leaflets, murmur, and gradient are all characteristic of HC, but the explanation is mechanistic and the resemblance to the genetic disorder (or disorders) is fortuitous. Similarly, left ventricular hypertrophy caused by hypertension was found to be asymmetrical, with at least one segment of the left ventricular wall 1.5 times the thickness of any other, in 34% of 102 patients.[79]

The early appearances of the left ventricle in older patients (usually women), who are first diagnosed in their 50s or 60s or later, are totally unknown. These people usually give no history of previously known heart disease and have been robustly healthy and active throughout their lives. Their conditions are detected because alert contemporary physicians are quick to detect the source of systolic murmurs heard during routine examinations. Such physicians will promptly order an echocardiographic study in patients with any unexplained electrocardiographic abnormality or mild hypertension. Some of these older patients who show the senile bent septum and narrow outflow tract with turbulence (with or without mitral annular calcification) but who have normal mitral and aortic valves have normal electrocardiograms. The latter is never seen in classic FHC, in which ECG abnormality is an early feature.

HYPERTROPHIED HEARTS IN ATHLETES

A further difficulty involves the distinction between adaptive and pathologic hypertrophy in the athlete.[80] Furthermore, there is the conflict between the functional diastolic abnormalities found in classical HC[81] (attributed variously to the hypertrophy itself, to disarray, to abnormalities in small coronary arteries, or to increased fibrous tissue replacement) and the overtly supernormal performance that is necessary for success in athletics. In HC the left ventricular cavity tends to be small. Isometric contraction is prolonged, as are relaxation and filling. The endurance-trained athlete with a maximum heart rate that is the same as that of his healthy but untrained peer, but with a maximum oxygen consumption (MVO_2) perhaps twice as high, must produce a massively higher left ventricular stroke volume during peak exercise. Diastolic relaxation must be

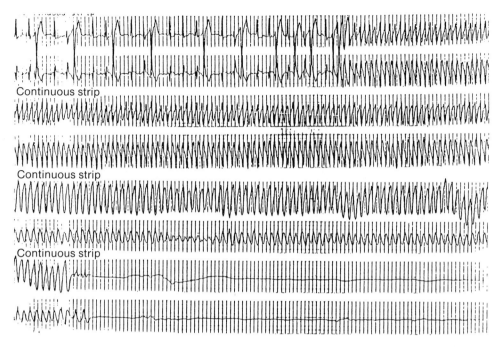

Continuous strip

Continuous strip

Continuous strip

Fig. 7-20. Holter ECG recording showing ventricular tachycardia degenerating into ventricular fibrillation in a patient with hypertrophic cardiomyopathy.

faster to accommodate the increased stroke volume during the short diastolic interval; ejection must also be fast. The athlete with HC cannot show any of the functional defects associated with HC while succeeding in his sport. How is it, then that almost half of competitive athletes under age 35 who suddenly die have HC?[41] Perhaps they just have more adaptive hypertrophy than we yet recognize, or perhaps function can be genuinely normal in HC at a young age. We do not know whether individuals who are able to generate a greater amount of adaptive hypertrophy in response to athletic training may both excel at their sport and put themselves at risk from sudden death. Hypertrophic cardiomyopathy is particularly likely to be found in black athletes who die suddenly during athletics. The clinical problem of whether such an athlete has adaptive hypertrophy or a cardiomyopathy is particularly common and difficult when the athlete in question is black.[82,83] It is also well known that black patients with hypertension or dilated cardiomyopathy tend to have thicker and heavier hearts than white subjects.

Some abnormality in the response of the myocardium to sympathetic stimuli has been suspected almost since the recognition of HC. The high level of sympathetic activity that drives athletes at their peak of performance might normalize the function even of defective myofibrils while increasing the risk of fatal arrhythmia. Enhanced vagal tone supervening on cessation of exercise occurs in athletes who demonstrate profound bradycardia or even atrioventricular block on resting. Ventricular tachycardia and fibrillation have occurred during exertion in athletes who,

after resuscitation, have shown no evidence of HC or other cardiac abnormality on comprehensive full investigation.[84]

SUDDEN DEATH

In classic familial hypertrophic cardiomyopathy, development of hypertrophy seems to be most rapid at puberty.[33] Sudden death is most common before age 20. It is noteworthy that children and young people with HC fail to show the typical nonsustained ventricular tachycardia (VT) so characteristic of HC in older individuals, yet are more at risk from sudden death.[85] It has been suggested that disarray may engender ventricular fibrillation (VF) rather than VT in young people. However, many such patients have survived a collapse outside the hospital and are in VF on arrival, but far later than would have been possible had the initial collapse been caused by VF. Ventricular tachycardia has been seen preceding VF on Holter recordings. Fig. 7-20 shows such a Holter ECG recording during the sudden death of a patient with hypertrophic cardiomyopathy. In older patients with HC, ventricular ectopy can be related to poor prognosis and is characterized by short bursts of self-terminating VT. In children and athletes, sudden death is almost always precipitated by exercise or emotion, which suggests that hemodynamic stress, sympathetic excess, tachycardia, and possibly a low input-low output state may be the ingredients for fatal arrhythmia. Certainly the propensity to sudden death cannot be related to the severity of any functional defect because this is usually notably absent in the young. In adults, such spontaneous arrhythmias do not correlate with the degree of left ventricu-

NATURAL HISTORY OF FAMILIAL HYPERTROPHIC CARDIOMYOPATHY

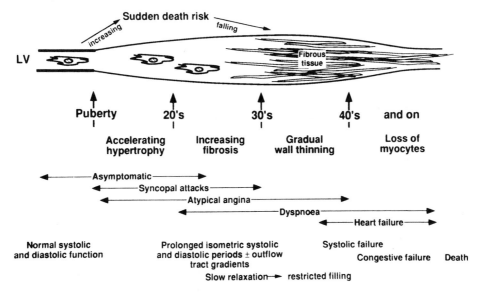

Fig. 7-21. The natural history of hypertrophic cardiomyopathy is depicted. The early asymptomatic phase with marked hypertrophy but still excellent systolic and diastolic function (a time when sudden death is most frequent) is followed by increasing diastolic dysfunction going on to progressive systolic dysfunction accompanied by wall thinning with fibrous replacement and the phase of terminal low output failure.

lar hypertrophy or with systolic or diastolic dysfunction. It seems most likely that myocardial disarray or fibrosis provides the substrate for reentrant VT in adults.

Deaths in older patients are less often sudden and usually occur in association with deteriorating symptoms and demonstrable hemodynamic abnormality. The latter may be raised left ventricular end-diastolic pressure, pulmonary hypertension, or poor exercise performance with low MVO_2.Surgical treatment does not prevent and may promote this.[86,87] The progression and hemodynamic deterioration that occur during the years of observation may be more an expression of the progression of a true myopathy than attributable to secondary phenomena. The myocyte fallout, replacement fibrosis, and functional and structural changes in the coronary resistance vessels may all be part of the progressive myopathic process and analogous to the changes in skeletal muscles seen in familial skeletal myopathies.

NATURAL HISTORY

In those patients who survive the enhanced risk of sudden death during their first decades, increasing diastolic abnormality[82,83] is the rule. The diastolic changes are followed by diminishing systolic function; end-systolic volume tends to increase with loss of outflow tract turbulence and gradients[6] (Fig. 7-21). However, the increase in end-diastolic volume is rather little. An increased residual volume with falling ejection fraction and stroke volume results in further elevation of left ventricular filling pressure.

Left atrial distension caused by a rise in its pressure leads first to a loss of left atrial contractile function and contribution to left ventricular filling, then to atrial fibrillation. Atrial fibrillation marks a major fall in hemodynamic performance[47] caused by loss of regularity, with stroke volume being maximal only at small ranges of RR-interval. At this stage, ventricular pacing after His' bundle ablation may be helpful simply through restoring regularity and optimization of ventricular rate. In other patients, time brings increasing structural changes in the mitral leaflets, leading to fixed mitral regurgitation or rarely stenosis. In such patients loss of forward flow and a further rise in left atrial pressure may lead to pulmonary edema even while sinus rhythm is preserved. Such patients may benefit from replacement of the mitral valve with a low profile prosthesis.[88]

The clinical course of familial hypertrophic cardiomyopathy varies from family to family, some families have a high incidence of sudden death in childhood and adolescence, whereas others experience a more benign course. The natural history has been pieced together by studying family members from different generations, as well as from following individual family members (Fig. 7-3). Symptoms are hard to evaluate; they may be more related to the diagnosis than to the disease. They also may be linked to detraining from inactivity, knowledge of the risk of sudden death following the loss of family members or from their reading, physicians' concern, and either no medication or changing medication, which seems to reflect the physician's uncertainty. Exercise testing at this time may reveal unfitness and chronic hyperventilation as the main determinants of poor exercise tolerance.[89] At the other extreme, exercise tolerance may remain excellent. The difficulty involves counseling against indulgence in sporting activities, particularly competitive ones. During these years careful sequential analysis of left ventricular diastolic filling may catch a gradual transition from a pattern of slow relaxation (with prolonged isometric relaxation, lengthened deceleration phase and time to peak filling with enhanced atrial contribution) to a restrictive pattern of shorter isometric relaxation, early completion of peak filling, and a reduced atrial contribution. This is best analyzed by a combination of Doppler echocardiography, M-mode imaging, and mechanical impulse recording.[90] The Doppler pattern will show a transition from an early enhanced A/E to a later increase in E/A, with a period of pseudonormalization in between. Lagging slightly behind are changes in systolic function, including a reduction in outflow tract velocity and gradients (though often with retention or even increase in mitral regurgitation), an increase in end-systolic dimension, and a gradual reduction in left ventricular wall thickness para passu with the decline in systolic ejection. Left atrial size increases and is followed by the onset of atrial fibrillation. This is likely to be associated with a rise in left atrial pressure, the development of pulmonary hypertension, and sometimes congestive failure. Diuretics are needed when the left atrial pressure starts to rise with the decline in left atrial ability to empty, which is caused by increasing left ventricular stiffness. Patients with FHC who go the whole course do so by avoiding the sudden death risk (perhaps by chance or through therapy) and eventually entering the final phase of low output failure. The latter usually includes a still undilated, poorly contracting left ventricle, atrial fibrillation, pulmonary hypertension, right ventricular dilatation, and congestive heart failure. At this stage transplantation is justified.

REFERENCES

1. Hallopeau M: Retrecissement ventriculo-aortique, *Gaz Med Paris* 24:683, 1869.
2. Schmincke A: Ueber linkseitige musckulose consusstenosei, *Dtsch Med Wochenschr* 33:2082, 1907.
3. Bernheim PI: De L'asystolic veinense dans i'hypertrophic du coeur gauche par stenose concomitante du ventricule droit, *Rev Med* 30:785, 1910.
4. Teare RD: Asymmetrical hypertrophy of the heart in young adults, *Br Heart J* 20:1, 1958.
5. Brock RC: Functional obstruction of the left ventricle, *Guys Hosp Rep* 106:221, 1957.
6. Fighali S, Krajcer Z, Edelman S et al: Progression of hypertrophic cardiomyopathy into a hypokinetic left ventricle: higher incidence in patients with midventricular obstruction, *J Am Coll Cardiol* 9:288, 1987.
7. Menges JR, Brandenburg RO, Brown AL Jr: The clinical haemodynamic and pathologic diagnosis of muscular subvalvular aortic stenosis, *Circulation* 24:1126, 1961.
8. Sasson Z, Rokowski H, Wigle E: Hypertrophic cardiomyopathy, *Cardiol Clin* 6:233, 1988.
9. Gordon E, Henderson M, Rakowski H et al: Midventricular obstruction with apical infarction and aneurysm formation, *Circulation* 70 (suppl 2): 145, 1984, abstract.
10. Sakamoto T, Tei L, Murayama M et al: Giant negative T-wave inversion as a manifestation of asymmetric apical hypertrophy (AAH) of the left ventricle. Echocardiographic and ultrasonocardiotomographic study, *Jpn Heart J* 17:611, 1976.
11. Sakamoto T, Amano K, Hada Y et al: Asymmetric apical hypertrophy: ten years experience, *Postgrad Med J* 62:567, 1986.
12. Koga Y, Haya M, Takahashi H et al: Apical hypertrophy and its genetic and acquired factors, *J Cardiol* 15 (suppl VI):VI-65-74, 1985.
13. Maron BJ: Apical hypertrophic cardiomyopathy: the continuing saga, *J Am Coll Cardiol* 15:91, 1990.
14. Lewis JF, Maron BJ: Hypertrophic cardiomyopathy characterized by marked hypertrophy of the posterior left ventricular free wall. Significance and clinical implications, *J Am Coll Cardiol* 18:421, 1991.
15. Olsen EGJ: Myocardial disarray revisited, *Br Med J* 285:991, 1982.
16. Tazelaar HD, Billingham ME: The Surgical pathology of hypertrophic cardiomyopathy, *Arch Pathol Lab Med* 111:257, 1987.
17. McKenna WJ, Stewart JT, Nihoyannopoulos P et al: Hypertrophic cardiomyopathy without hypertrophy: two families with myocardial disarray in the absence of increased myocardial mass, *Br Heart J* 63:287, 1990.
18. Alfonso F, Frenneaux MP, McKenna WJ: Clinical sustained uniform ventricular tachycardia in hypertrophic cardiomyopathy: association with left ventricular apical aneurysm, *Br Heart J* 61:178, 1989.
19. Factor SM, Butany J, Sole MJ et al: Pathologic fibrosis and matrix connective tissue in the subaortic myocardium of patients with hypertrophic cardiomyopathy, *J Am Coll Cardiol* 17:1343, 1991.
20. Maron BJ, Wolfson JK, Epstein SE et al: Intramural ("small vessel") coronary artery disease in hypertrophic cardiomyopathy, *J Am Coll Cardiol* 8:545, 1986.
21. Cannon RO, Rosing DR, Maron BJ et al: Myocardial ischaemia in patients with hypertrophic cardiomyopathy: contribution of inadequate vasodilator reserve and elevated left ventricular filling pressures, *Circulation* 71:234, 1985.
22. Camici P, Spessot M, Lorenzoni R et al: Evidence of generalized arteriolar dysfunction in patients with hypertrophic cardiomyopathy, *Circulation* 82(Suppl. III) 26, 1990.
23. Pasternac A: Myocardial stunning in hypertrophic cardiomyopathy? *J Am Coll Cardiol* 13:1419, 1989.
24. Pasternac A, Noble J, Streulens Y et al: Pathophysiology of chest pain in patients with cardiomyopathies and normal coronary arteries, *Circulation* 65:778, 1982.
25. Wagner JA, Sax FL, Weisman HF et al. Calcium-antagonist receptors in the atrial tissue of patients with hypertrophic cardiomyopathy, *N Engl J Med* 320:755, 1989.
26. Wigle ED, Sasson Z, Henderson MA et al: Hypertrophic cardiomyopathy. The importance of the site and extent of hypertrophy: a review, *Prog Cardiovasc Dis* 28:1, 1985.
27. Oakley CM: Clinical definition of the cardiomyopathies, *Circulation* 34 (Suppl): 152, 1974.
28. Lewis JF, Maron BJ: Elderly patients with hypertrophic cardiomyopathy: a subset with distinctive left ventricular morphology and progressive clinical course late in life, *J Am Coll Cardiol* 13:36, 1988.
29. Kronzon I, Glassman E: Mitral annulus calcification in idiopathic subaortic stenosis, *Am J Cardiol* 42:60, 1978.
30. Motamed HE, Roberts WC: Frequency and significance of mitral annular calcium in hypertrophic cardiomyopathy: analysis of 200 necropsy patients, *Am J Cardiol* 60:877, 1987.
31. Klues HG, Dollar AL, Woberts WC et al: Diversity of mitral valve structure in patients with hypertrophic cardiomyopathy: evidence for a primary mitral valve abnormality, *Circulation* 82 (suppl III):III-294, 1990.

32. Klues HG, Roberts WC, Maron BJ et al: Anomalous insertion of papillary muscle directly onto anterior mitral leaflet: a previously unrecognized mechanism of subaortic obstruction in hypertrophic cardiomyopathy, *Circulation* 82 (suppl III):III-400, 1990, (abstract).

33. Maron BJ, Spirito P, Wesley Y et al: Development and progression of left ventricular hypertrophy in children with hypertrophic cardiomyopathy, *N Engl J Med* 315:610, 1986.

34. Spirito P, Maron BJ: Absence of progression of left ventricular hypertrophy in adult patients with hypertrophic cardiomyopathy, *J Am Coll Cardiol* 9:1013, 1987.

35. Gravanis MB, Robinson PH, Hertzler GL: Hypertrophic cardiomyopathy evolving into a hypokinetic and dilated left ventricle: coronary embolization as a probable pathogenetic mechanism, *Clin Cardiol* 13:500, 1990.

36. Romeo F, Pelliccia F, Cristofani R et al: Hypertrophic cardiomyopathy: is a left ventricular outflow tract gradient a major prognostic determinant? *Eur Heart J* 11:233, 1990.

37. Spirito P, Chiarella F, Carrantino L et al: Clinical course and prognosis of hypertrophic cardiomyopathy in an outpatient population, *N Engl J Med* 320:749, 1989.

38. McKenna WJ, Kleinebenne A, Nihoyannopoulos P et al: Echocardiographic measurement of right ventricular wall thickness in hypertrophic cardiomyopathy: relation to clinical and prognostic features, *J Am Coll Cardiol* 11:351, 1988.

39. Maron BJ, Bonow RD, Cannon RO et al: Hypertrophic cardiomyopathy. Interrelations of clinical manifestations, pathophysiology and therapy (Part I), *N Engl J Med* 316:780, 1987.

40. Nienaber CA, Hiller S, Spielmann RF et al: Syncope in hypertrophic cardiomyopathy: multivariate analysis of prognostic determinants, *J Am Coll Cardiol* 15:948, 1990.

41. Maron BJ, Epstein SE, Roberts WC et al: Causes of sudden death in competitive athletes, *J Am Coll Cardiol* 7:204, 1986.

42. Spirito P, Maron BJ: Relation between extent of left ventricular hypertrophy and occurrence of sudden cardiac death in hypertrophic cardiomyopathy, *J Am Coll Cardiol* 15:1521, 1990.

43. Greenspan AM: Hypertrophic cardiomyopathy and atrial fibrillation: a change of perspective, *J Am Coll Cardiol* 15:1286, 1990.

44. Ciro E, Maron BJ, Roberts WC: Coexistence of asymmetric and symmetric left ventricular hypertrophy in a family with hypertrophic cardiomyopathy, *Am Heart J* 104:643, 1982.

45. Child JS, Perloff JK, Bach PM et al: Cardiac involvement in Friedreich's ataxia: a clinical study of 75 patients, *J Am Coll Cardiol* 7:1370, 1986.

46. Fitzpatrick AP, Emanuel RW: Familial neurofibromatosis and hypertrophic cardiomyopathy, *Br Heart J* 60:247, 1988.

47. Fiorito S, Autore C, Fragola PV et al: HLA-DR3 antigen linkage in patients with hypertrophic obstructive cardiomyopathy, *Am Heart J* III:91, 1986.

48. Wagner JA, Sax FL, Weisman HF et al: Calcium-antagonist receptors in the atrial tissue of patients with hypertrophic cardiomyopathy, *N Engl J Med* 320:755, 1989.

49. Braunwald E: Hypertrophic cardiomyopathy - continued progress, *N Engl J Med* 320:800, 1989.

50. Gwathmey JK, Copelas L, MacKinnon R et al: Abnormal intracellular calcium handling in myocardium from patients with end-stage heart failure, *Circ Res* 61:70, 1987.

51. Jarcho JA, McKenna W, Pare P et al: Mapping a gene for familial hypertrophic cardiomyopathy to chromosome 14ql, *N Engl J Med* 321:1372, 1989.

52. Solomon SD, Geisterfer-Lowrance AAT, Vosberg HP et al: A locus for familial hypertrophic cardiomyopathy is closely linked to the cardiac myosin heavy chain genes, CRI-L436, and CRI-L329 on chromosome 14 at q11-q12, *Am J Hum Genet* 47:389, 1990.

53. Nishi H, Kimura A, Sasaki M et al: Localization of the gene for hypertrophic cardiomyopathy to chromosome 18q, *Circulation* 80 (Suppl II):457, 1989, (Abstract).

54. Ferraro M, Scarton G, Ambrossini M et al: Coagulation of hypertrophic cardiomyopathy and a fragile site on chromosome 16 in a large Italian family, *J Med Genet* 27:363-366, 1990.

55. Epstein N, Fananapazir L, Lin H et al: Genetic heterogeneity in hypertrophic cardiomyopathy: evidence that HCM maps to chromosome 2p, *Circulation* 82 (suppl III):III-339, 1990, (abstract).

56. Geisterfer-Lowrance AAT, Kass S, Tanigwa G et al: A molecular basis for familial hypertrophic cardiomyopathy: a b cardiac myosin heavy chain gene missense mutation, *Cell* 62:999, 1990.

57. Zumo S, Nadal-Ginard B, Mahdavi V: Protooncogene induction and reprogramming of cardiac gene expression produced by pressure overload, *Proc Natl Acad Sci USA* 85:339, 1988.

58. Hejtmancik JF, Brink PA, Towbin J et al: Localization of gene for familial hypertrophic cardiomyopathy to chromosome 14ql in adverse US population, *Circulation* 83:1592-7, 1991.

59. Rosenzweig A, Watkins H, Hwang DS et al: Preclinical diagnosis of familial hypertrophic cardiomyopathy by genetic analysis of blood lymphocytes, *N Engl J Med* 325:1753-60, 1991.

60. Goodwin JF, Hollman A, Cleland WP, et al: Obstructive cardiomyopathy simulating aortic stenosis, *Br Heart J* 22:1403, 1960.

61. Braunwald E, Lambrew CT, Rockoff SD et al: Idiopathic hypertrophic subaortic stenosis, *Am Heart Assoc Monograph* No. 10, New York, 1964.

62. Cohen J, Effat H, Goodwin JF et al: Hypertrophic obstructive cardiomyopathy, *Br Heart J* 26:16, 1964.

63. Criley JM, Lewis KB, White RI et al: Pressure gradients without obstruction: a new concept of "hypertrophic subaortic stenosis", *Circulation* 22:881, 1965.

64. Murgo JP, Alter BR, Doretly JF et al: Dynamics of left ventricular ejection in obstructive and non-obstructive hypertrophic cardiomyopathy, *J Clin Invest* 66:1369-1382, 1980.

65. Davies LG: A familial heart disease, *Br Heart J* 14:206, 1952.

66. Henry WL, Clark CE, Epstein SE: Asymmetric septal hypertrophy (ASH), *Circulation* 47:225-233, 1973.

67. Maron BJ: Asymmetry in hypertrophic cardiomyopathy: the septal to free wall ratio revisited, *Am J Cardiol* 55:835, 1985.

68. Domenicucci S, Lazzeroni E, Roelandt J et al: Progression of hypertrophic cardiomyopathy. A cross sectional echocardiographic study, *Br Heart J* 53:405, 1985.

69. Shenov MM, Khanna A, Nejaj M et al: Hypertrophic cardiomyopathy in the elderly. A frequently misdiagnosed disease, *Arch Intern Med* 146:658, 1986.

70. Pelliccia F, Cianfroccac, Romeo F, et al: Natural history of hypertrophic cardiomyopathy in the elderly, *Cardiology* 78:329-33, 1991.

71. Shenov MM, Khanna A, Ansari M: Hypertrophic cardiomyopathy. Why is it often overlooked in elderly patients? *Postgrad Med J* 90:187-90, 1991.

72. Whiting RB, Powell WJ, Dinsmore RE, et al: Idiopathic hypertrophic subaortic stenosis in the elderly, *N Engl J Med* 285:196-200, 1971.

73. Lewis JF, Maron BJ: Elderly patients with hypertrophic cardiomyopathy: a subset with distinctive left ventricular morphology and progressive clinical course later in life, *J Am Clin Cardiol* 13:36-45, 1989.

74. Krasnow N, Stein RA: Hypertrophic cardiomyopathy in the aged, *Am Heart J* 96:326-36, 1978.

75. Pomerance A, Davies MD: Pathologic features of hypertrophic obstructive cardiomyopathy (HOCM) in the elderly, *Br Heart J* 37:305-12, 1975.

76. Topol EJ, Traill TA, Fortuin N: Hypertensive hypertrophic cardiomyopathy in the elderly, *N Engl J Med* 312:277-83, 1985.

77. Petrin TE, Tavel ME: Idiopathic hypertrophic subaortic stenosis as observed in a large community hospital in relation to age and history of hypertension, *J Am Geriat Soc* 27:43-46, 1979.

78. Pomerance A, Davies MD: Pathologic features of hypertrophic obstructive cardiomyopathy (HOCM) in the elderly, *Br Heart J* 37:305-12, 1975.

79. Lewis JF, Maron BJ: Diversity of patterns of hypertrophy in patients

with systemic hypertension and marked left ventricular wall thickening, *Am J Cardiol* 65:874-81, 1990.

80. Burke AP, Farb A, Virmani R et al: Sports related and non sports related sudden cardiac death in young adults, *Am Heart J* 121:568-75, 1991.

81. Bonow RO: Left ventricular diastolic function in hypertrophic cardiomyopathy, *Herz* 16:13-21, 1991.

82. Watkins LO, Williams RA: Cardiomyopathy in blacks, *Cardiovasc Clin* 21:279-96, 1991.

83. Lewis JF, Maron BJ et al: Preparticipation echocardiographic screening for cardiovascular disease in a large predominantly black population of collegiate athletes, *Am J Cardiol* 64:1029-33, 1989.

84. Bugu G, Meneghello MP, Bellotto F: Isolated episode of exercise related ventricular fibrillation in a healthy athlete, *Int J Cardiol* 24:121-3, 1989.

85. Fananapazir L, Tracy CM, Leon MB et al: Electrophysiological abnormalities in patients with hypertrophic cardiomyopathy. A consecutive study in 155 patients, *Circulation* 80:1259-68, 1989.

86. Blanchard DG, Ross J Jr: Hypertrophic cardiomyopathy. Prognosis with medical or surgical therapy, *Clin Cardiol* 14:11-19, 1991.

87. Seiler C, Hess OM, Schoenbeck M et al: Long term follow-up of medical versus surgical therapy for hypertrophic cardiomyopathy: a retrospective study, *J Am Coll Cardiol* 17:634-42, 1991.

88. McIntosh CC, Greenberg GJ, Maron BJ et al: Clinical and haemodynamic results after mitral valve replacement in patients with obstructive hypertrophic cardiomyopathy, *Ann Thorac Surg* 47:236-246, 1989.

89. Frenneaux MP, Porter A, Caforio ALP et al: Determinants of exercise capacity in hypertrophic cardiomyopathy, *J Am Coll Cardiol* 13:1521-1526, 1989.

90. Hess OM, Grimm J, Krayenbuhk HP: Diastolic function in hypertrophic cardiomyopathy: effects of propranolol and verapamil in diastolic stiffness, *Eur Heart J* 4 (suppl F):47056, 1983.

PART IV ENDOMYOCARDIAL BIOPSY

Before the introduction of the Konno bioptome in 1962, cardiac biopsy was hazardous. The procedure was carried out by either the transthoracic route or via thoracotomy. Refinement of the bioptome and its introduction via the percutaneous route by way of a long sheath made endomyocardial biopsy simply a part of the diagnostic catheterization of the patient with suspected myocardial disease. The procedure was found to be remarkably safe, but critics questioned the usefulness of the information derived from the very small pieces obtained.[1,2,3,4] Some carried out the biopsies from the arterial route, but the risks of left ventricular perforation and of systemic embolism made this approach less popular. Except for specific problems in which the pathology appeared to be confined to the left ventricle, biopsy of the right ventricular side of the septum by the venous route has been preferred. Studies have shown that the information obtained from the right or the left ventricle is usually similar in patients with cardiomyopathy. The biopsy material must be dropped immediately into Formalin for light microscopic examination, or into glutoraldehyde for electron microscopic examination. The biopsied material should be fast frozen in liquid nitrogen if histochemical studies are to be undertaken.

The main thrust of cardiac biopsy has been in the diagnosis of myocarditis and dilated cardiomyopathy because the former is extremely difficult to diagnose clinically and the latter is common. Recent investigations of possible viral and immunologic mechanisms for dilated cardiomyopathy have been much aided by the attaining of myocardial biopsy specimens.[5] The technique is not confined to adults and can be carried out safely in children.[6]

Disorders of the myocardium that have specific pathology and are generalized can be identified readily by endomyocardial biopsy. A good example is amyloidosis. Critics of cardiac biopsy suggest that amyloidosis can be diagnosed more safely by biopsy of other involved tissue or by echocardiography. However, rectal or gum biopsy may be negative in some patients with cardiac amyloidosis, and echocardiography does not provide a tissue diagnosis. Recent research has shown the many varieties of amyloidosis that exist. The genetic defects have been identified in a number of familial cases, thus paving the way for future gene therapy.

In focal disorders of the myocardium such as sarcoidosis, the sarcoid tissue may well be missed at biopsy event though ultrasound guidance of the bioptome can ensure that samples are obtained from the areas that seem to be abnormal. The same applies to tumors of the heart that can be biopsied. An appropriate therapeutic strategy can then be planned (e.g., excision, chemotherapy, irradiation, or cardiac transplantation).

Because the disarray present in cases of hypertrophic cardiomyopathy is not usually generalized, the pathologic diagnosis of the condition depends on examining the whole specimen. Thus there is no place for cardiac biopsy in the diagnosis of HC, except in the differential diagnosis between hypertrophic cardiomyopathy and amyloid heart disease. Recent advances in the unraveling of the genetic mutations responsible for hypertrophic cardiomyopathy may well give new impetus to obtaining biopsy specimens of myocardium.

MYOCARDITIS

Myocarditis is uncommon in hospital cardiologic practice. It tends to complicate otherwise mundane virus illnesses that are treated at home or when they are more serious, in hospital by specialists in infectious diseases or general physicians. Moreover, patients usually either die or get well quite quickly. The clinical features of myocarditis tend to be plebeian. Disproportionate tachycardia, hypotension, conduction defects on the electrocardiogram, or the development of an infarct pattern on the electrocardiogram provide obvious clues, although they are rarely present. The cardiac illness is often delayed too long after the initial infection for pharyngeal washings or stools to contain virus, and serologic evidence comes only from convalescent titers. Histologic criteria for myocarditis used to be widely variable until 1984 when a panel of cardiovascular pathologists met in Dallas to establish criteria for the pathologic diagnosis of myocarditis from biopsy specimens and thus ensure a uniform interpretation.[7] The Dallas criteria demand that a first biopsy must show myocytolysis and lymphocytic infiltration to meet criteria for acute myocarditis. Unless such changes are seen, diagnoses of healed or healing myocarditis are untenable because they are based on lesser changes that on their own are not specific.

Timing of the biopsy in myocarditis is an additional problem. Many physicians are loathe to submit an acutely ill patient for biopsy, preferring to wait for several days, by which time the acute changes may well have resolved. Furthermore, myocarditis is known to be focal often; therefore acute changes might be present in one part of the heart while apparently resolving changes are seen in another. Multiple biopsies are deemed essential because of this trait, and at least three are usually taken. About five or more biopsies need to be taken to reduce the variability.[8,9] Numerous additional studies have been made on biopsy material. Investigators have examined ultrastructural morphometry of the microvasculature in dilated cardiomyopathy, myofibrillar content, collagen amount and type, and immunologic features.[10] Distinction between dilated cardiomyopathy and alcoholic heart disease has proved impossible on morphologic studies, but some differences in myocardial enzyme activity have been suggested.[11]

The main thrust of research has involved trying to find out whether virus infection plays a part in the development of dilated cardiomyopathy.[12-15] Initial interrogation by hybridization probes were positive for virus RNA sequences in a considerable number of patients, not only those with myocarditis, but also patients with nonspecific dilated cardiomyopathy. The development of more sophisticated and more specific probes with utilization of polymerase chain reaction has revealed a much smaller proportion of patients with dilated cardiomyopathy showing virus RNA sequences. Because the morphologic changes in dilated cardiomyopathy are mainly nonspecific and more useful in excluding specific pathologies (including active myocarditis) than in positive recognition, these supplementary studies seem particularly important.[16,17,18]

In patients with restrictive hemodynamics, absence of an increase in left ventricular wall thickness and other features usually distinguish patients with amyloid heart disease from patients with a primary restrictive cardiomyopathy, who are usually younger and whose prognosis is much better. Cardiac biopsy should be carried out in cases of restrictive cardiomyopathy and sometimes in patients with unexplained arrhythmias.[19] Some patients will show a diffuse fine interstitial fibrosis. Others will show myocyte hypertrophy with interstitial fibrosis. Some of this group will have the family history of cardiomyopathy, progressive conduction system change, and skeletal myopathy. Others may show myocyte hypertrophy with disarray without wall thickening. It is uncertain so far whether such patients will show mutations (in the myosin heavy chain gene or at other sites) similar to those seen in patients with familial classic hypertrophic cardiomyopathy.

Endomyocardial biopsies will undoubtedly continue to play a role in research because of the many unanswered questions concerning the pathogenesis and treatment of myocarditis and dilated cardiomyopathy.

REFERENCES

1. Mackay EH, Littler WA, Sleight P: Critical assessment of diagnostic value of endomyocardial biopsy, *Br Heart J* 40:69-78, 1978.
2. Lie JT: Myocarditis and endomyocardial biopsy in unexplained heart failure: a diagnosis in search of a disease, *Ann Intern Med* 109:525-8, 1988.
3. Becker AR, Heijmans CD, Essed CE: Chronic non-ischaemic congestive heart disease and endomyocardial biopsies. Worth the extra? *Eur Heart J* 12(2):218-23, 1991.
4. Loire R: Is myocardial biopsy necessary in the diagnosis of myocardial diseases? *Arch Mal Coeur Vaiss* 82(11):1887, 1989.
5. Olsen EGJ: The value of endomyocardial biopsies in myocarditis and dilated cardiomyopathy, *Eur Heart J* 12(Suppl D):10-12, 1991.
6. Celiker A, Ozkutlu S, Ozer S et al: Endomyocardial biopsy in children. Usefulness in various myocardial disorders, *Jpn Heart J* 32(2):227-37, 1991.
7. Aretz HT, Billingham ME, Edwards ED et al: Myocarditis: a histopathologic definition and classification, *Am J Cardiovasc Pathol* 1:3-13, 1987.
8. Baadrup U, Olsen EGJ: Critical analysis of endomyocardial biopsies from patients suspected of having cardiomyopathy. I:Morphological and morphometric aspects, *Br Heart J* 45:475086, 1981.
9. Baandrup U, Florio RA, Rehahn M et al: Critical analysis of endomyocardial biopsies from patients suspected of having cardiomyopathy. II: Comparison of histology and clinical/hemodynamic information, *Br Heart J* 45:487-93, 1981.
10. Mosseri M, Schaper J, Admon D et al: Coronary capillaries in patients with congestive cardiomyopathy or angina pectoris with patent main coronary arteries. Ultrastructural morphometry of endomyocardial biopsy samples, *Circulation* 84(1):203-10, 1991.
11. Richardson PJ, Wodak AD, Atkinson L et al: Relation between alcohol intake, myocardial enzyme activity and myocardial function in dilated cardiomyopathy. Evidence for the concept of alcohol induced heart muscle disease, *Br Heart J* 56: 165-70, 1986.
12. Billingham M: Acute myocarditis: a diagnostic dilemma, *Br Heart J* 56:6-8, 1987.
13. Bowles NE, Olsen EGJ, Richardson PJ et al: Detection of coxsackie-B-virus specific RNA sequences in myocardial biopsy samples from patients with myocarditis and dilated cardiomyopathy, *Lancet* i:1120-3, 1986.
14. Kandolf R, Kirschner P, Ameis D et al: *Enteroviral heart disease: diagnosis by in situ hybridization.* In Schultheiss HP, ed: *New concepts in viral heart disease,* Heidelberg, 1988, Springer-Verlag.
15. Archard LC, Bowles NE, Olsen EGJ et al: Detection of persistent coxsackie B virus RNA in dilated cardiomyopathy and myocarditis, *Eur Heart J* 8:437-40, 1987.
16. Archard LC, Bowles NE, Cunningham L et al: Molecular probes for detection of persisting enterovirus infection of human heart and their prognostic value, *Eur Heart J* 12(Suppl D):56-9, 1991.
17. Camerini F, Salvi A, Sinagra G: Endomyocardial biopsy in dilated cardiomyopathy and myocarditis: which role? *Int J Cardiol* 31(1):1-8, 1991.
18. Figulla HR, Bardosi A, Dechant K et al: Enzyme histochemistry of endomyocardial biopsies in idiopathic dilated cardiomyopathy, *Cardiology* 78(3):282-90, 1991.
19. Frustaci A, Caldarulo M, Buffon A et al: Cardiac biopsy in patients with "primary" atrial fibrillation. Histologic evidence of occult myocardial diseases, *Chest* 100(2):303-6, 1991.

Chapter 8

PERICARDIAL DISEASE

I. Sylvia Crawley
Michael B. Gravanis

ANATOMY AND FUNCTION OF THE NORMAL PERICARDIUM

The pericardium is composed of a visceral and a parietal layer. The visceral layer of the pericardium is made up of mesothelial cells and fibrous tissue. This layer is continuous with the inner mesothelial layer of the parietal pericardium, forming a closed sac that envelops the heart.[1-3] The parietal pericardium also has a middle fibrosal layer made up of "variously oriented" collagen bundles, small elastic fibers, and an outer layer of connective tissue and collagen bundles.[4] This outer layer also contributes to the ligamentous attachments of the pericardium to the sternum and diaphragm. The mesothelial layers of the visceral and parietal pericardium form the pericardial space. These mesothelial cells contain cilia and microvilli that function to increase surface area for fluid transport and absorb friction of the two surfaces.[4] The pericardial space contains a small amount of fluid, 15 ml to 50 ml, which by content is an ultrafiltrate of the blood plasma.[5] The exact mechanism of its production is unclear.[5] Similarly, the lymphatic drainage of the pericardium is not clearly understood.

The mechanical properties of the human pericardium have been studied in vitro and in situ by various methods. Stretch-tension curves demonstrate that pericardial tissue is very compliant at low tension but will abruptly become inextensible with further stretch.[6] This phenomenon is thought to occur when the stretch capacity of the elastic fibers is exceeded and the collagen fibers become more parallel.[7]

The in situ behavior of the human pericardium has been studied by observing intracardiac and intrapericardial pressure changes during maneuvers that volume load the cardiac chambers. Inferences regarding effects of the pericardium can be made from studies before and after pericardiectomy or pericardiotomy. Ventricular interdependence is to a great extent modulated by the stretch characteristics of the intact pericardium.[6] Ventricular interdependence results from the sharing of the right and left ventricles of a common interventricular septum and intrapericardial space.[8] Thus any changes in diastolic volume of either ventricle will influence the other; this interdependence is modulated by the intact pericardium when intrapericardial pressure increases to the point of inextensible or noncompliant stretch.

Pericardial constraint is more effective on the right ventricle than it is on the left ventricle. Studies demonstrate that right ventricular filling pressure is equal to intrapericardial pressure, and that the compliance of the pericardium may be inferred from changes in the intrapericardial pressure as long as right ventricular pressure remains at physiologic levels (see later discussion).

There are a number of limitations to understanding the exact role the pericardium plays in this constraint of ventricular filling. Multiple variables may be in effect. The pericardium may not be equally compliant in all individuals. Aging may reduce compliance.[9] Pathologic processes that alter the structure of the pericardium and thus its distensibility may also reduce its compliance, resulting in a greater degree of constraint for any given ventricular filling pressure. A decrease in the diastolic compliance of either ventricle due to an independent variable may also vary the ability of the pericardium to modulate ventricular diastolic function.

There are inherent methodologic limitations in in vitro studies, and these studies do not duplicate the in situ processes. The measurement of in situ pericardial pressures varies with different techniques.[10] Both an open-ended catheter and a flat balloon placed in the pericardial space record pressures equal to right atrial pressure at high intrapericardial pressures, but at low pressures the open-ended catheter pressure falls below right atrial pressure while the intrapericardial pressure recorded with the flat balloon remains equal to right atrial pressure.[10]

The reasons for this discrepancy are not entirely clear. Several mechanisms have been postulated. In the normal pericardial space there is minimal fluid, and the parietal and visceral pericardium are in contact during variable periods of the cardiac cycle. In addition, the distribution of fluid in the pericardial space may be nonuniform.[10,11] Any measuring technique used in the in situ studies alters to varying degrees the integrity of the pericardium, and may influence the accuracy of the observations in reflecting the normal physiology.[12]

CLINICAL PRESENTATIONS

Pericardial disease is frequently associated with other disease processes in the body that may affect any organ system. A review of the *Index Medicus* listings regarding pericardial disease will emphasize these associations. The pathophysiologic mechanisms of the development of pericardial disease also allow for the simulation of other disease processes. Recognition of pericardial disease may be provided by symptoms, physical examination, electrocardiographic changes, echocardiographic findings, or hemodynamic alterations. An understanding of the pathogenesis and pathophysiologic mechanisms aids in the understanding and clinical recognition of pericardial disease. In some disease processes pericardial involvement may not become clinically apparent, and thus will be recognized only during postmortem examination. The more common clinical presentations and etiologies are discussed in this chapter.

Acute idiopathic or viral pericarditis

Acute pericarditis frequently presents with chest discomfort that is typically precordial and sharp and is aggra-

vated by breathing or the supine position. The pain may be aggravated by eating or relieved by sitting up and leaning forward.[13] The pain radiates to the interscapular area, neck or arms. Occasionally the pain may be entirely outside the thoracic area. Severe pain may be limited to the neck, arms, or epigastrium. In many cases the characteristics of the pain are the only diagnostic findings. A three-component pericardial friction rub on physical examination or characteristic electrocardiographic changes may be helpful for diagnosis.

The pericardial rub results from cyclic contact of the inflamed and irregular surfaces of the visceral and parietal pericardium and the adjacent pleura. There may be three components representing ventricular systole, ventricular diastole and atrial systole. The presence of all three components is most diagnostic. The presence of a pericardial effusion does not preclude a pericardial rub.[14]

Electrocardiographic changes may not be present. Diffuse ST segment elevation and resolution followed by diffuse T wave inversion, which may persist for years, characterize the evolutionary changes. These ST-T changes imply subepicardial myocardial involvement. PR segment depression may be present and reflects similar subepicardial involvement of the atria.[15] Other clinical findings may reflect the etiologic source or define hemodynamic alterations, including cardiac tamponade, constrictive pericarditis, or effusive constrictive physiology, which will be discussed later in this chapter.

An animal model of acute pericarditis and its progression has been demonstrated by Leak, et al.[16] An initial inflammatory response with increased microvascular permeability and exudation of neutrophils and macrophages is followed by an intense mesothelial response. There is contraction of the mesothelial cells, reduction in their surface microvilli and eventual desquamation. A fibrinous phase follows with newly formed connective tissue, which eventually contains lymphocytes, fibroblast and dense collagen bundles. This phase results in thickening of the layers of the pericardium and adhesions between the visceral and parietal layers, which may eventually obliterate the pericardial space.

The myocardium may be involved to a significant degree and is manifested clinically by elevation of creatine kinase MB fraction.[17] In more severe cases significant left ventricular dysfunction may develop. This myocardial involvement may manifest in the acute phases of pericarditis as acute viral myopericarditis. Any etiology of pericardial disease may eventually involve a significant amount of myocardium.

Most commonly, acute pericarditis develops without any identifiable cause. In some cases an antecedent viral syndrome is manifested by respiratory tract symptoms or influenza. The pericarditis becomes manifest 2 to 4 weeks later. The initial viral syndrome may be mild or severe. In most cases postviral pericarditis is benign but may be recurrent. An altered immune response is suggested as the mechanism of development of acute viral pericarditis, and may be genetically determined. With specific viral probes the presence of viral RNA has been found in the pericardium many years after the original infection, and may explain the often chronic nature of the condition and its liability to recurrence when reactivated by some triggering mechanism.[18] C1-binding immune complexes are frequently found in patients with postviral pericarditis; IgM is found most often, either alone or with IgG, and occasionally IgA.[19] The presence or absence of immune complexes does not correlate with the clinical fluctuations in the disease,[20] although among patients with acute pericarditis, the level of IgM antibody may be significantly higher in those who subsequently relapse.[21] Viral cultures and acute and convalescent viral titers may substantiate the diagnosis but are not necessary for the proper care of the patient.[22] Many patients will have recurrences over many years.[23] Although uncommon, tamponade may occur during the acute episode or during recurrences. Constrictive pericarditis is also an uncommon sequela.

Dressler syndrome

An acute inflammatory process in the pericardium during the course of acute myocardial infarction is not uncommon. It is reported in up to one third of cases examined in postmortem studies.[24] In the early postmyocardial infarction period pericardial involvement may be limited to the pericardium adjacent to the involved myocardium. It occurs in the majority of cases of transmural myocardial infarction but infrequently (10%) with subendocardial infarction. This form of involvement is responsible for what is clinically referred to as postinfarction pericarditis and becomes manifest within the first few days after myocardial infarction. Pericarditic chest pain, a pericardial friction rub, and a small pericardial effusion may be present. The early pericarditis usually does not alter the clinical course. The Multicenter Investigation of the Limitation of Infarct Size reported that 25% of 492 patients with transmural infarction had a pericardial rub, while only 18 of 211 patients with non-Q wave infarctions had a pericardial rub.[25] A recent echocardiographic study by Sugiura, et al,[26] demonstrated pericardial effusion in 25% of 330 patients on the third day after acute myocardial infarction. A pericardial rub was detected in 45% of the patients with pericardial effusion. Pericardial effusion or pericardial rub is more frequent in patients with more advanced left ventricular dysfunction,[25,26] which suggests that the altered hemodynamics, as well as the extent of myocardial damage, contribute to the pathogenesis. Thrombolytic therapy or heparin anticoagulation does not appear to influence the incidence of pericardial effusion early after myocardial infarction.[26,27]

A potentially more disabling form of postinfarction pericarditis, Dressler syndrome,[24] usually develops in 2 to 3 weeks after myocardial infarction and is associated with systemic signs and symptoms including fever, pericardial and pleural chest pain, pericardial and pleural effusions and pulmonary infiltrates. In these cases there is diffuse involvement of the pericardium, and the process may be hemorrhagic. The pericardial effusion is frequently much larger than in the early postinfarction period and rarely may cause cardiac tamponade. Recurrences may develop during years following the acute infarction. Constrictive pericarditis is a rare complication.

Tuberculous pericarditis

Until recently the incidence of tuberculous pericarditis in the United States had declined.[28] However, since tuberculous pericarditis is more frequent in patients with immunodeficiency states, the increased prevalence of AIDS may result in a increased incidence.[29] Tuberculous pericarditis may present as acute pericarditis, asymptomatic pericardial effusion, cardiac tamponade, or constriction. Symptoms of weight loss, cough, dyspnea, and chest pain may be present.[28]

Although tuberculous pericarditis is always associated with infection elsewhere in the body, the extracardiac involvement is not always apparent. Attention to these potential sources of tuberculous infection may aid in the diagnosis of involvement of the pericardium. Pulmonary involvement is apparent by chest radiogram in only one half of cases.[30] Pericardial involvement is the result of lymphatic extension from adjacent structures or hematogenous spread from adjacent or remote sites.[28]

The pericardial fluid may be clear to grossly bloody with exudative contents and predominant lymphocytes.[31] The tubercle bacilli are identified on stained smears in less than one half of cases and by culture in one half to three fourths of cases. In cases with negative smears and cultures a diligent search for a remote source becomes essential for diagnosis. Measurement of adenosine deaminase activity in pleural or pericardial fluid may improve diagnostic accuracy.[32,33] False positive and false negative results have been reported.[32]

Fibrin deposition occurs in the early stages. The pericardial fluid is serous or serosanguineous and contains polymorphonuclear cells. Later lymphocytes predominate. The pericardium is grossly thickened, with necrotic and fibrotic material covering the serosal surfaces of the visceral and parietal pericardium (Fig. 8-1). Pericardial effusion may be present with or without hemodynamic compromise. In later stages the pericardial space may be obliterated by the fibrotic process. Histologically, there is an extensive lymphocytic infiltration. The mesothelial cells of the serosal surface are replaced by a granulomatous reaction that involves all layers of the parietal pericardium (Fig. 8-2). Giant cells, caseation necrosis, epithelioid histocytes, and Langhans' giant cells may be present. Chronic constrictive pericarditis may develop, even in patients who survive without treatment. In such cases, depending on the chronicity, the visceral and parietal pericardium demonstrate dense fibrous adhesions without any in-

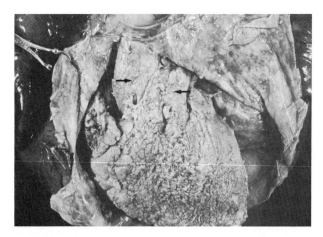

Fig. 8-1. Diffuse, exudative pericarditis involving both visceral and parietal pericardial surfaces. This tuberculous etiology pericarditis appears to extend over the great vessels *(arrows).*

flammatory reaction. Calcification may be scanty or severe.[34,35]

Bacterial pericarditis

The clinical presentation of bacterial pericarditis is variable. With a high index of suspicion it may be detected by appropriate diagnostic studies in the absence of the usual clinical manifestations of an acute pericarditis. Dyspnea, fever, and chest pain are the most common symptoms but they may be absent in some patients. Physical findings that suggest hemodynamic compromise are absent in nearly one-half of cases.[36] Cardiac tamponade may be the initial presentation, even with a small effusion. Bacterial pericarditis is more likely to occur in the immunocompromised patient. The bacterial organisms most commonly identified are *Staphylococcus aureus, Streptococcus pneumoniae* and gram-negative organisms such as Proteus, *Escherichia coli, Pseudomonas* and *Klebsiella*[36]. These organisms involve the pericardium by hematogenous or lymphatic dissemination from other foci of infection, such as pneumonia, osteomyelitis, septic arthritis or subdiaphragmatic abscess. In more recent years bacterial pericarditis is more commonly associated with underlying disease processes that may predispose the patient to infection.[37]

The gross and histologic findings in bacterial pericarditis reflect the duration of the process. An initial inflammatory process with polymorphonuclear leukocytes may rapidly progress with exudative to frankly purulent pericardial effusion. The volume of the pericardial effusion may be small or moderate and is frequently loculated due to the presence of fibrinous adhesions.[37] Grossly the pericardium is thickened and has a shaggy irregular surface due to fibrinopurulent exudate (Fig. 8-3). This fibrinous reaction may result in obliteration of the pericardial space. In the acute phase histologic findings include interstitial edema, hyperemia, and polymorphonuclear leukocytes (Fig. 8-4).

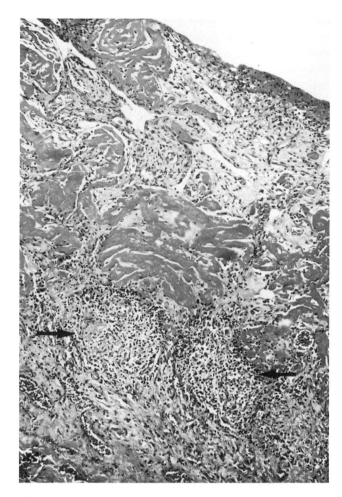

Fig. 8-2. Visceral pericardium showing non-caseating granulomas *(arrow),* edema, fibrosis, and fibrin deposition on the surface.

Destruction and desquamation of mesothelial cells and extensive fibrin deposition is present. In later stages the leukocytic infiltration resolves and there is evidence of organization with fibroblasts and collagen fibers. The offending organisms may be demonstrated by appropriate histologic examination or culture unless they have been eradicated by prior antibiotic therapy.[38]

Fungal pericarditis

Fungi, including *Histoplasma capsulatum, Blastomyces,* cryptococcosis, coccidioides, *Aspergillus, Candida albicans,* and *Nocardia asteroides* may cause infectious pericarditis. The most frequent causative organisms are *Candida, Aspergillus,* and *Nocardia.*[36] *Histoplasma capsulatum* is more likely in patients who have lived in areas endemic for histoplasmosis (Ohio Valley, Mississippi Valley, and western Appalachia). These cases may be chronic and subacute, and some may resolve without therapy. Calcific constrictive pericarditis may be a late presentation.[39] Patients with immunodeficiency or who are receiving im-

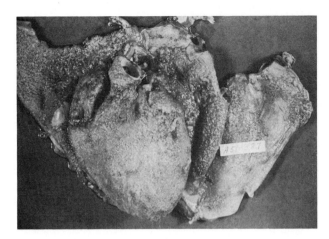

Fig. 8-3. Diffuse, purulent bacterial pericarditis involving both visceral and parietal layers.

munosuppressive or long-term antibiotic therapy are more susceptible, which suggests that the pericardium is relatively resistant to fungal infections.[40,41] Myocardial involvement may be present.[36] The infection may be indolent, and as with other forms of purulent pericarditis, the usual clinical manifestations of acute pericarditis may be absent. Thus a high index of suspicion is essential for recognition.

One of the predisposing factors for fungal pericarditis is postoperative inflammation of the pericardium, which often creates a posteriorly loculated pericardial effusion that may serve as a fertile medium. Other risk factors in the postoperative cardiac patient include immunosuppressive or cytotoxic drug therapy, and underlying debilitating conditions such as lymphoma or leukemia.[42] Medications such as glucocorticoids impair antifungal host defenses and effect the antifungal activity of phagocytes.[43]

Pericardial involvement occurs by direct spread from adjacent structures, including the esophagus, mediastinum, or lung. Hematogenous or lymphatic dissemination may also occur.[5]

The characteristics of the pericardial effusion are similar to other forms of purulent pericarditis. The pericardium is thickened (Fig. 8-5). The volume of pericardial fluid may be small. Analysis of pericardial fluid or tissue may aid in diagnosis. In histoplasmosis the pericardium may contain granulomas with or without caseation. Microabscesses and sulfur granules may be seen in actinomycosis.[5,30,31]

PERICARDIAL EFFUSION

The pericardial space normally contains up to 50 ml of clear fluid. The content is similar to plasma and contains lower concentrations of all elements. Pericardial effusion may be defined as the presence of greater than 50 ml of fluid in the pericardial space. Abnormal accumulation of pericardial fluid develops when there is an imbalance of

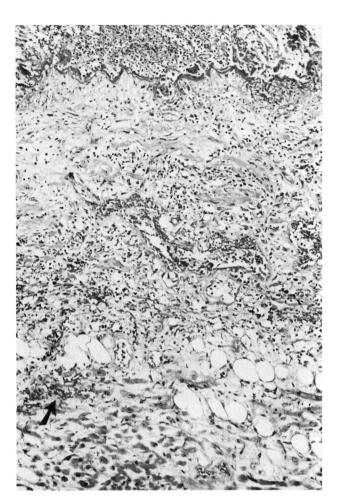

Fig. 8-4. Visceral pericardium showing severe edema, inflammatory infiltrates (predominantly polys), and fibrin deposition. Note extension of the inflammatory cells into the adjacent myocardium *(arrow)*.

fluid production and fluid drainage. With few exceptions pericardial effusion is associated with some form of pericardial disease.

The rate at which pericardial effusion develops, the compliance of the pericardium, and the compliance of the ventricles will determine the extent of any alterations in hemodynamics. Specific forms of pericardial disease cause thickening and fibrosis of the pericardium. In such cases the rapid accumulation of even small amounts of fluid may cause serious impairment of ventricular filling.

Clinical detection of pericardial effusion is usually based on evidence of a disease process known to cause pericardial disease and is easily documented by echocardiography. A very large pericardial effusion may cause a decrease in intensity of the heart sounds. Symptoms or physical findings associated with hemodynamic effects or etiology may be present. A pericardial rub may be present even with large effusions.[5] The electrocardiogram may show low voltage or decreased voltage compared with prior tracings. A slow heart rate may suggest hypothyroidism as an

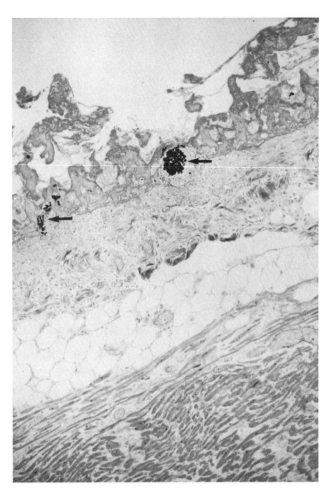

Fig. 8-5. Visceral pericardium showing moderate degree of edema, sparse round cell infiltrates, marked fibrin deposits on the epicardial surface and clusters of *Candida albicans (arrows).*

etiology. The chest x-ray film may be normal or demonstrate a large cardiac silhouette. The echocardiogram is an essential diagnostic tool.

Any process that involves the pericardium will cause some degree of pericardial effusion. Neoplastic, idiopathic, uremic, and postmyocardial infarction are the most common etiologic processes.[44] In certain situations the presence of pericardial effusion does not necessarily imply pericardial disease. Pericardial effusion may be present in congestive heart failure, volume overload, hypoalbuminemia[5,31] and pulmonary hypertension,[45] in which cases it does not cause any hemodynamic compromise. Pericardial effusion has also been demonstrated during the third trimester of pregnancy, possibly related to sodium and water retention.[46] Pericardial effusion has also been demonstrated in one-third of patients with bacteremia in the absence of any evidence for purulent pericarditis.[47] A small effusion is considered normal in utero but the detection of larger amounts may aid in the diagnosis of certain fetal problems.[48]

PERICARDIAL TAMPONADE

Pericardial tamponade may be defined as the development of hemodynamic alterations resulting from the accumulation of pericardial fluid at a rate which exceeds the distensibility of the pericardium. Intrapericardial pressure increases and ventricular filling is impaired throughout the diastolic filling period.[49-51]

With increasing pericardial pressures the right and left ventricular filling pressures equilibrate with the elevated intrapericardial pressure, cardiac output is reduced and pulsus paradoxus develops.[52] These hemodynamic alterations may develop over a spectrum of increasing severity.[53] In most situations, except for cardiac rupture or trauma, the clinical findings reflect this progression of severity. Reddy, et al,[53] have defined three phases of this progression by hemodynamic alterations and clinical findings.

The symptoms and physical findings are related to the severity of the hemodynamic compromise and are influenced by the presence of concomitant cardiac disease processes. Mild impairment may cause no symptoms at rest. With a progressive increase in ventricular filling pressures and reduction in cardiac output, weakness, diaphoresis, dyspnea, and near syncope may occur. In the most severe cases there may be a loss of consciousness.

On physical examination in mild cases there may be slight elevation of the jugular venous pressure. An exaggerated, but not abnormal, inspiratory decrease in systolic blood pressure may be present. In severe forms there is marked elevation of the jugular venous pressure with attenuation of the Y descent and pulsus paradoxus so pronounced that it obliterates the arterial pulse during inspiration.[53] Pulsus paradoxus may be absent despite severe tamponade when there is coexisting left ventricular failure, atrial septal defect, or aortic regurgitation.[1,52,54] In cases of acute cardiac tamponade associated with blood loss the jugular veins may not be distended, and the degree of pulsus paradoxus may be difficult to assess in the presence of hypotension.

The electrocardiogram may show low voltage and electrical alternans as a result of the "swinging" of the heart as demonstrated on echocardiography. The echocardiographic examination is useful to document pericardial effusion and to assess the hemodynamic changes. In addition to pericardial effusion, the findings associated with cardiac tamponade include: the heart "swinging in" a large effusion, right ventricular and right atrial collapse, and premature opening of the pulmonic valve.[55-58] The sensitivity of right atrial collapse is reported to be 70% to 100% sensitivity of right ventricular collapse is reported to range from 60% to 90%. The specificity of either right atrial or right ventricular collapse is 80% to 100%.[59] Collapse of either chamber is a reflection of several factors. The severity of tamponade as measured by hemodynamic alterations influences the development of these changes; right atrial collapse seems to occur earlier in the progression of hemodynamic deterioration.[59] Left ventricular collapse occurs infrequently, even with severe tamponade. Right ventricular collapse occurs with a much greater frequency than left ventricular collapse because the right ventricle is normally a lower pressure chamber. However, in the presence of right ventricular hypertrophy, right ventricular collapse may occur later in the progression of the severity of tamponade. Right ventricular systolic hypertension, ventricular rhythms including ventricular paced rhythm,[59] and acute right ventricular dysfunction[60] may also delay the development of right ventricular collapse. Left atrial collapse may be observed, especially with very large pericardial effusions.[59,61] Left ventricular diastolic collapse is more likely to occur in pericardial effusion that is loculated over the left ventricle.[61,62] Two-dimensional echocardiography is sometimes more sensitive in identifying milder forms of cardiac tamponade prior to the development of significant hypotension, pulsus paradoxus, and reduced cardiac output.[63]

Doppler echocardiography has also demonstrated some of the hemodynamic alterations, including diminished diastolic flow in the superior vena cava,[64] and across the tricuspid valve.[65] Doppler studies of tricuspid and mitral flow velocities have demonstrated a marked respiratory variation in diastolic flow velocities with a significant inspiratory decrease in early diastolic flow velocities.[66] Neither the sensitivity and specificity of these observations nor their correlation with severity of hemodynamic compromise have been established.[67]

The hemodynamics of cardiac tamponade have been elucidated by Reddy, et al, as developing over a spectrum of hemodynamic deterioration.[53] When intrapericardial pressure rises to equilibrate with both right and left ventricular diastolic pressures, ventricular filling becomes severely impaired, cardiac output is markedly reduced, and pulsus paradoxus appears. Pericardial effusion may develop gradually and allow the pericardium to stretch, in which case the rise in intrapericardial pressure is minimal and does not equilibrate with either the right or left ventricular diastolic pressures. When pericardial fluid accumulates at a more rapid rate to exceed the limit of pericardial extensibility, intrapericardial pressure rises more steeply to first equilibrate with right ventricular and then left ventricular diastolic pressure. As intrapericardial pressure equilibrates with right atrial and right ventricular diastolic pressures, right heart collapse may be appreciated on echocardiography. Impairment of early ventricular filling is reflected in attenuation of the Y descent of the right atrial pressure curve and Doppler flow studies of the atrioventricular valves and vena cavae.

A number of factors contribute to the pathophysiology of cardiac tamponade: the rate of accumulation of pericardial fluid, the distensibility of the pericardium, ventricular diastolic compliance, and intraventricular volume.[1,52,53,67] Ventricular interdependence also influences the hemody-

namic findings, especially at higher intrapericardial pressures.

Minimal reductions in ventricular filling and cardiac output may occur without significant elevations of filling pressures. Slight exaggeration of the normal inspiratory decline in systolic blood pressure may be present.[53] As intrapericardial pressure increases to equilibrate with right ventricular filling pressure there is a further increase in systemic venous pressure and reduction in cardiac output. The inspiratory decline in systolic blood pressure is greater and may exceed the normal 10 mm Hg to 12 mm Hg. As intrapericardial pressure equilibrates with left ventricular filling pressure, and as compensatory mechanisms increase intravascular volume, the effects of ventricular interdependence contribute to produce more marked inspiratory decrease in systolic blood pressure. Pulsus paradoxus is also present.[51,53]

The mechanism of pulsus paradoxus is incompletely understood. It is defined as an inspiratory decrease in systolic blood pressure of greater than 10 mm Hg. Some authors have used 12 mm Hg to 20 mm Hg as a diagnostic criterion. In some cases a percentage decrease (as compared with expiratory systolic pressure) may be useful; the normal percentage decrease is considered to be less than 9%. Moderate to severe tamponade may cause a 15% or greater decline in systolic pressure on inspiration.[49] Ventricular interaction is thought to be a major determinate of pulsus paradoxus.[51] When pericardial tamponade results in equilibration of pericardial pressure with both right and left ventricular filling pressures, then ventricular filling becomes interdependent within the confines of a noncompliant pericardium, and the interventricular septum becomes an important modulating structure. The exaggerated respiratory variations in ventricular filling, stroke volume and systolic blood pressure are hallmarks of cardiac tamponade and are in part due to this modulation of ventricular filling. An inspiratory increase in right ventricular filling producing reciprocal changes in left ventricular filling is necessary for the production of pulsus paradoxus.[66] Simultaneous with this inspiratory reduction in left ventricular filling, the inspiratory fall in intrathoracic pressure may also have an exaggerated negative effect on left ventricular filling.[67]

Pulsus paradoxus requires both ventricles to fill against a common resistance from systemic and pulmonary venous return. Factors that independently affect left ventricular filling may prevent its presence. Preexisting left ventricular failure or left ventricular hypertrophy may independently increase diastolic compliance to an extent exceeding the degree of impairment caused by the elevated intrapericardial pressure. Consequently, equilibration of filling pressures and pulsus paradoxus will not occur.[54] Aortic regurgitation provides an independent source of ventricular filling at the level of systemic arterial diastolic pressure that exceeds the level of restraint provided by the tamponading pericardium.

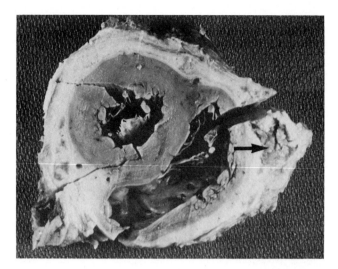

Fig. 8-6. Cross heart section, midventricular level, shows complete obliteration of the pericardial space by dense fibrous connective tissue, focally necrotic *(arrow)* and in areas calcified. Constrictive pericarditis of tuberculous etiology in a middle-age man.

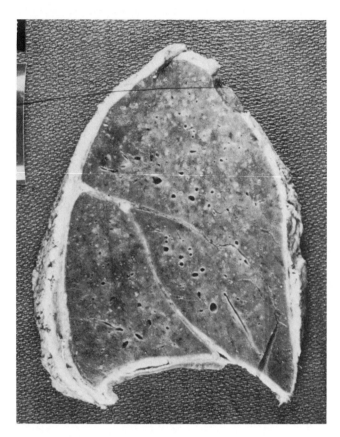

Fig. 8-7. Tuberculous pleurisy from the same patient as in Fig. 8-6.

Severe right ventricular hypertrophy may also impede equilibration of filling pressures in cardiac tamponade and delay or prevent the development of pulsus paradoxus.[68] Inspiratory decline in systolic blood pressure may be difficult to detect in cases of severe tamponade causing marked hypotension and a narrow pulse pressure, or in cardiac tamponade associated with hypovolemia. Echocardiographic findings of right heart collapse may be present without pulsus paradoxus in such cases.

Neither the presence of pulsus paradoxus nor left heart collapse are necessary parameters for cardiac tamponade. Fowler, et al, have demonstrated in an animal model that right-sided cardiac compression has greater significance than left-sided cardiac compression in the production of cardiac tamponade.[69]

CONSTRICTIVE PERICARDITIS

Constrictive pericarditis results from a marked reduction in compliance of the visceral and/or parietal layers of the pericardium. Intrapericardial pressure is not elevated. The severity of the clinical features and hemodynamic changes are determined by the extent of this constraint imposed on ventricular filling against a rigid pericardium.

Pericarditis due to any cause may cause constrictive pericarditis. Infectious agents, connective tissue diseases, neoplastic disease, metabolic abnormalities, and trauma are the most common causes.[70] Tuberculosis continues to be an important cause (Figs. 8-6 & 8-7). Trauma secondary to cardiac surgery or radiation therapy is becoming more frequent. Constrictive pericarditis may develop gradually over many years or subacutely over a period of weeks and months.

The clinical features are variable and are determined by the severity and chronicity of the process. With mild constrictive pericarditis there may be no symptoms or a minimal decrease in exercise tolerance. As the hemodynamic changes become more severe there is a progressive worsening of exercise tolerance, dyspnea, abdominal distention, and peripheral edema.[70] Palpatations, syncope, and epigastric or right upper quadrant pain are additional symptoms.

On physical examination the jugular veins are distended with a prominent Y descent or equal X and Y descents.[5] The systolic apical pulse may be attenuated, absent, or replaced with an early diastolic outward motion. A pericardial knock is present in up to one-half of cases.[70] In severe long-standing cases there may be massive ascites with minimal to severe peripheral edema.[70] The liver is frequently enlarged and pulsatile synchronously with the jugular veins.[16]

The electrocardiogram may be normal. In severe cases of long-standing, low voltage and atrial fibrillation may be present. The chest x-ray film may show a normal-to-enlarged cardiac silhouette. Pericardial calcification may be present but is not specific for constrictive physiology.

M-mode, two-dimensional, and Doppler echocardiography may show findings that reflect physiologic changes but are not specific for the diagnosis of constrictive pericarditis. Two-dimensional echocardiography is helpful in excluding left ventricular dilatation and valvular problems as the cause of the clinical presentation. Echocardiographic findings in constrictive pericarditis may include a calcified pericardium, reduced left ventricular diastolic posterior wall motion, abnormal septal motion, premature opening of the pulmonic valve, a rapid EF slope of the mitral valve and dilated atria, vena cavae, and hepatic veins. Septal motion may be paradoxic or demonstrate early diastolic motion (notching).[70,71]

Doppler flow patterns may demonstrate exaggerated diastolic flow velocity in the superior vena cava,[64] a W-wave pattern of flow in the hepatic veins with abrupt reversal of flow late in systole and in diastole before the A wave,[72] enhanced early diastolic mitral flow velocity, or diastolic tricuspid or mitral regurgitation.[70] These echocardiographic findings reflect anatomic and physiologic changes of constrictive pericarditis but may also be found in other forms of heart disease that cause impairment of ventricular filling and elevation of atrial pressures. Further observations are necessary to define their sensitivity and specificity in differential diagnosis.

The pericardium becomes rigid and noncompliant as a result of thickening by inflammation, fibrosis, calcification, or tumor invasion. Further filling is impeded when ventricular diastolic volume reaches the confines of the pericardial shell. Early diastolic filling, unlike pericardial tamponade, is not impaired and will become exaggerated as a compensation for restricted filling in mid and late diastole. This exaggerated early diastolic filling is followed by an abrupt halt in filling as the ventricular diastolic volume exceeds the fixed capacity of the pericardium. Further diastolic filling is accomplished by elevations in atrial and diastolic ventricular pressures. This sudden cessation of rapid early diastolic filling is reflected in the exaggerated Y descent of the right atrium and the early diastolic dip of the right ventricular pressure wave form. In most cases the constrictive process involves the right and left ventricles to an equal degree; right and left heart filling pressures equalize.[1] In some cases constriction may be localized.[5,73] Pre-existing left ventricular dysfunction with elevated diastolic pressure may also prevent equilibration of filling pressures. Although systolic ventricular function may remain normal, stroke volume and cardiac output become compromised. The heart rate may increase as a compensatory mechanism. Sodium and water retention increase intravascular volume. Atrial pressures are further elevated to improve ventricular filling and cardiac output. These hemodynamic alterations and compensatory mechanisms results, over time, in the clinical findings of jugular venous distention, pulsatile liver, ascites, and edema with symptoms of pulmonary venous congestion and inadequate cardiac output (dyspnea and fatigue).

The mechanism of sodium and water retention in pa-

tients with constrictive pericarditis may be somewhat different from patients with similar congestive changes and reduction in cardiac output due to myocardial failure. Anand et al[74] have demonstrated that secretion of atrial natriuretic peptide (ANP) is less with constrictive pericarditis; they postulate that this is due to diminished distensibility of the atria, which mediates the release of ANP.

Pulsus paradoxus does not occur in constrictive pericarditis unless associated with tamponading pericardial effusion (see effusive constrictive pericarditis). Kussmaul's sign may be present. The normal inspiratory decline in systemic venous pressure reflected in the jugular venous pressure does not occur and may actually increase. This phenomenon is a reflection of the inability of the right ventricle to enhance ventricular filling.[22]

Long-standing constrictive pericarditis may be associated with significant left ventricular dysfunction. The inflammatory and fibrotic process in the visceral pericardium may involve the subepicardial myocardium to a significant depth, and impair overall myocardial systolic function. Patients who have received radiation therapy are especially at risk because the myocardium is also sensitive to radiation injury.

Severe chronic constrictive pericarditis associated with ascites and passive congestion of the liver may cause significant hepatic dysfunction and masquerade as Budd-Chiari syndrome[75] or cirrhosis.

EFFUSIVE CONSTRICTIVE PERICARDITIS

Effusive constrictive pericarditis is the result of tamponading pericardial effusion with a constricting pericardium. Since constrictive pericarditis does not always obliterate the pericardial space, pericardial effusion may be present. When this effusion accumulates at a rate that exceeds the compliance of the stiff pericardium, intrapericardial pressure rises and tamponade physiology is superimposed. The net alterations cause clinical features that may be a combination of those of cardiac tamponade and cardiac constriction.

The pathophysiology is usually more like that of tamponade. Early diastolic filling is attenuated, and pulsus paradoxus is more likely.[1-2,76] When the pericardial fluid is removed to alleviate the tamponade, filling pressures decline but remain elevated to a degree determined by the severity of the constrictive process. Similarly, early diastolic filling improves and the Y descent becomes more prominent. The ventricular pressure contour demonstrates return of the rapid filling wave.

PERICARDITIS ASSOCIATED WITH OTHER PROBLEMS
Connective tissue diseases

Pericardial disease may be a part of the clinical presentation of systemic lupus erythematosus (SLE), rheumatoid arthritis (RA), and scleroderma. Other less common con-

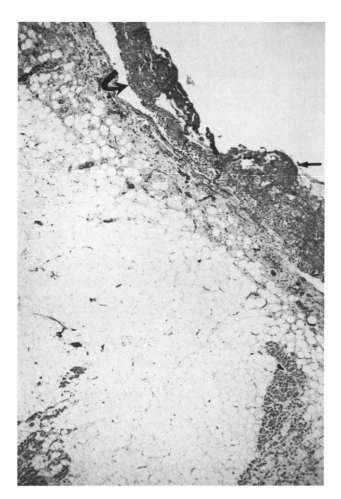

Fig. 8-8. Visceral pericardium showing round cell infiltration, fibrin deposition *(arrow)* and fibrous adhesions *(curved arrow)*.

nective tissue diseases may also involve the pericardium (see references 5 and 36).

With rheumatoid arthritis, evidence of pericardial disease is demonstrated in postmortem findings in one-third of cases (16% to 54% in various reported series).[77] Echocardiographic findings are reported in 22% of cases (3% to 46%). Clinically, pericardial disease is manifest in 2% to 10% of patients. The clinical presentations include acute pericarditis, cardiac tamponade, constrictive pericarditis and effusive constrictive pericarditis. Compressive physiology is thought to occur in less than 1% of patients with seropositive rheumatoid arthritis. Pericardial disease is more likely in patients who have had RA for years, are seropositive, and have extraarticular features.[77-79] The pathogenesis of RA appears to be similar to the pathogenesis of other extraarticular manifestations. Immune complexes bind to complement and activate the complement cascade. This in turn results in an influx of inflammatory cells (chemotaxis) that digest the immune complexes while releasing lysosomal enzymes capable of tissue damage. Whether the initial antigen is a autoantigen or is introduced from the environment remains unclear.

Pleural effusions are common, and pulmonary involvement may be present. Pericarditis is more likely to present during an exacerbation of arthritis, after abrupt steroid withdrawal, or during anticoagulant therapy. In rare cases pericardial involvement is manifest prior to the development of arthritis.[77]

The pericardial fluid is serosanguineous or hemorrhagic with elevated white blood cells, protein and lactate dehydrogenase (LDH).[77,80] The fluid may also be chylous. Glucose and complement levels are low. Cholesterol crystals may be present.[77,80] Immunofluorescence may demonstrate granular deposits of immunoglobulins, including IgG, IgM, and IgE.[77,80] The presence of the immune complexes are thought to contribute to the pathogenesis of rheumatoid pericarditis.[80,81]

The pericardium is fibrous and grossly thickened. Fibrinous adhesions in the pericardial space are common.[82] Microscopically there may be polymorphonuclear or mononuclear cells and plasma cells as well as extensive fibrosis.[35,82]

Pericardial disease is relatively common during the course of systemic lupus erythematosus and more frequent than in rheumatoid arthritis. It is also more frequently detected at autopsy than by clinical manifestations. In contrast to RA, cardiac compression is less common in SLE.[83] Acute pericarditis may be recognized during the clinical course in nearly one-half of cases.[84] and rarely as the initial manifestation of SLE.[78] Drug-induced SLE may also cause pericarditis with effusion and can present as cardiac tamponade. Unlike SLE, pericarditis may be the major manifestation of drug-induced lupus erythematosus.[78]

The pericardial fluid is a nonspecific exudate. Lupus cells, antinuclear antibodies, and rheumatoid factor are present. The drug-induced form may have low complement levels.[84] The pericardium is thickened with fibrous adhesions in the pericardial space (Fig. 8-8). Histologically, hematoxylin bodies, vasculitis, and fibrinoid necrosis may be seen.[85] Immune complexes support an immune response in the pathogenesis.[86]

The majority of cases of scleroderma will demonstrate pericardial involvement in postmortem examination (50% to 70%), while only 5% to 10% of patients will have clinically manifest pericardial disease.[78] Acute pericarditis or pericardial effusion are the most common clinical manifestations. Constrictive pericarditis is rare. Echocardiographic detection of pericardial effusion is reported in over one-third of patients but its presence may be related to other causes, including cardiomyopathy with congestive heart failure, or renal failure.[78]

The pericardial fluid may be a transudate or exudate. In comparison with SLE and RA the white cell count is lower and immune complexes are unlikely.[78] Autoantibodies are absent and the glucose content and complement levels are normal. The pathology is nonspecific. The pericardium may be thickened, but the fibrosis and inflammatory reaction is usually minimal.

Renal failure

Pericardial disease may occur during acute or chronic renal failure, or during chronic peritoneal dialysis or hemodialysis. Earlier treatment of renal failure has considerably reduced the incidence of uremic pericarditis prior to the development of dialytic therapy.[87] Pericarditis developing during the course of dialytic therapy occurs in 8% to 12% of patients.[87] The use of more frequent and more effective dialysis techniques may reduce this incidence.[87] Acute pericarditis, chronic asymptomatic pericardial effusion, cardiac tamponade, or constrictive pericarditis may also occur in cases of renal failure.

The pathogenesis of pericardial disease during the course of renal failure is uncertain and may be attributed to multiple factors. Inadequate dialysis by unknown mechanisms is associated with an increased frequency of pericarditis and can be independent of the blood levels of urea nitrogen or creatinine. Intrapericardial hemorrhage, unrecognized viral infections, and immunologic mechanisms have been implicated.[34] Other causes of pericardial disease may be present and there is greater susceptibility to infectious agents.

The pericardial fluid is usually hemorrhagic but may be serous or serosanguineous, and is frequently loculated due to prominent fibrous adhesions, which may be appreciated on gross examination. The pericardial reaction is hemorrhagic and fibrinous. The histology is nonspecific. Serosal hyperplasia, parietal pericardial vascular granulation tissue, and fibrosis may be present. The process may progress to a thickened fibrotic visceral and parietal pericardium and cause constrictive pericarditis.[34,39]

Neoplasms

Neoplastic involvement of the pericardium is most commonly associated with cancer of the lungs (36%), breast (22%), and hematologic malignancies (17%).[88] Of all patients who die of cancer, 8% to 12% have metastatic disease of the pericardium.[88,89] Primary neoplasms of the pericardium are rare, and mesothelioma is the most common.[31] Pericardial metastasis occurs by retrograde lymphatic spread, hematogenous dissemination or by direct invasion from adjacent tumor.[88] Pericardial effusion may be the result of impaired lymphatic drainage or increased production of abnormal pericardial fluid secondary to metastatic involvement of the serosal pericardium.[88] Acute pericarditis, cardiac tamponade, or effusive constrictive pericarditis may develop. Radiation therapy (see discussion on p. 000) or chemotherapy may be additional causes of pericardial disease in such patients.

The pericardial fluid is exudative and frequently hemorrhagic. Fluid cytology demonstrates malignant cells in the majority of cases.[90,91] Monoclonal antibody in the pericardial fluid has been demonstrated in metastatic adenocarcinoma of the breast.[92] In primary mesothelioma, determination of hyaluronic acid in the pericardial fluid may be diagnostic.[93] The gross appearance of the pericardium may be focal and nodular, or show diffuse neoplastic infiltration.[35] The surface may contain granulation tissue. Fibrous exudation may cover the serosal layer, and fibrous adhesions may cause variable fusion of the visceral and parietal layer. A diffuse or focal pattern of infiltration of tumor cells is demonstrated by histologic examination.

After cardiac surgery

During the perioperative period, pericarditis related to the trauma of surgery is common. Excessive bleeding may lead to cardiac tamponade being reported in .4% to 6% of cardiac surgery cases.[94] A postpericardiotomy syndrome may develop late after cardiac surgery and is similar to Dressler's syndrome. This condition may become manifest from 1 week to months and possibly years after cardiac surgery[95] and has been reported to occur in 1.6% to 34% of cases. It may be recurrent and can cause cardiac tamponade or constrictive pericarditis. The incidence of constrictive pericarditis following cardiac surgery is probably no more than .12% to .13% of all patients.[96] It does represent an increasing percentage of patients undergoing surgery for constrictive pericarditis because the incidence of other causes, especially tuberculosis, has lessened.[39] Constrictive pericarditis following cardiac surgery may present months to years later, but the average period is reported to be 8 months to 1 year.[39]

The pathogenesis is uncertain and possibly multifactorial. Exposure to foreign irritant material (povidone-iodine for example), hemorrhage, or an autoimmune process related to the postpericardiotomy syndrome are considered the most likely contributing factors.[39]

The pericardial fluid is grossly bloody in the perioperative period. The effusion of the postpericardiotomy syndrome is sanguineous or serosanguineous and is exudative with an elevated protein content and elevated white count that results from a predominance of lymphocytes. The pathology is nonspecific and includes fibrosis, adhesions, and organizing hematoma.[39] The fluid may be loculated and cause localized tamponade.

Radiation

Pericardial disease is the most common manifestation of radiation-induced heart disease. Myocardial, coronary artery or valvular problems may occur, but the pericardium is most sensitive. Acute pericarditis or asymptomatic pericardial effusion may present within months of radiation therapy or sometimes much later.[97] Pericardial effusion is the most common manifestation and has been reported to occur in up to one-third of patients.[98] It may resolve spontaneously, or persist for long periods without symptoms or significant hemodynamic compromise. Pericardial tamponade, constrictive pericarditis, and effusive constrictive pericarditis may develop.[97] These hemodynamic complications usually develop within 1 to 2 years but have been reported to become manifest many years later.[97,99] New techniques that decrease cardiac exposure to radiation have reduced the reported incidence of radiation pericarditis to 2.5% down from earlier reports of up to 40%.[97,100]

The pericardial effusion is usually serous or serosanguineous, but may be grossly bloody. The protein content is elevated and lymphocytes predominate.[98] Pericardial disease after exposure to radiation involves cellular damage or obstruction of lymphatic drainage due to fibrosis. An autoimmune response may also contribute to the pathogenesis. Animal studies have demonstrated that the early acute effects of radiation include a nonspecific inflammatory reaction with fibrinous exudation and hemorrhage that involves the parietal and visceral pericardium and subepicardial myocardium.[101,102] There are membrane abnormalities, cytoplasmic swelling of endothelial cells, platelet and fibrin deposition, thrombus formation, capillary rupture, and perivascular inflammation. This distortion and disruption of the microcirculation may impair the function of phagocytic and cytotoxic cells. In later stages there is gross thickening of all layers of the pericardium; the outer layer of the pericardium adheres densely to adjacent structures, including the sternum. These changes are more marked in the anterior portions of the pericardium because they are more exposed to an anterior port of radiation. Microscopic findings in the late stages include dense hyalinization and fibrosis without cellular components.[34,98]

Drugs

Drug-induced pericardial disease is most commonly caused by procainamide or hydralazine. These drugs produce a lupus-like syndrome with fever, arthralgias, pleuritis, and pericarditis. Unlike SLE there is no renal involvement[103] and pericardial effects may present without other clinical manifestations. Acute pericarditis with pericardial effusion occurs and cardiac tamponade and constrictive pericarditis may develop.[80,104,105]

Daunorubicin and doxorubicin have been reported to cause pericarditis usually in association with myocarditis.[106] Minoxodil may cause pericardial effusion.[5,13] Penicillin and cromolyn sodium produce a hypersensitivity reaction and pericarditis.[5]

Isoniazid, psicofuranine, phenylbutazone, and amiodarone have been implicated in the development of pericarditis.[22,84,107] Methysergide has been reported to cause constrictive pericarditis.[22]

The pericardial effusion in drug-induced pericarditis is a nonspecific exudate. In patients receiving procainamide, IgG antiguanosine antibodies may be associated with lupus-like pericarditis.[108] The pericardium shows nonspecific changes of fibrosis and thickening. Exudative, hemorrhagic, and fibrous reactions may be present. The pericardial space may be obliterated.[34]

CONGENITAL PERICARDIAL DEFECTS

Congenital defects of the pericardium are rare. Partial or complete absence of the left parietal pericardium is most common. Rarely is there absence of the entire pericardium. Most patients are asymptomatic, and the defect is suspected by characteristic x-ray findings. With complete absence of the left pericardium the heart is shifted to the left, the pulmonary artery segment is prominent, and there is interposition of lung between the left hemidiaphragm and inferior border of the heart.[109] In partial absence of the left pericardium there are varying degrees of prominence of the pulmonary artery or left atrial appendage. In these cases sudden death due to herniation of the heart has been reported.[109]

The effects of absence of the pericardium on cardiac function are not completely defined. An exaggerated dilation of the ventricles, especially the right ventricle, occurs with small increases in venous return.[110]

Echocardiographic findings are nonspecific. Dilation of the right ventricle and paradoxic septal motion characteristic of right ventricular volume overload may be demonstrated. Herniation of the left atrial appendage and an abnormal contour of the left ventricle secondary to partial herniation have been reported.[71] Computed tomography is more reliable in demonstrating the extent of the pericardial defect.[71]

MISCELLANEOUS ASSOCIATIONS

An association of atrial septal defect with pericardial effusion has been recognized. Pericardial adhesions with or without constriction have been reported. The severity of the atrial septal defect does not correlate with the presence of the effusion. The clinical course may be benign.[111]

Cholesterol pericarditis is usually associated with systemic disease such as rheumatoid arthritis, tuberculosis, or myxedema. It may occur in the absence of associated illnesses. Cardiac tamponade may develop. The mechanism is uncertain but is thought to occur after recurrent attacks of idiopathic pericarditis. The pericardium may be grossly thickened with a yellow appearance. Histologically there are cholesterol clefts and a foreign body granulomatous reaction.[112,113]

Pericardial effusion is uncommon in hypothyroidism[106] but with clinical myxedema it is more likely to occur. Cardiac tamponade or constrictive pericarditis may develop. The pericardial fluid may have a high cholesterol content. Cholesterol clefts and foam cells containing lipid have been described in the pericardium.[114]

Dermatitis herpetiformis has been reported to be associated with an immune complex mediated pericarditis. Deposition of complement (IgG and IgA) in the pericardium has been documented.[115]

Ulcerative colitis and Crohn's disease may be associated with recurrent pericarditis. Cardiac tamponade has been reported.[116] Acute pericarditis usually becomes manifest during an acute phase of colitis, but may occur when the bowel disease is inactive.[117]

Patients with acquired autoimmunodeficiency syndrome

(AIDS) are at risk of pericardial disease. Pericardial effusion is reported at postmortem examination in 32% of patients.[118] In the majority of these cases the effusion was not clinically significant and is thought to be related to metabolic changes with associated pleural effusions and ascites.[119] It is uncertain whether a primary infection by the HIV in the pericardium and myocardium can occur. The HIV has been demonstrated in the myocytes of HIV positive patients. The relationship of this finding to clinical cardiac problems is uncertain.[120] Cardiac tamponade due to *Staphylococcus aureus, Mycobacterium avium,* and *M. intracellulare,* and malignancy has been reported in HIV-infected patients.[121]

REFERENCES

1. Shabetai R, Mangiardi L, Bhargave V, et al: The pericardium and cardiac function, *Prog Cardiovasc Dis* 22:107, 1979.
2. Hancock EW: On the elastic and rigid forms of constrictive pericarditis, *Am Heart J* 100:917, 1980.
3. Shabetai R: The pericardium: An essay on some recent developments, *Am J Cardiol* 42:1036, 1978.
4. Ishihara T, Ferrans VJ, Jones M et al: Histologic and ultrastructural features of normal human parietal pericardium, *Am J Cardiol* 46:744, 1980.
5. Shabetai R: *The pericardium.* New York, 1981, Grune Stratton.
6. Freeman GL: The effects of the pericardium on function of normal and enlarged hearts, *Cardiol Clin* 8:579, 1990.
7. Hoit BD, Dalton N, Bhargava V et al: Pericardial influences on right and left ventricular filling dynamics, *Circ Res* 68:197, 1991.
8. Santamore WP, Shaffer T, Papa L: Theoretical model of ventricular interdependence: pericardial effects, *Am J Physiol* 259:H181, 1990.
9. Lee MC, Fung YC, Shabetai R et al: Biaxial mechanical properties of human pericardium and canine comparisons, *Am J Physiol* 253:H75, 1987.
10. Smiseth OA, Frais MA, Kingma I et al: Assessment of pericardial constraint: the relation between right ventricular filling pressure and pericardial pressure measured after pericardiocentesis, *J Am Coll Cardiol* 7:307, 1986.
11. Santamore WP, Constantinescu MS, Bogen D et al: Nonuniform distribution of normal pericardial fluid, *Basic Res Cardiol* 85:541, 1990.
12. Shabetai R: Measuring pericardial constraint, *J Am Coll Cardiol* 7:315, 1986.
13. Fowler NO: *Acute pericarditis.* In Fowler NO, ed: *The pericardium in health and disease,* Mount Kisco, NY, 1985, The Futura.
14. Spodick DH: Pericardial rub: prospective, multiple observer investigation of pericardial friction in 100 patients, *Am J Cardiol* 35:357, 1975.
15. Spodick DH: *Electrocardiographic changes in acute pericarditis.* In Fowler NO, ed: *The pericardium in health and disease,* Mount Kisco, NY, 1985, Futura.
16. Leak LV, Ferrans VJ, Cohen SR et al: Animal model of acute pericarditis and its progression to pericardial fibrosis and adhesions: ultrastructural studies, *Am J Anat* 180:373, 1987.
17. Karjalainen J, Heikkila J: "Acute pericarditis": myocardial enzyme release as evidence for myocarditis, *Am Heart J* 111:546, 1986.
18. Easton AJ, Eglin RP: The detection of Coxsackie virus RNA in cardiac tissue by in situ hybridization, *J Gen Virol,* 69:285, 1988.
19. Alkadiry WA, Gold RG, Bechan PO et al: Analysis of antigens in the circulating immune complexes of patients with Coxsackie infections, *Prog Brain Res* 61:37, 1983.
20. Gold RG: Post-viral pericarditis, *Eur Heart J* 9:175, 1988.
21. Muir P, Tilzeg AJ, English TAH et al: Chronic relapsing pericardi-

tis and dilated cardiomyopathy: serological evidence of persistent enterovirus infection, *Lancet* 1:804, 1989.
22. Shabetai R: *Acute Pericarditis.* In Shabetai R, ed: Diseases of the Pericardium, *Cardiol Clin* 8:639, 1990.
23. Fowler NO: *Recurrent pericarditis.* In Shabetai ed: *Cardiol Clin* 8:621, 1990.
24. Gregoratos G: *Pericardial involvement in acute myocardial infarction.* In Shabetai R, ed: Diseases of the Pericardium, *Cardiol Clin* 8:601, 1990.
25. Tofler GH, Muller JE, Stone PH et al: Pericarditis in acute myocardial infarction: characterization and clinical significance, *Am Heart J* 117:86, 1989.
26. Sugiura T, Iwasaka T, Takayama Y et al: Factors associated with pericardial effusion in acute Q wave myocardial infarction, *Circulation* 81:477, 1990.
27. Belkin RN, Mark DB, Aronson L et al: Pericardial effusion after intravenous recombinant tissue-type plasminogen activator for acute myocardial infarction, *Am J Cardiol* 67:496, 1991.
28. Fowler NO: Tuberculous pericarditis, *JAMA* 266:99, 1991.
29. Monsuez JJ, Kinney EL, Vittecoq D et al: Comparison among acquired immune deficiency syndrome patients with and without clinical evidence of cardiac disease, *Am J Cardiol* 62:1311, 1988.
30. Fowler NO: *Infectious pericarditis.* In Fowler NO, ed: *The pericardium in health and disease,* Mount Kisco, NY, 1985, Futura.
31. Roberts WC, Spray TL: *Pericardial heart disease: a study of its causes, consequences and morphologic features.* In Spodick DH, ed: Pericardial diseases, *Cardiovasc Clin* 7/3, 1976.
32. Soler-Soler J, Permanyer-Miralda G, Sagrista-Sauleda J: *A systematic diagnostic approach to primary acute pericardial disease. The Barcelona experience.* In Shabetai R ed: Diseases of the pericardium, *Cardiovasc Clin* 8:609, 1990.
33. Isaka N, Tanaka R, Nakamura M et al: A case of tuberculous pericarditis—use of adenosine deaminase activity (ADA) in early diagnosis, *Heart Vessels* 5:247, 1990.
34. El-Maraghi NRH: *Disease of the pericardium.* In Silver MD, ed: *Cardiovascular pathology, vol 1,* New York, 1983, Churchill Livingstone.
35. Mambo NC: Diseases of the pericardium: morphologic study of surgical specimens from 35 patients, *Hum Pathol* 12:978, 1981.
36. Hall IP: Purulent pericarditis, *Post Grad Med J* 65:444, 1989.
37. Klacsmann PG, Bulkley BH, Hutchins GM: The changed spectrum of purulent pericarditis. An 86 year autopsy experience in 200 patients, *Am J Med* 63:666, 1977.
38. Majid AA, Omar A: Diagnosis and management of purulent pericarditis. Experience with pericardiectomy, *J Thorac Cardiovasc Surg* 102:413, 1991.
39. Cameron J, Oesterle SN, Baldwin JC et al: The etiologic spectrum of constrictive pericarditis, *Am Heart J* 113:354, 1987.
40. Rubin RH, Moellering RC: Clinical, microbiologic and therapeutic aspects of purulent pericarditis, *Am J Med* 59:68, 1975.
41. Kraus, WE, Valenstein PN, Corey GR: Purulent pericarditis caused by *Candida:* report of three cases and identification of high-risk populations as an aid to early diagnosis, *Rev Infect Dis* 10:34, 1988.
42. Carrel JP, Schaffner A, Schmid ER et al: Fatal fungal pericarditis after cardiac surgery and immunosuppression, *J Thorac Cardiovasc Surg* 101:161, 1991.
43. Schaffner A, Douglas H, Braude A: Selective protection against conidia by mononuclear and against mycelia by polymorphonuclear phagocytes in resistance to aspergillus, *J Clin Invest* 69:617, 1982.
44. Colombo A, Olson HG, Egan J et al: Etiology and prognostic implications of a large pericardial effusion in men, *Clin Cardiol* 11:389, 1988.
45. Park B, Dittrich HC, Polikar R et al: Echocardiographic evidence of pericardial effusion in severe chronic pulmonary hypertension, *Am J Cardiol* 63:143, 1989.

46. Haiat R, Halphen C: Silent pericardial effusion in late pregnancy: a new entity, *Cardiovasc Intervent Radiol* 7:267, 1984.

47. Stratton JR, Werner JA, Pearlman AS et al: Bacteremia and the heart. Serial echocardiographic findings in 80 patients with documented or suspected bacteremia, *Am J Med* 73:851, 1982.

48. Jeanty P, Romero R, Hobbins JC: Fetal pericardial fluid: a normal finding in the second half of gestation, *Am J Obstet Gynecol* 149:529, 1984.

49. Curtiss EI, Reddy PS, Uretsky BF et al: Pulsus paradoxus: definition and relation to the severity of cardiac tamponade, *Am Heart J* 115:391, 1988.

50. Janicki JS, Weber KT, Loscalzo J et al: Extracardiac pressure and ventricular haemodynamics, *Cardiovasc Res* 21:230, 1987.

51. Reddy PS, Curtiss EI: *Cardiac tamponade.* In Crawford MH, ed: Diseases of the pericardium, *Cardiovasc Clin* 8/4, 1990.

52. Reddy PS, Curtiss EI, Uretsky BF et al: Cardiac tamponade: hemodynamic observations in man, *Circulation* 58:265, 1978.

53. Reddy PS, Curtiss EI, Uretsky BF: Spectrum of hemodynamic changes in cardiac tamponade, *Am J Cardiol* 66:1487, 1990.

54. Hoit BD, Gabel M, Fowler NO: Cardiac tamponade in left ventricular dysfunction, *Circulation* 82:1370, 1990.

55. Engle PJ: *Echocardiographic findings in pericardial disease.* In Fowler NO, ed: *The pericardium in health and disease,* Mount Kisco, NY, 1985, Futura.

56. Singh S, Wann LS, Schuchard GH et al: Right ventricular and right atrial collapse in patients with cardiac tamponade—a combined echocardiographic and hemodynamic study, *Circulation* 70:966, 1984.

57. Klopfenstein HS, Schuchard GH, Wann LS et al: The relative merits of plusus paradoxus and right ventricular diastolic collapse in the early detection of cardiac tamponade: An experimental echocardiographic study, *Circulation* 71:829, 1985.

58. Singh S, Wann LS, Klopfenstein HS et al: Usefulness of right ventricular diastolic collapse in diagnosing cardiac tamponade and comparison to pulsus paradoxus, *Am J Cardiol* 57:652, 1986.

59. Reydel B, Spodick DH: Frequency and significance of chamber collapses during cardiac tamponade, *Am Heart J* 119:1160, 1990.

60. Hoit BD, Fowler NO: Influence of acute right ventricular dysfunction on cardiac tamponade, *J Am Coll Cardiol* 18:1787, 1991.

61. Fast J, Wielenga RP, Jansen E et al: Abnormal wall movements of the right ventricle and both atria in patients with pericardial effusion as indicators of cardiac tamponade, *Eur Heart J* 7:431, 1986.

62. Chuttani K, Pandian NG, Mohanty PK et al: Left ventricular diastolic collapse. An echocardiographic sign of regional cardiac tamponade, *Circulation* 83:1999, 1991.

63. Levine MJ, Lorell BH, Diver DJ et al: Implications of echocardiographically assisted diagnosis of pericardial tamponade in contemporary medical patients: detection before hemodynamic embarrassment, *J Am Coll Cardiol* 17:59, 1991.

64. Byrd BF III, Linden RW: Superior vena cava doppler flow velocity patterns in pericardial disease, *Am J Cardiol* 65:1464, 1990.

65. Borganelli M, Byrd BF: *Doppler echocardiography in pericardial disease.* In Shiller NB, ed. *Cardiovasc Clinics* 8/2, 1990.

66. Burstow DJ, Oh JAE K, Bailey KR et al: Cardiac tamponade: characteristic doppler observations, *Mayo Clin Proc* 64:312, 1989.

67. Gonzalez MS, Basnight MA, Appleton CP et al: Experimental pericardial effusion: relation of abnormal respiratory variation in mitral flow velocity to hemodynamics and diastolic right heart collapse, *J Am Coll Cardiol* 17:239, 1991.

68. Shabetai R: Changing concepts of cardiac tamponade, *J Am Coll Cardiol* 12:194, 1988.

69. Fowler NO, Gabel M, Buncher C: Cardiac tamponade: a comparison of right versus left heart compression, *J Am Coll Cardiol* 12:187, 1988.

70. Brockington GM, Zebede J, Pandian NG: *Constrictive pericarditis.* In Shabetai R, ed: Diseases of the pericardium, *Cardiovasc Clin* 8/4, 1990.

71. Crawley IS: *Noninvasive diagnosis of pericardial disease.* In Miller DD, ed: *Clinical cardiac imaging,* New York, 1988, McGraw-Hill.

72. Von Bibra H, Schober K, Jenni R et al: Diagnosis of constrictive pericarditis by pulsed doppler echocardiography of the hepatic vein, *Am J Cardiol* 63:483, 1989.

73. Spodick DH: *Chronic and constrictive pericarditis.* New York, 1964, Grune and Stratton.

74. Anand IS, Ferrari R, Kalra GS, et al: Pathogenesis of edema in constrictive pericarditis, *Circulation* 83:1880, 1991.

75. Arora A, Tandon N, Sharma MP et al: Constrictive pericarditis masquerading as Budd-Chiari syndrome, *J Clin Gastroenterol* 13:178, 1991.

76. Hancock EW: Subacute effusive-constrictive pericarditis, *Circulation* 43:183, 1971.

77. Escalante A, Kaufman RL, Quismorio FP Jr et al: Cardiac compression in rheumatoid pericarditis, *Semin Arthritis Rheum* 20:148, 1990.

78. Spodick DH: *Pericarditis in systemic disease.* In Shabetai R, ed: Diseases of the pericardium, *Cardiovasc Clin* 8:709, 1990.

79. Kelly CA, Bourke JP, Griffiths ID: Chronic pericardial disease in patients with rheumatoid arthritis: a longitudinal study, *Q J Med* 75(277):461, 1990.

80. Van Offel JF, de Clerck LS, Kersschot IE: Cholesterol crystals and IGE-containing immune complexes in rheumatoid pericarditis, *Clin Rheumatol* 10:78, 1991.

81. Spodick DH: Low atrial natriuretic factor levels and absent pulmonary edema in pericardial compression of the heart, *Am J Cardiol* 63:1271, 1989.

82. Goldman AP, Kotler MN: Heart disease in scleroderma, *Am Heart J* 110:1043, 1985.

83. Doherty NE, Siegel RJ: Cardiovascular manifestations of systemic lupus erythematosus, *Am Heart J* 110:1257, 1985.

84. Cohen AS, Canoso JJ: *Pericarditis in the rheumatologic disease.* In Spodick DH, ed: Pericardial diseases, *Cardiovasc Clin* 7/3, 1976.

85. Bulkley BH, Roberts WC: The heart in systemic lupus erythematosus and the changes induced in it by corticosteroid therapy: A study of 36 necropsy patients, *Am J Med* 58:243, 1975.

86. Bidani AK, Roberts JL, Schwartz MM et al: Immunopathology of cardiac lesions in fatal systemic lupus erythematosus, *Am J Med* 69:849, 1980.

87. Rostand SG, Rutsky EA: *Pericarditis in end-stage renal disease.* In Shabetai R ed: Diseases of the pericardium, *Cardiovasc Clin* 8/4, 1990.

88. Press OW, Livingston R: Management of malignant pericardial effusion and tamponade, *JAMA* 257:1088, 1987.

89. Olopade OI, Ultmann JE: Malignant effusions. CA Cancer, *J Clin* 41:166, 1991.

90. Edoute Y, Malberger E, Kuten A et al: Symptomatic pericardial effusion in lung cancer patients: the role of fluid cytology, *J Surg Oncol* 45:121, 1990.

91. Wiener HG, Kristensen IB, Haubek A et al: The diagnostic value of pericardial cytology. An analysis of 95 cases, *J Clin Cyto Cytopath* 35:149, 1991.

92. Johnston WW, Szpak CA, Lottich SC et al: Use of a monoclonal antibody (B72.3) as an immunocytochemical adjunct to diagnosis of adenocarcinoma of human effusions, *Cancer Res* 45:1894, 1985.

93. Takeda K, Ohba H, Hyodo H et al: Pericardial mesothelioma: hyaluronic acid in pericardial fluid, *Am Heart J* 110:486, 1985.

94. Sahni A, Ivert T, Herzfeld I et al: Late cardiac tamponade after open-heart surgery, *Scand J Thorac Cardiovasc Surg* 25:63, 1991.

95. Schiavone WA: The changing etiology of constrictive pericarditis in a large referral center, *Am J Cardiol* 58:373, 1986.

96. Cimino JJ, Kogan AD: Constrictive pericarditis after cardiac surgery: report of three cases and review of the literature, *Am Heart J* 118:1292, 1989.

97. Arsenian MA: Cardiovascular sequelae of therapeutic thoracic radiation, *Prog Cardiovasc Dis* 33:299, 1991.

98. Martin RG, Ruckdeschel JC, Chang P et al: Radiation-related pericarditis, *Am J Cardiol* 35:216, 1975.

99. Pohjola-Sintonen S, Tötterman K-J, Salmo M et al: Late cardiac effects of mediastinal radiotherapy in patients with Hodgkin's disease, *Cancer* 60:31, 1987.

100. Crawley IS: *Effect of noncardiac drugs, radiation, electricity, and poisons on the heart.* In Hurst JW ed: *The heart,* ed 6, New York, 1986, McGraw-Hill.

101. Stewart JR, Fajardo LF: Radiation-induced heart disease. Clinical and experimental aspects, *Radiol Clin North Am* 9:511, 1971.

102. Ni Y, von Segesser LK, Turina M: Futility of pericardiectomy for post irradiation constrictive pericarditis, *Ann Thorac Surg* 49:445, 1990.

103. Blomgren SE, Condemi JJ, Vaughan JH: Procainamide-induced lupus erythematosus. Clinical and laboratory observations, *Am J Med* 52:338, 1972.

104. Sunder SK, Shan A: Constrictive pericarditis in procainamide-induced lupus erythematosus syndrome, *Am J Med* 36:960, 1975.

105. Carey RM, Coleman M, Feder A: Pericardial tamponade: a major presenting manifestation of hydralazine-induced lupus syndrome, *Am J Med* 54:84, 1973.

106. Bristow MR, Thompson PD, Martin RP et al: Early anthracycline cardiotoxicity, *Am J Med* 65:823, 1978.

107. Clarke B, Ward DE, Honey M: Pneumonitis with pleural and pericardial effusion and neuropathy during amiodarone therapy, *Int J Cardiol* 8:81, 1985.

108. Weisbart RH, Yee WS, Colburn KK et al: Antiguanosine antibodies: A new marker for procainamide-induced systemic lupus erythematosus, *Ann Intern Med* 104:310, 1986.

109. Nasser WK, Helmen C, Tavel ME et al: Congenital absence of the left pericardium. Clinical, electrocardiographic, radiographic, hemodynamic and angiographic findings in six cases, *Circulation* 41:469, 1970.

110. Beppu S, Naito H, Matsuhisa M et al: The effects of lying position on ventricular volume in congenital absence of the pericardium, *Am Heart J* 120, 1159, 1990.

111. Pietras RJ, Lam W: Large pericardial effusions associated with congenital heart disease: Five and eight year follow-up. *Am Heart J* 115:1334, 1988.

112. Ford EJ, Bear PA, Adams RW: Cholesterol pericarditis causing cardiac tamponade, *Am Heart J* 122:877, 1991.

113. Kabadi UM, Kumar SP: Pericardial effusion in primary hypothyroidism, *Am Heart J* 120:1393, 1990.

114. Van Buren PC, Roberts WC: Cholesterol pericarditis and cardiac tamponade with congenital hypothyroidism in adulthood, *Am Heart J* 119:697, 1990.

115. Afrasiabi R, Sirop PA, Albini SM et al: Recurrent pericarditis and dermatitis herpetiformis. Evidence for immune complex deposition in the pericardium, *Chest* 97:1006, 1990.

116. Breitenstein RA, Salel AF, Watson DW: Chronic inflammatory bowel disease: acute pericarditis and pericardial tamponade, *Arch Intern Med* 81:406, 1974.

117. Gould L, Patel C, Betzu R et al: Pericarditis and ulcerative colitis, *Am Heart J* 111:802, 1986.

118. Lewis W: AIDS: Cardiac findings from 115 autopsies, *Prog Cardiovasc Dis* 32:207, 1989.

119. Dasco CC: *Pericarditis in AIDS.* In Shabetai R, ed: Diseases of the pericardium, *Cardiovasc Clin* 8:697, 1990.

120. Rodriguez ER, Nasim S, Hsia J et al: Cardiac myocytes and dendritic cells harbor human immunodeficiency virus in infected patients with and without cardiac dysfunction: Detection by multiplex, nested, polymerase chain reaction in individually microdissected cells from right ventricular endomyocardial biopsy tissue, *Am J Cardiol* 68:1511, 1991.

121. Turco M, Seneff M, McGrath BJ et al: Cardiac tamponade in the acquired immunodeficiency syndrome, *Am Heart J* 120:1467, 1990.

Chapter 9

TUMORS OF THE HEART

Nanette K. Wenger

CARDIAC TUMORS: CLINICALLY UNCOMMON, ANATOMICALLY LESS SO

The categorization of cardiac tumors as rare relates more to their clinical presentation than to their morphologic presence, hence our preference for the designation "tumors of the heart" rather than "neoplastic heart disease."

Background information

Fewer than 10% of all cardiac tumors are symptomatic; the majority, in prior years, were diagnosed as incidental findings at autopsy examination or unexpected findings at surgery. Antemortem diagnosis of cardiac tumor is predominantly a phenomenon of the past 4 decades. It has been spurred to a great extent by the possibility of surgical intervention, and aided initially by cardiac catheterization and subsequently by a variety of noninvasive imaging techniques. The first reported correct antemortem diagnosis of cardiac tumor was in 1913. Since then, a combination of the new technologies and heightened clinical awareness has substantially increased the consideration and recognition of cardiac tumors. Successful surgical removal of a primary cardiac tumor was first described in 1954.[1]

Contribution of imaging techniques

Contemporary imaging techniques: echocardiography, computer tomography (CT) of the chest, positron emission tomography (PET), and magnetic resonance imaging (MRI) (Fig. 9-1), among others, have increased the diagnosis of cardiac tumors during life and enabled their differentiation from other heart-related masses. Newer noninvasive imaging techniques are of particular value when the less expensive and more rapidly performed echocardiography is not technically adequate, e.g., in obese or emphysematous patients. The role of transesophageal echocardiography has not been fully examined, but is likely to be of greater value with atrial than with ventricular intracavitary tumors. The importance of diagnostic and preoperative invasive procedures has declined with the improvement and increased availability of noninvasive imaging techniques.

Incidence of primary cardiac tumors

Some have attributed the relative rarity of primary tumors of the heart to the limited mitotic activity of cardiac muscle, i.e., cardiac muscle reacts to injury by degenera-

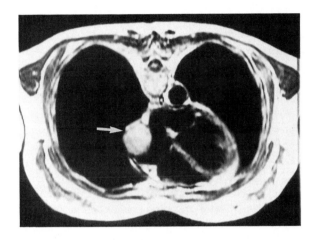

Fig. 9-1. Right atrial rhabdomyoma *(arrow)* demonstrated by magnetic resonance imaging (MRI). (Courtesy of Department of Radiology, Emory University School of Medicine.)

tion and fibrosis rather than by regenerative phenomena. However, when the heart percentage of total body weight, 0.4% to 0.5%, is considered, primary cardiac tumors are not disproportionately rare. Cardiac tumors occur more commonly at the base than the apex of the heart. The majority of primary tumors are benign.[2] Atrial myxomas accounted for approximately 42% of all tumors and 50% of primary benign cardiac neoplasms at the University of Minnesota; the histologic distribution of benign tumors, listed in order of frequency, was: myxomas 50%, rhabdomyomas 13%, papillomas 11%, fibromas 9%, hamartomas 4%, teratomas 2%, glomangiomas 2%, and others including lipomas, mesotheliomas, fibroelastomas, and hemangiomas (Fig. 9-2) totalling 9%. All 21 primary malignant neoplasms were sarcomas; in order of frequency, there were six rhabdomyosarcomas, four angiosarcomas, three myosarcomas, three spindle cell sarcomas, two fibrosarcomas, and one each of leiomyosarcoma, reticulum cell sarcoma, and liposarcoma.[2] In our experience and in other series, angiosarcomas were the most commonly encountered primary malignant tumors.

Tumor metastases to the heart: mechanisms and pathways

Regarding tumor metastases to the heart, there appears to be relative resistance of the cardiac valves, the arteries and the conducting tissue to tumor invasion. Metastatic cardiac tumor involves the pericardium, myocardium, and endocardium in descending order of frequency. Tradition-

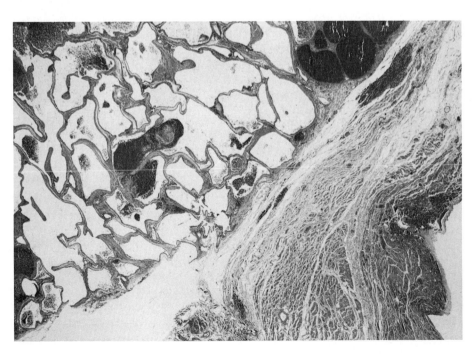

Fig. 9-2. A right atrial tumor in a 54-year-old woman. The tumor measured 5 cm × 4 cm × 3 cm, was spongy in consistency, grayish-red in color, and was attached to the lateral atrial wall. Microscopic section showing large cavernous vascular channels characteristic of a hemangioma.

ally, and probably inappropriately simplistically, the relative infrequency of metastatic disease to the myocardium has been attributed, at least in part, to: (1) rapid intracardiac blood flow, (2) the strong kneading action of the myocardium, (3) the restricted cardiac lymphatic channels through which metastases to the heart via lymphatics must invade in a retrograde fashion, and (4) the metabolic characteristics of myocardium, which requires virtually completely aerobic metabolism. Tumor metabolism, on the other hand, is highly anaerobic, requiring much glucose and little oxygen, and producing lactate (which can be used by cardiac muscle for its metabolism), rendering myocardium and its tumor metastases partly symbiotic. Also suggested is the right-angle takeoff of the coronary arteries from the aorta, which restricts tumor cell entry. Other theories about the biology of human neoplastic disease may be relevant. A century ago, Paget[3] suggested that certain tumors were predisposed to spread to particular tissues, based on the tissue's ability to support tumor growth. Ewing considered that preferential colonization of certain organs could be attributed entirely to routes of blood flow that carried tumor cells away from the primary site.[4] According to this mechanical theory of metastatic spread, body tissues are passive receptacles for tumor cells.

Contemporary concepts of metastasis suggest that it is a highly selective process, regulated by a number of mechanisms. Recent experimental studies have shown that specific organs contain determinants that affect specific types of tumor cells.[5] Phenomena occurring at the primary tumor site may facilitate tumor cell motility and enhance its ability for intravasation. Recent evidence also indicates that passive cell trapping is not sufficient to promote formation of metastatic colonies.[6] A specific cellular adhesive interaction may initiate recognition of a favored secondary site by a circulating metastatic cell.[7] The working hypothesis is that tumor/endothelial cell recognition may represent an important determinant of site-specific metastasis.[8] Preferential metastatic tumor adherence may be due to organ-specific adhesion molecules, resulting in an initial bond between tumor cells and adhesive molecules on the luminal side of the vascular endothelium. It is not known if the molecules involved in initial adhesion are the same molecules that support tumor cell growth after traversing the endothelial cell barrier. However, tumor cell death in the microcirculation may occur quickly, because of lack of specialized structures of blood cells to render them sufficiently deformable to survive transcapillary passage.[9]

Tumor cells lodged in capillaries may cause retraction of endothelial cells, exposure of the basement membrane, and adhesion of tumor cells to the subendothelial matrix. Adhesion molecules in the basement membrane include fibronectin, laminin, type IV collagen, heparan sulfate proteoglycan and vitronectin.[10] Tumor cell surface receptors have been identified for fibronectin, type IV collagen, vitronectin, and laminin,[11] so organ specificity of blood-borne tumor metastases could relate to interaction of cell receptors with the adhesion molecules of the target organ. Endothelia from different tissues may differ and may express different adhesive determinants, contributing to the organ specificity of metastasis.[12] The adhesive elements of the extracellular matrix may also vary from organ to organ.[13] For example, malignant cells with higher affinity for laminin than fibronectin tend to metastasize predominantly to lung. Organ site specificity may also relate to antibodies that block the attachment process, thus blocking metastases in those tissues.[13]

Migration of recirculating lymphocytes from blood to lymphoid sites has been termed *homing*. Specific lymphocytes, cell-surface molecules that mediate this process, are referred to as *homing receptors*. Theoretically, metastatic cells that express lymphocyte homing receptors could use this mechanism to enter tissues that lymphocytes enter.[12] Experimental fusion of normal lymphocytes with nonmetastatic tumor cells confers metastatic capacity on the resulting hybrids; such fusion may occur spontaneously in vivo and result in enhanced metastatic capacity for the tumor.[14]

The metastatic potential of tumor cells also depends on their ability to degrade extracellular matrix and connective tissue, a task accomplished by elaboration of degradative enzymes such as cathepsin B, type IV collagenase, elastase, heparitinase and plasminogen activator.[7] Different tissues have different molecular distribution and localization in their extracellular matrix. Therefore specific degradative enzymes on the surface of tumor cells may dictate their ability to invade specific tissues. After tumor cells have penetrated the vessel wall, parenchymal invasion may be accomplished passively (by cell growth) or actively by increased motility related to an autocrine motility factor, although a variety of tissues possess chemotactic factors for metastatic tumors.[15] Many chemotactic factors are fragments of extracellular matrix molecules that are produced by the action of tumor-derived enzymes. Thus there is evidence for tissue specificity of tumor invasion at secondary sites. Loose connective tissue and bone are readily invaded by many malignant tumors, whereas cartilage, cornea, lens, aorta and other tissues resist invasion.[16] Resistance to invasion has been attributed to tissue structural properties and/or tissue substances that directly inhibit tumor cell invasion. In the selective invasion of a target tissue, selective target tissue adhesion and selective destruction of target tissue may be important mechanisms in addition to chemotaxis.

Multiple mechanisms may be responsible for different steps of the metastatic process. Growth of tumor cells at sites distant from the primary site appears related to their ability to respond to the site's microenvironment. Tumor cells can synthesize and secrete active growth factors (autocrine function).[17] The host response that kills neoplastic cells or prevents their growth is an important factor in metastasis. Some host cells may stimulate tumor growth, while other host effector cells may inhibit tumor growth. Activated macrophages, for example, may release substances that have natural antitumor activities.[18] Further, tumor cells may achieve organ specificity by unique responses to host microenvironments. With neoplastic progression, tumor cell diversification may result in increased multisite metastasis with less organ specificity. This malignant progression could be due to increased tumor autocrine molecules that modulate adhesion, invasion and growth.[10]

Although many cancer cells from primary tumors are released in the blood stream in humans and in animal models, comparatively few metastases result. This metastatic inefficiency is attributed to the destruction of cancer cells in the microcirculation.[19] Metastatic inefficiency appears striking in the heart, skin, spleen, intestine, and muscle; these collectively account for most of the total arterial output of the heart, yet are only sporadically the site of metastases. Cardiac metastasis is uncommon, particularly in the absence of metastases elsewhere.

In animal experiments (mice), injection of cancer cells, followed by bioassays of the lungs, liver, myocardium, and skeletal muscle, indicates that the majority of cancer cells are killed in the microcirculation of these organs within 2 to 3 minutes. Rapid tumor cell destruction suggests mechanical trauma,[11] although a variety of cellular and humoral host defense factors may also be involved. Cancer cells in the arterial circulation that pass the capillaries may emerge in venous blood in a viable state, may be arrested in the microvasculature and give rise to few metastases, or may be released slowly with loss of ability to grow. The percentage in any of these three groups depends on the type of cancer cell and the organ involved.[20] The diameter of myocardial capillaries ranges from $4.4/\mu$ in systole to $5.2/\mu$ in diastole, and myocardial blood flow during systole is greatly reduced by compressive forces within the myocardium. Rapid tumor cell destruction in the microvasculature may result from change in cell shape from spherical to sausage-shaped to pass through capillaries with smaller diameters than the cells. At constant cell volume, shape changes are accompanied by an increase in surface area. At the beginning, this is accomplished by unfolding the pleated surface membranes and later (true increase) by stretching the unfolded membranes. Stretching to achieve a 4% increase in surface area can result in an increase in membrane tension sufficient to produce membrane rupture.[19] Deformation of cancer cells in myocardial capillaries also depends on the external pressures during ventricular contraction. At approximately 4 dyne $\cdot$ cm^{-1}, 50% of some cell populations rupture.[21] Intramyocardial pressures are 120 mm Hg near the endocardium and 90 mm Hg at the epicardium in the dog, (corresponding to 3.3 and 2.2×10^5 dynes, respectively), 4 to 5 times higher than tensions required to rupture cancer cell membranes.[11]

Thus systolic compression of intraluminal cells tends to lead to their expulsion; if they remain because of adhesion to the vessel, increases in membrane tension may cause eventual rupture. Similar trauma to cancer cells has been observed in the microvasculature of skeletal muscles, supporting the hypothesis that muscle contraction can act as a rate regulator for metastasis.[11] In experimental animals, despite receiving more than twice the dose of cancer cells than the lungs, significantly fewer cancer cells survived in myocardium. Rapid cancer cell death could not be attributed to any inherent toxicity of cardiac muscle.[19] Given the biomechanical trauma to cancer cells in the myocardial microvasculature, one wonders how any metastases develop. Perhaps metastases develop in the subepicardial myocardium where mechanical trauma is minimal. Causes other than biomechanical for cancer cell trauma are not known. Organ-specific metastasis in the heart (adhesion molecules, growth factors, inhibitory host influences, etc.) is under active experimental study.

There is no consensus as to whether right-sided or left-sided, atrial or ventricular metastases predominate.[22] Nevertheless, metastatic cardiac tumors are 20 to 40 times more common than are primary tumors, and myocardial invasion by carcinoma is more frequent than by sarcoma. Carcinoma of the lung (Fig. 9-3) and of the breast, malignant melanoma, leukemia, and malignant lymphoma are encountered most often.

Tumor cells may gain access to the heart[22] through the coronary arteries, through the great veins (to implant on endocardium), via retrograde flow through cardiac lymphatic channels, and by direct extension from mediastinal tumors. Blockage of cardiac lymphatic channels by mediastinal tumor facilitates retrograde flow. Cardiac metastases from carcinoma of the lung are postulated to enter the pulmonary veins, traverse the left-sided cardiac chambers, enter the coronary arteries and subsequently implant in the myocardium; left atrial extension of bronchial carcinoma has been demonstrated with two-dimensional echocardiography[23] and MRI.[24] Alternatively, invasion of the thoracic duct with extension into the azygos septum and superior vena cava may involve the right side of the heart, and may spread through the inferior vena cava.[25]

Cardiac metastatic disease is far more common at older age; the increasing prevalence in recent years probably reflects improved tumor therapy that allows greater prolongation of life for cancer patients, with the potential for increased tumor dissemination. Additionally, more precise noninvasive diagnostic techniques may better identify cardiac metastases during life. Metastatic cardiac tumors have been described in from .1% to 6% or 7% of consecutive unselected autopsies, with the age of the population involved a major determining factor. In patients with known malignant tumor, the autopsy incidence of cardiac metastases has varied from 1% to 2% to as high as 25%.[26] Cardiac metastases are commonly associated with widespread involvement of many other organs by cancer.

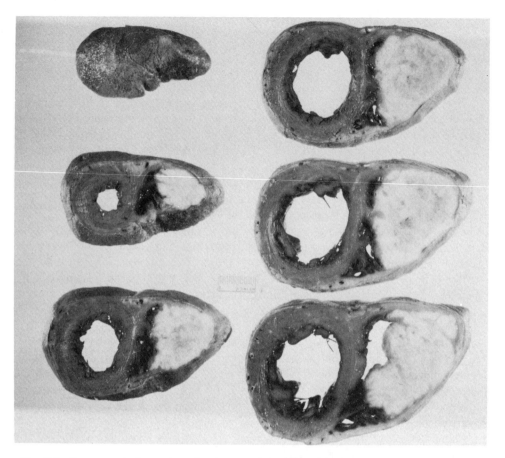

Fig. 9-3. Cross ventricular sections showing complete obliteration of the right ventricle by a metastatic bronchogenic carcinoma.

DETECTION OF TUMORS OF THE HEART

Tumors of the heart become symptomatic when they interfere with cardiac function; thus the clinical manifestations relate predominantly to the location of the tumor. Primary cardiac tumors,[27] whether benign or malignant, and metastatic cardiac tumors produce virtually identical clinical manifestations when located in comparable sites.[28,29] The presence or absence of symptoms, in a number of series, is more dependent on the location and tendency to embolize than on the size of the tumor. Extensive cardiac involvement with tumor may be present with few or no symptoms. Therefore, discussion of the pathogenesis and pathophysiology of tumors of the heart is best categorized by tumor location[30]: intracavitary (including valvular); myocardial; pericardial; and the rare but often highly symptomatic cardiac conduction system tumors.

Prior to the availability of contemporary imaging techniques, radiographic clues suggestive of cardiac tumor included an unusual or irregular cardiac silhouette (Fig. 9-4), both with and without abnormal pulsations; ectopic or unusual location of calcium deposits within the cardiac silhouette; displacement or distortion of the cardiac chambers; and intracardiac filling defects at invasive angiographic studies.

The term *benign* for a cardiac tumor refers to its histologic characteristics. Histologically benign tumors, when clinically evident, may be highly symptomatic or even lethal, related to their potential to engender arrhythmias obstruct or obliterate cardiac chambers block valvular orifices with resultant inflow or outflow obstruction to cause embolic phenomena to produce mechanical hemolysis, biochemical effects, and constitutional symptoms and produce pericardial effusion, at times with cardiac tamponade. The development of unexplained and intractable cardiac failure warrants consideration of cardiac tumor as causal.

Malignant primary tumors of the heart, when symptomatic, often have a rapid clinical course characterized by combinations of cardiac enlargement, cardiac failure, bizarre and varying arrhythmias, chest pain, hemopericardium, and occasionally sudden death. Metastatic cardiac tumors are no more frequently symptomatic than are primary tumors and are more likely to be overshadowed by

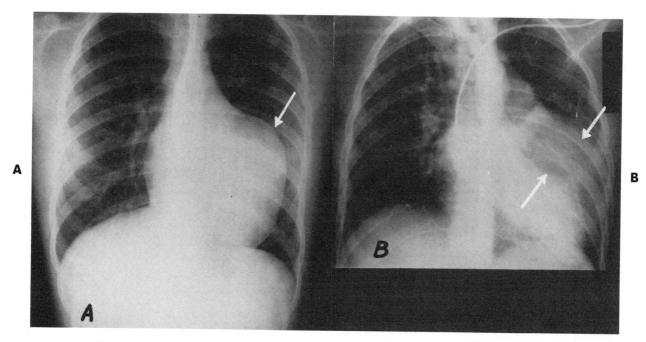

Fig. 9-4. Hamartoma of the myocardium. **(A)** Alteration of the cardiac configuration by a tumor projecting from the border of the left side of the heart *(arrow)*. **(B)** Left-sided opacification following superior vena cava injection of contrast material. A filling defect of the left atrium and left ventricle is produced by encroachment of the tumor mass *(arrow)*. (Courtesy of Department of Radiology, Emory University School of Medicine.) (From Wenger NK: *Rare causes of heart disease.* In Hurst JW, ed: *The heart*, New York, 1966, McGraw-Hill.

the systemic manifestations of the metastatic illness. Arrhythmias appear to occur more frequently with metastatic than with primary cardiac tumors and are often poorly responsive to standard antiarrhythmic therapies.

Cardiac tumors can imitate the clinical and hemodynamic presentations of a variety of cardiovascular disorders. Intracavitary tumors may present as new cardiac murmurs, nonexertional and often positional dizziness or syncope, or as evidence of pulmonary or systemic embolization. Myocardial tumors may produce unexplained heart failure (as may intracavitary tumors secondary to obstruction of blood flow), with pulmonary congestion, elevated jugular venous pressure, edema and ascites. The tumors involving the pericardium present predominantly with pericardial pain, pericardial effusion (often with a rapid increase in heart size), pericardial tamponade, or pericardial constriction when tumor fills the pericardial space. Many types of tumors may produce atrial and ventricular arrhythmias, atrioventricular block, and a variety of electrocardiographic abnormalities. However, the duration of symptoms is often short and the progression of severity more rapid than usual for the disease process that is simulated.[29]

Early tumor detection and identification is important, given the good prognosis when benign tumors are resected. Even with extensive resection, the prognosis for malignant tumors is uniformly poor.[2] Once tumor is suspected by noninvasive imaging techniques, endomyocar-dial biopsy may enable a histopathologic diagnosis that is needed to guide therapy.[31]

GENERAL CLUES SUGGESTING CARDIAC TUMORS

Combinations of symptoms, physical findings, and laboratory data incompatible with usual cardiovascular lesions, e.g., a bizarre or atypical clinical presentation, warrants inclusion of cardiac tumor in the differential diagnosis. Otherwise, unexplained cardiac findings in a patient known to have a malignant neoplasm makes the consideration of cardiac tumor a less obscure possibility.

Further, sudden onset of severe, unrelenting, and rapidly progressive cardiac failure without apparent cause should suggest cardiac tumor, often malignant. The fulminant illness often terminates with sudden death.

INTRACAVITARY TUMORS
General presentations
Primary tumors

The majority of benign primary cardiac tumors are intracavitary in location[27] recognition of their clinical and hemodynamic presentations is important because surgical cure is often possible. Myxomas are the most common primary tumor type and account for about half of all benign tumors of the heart. Intracavitary cardiac tumors occur predominantly in the atria; the clinical manifestations reflect either acute or chronic impairment of either filling or

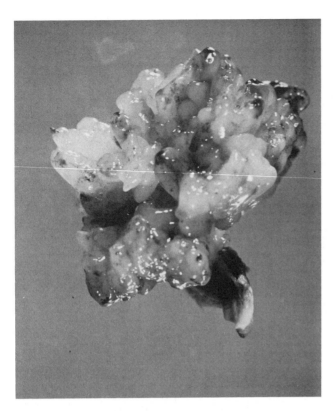

Fig. 9-5. Left atrial myxoma with irregular variegated surface and multiple finger-like projections.

emptying of a cardiac chamber.[32] As such, clinical findings of intracavitary tumors may mimic valvular heart disease (predominantly valvular blockade), or obstruction of flow through a cardiac chamber. The symptoms and murmurs often vary more with position than do classical valvular lesions and the speed of development of hemodynamically significant disease is typically more rapid. The de novo appearance of what is characteristically a congenital cardiac lesion, e.g., pulmonic stenosis, should suggest cardiac tumor. Intracavitary tumors are associated with a high incidence of pulmonary and systemic thromboembolic complications. The clinical manifestations (symptoms and physical findings) are unique to the specific intracavitary location of the tumor. Venous thrombosis may occur, as may pulmonary hypertension, depending on the intracavitary location of the tumor; pulmonary emboli from right heart tumors and pulmonary venous hypertension from left atrial or left ventricular obstruction may be causal. Pulmonary infarction secondary to pulmonary venous occlusion by left atrial myxoma has also occurred.[33] Although embolic phenomena suggest an intracavitary tumor, the symptoms may also mimic infectious endocarditis. Multiple embolic episodes in patients with sinus rhythm should suggest intracavitary tumor. Less commonly, microscopic examination of an arterial embolus may identify its source as a cardiac tumor.

Primary atrial tumors, other than myxomas, are typically sessile. Fibromas, lipomas, angiomas, and teratomas, are either asymptomatic or produce evidence of obstruction to blood flow dependent on their location. An exception is sarcoma, which is discussed subsequently (see right atrial tumors).

Nonprolapsing intracavitary tumors may produce symptoms by obstructing semilunar valve orifices or pulmonary venous inflow, often in the absence of cardiac murmurs. In this instance, the clinical presentation is that of heart failure, occasionally in association with arrhythmias, with characteristic elevation of the jugular venous pressure, edema, hepatomegaly, ascites, and at times evidence of pulmonary and systemic embolism. Echocardiography and other imaging techniques can provide the diagnosis.

Metastatic tumors

Metastatic tumor situated on the endocardium or the cardiac valves is less common because, these areas are relatively avascular; however, a papilloma of the right aortic valve cusp is described to occlude the right coronary ostium, producing chest pain and sudden death.[34] Metastatic tumor, when present, probably occurs by direct implantation, possibly on an abnormal endothelium. Intracavitary metastases may embolize, mimicking both myxoma and infectious endocarditis. The pattern of blood flow typically determines the location of intracavitary metastatic tumors, which probably are implanted via the great veins. Right atrial metastases from carcinoma of the thyroid, the bronchus, the testis and the kidney commonly invade via the vena cavae; whereas metastases to the left atrium, typically from bronchogenic carcinoma, characteristically invade via the pulmonary veins. When there is metastatic involvement of the atria, supraventricular tachyarrhythmias which are often resistant to antiarrhythmic drugs, may be present. Progression of symptoms with intracavitary metastatic tumors is typically more rapid and relentless than with primary benign tumors.

Left atrial tumors

Left atrial tumors are clinically manifested by signs and symptoms of obstruction of the pulmonary circulation. Myxomas, which constitute one-third to one-half of all primary cardiac tumors, are the most common intracavitary tumors and the prototype for left atrial obstruction.

Myxomas: age relationships

About three fourths of myxomas are located in the left atrium, with most others occurring in the right atrium, although biatrial tumors can occur.[2] Myxomas are rare in childhood and almost unknown in infancy. Among adults, sporadic cardiac myxomas occur three times more commonly in women. Familial occurrence is reported with greater likelihood of multiple tumors when there is familial incidence.[35] Atrial myxoma has also been described in elderly patients[36] in whom it is often misdiagnosed as a more common etiology of heart failure and stroke.

Myxomas: anatomic characteristics

The anatomic characteristics of the tumor explain the clinical manifestations. Myxomas are typically gelatinous, mucoid tumors that arise on a pedicle from the interatrial septum, usually originating near the fossa ovalis, but at times arising from other sites in the atrium. (Figs. 9-5 and 9-6) Thrombi may be present on the tumor surface. The gross appearance of a myxoma is characterized by a smooth surface, gray to white in color, with focal hemorrhagic areas and a gelatinous lucent cut surface. However, on scanning electron microscopy, the myxoma surface has numerous clefts and crevices and is covered by a continuous cellular lining apparently derived from underlying myxoma cells. By scanning electron microscopy, the cut surface reveals a stroma with a sponge-like architecture permeated by mucopolysaccharides in which reticular fibers form lacunae.[37] Light microscopic features include a myxomatous stroma, with varying cellularity and stromal cells of either stellate or polygonal shape. The cells are arranged singly or in groups, often in close apposition to vascular structures. Cellular cords or clusters usually reveal delicate interdigitating cell processes. The nuclei of myxoma cells are often round or oval and generally uniform; the cytoplasm is scant, eosinophilic and often vacuolated (lipidic cells) (Fig. 9-7). Mitoses are extremely rare. Lymphocytes, macrophages, neutrophils, foci of hematopoiesis, and areas of calcification are often present. Rarely, myxoma cells form glandular or cyst-like spaces filled with amorphous material. The stroma is composed of

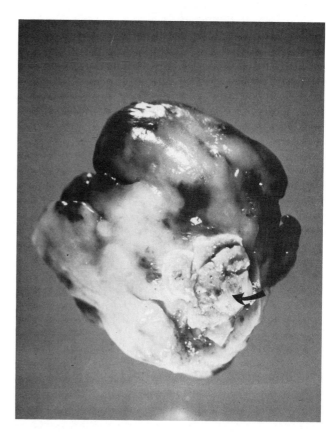

Fig. 9-6. Left atrial myxoma (5.5 cm × 5 cm × 4.5 cm) attached to the interatrial septum with a relatively broad-based pedicle *(arrow).*

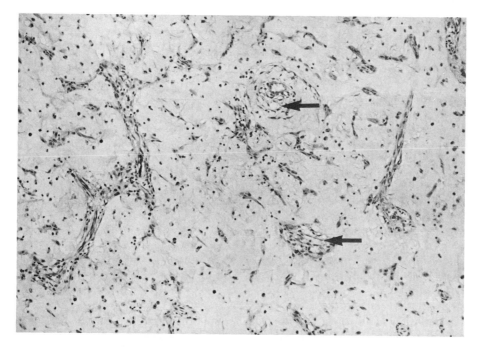

Fig. 9-7. Section from an atrial myxoma showing abundance of ground substance, stellate cells, and lipidic cells *(arrows)* forming pseudochannels.

mucopolysaccharides, collagen, and reticular and elastic fibers. The mucopolysaccharides consist primarily of chondroitin sulfate A and/or C, not hyaluronic acid. There is evidence that myxoma cells can actively synthesize glycosaminoglycans and proteoglycans intracellularly.[38]

Myxoma cells have abundant cytoplasmic organelles on electron microscopy, prominent rough endoplasmic reticulum and Golgi apparatus, intracytoplasmic filaments and discontinuous basement membranes. Stromal myxoma cells do not stain positive for factor VIII. Immunohistochemical studies have shown myxoma cells to be positive for vimentin and S100 (a marker for chondromatous differentiation) and negative for myoglobin; apparently only the myxoma cells are neoplastic.[39] Based on immunohistochemical studies, myxomas probably arise from multipotential mesenchymal cells with the potential to differentiate along several cell lines,[40] including endothelial cells, smooth muscle cells, fibroblasts, myofibroblasts, chondroid cells and lipidic cells. However, such potential is evidence of differentiation rather than histogenesis.

Myxomas: evidence of neoplasia

Overwhelming evidence indicates that myxomas are true neoplasms rather than organized thrombi, but uncertainty remains about their histogenesis. Tissue culture studies of myxoma cells showed them to have neoplastic characteristics, further negating the concept that myxomas were highly organized thrombi.[41] Histochemical studies and immunoreactivity of myxomas confirm the cellular heterogeneity of these tumors, compatible with their origin from primitive multipotential mesenchymal cells.[42] Although the overwhelming majority of cardiac myxomas are benign, a few may present a wide spectrum of malignancy manifested either by recurrence, metastasis or both. While repeated embolic episodes may not necessarily result in metastasis, local growth of a myxoma embolus through the arterial wall of a distant organ, resulting in the formation of metastasis, has been reported.[43] "Metastases" of cardiac myxomas are described particularly in those arising from sites other than the interatrial septum.[44]

Myxomas: anatomic—clinical correlations

The friable character of the tumor, coupled with the pedunculated attachment that renders the tumor mobile, are the basis for the high prevalence of systemic tumor emboli; the length of the pedicle determines the extent of tumor mobility. The tumors vary greatly in size, from 1/2 cm to 8 cm, averaging 5.5 cm, and calcification of the tumor may occur. In one series, large tumor size best correlated with the number and type of associated clinical and laboratory abnormalities,[45] although embolism correlated best with tumor consistency. Because of the pedunculated character of the myxoma, ball-valve obstruction of the mitral valve is frequent, with the resulting symptoms and signs simulating mitral stenosis. Smaller tumors, prolapsing between the atrium and ventricle, may deform the mitral valve or mitral annulus with resultant mitral regurgita-

tion. A mobile calcified atrial myxoma may destroy the mitral valve leaflet or cause chordae tendineae rupture with resultant severe mitral regurgitation. The mobility of calcified myxomas can be appreciated at fluoroscopy. Occasionally, myxomas can rapidly increase in size, due to hemorrhage within the tumor. Diagnosis of myxoma has occasionally been made by histologic examination of an arterial embolus.

Myxomas: symptom triad

A classic triad of obstructive, embolic, and constitutional symptoms is described with atrial myxoma.[46,47] This broad spectrum of manifestations requires differentiation from a large number of clinical problems. Acute paroxysmal dyspnea, cough, hemoptysis, and pulmonary edema, often with acute circulatory failure and shock, may occur from blockage of the mitral orifice. Other presenting clinical manifestations of sudden valvular obstruction include syncope, at times with seizures, related to cerebral hypoperfusion; coma; cyanosis; gangrene of the extremities; and less commonly, episodic bizarre behavior. The episodic nature of the dyspnea, dizziness, syncope, or seizures, often varying with positional change and relieved by recumbency, without relationship to physical effort, constitutes an important clue. Angina may result from the decrease in cardiac output, with episodic symptoms more related to changes in the patient's posture than to activity intensity; particularly syncope, but also angina, appears ominous, warning of sudden cardiac death.[48] Rarely, sudden death is the initial presentation. Palpitations, as evidence of arrhythmia, may not be positionally related.

Tumor embolization occurs in about half of patients with atrial myxoma; rarely there is embolization of the complete tumor. Tumor emboli, at least in part, appear related to contact of the tumor with the mitral valve leaflet and, on occasion, with the ventricular septum. Some embolic manifestations may mimic infectious endocarditis, because of the associated fever, cardiac murmur and elevated sedimentation rate. Tumor embolism to the coronary artery may cause myocardial infarction or coronary arterial aneurysmal dilatation. Tumor embolism to the central nervous system[49] causes stroke, with a resultant neurologic deficit; embolic stroke in a young adult with sinus rhythm should raise suspicion of a left atrial myxoma. Monocular blindness or visual defects have occurred from tumor emboli to the retinal artery, predominantly left-sided, related to the branching pattern of the left internal carotid artery from the aorta. Intracranial arterial aneurysms have resulted from myxomatous emboli, and late rupture has been described, even after tumor resection.

The nonspecific or constitutional manifestations that occur in most patients with atrial myxoma may relate to multiple emboli or may reflect an autoimmune response to the tumor. Fatigue, malaise, anorexia, weight loss, occasional cachexia, low-grade fever, arthralgia, clubbing, Raynaud's phenomenon and the like may erroneously suggest the diagnosis of infectious endocarditis, collagen vascular disease or other vasculitis, or myocarditis. The presence of a cardiac murmur often leads to an incorrect diagnosis of acute rheumatic fever.

As is the case with many clinical symptoms, the physical findings: heart rate, blood pressure, and auscultatory findings of the cardiac murmurs, may vary with change in position. The first heart sound is accentuated (as with mitral stenosis), but is frequently widely split, with the second component delayed. The delay in mitral valve closure corresponds to the time of tumor expulsion from the ventricle through the mitral orifice to return to the left atrium. There is an accentuated pulmonic component of the second heart sound when pulmonary hypertension is present. Both the apical systolic and diastolic murmurs often vary in character with time and particularly with change in position. With pulmonary hypertension, the "a" wave of the jugular venous pulse may become prominent. The apical diastolic murmur may vary from a rumble to a high-pitched whoop, but most important is the disproportionate intensity of the cardiac murmur to the degree of functional impairment. An early diastolic sound, the so-called "tumor plop," (Fig. 9-8) is heard from 80 ms to 120 ms after aortic closure. It may be confused with an opening snap of mitral stenosis, exhibit disparity between the timing of the tumor plop and severity of the clinical symptoms, or may be confused with an S_3 because of its low pitch and timing following A_2 (intermediate between that usual for an opening snap and a third heart sound). It remains controversial whether this sound is due to sudden tension on the tumor stalk at the end of its excursion or whether it reflects the impact of the tumor against the myocardium. Endocardial sounds are described, presumably reflecting contact of the tumor with either the atrial or ventricular endocardium; these may mimic a friction rub. A tricuspid valve honk due to severe pulmonary hypertension and secondary tricuspid regurgitation disappeared with removal of a left atrial myxoma and resolution of the pulmonary hypertension.[50] If the tumor prevents valve closure, a murmur of mitral regurgitation may be heard. The occurrence of clubbing may factitiously suggest congenital heart disease.

Myxomas: differentiation from mitral stenosis

To summarize, the important clinical features that help differentiate left atrial myxoma from mitral stenosis[1] include absence of a history of rheumatic fever, intermittency of the signs and symptoms, relatively short clinical history with sudden onset and rapid progression of symptoms, absence of atrial fibrillation, and particularly the lack of correlation between severity of symptoms, physical findings, and roentgenologic examination. Further features suggesting myxoma include prominent positional variations in the murmurs, blood pressure, heart rate, and symptoms; often there is marked and immediate symptomatic improvement on assuming the recumbent position. Similarly, syncope is positional. An opening snap is either

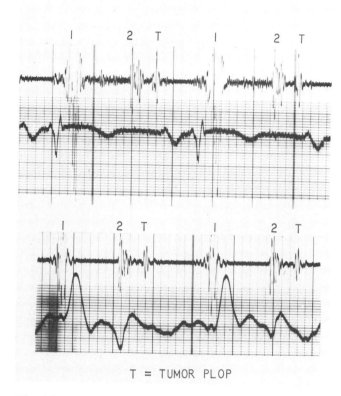

LEFT ATRIAL MYXOMA

T = TUMOR PLOP

Fig. 9-8. "Tumor plop," or opening snap, in a case of left atrial myxoma. (Courtesy of Dr. B.W. Cobbs, Jr.) (From Wenger NK: *Rare causes of heart disease.* In Hurst JW, ed: *The heart,* New York, 1966, McGraw-Hill.).

absent or there is disparity between the timing of the opening snap (tumor plop) and the clinical symptoms, and the "tumor plop" may be far more low-pitched than a usual opening snap. Incongruities such as an inordinately early third heart sound associated with apical systolic murmur of mitral regurgitation, or an unusually late and low pitched "opening snap" associated with an apical diastolic rumble compatible with severe mitral stenosis, should suggest that the sound is a "tumor plop" of atrial myxoma. The persistence of sinus rhythm in association with symptoms suggesting severe mitral stenosis, and often a third heart sound, belie the diagnosis of mitral stenosis. Intracardiac calcification, when present, is not in the area of the mitral valve as seen with mitral stenosis, but in an unusual location within the cardiac silhouette.

Myxomas: laboratory data

Laboratory test abnormalities of an elevated erythrocyte sedimentation rate, leukocytosis, anemia, and an elevated serum immunoglobulin concentration, predominantly IgG, may reflect autoimmune responses[51] either to tumor emboli, to degenerative changes in the tumor, or to myocardial changes related to the tumor. Anemia is likely due to mechanical hemolysis. Polycythemia, paradoxically, may

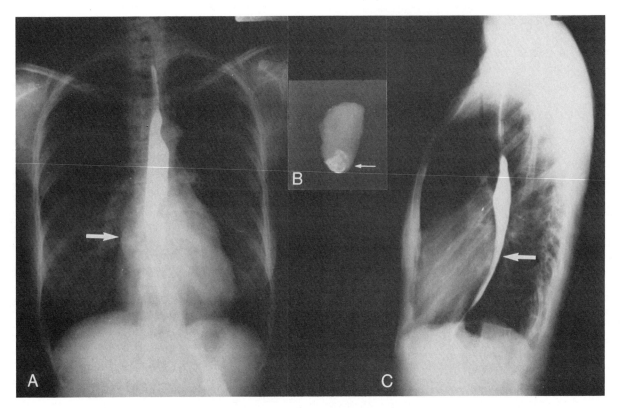

Fig. 9-9. Mitral configuration of the heart due to a calcified left atrial myxoma. **(A)** Left atrial enlargement, with visible right border of the left atrium *(arrow)*. **(B)** X-ray of surgical specimen, showing calcification of the myxoma *(arrow)*. **(C)** Indentation of the esophagus by the enlarged left atrium *(arrow)*. (Courtesy of Department of Radiology, Emory University School of Medicine.) From Wenger NK: *Rare causes of heart disease*. Hurst JW, ed: *The heart*, New York, 1966, McGraw-Hill.

be present if the tumor produces erythropoietin.[52] The chest roentgenogram may show left atrial enlargement, changes of pulmonary hypertension or pulmonary venous congestion, and at times intermittent pulmonary edema, all equally compatible with mitral stenosis (Fig. 9-9). An abnormal cardiac silhouette, at times with ectopic calcification, may suggest the presence of an intracardiac tumor (Fig. 9-10). Electrocardiographic changes are frequent but nonspecific; there may be intermittent arrhythmias, particularly atrial fibrillation or flutter, abnormal P waves, conduction defects, repolarization abnormalities, and the like.

Myxomas: imaging techniques and diagnosis

Initial diagnosis is typically made by an echocardiogram[53] that shows an essentially normal mitral valve, although mitral regurgitation can occasionally be present. With a mobile myxoma, there may be a decreased E-F slope of the anterior mitral leaflet, and a dense mass of tumor echoes may be evident behind the mitral leaflet on M-mode echocardiography. A characteristic echo-free space at the onset of diastole reflects the time needed for the myxoma to prolapse through the mitral orifice (Fig. 9-11). Tumor echoes can be seen in the left atrium during ventricular systole. The two-dimensional echocardiogram[45] (Fig. 9-12) can identify not only mobile left atrial myxo-

mas but also nonprolapsing ones. Two-dimensional echocardiography aids in identifying multiple atrial myxomas, defining the relationship to the atrial septum, and helps differentiate other left atrial masses from atrial myxomas. Doppler echocardiography, which can delineate the hemodynamic consequences, has shown mild mitral regurgitation to be common following surgical removal of the tumor.[54] Precise identification comparable to two-dimensional echocardiography, with characterization of tumor size, shape, mobility, and site of attachment, can be obtained with gated radionuclide imaging, cine-computed tomography (CT),[55] and magnetic resonance imaging. MRI enables high-resolution tomography in three dimensions and can generate intravascular and soft tissue contrast without the need for contrast medium (Fig. 9-13). Both echocardiography and MRI have limitations; with echocardiography, there is significant interference by bone and lungs, particularly in patients with obstructive pulmonary disease or narrow rib spaces. MRI cannot identify calcium, therefore calcification of a mass or other mediastinal structures is better identified by computed tomography.[56] Preoperative cardiac catheterization is indicated only to exclude concomitant coronary atherosclerosis in patients of the appropriate age group; occasionally, coronary occlu-

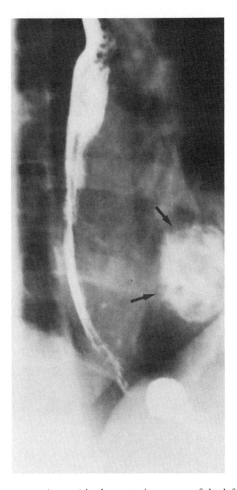

Fig. 9-10. Calcified tumor mass *(arrow)* in the posterior aspect of the left atrium. At fluoroscopy this mass moved freely in a superior-inferior axis within the cardiac silhouette. The tumor has been known to be present for at least 15 years and is thought to represent a calcified myxoma in a completely asymptomatic patient. (Courtesy of Department of Radiology, Emory University School of Medicine.) (From Wenger NK: *Rare causes of heart disease.* In Hurst JW, ed: *The heart, New York,* 1966, McGraw-Hill.

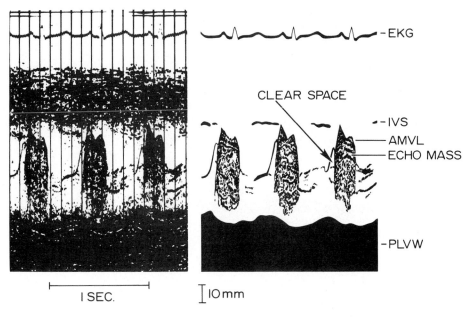

Fig. 9-11. M-mode echocardiogram: left atrial myxoma. Note mass of echoes behind the anterior mitral valve leaflet, preceded by the characteristic clear or echo-free space. (Courtesy of Dr. J. Ferlner.) From Wenger NK: *Cardiac tumors.* In Hurst JW, ed: *The heart,* New York, 1978, McGraw-Hill.

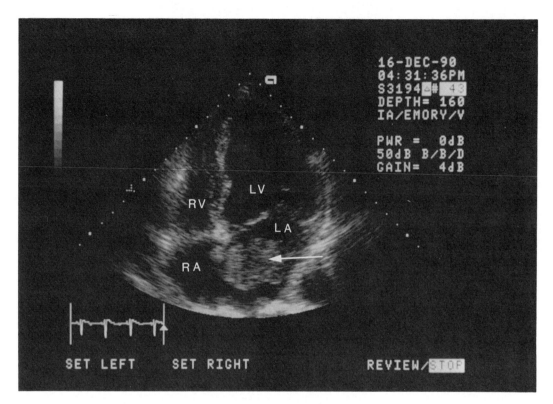

Fig. 9-12. Two-dimensional echocardiogram of a 32-year-old woman. This apical four-chamber view during diastole shows a large mass *(arrow)* within the left atrium attached to the interatrial septum. LA = left atrium; RA = right atrium; LV = left ventricle; RV = right ventricle.

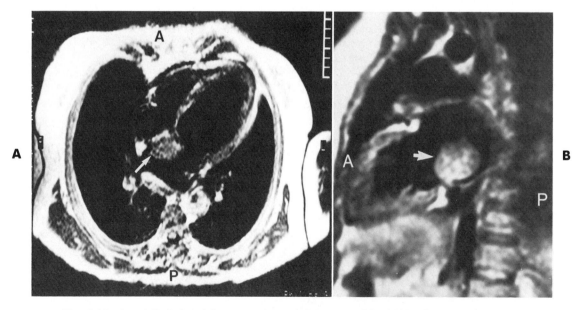

Fig. 9-13. A and **B,** Left atrial myxoma *(arrow)* demonstrated by MRI. (Courtesy of Dr. R.I. Pettigrew, Department of Radiology, Emory University School of Medicine)

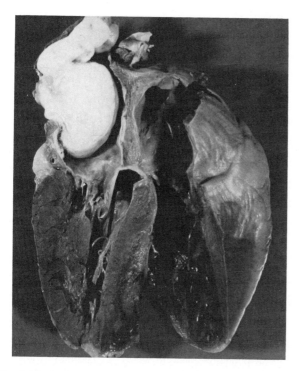

Fig. 9-14. A 38-year-old woman presenting with uncontrollable epistaxis found to have pulmonary hypertension. She died from cardiopulmonary arrest. A firm, grayish-white tumor arising from the posterolateral left atrial wall was present, filling the entire atrial chamber. Note extension of the neoplasm (leiomyosarcoma) to the pulmonary veins.

sion or aneurysm secondary to tumor emboli may be evident. It is more difficult to diagnose a nonprolapsing intracavitary atrial myxoma, which either impedes flow across the mitral valve[57] or obstructs pulmonary venous return; both may result in left atrial hypertension, pulmonary venous hypertension, pulmonary congestion, and eventually pulmonary arterial hypertension and right-sided cardiac failure, clinically indistinguishable from valvular mitral stenosis. Wide resection of the tumor stalk is recommended to limit the risk of tumor recurrence.

Myxomas: characteristics of recurrent types

Although myxomas are generally curable by surgical resection, recurrence rates of 5% to 14% have been reported.[58,59] Earlier data about recurrence rates did not discriminate between sporadic myxomas and those of the familial types. Recurrences are more likely and may occur rapidly with what has been termed "syndrome" cardiac myxoma, rather than the sporadic type.[60] In recent years, two types of cardiac myxoma have been recognized: a sporadic type occurs in patients older than 40 years of age and is characterized by a single left atrial tumor; a "syndrome myxoma" occurs in a unique subset of patients and constitutes 5% to 7% of all patients with cardiac myxoma.[61] These syndrome myxomas tend to have multicentric origin of the myxomas and have more recurrent myxomas. Familial myxoma may be one expression of syndrome myxoma;

both appear to be transmitted as an autosomal dominant trait. This syndrome is characterized by a complex of multiple cardiac myxomas, often familial occurrence and occurrence at younger age, equal sex distribution, spotty skin pigmentation, endocrine overactivity with endocrine tumors, cutaneous myxomas and myxoid breast fibroadenomas. Close surveillance of the patient with serial echocardiography and laboratory testing for serum protein levels, hemoglobin concentration and erythrocyte sedimentation rate abnormalities, as well as screening of family members or cardiac myxoma is recommended.[61-64]

Osteosarcomas

Cardiac osteosarcomas are prone to locate in the left atrium or mitral valve, (also a common site for myxomas), in contrast to angiosarcomas of the heart, which have a predilection for the right atrium or ventricle. Several osteosarcomas have been clinically mistaken for myxomas with calcification, although the amount of calcification in some osteosarcomas was minimal.[65]

Right atrial tumors

Clinical presentations

Right atrial intracavitary tumors present evidence of inflow obstruction (Fig. 9-14). Dyspnea is common, and intermittent cyanosis may be present, often varying with body position. Similarly, dizziness and syncope, as evidence of a decreased cardiac output, may be intermittent and posturally related. The evaluation of unexplained pulmonary emboli or unexplained pulmonary hypertension should include consideration of right heart tumors and their embolization. The rapid progression of right-sided cardiac failure, unresponsive to usual therapy, should suggest right atrial tumor. With pulmonary and right-sided hypertension, right-to-left (at times intermittent) shunting may occur through a patent foramen ovale, with resulting cyanosis.

Myxomas: anatomic—clinical relationships

Right atrial myxomas can originate from a variety of atrial sites, often have a broader attachment to the atrial wall (Fig. 9-15), and are generally larger and more solid than left atrial myxomas. There may be evidence of pulmonary embolization and constitutional symptoms including fever, sweating, and weight loss, although the systemic manifestations are less prominent than with left atrial myxoma. This distinction has raised speculation that substances released from the tumor into the circulation are in some way inactivated during passage through the lung. The classical findings are those of severe right-sided heart failure with systemic venous hypertension, often mimicking constrictive pericarditis. There is elevation of the jugular venous pressure, often with a prominent "a" wave, with pleural effusion, hepatomegaly, ascites, and peripheral edema. Virtually all patients have a cardiac murmur and some have a friction rub. The murmur typically simulates tricuspid stenosis, with the diastolic rumble often ac-

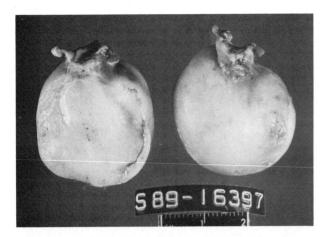

Fig. 9-15. A 74-year-old woman was evaluated for symptoms of coronary heart disease. An echocardiogram revealed a right atrial tumor attached to the right atrial wall by a broad base pedicle. It measured 4 cm × 3.5 cm × 2.5 cm, was moderately firm and encapsulated.

centuated by inspiration. Early systolic tricuspid regurgitation, due to tumor keeping the tricuspid valve open, may also manifest inspiratory accentuation. Palpable tumor shocks and concomitant audible tumor plops at the lower left sternal border and xiphisternum probably reflect tumor impact against a cardiac chamber wall or cardiac valve; this may be associated with a loud early systolic sound, corresponding to tumor expulsion from the right ventricle.[66] The murmurs of both tricuspid stenosis and regurgitation are produced de novo by a large, mobile right atrial metastatic tumor that extends into the right ventricular outflow tract in diastole.[67] Both the murmur and the elevation of the jugular venous pressure may vary with changes in posture. However, the acute onset of tricuspid stenosis is unusual, and acute development of isolated tricuspid stenosis should suggest right atrial myxoma. Occurrence of right-sided heart failure, often with arrhythmias, may mimic the Ebstein anomaly, but this diagnosis is usually suspected earlier in life and the progression of symptoms is more gradual. Alternately, there may be confusion with a superior vena caval syndrome because of the facial edema, cyanosis, distended neck veins, dilated superficial collateral veins, and edema of the upper extremities. Congenital heart disease may be erroneously diagnosed when both cyanosis and clubbing are present.[68] Carcinoid tumor may be suggested by the paroxysmal symptoms and the new right-sided cardiac murmurs. Even without damage to the tricuspid valve, a systolic murmur of tricuspid regurgitation may be present when the tumor mass interferes with tricuspid valve closure. Alternately, a prolapsing calcified or very large right atrial myxoma may cause destruction of the tricuspid valve leaflet or leaflets,[69] producing massive tricuspid regurgitation evident by a large "v" wave in the jugular venous pulse. Valve repair may be required when the tumor is excised.

Myxomas: laboratory data

Suggestive laboratory test abnormalities are as with left atrial myxoma, except that hemolytic anemia is more common, caused by the often calcified right atrial myxomas. Electrocardiographic abnormalities include evidence of right atrial abnormality, typically with either right ventricular hypertrophy or right bundle branch block. Early postoperative disappearance of the right atrial abnormality on the electrocardiogram is described. Both right atrial and right ventricular enlargement are characteristic on the chest roentgenogram, but pulmonary vascular congestion is absent despite the clinical manifestations of severe right-sided heart failure. As with left atrial myxoma, ectopic intracardiac calcification is not unusual.

Myxomas: imaging techniques and diagnosis

Echocardiography can document the presence and behavior of the right atrial tumor, with M-mode echocardiography showing a dense mass of echoes behind the tricuspid valve in diastole. At times, the myxoma may not return to the right atrium until early systole. Delineation of both tumor size and tumor movement is best accomplished by two-dimensional echocardiography, or can be documented with other imaging techniques such as radionuclide studies or magnetic resonance imaging (Fig. 9-16).

In one patient with a right atrial mass on transthoracic echocardiography, an attachment to the septal leaflet of the tricuspid valve was evident on transesophageal echocardiography[70] the tumor was a valvular hamartoma.

Sarcomas: anatomic characteristics

Primary cardiac sarcomas occur preponderantly on the right side of the heart, with a predilection for the right atrium. They occur more commonly in men. They differ from myxomas (which occur more commonly in the left atrium), in that they more frequently fill the entire atrial chamber, obstruct the superior vena cava or tricuspid valve, extend into the pericardium and cause pericardial tamponade, and less often have the ball-valve type obstruction seen with myxomas. In addition, inferior vena caval obstruction is less frequent.

Histologic variations of angiosarcomas are common (Figs. 9-17, and 9-18). Although some appear anaplastic or non-vasoformative variants, others may present a deceptively innocuous appearance difficult to differentiate from a benign hemangioma. Myxosarcomas are usually intracavitary and do not exclusively originate from the right atrium. Identification of myxosarcomas is difficult because they may simulate benign atrial myxomas preoperatively. Furthermore, a myxomatous gross appearance does not necessarily indicate myxosarcoma or myxoma, because other sarcomas may contain a myxomatous matrix (as occurs with leiomyosarcomas). Thus the preoperative diagnosis does not always indicate malignancy, although most myxosarcomas, which are sessile, are symptomatic because of invasion of underlying structures.[71] Microscopically, they resemble cardiac myxomas, although they ex-

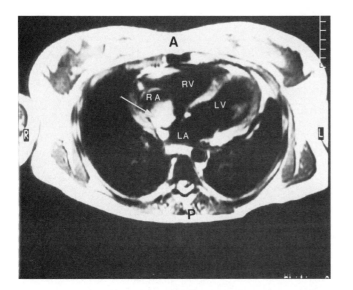

Fig. 9-16. Right atrial myxoma *(arrow)* demonstrated by MRI. (Courtesy of Department of Radiology, Emory University School of Medicine.)

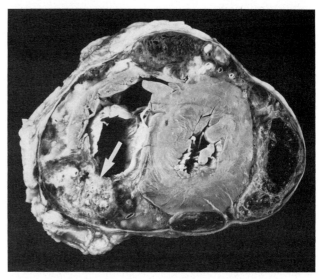

Fig. 9-17. Cross section of the heart (midventricle level) shows a hemorrhagic, partially necrotic neoplasm completely encasing the heart. This angiosarcoma most probably arose from the right ventricle *(arrow)*. (Courtesy of Dr. William D. Edwards, Mayo Clinic).

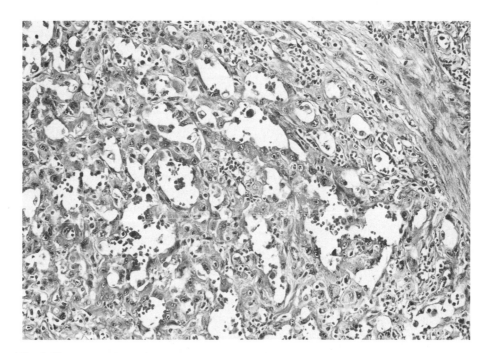

Fig. 9-18. Poorly differentiated mesenchymal neoplasm forming vascular channels. In areas, this angiosarcoma consisted of bands of spindle cells *(right upper corner)*.

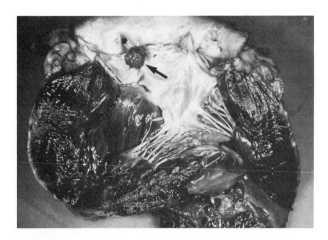

Fig. 9-19. Left ventricular view showing a round mulberry-like fibroelastoma (approximately 1.5 cm) attached to the left coronary cusp of the aortic valve.

hibit mitotic activity, cellular atypia, and foci of necrosis. It is generally agreed that sarcomas with myxomatous features arise de novo and do not represent malignant transformation of a myxoma to myxosarcoma.

Sarcomas: clinical characteristics

The typical clinical presentation includes chest pain and heart failure, at times with hemoptysis, and evidence of cardiac enlargement. These manifestations require differentiation from conditions such as myocardial infarction, pericarditis of varied etiology, pulmonary embolism, and aortic dissection. Sarcomas grow extremely rapidly, and the heart failure has an accelerated and relentless course. These tumors often produce rapidly changing cardiac contours on the chest roentgenogram. Unfortunately, metastatic disease is often already present at the time of tumor diagnosis.[2]

Left ventricular tumors

Tumor types

Intracavitary left ventricular tumors may mimic left ventricular outflow tract obstruction or aortic valve stenosis. Myxomas and fibromas, (which more commonly arise from the heart valves), are the most common tumors. Valvular fibromas or fibroelastomas are more commonly recognized after age 50. Mitral valve (ventricular aspect) rhabdomyoma has also caused evidence of subaortic stenosis.[72] A papillary fibroelastoma of the aortic valve, prolapsing into the right coronary ostium, has resulted in myocardial ischemia and infarction.[73] Other such tumors, (which more often involve the aortic valve), have, despite their small size, produced angina or sudden death; cerebral and other embolic complications are also described. The mechanism for systemic embolization is speculated to be detachment of delicate fronds; alternately, the tumor may serve as a nidus for platelet-fibrin aggregation that subsequently embolizes.

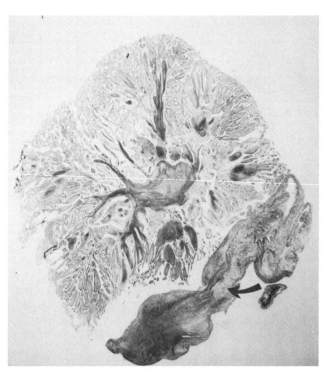

Fig. 9-20. A section from a papillary fibroelastoma attached to a pulmonary cusp *(arrow)*. Note that the lesion resembles a sea anemone, has a central fibroelastic core, and multiple arborizations. From a 58-year-old man with pulmonary hypertension.

Fibroelastomas

Papillary fibroelastomas constitute 5% to 10% of all benign cardiac tumors and most frequently arise from heart valves, but may originate from any endocardial surface. In one autopsy series, the distribution of 45 fibroelastomas was: aortic valve 15 (Fig. 9-19), tricuspid valve 9, pulmonic valve 8, mitral valve 7, right atrium 2, right ventricle 2, left ventricular septum 1, and left atrium 1. Multiple fibroelastomas have been repeatedly reported. Although *papillary fibroelastoma* is the accepted term that accurately describes the gross and histologic appearance, terms used in the past include *cardiac papilloma papillary endocardial fibroma, papillary myxoma,* and *myxofibroma.* Papillary fibroelastomas are composed of many fronds with minute filiform surface projections and are attached to the valvular or mural endocardium by a short stalk (Fig. 9-20). They vary in size from less than 1 cm to as large as 2 cm to 3 cm. Microscopically, a fibroelastic core is surrounded by a myxomatous-appearing ground substance (Alcian-positive) and covered by endothelial cells. Occasional scattered smooth muscle cells may be present within the mucopolysaccharide matrix.

Theories about the histogenesis of valvular tumors (hamartomatous, neoplastic, congenital, thrombogenic) remain controversial. Some authors have suggested that fibroelastomas are hamartomas, whereas others believe they are true neoplasms. Perhaps another pathogenetic mechanism for formation of these papillary lesions should be considered. In one of our cases, histochemical studies with the immunoperoxidase method demonstrated fibrin within the core of the fronds, suggesting a possible thrombogenic origin. Our patient, who had pulmonary hypertension, had a fibroelastoma on one cusp of the pulmonary valve. We hypothesized that hemodynamic turbulence may have been the initiating factor.

Clinical presentation

The clinical presentation of left ventricular tumors characteristically involves combinations of chest pain, syncope, otherwise unexplained neurologic deficits, and/or heart failure. Syncope is described as more frequent with left ventricular myxomas than with other cardiac tumors. Evidence of hemodynamic obstruction is often less prominent than with atrial tumors; constitutional symptoms are also less evident. Peripheral arterial embolus occurs occasionally.[74] There are rare reports of coronary embolism; relapsing and remitting neurologic symptoms due to cerebral emboli mimicked multiple sclerosis in one patient.[75] With mobile left ventricular tumors, the evidence of left ventricular outflow obstruction, the intensity of the murmur, and often the blood pressure, will vary with position. Left ventricular hypertrophy is often evident on the electrocardiogram, and less often abnormalities suggesting myocardial ischemia. Occasionally left ventricular enlargement is present on the chest x-ray. Sarcoma has been described as resulting in both inflow and outflow left ventricular obstruction, and also in fatal obstruction of the the coronary ostia.[76] Echocardiography and other noninvasive imaging techniques with high resolution can delineate tumor movement and confirm the diagnosis.[77] Differentiation from left ventricular thrombi is challenging; a combination of imaging techniques can produce supplementary information.

Right ventricular tumors

Tumor types and clinical presentation

Right ventricular tumors may also present with syncope (often postural) related to intermittent right ventricular outflow obstruction. Otherwise, unexplained fever may be present, again raising question of infectious endocarditis when a new murmur is also heard. Myxomas can simulate pulmonic stenosis, but the onset of a murmur late in life is unusual with congenital heart disease, and the severity of symptoms is excessive compared with the clinical signs of right ventricular outflow obstruction. Rhabdomyoma, the most common cardiac tumor in infancy, may also cause right ventricular outflow tract obstruction and simulate pulmonic stenosis. Rhabdomyosarcoma, malignant mesenchymoma, and fibrosarcoma have had comparable presentations,[78,79] but tumor growth and metastatic spread are typically rapid.[80] The constitutional systems common with atrial tumors are unusual with right ventricular tumors. Right ventricular outflow tract obstruction due to metastatic disease is rare, although both right ventricular inflow and outflow obstruction have been described with metastatic malignant melanoma[81]; extrinsic compression more commonly blocks right ventricular outflow.

Physical findings

Physical findings vary with the location of the tumor; as with most right-sided events, the murmur increases in intensity with inspiration. The murmurs may be those of tricuspid valve obstruction or of pulmonic valve obstruction. With extrinsic compression by tumor simulating pulmonic stenosis, the murmur may virtually disappear at peak inspiration[82] when the tumor is lifted off the pulmonary artery. One report[83] describes a mid-diastolic vibration (tumor "plop") coinciding with the most anterior retrograde excursion of the tumor into the right ventricular outflow tract and its impact on the right ventricular wall. An accentuated and delayed pulmonic component of the second heart sound and a variety of clicks and rubs, some varying with position, suggest the diagnosis.[84] Rarely, right ventricular mobile tumors can prolapse into the main pulmonary artery during ventricular systole.[85]

Laboratory data

The chest roentgenogram may show right ventricular enlargement and ectopic intracardiac calcification; calcium deposition is described in the right ventricular outflow tract. New right axis deviation, a right ventricular conduction delay, or right bundle branch block, right ventricular hypertrophy, and/or a right atrial abnormality on the electrocardiogram, particularly in association with pericardial effusion,[86] suggest right ventricular tumor. Non-invasive imaging techniques can define the extent and potential respectability of the tumor.[81]

TUMORS OF THE MYOCARDIUM

Primary tumors of the ventricular myocardium, albeit unusual, may arise from a wide variety of cell types. Common myocardial tumors include rhabdomyomas, fibromas, angiomas, hamartomas, and mesotheliomas.

Rhabdomyomas

Rhabdomyomas comprise approximately 13% of all benign cardiac neoplasms. The gross morphologic appearance is of a white fibrous-looking tumor with a reddish-tan cut surface (Fig. 9-21). Light microscopy shows vacuolated myocytes divided in groups by connective tissue septae. The degree of vacuolization is extreme in some cells, revealing intervening cytoplasmic processes extending to the cell membrane in a spoke-like fashion; these cells are known as "spider cells" (Fig. 9-22). Extensive deposits of glycogen are present in the vacuolated myocytes, which are positive by periodic acid-Schiff stain with and without diastase treatment. Ultrastructural studies confirm the myocytic origin of the tumor cells, revealing pools of b-particle-type glycogen, prominent myofibrils, leptomeric fibrils, and junctional complexes resembling intercalated disks.[87] Rhabdomyomas are the most common cardiac tumor of infancy, and more than 50% of them occur in infants less than 2 weeks old.[2] Their size varies from a few millimeters to large and multicentric, encroaching on ventricular chambers. As ultrasound examinations have become routine procedures during pregnancy, rhabdomyomas have been diagnosed in the fetus, thus cre-

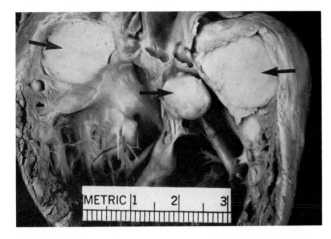

Fig. 9-21. Left ventricular view shows multiple well-circumscribed, white, fleshy, appearing rhabdomyomas at the outflow tract. One appears to be resting on the atrial side of the anterior mitral leaflet. (Courtesy of Dr. William D. Edwards, Mayo Clinic).

ating the potential for surgical removal in the early neonatal period.[88] Other reports described stillborn infants due to obstructing rhabdomyomas; a more favorable outcome of a prenatally detected rhabdomyomas involved successful surgical excision in the second year of life.[89]

Rhabdomyomas are associated with tuberous sclerosis in about half of patients. Coexistence of rhabdomyomas with congenital malformations of the heart also adversely affects prognosis. In two cases of malformation of the tricuspid valve (one Ebstein anomaly) associated with myocardial rhabdomyomas, the authors advanced the hypothesis that tumors within the heart might interfere with normal development if present at an early stage.[90] Controversy exists regarding the exact nature of rhabdomyomas (which most believe to be a form of hamartoma), because of the low mitotic rate and lack of tendency to generate metastases, rather than representing glycogen storage disease or a true neoplasm. The rhabdomyoma "spider cell" has features in common with cardiac muscle cells; glycogen, intracytoplasmic myofibers and cross-striations have been identified using special stains. A recent report describes the usefulness of MRI in detecting cardiac tumors in patients with tuberous sclerosis.[91]

Rhabdomyomas in the ventricular myocardium are often multiple and may project into the cardiac chambers, mimicking subpulmonic or subaortic stenosis[92] surgical resection is recommended for symptomatic obstructing lesions[93] and is often feasible because rhabdomyomas are slowly growing tumors.

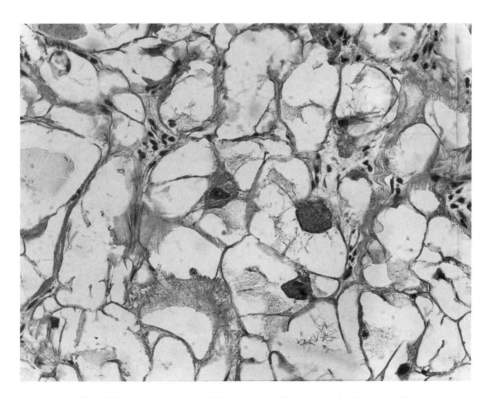

Fig. 9-22. Section from a rhabdomyoma. Note the typical spider cells.

Fibromas

Cardiac fibromas comprise about 9% of all benign cardiac tumors. They usually occur in children, predominantly under 2 years of age, without sexual preponderance. Fibromas are circumscribed, firm, whitish tumors occurring within the ventricular myocardium, particularly the septum; approximately half are located close to the endocardial surface.[2] Microscopically, they consist of interlocking bundles of dense collagen (with or without elastin) and variable numbers of fibroblasts; foci of calcification may be present. Because of their multicentric features and expansile growth, fibromas may result in obstruction of blood flow, valvular dysfunction and arrhythmias. Cardiac fibroma may mimic a broad spectrum of disease. The most usual presentation is with the murmurs of subaortic stenosis or pulmonary stenosis, although congestive heart failure or sudden death also occur.[94] Although the tumor may appear grossly well-circumscribed or even encapsulated, the periphery of the neoplasm may intermingle with myocardial tissue to such a degree that resection cannot be accomplished.[95]

Teratomas

Only 2% of the benign neoplasms reported by Molina[2] were teratomas. Despite their benign nature, teratomas may present serious risk because of their size and location.[96]

Lipomas

Lipomas constitutes approximately 8% of cardiac tumors, and may present with signs and symptoms consistent with compression or displacement of the heart. Some lipomas, although of epicardial origin, may present as intracavitary masses (Figs. 9-23 and 9-24)[97]. Cardiac lipomas in the ventricular septum have been diagnosed by echocardiography and MRI.[98] Approximately 50% of lipomas may be subendocardial.

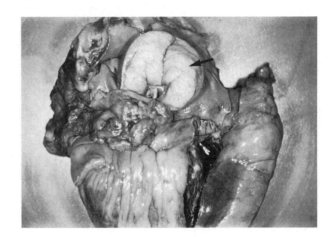

Fig. 9-23. Posterior view, base of the heart, shows a tumor in the interatrial septum (bisected). The tumor measured 6 cm × 4.5 cm × 4 cm, appeared well-circumscribed and yellow; lipomatous infiltration of the atrial septum. (From Wenger NK: *Cardiac tumors* Hurst JW, ed: In *The heart,* New York 1978, McGraw-Hill.)

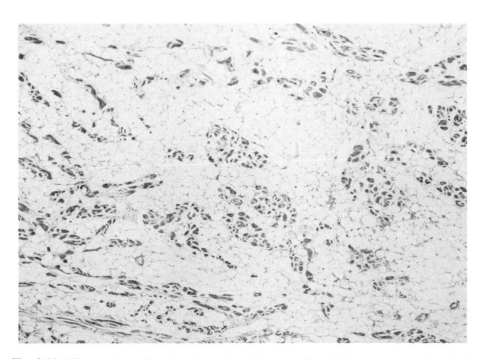

Fig. 9-24. Microscopic section from the right atrial tumor (Fig. 9-23) shows mature fat, blood vessels, and islands of myocytes.

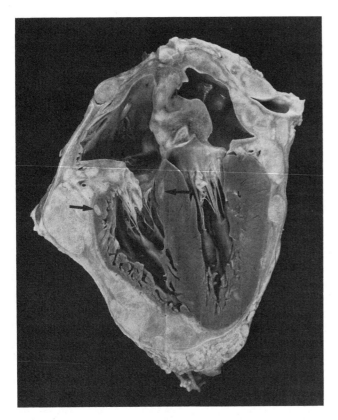

Fig. 9-25. Multiple tumor nodules encase the heart and cause marked thickening of the left atrial wall and interatrial septum. This diffuse large-cell lymphoma occurred in a patient with AIDS. (Courtesy of Dr. Robert Siegel, Department of Pathology, Emory University School of Medicine.)

Hemangiomas

Rare hemangiomas of the left ventricular wall have produced heart failure.[2]

Sarcomas

Myocardial sarcomas are rare. Myocardial invasion with Burkitt lymphoma is frequent and typically has a rapidly progressive course.

Clinical presentations

Myocardial mural tumors are characteristically asymptomatic.[99] When symptoms occur, those of arrhythmias or conduction abnormalities are most frequent, and manifest as palpitations, tachycardias, or Stokes-Adams syncope. Arrhythmias may be due to interference with the conduction system, creation of an automatic focus, or vulnerability to reentrant arrhythmias. Worthy of emphasis is the fact that the occurrence of arrhythmia in a patient with known malignant disease suggests metastatic involvement of the heart. Unexplained arrhythmias, both ventricular[100,101] and supraventricular, may be due to myocardial involvement by tumor, although these arrhythmias may occur with pericardial tumor invasion as well. Arrhythmias

are frequently refractory to conventional therapy and may prove fatal. Incessant ventricular tachycardia in infants is most often associated with cardiac tumor, even when echocardiography and angiocardiography fail to confirm the diagnosis.[101] Electrophysiologic study and intraoperative mapping enables localization, surgical excision, and long-term cure of myocardial hamartomas and, less often, rhabdomyomas that cause symptomatic rapid ventricular tachycardia in infancy and childhood, unresponsive to medical therapy.[100,101]

Angina pectoris may be due either to myocardial tumor compressing a coronary artery or to intracardiac tumor coronary embolus leading to myocardial infarction. Many myocardial tumors are "signomatic," rather than symptomatic, i.e., the absence of tissue generating electromotive force in the tumor mass produces electrocardiographic changes of a "dead zone," mimicking myocardial infarction. Both heart failure and myocardial infarction are unusual, but sudden death occurs frequently.[102] Successful surgical resection of symptomatic myocardial tumors has been described.[103,104] Cardiac transplantation may be considered for nonresectable, symptomatic, benign ventricular tumors.

Lymphoma—immunosuppression relationships

Extranodal, highly aggressive non-Hodgkin's lymphoma in immunosuppressed patients has been attributed to impaired immune surveillance, chronic antigenic stimulation, reactivation of latent oncogenic herpes-group viruses, and direct oncogenic effects of immunosuppressive drugs.[105] The usual histologic type is that of a diffuse, large B-cell lymphoma. It has been suggested that these tumors begin as virally induced polyclonal B cell hyperplasia, with progression to monoclonal B-cell lymphoma. Malignant lymphoma, probably originating in the heart, is described in patients with acquired immune deficiency syndrome (AIDS) (Fig. 9-25),[105,107] as well as in other immunocompromised patients, e.g., after renal or cardiac transplantation. A possible predilection of large-cell lymphomas for myocardial sites is suggested, both with and without an immunosuppressed state. Metastatic malignant lymphomas to the heart are far more common than primary malignant lymphoma. The most common presenting features are congestive heart failure, pericardial effusion and superior vena caval obstruction. In rare cases, extensive myocardial spread of lymphoma and damage to the conduction system can lead to complete heart block.[108]

Metastatic tumors: anatomic features

No malignant tumor tends particularly to metastasize to myocardium, except for malignant melanoma,[109] where myocardial involvement occurs in more than half of all cases; the multifocal myocardial metastases, with more frequent myocardial than epicardial location, suggest hematogenous spread. Cardiac metastases frequently occur from bronchogenic carcinoma and carcinoma of the breast,

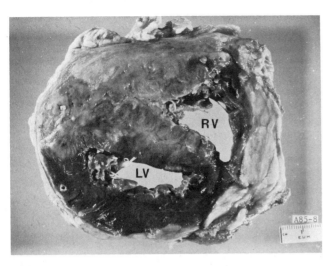

Fig. 9-26. Cross section of the heart (midventricle level) showing extensive metastatic infiltration of the anterior wall of both ventricles and the septum, in a patient with primary laryngeal carcinoma.

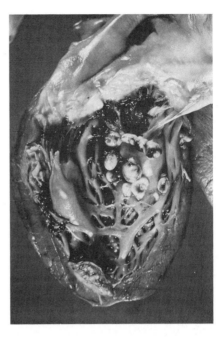

Fig. 9-27. Left ventricular view showing multiple metastatic endocardial nodules from a primary lung carcinoma.

being evident in about one third of cases (Fig. 9-26) Other common cardiac metastases are from carcinomas, sarcomas, leukemia, lymphoma, myeloma, and Kaposi's sarcoma. Cardiac involvement is occasionally the initial presentation of malignant non-Hodgkin's lymphoma.[107,110] Clinical manifestations have included heart failure, pericardial effusion, and progressive atrioventricular (AV) block.

Macroscopic myocardial infiltration may be present in up to half of autopsy cases of leukemia, and grossly visible cardiac infiltration often occurs with lymphoma, particularly with reticulum cell sarcoma. Leukemic infiltration has caused cardiac rupture. It remains uncertain whether the electrocardiographic changes that suggest myocardial infarction reflect extensive myocardial infiltration with tumor or are due to invasion and occlusion of a major coronary artery. Metastatic tumor can reach the heart by embolic hematogenous spread, by lymphatic spread, or by direct invasion, in descending order of likelihood. Cardiac lymphatics are considered to be the major pathway for tumor metastasis to the heart, particularly carcinoma of the bronchus and carcinoma of the breast. The proximity of the heart to the major mediastinal lymphatic channels accounts for the high incidence of cardiac metastases from tumors that involve the mediastinum. Myocardial tumors may spread to involve the pericardium and less commonly erode onto the endocardium (Fig. 9-27).

Metastatic tumors invade the myocardium more frequently than do primary myocardial tumors. In many reports, all areas of myocardium seem equally likely to be invaded by tumor in proportion to their bulk, accounting for the preponderance of left ventricular metastases. Other reports describe a greater incidence of right-sided metastases, presumably because 75% of the coronary blood flow returns to the right side of the heart, allowing more

embolic tumor cells to lodge in this area. A reason offered for common atrial invasion is its relative lack of mobility.

Metastatic tumors: ECG abnormalities

Metastatic disease to myocardium commonly produces pronounced persistent ST segment elevation in the absence of Q waves[111] both this abnormality and complete AV block, simulating myocardial infarction, were also described with malignant lymphoma.[112] Arrhythmias are more often associated with metastatic tumors than with benign tumors of the myocardium; metastatic tumor invading myocardium may result in myocardial necrosis and electrocardiographic changes that mimic myocardial infarction. A progressive and prolonged "current of injury," ST displacement, was described[113] in a patient with myocardial metastases from bronchogenic carcinoma; myocardial necrosis was prominent in areas of tumor infiltration. On occasion, the characteristics of the electrocardiographic abnormalities may even suggest the location of a neoplasm in the myocardium.[114] Metastatic tumor to the atrium has mimicked atrial infarction.[115] True myocardial infarction, at times with a typical clinical presentation, has occurred when metastatic tumor compresses or invades the epicardial coronary arteries.[116]

Metastatic tumors: clinical and laboratory manifestations

On physical examination there may be evidence of the two most common rhythm disturbances, atrial flutter and atrial fibrillation, seen most commonly when there is tumor invasion of the atrium. Carcinoma of the lung is most frequent tumor type. Cardiac enlargement and heart fail-

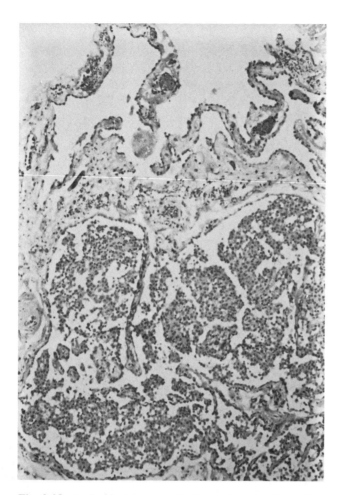

Fig. 9-28. An incidental autopsy finding in the epicardium of an explanted heart. Note a well-circumscribed lesion beneath the epicardial surface that consisted of uniform benign mesothelial cells.

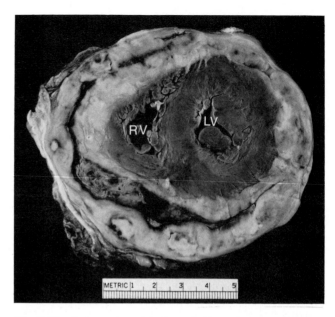

Fig. 9-29. Cross section of the heart (midventricular level) shows a fleshy, solid neoplasm completely surrounding both ventricles and obliterating the pericardial space; histologically mesothelioma. (Courtesy of Dr. William D. Edwards, Mayo Clinic).

TUMORS OF THE PERICARDIUM

Primary pericardial tumors such as teratoma,[120] leiomyoma, mesothelioma, lipoma, fibroma, neurofibroma, and hemangioma are less common than are myocardial tumors. Sarcoma is one of the most frequent malignant pericardial tumors.

Mesotheliomas

Mesothelioma is probably the most common pericardial neoplasm, followed by sarcoma and teratoma. The clinical diagnosis of mesothelioma is usually made at a late stage when serous or hemorrhagic pericardial effusion is present, or when constriction is caused by tumor expansion. Most cases reveal cardiomegaly, low voltage QRS complexes with nonspecific T-wave changes on the ECG, and evidence of a thickened pericardium at echocardiography. MRI is described as better than echocardiography in the diagnosis of pericardial infiltrations.[121] Pericardial mesotheliomas (Fig. 9-28) may be localized solid or cystic masses, or may consist of diffuse nodules. Complete encasement of the heart is rare (Fig. 9-29), but may present as constrictive pericarditis.[122] The tumor may invade the myocardium, including the conduction system or coronary arteries, and compress the great vessels. While local spread is common, extrathoracic metastasis is rare. Whether there is an association between asbestos exposure and pericardial mesothelioma is not clear.

Metastatic tumors

On the other hand, tumor metastases to the pericardium[123] occur more frequently than do myocardial metastases. About 85% of patients with malignant cardiac tu-

ure, occasionally with angina pectoris and even with associated pericarditis, may be encountered on rare occasions, when there is extensive myocardial infiltration with tumor. The electrocardiogram, in addition to arrhythmias, may show a variety of conduction defects including bundle branch block; abnormal P waves may be present when there are atrial tumors; and there may be changes of myocardial ischemia or myocardial infarction. There is often an abnormal, but rarely a diagnostic, alteration of the cardiac silhouette on chest roentgenogram, but at times the cardiac contour may be normal, and even angiocardiography may be unrevealing. Echocardiography[117] is of diagnostic value only when the tumor alters the echocardiographic characteristics of the ventricular wall. However, preferential involvement of the ventricular system by a primary cardiac sarcoma simulated asymmetric septal hypertrophy at echocardiography.[118] Radioisotopic and other noninvasive imaging procedures may safely help identify myocardial tumors without need for intravenous contrast studies; MRI use avoids radiation exposure.[119]

mors are estimated to have pericardial involvement. Tumor metastases involve the pericardium, probably more often by direct extension from mediastinal lesions; retrograde lymphatic or hematogenous metastases occur less frequently. When retrograde lymphatic metastatic spread occurs, the tumor typically has first metastasized to the mediastinal lymph nodes. This is in contrast to the myocardium, which is invaded predominantly via hematogenous tumor dissemination. Pericardial metastases are particularly frequent with intrathoracic tumors; tumors metastatic to the pericardium are likely to invade the epicardium and myocardium as well. When pericardial metastatic disease is present, systemic evidence of metastatic disease is characteristic. Both myocardial and pericardial lymphoma also result in pericardial effusion.

Sarcomas

Pericardial sarcomas encompass a variety of pathologic entities, but all tend to be diffuse, to encase the pericardium, or to deform or obliterate the cardiac contour. Many sarcomas appear to have originated in the right atrium with wide extension to the pericardium.[124] Mesothelioma, the third most frequent malignant cardiac tumor, has a variety of life-threatening presentations, including pericarditis with hemopericardium and pericardial tamponade[125] obliteration of the pericardial cavity simulating constrictive pericarditis; and tumor invasion of a coronary artery, resulting in myocardial infarction. Erosion of an artery causing pericardial tamponade; invasion of the conduction system; and compression of the great vessels as they enter the pericardium are also potentially deadly presentations.

Kaposi sarcoma of the heart in association with skin and other visceral involvement has been described in the classical, African, and AIDS-associated forms.[126,127] However, irrespective of the clinical form, lesions are usually in the epicardium or pericardium, quite small and localized, and are often asymptomatic. Epicardial Kaposi sarcoma, associated with AIDS, has resulted in fatal acute hemorrhagic pericardial tamponade.[128]

Clinical presentations

Pericardial tumors may present as acute pericarditis, both with and without effusion. The clinical presentation, particularly with malignant pericardial tumors, may include acute pericarditis with pain, a friction rub, and often, the electrocardiographic changes of pericarditis. At times the pain may be dull and without symptomatic relief by sitting upright and leaning forward; such may be the case when chest pain is due to myocardial infiltration, as is often seen with angiosarcoma. Dyspnea, cough, hoarseness or dysphagia, orthopnea, pulmonary congestion, right upper quadrant discomfort secondary to hepatomegaly, en-

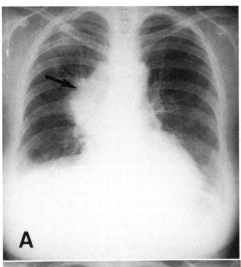

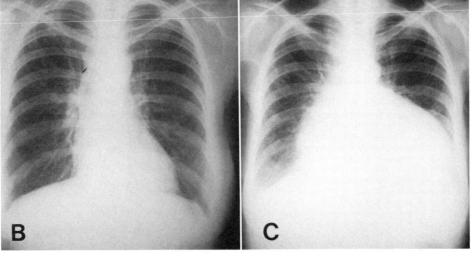

Fig. 9-30. A, Bronchogenic carcinoma with mediastinal extension *(arrow).* **B,** Four months later: regression of the bronchogenic carcinoma after x-ray therapy. **(C)** Nine months later: massive pericardial effusion due to pericardial metastases from the bronchogenic carcinoma. (Courtesy of Department of Radiology, Emory University School of Medicine.) Reproduced from Wenger NK: *Rare causes of heart disease.* In Hurst JW, ed: *The heart,* New York, 1966, McGraw-Hill.

gorgement of the neck veins, and leg edema are often present when there is large pericardial effusion. Metastases to the pericardium often cause a rapidly increasing size of pericardial effusion, often with a persistent pericardial friction rub that may progress to cardiac tamponade. Pericardial effusion (Fig. 9-30), particularly if hemorrhagic or rapidly accumulating, suggests pericardial tumor. Cardiac arrhythmias, particularly atrial arrhythmias, are frequent. The effusion is frequently large and compresses the right atrium and right ventricle, limiting diastolic filling. At times it produces a superior vena caval syndrome, and frequently results in pulsus paradoxus, tachycardia, diminished heart sounds, and hypotension as evidence of impending pericardial tamponade. Pulsus paradoxus is not a paradoxical change, but rather an accentuation of a normal finding, i.e., an inspiratory decrease in the systolic blood pressure in excess of 10 to 12 mm Hg. Constrictive pericarditis is most often caused by metastases from bronchogenic carcinoma and carcinoma of the breast. Effusive-constrictive hemodynamic changes can occur with neoplastic invasion of the pericardium.[129] Unexplained pericarditis, often with a persistent pericardial friction rub, is also suggestive.

Laboratory data

The electrocardiogram can confirm the atrial arrhythmias and decreased ECG voltage may be evident when pericardial effusion is present. Large size malignant pericardial effusions are often associated with electrical alternans on the electrocardiogram, as well as low voltage, when pericardial tamponade is imminent. The chest roentgenogram often suggests tumor, because of the bizarre cardiac contour related to an epicardial tumor mass; atypical or bizarre calcification may also be present. When large effusion is present, the rapidly enlarging cardiac silhouette often assumes a water bottle shape. Pleural effusion and thoracic metastatic lesions are often evident.

Hemorrhagic pericardial effusion with an increased protein content ($>$ 3 mg/dl) and high specific gravity ($>$ 1.016) suggest malignant effusion. The histologic diagnosis is often provided by examination of the fluid at pericardiocentesis, which often is necessary to avert tamponade. Because malignant effusion characteristically recurs rapidly following pericardiocentesis, surgical drainage of the effusion into the thoracic cavity (pericardial "window") is advisable. Echocardiography may also be helpful; strands of fibrin in the effusion and pericardial masses may be demonstrated. Transesophageal echocardiography may be particularly helpful.[129a] MRI or CT may also detect pericardial metastases. At times, pericardial biopsy may be required for a tissue diagnosis.

TUMORS INVOLVING THE CARDIAC CONDUCTION SYSTEM

Tumor invasion of the AV node or the ventricular septum may result in atrioventricular block with Stokes-Ad-

ams syncope.[130] Otherwise, unexplained complete atrioventricular block, often with Stokes-Adams syncope, should suggest tumor involvement of the conduction system. Complete heart block has been described as the initial presentation of Burkitt lymphoma.[131] Sudden death may be the initial or subsequent presentation of a cardiac tumor.

Similarly, primary mesotheliomas of the AV node, typically slow-growing cystic tumors, may produce partial or complete heart block, Stokes-Adams syncope,[132] and even sudden death. Sudden death is described as due to ventricular tachycardia/fibrillation; the illustration in one report showed what is now recognized as torsade de pointes.[133] Because of the combination of AV block and ventricular tachyarrhythmias, isolated pacemaker insertion may be inadequate. Most of these tumors are diagnosed at autopsy; they characteristically invade the AV node and its approaches but spare the AV bundle and its branches.[134] These tumors occur predominantly in women. Although earlier reports indicated an endodermal origin of this neoplasm, perhaps representing the missing link between the foregut and the heart, other reports have repeatedly stressed the mesothelial origin of this tumor or suggested an endodermal heterotopia hypothesis, supported by histochemical and immunoperoxidase studies.[135]

A deposit of myeloma involving the sinoatrial node has resulted in digitalis-resistant atrial fibrillation.[136] A case of non-Hodgkin's lymphoma in a patient with AIDS showed cardiac involvement at initial presentation, with pericardial effusion, atrial tumor, tumor of the AV node, and atrioventricular block; complete remission with cytotoxic chemotherapy is described.[137] Bundle branch block has occurred with tumor infiltration of the conducting system. Generally, primary malignant schwannoma of the heart are thought to arise from the cardiac branch of the vagus nerve. A recent report stressed the rarity of primary malignant cardiac schwannomas and reported a case with significant pericardial effusion and a tumorous mass at the left atrioventricular groove.[138]

NON-NEOPLASTIC LESIONS THAT MIMIC CARDIAC TUMOR

A mass or thrombus in a cardiac cavity, in the myocardium, or in the pericardium may simulate a tumor, hence the designation *pseudotumor*.[139] Intracavitary tumors are more commonly mimicked by thrombi, an abscess, or a foreign body. A large Libman-Sacks vegetation with cerebral embolism, as the presenting feature of systemic lupus erythematosus, mimicked an intracardiac tumor.[140] Ectopic thyroid tissue has been described in the right ventricle of a symptomatic patient during surgical removal of a lesion obstructing the right ventricular outflow tract.[141] Lipomatous infiltration of the heart, most often of the atrial septum and continuous with the epicardial fat, is probably not a true tumor. Rare reports describe right atrial lipomatous hypertrophy and obstruction of the superior vena cava.[142] This entity occurs primarily in the elderly and is associated with generalized obesity and increased epicardial fat. Lipomatous infiltration of the heart by an unencapsulated mass of fatty tissue in the myocardium and containing varying amounts of cardiac muscle is also described.[143] Supraventricular arrhythmias, conduction abnormalities, and sudden death are described; MRI imaging can better characterize the tissue.[144] An abscess, hematoma, or cyst may mimic an intramural myocardial tumor; pericardial tumor may be simulated by such conditions as a diverticulum of the pericardium, pericardial cyst, ventricular aneurysm, or coronary artery aneurysm.

SUMMARY

Clinical recognition[30] of cardiac tumors requires a high index of suspicion based on the compatible clinical findings delineated previously in this chapter. A number of noninvasive diagnostic procedures provide confirmatory evidence. Early surgery can be lifesaving and can effect cures for most benign primary cardiac tumors; palliation can be achieved for some malignant and metastatic tumors.

REFERENCES

1. Griffiths GC: A review of primary tumors of the heart, *Prog Cardiovasc Dis* 7:465, 1965.
2. Molina JE, Edwards JE, Ward HB: Primary cardiac tumors: experience at the University of Minnesota, *Thorac Cardiovasc Surg* 38:183, 1990.
3. Paget S: The distribution of secondary growths in cancer of the breast, *Lancet* i:571, 1889.
4. Ewing J: *A treatise on tumors,* ed 3, Philadelphia, 1928, WB Saunders.
5. Graf A-H, Buchberger W, Langmayr H, et al: Site preference of metastatic tumours of the brain, *Virchows Arch A Pathol Anat Histopathol* 412:493, 1988.
6. Tarin D: Clinical and experimental studies on the biology of metastasis, *Biochim Biophys Acta* 780:227, 1985.
7. Zetter BR: The cellular basis of site-specific tumor metastasis, *N Engl J Med* 322:605, 1990.
8. Auerbach R, Alby L, Morrissey LW, et al: Expression of organ-specific antigens on capillary endothelial cells, *Microvasc Res* 29:401, 1985.
9. Nicolson GL, Poste G: Tumor cell diversity and host response in cancer metastasis. Part I - properties of metastatic cells, *Curr Probl Cancer* 7:1, 1982.
10. Nicolson GL: Organ specificity of tumor metastasis: role of preferential adhesion, invasion and growth of malignant cells at specific secondary sites, *Cancer Metastasis Rev* 7:143, 1988.
11. Weiss L, Orr FW, Honn KV: Interactions between cancer cells and the microvasculature: a rate-regulator for metastasis, *Clin Exp Metastasis* 7:127, 1989.
12. Sher BT, Bargatze R, Holzmann B, et al: Homing receptors and metastasis, *Adv Cancer Res* 51:361, 1988.
13. Doerr R, Zvibel I, Chiuten D, et al: Clonal growth of tumors on tissue-specific biomatrices and correlation with organ site specificity of metastases, *Cancer Res* 49:384, 1989.
14. De Baetselier P, Roos E, Brys L, et al: Generation of invasive and metastatic variants of a non-metastatic T-cell lymphoma by *in vivo* fusion with normal host cells, *Int J Cancer* 34:731, 1984.
15. Liotta LA, Schiffmann E: Tumour motility factors, *Cancer Surv* 7:631, 1988.
16. Pauli BU, Schwartz DE, Thonar EJ-M, et al: Tumor invasion and host extracellular matrix, *Cancer Metastasis Rev* 2:129, 1983.
17. Sporn MB, Roberts AB: Peptide Growth factors and inflammation, tissue repair, and cancer, *J Clin Invest* 78:329, 1986.
18. Fidler IJ: Macrophages and metastasis - a biological approach to cancer therapy: Presidential address, *Cancer Res* 45:4714, 1985.
19. Weiss L: Biomechanical destruction of cancer cells in the heart: a rate regulator for hematogenous metastasis, *Invasion Metastasis* 8:228, 1988.
20. Weiss L, Dimitrov DS, Angelova M: The hemodynamic destruction of intravascular cancer cells in relation to myocardial metastasis, *Proc Natl Acad Sci USA* 82:5737, 1985.
21. Weiss L, Dimitrov DS: A fluid mechanical analysis of the velocity, adhesion, and destruction of cancer cells in capillaries during metastasis, *Cell Biophys* 6:9, 1984.
22. Smith C: Tumors of the heart, *Arch Pathol Lab Med* 110:371, 1986.
23. Popovic AD, Harrigan P, Sanfilippo AJ, et al: Echocardiographic detection of left atrial extension of bronchial carcinoma, *JAMA* 261:1478, 1989.
24. Cheung EH, Ziffer JA, Felner JM, et al: Diagnosis and surgical treatment of a primary lung carcinoma extending into the left atrium, *Emory University J Med* 5:118, 1991.
25. Akhtar MJ, Al-Aska AK, Al-Siddique A, et al: Primary hepatic carcinoma presenting as atrial myxoma with review of the literature, *J Saudi Heart Assoc* 3:113, 1991.
26. Bisel HF, Wroblewski F, LaDue JS: Incidence and clinical manifestations of cardiac metastases, *JAMA* 153:712, 1953.
27. Fine G: Primary tumors of the pericardium and heart, *Cardiovasc Clin* 5:207, 1973.
28. Goodwin JF: The spectrum of cardiac tumors, *Am J Cardiol* 21:307, 1968.
29. Tillmanns H: Clinical aspects of cardiac tumors, *Thorac Cardiovasc Surg* 38:152, 1990.
30. Harvey WP: Clinical aspects of cardiac tumors, *Am J Cardiol* 21:328, 1968.
31. Flipse TR, Tazelaar HD, Holmes DR, Jr: Diagnosis of malignant cardiac disease by endomyocardial biopsy, *Mayo Clin Proc* 65:1415, 1990.
32. Nasser WK, Davis RH, Dillon JC, et al: Atrial myxoma. I. Clinical and pathologic features in nine cases, *Am Heart J* 83:694, 1972.
33. Stevens LH, Hormuth DA, Schmidt PE, et al: Left atrial myxoma: pulmonary infarction caused by pulmonary venous occlusion, *Ann Thorac Surg* 43:215, 1987.
34. Butterworth JS, Poindexter CA: Papilloma of cusp of the aortic valve. Report of a patient with sudden death, *Circulation* 58:213, 1973.
35. Siltanen P, Tuuteri L, Norio R, et al: Atrial myxoma in a family, *Am J Cardiol* 38:252, 1976.
36. Davison ET, Mumford D, Zamam Q, et al: Left atrial myxoma in the elderly: report of four patients over the age of 70 and review of the literature, *J Am Geriatr Soc* 34:229, 1986.
37. Zhang P-f, Jones JW, Anderson WR: Cardiac myxomas correlative study by light, transmission, and scanning electron microscopy, *Am J Cardiovasc Pathol* 2:295, 1989.
38. Lam RMY, Hawkins ET, Roszka J: Cardiac myxoma: histochemical and ultrastructural localization of glycosaminoglycans and proteoglycans, *Ultrastruct Pathol* 6:69, 1984.
39. Johansson L: Histogenesis of cardiac myxomas. An immunohistochemical study of 19 cases, including one with glandular structures, and review of the literature, *Arch Pathol Lab Med* 113:735 1989.
40. Landon G, Ordonez NG, Guarda LA: Cardiac myxomas. An immu-

nohistochemical study using endothelial, histiocytic, and smooth-muscle cell markers, *Arch Pathol Lab Med* 110:116, 1986.

41. Symbas PN, Hatcher CR, Jr, Gravanis MB: Myxoma of the heart: clinical and experimental observations, *Ann Surg* 183:470, 1976.

42. Boxer ME: Cardiac myxoma: an immunoperoxidase study of histogenesis, *Histopathology* 8:861, 1984.

43. de Morais CF, Falzoni R, Alves VAF: Myocardial infarct due to a unique atrial myxoma with epithelial-like cells and systemic metastases, *Arch Pathol Lab Med* 112:185, 1988.

44. Kotani K, Matsuzawa Y, Funahashi T, et al: Left atrial myxoma metastasizing to the aorta, with intraluminal growth causing renovascular hypertension, *Cardiology* 78:72, 1991.

45. Fyke EF III, Seward JB, Edwards WD, et al: Primary cardiac tumors: experience with 30 consecutive patients since the introduction of two-dimensional echocardiography, *J Am Coll Cardiol* 5:1465, 1985.

46. Goodwin JF: Diagnosis of left atrial myxoma, *Lancet* i:464, 1963.

47. Peters MN, Hall RJ, Cooley DA, et al: The clinical syndrome of atrial myxoma, *JAMA* 230:695, 1974.

48. Wight RP Jr, McCall MM, Wenger NK: Primary atrial tumor. Evaluation of clinical findings in ten cases and review of the literature, *Am J Cardiol* 11:790, 1963.

49. Knepper LE, Biller J, Adams HP Jr, et al: Neurologic manifestations of atrial myxoma. A 12-year experience and review, *Stroke* 19:1435, 1988.

50. Cecil MP, Silverman ME: Tricuspid valve honk due to pulmonary hypertension secondary to left atrial myxoma, *Am J Cardiol* 67:321, 1991.

51. Maisch B: Immunology of cardiac tumors, *Thorac Cardiovasc Surg* 38:157, 1990.

52. Burns ER, Schulman IC, Murphy MJ Jr: Hematologic manifestations and etiology of atrial myxoma, *Am J Med Sci* 284:17, 1982.

53. Nasser WK, Davis RH, Dillon JC, et al: Atrial myxoma. II. Phonocardiographic, echocardiographic, hemodynamic, and angiographic features in nine cases, *Am Heart J* 83:810, 1972.

54. Panidis IP, Mintz GS, McAlister M: Hemodynamic consequences of left atrial myxomas as assessed by Doppler ultrasound, *Am Heart J* 111:927, 1986.

55. Bateman TM, Sethna DH, Whiting JS, et al: Comprehensive non-invasive evaluation of left atrial myxomas using cardiac cine-computed tomography, *J Am Coll Cardiol* 9:1180, 1987.

56. Freedberg RS, Kronzon I, Rumancik WM, et al: The contribution of magnetic resonance imaging to the evaluation of intracardiac tumors diagnosed by echocardiography, *Circulation* 77:96, 1988.

57. Sung RJ, Ghahramani AR, Mallon SM, et al: Hemodynamic features of prolapsing and nonprolapsing left atrial myxoma, *Circulation* 51:342, 1975.

58. Markel ML, Waller BF, Armstrong WF: Cardiac myxoma. A review, *Medicine* 66:114, 1987.

59. Croxson RS, Jewitt D, Bentall HH, et al: Long-term follow-up of atrial myxoma, *Br Heart J* 34:1018, 1972.

60. Vatterott PJ, Seward JB, Vidaillet HJ, et al: Syndrome cardiac myxoma: more than just a sporadic event, *Am Heart J* 114:886, 1987.

61. McCarthy PM, Piehler JM, Schaff HV, et al: The significance of multiple, recurrent and "complex" cardiac myxomas, *J Thorac Cardiovasc Surg* 91:389, 1986.

62. Read RC, White HJ, Murphy ML, et al: The malignant potentiality of left atrial myxoma, *J Thorac Cardiovasc Surg* 68:857, 1974.

63. Meyer BJ, Weber R, Jenzer HR, et al: Rapid growth and recurrence of atrial myxomas in two patients with Swiss syndrome, *Am Heart J* 120:220, 1990.

64. Carney JA, Toorkey BC: Myxoid fibroadenoma and allied conditions (myxomatosis) of the breast. A heritable disorder with special associations including cardiac and cutaneous myxomas, *Am J Surg Pathol* 15:713, 1991.

65. Burke AP, Virmani R: Osteosarcomas of the heart, *Am J Surg Pathol* 15:289, 1991.

66. Massumi R: Bedside diagnosis of right heart myxomas through detection of palpable tumor shocks and audible plops, *Am Heart J* 105:303, 1983.

67. Esper RJ, Machado RA, Schapira L, et al: Loud systolic and diastolic murmurs originating on a right atrial metastatic tumor, *Chest* 91:926, 1987.

68. Talley RC, Baldwin BJ, Symbas PN, et al: Right atrial myxoma. Unusual presentation with cyanosis and clubbing, *Am J Med* 48:256, 1970.

69. Turlapati RV, Jacobs LE, Kotler MN: Right atrial myxoma causing total destruction of the tricuspid valve leaflets, *Am Heart J* 120:1227, 1990.

70. Crotty TB, Edwards WD, Oh JK, et al: Lipomatous hamartoma of the tricuspid valve: echocardiographic-pathologic correlations, *Clin Cardiol* 14:262, 1991.

71. Klima T, Milam JD, Bossart MI, et al: Rare primary sarcomas of the heart, *Arch Pathol Lab Med* 110:1155, 1986.

72. Pillai R, Kharma N, Brom AG, et al: Mitral valve origin of pedunculated rhabdomyomas causing subaortic stenosis, *Am J Cardiol* 67:663, 1991.

73. Israel DH, Sherman W, Ambrose JA, et al: Dynamic coronary ostial obstruction due to papillary fibroelastoma leading to myocardial ischemia and infarction, *Am J Cardiol* 67:104, 1991.

74. McFadden PM, Lacy JR: Intracardiac papillary fibroelastoma: an occult cause of embolic neurologic deficit, *Ann Thorac Surg* 43:667, 1987.

75. Albers GW, Avalos SM, Weinrich M: Left ventricular tumor masquerading as multiple sclerosis, *Arch Neurol* 44:779, 1987.

76. Calvelo MG, Korns ME: Left ventricular obstruction caused by metastatic sarcoma, *Arch Pathol Lab Med* 21:222, 1971.

77. Camesas AM, Lichtstein E, Kramer J, et al: Complementary use of two-dimensional echocardiography and magnetic resonance imaging in the diagnosis of ventricular myxoma, *Am Heart J* 114:440, 1987.

78. Goldstein S, Mahoney EB: Right ventricular fibrosarcoma causing pulmonic stenosis, *Am J Cardiol* 17:570, 1966.

79. Ceretto WJ, Miller ML, Shea PM, et al: Malignant mesenchymoma obstructing the right ventricular outflow tract, *Am Heart J* 101:114, 1981.

80. Brown BC, Mason TE, Ballard WP, et al: Cardiac angiosarcoma: a case report, *J Med Assoc Ga* 80:435, 1991.

81. Emmot WW, Vacek JL, Agee K, et al: Metastatic malignant melanoma presenting clinically as obstruction of the right ventricular inflow and outflow tracts: characterization by magnetic resonance imaging, *Chest* 92:362, 1987.

82. Littler WA, Meade JB, Hamilton DI: Acquired pulmonary stenosis, *Thorax* 25:465, 1970.

83. Hada Y, Wolfe C, Murray GF, et al: Right ventricular myxoma. Case report and review of phonocardiographic and auscultatory manifestations, *Am Heart J* 100:871, 1980.

84. Snyder SN, Smith DC, Lau FYK, et al: Diagnostic features of right ventricular myxoma, *Am J Cardiol* 91:240, 1976.

85. Nanda NC, Barold SS, Gramiak R, et al: Echocardiographic features of right ventricular outflow tumor prolapsing into the pulmonary artery, *Am J Cardiol* 40:272, 1977.

86. Firmin R, Lowes A, Hickson B: A case of rhabdomyosarcoma of the right ventricle, *Br Heart J* 40:1426, 1978.

87. Howanitz EP, Teske DW, Qualman SJ, et al: Pedunculated left ventricular rhabdomyoma, *Ann Thorac Surg* 41:443, 1986.

88. Brezinka C, Huter O, Haid C, et al: Prenatal diagnosis of a heart tumor, *Am Heart J* 116:563, 1988.

89. Boxer RA, Seidman S, Singh S, et al: Congenital intracardiac rhabdomyoma: prenatal detection by echocardiography, perinatal management, and surgical treatment, *Am J Perinatol* 3:303, 1986.

90. Russell GA, Dhasmana JP, Berry BP, et al: Coexistent cardiac tumours and malformations of the heart, *Int J Cardiol* 22:89, 1989.

91. Matsumura M, Nishioka K, Yamashita K, et al: Evaluation of cardiac tumors in tuberous sclerosis by magnetic resonance imaging, *Am J Cardiol* 68:281, 1991.

92. Kuehl KS, Perry LW, Chandra R, et al: Left ventricular rhabdomyoma: a rare cause of subaortic stenosis in the newborn infant, *Pediatrics* 46:464, 1970.

93. de Loma JG, Villagra F, de Leon JP, et al: Rhabdomyoma of the heart. Surgical treatment, *J Cardiovasc Surg* 23:149, 1982.

94. Brown IW, McGoldrick JP, Robles A, et al: Left ventricular fibroma: echocardiographic diagnosis and successful surgical excision in three cases, *J Cardiovasc Surg* 31:536, 1990.

95. Tahernia AC, Bricker JT, Ott DA: Intracardiac fibroma in an asymptomatic infant, *Clin Cardiol* 13:506, 1990.

96. Farooki ZQ, Chang CH, Jackson WL, et al: Intracardiac teratoma in a newborn, *Clin Cardiol* 11:642, 1988.

97. Graham TR, Chalmers JAC, Aldren C: A large epicardial lipoma - an insight into the surgical anatomy of the interatrial septum, *Int J Cardiol* 25:119, 1989.

98. Kamiya H, Ohno M, Iwata H, et al: Cardiac lipoma in the interventricular septum: evaluation by computed tomography and magnetic resonance imaging, *Am Heart J* 119:1215, 1990.

99. Roberts WC, Glancy DL, DeVita VT Jr: Heart in malignant lymphoma (Hodgkin's disease, lymphosarcoma, reticulum cell sarcoma and mycosis fungoides). A study of 196 autopsy cases, *Am J Cardiol* 22:85, 1968.

100. Kearney DL, Titus JL, Hawkins EP, et al: Pathologic features of myocardial hamartomas causing childhood tachyarrhythmias, *Circulation* 75:705, 1987.

101. Garson A Jr, Smith RT Jr, Moak JP, et al: Incessant ventricular tachycardia in infants: myocardial hamartomas and surgical cure, *J Am Coll Cardiol* 10:619, 1987.

102. Violette EJ, Hardin NJ, McQuillen EN: Sudden unexpected death due to asymptomatic cardiac rhabdomyoma, *J Forensic Sci* 26:599, 1981.

103. Geha AS, Weidman WH, Soule EH, et al: Intramural ventricular cardiac fibroma. Successful removal in two cases and review of the literature, *Circulation* 36:427, 1967.

104. Childress RH, King RD, Aldrich DD, et al: Successful resection of a benign right ventricular mesenchymoma, *Am J Cardiol* 20:255, 1967.

105. Guarner J, Brynes RK, Chan WC, et al: Primary non-Hodgkin's lymphoma of the heart in two patients with the acquired immunodeficiency syndrome, *Arch Pathol Lab Med* 111:254, 1987.

106. Balasubramanyam A, Waxman M, Kazal HL, et al: Malignant lymphoma of the heart in acquired immune deficiency syndrome, *Chest* 90:243, 1986.

107. Cairns P, Butnay J, Fulop J, et al: Cardiac presentation of non-Hodgkin's lymphoma, *Arch Pathol Lab Med* 111:80, 1987.

108. Chou S-T, Arkles LB, Gill GD, et al: Primary lymphoma of the heart. A case report, *Cancer* 52:744, 1983.

109. Glancy DL, Roberts WC: The heart in malignant melanoma. A study of 70 autopsy cases, *Am J Cardiol* 21:555, 1968.

110. Gill PS, Chandraratna PAN, Meyer PR, et al: Malignant lymphoma: cardiac involvement at initial presentation, *J Clin Oncol* 5:216, 1987.

111. Hartman RB, Clarke PI, Schulman P: Pronounced and prolonged ST segment elevation. A pathognomonic sign of tumor invasion of the heart, *Arch Intern Med* 142:1917, 1982.

112. Nishikawa Y, Akaishi M, Handa S, et al: A case of malignant lymphoma simulating acute myocardial infarction, *Cardiology* 78:357, 1991.

113. Harris TR, Copeland GD, Brody DA: Progressive injury current with metastatic tumor of the heart. Case report and review of the literature, *Am Heart J* 69:392, 1965.

114. Swirsky MH, Roth O, Celentano L: Electrocardiographic diagnosis of a metastatic heart tumor, *Conn Med* 40:375, 1976.

115. Rothfeld EL, Zirkin RM: Unusual electrocardiographic evidence of metastatic cardiac tumor resembling atrial infarction, *Am J Cardiol* 10:882, 1962.

116. Franciosa JA, Lawrinson W: Coronary artery occlusion due to neoplasm, *Arch Intern Med* 128:797, 1971.

117. Duncan WJ, Rowe RD, Freedom RM, et al: Space-occupying lesions of the myocardium: role of two-dimensional echocardiography in detection of cardiac tumors in children, *Am Heart J* 104:780, 1982.

118. Isner JM, Falcone MW, Virmani R, et al: Cardiac sarcoma causing "ASH" and simulating coronary heart disease, *Am J Med* 66:1025, 1979.

119. Boxer RA, LaCorte MA, Singh S, et al: Diagnosis of cardiac tumors in infants by magnetic resonance imaging, *Am J Cardiol* 56:831, 1985.

120. MacDonald S, Fay JE, Lynn RB: Intrapericardial teratoma: a continuing challenge, *Can J Surg* 26:81, 1983.

121. Vogel HJ Ph, Wondergem JHM, Falke THM: Mesothelioma of the pericardium: CT and MR findings, *J Comput Assist Tomogr* 13:543, 1989.

122. Llewellyn MJ, Atkinson MW, Fabri B: Pericardial constriction caused by primary mesothelioma, *Br Heart J* 57:54, 1987.

123. Kralstein J, Frishman W: Malignant pericardial diseases: diagnosis and treatment, *Am Heart J* 113:785, 1987.

124. Janigan DT, Husain A, Robinson NA: Cardiac angiosarcomas: a review and a case report, *Cancer* 57:852, 1986.

125. El Allaf D, Burette R, Pierard L, et al: Cardiac tamponade as the first manifestation of cardiothoracic malignancy: a study of 10 cases, *Eur Heart J* 7:247, 1986.

126. Templeton AC: Studies in Kaposi's sarcoma, *Cancer* 30:854, 1972.

127. Silver MA, Macher AM, Reichert CM, et al: Cardiac involvement by Kaposi's sarcoma in acquired immune deficiency syndrome (AIDS), *Am J Cardiol* 53:983, 1984.

128. Steigman CK, Anderson DW, Macher AM, et al: Fatal cardiac tamponade in acquired immunodeficiency syndrome with epicardial Kaposi's sarcoma, *Am Heart J* 116:1105, 1988.

129. Mann T, Brodie BR, Grossman W, et al: Effusive-constrictive hemodynamic pattern due to neoplastic involvement of the pericardium, *Am J Cardiol* 41:781, 1978.

129a. Frohwein SC, Karalis DG, McQuillan JM et al: Preoperative detection of Pericardial angiosarcoma by transesophageal echocardiography, *Am Heart J* 122:874, 1991.

130. Lenegre J, Moreau Ph, Iris L: Deux cas de bloc auriculo-ventriculaire complet par sarcome primitif du coeur, *Arch Mal Coeur Vaiss* 56:361, 1963.

131. Cole TO, Attah EdB, Onyemelukwe GC: Burkitt's lymphoma presenting with heart block, *Br Heart J* 37:94, 1975.

132. Hellemans IM, van Hemel NM, Kooyman CA: Atrioventricular block in childhood caused by mesothelioma, *PACE* 4:216, 1981.

133. Manion WC, Nelson WP, Hall RJ, et al: Benign tumor of the heart causing complete heart block, *Am Heart J* 83:535, 1972.

134. James TN, Galakhov I: De Subitaneis Mortibus. XXVI. Fatal electrical instability of the heart associated with benign congenital polycystic tumor of the atrioventricular node, *Circulation* 56:667, 1977.

135. Sheffield EA, Corrin B, Addis BJ, et al: Synovial sarcoma of the heart arising from a so-called mesothelioma of the atrioventricular node, *Histopathology* 12:191, 1988.

136. Atkinson K, McElwain TJ, Mackay AM: Myeloma of the heart, *Br Heart J* 36:309, 1974.

137. Kelsey RC, Saker A, Morgan M: Cardiac lymphoma in a patient with AIDS, *Ann Intern Med* 115:370, 1991.

138. Morishita T, Yamazaki J, Ohsawa H, et al: Malignant schwannoma of the heart, *Clin Cardiol* 11:126, 1988.

139. Wollenweber J, Giuliani ER, Harrison CE Jr, et al: Pseudotumors of the right heart, *Arch Intern Med* 121: 169, 1968.

140. Appelbe AF, Olson D, Mixon R, et al: Libman-Sacks endocarditis mimicking intracardiac tumor, *Am J Cardiol* 68:817, 1991.

141. Pollice L, Caruso G: Struma cordis. Ectopic thyroid goiter in the right ventricle, *Arch Pathol Lab Med* 110:452, 1986.

142. McNamara RF, Taylor AE, Panner BJ: Superior vena caval obstruction by lipomatous hypertrophy of the right atrium, *Clin Cardiol* 10:609, 1987.

143. Izumi T, Matsuoka A, Nagai K, et al: Massive lipomatous infiltration to the left ventricle mimicking a cardiac tumor, *Jpn Heart J* 27:273, 1986.

144. Levine RA, Weyman AE, Dinsmore RE, et al: Noninvasive tissue characterization: diagnosis of lipomatous hypertrophy of the atrial septum by nuclear magnetic resonance imaging, *J Am Coll Cardiol* 7:688, 1986.

Chapter 10

AGING AND THE CARDIOVASCULAR SYSTEM: IMPLICATIONS IN HEALTH AND DISEASE

Gottlieb C. Friesinger
Michael B. Gravanis

Our older population, arbitrarily defined as Americans more than 65 years of age, is increasing at a remarkable rate. Between 1900 and 1985, Americans over the age of 65 increased from about 3 million to 28 million. By 2020, this population will reach 64 million. Older persons make more extensive use of the health care system than does any other group. Health care costs are increasing at a much greater rate than the increase in numbers of older citizens.

An important problem in the delivery of health care to this population is the heterogeneity of older persons. Most remain self-sufficient. Unfortunately, many do not. Approximately one third of health care expenditures (more than $800 billion annually) is committed to care of older citizens. These features have particularly attracted the attention of federal agencies responsible for providing payment for most of the care through Medicare programs.[1-6] The lay press and interested, politically active organizations of older citizens, also have shown great interest and concern.

During the last several years, segments of the medical profession have become increasingly alerted to and involved in the special problems related to medical care of older persons. Cardiovascular disease constitutes, by a large margin, the most frequent and important morbid condition among older persons. More than 50% of persons over the age of 65 will die of cardiovascular diseases.[7] In addition, the rate of increase in cardiovascular services provided by cardiologists to the Medicare population, including technical services (e.g., cardiac catheterization, echocardiography, electrocardiography, and percutaneous transluminal coronary angioplasty), increased in excess of 50% (some as much as 143%) between 1986 and 1989. Visits to hospitalized patients, as well as office visits, were similarly increased.[8]

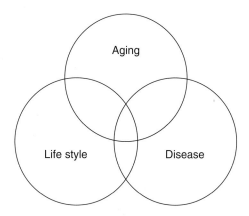

Fig. 10-1. The Venn diagram illustrates the dilemma in attempting to differentiate the changes of aging from those of disease and life-style changes. See text for discussion.

Fries[9] developed a controversial hypothesis that states that the increase in the older population is related primarily to an increase in the average life expectancy and not to an increase in maximum length of life.[9,10] The "average maximum length of life" has remained constant in the United States at 85 years to 87 years of age during this century, while the average length of life has increased from 47 years to about 75 years. If this is true, there are important implications regarding the allocation of resources and the philosophy of care for cardiovascular disease—and all other health conditions—in older persons. As will be mentioned repeatedly, the overwhelming problem with aging in reference to cardiovascular illness is the heterogeneity of the older population; chronology is a very poor surrogate for biology (or physiology) in older persons—particularly those over the age of 75.

Another important and intriguing conceptual and practical problem is demonstrated by the Venn diagram (Fig. 10-1). It is often difficult to separate the effects of aging from those related to changes in lifestyle and concomitant disease. Alterations in lifestyle, including loss of muscle mass due to poor nutrition, lack of exercise and deconditioning, and altered mood and mental states, can produce weight loss and symptoms that lead to the perception that the aging process is accelerating and/or important disease is present. In addition, medications (discussed below), which are used with much greater frequency and produce a higher incidence of side effects in the old than in the young, can also produce symptoms and findings mistakenly attributed to aging and disease. Finally, much of our data about aging are fragmentary, since only limited longitudinal studies have been carried out, and most clinical trials have excluded older persons.

On the basis of the background briefly cited in the above paragraphs, this chapter will have three sections. The first section will be a resumé of the *cardiovascular changes* that have been reasonably characterized and *can*

be related to aging per se and always occur with aging, but not predictably at a specific age. Included in this section are brief comments on the important matter of drug metabolism alteration(s) with aging. The second section discusses *cardiovascular changes that may occur in other settings but that are primarily related to aging,* yet do not occur in all aged persons. Isolated systolic hypertension, calcific aortic stenosis, and degenerative changes in the cardiac conduction system are examples of these phenomena. The third section reviews the *common cardiovascular diseases that may occur earlier in life but are increasingly frequent with aging.* The emphasis will be on pathophysiology, with only brief mention of the pathology underlying the changes. Therapy is not discussed comprehensively, but the background pathophysiology provides clues and guidelines to therapeutic approaches, and potential problems related to treatment of older persons with cardiovascular disease.

CARDIOVASCULAR CHANGES RELATED TO AGING

Alterations in the cardiovascular system related to aging are parallel to age-related changes in the entire person; i.e., age-related changes in a single organ or group of organs, such as the joints, brain, lungs, or kidneys, may be responsible for the limitations and deterioration of aging, while all other organs remain functionally intact. Similarly, aging alterations, unrelated to any disease process in the cardiovascular system, are also selective. The box on page 301 lists a number of cardiovascular changes that occur with aging. Not included in the box, because these functions are not altered, are items such as systolic ventricular function (the inherent ability of the myocardium to shorten and develop tension), and the ability of the heart muscle to extract oxygen and produce adenosine triphosphate as the source for myocardial energy. Because these functions, in the absence of cardiovascular disease, are not impaired, we can assume that an old, healthy heart does not impose the primary limitation on the ability to exercise, nor is it more susceptible to ischemia. The features in the box, each of which will be discussed briefly, do alter cardiovascular performance; e.g., an old heart must utilize alternative mechanisms, compared with hearts in younger persons, to achieve a high cardiac output as discussed subsequently.

There is lack of consensus regarding the gross and microscopic findings in the senescent heart. However, most studies indicate that the weight of the heart increases at a rate of 1 g to 1.5 g per year between 30 years and 90 years of age.[11,12]

The ventricular septal thickness increases between the third and tenth decades of life while there is a decrease of the base-to-apex dimension, creating a reduced ventricular chamber. Another morphologic change in the senescent heart is the so-called "sigmoid septum," probably resulting

---

Cardiovascular changes related to aging.

Decreased aortic elasticity—mild LV hypertrophy
Decreased myocardial relaxation
Decreased sensitivity to beta-agonists
Loss of pacemaker cells and Purkinje fibers
Diminished reactivity to chemo- and baroreceptor reflexes
Increased vagal tone and sensitivity
Fibrosis and calcification of the cardiac "skeleton"
Altered pharmacokinetics/pharmacodynamics

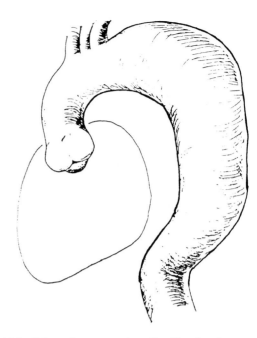

Fig. 10-2. Schematic presentation of a dilated and tortuous descending thoracic aorta. (Reprinted from Gravanis, Holland: *Cardiovascular pathophysiology*. New York, 1987, McGraw-Hill.)

from the reduction in the ventricular size and the rightward shift of the dilated ascending aorta.[13] The curved ventricular septum has no hemodynamic significance, although it may simulate echocardiographically asymmetric hypertrophic cardiomyopathy.

Elderly hearts reveal relative myocyte hypertrophy, most marked in the midmyocardial zone, and a distinct increase of connective tissue matrix, particularly in the posterior left ventricular region.[14]

Some studies suggest that with aging there is a progressive reduction of the more distensible form of collagen with an augmentation of the more rigid type. Such an alteration in the connective tissue matrix may be responsible for the greater stiffness of the senescent heart, which requires higher filling pressures to adapt to an increased preload by the Frank-Starling mechanism.[15]

Age-related change in the arteries, especially the aorta, has long been the focus of investigative efforts. Changes in elasticity and distensibility, as well as dilatation, which are believed to be independent of atherosclerosis and hypertension (although exacerbated by those processes), commence in middle life and accelerate in old age.

Morphologic changes first appear in the thoracic aorta and involve the intima and media. Dilatation of the ascending aorta and the sinuses of Valsalva is usually mild or moderate and thus is not associated with overt cardiac dysfunction. However, severe sinotubular stretching may effect the complete coaptation of the cusps, resulting in valvular regurgitation. Figure 10-2 illustrates these abnormalities diagramatically.

Age-related changes in the aortic intima consist of irregularity in size and shape of endothelial cells and increased numbers of multinucleated endothelial giant cells. The subendothelial layer is thick and contains increased numbers of smooth muscle cells, elastic lamellae, lipids, and foci of calcification.

Reduced prostacyclin synthesis by endothelial cells in advanced age has been reported. It is not clear whether this decrease functions in the development of thrombosis and atherosclerosis in the elderly.[16] Functional changes in small vessels are more difficult to study, but data are accumulating that indicate endothelial-derived relaxation factor is not elaborated as effectively in the old as in the young.

The endothelial-dependent responses to an agonist such as acetylcholine are reduced.[17-19] Such alterations, if confirmed, have important clinical implications in response to stresses and disease. It is difficult to separate changes of aging endothelium from the same alteration (reduced endothelial-dependent relaxation) that is known to result from hypertension, atherosclerosis, and hypercholesteremia per se. However, age is an independent risk factor for loss of endothelial-dependent relaxation in the studies cited.

The media, besides the fragmentation of elastic lamellae, reveals increased amounts of collagen and mucopolysaccharides, and thus appears thick despite the concomitant dilatation.[20]

These processes are undoubtedly modified by genetics and concomitant disease(s). The consequences of these changes—loss of elasticity and distensibility, progressive dilatation and elongation of the aorta—result in a loss of the diastolic contraction of the aorta (which serves as a kind of secondary pump in the young), a higher systolic pressure, and widened pulse pressure.[21-24] The left ventricle has a greater afterload, which results in mild but definite thickening of the left ventricle and increased left ventricular muscle mass in active older patients.

Myocardial function in relation to aging has been studied extensively. Much of the pertinent data has been summarized by Weisfeldt[25] and his colleagues, who have been major contributors to our understanding of this aspect of aging. In a wide variety of animal preparations of different species, as well as in humans, systolic myocardial function (the ability of heart muscle to shorten and/or develop tension) remains essentially normal. There have been extensive investigations of systolic and diastolic myocardial function in reference to aging at the cellular and subcellular level, including study of the availability and use of energy stores, intracellular calcium handling, and evaluation of the transmembrane action potential.

The more intriguing features of direct clinical pertinence are provided by studies in isolated cardiac muscle. Muscles from older animals show a reduction in inotropic response to catecholamines and digitalis, but the response of myofibrils to direct exposure of calcium (following chemical removal of the cell membrane) is maintained. In addition, the post-extrasystolic potentiation phenomenon is maintained in senescent animals, a response that would be predicted on the basis of the calcium observations. A diminished response to digitalis is seen both in old rats and old dogs.[26] Whether these observations can be directly transposed to humans is not clear, but observational and anecdotal evidence would suggest such changes with aging do occur. Older persons have higher levels of catecholamines and greater elaboration of catecholamines with stress, but show reduced chronotropic and inotropic responses.

In contrast to systolic function, which, overall, is preserved although modified in its response to various agonists, diastolic dysfunction is impaired. The changes are not dramatic, but definite and of potential clinical importance. From study of a variety of senescent animal models, the most striking and predictable change in the function of cardiac muscle is the prolonged duration of relaxation.[25] This *inherent property of senescent myocardium* is likely attributable both to a decrease in the velocity of intracellular handling of calcium and to the prolongation of the action potential duration that occurs with aging. This delayed relaxation in senescent myocardium is further enhanced in the intact heart by left ventricular *chamber characteristics* and, possibly, structural changes in the mitral valve. The thickening of the left ventricle, as well as age-specific changes in some patients (e.g., infiltration of amyloidosis which will be discussed later), could cause further diastolic dysfunction. A number of studies in humans using echocardiographic Doppler techniques to estimate the rate and time course of ventricular relaxation with these noninvasive techniques confirm a slower relaxation phase and diastolic dysfunction in normal old persons when compared with young persons.[27-29]

The changes in myocardium and ventricular performance with aging can be summarized. Peak contractile force and the ability of heart muscle to shorten is not impaired; systolic function is preserved. Agonists such as digitalis and beta-adrenergic stimuli have diminished effect, whereas stimulating the muscle directly with calcium produces no diminution in effect. The most consistent change in aging myocardium, which is manifested both at the myocardial as well as the organ level, is a diminution in myocardial relaxation, producing diastolic dysfunction.

Overall integrated cardiovascular performance

The age-related changes in the heart and peripheral vasculature alter considerably the integrated response to stress, including daily activities such as exercising, standing, and eating. Differentiating the effects of aging on integrative cardiovascular performance from those related to disease and lifestyle changes is not always possible. Even motivational and psychologic problems may make interpretation of studies difficult. Early studies indicated there was a steady decline in overall cardiovascular performance, as judged by exercise, with aging.[30] All studies show a decline in maximum oxygen consumption, but this could be the result of a decrease in muscle mass with aging, and not related to a reduction in overall cardiovascular performance or cardiac output.[31] On the basis of the changes that are known to be age-related, we know that afterload will be increased by the changes in the aorta, and contractility during stress and exercise must be reduced because of the altered response of the myocardium to beta-adrenergic stimulation. The changes in afterload have been studied most elegantly by Yin[32] et al. in an evaluation of aortic input impedance in exercising young and old beagles. Except at the highest levels of exercise, old dogs had stroke volume increases limited by increase in the characteristic aortic impedance. Port[33] et al. studied 77 healthy volunteers selected because they had no evidence of disease by history, physical, chest radiogram, electrocardiogram, and normal resting left ventricular ejection fraction by radionuclide ventriculography. They concluded exercise ejection fraction diminished with aging and that the .05 increase that occurs in normal people less than 60 years of age did not occur in older subjects. However, this study, although carefully done, reflects the dilemma in differentiating exercise changes related to aging from those that might result from occult disease. Subjects over the age of 60—of whom 21 of 29 had a reduction in ejection fraction with exercise—frequently had regional wall motion abnormalities that could be assumed to be the result of subtle coronary arteriosclerosis and ischemia (or other myocardial disease) during exercise, despite the attempts to exclude patients with overt cardiovascular disease.

The most carefully done study has been reported by Rodeheffer,[34] who studied 61 patients age 25 years to 79 years in the Baltimore longitudinal study. However, only a small number (less than 10) were over 70 years of age. These subjects had no evidence of cardiovascular disease by any criteria, including the thallium exercise test to search for occult ischemia. The group did vigorous exercise at 125 watts and to the point of exhaustion. This allows the assumption that the group was well-conditioned physically and highly motivated. Cardiac output did not decrease with advancing age, but the manner in which the increase in output was achieved was modified. A particularly important aspect of this study was the very careful measurement of ventricular volumes. Considering the four primary determinants of cardiac output during exercise, there was an age-related decrease in heart rate, an age-related decrease in the increased contractility expected with exercise, and an increase in impedance to ejection (afterload), which was offset by an increase in end diastolic volume. The larger diastolic volume in the older subjects allowed an increase in stroke volume to maintain cardiac output by utilizing the Frank-Starling mechanism.

Although it would be desirable to have additional studies utilizing other methods, it is reasonable to conclude on the basis of all of the available data that cardiac output is maintained in normal older persons *provided* they are motivated and physically fit, but the output increases are achieved by different mechanisms that are completely consistent with the data from a variety of muscle preparations and animal studies of young vs. old. Longitudinal studies on people as they age are needed to confirm these concepts in the most rigorous fashion. Finally, there are abundant data that demonstrate that older individuals can successfully undergo physical training and benefit in the same ways as do younger persons in reference to increasing exercise tolerance and muscle mass.[35-37]

The differences between younger and older patients in reference to hemodynamic changes on standing and eating are usually of no clinical importance except when blood volume may be decreased and/or drugs that alter reflexes or blood volume distribution (such as nitrates, diuretics, and antihypertensive agents) are being used, but these drugs are prescribed very frequently. Age-related attenuation of baroreflexes make older persons much less able to respond to increases or decreases in arterial pressure on changing position than younger persons.[38] This inability to respond promptly will be exaggerated not only by medications, but also by alteration in sodium intake. Similarly, although younger persons have no change, or even sometimes a slight rise, in systemic blood pressure after eating a meal, older persons may have postprandial hypotension, possibly related to inability to compensate for the splanchnic vasodilatation related to food ingestion.

Use of drugs in the aged

It is beyond the scope of this brief resumé to discuss the details of drug use, altered drug distribution and sensitivity, and the high incidence of important side effects in older persons. However, these matters are of such enormous importance in considering cardiovascular problems in health and disease in the aged that brief mention must be made. The box above outlines some of the major considerations. Many older persons with relatively minor and well-controlled cardiovascular conditions may take four or five drugs. It is not uncommon for older patients with some combination of coronary heart disease, hypertension,

---

Drugs in the elderly

General considerations

Three times as many drugs prescribed over age 65
Multiple drugs are usual
Tendency to use "own" drugs
Memory problems and confusion (or lack of patient education)

Pharmacokinetics

Absorption
Drug distribution
   Less lean body mass and blood volume
     e.g., more hypotension with TNG
   Volume of distribution changes depend on lipid solubility
Metabolism (biotransformation)
   Less liver mass—reduced blood flow
   Reduce cellular enzyme activity (primarily affects oxidation)
     e.g., T ½ increased for Digoxin, lidocaine, quinidine, propranolol, phenytoin, prazosin
Elimination
   GFR and tubular secretion reduced
     Reduced dosage for digoxin, procainamide, disopyramide, hydralazine
Protein binding
   Higher alpha acid glycoprotein (AAG)
     e.g., more propranolol available

Altered sensitivity to drugs (pharmacodynamics)

Receptor change(s)
Blunted reflex responses

---

diabetes, peripheral vascular disease, lipid abnormalities, and associated problems to take 8 to 15 drugs. This, coupled with the universally acknowledged increased incidence of drug toxicity in older people, presents major problems. Differentiating side effects and toxicity of drugs from symptoms and findings related to the disease processes being treated can be difficult. Alterations occur in both pharmacokinetics—the bioavailability of a drug—as well as in pharmacodynamics—the sensitivity of the patient to any given level of drug available.

It is convenient to think of pharmacokinetics in reference to drug absorption, distribution, biotransformation, tissue and protein binding, and rate of elimination. All of these processes may be altered with aging. Gerber and Brass[39] have comprehensively reviewed these matters.

Drug absorption has not been convincingly shown to be altered, although studies related to aging and absorption are limited. Absorption abnormalities might be anticipated on the basis of an estimated 30% decrease in mucosal absorptive surface in the small bowel, as well as decrease in gastrointestinal motility.[40-42] Small intestinal blood flow is reduced by an estimated 40%. Although drug absorption is not convincingly reduced because of these abnormalities, drug interactions can play a major role in the bioavailability of drugs. It is in this respect that the multiple drugs used by old people can influence bioavailability. Antacids decrease the absorption of a number of drugs, including chlorpromazine and tetracycline, whereas cholestyramine can bind, and therefore decrease, the absorption of warfarin, thiazides, digitalis, aspirin, and acetaminophen. Drugs with anticholinergic effects can decrease motility and delay absorption. These interactions can occur in patients of all age groups, but assume greater importance in the aged because of the propensity of older people to use multiple drugs.

Because aging decreases the metabolic capacity of the liver, drugs that are extensively metabolized during their first pass after absorption will have their bioavailability increased. Drug distribution may undergo major alterations with advancing age because lean body mass and total body water content are reduced, and body fat as a proportion of body weight increases with aging. These alterations in body composition, together with the propensity for plasma concentration of albumin to decrease with aging, can result in a decrease in plasma protein binding for acidic drugs such as phenytoin, phenylbutazone, and warfarin. The complexities of drug availability in aging is emphasized by the fact that drugs such as lidocaine and propranolol bind mainly to α_1-acid glycoproteins, and their concentration increases with age. These considerations emphasize that drug availability can be altered in a variety of ways, depending on whether drugs are distributed mainly in body water or body fat, are protein bound, or are subject to a major first pass effect. Because the volume of distribution of a drug, together with the plasma clearance, is a key determinant of the half-life of a drug, it can be anticipated that many drugs will have their half-lives altered on the basis of aging per se.

Many drugs are eliminated primarily through the kidneys. Digoxin, procainamide, thiazide, diuretics, and beta-adrenergic blockers (atenolol, nadolol, disopyramide, and hydralazine) are such drugs. Although it is highly variable, glomerular filtration rate at age 70 is only about 60% of that at age 20. In addition, renal blood flow is decreased by 40%, and maximum sodium and water conservation is impaired in older persons. Because muscle is the principal source of creatinine, a conventionally calculated creatinine clearance does not indicate the same glomerular filtration rate in the old as in the young. Hence, even when the serum creatinine concentration is normal, a substantial reduction in renal function, as much as 40%, can be assumed. Half-lives of all drugs eliminated primarily by the kidney will be substantially lengthened, and the dose of the drug must be reduced to prevent toxicity.

When drug metabolism primarily takes place in the liver, major alterations occur with aging because liver mass, cellular microsomal enzyme activity (such as the cytochrome P-450 system), and hepatic blood flow all reduce with age. These alterations will prolong the half-lives of drugs that are inactivated by hepatic metabolism, including digoxin, lidocaine, quinidine, phenytoin, and propranolol. Any drug that undergoes extensive first pass effect will have its bioavailability increased. On the other hand, as is true with all aspects of aging, not all metabolic pathways in the liver are uniformly affected. Oxidation is the principal metabolic pathway affected by age, while drug conjugation is relatively spared. This means a benzodiazepine, such as lorazepam, is relatively unaffected by age, because its principal route of metabolism is glucuronidation.

In general, the aging changes described above tend to enhance drug availability and result in the need to administer lower doses of drugs, although there is great variability. To complicate further these pharmacokinetic alterations, which tend to result in excessive blood levels, there may also be changes in end organ responsiveness (pharmacodynamic alterations) that can result from alteration in receptor number or affinity, changes in the enzymes that eventually translate the effect of the drug, or structural changes in the end organ that reduce the organ's ability to respond.

The older person has a reduced responsiveness to intravenously administered isoproterenol, although the exact mechanism whereby this occurs is not clear. The aged have an enhanced orthostatic response to antihypertensive agents and nitroglycerin because aging is associated with an abnormal baroreceptor response to hypotension. Older persons frequently take diuretics, providing another potential for orthostatic hypotension related to reduced circulating blood volume and increased sodium loss resulting from age-related diminished reflex response.

The effect of age on drug use for cardiovascular disease(s) can be summarized. Overall, there is a propensity to increase free drug in the blood as a result of reduced metabolism, decreased tissue and protein binding, and slower excretion. This propensity, coupled with potential alterations in end organ response, reduced blood volume, and altered reflux responses, emphasizes the need for ordinarily administering the drug in lower doses, monitoring the patient critically, alerting the patient to side effects and possible need for dose adjustment, and minimizing the use of multiple drugs.

Drugs can improve function and make patients more comfortable, but adverse reactions are so frequent and drug interactions so common that constant vigilance is essential. Finally, confusing drug effects with manifestation of disease is a special problem in the aged.

CARDIOVASCULAR CONDITIONS RELATIVELY SPECIFIC IN THE AGED POPULATION
Valvular heart disease

Systolic murmurs are extremely common in persons over 65 years of age, with a prevalence as high as 60% or greater in some reports. Most of these murmurs do not

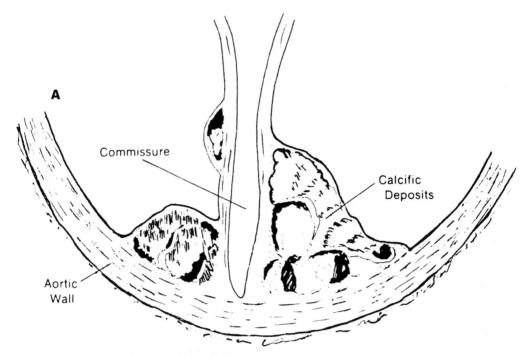

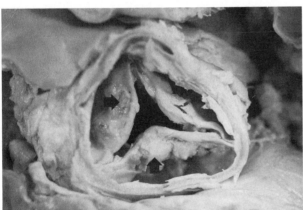

Fig. 10-3. A Schematic presentation of early calcific deposits at the junction of the cusps with the aortic wall. Note that the process does not induce commissural adhesions. (Reprinted from Gravanis, Holland: *Cardiovascular pathophysiology*. New York, 1987, McGraw-Hill. **B,** Photograph of senile calcific aortic stenosis from above the valve. There are heavy calcific deposits at the depths of the sinuses *(arrows)* and no commissural fusion is present.

carry important clinical implications and are related to thickening and sclerosis caused by long-term wear and tear on the aortic valve, or a minor degree of mitral regurgitation related to papillary muscle dysfunction as a result of ischemic heart disease, or hypertensive or idiopathic cardiomyopathy. The most frequent cause of important and potentially serious valvular heart disease in older persons is calcific aortic stenosis. The murmur resultant from important calcific aortic stenosis may not be prominent, often not greater than grade 2, and the associated findings of striking left ventricular hypertrophy, delayed carotid upstroke, and narrow pulse pressure and basal thrill, so frequent in younger persons, are often absent in older persons who have accompanying conditions, such as hypertension or pulmonary disease. A congenitally bicuspid aortic valve with acquired calcification and stenosis is the most frequent cause of calcific aortic stenosis until into the sixth decade. By the seventh decade, the aging changes of the

aortic valve can often result in calcific deposits and important stenosis of an initially anatomically normal tricuspid valve.[43,44] Figure 10-3, illustrates the gross pathologic changes. Although rheumatic heart disease that has been present since childhood or early adult life may manifest itself initially in older persons, such occurrences are now extremely uncommon in our society because acute rheumatic fever is very rare.

Because significant calcification is always present when clinically important stenosis is present, diminution or absence of the aortic valve closure sound regularly occurs. In addition, it is possible that compensatory hypertrophy, which is so prominent in children and young adults with aortic stenosis, may not occur in elderly patients; at least hypertrophy has been demonstrated to be age-dependent in the rat model.[45] Overall, senile calcific aortic stenosis can be difficult to diagnose, but a high level of suspicion, a very careful search for subtle physical findings, and the

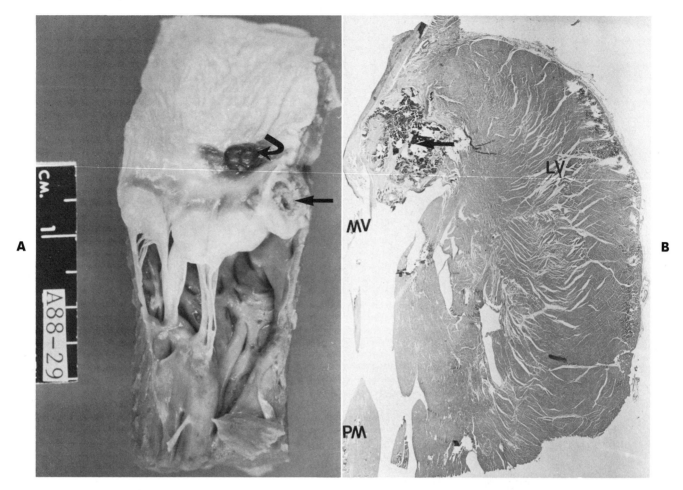

Fig. 10-4. A Photograph of a longitudinal section of the posterior wall of the left atrium, posterior mitral leaflet, and posterior left ventricular wall. Note massive calcification of the mitral annulus *(arrow)*, and the ulceration through the atrial endocardium. The latter is covered by a thrombus *(curved arrow)*. **B** Microscopic longitudinal section of posterior left ventricular wall, posterior mitral leaflet, and posteromedial papillary muscle. There is massive calcification of the mitral annulus *(arrow)* extending also into the adjacent myocardium. LV = left ventricle, MV = mitral valve, PM = papillary muscle.

use of a Doppler echocardiogram when the suspicion is high will allow diagnosis to be established and the severity of the stenosis rather accurately assessed.

It has been estimated that senile aortic stenosis accounts for approximately 10% to 30% of all cases of aortic stenosis.[46] The figures may be low, however, because statistics most often are derived from surgically excised valves. Understandably, many elderly people with calcified stenosis are not candidates for surgery, and therefore are not included in the statistical analysis.

An autopsy study of normal hearts found no correlation between aortic valvular thickness and sex, height, weight, body surface area, or heart weight, after the effect of age was removed.[47] The age-related changes of wear and tear are often seen at the sites of contact of cusps. Early changes are characterized by fibrosis followed by calcium deposition initially within the fibrosa at the base of the

cusps, resulting in cuspal stiffness. Calcium deposits do not extend beyond the linea alba and do not involve and/or compromise the commissures. Mild or even moderate calcific deposits may reduce the cuspal mobility, but impose minimal hemodynamic alterations. However, heavy deposits may completely immobilize all three cusps with resultant stenosis.

Age-related changes are also observed in the aortic ring. The collagen of the ring reveals loss of parallel orientation of fibrils, takes a fatty character, and finally calcifies. This histologic alteration of the aortic ring may lead to annuloaortic ectasia and mild to moderate aortic regurgitation.

Aortic regurgitation is much less common than aortic stenosis in elderly patients, usually is of a trivial degree, and usually results from hypertension and/or atherosclerotic valvular deformation. On the other hand, rare but very important causes, such as infectious endocarditis and aortic dissection, must be kept in mind. Although such causes of aortic regurgitation in older persons often present with rather major acute illnesses, the presentations might be subtle. If the patient has received antibiotics and/or antihypertensive drugs for other problems, chronic aortic regurgitation may occur, without dramatic clinical presentation.

As indicated in the introductory paragraph of this section, a minor degree of mitral regurgitation caused by papillary muscle dysfunction is common. Of increasing interest as so many of our population reach old age is the mitral regurgitation that occurs with mitral valve prolapse. The condition is quite common in the young, more so in women than in men, and seems less frequent in older persons. A small minority of patients with mitral valve prolapse will develop progressive regurgitation and in older age (frequently in their 60s and more so in their 70s) develop chordal rupture and marked mitral regurgitation, often associated with the onset of congestive heart failure. This process, always associated with myxomatous degeneration of the mitral valve, is an increasingly common indication of the need for mitral valve replacement in older patients. Mitral prolapse in the elderly is generally associated with a greater severity of insufficiency and has poorer prognosis than in younger individuals.[48] The underlying morphologic changes, namely expansion of the leaflets, stretching and thinning of the chordae tendineae, and increased mucopolysaccharides in the spongiosa layer of the leaflets are similar to those observed in younger individuals. A more specific form of mitral valve disease, usually associated with only mild or moderate regurgitation, and almost exclusively limited to the elderly population, is mitral annular calcification. It occurs in young patients with specific disease entities, such as Marfan's syndrome. Mitral annular calcification can be seen easily on chest radiogram, is always diagnosed by echocardiography, and should always be considered in a differential diagnosis of a systolic murmur in older persons, particularly women.[49] In rare instances, the regurgitation can be marked, and extremely uncommonly, the calcification can be so extensive that mitral inflow will be impeded and functional mitral stenosis be present.

Age-related changes in the mitral valve leaflets are more striking in the anterior leaflet, where they are characterized by fragmentation and disorganization of elastic and collagen fibers, and deposition of lipid and calcium. Similar degenerative changes in the fibrous ring of the mitral valve lead to calcification. Severe calcification abolishes the sphincteric function of the mitral ring, may immobilize the posterior mitral leaflet, and results in moderate mitral regurgitation. Extensive calcific deposits in the mitral ring may impinge on the conduction system and produce heart block, or may ulcerate and embolize, or become the site of infectious endocarditis (Fig. 10-4).

Degenerative conduction system disease

A wide variety of electrocardiographic and electrophysiologic abnormalities, sometimes associated with important clinical manifestations caused by degenerative changes in the conducting system, may occur.[50-54] When the electrophysiologic and/or clinical manifestations exclusively, or principally, involve the sinus node, the term *sick sinus syndrome* is used. The most frequent manifestations are sinus pauses, sinus bradycardia, atrial fibrillation, and other varieties of atrial ectopy and arrhythmias. Very frequently, no symptoms result, although the electrocardiographic manifestations frequently excite major clinical interest, and on occasions result in drug or even pacemaker treatments. In general, the extent of underlying cardiac disease is of major importance in producing symptoms. Symptoms, not the presence of the electrocardiographic abnormalities caused by degenerative conduction system disease, should dictate the therapy. "Sick sinus syndrome" is a misnomer because additional manifestations of degenerative conduction system disease can usually be uncovered when specifically sought. In many instances, the routine electrocardiogram will also show infranodal conduction abnormalities such as left anterior hemiblock, on right or left bundle branch block. These changes in the His-Purkinje system are sometimes, but unpredictably, the harbingers of progressive degeneration of the conduction system and the development of heart block, frequently with syncope. Electrophysiologic studies in older persons with conduction defects undertaken in an effort to predict who might develop progressive changes and important clinical manifestations, have been disappointing.

Drugs that are commonly used in older patients, including beta-blockers, calcium channel blockers, digitalis, and antihypertensives (such as alpha-methyldopa), can produce the same electrocardiographic changes as degenerative conduction system disease. This, then further illustrates the need to differentiate carefully abnormalities caused by drugs from those related to aging.

Information about morphologic changes in the conduction system has been collected primarily from human studies. The number of sinus node cells decreases with age, particularly after the age of 60, and there is a greater irregularity in the shape of these cells. In addition, there is an increase in fat, elastic fibers, and collagen within the nodal tissue with aging. However, in spite of the significant cellular reduction, particularly after the age of 75, the nodal pacemaker activity may be remarkably normal.[55] Vascular disease in the nodal artery is not considered the cause of the histologic changes in the sinus node (e.g., reduction in cells, and fibrosis). As discussed in the subsequent section, the frequency of amyloid deposits in the sinus node of the normal senescent heart is very low.

Besides the histologic changes in the sinus node, all three components of the atrioventricular junction (the AV node, His bundle, and bundle branches) are reduced in

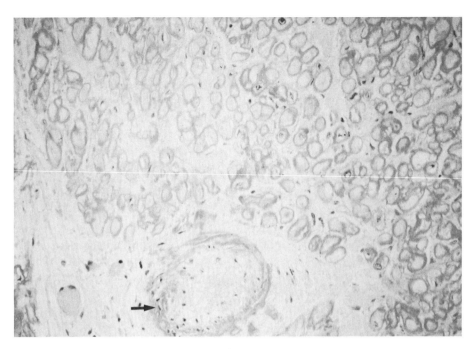

Fig. 10-5. Diffuse amyloid deposition on myocardial fibers. Amyloid deposits are present in the wall of a small intramyocardial artery *(arrow)*.

size with increasing age. Detailed histologic studies have shown that the number of conducting cells in the AV node decrease in subjects over the age of 70, in the His bundle over the age of 40, in the left bundle over the age of 70, and in the right bundle over the age of 50.[55]

Senile amyloidosis

Although amyloid deposits were first described in elderly patients in 1876,[56] the frequency with which they occur and their potential importance in reference to pathophysiology is still being clarified. The biochemical properties of amyloid in old hearts is being defined; the relationship of these amyloid deposits to the amyloid in familial amyloidosis and that associated with multiple myeloma is being clarified. In an early report by Pomerance,[56] 21 patients were described. Ten percent of patients over the age of 80 and 50% over the age of 90 had amyloid deposits. Congestive heart failure was present in half the cases and was judged attributable to the amyloidosis, entirely so in five of the cases. In a recent study of hearts from 12 patients, detailed immunohistochemical studies were performed.[57] The patients were from 82 years to 92 years of age. Convincing clinical evidence that the amyloid deposits contributed to their deaths, despite the fact that amyloidosis was not diagnosed antemortem in any of the cases, was found on retrospective review. Although senile amyloidosis is rarely diagnosed clinically, postmortem studies indicate it is frequently present in patients over the age of 75 and particularly in the oldest of the old, i.e., patients more than 85 years old. Definitive diagnosis has been

made by biopsy.[58] Figure 10-5 illustrates the histology of the condition. As the severity of the amyloid deposits increases, diastolic dysfunction will occur, leading to pulmonary congestion caused by the increased left ventricular filling pressure required to distend the noncompliant left ventricle to produce adequate systolic function, and right-sided failure with edema. An interesting feature is that conduction defects and atrial fibrillation, although common in these older patients with amyloid deposits, do not seem to be related to amyloid infiltration into the conducting system. This is in striking contrast to the conduction system disease, which occurs because of deposits in patients with familial amyloidosis with polyneuropathy.[59]

There is a strong clinical suspicion that patients with senile amyloidosis are more sensitive to the effects of digitalis and have more frequent episodes of digitalis toxicity. However, in light of the complexities in the handling of digitalis preparations—and all other drugs—in the elderly, this impression has not been convincingly proved. There remains much to be learned about senile amyloidosis in reference to its characteristics, occurrence, and particularly, the pathophysiologic effects in reference to heart failure in older persons. However, the data support the idea that this is an important finding in substantial numbers of patients. Whether its occurrence is somehow genetically determined or is only related to aging with its associated immunologic changes is not clear.

In recent years, immunohistochemical studies have recognized three distinct types of senile cardiovascular amyloidosis; isolated atrial amyloidosis, senile aortic amyloidosis, and senile systemic amyloidosis in which besides the cardiac involvement, other organs such as lungs, liver, and kidneys are involved.[60] The latter, although uncommon, may cause significant cardiovascular morbidity. The histologic distinction between the nonsecretory immunoglobulin-derived primary amyloidosis with cardiac involvement and senile systemic amyloidosis is only possible with immunohistochemical techniques.

Postmortem studies of patients above 90 years of age have revealed that two thirds had senile cardiac amyloidosis, one third had extensive ventricular involvement, and amyloidosis was the primary cause of death in approximately one fourth of the cases.[61] In rare cases of senile cardiac amyloidosis, partial characterization of the amyloid protein has shown a relationship to transthyretin (prealbumin).[62]

Isolated systolic hypertension (ISH)

Isolated systolic hypertension (ISH) is a good illustration of the kinds of problems that exist in assessing and treating medical conditions in older persons.

ISH raises issues about what is normal, inevitable, and innocent aging, what drugs might be used to treat a common condition considering the high incidence of adverse effects and expected costs and benefits. As discussed in an earlier section, the morphologic changes in the aorta and the peripheral vasculature, including stiffening, failure of relaxation to beta agonists, and the reduced ability of endothelium to respond to vasodilatory stimuli makes systolic hypertension inevitable and, at least in part, a consequence of aging per se. Diastolic hypertension has long been considered an abnormality that enhances significantly the risk for cardiovascular disease and that should be treated. ISH in older persons was long debated as a normal phenomenon that need not be treated. In fact, anecdotal experiences suggested lowering blood pressure might increase the incidence of such cardiovascular events as stroke and myocardial infarction.

ISH is defined as a systolic blood pressure in excess of 160 mm Hg and a diastolic pressure of 90 mm Hg. The prevalence of ISH varies from population to population and study to study, but the very carefully done study of Systolic Hypertension in the Elderly Program (SHEP) found a 6% incidence in individuals age 60 to 69, increasing to 18% for those age 80 and older. In the SHEP study, nearly 450,000 patients over the age of 60 were screened and 4736 randomized to treatment or placebo.[63] The follow-up period was about 5 years. The results were unequivocal and showed a favorable benefit for the primary endpoint of stroke as well as the secondary endpoint of myocardial infarction. There was also a trend toward a favorable benefit for treatment in reference to total mortality and cardiovascular deaths, but it was not statistically significant. Of particular importance is the fact that adverse drug effects were not a problem. This likely relates to the

fact that the dose of medications, primarily a thiazide diuretic, or a beta blocker in patients where the response was inadequate, were quite low. This fact is consistent with discussion concerning drug metabolism in older persons and emphasizes the need to use a low dose. Blood pressure was lowered to an average of 143/68 in the treatment group. Although there was some metabolic abnormality, the major concerns about hypokalemia, increased lipids and glucose, and hyperuricemia were not realized. This study tends to confirm an earlier report from Great Britain concerning ISH.[64]

Hence, although ISH is clearly a risk factor for cardiovascular events and merits treatment, many problems remain unresolved because the SHEP study selected only one of 1000 patients over the age of 60 who were screened, and represented a relatively uncomplicated group of patients. Expanding the treatment to a much larger group of older patients with more advanced cardiovascular disease and additional comorbidity will likely lead to greater complications from drug therapy and possibly less benefit. In addition, the health policy implications of treating all older patients with ISH are enormous because the costs of treatment would be profound. The drugs used in the SHEP trial, particular the diuretic, are quite inexpensive; however, there is strong opinion that newer drugs, such as angiotensin-converting enzyme inhibitors and calcium channel blockers, would be more appropriate treatments for ISH in older persons. These drugs would be much more expensive. The ISH problem represents a microcosm of all the issues related to common conditions in older persons. Differentiating inevitable and relatively unimportant consequences of aging per se from diseased conditions, screening large populations for the condition being studied, designing complex randomized trials to test interventions, selecting the drug to be utilized and the appropriate dose, adding adequate endpoints, and designing sensible, affordable health policy are among the issues relevant to the evaluation of ISH. Similar problems exist with the other cardiovascular risk factors in older persons.

CARDIOVASCULAR DISEASES INCREASINGLY COMMON WITH AGING

This section is a brief review of diseases that occur at younger ages but that are of increasing frequency and importance in the aged. Virtually all diseases may occur in the elderly, including even some congenital lesions (such as atrial septal defect, coarctation of the aorta, ventricular septal defects, and pulmonary stenosis) when congenital abnormalities are mild. These very interesting but quite uncommon problems will not be discussed in this section.

Coronary arteriosclerosis and coronary heart disease

Coronary arteriosclerosis, of varying degree but often severe, is found with increasing frequency with aging. Of persons over the age of 60, 50% to 80% have coronary arteriosclerosis at postmortem examination.[65] Coronary heart disease, the ischemic manifestation of coronary arteriosclerosis, is much less frequent. However, the frequency at which coronary heart disease is diagnosed will be directly related to the methods used to detect it. Exercise testing, particularly utilizing nuclear cardiology methods, will uncover many cases not apparent on routine clinical examination. A substantial proportion of older persons will have silent myocardial ischemia. Even in patients who have clinically manifest ischemia in the form of angina and/or past myocardial infarction, silent ischemia is often present and may constitute a majority of episodes.

In considering coronary arteriosclerosis, it is important to differentiate coronary arteriosclerosis without any ischemic manifestations from coronary arteriosclerosis that has resulted in coronary heart disease with silent and/or clinically manifest ischemia.

Regardless of the precise definitions or frequency of manifestations, coronary arteriosclerosis is quite uncommon in younger women. However, more women than men will have coronary heart disease over the age of 70. Cardiovascular diseases, primarily coronary heart disease, are the leading causes of death in women—an important fact that is not yet widely appreciated.[7]

Epicardial coronary arteries in the elderly may reveal tortuosity, dilatation, and atheromatous plaques characterized by dense collagenous tissue with calcification (hard lesions). However, the distribution of occlusive coronary disease in the elderly is not dissimilar to the one recorded in the general population. In one autopsy study of patients 90 to 105 years old, more than half of the hearts did not reveal critical occlusive disease in any of the four major arteries. Although coronary calcification was present in the great majority of the cases, only one third of the cases with calcification was associated with significant occlusive disease.[66]

The senescent heart may also reveal a capillary network deficit in view of the myocardial hypertrophy observed in aging. Age-related changes are also noted in the sinusoids of the heart. The sinusoids and venous channels become larger, and after the age of 40 the number of sinusoids increases significantly.[66]

Myocardial infarction

Myocardial infarction is of particular importance because of its frequency and extremely high mortality in older persons.[67-70] As in younger patients, the presentations of myocardial infarction may be typical, painless, or atypical (e.g., dyspnea, central nervous system findings, and arrhythmias, or silent. Although the data are less adequate than desirable, there are strong reasons to believe that silent and atypical presentations are increasingly frequent with age. In a prospective study of 390 older persons[69] age 75 to 85 years, 115 new Q-wave infarctions were diagnosed by serial electrocardiographic study. Thir-

ty-five percent of these were silent; i.e., there were no clinical manifestations. In other less rigorously done studies, one-third to one-half of infarct presentations in older persons were atypical and/or painless. It is possible that mental deterioration, including memory loss, which often accompanies aging, and comorbidity are the reasons for the high incidence of atypical and silent presentations. These matters result in diagnostic errors and inadequate diagnosis of the condition. Regardless of presentation, the mortality of myocardial infarction is extremely high and not closely related to presentation except for the fact that patients presenting primarily with new onset heart failure and/or central system manifestations have the highest mortality. Figure 10-6 illustrates the relationship between mortality and age.

This high mortality becomes even more intriguing when the complications related to myocardial necrosis, cardiogenic shock, and congestive heart failure are considered. These complications occur with increasing frequency with age despite the fact that myocardial infarct size, as judged by CK enzyme release, is less in older patients than in younger patients.[70] The high mortality and the increasing frequency of complications in the absence of clinical evidence of larger infarctions in the elderly suggests that age per se may constitute a major risk in older persons with myocardial infarction. The features discussed in the opening section on age-related changes may be pertinent. "Cardiac reserve" is diminished, as is discussed in the description of exercise maintenance of cardiac output in the elderly. The older person's inability to respond to stress by increased contractility, vulnerability to alterations in loading conditions (either preload or afterload), as well as other aging changes in the lungs, kidneys, and liver, make the stress of myocardial infarction much less tolerable to the healthy old person than to the young. In addition to the interesting data suggesting that enzyme release is less in old persons with complications than in the young, the important mortality difference in relation to myocardial infarction location tends to disappear. In young patients, large infarcts, as judged by anterior location, or complex inferior infarcts (changes in right-sided leads, reciprocal ST-segment depression in the anterior leads, or heart block) have higher mortality than uncomplicated inferior infarction. These differences tend to disappear, and inferior infarction carries a high—and similar, albeit less risk—than anterior infarction in older persons.[71] The age-related changes in the conduction system make the old heart more vulnerable to heart block and, for the reasons cited, less able to tolerate the consequences of heart block.

Stable and unstable angina pectoris

The other common clinical presentations for coronary heart disease, stable and unstable angina, are fraught with similar complexities in relation to clinical diagnosis, because atypical symptomatology is common (although the

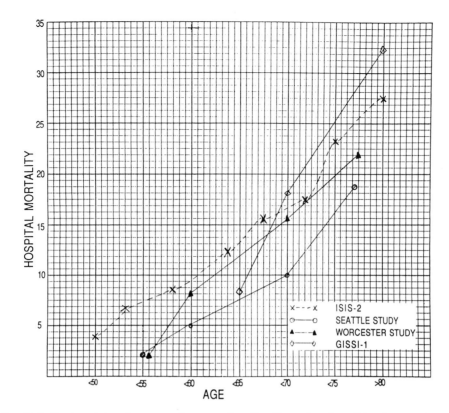

Fig. 10-6. Replotted data from recently reported studies illustrating the striking increase in mortality of myocardial infarction with advancing age. All reports include a large number of patients (at least several thousand in each study). (Modified from Lancet 1988; 2:526 (x—x); J. Am. Coll. Cardiol. 1991; 18:657; (o—o); Am. Heart J. 1989; 117:543(▲—▲); Lancet 1986; 1:397 (◇—◇).

true frequency is unknown). Of particular importance, standard diagnostic studies involving exercise testing have not been systematically evaluated in older persons, particularly in those over the age of 70 or 75 years. A fundamental problem in the use of exercise testing is the fact that a large number (often a sizable minority or even majority) of older persons cannot exercise adequately to reach a satisfactory endpoint for ischemia. Inability to exercise may be related to cardiac disease, orthopedic problems, or the less specific frailties of being old. Ischemic complaints and/or association of exercise with striking ST-segment depressions, which carries a poor prognosis in younger patients, may not do so in the old. The ability to exercise and duration of exercise are important prognostic features in the old. Much more data, systematically collected and thoughtfully analyzed, is needed regarding older persons in reference to stable/and unstable angina syndromes. It is surprising that only fragmentary and incomplete data are available for these very common and important clinical problems of coronary heart disease in older persons.[72]

Hypertrophic cardiomyopathy in the elderly

Whether hypertrophic cardiomyopathy in the elderly has the same genetic basis, pathophysiology, or carries the same prognosis with the one seen in young individuals is not clear. Figure 10-7 illustrates the unusual histology of the condition. However, echocardiographic studies in both young and old with hypertrophic cardiomyopathy have shown similar asymmetric hypertrophy of the septum, systolic anterior motion of the mitral valve, and severity of an outflow tract gradient, although the younger group had more severe hypertrophy.[73] Furthermore, different ventricular cavity contours were noted between the two groups; the septum in the young is more hypertrophied, has reversed curvature, and thus creates a crescent-shaped left ventricular cavity. The elderly group with hypertrophic cardiomyopathy has normally shaped left and right ventricles and overall less severe hypertrophy.

A subgroup of elderly patients with obstructive hypertrophic cardiomyopathy, most of whom were women (87%), revealed an atypical systolic contact between the mitral valve and the interventricular septum, producing a dynamic subaortic obstruction. In this subgroup the systolic contact of the mitral valve with the septum was also the result of a posterior excursion of the ventricular septum toward the mitral valve. Sizeable calcium deposits in the mitral valve annulus in these elderly patients probably contributed to the outflow tract narrowing.[74] In another subset

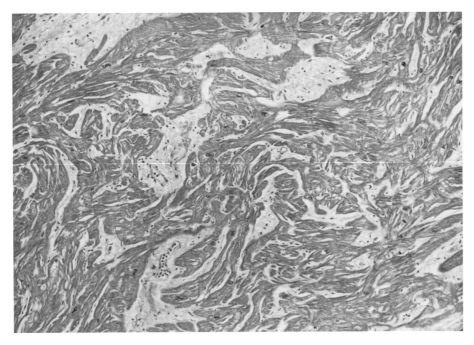

Fig. 10-7. Histology of myocardial section from a patient with hypertrophic cardiomyopathy. Myocyte hypertrophy, interstitial fibrosis, and myocyte disarray are present.

of patients, most of whom were black, severe concentric hypertrophy with small LV cavity, increased ejection fraction (80%), and diastolic dysfunction occurred. In these patients hypertension has been present, and it is suspected the increased blood pressure in some unknown way serves as the stimulus to unusual and severe hypertrophy.[75] The association of hypertrophic cardiomyopathy with systemic hypertension in some elderly patients has prompted some authors to suggest an etiologic link between these two entities. Others, however, although they recognize that hypertension may aggravate the underlying cardiomyopathy by leading to an increase in myocardial mass, have stressed that hypertension is not the primary cause of hypertrophic cardiomyopathy.[76]

Follow-up studies of elderly patients with hypertrophic cardiomyopathy indicate that their survival rate is quite similar to that of an age and gender-matched control group.[77] Although studies on the genetic transmission of hypertrophic cardiomyopathy in the elderly are lacking, one may state that this disease entity in advance age is rather benign in comparison with the more malignant stigmata seen in younger patients.

Congestive heart failure

Congestive heart failure is not a disease, but a syndrome of diverse etiologies and well-known signs and symptoms. Although not easily defined, the syndrome results from the inability of the heart to supply adequately the oxygen needs of the body, at rest and with exercise, at normal intracardiac filling pressures. This definition indicates the syndrome can occur in instances where myocardial dysfunction may be systolic or diastolic in origin, when myocardial function may be normal but loading conditions are abnormal (such as valvar disease and hypertension), and in instances where restrictive processes (such as pericarditis) are present. In fact, there may or may not be congestion, so the term *heart failure* might be more appropriate in many instances. In this discussion, we will use the generic term *congestive heart failure*.

In reference to older patients, congestive heart failure is of extraordinary importance because it is so common, diverse in its etiologies, and generates huge medical costs for hospitalization and care. It is the most frequent diagnosis related group (DRG) recorded in the Medicare population. In addition to the increased prevalence and incidence of congestive heart failure with advancing age, there is also a marked increased mortality, even when allowing for such independent determinants of mortality as etiology of heart failure and ejection fraction.[78-80]

The etiology of congestive heart failure in older patients is often multifactorial and sometimes uncertain. As discussed, the incidence of coronary arteriosclerosis is high in older persons, but the presence of congestive heart failure should not be equated with the presence of coronary heart disease when no evidence of past infarction, scarring, or ischemia is present. Although coronary heart disease may be the cause of or a contributor to congestive heart failure, hypertension and left ventricular hypertrophy with systolic and diastolic dysfunction also may be a contributor, as well as aortic and/or mitral valvar disease. Older patients may have cardiomyopathy of the hypertrophic or dilated type as is seen in younger persons.

Regardless of the etiology(ies) of the congestive heart failure, the age-related changes in the cardiovascular system enhance the propensity to develop congestive heart failure, particularly in reference to problems of diastolic dysfunction. A sizable proportion of elderly patients with congestive heart failure have well-preserved systolic function, and their principal abnormality is in diastolic dysfunction. As discussed, age-related diastolic dysfunction related to both myocardial properties and left ventricular chamber properties is present. In a substantial number of persons between the age of 75 and 80, amyloid deposits may be sufficient to add further to the problems of diastolic dysfunction. Finally, the aging changes in the lungs with both airway and compliance changes adds to the propensity for dyspnea, and renal mechanisms altering the handling of sodium also contribute to the syndrome of congestive heart failure.

Age-related changes also have important implication in reference to treatment. Diastolic dysfunction and the decreased responsiveness of old myocardium to beta-adrenergic stimulation combine to make preload (and the use of the Frank-Starling mechanism to maintain cardiac output) of utmost importance. Hence, older persons with congestive heart failure may be prone to have adverse effects when given diuretics to lessen congestion because reducing preload may compromise systolic function, which may be unduly dependent on high filling pressures. Although animal study results cited in reference to diminished responsiveness to digitalis glycosides and a greater propensity to toxic effects may not be directly transferrable to older human patients, the suspicion that such is true exists. The availability of vasodilators has helped considerably with treatment by improving the symptomatic state and convincingly reducing mortality.[81] This was most strikingly demonstrated in a randomized, controlled trial of advanced congestive heart failure in patients with a mean age of 70. A 31% reduction in mortality was shown at 1 year.

Syncope

Syncope or near-syncope increases in prevalence with age, and the etiology alters. In young persons, vasovagal episodes are frequent and often provide the explanation for syncope in a majority of cases. In elderly patients, vasovagal episodes are rare, and a large number—30% to 40% of cases—are attributable to cardiovascular causes.[82] Many syncopal episodes are unexplained in older persons, which is perhaps not surprising because they may be multifactorial, involving both cardiac, CNS, and other organ dysfunctions. Much of the syncope attributable to cardiovascular causes has its explanation in age-related changes.

As described, loss of pacemaker and conducting cell function as a part of normal aging predisposes the elderly to sinus node dysfunction, with pauses and abnormalities

of conduction in the atrio-ventricular node and His-Purkinje system, leading to heart block as well as tachycardias, particularly related to atrial fibrillation and ventricular mechanisms. Because older patients have a high incidence of carotid and cerebrovascular disease, they are very sensitive to alterations in preload (ventricular filling pressure) because of diastolic dysfunction, and have blunted baroreceptor reflexes. As a result, syncope of cardiovascular origin, primarily related to the changes of aging per se, is easily understood. Normal physiologic stresses, such as defecation, micturition, coughing and swallowing, may produce syncope or near-syncope in susceptible older persons. In addition, there is a propensity for older persons to develop adverse effects in response to multiple cardiovascular drugs, including inordinate reduction in preload with diuretics and sensitivity to a variety of antihypertensive agents that are commonly prescribed. Further the kidneys' capacity to conserve salt declines with age. Hypovolemia related to poor eating habits and diminished food intake (many elderly persons have impaired thirst response), and even modest and subtle fluid losses related to intercurrent illnesses with vomiting and diarrhea, enhance the propensity to syncope.[83]

Risk factors in cardiovascular disease

The role of conventional cardiovascular risk factors in older persons is not well understood because only fragmentary and inadequate data are available in most instances. During the last few years there has been increasing concern about the role of risk factors, especially lipids and isolated systolic hypertension (ISH). The hypothesis that conventional risk factors are not important in the aged, because age per se becomes such a powerful risk factor, is giving way to the idea that we need more and better data concerning matters such as smoking and lipids. Data on ISH are becoming increasingly clear, as was discussed in an earlier section.

The data available regarding the effects of smoking as a risk in older persons are fragmentary and inconsistent. An observational study from the Coronary Artery Surgical Study Registry involved 1800 patients in two groups felt to be reasonably well matched except for smoking.[84] One group continued smoking after entering the study while the "matched group" abstained. Although this study included the oldest patients in the database, (all patients older than 55 years), the mean age of the 1800 patients was only 60 years, and there were extremely few over the age of 75. Regardless, this study demonstrated a statistically significant reduction in the risk of myocardial infarction or death in these patients with advanced coronary heart disease if they quit smoking. Beneficial effect was the same in patients 55 to 64 years and 65 years and older. Dividing patients into risk quartiles, the benefits of smoking cessation were greatest in those with a moderate risk (for infarction or death) and barely discernible for the two quartiles with minimal risk or with the highest risk. More data are needed, but it is rational to believe that smoking cessation will benefit patients at risk in all age groups. Randomized, controlled trials would be required to prove the point definitively.

The importance of elevated blood lipids in relation to cardiovascular risk is currently very controversial, studies are underway to clarify these issues in older persons. This matter is complicated by the need to screen older persons for blood lipid abnormalities, which involves considerable expense, important problems related to laboratory quality control, and scientific issues related to the importance of the various blood lipid fractions that might be the risk factors in this age group.

Reviews and position papers[85,86] have summarized the data. Epidemiologic studies tend to show that hypercholesterolemia is not a risk factor, but these studies are confounded by including frail and ill old people who may have low cholesterol levels because of these noncardiac conditions and who live for only a short period of time because of these conditions. In addition, because coronary heart disease is frequent and the leading cause of death in older people, a modest effect achieved by lipid lowering could have a very significant mortality and morbidity benefit. (This emphasizes the need to consider attributable risks, not merely relative risks when the disease condition is frequent.)

Much more epidemiologic, clinical, and basic research is needed before the importance of lipids can be known and general recommendations made.

Diabetes mellitus is common in older persons, occurring in nearly 20% of people over the age of 70, and often cited as a risk factor in identifying the progression of cardiovascular disease. The overwhelming development of diabetes in older persons is of the type II, or non-insulin-dependent, diabetes mellitus (NIDDM). There are hereditary associations, and the condition can be aggravated by obesity and a variety of drugs. As with cardiovascular function, age-related deterioration and carbohydrate tolerance occurs, increasing the propensity to the development of NIDDM because of the lack of reserve mechanisms to handle hyperglycemia. Although discussion of these is beyond the scope of this brief resumé, it is essential to remember that the diabetic state can, and often will, influence a wide variety of metabolic processes and fluid balance, which can have major implications in reference to the presentation and treatment of cardiovascular conditions in older persons. However, its importance as a risk factor independent of all other confounding features of the aged is uncertain.

SUMMARY

The extraordinary rate of increase in our older population, coupled with the inevitable age-related changes in the cardiovascular system, make the study and understanding of these matters one of the most important and intriguing endeavors in all of medicine. The cardiovascular system does not age and degenerate in a uniform fashion but rather in specific ways, as does the human organism itself. For example, diastolic but not systolic ventricular function may be influenced. The conduction system and left-sided cardiac valves, as well as portions (but not all) of the aorta undergo easily discernable anatomic degenerative changes. The situation is made much more complicated by the enormous heterogeneity of the aging process in our society. Chronology, in general, very poorly predicts biologic aging and the accompanying physiologic changes that occur. Most people will die before they reach their early 80s, and many will be incapacitated by the changes of disease or aging. However, some will remain vigorous and even be able to develop a cardiac output (albeit by different mechanisms) equivalent to that of their younger peers. Although this tremendous heterogeneity in aging must be in large part genetically determined, a variety of physical, emotional, and mental factors must also be involved. Pfaffenbarger's[87] studies convincingly demonstrate that a lifelong exercise habit not only enhances survival, but also makes cardiovascular events, such as myocardial infarction, less morbid. Depression has been demonstrated to be an adverse feature for survival in older persons when other important determinants of longevity are matched among patient groups.[88]

Particular attention must be paid to the interaction between disease, aging, and lifestyle, as well as to the role that medications may be playing in patient complaints and altered functional capacity. A highly individualistic and comprehensive approach must be taken to all older persons, keeping in mind complex and multiple interactions that will exist in every individual. Although all interventions, whether diagnostic or therapeutic (e.g., drug, surgical, or invasive catheterization), tend to have a higher morbidity and mortality in the old than they do in the young, such problems do not constitute contraindications to such methods. They only additionally emphasize the need for a particularly thoughtful and individualized approach.

REFERENCES

1. Cluff LE: The meaning of being old in America: the responsibilities of the medical profession, *Trans Am Clin Climatol Assoc* 96:185, 1984.
2. Callahan D: *Setting limits: medical goals in an aging society.* New York, 1987, Simon and Schuster.
3. Council on Scientific Affairs : American Medical Association white paper on elderly health, *Arch Intern Med* 150:2459, 1990.
4. 18th Bethesda Conference, Cardiovascular disease in the elderly, *J Am Coll Cardiol* 10:A-1, 1987.
5. Schneider EL, Guralnik JM: The aging of America, *JAMA* 263:2333, 1990.
6. Demographics and socioeconomics (aspects of aging in the United States), *U S Bureau of the Census* 138:23, 1984.
7. DHHS PUB# (PHS) 90-1231 Catalogue #76-641 498, *Library of Congress* 1989.

8. Frye RL: President's Page, *JACC* 19:468, 1992.

9. Fries JF: Aging, natural death, and the compression of morbidity, *N Engl J Med* 303:130, 1980.

10. Fries JF: The Compression of mortality. Near or far, *The Millbank Quarterly* 67:2, 1989.

11. Harris R, ed: Clinical geriatric cardiology: management of the elderly patient. Philadelphia, 1986, J.B. Lippincott.

12. Kitzman DW, Scholz DG, Hagen PT, et al: Age-related changes in normal human hearts during the first 10 decades of life, Part II (Maturity). A quantitative anatomic study of 765 specimens from subjects 20 to 99 years old, *Mayo Clin Proc* 63:137, 1988.

13. Goor D, Lillehi CW, Edwards JE: The "sigmoid septum": variation in the contour of the left ventricular outlet, *Am J Roentgenol* 107:366, 1969.

14. Burns RT, Klima M: Morphometry of the aging heart, *Mod Pathol* 3:336, 1990.

15. Nixon JV, Hallmark H, Page K, et al: Ventricular performance in human hearts age 61 to 73 years, *Am J Cardiol* 56:932, 1985.

16. Tokunaga O, Yamada T, Fan J, et al: Age-related decline in prostacyclin synthesis by human aortic endothelial cells. Qualitative and quantitative analysis, *Am J Pathol* 138:941, 1991.

17. Lee TJF, Shirasaki Y, Nickols GA: Altered endothelial modulation of vascular tone in aging and hypertension, *Blood Vessels* 24:132, 1987.

18. Yasue H, Matsuyama K, Okumura K, et al: Responses of angiographically normal human coronary arteries to intracoronary injection of acetylcholine by age and segment: Possible role of early coronary atherosclerosis, *Circulation* 81:482, 1990.

19. Vita JA, Treasure CB, Nabel EG, et al: Coronary vasomotor response to acetycholine relates to risk factors for coronary artery disease, *Circulation* 81:491, 1990.

20. Yin FCP: *The Aging vasculature and its effects on the heart.* In Weisfelt ML, ed: *The aging heart: its function and response to stress,* New York, 1980, Raven.

21. Movat HZ, More RH, Haust MD: The diffuse intimal thickening of the human aorta with aging, *Am J Pathol* 34:1023, 1958.

22. Hutchins GM, Bulkley BH, Miner MM: Correlation of age and heart weight with tortuosity and caliber of normal human coronary arteries, *Am Heart J* 94:196, 1977.

23. Avolio AP, Chen S, Wang R, et al: Effects of aging on changing arterial compliance and left ventricular load in a northern Chinese urban community, *Circulation* 68:50, 1983.

24. Virmani R, Avolio AP, Mergner WJ, et al: Effect of aging on aortic morphology in populations with high and low prevalence of hypertension and atherosclerosis, *Am J Pathol* 139:1119, 1991.

25. Weisfeldt ML, Lakatta EG, Gerstenblith G: *Aging and cardiac disease.* In Braunwald EB, ed: *Heart disease,* Philadelphia, 1988, WB Saunders.

26. Guarnieri T, Spurgeon H, Froehlich JP, et al: Diminished inotropic response but unaltered toxicity to acetylstrophanthidin in the senescent beagle, *Circulation* 60:1548, 1979.

27. Spirito P, Maron BJ: Influence of aging on Doppler echocardiographic indices of left ventricular diastolic function, *Br Heart J* 59:672, 1988.

28. Gerstenblith G, Frederiksen J, Yin FCP, et al: Echocardiographic assessment of a normal adult aging population, *Circulation* 56:273, 1977.

29. Miyatake K, Okamoto M, Kinoshita N, et al: Augmentation of the atrial contribution to left ventricular inflow with aging as assessed by intracardiac Doppler flowmetry, *Am J Cardiol* 53:586, 1984.

30. Brandfonbremer M, Landowne M, Shock MW: Changes in cardiac output with age, *Circulation* 12:557, 1955.

31. Fleg JL, Lakatta EG: Role of muscle loss in the age-associated reduction in VO2max, *J Appl Physiol* 65:1147, 1988.

32. Yin FCP, Weisfeldt ML, Milnor WR: The role of aortic input impedance in the decreased cardiovascular response to exercise with aging in the dog, *J Clin Invest* 68:28, 1981.

33. Port S, Cobb FR, Coleman RE, et al: Effect of age on the response of the left ventricular ejection fraction to exercise, *N Engl J Med* 303:1133, 1980.

34. Rodeheffer RJ, Gerstenblith G, Becker LC, et al: Exercise cardiac output is maintained with advancing age in healthy human subjects: cardiac dilatation and increased stroke volume compensate for a diminished heart rate, *Circulation* 69:203, 1984.

35. Robinson S, Dill DB, Tzankoff SP, et al: Longitudinal studies of aging in 37 men, *J Appl Physiol* 38:263, 1975.

36. Haber P, Honiger B, Klicpera M, et al: Effects in elderly people 67-76 years of age of three-month endurance training on a bicycle ergometer, *Eur Heart J* 5:537, 1984.

37. Hagberg JM: Effect of training on the decline of VO$_{2max}$ with aging, *Federation Proc* 46:1830, 1987.

38. Lipsitz LA, Nyguist BP, Wei JY, et al: Postprandial reduction in blood pressure in the elderly, *N Engl J Med* 309:81, 1983.

39. Gerber JG, Brass EP: *Drug use.* In Schrier RW, ed: *Geriatric medicine,* Philadelphia, 1990, WB Saunders.

40. Montgomery RD, Haeney MR, Ross IN, et al: The ageing gut: a study of intestinal absorption in relation to nutrition in the elderly, *Q J Med* 47:197, 1978.

41. Weiling PG: Interactions affecting drug absorption, *Clin Pharmacokinet* 9:404, 1984.

42. Plein JB, Plein EM: Ageing and drug therapy, *Ann Rev Gerontol Geriatr* 2:211, 1981.

43. Roberts WC: The structure of the aortic valve in clinically isolated aortic stenosis. An autopsy study of 162 patients over 15 years of age, *Circulation* 42:91, 1970.

44. Pomerance A: *Age-related cardiovascular changes and mechanically induced endocardial pathology.* In Silver MD, ed: *Cardiovascular pathology,* ed New York, 1992, Churchill Livingstone.

45. Isoyama S, Wei JY, Isumo S, et al: Effect of age on the development of cardiac hypertrophy produced by aortic constriction in the rat, *Circ Res* 61:337, 1987.

46. Edwards WD: *Surgical pathology of the aortic valve.* In Waller BF, ed: *Pathology of the heart and great vessels,* New York, 1988, Churchill Livingstone.

47. Sahasakal Y, Edwards WD, Naessens JM, et al: Age-related changes in aortic and mitral valve thickness: implications for two-dimensional echocardiography based on an autopsy study of 200 normal human hearts, *Am J Cardiol* 62:424, 1988.

48. Leibovitch ER: Cardiac valve disorders: growing significance in the elderly, *Geriatrics* 44:91, 1989.

49. Korn D, DeSanctis RW, Sells S: Massive calcification of the mitral annulus: A clinico-pathological study of 14 cases, *N Engl J Med* 267:900, 1962.

50. Agruss NS, Rosin EY, Adolph RJ, et al: Significance of chronic sinus bradycardia in elderly people, *Circulation* 46:924, 1972.

51. Gann D, Tolentino A, Samet P: Electrophysiologic evaluation of elderly patients with sinus bradycardia, *Ann Intern Med* 90:24, 1979.

52. Fleg JL, Kennedy HL: Cardiac arrhythmias in a healthy elderly population: detection by 24-hour ambulatory electrocardiography, *Chest* 81:302, 1982.

53. Lenegre J: Etiology and pathology of bilateral bundle branch block in relation to complete heart block, *Prog Cardiovasc Dis* 6:409, 1964.

54. Lev M: The pathology of complete atrioventricular block, *Prog Cardiovasc Dis* 6:317, 1964.

55. Fugino M, Okada R, Arakawa K: The relationship of aging to histological changes in the conduction system of the normal human heart, *Am Heart J* 24:13, 1983.

56. Pomerance A: Senile cardiac amyloidosis, *Br Heart J* 27:711, 1965.

57. Johansson B, Westermark P: Senile systemic amyloidosis: A clinico-pathological study of twelve patients with massive amyloid infiltration, *Int J Cardiol* 32:83, 1991.

58. Olson LJ, Gertz MA, Edwards WD, et al: Senile cardiac amyloidosis with myocardial dysfunction: Diagnosis by endomyocardial biopsy and immunochemistry, *N Engl J Med* 317:738, 1987.

59. Kyle RA, Gertz MA: Cardiac amyloidosis, *Int J Cardiol* 28:139, 1990.

60. Pitkanen P, Westermark P, Cornwell GG III: Systemic senile amyloidosis, *Am J Pathol* 117:391, 1984.

61. Lie JT, Hammond PT: Pathology of the senescent heart: anatomic observation of 237 autopsy studies of patients 90 to 105 years old, *Mayo Clin Proc* 63:551, 1988.

62. Goreric PD, Prelli FC, Wright J, et al: Systemic senile amyloidosis. Identification of a new prealbumin (transthyretin) variant in cardiac tissue: immunologic and biochemical similarity to one form of familial amyloidotic polyneuropathy, *J Clin Invest* 83:836, 1989.

63. SHEP Cooperative Research Group : Prevention of stroke by antihypertensive drug treatment in older persons with isolated systolic hypertension: Final results of the Systolic Hypertension in the Elderly Program (SHEP), *JAMA* 265:3255, 1991.

64. Amery A, Birkenhager W, Brixko P, et al: Mortality and morbidity results from the European working party on high blood pressure in the elderly trial, *Lancet* 1:1349, 1985.

65. White NK, Edwards JE, Dry TJ: Relationship of the degree of coronary atherosclerosis with age, in women, *Circulation* 1:1345, 1950. For men: *Circulation* I:645:1950.

66. Hadziselimovic H: Age characteristics of blood vessels of the human heart, *Act Anat* 109:231, 1981.

67. GISSI Gruppo Italiano per lo Studio della Streptochinasi nell' Infarto Miocardico: Effectiveness of thrombolytic treatment in acute myocardial infarction, *Lancet* 1:397, 1986.

68. ISIS-2 (Second International Study of Infarct Survival) : Collaborative Group: Randomized trial of intravenous streptokinase, oral aspirin, both, or neither among 17,187 cases of suspected acute myocardial infarction: ISIS-2, *Lancet* 2:349, 1988.

69. Nadelmann J, Frishman WH, Ooi WL, et al: Prevalence, incidence and prognosis of recognized and unrecognized myocardial infarction in persons age 75 years or older: The Bronx Aging Study, *Am J Cardiol* 66:533, 1990.

70. Goldberg RJ, Gore JM, Gurwitz JH, et al: The impact of age on the incidence and prognosis of initial acute myocardial infarction: The Worcester Heart Attack Study, *Am Heart J* 117:543, 1989.

71. Friesinger GC, Goldman L: Unpublished data 1992.

72. Podczeck A, Frohner K, Foderler G, et al: Exercise test in patients over 65 years of age after the first myocardial infarction, *Eur Heart J* 5:89, 1984.

73. Lever HM, Karam RF, Currie PH, et al: Hypertrophic cardiomyopathy in the elderly. Distinctions from the young based on cardiac shape, *Circulation* 79:580, 1989.

74. Lewis JF, Maron BJ: Elderly patients with hypertrophic cardiomyopathy: A subset with distinctive left ventricular morphology and progressive clinical course late in life, *J Am Coll Cardiol* 13:36, 1989.

75. Topol EJ, Taarill TA, Fortuin NJ: Hypertensive hypertrophic cardiomyopathy in the elderly, *N Engl J Med* 312:277, 1985.

76. Karam R, Lever HM, Healy BP: Hypertensive hypertrophic cardiomyopathy or hypertrophic cardiomyopathy with hypertension? A study of 78 patients, *J Am Coll Cardiol* 13:580, 1989.

77. Fay WP, Taliercio CP, Ilstrup DM, et al: Natural history of hypertrophic cardiomyopathy in the elderly, *J Am Coll Cardiol* 16:821, 1990.

78. Kannel WB, Belanger AJ: Epidemiology of heart failure, *Am Heart J* 121:951, 1991.

79. Smith WM: Epidemiology of congestive heart failure, *Am J Cardiol* 55:3A, 1985.

80. Yusuf S, Bourassa M, Friesinger G: Studies on left ventricular function (SOLVD) registry of 6,152 patients with congestive heart failure, *Unpublished studies* 1992.

81. CONSENSUS Trial Study Group : Effects of enalapril on mortality in severe congestive heart failure, *N Engl J Med* 316:1429, 1987.

82. Jonsson PV, Lipsitz LA: *Syncope*. In Schrier RW, ed: *Geriatric medicine*, Philadelphia, 1990, WB Saunders.

83. Shannon RP, Wei JY, Rosa RM, et al: The effect of age and sodium depletion on cardiovascular responses to orthostasis, *Hypertension* 8:438, 1986.

84. Hermanson B, Omenn GS, Kronmal RA, et al: Beneficial six-year outcome of smoking cessation in older men and women with coronary artery disease, *N Engl J Med* 319:1365, 1988.

85. Denke MA, Grundy SM: Hypercholesterolemia in elderly persons: resolving the treatment dilemma, *Ann Intern Med* 112:780, 1990.

86. Garber AM, Littenberg B, Sox HC Jr.: Costs and effectiveness of cholesterol screening in the elderly, *Health Program, Office of Technology Assessment, Congress of the United States*, Washington 1-57, 1989.

87. Paffenbarger RS, Wing AL, Hyde RT: Physical activity as an index of heart attack risk in college alumni, *Am J Epidemiol* 108:161, 1978.

88. Mossey JM, Shapiro E: Self-rated health: A predictor of mortality among the elderly, *Am J Public Health* 72:800, 1982.

Chapter 11

CARDIOVASCULAR MANIFESTATIONS IN SYSTEMIC DISEASES

Michael B. Gravanis
Stephen D. Clements, Jr.

Systemic autoimmune diseases
    Systemic lupus erythematosus
    Mixed connective tissue disease
    Systemic sclerosis (scleroderma)
    Rheumatoid arthritis
    Polymyositis and dermatomyositis
Systemic disorders with multiorgan involvement
    Wegener granulomatosis
    Whipple disease
    Thrombotic thrombocytopenic purpura
Seronegative spondylarthropathies
    Ankylosing spondylitis
Heritable connective tissue disorders
    Marfan syndrome
    Osteogenesis imperfecta
    Ehlers-Danlos syndrome
    Pseudoxanthoma elasticum
    Cutis laxa
    Combined Marfan and Ehler-Danlos syndrome
    Adult polycystic kidney disease
    Annuloaortic ectasia
Endocrine disorders
    The thyroid and the cardiovascular system
    Thyrotoxicosis
    Hyperthyroidism
    Hypothyroidism (myxedema)
Adrenal disorders
    Cushing syndrome
    Addison disease
    Pheochromocytoma
Pituitary disorders
    Hypopituitarism
    Acromegaly

Effects of parathyroid hormone on the cardiovascular system
    Hyperparathyroidism
    Hypocalcemia
Diabetes mellitus
Carcinoid heart disease
Infiltrative systemic disorders and depositions
    Amyloidosis
    Cardiac sarcoidosis
    Gout
Immune deficiency diseases
    Human immunodeficiency virus infection

A large number of heterogeneous disorders have been included in this chapter. The common denominator regarding their selection is involvement of the heart and blood vessels. These systemic disease entities may involve different anatomic sites within the heart (e.g., pericardium, myocardium, endocardium, valves, or coronary arteries) and/or various sizes of arteries or veins in different locations.

It is important to emphasize, however, that in this wide spectrum of systemic disorders, the pathophysiologic derangements (and thus the patient's symptoms) depend primarily on the anatomic location and extent of the lesions rather than on the specific histopathologic changes.

Although several systemic diseases may induce pericarditis with or without effusion, the histologic features of such pericardial involvement are often not pathognomonic, except in rare cases in which a characteristic lesion is identified (e.g., rheumatoid or sarcoid granuloma). Similarly, myocardial or conduction system involvement may not reveal the exact nature of an inflammatory infiltrate. Therefore a definitive clinical entity may not be recognized. However, in a given patient with cardiovascular involvement, additional laboratory data may distinguish between several potential causes for such involvement.

The higher incidence of cardiovascular involvement in systemic diseases reported from autopsy studies should not come as a surprise because the cardiovascular pathophysiologic derangement is often mild, and therefore unrecognized clinically. However, new invasive diagnostic techniques (endomyocardial biopsy) have somewhat increased the rate of detection in certain systemic disorders (e.g., myocardial infiltrates and depositions).

SYSTEMIC AUTOIMMUNE DISEASES

Previously called the connective tissue diseases or the collagen vascular diseases, the systemic autoimmune diseases include systemic lupus erythematosus (SLE), rheumatoid arthritis, polymyositis, dermatomyositis, Sjögren's syndrome, polychondritis, and Behcet syndrome. All of these diseases are characterized by multiorgan dysfunction. All of them, except for Behcet syndrome and relapsing polychondritis, have specific autoantibodies that have been identified; this may help with diagnosis and monitoring of disease activity. The role of these autoantibodies in the autoimmune process remains undefined, although the pathogenesis may involve genetic, immunologic, hormonal, and environmental factors and their interactions, resulting in B-cell activation.

In cases of SLE, end organ damage appears to be primarily mediated by immune complex deposition. Disease markers include anti-double–stranded DNA antibodies, and titers that may correlate with disease activity (as is the case with the glomerulonephritis of SLE, in which there is a direct correlation). The etiology of the systemic autoimmune diseases is unclear, although the cardinal defect in SLE is believed to be a failure of the regulatory mechanisms that sustain self-tolerance. Rheumatoid arthritis, polymyositis, and Sjögren syndrome are thought to be mediated by T-lymphocytes of the helper/inducer type. Scleroderma is a systemic fibrosing disease with evidence of cytosine activation of fibroblasts, as well as toxicity to endothelial cells, leading to vasculopathy and tissue fibrosis.

Systemic lupus erythematosus (SLE)

The availability of noninvasive cardiac evaluations, the routine use of corticosteroids, and the significant prolongation of life-spans of patients with SLE have all contributed to the increased recognition of cardiovascular involvement in this disease. The frequency of pericarditis in SLE patients was appreciated after the increased use of echocardiography. Similarly, the incidence of coronary arteritis and high rate of atherogenesis in patients treated with corticosteroids was noted after the growing use of cardiac catheterization. Nevertheless, in spite of the new and sophisticated diagnostic modalities, the diagnosis of lupus carditis is made by exclusion, as well as by association with extracardiac features of SLE. In addition, the longer life-span of patients treated with corticosteroids had a significant effect on the type, frequency, and morphology of cardiovascular lesions in SLE.

Pathogenesis of SLE. The basic underlying pathogenetic mechanism in the induction of the various cardiovascular lesions in SLE is believed to be the excessive formation of autoantibody, resulting in generation of antigen/antibody complexes that may deposit on small vessels, bind to complement, and initiate a chain reaction with damaging local effects. The complexes are phagocytosed by polys which then release lysosomal enzymes capable of producing fibrinoid necrosis. Moreover, release of vasoactive amines and prostaglandins may cause increased vascular permeability and thus exudation of serum from the injured vessels.

Systemic lupus erythematosus is the paradigmatic systemic autoimmune disease, affecting multiple organ systems including the skin, kidneys, CNS, and lungs. Cardiovascular involvement includes the heart and blood vessels. Cutaneous small vessel vasculitis (leukocytoclastic vasculitis) may occur in up to 20% of patients at some time during their disease course. A systemic vasculitis similar to polyarteritis nodosa involving larger vessels may also occur. The pathogenesis of both types is thought to be related to immune complexes deposition.

Clinical and laboratory criteria in the diagnosis of SLE. The American Rheumatism Association has published 11 revised criteria for the diagnosis of systemic lupus erythematosus. The presence of any 4 of the 11, simultaneously or serially, is believed to be diagnostic for SLE.[1] However, as new expressions of this disorder become known, the critiera listed below may not identify all cases of SLE:

1. Malar rash
2. Discoid rash
3. Photosensitivity
4. Oral ulcers
5. Arthritis (nonerosive, or two or more joints)
6. Serositis
7. Renal disorder (proteinuria or casts)
8. Neurologic disorder
9. Hematologic disorder
10. Immunologic disorder (Positive LE test; anti-DNA and other antibodies)
11. Antinuclear antibody

Cardiovascular manifestation in SLE. The cardiovascular manifestations of SLE are well defined, consisting mainly of pericarditis, myocarditis, and endocarditis. These manifestations are well recognized, but they are uncommon as isolated presenting problems. More commonly, cardiac symptoms are associated with other manifestations, such as arthritis, dermatitis, or renal dysfunction. It is well recognized that clinically obvious cardiac involvement is present in more than 50% of cases of SLE.[2,3] Earlier postmortem studies have reported some type of cardiac abnormality in nearly all cases.

Pericarditis in SLE. Immune complexes are found in the pericardial tissue regardless of the type of pericarditis in patients with SLE. Clinical pericarditis is estimated to occur in 20% to 30% of all patients and in as much as 75% of those studied echocardiographically.[4]

The pericarditis symptoms and signs may occur acutely, may be intermittent, or may be a recurring problem. The typical location of the discomfort is retrosternal, in the neck or left shoulder. It usually is a sharp or pressure pain aggravated by deep breathing, supine position, coughing, and sometimes swallowing. A three-component friction rub noted at the left sternal border often accompanies the discomfort. The absence of a friction rub does not exclude the diagnosis.

The electrocardiogram shows S-T segment elevation with a mean vector toward the apex writing, S-T elevation in the appropriate leads, and P-R segment depression. These changes evolve over a few days to T-wave changes. If pericardial effusion is present, low voltage may be present, and even electrical alternate may be observed in cases of cardiac tamponade. However, only occasionally large effusions may result in cardiac tamponade.[5] Rarely, constrictive pericarditis may become a clinical problem, although this complication has been observed more often in drug-induced lupus.[6] Furthermore, it has been suggested that corticosteroids may convert fibrinous pericarditis to a more fibrous type.[7]

Morphologic findings in lupus pericarditis. The morphologic findings of lupus pericarditis are not pathognomonic, except perhaps for the presence of hematoxylin bodies (tissue counterparts of the LE cell).

The acute phase pericarditis may be either focal or diffuse with fibrinous or serous effusions. Both pericardial surfaces are edematous and inflamed and may reveal foci of fibrinoid necrosis. The pericardial fluid is either pale or slightly serosanguineous and reveals marked leukocytosis (95% polymorphonuclear cells), low glucose and complement levels, and contains antinuclear antibodies.[8] In the chronic stage fibrous adhesions with obliteration of the pericardial space are observed, but calcium deposits are rarely found.

Myocardial involvement in SLE. Myocarditis has been a common finding at postmortem, but myocardial dysfunction from myocarditis is seldom evident clinically.[3]

The availability of endocardial biopsy may allow early detection of myocarditis and recognition of milder disease.[4]

Myocarditis in SLE has been associated with the anti-RNP autoantibodies and may occur anytime in the course of the illness. The usual histologic finding is nonspecific perivascular infiltration of lymphocytes and neutrophils. Edema, foci of fibrinoid necrosis, and occasional hematoxylin bodies are also noted.

Demonstration of immunoglobulin and complement components in the myocardium is not always accompanied by significant morphologic alterations comparable to the skin biopsy, which may reveal immunoglobulin deposition of the dermal-epidermal junction despite the absence of cutaneous lesions.[3] This lack of correlation may suggest that deposition of immune reactants alone is not sufficient for the initiation of a pathologic response.

Patchy fibrosis and scarring of the interstitium are observed in the chronic phase of the myocardial involvement.

Despite the high frequency of myocardial findings in SLE patients, many investigators are reluctant to accept the concept of a mild cardiomyopathy in this population. However, evidence in favor of a cardiomyopathy in SLE is provided by the often observed thrombotic or inflammatory microvascular coronary disease.

Conduction abnormalities in SLE. High grade atrioventricular block in SLE occurs rarely but is well documented. The heart block may be a manifestation of myocarditis and may spontaneously resolve with treatment. Histologic studies of the conduction system in SLE reveal foci of chronic inflammation, vasculitis of small vessels, and fibrosis along the conduction system. However, the sinoatrial node is involved more frequently than the AV node, perhaps because of the frequency of pericarditis.[9,10]

A well-known correlation exists between maternal SLE and congenital complete heart block (CHB) in children. According to recent reports CHB is often associated with other congenital heart abnormalities, structural valvular changes, and cardiomyopathy.[11]

Antinuclear antibody anti-Ro (SS-A) in the sera of women who delivered infants with CHB has been demonstrated, although this association is not universal because mothers with anti-Ro may give birth to nonaffected infants.[12] Only the minority of SS-A-positive or SS-B-positive women have pregnancies complicated by neonatal lupus.[13]

Coronary artery involvement in SLE. Intimal proliferation and/or recanalization of vessels is commonly observed in the small intramyocardial arteries, and is a possible indication of healed arteritis or primary thrombosis.[14] Embolism, thrombosis, or arteritis of extramural coronary arteries may occur in SLE, but is considered rare. Atherosclerotic disease of these arteries is not unusual, although the role of the corticosteroids in this vascular complication of SLE is not yet elucidated. A recent autopsy study suggested that disease activity and duration contributes more than corticosteroids to coronary atherosclerosis.[15] Others have pointed out that besides hypertension and hyperlipidemia, immune complex deposition plays an important role in the development of accelerated coronary atherosclerosis in SLE patients.[4] Intimal proliferation resulting from stimulation of the vascular endothelium by immunologic factors may initiate the atherosclerotic change. Both lupus anticoagulants and antiphospholipid antibodies are associated with increased thrombosis and may directly stimulate vascular endothelial cell proliferation.[16,17] Myocardial ischemia and rarely infarction may occur as the result of either arteritis or occlusive atherosclerotic lesions.

Valvular manifestations in SLE. Although symptomatic valvular heart disease caused by SLE was considered rare in the past, recent reports indicate an increase in cases with hemodynamically significant regurgitant or stenotic valvulopathies in SLE. Furthermore, echocardiography has identified lesions other than verrucous endocarditis, such as valvular thickening and dysfunction, that are prone to hemodynamic deterioration.[18]

The exact prevalence of valvular involvement in SLE is not known. Autopsy series have shown a high proportion (13% to 50%) which, however, does not necessarily reflect the degree of prevalence in the living population of SLE patients. An overall prevalence of valvular disease in SLE of 18% was reported in a study based on echocardiographic data.[19]

The verrucous nonbacterial valvular and mural endocarditis of the Libman-Sacks variety is the best known and most specific type of valvular involvement in systemic lupus. This lesion has a greater propensity in young patients during the active phase of the disease and is associated with mild valvular regurgitation in some patients, and no symptomatology in others. The verrucae are often found on the ventricular undersurface of the posterior mitral leaflet, the ventricular mural endocardium, chordae tendineae, and papillary muscles. They are usually single and measure 3 mm to 4 mm, or conglomerate in mulberry-like structures (Figs. 11-1, 11-2). Rarely, they can be large to simulate intracardiac tumors. The term endocardoma has been used for such large vegetations.[20] Systemic embolization of Libman-Sacks lesions is rather rare but may occur.

Morphologic features of verrucous nonbacterial endocarditis. Microscopically, verrucae may reveal a zoning arrangement: the superficial zone consisting of amorphous protein, fibrin, and hematoxylin bodies; a middle zone of proliferating fibroblasts and capillaries; and the innermost zone of more mature connective tissue with neovascularization (Fig. 11-3). The leaflet substance appears edematous, contains foci of fibrinoid necrosis (which may result in cusp perforation), and hematoxylin bodies at the early stages, and more fibrotic features at the healing stage. De-

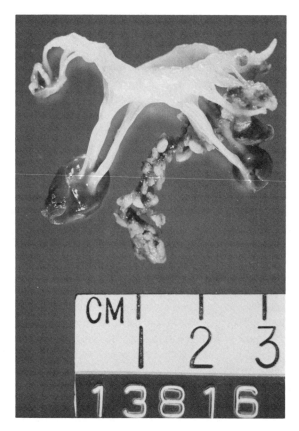

Fig. 11-1. Surgically excised mitral valve of a patient with SLE. Multiple verrucae are present on the ventricular undersurface of the leaflet and chordae in a mulberry-like formation (endocardoma).

posits of IgG and complement components may be demonstrated by immunofluorescence.

In some patients, however, echocardiography reveals valvular thickening and stiffness, resulting in either stenosis or regurgitation. These are usually patients with longer duration of the disease who had received large dosages of corticosteroids.[18] The morphologic features in this group of patients are characterized by leaflet thickening, deformity, and commissural fusion reminiscent of rheumatic valvulitis. Severe scarring, hyalinization, and calcification are the usual microscopic features.

Although the specificity of these valvular lesions in lupus can be questioned, it is believed that changes such as valvular scarring, retraction, and calcification may be facilitated by the corticosteroid therapy.[18] Furthermore, vegetations in patients under steroid therapy are often single and smaller, an indication that corticosteroids interfere with the pathogenic sequence responsible for the growth and healing of these verrucae. However, it is difficult to attribute all the differences in the clinical expression of SLE-related valvular disease to the steroid use. Perhaps factors such as active disease or concurrent renal failure

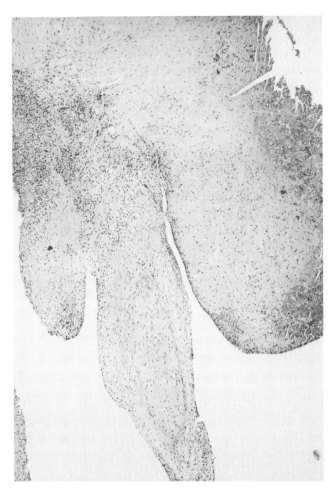

Fig. 11-2. Healing stage of Libman-Sacks endocarditis. Note encasing of chordae by loose, moderately cellular connective tissue, focal fibrinoid necrosis, and deposition of fibrin on the surface of the verrucae.

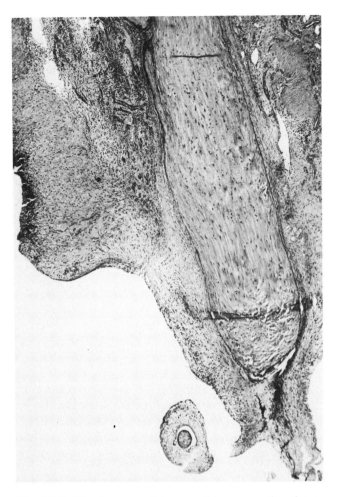

Fig. 11-3. Chorda wrapped by organizing connective tissue. Note the zoning arrangement: a superficial zone of fibrin, middle zone of proliferating fibroblasts and capillaries, and an innermost zone of mature connective tissue with neovascularization.

may also account for the different SLE valvulopathies during life.[21]

Lupus anticoagulant and antiphospholipid antibodies are known to be associated with thromboembolic phenomena in patients with or without SLE. Association of lupus anticoagulant and antiphospholipid antibodies with severe valvular heart disease in patients with SLE has been reported.[22] According to those reports, organizing thrombi on the surface of the valve may cause distortion and subsequent dysfunction. However, lupus anticoagulant also occurs in individuals without SLE who exhibit an increased tendency to thrombosis. The pathogenesis of the associated prothrombotic tendency is not clear, although suggested mechanisms include direct endothelial injury by antiphospholipid antibodies, which may lead to activation of coagulation factors, platelet consumption, or inhibition of prostacyclin production, resulting in enhanced platelet aggregation.[22,23]

Whether antibodies against phospholipids are the cause of the valvular lesions in SLE or simply accompany more basic underlying immunologic disturbances such as deposition of immune complexes has not been fully assessed.

Pulmonary vascular manifestations in SLE. Pulmonary hypertension has been clinically well documented in SLE, although morphologic studies of pulmonary vessels often reveal absence or only minimal inflammatory reaction despite the demonstrated deposition of immune complexes.[24,25] Whether a "hypercoagulable state" associated with SLE may be responsible for multiple vascular occlusions and subsequent pulmonary hypertension remains unknown.

Mixed connective tissue disease (MCTD)

Mixed connective tissue disease is a syndrome of a lupus-like disorder often having in common features with polymyositis and scleroderma. Serologically it is characterized by high titers of antibodies to nuclear ribonucleoprotein (RNP). MCTD presents clinically with a mixture of features such as polyarthritis, Raynaud's phenomenon, sclerodactyly, and proximal muscle weakness. However, the more serious cerebral and renal lesions of SLE are uncommon.

Cardiac involvement in MCTD is characterized by pericarditis with occasionally large effusions or tamponade. Cases of myocarditis with heart block have been reported in both adults and children.[26]

Whether MCTD constitutes a distinct entity or is a heterogeneous mixture of subsets of SLE, scleroderma, or polymyositis is still actively debated. Those supporting the idea of MCTD being a distinct disease argue that, although the presence of anti-RNP antibody by itself is not diagnostic, the absence of antibodies to native DNA and Sm antigen, characteristic for SLE, is important in defining MCTD.[27]

Systemic sclerosis (scleroderma)

Systemic sclerosis is a multisystem disease characterized by cutaneous features and visceral involvement. The latter, which are serious and life-threatening, may effect the kidneys, lungs, heart, and gastrointestinal tract.

The onset of scleroderma is often insidious, develops usually in middle or later adult life, and affects more women than men. The CREST syndrome (Calcinosis, Raynaud's phenomenon, Esophageal dysfunction, Slcerodactyly, and Telangiectasia) is a milder and more slowly evolving form of systemic sclerosis. There are fewer visceral lesions in the CREST syndrome, and cardiac and re-

nal involvement is rare. The anticentromere antibody is found in the sera of more than 50% of patients with the CREST syndrome.[28] Although scleroderma generally is not considered to be an inherited disease, reports of familial aggregation of cases suggests a possible genetic predisposition.[29] However, familial aggregation does not necessarily imply a genetic etiology.

Cardiac manifestations in scleroderma. Cardiac disease is a common manifestation of diffuse systemic sclerosis and can be life-threatening if significant myocardial or conduction system involvement is present. However, a number of clinical symptoms that may suggest cardiac involvement in scleroderma may reflect underlying pathologic processes of restrictive lung disease, pulmonary hypertension, renal disease with systemic hypertension, or uremic pericarditis.

Primary involvement of the heart in systemic sclerosis may include the pericardium, myocardium, coronary arteries, conduction system, and very rarely, the valves.

Pericardial findings in scleroderma. Pericardial disease is frequently detected on echocardiography in patients with systemic sclerosis, but is clinically apparent in only a minority of patients.[30]

An active fibrinous pericarditis, most commonly chronic, with or without effusion, is present. The pericardial fluid reveals moderate pleocytosis, normal glucose levels, low protein content, and lack of evidence of autoantibodies, immune complexes, or complement deple-

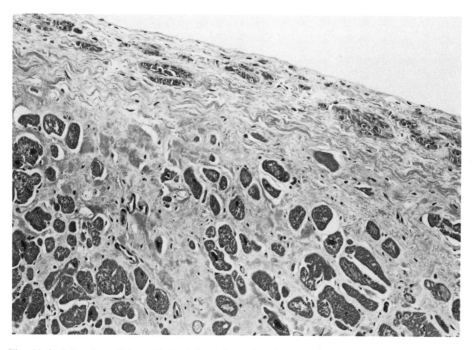

Fig. 11-4. Subendocardial scar (microinfarct) in a scleroderma patient. Note reactive myocyte hypertrophy.

tion.[31] Constrictive pericarditis is virtually unknown in systemic sclerosis.

Myocardial involvement in scleroderma. Of all the cardiac lesions in systemic sclerosis, the myocardial involvement appears to be the most intriguing. The pathogenesis of the myocardial lesions remains speculative, although transient ischemia at the microvascular level is the most attractive hypothesis.

Myocardial lesions in systemic sclerosis are characterized by focal myocyte degeneration and/or necrosis accompanied by focal fibrosis in both ventricles and atria, from the subendocardium to the subepicardium. The direct extension of the fibrotic lesions to the endocardium may create visible endocardial depressions, or "pockmarks," (Fig. 11-4). This is in contrast to the scars resulting from occlusive epicardial coronary disease, in which the subendocardial myocardium is spared. Furthermore, the fibrotic lesions do not appear to correspond to a particular distribution of a major coronary artery.

Although structural changes in small intramyocardial arteries, such as intimal proliferation and fibrosis, and medial hypertrophy have been noted, the frequency of these findings is relatively low, and the extent of the surrounding myocardial fibrosis appears out of proportion to the vascular lesions.

Contraction band necrosis of myocytes has been seen with significant frequency in hearts of patients with systemic sclerosis (Fig. 11-5). This type of myocyte injury

has been associated with temporary obstruction of blood flow followed by reperfusion. Similar intermittent obstruction and reperfusion has been hypothesized as the underlying pathogenetic mechanism in scleroderma, that is, coronary spasm analogous to the Raynaud's phenomenon of the skin.[32] Such an intermittent spasm besides that may be cumulative is apparently in line with other known scleroderma phenomena of spasm in the digits and kidneys. This hypothesis, however, was advanced before our current understanding of myocardial preconditioning by intermittent interruptions of coronary blood flow, and its protective effects on the myocardium.[33]

Vascular pathophysiology in scleroderma. Recent studies have demonstrated that coronary reserve is greatly impaired in progressive systemic sclerosis, and it may be an important contributor to the pathogenesis of scleroderma myocardial disease.[34] These studies suggested that the decreased coronary reserve in scleroderma is caused by primary abnormalities of small coronary vessels, and that immune-mediated injury may also play a role.

Reversible defects in myocardial perfusion in patients with normal epicardial vessels were demonstrated by thallium and PET scanning at rest and during exercise. The results of these studies suggest that the myocardial lesions (fibrosis) seen in systemic sclerosis probably result from vasospasm of small intramyocardial arteries, inducing transient ischemia.[35]

Other researchers have shown that transient reduction in

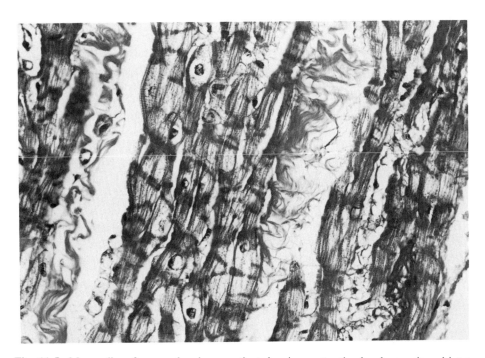

Fig. 11-5. Myocardium from a scleroderma patient showing contraction band necrosis and intracellular (myocyte) edema.

perfusion of different regions of the ventricular myocardium can be induced by a cold stimulus in patients with no signs of previous myocardial defect. These results further support the concept of a form of Raynaud's phenomenon affecting the myocardium.[36]

Although angina pectoris may be a feature in this entity, the extramural coronary arteries are usually patent.[32] Heart failure usually takes the form of a congestive or dilated cardiomyopathy, but sometimes may be that of a restrictive cardiomyopathy.[37]

Valvular manifestations in scleroderma. Primary valvular lesions caused by systemic sclerosis are considered to be rare. However, hemodynamic derangement of a valve may be a secondary result of systemic sclerosis, such as aortic incompetence caused by severe systemic hypertension or pulmonary valve incompetence in a patient with severe pulmonary hypertension. Autopsy studies have failed to establish an association between systemic sclerosis and mitral valve prolapse, although echocardiographic studies have shown a disproportionately high incidence of mitral valve prolapse in both the CREST and nonCREST forms of systemic sclerosis.[38]

Arrhythmias and conduction abnormalities in scleroderma. Electrocardiographic abnormalities are common in systemic sclerosis and may be present before the cutaneous manifestations. Changes in rhythm and in conduction are frequent such as S-T and T-wave changes, or low voltage ventricular complexes indicative of myocardial damage. More than 50% of monitored patients revealed some form of ECG abnormality.[39,40]

First degree block or bundle-branch block are relatively common in systemic sclerosis. However, complete heart block is considered rare.[41] Autopsies of patients with systemic sclerosis have shown that the nodal (SA and AV) or Purkinje tissue may be atrophic or replaced by fibrous connective tissue. In rare cases, the arteries perfusing the nodes may be partially or totally occluded. Some reports indicate that the SA node is affected more frequently than the AV node, probably because of the close proximity of the SA node to the overlying pericarditis.[42]

Pulmonary hypertension in scleroderma, and particularly in the CREST syndrome, is discussed in Chapter 5 (Pulmonary Hypertension and Cor Pulmonale).

Rheumatoid arthritis (RA)

The major clinical feature of rheumatoid arthritis is chronic synovitis. The effects of this disease, however, are by no means confined to the joints or even to the musculoskeletal system. Cardiac involvement is one of the many extraarticular manifestations of rheumatoid arthritis (RA). RA may begin acutely or insidiously, and its clinical course is extremely variable. Exacerbations and remissions are frequent, although in most cases the disease eventually becomes progressive.

Patients with RA may reveal mild anemia, polyclonal hyperglobulinemia, increased sedimentation rate, and other acute-phase reactants. Rheumatoid factor, an immunoglobulin M (IgM) that reacts with aggregated gamma globulin, is found in about 70% to 75% of patients.

Although the presence of rheumatoid factor is not necessary for the diagnosis of RA, it is associated with more severe disease and therefore has a certain prognostic significance. For instance, the cardiac and vascular manifestations of RA are almost exclusively found among patients with seropositive disease.

Evidence accumulated in recent years indicates that there is a genetic predisposition to RA linked with the presence of cell surface antigens of the HLA-D series, encoded by the major histocompatability complex (MHC) that is part of chromosome 6. Although there are ethnic variations, the cell marker HLA-DR4 is present in approximately 70% of patients with RA, compared with 28% of patients in control groups.[43] Some antigens in the series may influence the severity of the disease and the development of extraarticular lesions and vasculitis.[44]

Pathogenesis of RA. Data about the pathogenesis of RA indicate that in the continuing proliferative inflammation (synovium) globulin antibodies themselves become antigenic, and antibodies are formed against them. Those antibodies are the rheumatoid factors found in IgG and IgM classes of globulin. The immune complexes bind to complement and activate the complement cascade. This in turn results in an influx of inflammatory cells (chemotaxis) that ingest the immune complexes while releasing lysosomal enzymes capable of tissue damage. In this hypothesis, it is not clear whether the initial antigen is an autoantigen or an antigen introduced from the environment (e.g., virus).

Cardiac manifestations in RA. Cardiac involvement is one of the many extraarticular manifestations of RA. The proliferative inflammatory process characteristic of RA may involve the pericardium, valves, myocardium, conduction system, and coronary arteries.

Pericarditis in RA. Evidence of active or past pericarditis is a frequent autopsy finding in as many as 50% of the cases,[45] whereas pericardial effusion has been noted in approximately 30% of patients in echocardiographic screening studies,[46] although only 1 in 10 patients develops symptomatic pericarditis during the course of their illness. The most significant physical sign of the pericardial involvement is a pericardial friction rub, which may not always be present and may not necessarily be associated with pain. Fever is not uncommon during the active phase of pericarditis.

The pathogenesis of pericarditis in RA appears to be similar to the pathogenesis of other extraarticular manifestations. In the active phase of pericarditis both the visceral and parietal surfaces of the pericardium appear edematous and are infiltrated by lymphocytes and plasma cells. The pericardial effusion consists of a serofibrinous exudate with a predominance of polymorphonuclear cells, low glucose and complement levels, and elevated amounts of IgG, rheumatoid factor, and immune complexes.

Constrictive pericarditis or tamponade are unusual complications of RA. Constriction occurs more frequently in males and is often associated with rheumatoid granulomas.[47] In constrictive pericarditis, the pericardium may be up to 5 mm thick and contains a quantity of loculated fluid.

Myocardial involvement in RA. Myocyte damage occasionally found in RA is usually focal and most commonly seen near valvular rings. Intracardial rheumatoid nodules may also be present, although they have a propensity for valvular rings and the conduction system. Whether the myocyte damage results from the inflammatory infiltrate, vasculitis, or atherosclerosis accelerated by vasculitis is not clear. The collagenous cardiac skeleton is also involved by the autoimmune process. A cell-mediated immunity directed against collagen has been suggested.[48]

Conduction abnormalities in RA. Conduction abnormalities such as high grade AV block may occur in seropositive RA. In some cases, a rheumatoid granuloma may be at or near the AV node or bundle of His. In most of the cases, however, there is no granuloma; only round cell infiltration, histiocytes, and fibrosis are noted.

In some studies a high frequency (more than two thirds of patients) of cardiac conducting tissue antibodies was detected in RA patients with conduction abnormalities. However, the precise pathogenetic mechanism involved in the mediation of an in vivo lesion in the conduction system has not been established.[49]

Amyloid deposits within the myocardium and the conduction system may lead to diastolic myocardial dysfunction and atrioventricular conduction disturbances.[50]

Vascular involvement in RA. A systemic vasculitis may occur in active RA in the form of a small vessel leukocytoclastic type or occasionally a vasculitis of larger vessels quite similar to polyarteritis nodosa. The pathogenetic mechanism for these vascular lesions is believed to be immune complex deposition in the arterial wall.

Coronary arteritis is often clinically silent, except when accompanied by luminal thrombus. At the acute stage, the coronary arteries reveal massive medial and adventitial infiltration by lymphocytes, plasma cells, and histiocytes, and disruption of the internal elastica. In some cases, the inflammatory infiltrate is strictly perivascular, whereas in other cases necrotizing areas in the arterial wall are present and surrounded by acute inflammatory cells. Intimal thickening by fibromuscular tissue proliferation may produce marked luminal narrowing. Thrombosis is not a common complication in these vessels.

Besides the involvement of the large epicardial coronary arteries, vasculitis of the small intramyocardial coronary arteries has been described. Patients with small coronary vasculitis may be asymptomatic, particularly those

who have severe arthritic changes and are relatively immobile. Occasionally, myocardial biopsy may reveal IgM deposits in the small intramyocardial vessels without evidence of an inflammatory response. However, in some cases luminal compromise may effect myocardial perfusion. It is of considerable interest that some reports indicate that antiinflammatory therapy may improve symptoms of congestive heart failure and improve ejection fraction in some patients with cardiac rheumatoid involvement.[51]

Valvular manifestations in RA. Valvular lesions caused by rheumatoid arthritis have been well recognized. The usual underlying morphologic lesion in such cases is either a nonspecific inflammation or rheumatoid granulomas involving the valvular apparatus and most specifically, the valvular annulus.

Valvular lesions in RA, although uncommon, may produce significant aortic regurgitation and less often, mitral regurgitation. Rheumatoid granulomas may be present at the base and annulus of both valves, thereby interfering with the proper closing of the cusps (Fig. 11-6). A rheu-

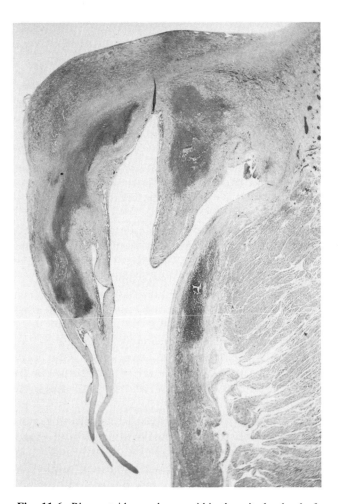

Fig. 11-6. Rheumatoid granulomas within the mitral valve leaflet, base of valve, and subendocardial region of the left ventricular wall.

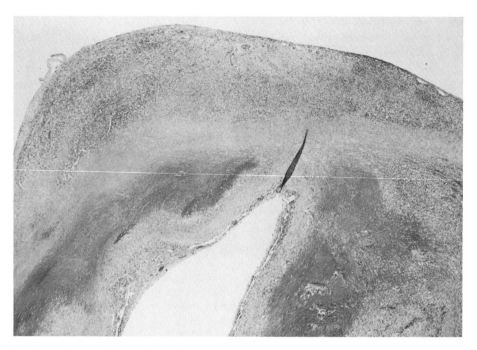

Fig. 11-7. Rheumatoid granulomas; base mitral valve showing a necrotic center (fibrinoid necrosis) surrounded by epithelioid cells, lymphocytes, and fibroblasts.

matoid nodule is a round or oval structure of approximately 1 mm to 10 mm in its greatest diameter. It reveals a necrotic center of fibrinoid material surrounded by palisading epithelioid cells and a rim of lymphocytes and fibroblasts at the periphery (Fig. 11-7). Granulomas may perforate the cusps, and therefore contribute to the regurgitant phenomena. Healing of these granulomas may result in more diffuse fibrosis, scarring, retraction, and occasionally, calcification.

Aortitis in RA. Aortitis in classic rheumatoid arthritis has been reported only sporadically and is considered rare. The usual gross finding in rheumatoid aortitis is aneurysmal dilatation of the aortic root and the ascending aorta.[52] In addition, thickening and irregularity of the cusps may be seen grossly, but commissural fusion or widening is not a feature of rheumatoid disease.

The aorta is usually affected in the proximal 3 cm to 5 cm, although occasionally its entire length may be involved. Rheumatoid granulomas may be present, or the morphologic appearance may be that of a nonspecific panaortitis.

Morphology of aortitis in RA. When rheumatoid granulomas are present they are usually found in the adventitia, outer media, the aortic ring, and within the basal half of the cusps. Vasculitis and fibrinoid necrosis of vessels exiting the aorta is occasionally seen. An inflammatory infiltrate of predominantly lymphocytes, plasma cells, occasional histiocytes, and polymorphs extends through the entire thickness of the aortic wall, although the intensity is

greater in the adventitia and media. Necrosis of medial smooth muscle and disruption of the elastic lamina results in medial fibrosis. The vasa vasora reveal a perivascular cuffing of mononuclear cells, but contrary to the classic obliterative endarteritis seen in syphilis, those vessels are dilated and patent.

Although there are some superficial similarities between the aortitis of ankylosing spondylitis and that of rheumatoid arthritis, a number of important distinguishing features separates them. The aortitis of ankylosing spondylitis primarily involves the adventitia with secondary medial involvement, extends only a few centimeters (3 to 4) above the aortic ring, and contains no rheumatoid granulomas.

Polymyositis and dermatomyositis (PM/DM)

Polymyositis and dermatomyositis are inflammatory diseases primarily involving proximal striated muscles, but may also involve the skin, (dermatomyositis), serosal surfaces, joints, kidneys, eyes, and heart. Although these syndromes can occur in isolation, they may occasionally be associated with other autoimmune diseases, such as lupus erythematosus, rheumatoid arthritis, or systemic sclerosis. However, it is only dermatomyositis that truly overlaps with systemic sclerosis and mixed connective tissue disease. Additionally, these two entities (PM/DM) may be associated with infections (usually viral) and malignancies in various organs (e.g., breast, lung, ovary, and stomach). Both entities affect females more frequently than males.

Clinical manifestations in PM/DM. The early clinical

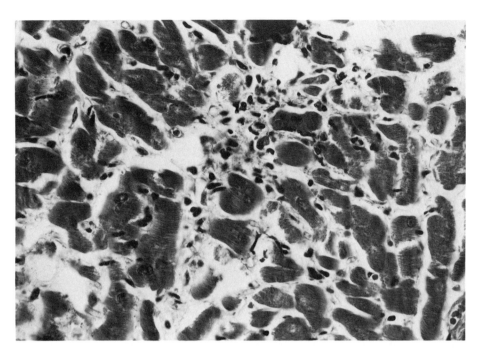

Fig. 11-8. Cardiac explant from a patient with polymyositis. Note focal lymphocytic and plasmacytic infiltrate and individual myocardial cell necrosis.

features consist primarily of muscle weakness and wasting of proximal limb muscles, resulting in difficulty with simple maneuvers (e.g., getting up from a chair, or climbing stairs). At later stages, however, the trunk muscles, including the respiratory ones, may be involved. In dermatomyositis the muscle involvement is combined with skin lesions that characteristically consist of a lilac discoloration (heliotrope) of the eyelids with edema and an erythema and scaling on the limbs (e.g., knuckles) and upper trunk. In contrast, polymyositis has no unique clinical features and its diagnosis is often made by exclusion.

Cardiac involvement in PM/DM. Data from conventional and contemporary noninvasive methods indicate that cardiac involvement in polymyositis/dermatomyositis is relatively common (50% to 75%) and may possibly be the most common cause of death in these entities. However, although there is an apparent correlation between the duration and severity of skeletal muscle involvement, and the cardiac manifestations, the exact relationship between them is not established. Although the total CK level has a fair correlation with cardiac involvement, an MB fraction over 3% is highly suggestive of cardiac involvement in patients with PM/DM.[53]

The cardiac clinical features include arrhythmias, conduction disturbances, low ejection fractions, cardiac dilatation, and heart failure. EKG abnormalities have been noted in as many as 70% of the patients.

An increase prevalence for mitral insufficiency in polymyositis has been observed, although the underlying pathogenesis for this valvular dysfunction has not been elucidated. Whether the mitral incompetence is the result of a poorly defined congestive cardiomyopathy in polymyositis (e.g., chamber dilatation on papillary muscle lateral displacement) or caused by some other mechanism is not clear.

Pericardial and myocardial manifestations in PM/DM. Pericardial involvement may also occur, but it is less frequent than in SLE and rheumatoid arthritis. Rare cases of constrictive pericarditis complicating dermatomyositis have been reported.[54] However, myocardial involvement, including that of the conduction system, is the most important occurrence in PM/DM, because of its frequency and because it is the leading cause of death in these two entities.[53] It has been estimated on the basis of clinical and postmortem studies that approximately one third of patients with PM/DM develop myocarditis, although such an underlying pathologic condition may be clinically inapparent.

Morphologic features of PM/DM. The usual histopathologic findings in the myocardium are interstitial edema, round cell infiltration (lymphocytes and plasma cells), and patchy myocyte necrosis (Fig. 11-8). These features of myocarditis are often accompanied by patchy myocardial fibrosis, which also involves the conduction system. The coexistence of myocarditis and fibrosis perhaps denotes relapsing episodes of cardiac involvement. Although anatomic alterations have been observed in several regions of the conduction system, the most common site for fibrous replacement is the distal segment of the His bundle and its branches.[55] Such fibrosis of the His bundle has been documented at postmortem in patients who died following complete heart block.

An intriguing observation has been that the conduction system in polymyositis reveals histopathologic changes that closely resemble the lesions described in neonatal lupus syndrome, in which a maternal autoantibody to tissue ribonucleoproteins (anti-Ro) passes the placenta and causes injury to the conduction system of the fetus.[56]

Pathogenesis and etiology of PM/DM. Although the cause of the inflammatory myopathies remains unknown, the serologic findings strongly suggest an autoimmune basis. Several antibodies against nuclear and cytoplasmic antigens have been found in the sera of patients with inflammatory myopathies. However, autoantibodies against nuclear antigens, such as antinuclear antibody and antinuclear ribonucleoproteins, are not myositis-specific. Similarly, the pathogenetic role of the autoantibodies against cytoplasmic ribonucleoproteins involved in translation and protein synthesis found in inflammatory myopathies remains uncertain.[57] The possibility of viruses triggering the inflammatory myopathies, although attractive, is largely unconfirmed.

The mononuclear endomyocardial infiltrates in DM reveal a high percentage of B cells and a higher ratio of CD4+ cells to CD8+ cells. Such a cellular composition suggests a pathogenetic mechanism mediated primarily by humoral processes directed against the intramuscular microvasculature. This immune process is mediated by the complement C5b-9 membranolytic attack complex.[58] Focal deposits of IgG, IgM, and complement have been demonstrated by direct immunofluorescence within the walls of cutaneous and muscle vessels.[59]

In PM, however, there is no evidence of microangiopathy, but there is evidence of an antigen-directed cytotoxicity mediated by cytotoxic T-cells.

To gain a better insight on the pathogenesis of PM, investigators have analyzed the phenotypes of mononuclear cells (lymphocytes) in affected muscle tissue. In PM, endomysial mononuclear cells appear to surround, invade, and destroy nonnecrotic muscle fibers. These autoaggressive mononuclear cells are mostly CD8+ T-cells.[60] The invading CD8+ T-cells appear to be cytotoxic rather than suppressor cells. In contrast to PM, the inflammatory infiltrates in DM are predominantly perivascular or in the interfascicular septa.

The fact that MCH-I antigens have been detected on fibers invaded by mononuclear cells indicates that the T cell-mediated cytotoxicity is antigen-specific.[61] Furthermore, it has been proposed that the increased MCH-I expression in muscle fibers in inflammatory myopathies is mediated by α-, β-, and γ-interferon (IFN) released from inflammatory cells.[62] Others, however, have failed to verify the interferon hypothesis of cell-mediated cytotoxicity

in PM and have found that increased MHC-I expression precedes fiber invasion; therefore enhanced MHC-I expression may be a nonspecific reaction to fiber injury.[63] However, regardless of whether the interferon hypothesis is correct or not, the hallmark of PM is considered to be the invasion and destruction of nonnecrotic muscle fibers by autoaggressive CD8+ cytotoxic T-cells. Although in the vast majority of cases, the CD8+ cells use the common a/b T-cell receptor for the recognition of antigen T-cells, expression of a gamma/delta (γ/δ) receptor has also been recognized.[64] Such gamma delta/T-cells accumulate in chronic inflammations and are known to recognize heat-shock proteins. Furthermore, it has been speculated that γ/δ T-cells reacting against heat-shock proteins could participate in autoimmune reactions.[65]

In a recently reported case of PM all muscle fibers were highly reactive for MHC class I antigen and the 65-kd heat-shock protein, and were invaded by γ/δ T-cells. According to the authors this diversity of T-cell receptors (γ/δ instead of α/β T-cell receptor) supports the concept that PM is a heterogeneous group of disorders.[66]

It is important to emphasize, however, that all of the studies (regarding the pathogenetic role of CD8+ cytotoxic T-cells in polymyositis) mentioned above have been conducted on samples of skeletal muscle. Whether similar pathogenetic mechanisms are also involved in the induction of myocarditis in patients with PM remains unclear. It is logical to assume, though, that in a systemic disorder such as polymyositis, the underlying pathogenesis is uniform regardless of the site of tissue injury.

SYSTEMIC DISORDERS WITH MULTIORGAN INVOLVEMENT

Wegener granulomatosis, Whipple disease, and thrombotic thrombocytopenic purpura are systemic diseases with multiorgan involvement that includes the cardiovascular system. Although these entities are not characterized as autoimmune diseases, their clinical and morphologic manifestations may simulate disorders of autoimmune etiology.

Wegener granulomatosis

Wegener granulomatosis is primarily a systemic necrotizing vasculitis, therefore in this chapter only the cardiac involvement, which may be found in one third of patients at autopsy,[67] will be discussed. In rare cases isolated kidney involvement may be the first manifestation of this entity. Occasionally, this vascular disorder may present as microangiopathic hemolytic anemia with consumptive coagulopathy.[68]

Cardiac manifestations. The most common cardiac lesion in Wegener granulomatosis is pericarditis, which is usually fibrinous and with or without pericardial effusion. Other cardiac lesions include coronary necrotizing arteritis and intramyocardial granulomas. Arteritis of the coronary arteries may result in myocardial infarction or other ischemic sequelae. Complete heart block caused by Wegener's granulomatosis has been observed in rare cases. It is assumed that in those cases the conduction system was involved by granulomata, or the conduction abnormality was caused by an arteritis of the AV nodal artery.[69]

Morphologic features. The lesions in Wegener granulomatosis have a morphologic resemblance to tubercles and may be found in the nasal and paranasal sinuses, larynx, trachea, and throughout the lung parenchyma. Some lesions, particularly in the lungs, may become cavitary; others undergo organization and eventually fibrosis. Small arteries and veins reveal evidence of inflammation that is fairly similar to that seen in polyarteritis nodosa. However, occasional granulomas are present either within the arterial wall or adjacent to it.

The discovery of antibodies to cytoplasmic components of neutrophils (ANCA) has been extremely helpful in making an early diagnosis of Wegener granulomatosis.[70] These antibodies are directed against constituents of lysosomes in neutrophilic primary (azurophilic) granules. The exact pathogenetic role of these antibodies has not been elucidated. One possible mechanism proposed is that they may activate neutrophils by binding to their respective antigens. This could occur either by internalization of the antibody or by surface expression of these lysosomal antigens, presumably occurring in neutrophils "primed" by cytokines.[71]

Whipple disease

Whipple disease, also known as intestinal lipodystrophy, is a rare infectious multisystem disorder characterized by the absence of pathognomonic laboratory findings. Although the majority of patients present with chronic steatorrhea (with or without protein loss), weight loss, arthritis, generalized lymphadenopathy, and fever, symptoms pertaining to the pulmonary and cardiovascular systems may also be present.

The exact incidence and prevalence of Whipple disease is not known. Most patients are Caucasian, male, and middle-aged[72] (40-49).

Cardiovascular involvement in Whipple disease. Cardiac involvement is common in Whipple disease and the underlying pathologic mechanism may be that of endocarditis, myocarditis, pericarditis, and coronary arteritis. Patients with cardiac involvement usually reveal nonspecific ECG findings such as flattening of the T-waves, lengthening of the Q-T interval and a lower level of the S-T segment. Sudden death, probably caused by conduction abnormalities, is estimated to occur in about one fifth of patients with Whipple disease.[73]

A triad of hypotension, pericardial friction rub, and congestive heart failure may be the clinical manifestations. Heart murmurs resulting from valvular disease are most often heard in the mitral valve and to a lesser extent in the aortic valve. Endocardial vegetations of the involved

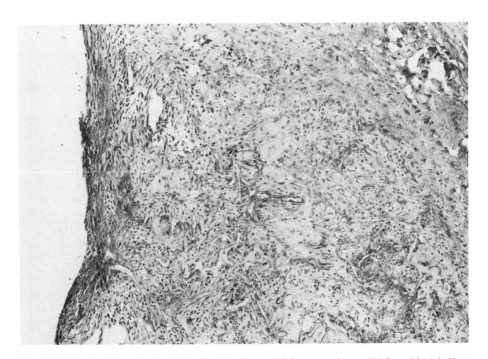

Fig. 11-9. Surgically excised mitral valve showing multiple macrophages (PAS-positive) infiltrating the valvular tissues. Valvular vegetations of nonbacterial nature were also present on the leaflets.

valves are seen in approximately one third of the cases of Whipple disease. Aortic involvement presents clinically as regurgitation, whereas the clinical picture of mitral involvement is that of stenosis.

Cardiac morphology in Whipple disease. The basic histopathologic lesion in all cardiac locations (pericardium, myocardium, valves, and coronary arteries) contains similar components, namely PAS-positive macrophage infiltrate and a sparse round cell infiltrate (Fig. 11-9).

The pericardium often reveals fibrous adhesions and occasional non-necrotizing granulomas containing PAS-positive debris. Yellow vegetations may be present along the lines of closure of cardiac valves, whereas the macrophage infiltrate within the valve substance and the valvular ring may severely distort the valvular apparatus. The overall anatomic configuration of an involved mitral valve might be similar to that seen in rheumatic mitral disease.[74]

The myocardium may be infiltrated by PAS-positive macrophages and rarely may reveal an interstitial lymphocytic myocarditis without evidence of fibrosis.[75]

Vasculitis with or without fibrinoid necrosis may be present in arterioles and venules and less commonly in large coronary arteries. Both the endothelium and the tunica media are involved, and the lumen may be occluded by a thrombus, resulting in a microinfarct. Rare cases of involvement of the aorta and pulmonary artery have been observed.[72]

Ultrastructural studies have revealed "bacillary bodies" within the abnormal macrophages. The rod-shaped organisms have a dense cell wall, a distinct double membrane, and a intracellular fibrillary structure.[76]

Pathogenesis and etiology of Whipple disease. The causative role of bacteria-like forms in Whipple disease is widely accepted after their discovery in tissue specimens by electron microscopy. However, the precise pathogenetic mechanisms involved and the reason(s) for the susceptibility of certain individuals remain uncertain. Some hypotheses suggest a reduced immune function as a primary event in Whipple disease, whereas others stress that the reduced immune function is secondary to the intestinal disease.

Immunologic abnormalities in various reports include polyclonal hypergammaglobulinemia, deficiencies of the fourth component of complement, and panhypogammaglobulinemia.[74] Cutaneous anergy is present in some patients. However, although no significant humoral abnormality is detected, defective cell-mediated immunity has been reported in Whipple disease.

Several investigators have stressed that the invading microbe in Whipple disease is not highly virulent and a rather poor immunogen because tissue injury is usually minimal and an inflammatory response is lacking. Cultures from intestinal biopsies have yielded a variety of organisms, but most frequently gram-positive rods (with similar dimensions to bacilliform bodies) of *Corynebacterium* species. A common argument against the bacterial etiology of Whip-

ple has been that the disease is not transmissible to experimental animals, and therefore does not fulfill the Koch postulates.[77]

A genetic predisposition for Whipple disease has been suggested in several reports. At least two sets of brothers have been affected by Whipple disease. Furthermore, there is a higher than normal incidence (27% vs. 8%) of the histocompatibility antigens HLA-B27 in patients with Whipple disease.[78]

Thrombotic thrombocytopenic purpura

Thrombotic thrombocytopenic purpura (TTP) is a multisystem disease presented by the classic pentad of thrombocytopenia, hemolytic anemia, neurologic abnormalities, renal disease, and fever. During the past decade it has become clear that TTP and hemolytic uremic syndrome (HUS) are the same disease process.[79]

The symptoms and signs of TTP are believed to be caused by microthrombi composed of agglutinated platelets and fibrin, within arterioles and capillaries throughout many organs (Fig. 11-10).

Although there is no underlying disease or precipitating cause in the majority of patients with TTP, in some there is an associated infection, pregnancy, cancer, organ transplantation, collagen vascular disorder or drug abuse.[80]

There is no laboratory test or group of tests pathognomonic for TTP-HUS; therefore the diagnosis of this entity is usually made by exclusion. The morphologic changes of the RBCs (fragmentation, polychromatophilia, basophilic stippling, microcytosis, nucleated RBCs) are caused by membrane damage sustained during their attempt to traverse arterioles and capillaries partially obstructed by hyaline thrombi.[81]

Cardiac manifestations in TTP. Cardiac involvement in TTP results from microvascular thrombosis, hemorrhage, or myocarditis. From the few reported cases, the cardiac symptoms and signs were fairly nonspecific. Atrial fibrillation, sustained ventricular tachycardia, moderate to severe global left ventricular dysfunction with akinesis, and pericardial effusion are the most commonly reported clinical manifestations.

The heart grossly may reveal intramyocardial and subepicardial hemorrhages, some of which are confluent. Focal mononuclear cell infiltrates may be seen in association with myocyte necrosis. Evidence of healing and focal myocyte hypertrophy are also present.

Pathogenesis of TTP. There is strong evidence against a primary RBC abnormality in TTP-HUS. There is, however, evidence suggesting that the target organ damaged in TTP-HUS is the endothelial cell. As a result of the endothelial injury, there may be changes in the synthesis and release of PGI_2, von Willebrand factor, plasminogen activators and tissue plasminogen activator inhibitor, and in the expression of thrombomodulin by the endothelial cells.[82]

The pathogenetic significance of PGI_2 remains unclear.

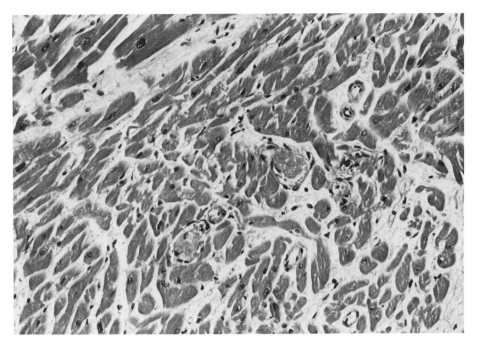

Fig. 11-10. Microthrombi in intramyocardial arterioles composed of agglutinated platelets and fibrin, from a patient with TTP.

Similarly, the abnormally large von Willebrand factor multimers, which may agglutinate platelets, are not considered to be the primary initiating event.

In the plasma of some patients with TTP-HUS, a substance designated *platelet aggregating factor* (PAF) has been identified. This factor, however, is present only in a subset of patients with TTP. Exotoxins (verotoxin), drug hypersensitivity, or immune-mediated mechanisms have also been considered as possible triggering events in TTP-HUS. While the primary mover in TTP-HUS is yet to be identified, the present belief is that endothelial damage is the primary event, and the plasma alterations are secondary.[81]

SERONEGATIVE SPONDYLARTHROPATHIES

Entities such as ankylosing spondylitis, Reiter syndrome, psoriatic arthropathy, arthritis of inflammatory bowel disease, Whipple disease, and Behcet syndrome, although they reveal minor clinical and radiologic differences, are all termed *seronegative spondylarthropathies*. These disorders are characterized by absence of rheumatoid factor and rheumatoid nodules, familial aggregation, sacroiliitis with or without spondylitis, and peripheral arthritis. An important biologic link of these entities is the presence of HLA-B27, although with different frequencies in different members of the group.

Ankylosing spondylitis (AS)

Ankylosing spondylitis (AS), which affects primarily young male adults or adolescents, is a chronic inflammatory disease, characteristically involving the sacroiliac joints and the axial skeleton. The extraspinal manifesta-

tions of ankylosing spondylitis include cardiac, pulmonary, and neurologic involvement, and occasional amyloidosis. The patients often present with low-grade fever, fatigue, and weight loss.

Approximately 8% to 10% of Caucasians carry the HLA-B27 antigen. It is estimated that the incidence of ankylosing spondylitis in this population is about 1%, although in some individuals the sacroiliitis is too mild to meet the New York diagnostic criteria.[83]

Pathogenesis of AS. The precise role of the HLA-B27 antigen in the pathogenesis of the spondylarthropathies is not clear. Some of the proposed hypotheses suggest a pathogenetic mechanism similar to that of the streptococcus in rheumatic heart disease, or a molecular mimicry between an unknown antigen and the B27 antigen as the cause of the chronic inflammatory process.[84]

Cardiac manifestations in AS. The most common cardiac manifestations are valvular lesions, such as aortic insufficiency, aortic insufficiency and stenosis, mitral insufficiency, and conduction disturbances.[85]

Most of the cardiovascular complications appear to occur in patients above 40 years of age, but the exact frequency of the valvular and conduction system involvement in AS varies considerably in different series. In one recent series of 40 patients with AS, aortic insufficiency, a feature of longstanding disease, was diagnosed in 12.5% of the cases and AV block and bundle branch block were diagnosed in 7.5% and 12.5% respectively.[86]

Characteristically, the patient with aortic insufficiency is a male with ankylosing spondylitis of 10 or more years duration. He may be asymptomatic initially, but gradual

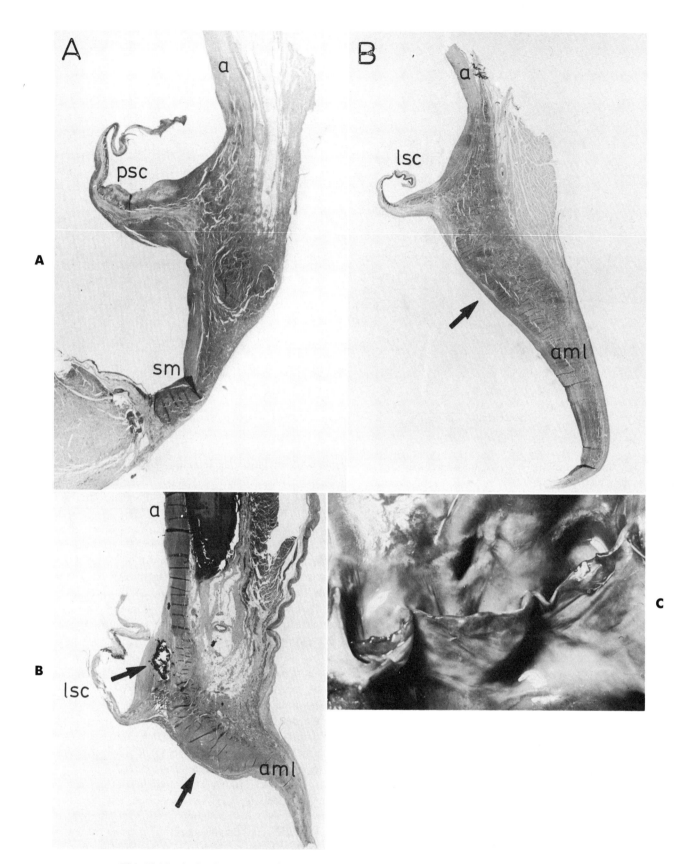

Fig. 11-11. A, Sections through the posterior **(A)** and left **(B)** sinus of Valsalva. Note fibrous and nodular thickening of the base of the aortic cusps, particularly the posterior cusp, and the mitral leaflet, which bends inwards to the subaortic area *(arrow)*. The free margins of the aortic cusps are rolled. (*a* = aorta; *aml* = anterior mitral leaflet; *lsc* = left semilunar cusp; *psc* = posterior semilunar cusp; *sm* = septum membranaceum.) **B,** Section through the aortic root, left semilunar cusp *(lsc),* and anterior mitral leaflet *(aml)*. The base of the cusp and leaflet show marked fibrous thickening, calcification *(upper arrow),* and a protrusion toward the subaortic area *(lower arrow).* The free margin of the aortic cusp is rolled. Hemorrhage is noted between the aorta *(a)* and atrial wall. **C,** Aortic valve showing significant thickening of the base of the cusps. The ostium of the right coronary artery is distorted. (Reprinted by permission of Jovan Rajs, MD and *Am J Med* 77:961, 1984).

progression of the aortic incompetence results in left ventricular dilatation, dyspnea, angina, and ultimately congestive heart failure.

Morphologic findings. The aortic involvement in AS is mainly confined to the area behind the sinuses of Valsalva and the first few centimeters of the ascending aorta. In the active phase of aortitis, there is an endarteritis obliterans of small adventitial vessels, which reveals perivascular cuffing by lymphocytes and plasma cells (similar to that seen in syphilitic aortitis). At the chronic phase, there is adventitial fibrosis, which may also extend into the outer media, and may reveal focal calcification. The intima also reveals fibrosis and longitudinal wrinkling, and the aortic diameter is increased. The valvular cusps are thickened at the base, as well as at the free margins, where they appear somewhat rolled and inverted (Fig. 11-11, *A,B*).

Valvular abnormalities in AS. The adventitial fibrosis often extends into the groove between the anterior mitral leaflet and the aortic cusps, producing a fibrous ridge that may impinge on the conduction system. In some cases of ankylosing spondylitis, the aorta may be spared; the only morphologic changes are seen in the vicinity of the central fibrous body and the conduction system. In rare atypical cases, the disease may present as aortic arch syndrome, with one or more branches of the aorta being partially or totally obstructed at their origins.[87]

Mitral valve insufficiency in ankylosing spondylitis is rather rare. It has been attributed to a protrusion created by the extension of the fibrosis of the adventitia of the proximal aorta into the subaortic area adjacent to the base of the anterior mitral leaflet[88] (Fig. 11-11, *C*). It is likely, however, that ventricular dilatation secondary to aortic insufficiency may also contribute to the mitral regurgitation.

Myocardial abnormalities in AS. Although early diastolic abnormalities of the left ventricle were demonstrated on echocardiography in half of the patients with AS, the histopathologic findings in the myocardium are usually nonspecific and often minimal.[89] Mild increase of interstitial connective tissue is present, but there are no inflammatory changes, although occasional inflammatory cells may be seen in the vicinity of the central fibrous body and the AV node. In contrast, myocarditis has been a common finding in Reiter's disease and yersinia arthritis, two entities closely associated with ankylosing spondylitis.

Systolic myocardial dysfunction was observed by some investigators in patients whose basic disease had existed for more than 10 years.[90] Echocardiographic evidence of hypertrophy and hypokinesis of the septum and the posterior wall of the left ventricle were noted.

Conduction abnormalities in AS. Ankylosing spondylitis patients with AV block have revealed, in electrophysiologic studies, that the site of the block is proximal to the bundle of His. Right bundle branch block appears to be the most frequent conduction disturbance, and

ventricular ectopy the most common arrhythmia in AS.[90]

Although lung complications (pulmonary fibrosis, emphysema, pleural effusions) may occur in AS, their frequency is relatively limited, and they are usually a late complication of the disease.

HERITABLE CONNECTIVE TISSUE DISORDERS

Recent advances in molecular genetics have significantly improved understanding of the pathogenesis of the inherited connective-tissue disorders, including the most common of those, Marfan syndrome.

Current data have shown that collagen genes may harbor mutations that can lead to a wide spectrum of human diseases. Similarly, recent studies have revealed that there is some phenotypic variability among patients with connective tissue diseases.

Sophisticated techniques, such as linkage analysis with polymorphic markers, are currently used to pinpoint the locus of mutations in Mendelian disorders. However, recent successes in unraveling the mysteries of heritable connective-tissue disorders have also reemphasized that linkage analysis between a candidate gene and a disease locus, although highly suggestive, does not constitute final proof of causal relationship. Furthermore, investigators have become aware that definition of the gene lesion responsible for a syndrome does not invariably lead to design of definitive diagnostic tests. A single mutant gene may promote many end effects (pleiotropism), and mutations of several genetic loci may produce the same trait (genetic heterogeneity).

Marfan syndrome

This autosomal dominant inherited disorder affects the musculoskeletal, cardiovascular, and ocular systems. A set of rigid criteria for the diagnosis of Marfan syndrome have been proposed. Those are: (1) ocular manifestations (ectopia, lentis, myopia); (2) skeletal manifestations (pectus deformity, dolichostenomelia, arachnodactyly, kyphoscoliosis, high arched palate, hyperextensible joints); (3) cardiovascular manifestations (aortic root dilatation, aneurysm, dissection or regurgitation, and mitral valve prolapse with or without regurgitation); and (4) positive family history.[91]

Marfan syndrome, which has an incidence of about 1 in 20,000, reveals no differences in prevalence between races, ethnic groups, and genders.

The phenotypic variability of Marfan syndrome is considerable, thus not all patients present the classic form with ocular, cardiovascular, and skeletal abnormalities. Furthermore, the autosomal mode of inheritance is not obvious in all patients. In approximately 30% of patients, Marfan syndrome may be the result of new mutations.[92]

The mutant gene, whatever protein it encodes, exerts a pleiotrophic effect. Patients who share the same mutant gene, such as relatives, may exhibit the effect of the gene differently. This is referred to as *intrafamilial variation*.[93]

Genetic heterogeneity can be the result of different mutant alleles or mutations at different loci.

Cardiovascular findings in Marfan syndrome. Although early reports have indicated that cardiovascular abnormalities in Marfan syndrome patients occurred only in about half of the cases, the advent of echocardiography and other diagnostic techniques have raised the rate of cardiovascular involvement to less than 95% of adults with Marfan syndrome and 100% of children with this syndrome.[94]

Valvular manifestations in Marfan syndrome. The most striking cardiovascular lesions in Marfan syndrome are dilatation of the aortic root associated with aortic regurgitation and mitral regurgitation. However, although mitral valve prolapse is frequent in Marfan syndrome and can occur early in infancy, significant mitral regurgitation is rare before adolescence. This is also true for significant aortic regurgitation.

Left atrial and left ventricular end-diastolic diameter and posterior left ventricular wall thicknesses are usually within normal limits in children with Marfan syndrome from about 6 to 14 years of age.[95] However, aortic dilatation is the major life-threatening cardiovascular abnormality of the syndrome in adulthood. Evidence indicates that aortic dilatation is positively correlated to body growth during infancy and adolescence.[95] Aortic regurgitation in Marfan syndrome may be the result of dilatation of the sinuses of Valsalva and the aortic annulus, redundancy of the aortic cusps and cusp eversion resulting from myxoid change, aortic dissection, and cusp perforation.[96] (The hemodynamic and clinical manifestations of aortic and mitral regurgitation are discussed in Chapter 3).

Although there is a definite association between mitral valve prolapse and skeletal abnormalities (thoracic), there is no support for the hypothesis that in certain individuals

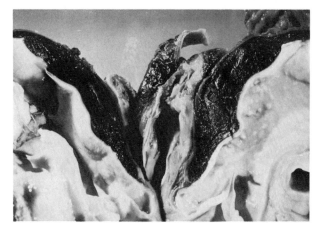

Fig. 11-12. Proximal aortic dissection in a patient with Marfan syndrome.

mitral valve prolapse represents a "forme fruste" of Marfan syndrome.[97]

Aneurysms in Marfan syndrome patients. Aneurysms of the ascending or descending thoracic aorta, abdominal aorta, pulmonary artery, cerebral vessels, and coronary arteries have all been reported in Marfan syndrome.[96] Dissection of the aorta (Fig. 11-12) or rupture of an aneurysm in Marfan syndrome are the other catastrophic events contributing to the decreased life expectancy of these individuals. Recent developments in echocardiography using the esophageal transducer have greatly facilitated the diagnosis and classification of these problems in the acute setting.[98] These studies seem to have displaced aortography and computerized tomography as a diagnostic modality.

Comparative studies of individuals with Marfan syndrome and normal subjects have shown decreased aortic distensibility in the ascending and abdominal aorta in those with Marfan syndrome. Moreover, an inverse correlation was noted between the ascending aortic diameter and aortic distensibility, a clear indication that as the aorta becomes wider it loses its elasticity. This inverse correlation, however, was not applicable to the abdominal aorta.[99] This study also disclosed an increased aortic stiffness index in the ascending and the abdominal aorta, and rapid pulse wave velocity in patients with Marfan syndrome compared with normal patients. The stiffness index obtained from the logarithmic value of the ratio of the systolic and diastolic blood pressure and changes in the diameter of the vessel was independent of blood pressure.[99]

In general, cardiovascular manifestations account for approximately 93% of the deaths in Marfan syndrome.[100] Other causes of death are congestive heart failure and myocardial infarction.

Morphologic findings in Marfan syndrome. The morphologic findings in the walls of arteries, particularly large elastic vessels, in Marfan syndrome are characterized by severe fragmentation, atrophy, and loss of elastic fibers, an increase in collagen, and a marked increase in acid mucopolysaccharide material forming pools between the fragmented elastic lamellae.[96]

Electron microscopy studies have revealed that elastic fibers have a moth-eaten appearance, increase in electron density, and appear to degenerate into masses of dark granules.[101]

Biochemical studies in Marfan syndrome. The precise biochemical defect in Marfan syndrome is not known, although several reports have suggested a defect either in collagen or elastin or both. Reports of decreased amounts of nonreducible collagen cross-links in the aorta and skin of patients with Marfan syndrome compared with those of normal persons have been published. This reduction was attributed to genetic defect in the COL1A2 (type I) gene, which encodes for the alpha chain of type I collagen.[102] However, in spite of some reported abnormalities in collagen, conclusive evidence that a defect in collagen is the major cause of Marfan syndrome is still lacking.

Studies of COL3A1 (type III) gene on chromosome 2, which is responsible for encoding type III collagen (a protein that is an important component of the adventitia and media of the aortic wall), have excluded the possibility that this particular gene is the mutant locus involved in the syndrome.[103]

Exclusion of possible defects in collagen type I (COL1A2 gene) and type III (COL3A1 gene) has directed the search for a biochemical abnormality in Marfan syndrome to other connective tissue proteins. One such protein is elastin, a defect of which could be the underlying molecular abnormality in Marfan syndrome. This reasoning was prompted by the fact that biochemical studies have demonstrated that the content of elastin in the aorta from patients with Marfan syndrome is reduced.[104] Elastin isolated from aortas of Marfan syndrome patients revealed that the elastin-specific cross-links, desmosine and isodesmosine, were reduced.

A study applied biochemical, structural, and mechanical analysis of the aortic media from patients with Marfan syndrome concluded that the tensile strength of the aorta in Marfan syndrome patients is lower than that in control subjects; the solubility of collagen is within normal levels; and the relative ratio of collagen types I, III, and V was normal. Furthermore, deficiencies in desmosine and isodesmosine were present in these patients, and the amount of elastin in the aorta decreased. The arrangement of elastin fibers in the media was found to be abnormal in that the fibers were widely separated by spaces and deficient in connecting interlaminar fibers. The latter findings are consistent with the so-called cystic medial necrosis seen in Marfan syndrome.[105] However, the above study could not explain the skeletal manifestations, if indeed the only underlying abnormality in Marfan syndrome is in elastin.

Genetic studies in Marfan syndrome. Recently, investigators using linkage analysis with polymorphic markers of the human genome have mapped the genetic defect to chromosome 15q 15-21 in five families with Marfan syndrome. These investigators suggested that the most probable location of the gene for the disease was D15S45.[106]

Chromosome 15 is known to contain genes associated with connective tissue disorders. The genes coding for type I collagen receptor,[107] chrondroitin sulfate proteoglycan I core protein,[108] and cardiac muscle α-actin[109] are all located in chromosome 15 and are also candidate genes for the mutation in Marfan syndrome.

Recently, immunohistologic studies have revealed that fibrillin, a connective tissue glycoprotein (relative molecular mass 350,000), may be defective or deficient in Marfan syndrome.[110] Fibrillin is an element of elastic tissue and the periosteum, which are tissues often involved in Marfan syndrome.

Genetic linkage data localizing the Marfan gene to chromosome 15, and the in situ hybridization of fibrillin complementary DNA to 15q 21.1, strongly support fibrillin as a candidate for the Marfan gene involvement.[111] After the identification of fibrillin, studies of immunohistopathologic quantification of this protein in skin and fibroblast culture, fibrillin synthesis, extracellular transport, and incorporation into the connective tissue matrix, have revealed certain abnormalities of fibrillin metabolism in most Marfan syndrome patients. Furthermore, a de novo missense mutation in the fibrillin gene in patients with sporadic Marfan disease has been recently reported.[112]

A second fibrillin gene mapped to chromosome 5q 23-31 was recently identified. This new gene is apparently linked to congenital contractural arachnodactyly, a condition that shares some of the features of Marfan syndrome. These two related syndromes by two related genes indicate that fibrillin mutations may be responsible for different Marfan syndrome phenotypes.[113]

The above findings demonstrate that fibrillin is probably a family of connective tissue proteins, perhaps comparable to collagens. However, accumulated evidence with mutations in the collagen and other large genes discloses that mutations at different sites in the gene (allelic mutations) may result in a clinical presentation that is quantitatively and even qualitatively distinctive.[114]

Osteogenesis imperfecta (OI)

This entity comprises a heterogeneous group of heritable connective tissue disorders. The clinical presentation includes brittle bones, blue sclerae, dental malformations, deafness, hyperextensible ligaments, and cardiovascular abnormalities.

Sillence's[115] classification (types I-IV) is based on the age of onset, associated phenotypic signs, mode of inheritance, severity of bone fragility, and resultant skeletal deformity.

Types I and IV have a relatively mild clinical course and an autosomal dominant mode of inheritance. Type II is the most severe form and is lethal in the perinatal period. Type III is an autosomal recessive form with a severe clinical course. However, a considerable number of patients cannot be assigned to any of the four subtypes.

Genetic studies in OI. Several mutations (more than 70) in the two structural genes for type I procollagen (COL1A1 and COL1A2) have been found in probands with osteogenesis imperfecta. The mutations include deletions, insertions, RNA splicing mutations, and single-base substitutions that convert a codon for glycine to a codon for an amino acid with a bulkier side chain.[116]

Severe phenotypes of this condition are thought to result from synthesis of structurally defective pro α1 and pro α2 chains of type I procollagen that either interfere with the folding of the triple helix or with self-assembly of collagen into fibrils.[116] It has also been stressed that the zipper-like folding of the collagen triple helix and the self-assembly of collagen fibrils depend on the principle of nucleated growth. By this process a few subunits form a nucleus that is then propagated to form a large structure with a precisely defined architecture. This is a very efficient mechanism for the assembly of large structures. However, biologic systems that depend extensively on nucleated growth are highly prone to mutations that cause synthesis of structurally abnormal but partially functional subunits.[116]

Cardiovascular manifestations in OI. Cardiovascular lesions in osteogenesis imperfecta are relatively similar to those in Marfan syndrome, with aortic regurgitation, valvular lesions, and vascular aneurysms being the most common.

Aortic regurgitation is the most common valvular lesion; mitral regurgitation is less common. Dilatation of the aortic root and deformity of the valvular cusps result from abnormally translucent weak and elongated valves. The mitral annulus is usually dilated, the leaflets are redundant and tend to prolapse, and the chordae tendineae attenuate and may rupture. There has been a rare report of left atrial rupture in an individual with osteogenesis imperfecta and mitral prolapse.[117]

The valves and the aorta may reveal reduced amounts of fibrous connective tissue and elastic fibers, and accumulation of acid mucopolysaccharides.[96]

Aortic root dilatation seems to present a distinct phenotypic trait in patients with osteogenesis imperfecta that is nonprogressive and occurs in about 12% of affected individuals. Whether mitral valve prolapse should also be considered as a part of the cardiovascular phenotype in osteogenesis imperfecta, or as an entity that segregates as an independent autosomal dominant trait, has yet to be determined because the incidence of this abnormality is about the same as in the general population.[118]

Ehlers-Danlos syndrome

This syndrome comprises a heterogeneous group of disorders of collagen metabolism that share certain phenotype expressions. The most characteristic clinical findings are hypermotility of joints, cutaneous hyperextensibility, easy bruisability, and extreme tissue fragility.

Genetic studies in Ehlers-Danlos syndrome. More than 11 types of Ehlers-Danlos syndrome have been defined by clinical, biochemical, and genetic criteria. Mutations in the type I procollagen genes have been found in some subtypes of Ehlers-Danlos syndrome, such as type VII. Mutations in the type III procollagen gene have been found in families with the type IV variant of Ehlers-Danlos syndrome, which is the most severe form, characterized by sudden death from rupture of large arteries or other hollow organs.[119]

Inheritance in Ehlers-Danlos syndrome is autosomal dominant in types I-IV, X-linked recessive in type V, and autosomal recessive in types VI and VII. Types I-III are caused by unknown biochemical defects; type V is caused by lysyl oxidase deficiency; type VI is caused by lysyl hydroxylase deficiency; and type VII results from a procollagen peptidase deficiency.[96]

Cardiovascular manifestations in Ehlers-Danlos syndrome. Cardiovascular lesions have been best described for type I (the gravis form), type III (the benign familial hypermotility syndrome), and type IV (the ecchymotic, or arterial form). Dissection of the aorta and tears in peripheral arteries have been described in type I. In type II, the mitis form, atrial septal defect, congenital AV block, aneurysms of the ascending aorta, brachial artery, and abdominal aorta have been reported. In type I and III, mitral valve prolapse, and aortic root or sinus of Valsalva enlargement occur, whereas in type IV (arterial, or Sack type), major complications such as rupture of the aorta or other major arteries or veins have been reported.[96] Vascular morphologic observations in Ehlers-Danlos syndrome consist of a diffuse decrease in medial elastic tissue, accumulation of acid mucopolysaccharides between medial elastic lamellae, and a decrease in adventitial and medial collagen.

Pseudoxanthoma elasticum (PE)

PE, also known as Grönbland-Strandberg syndrome, is a rare, autosomal recessive, heritable connective tissue disorder. It primarily involves the skin, cardiovascular system, and eyes, with rare manifestations from the central nervous system, skeleton, and gastrointestinal tract.[120] Although rare, it is more common in females, but the syndrome reveals no ethnic predilection. Five phenotypically distinct forms of the syndrome have been described:[121] (1) autosomal recessive type I, in which patients reveal vascular and retinal degeneration and peau d' orange skin lesions; (2) autosomal recessive type II, a rare form characterized only by generalized skin manifestations; (3) autosomal dominant type I, which presents with severe retinal and cardiovascular degeneration and typical cutaneous features; (4) autosomal dominant type II, with mild cardiovascular and retinal lesions together with Marfanoid features; and (5) a recently described autosomal recessive form in an Afrikaner community in South Africa, with mild to moderate skin and cardiovascular manifestations and severe ophthalmologic lesions.

Cardiovascular manifestations in pseudoxanthoma elasticum. Although the underlying biochemical defect of pseudoxanthoma elasticum has not yet been defined, the cardiovascular and other manifestations result from degeneration and calcification of elastic fibers (deranged metabolism and synthesis). Some experimental studies have shown abnormalities in sulfated proteoglycans, substances that may in part be responsible for the inhibition of mineralization of normal tissue.[122] Premature obliterative arteriosclerotic changes occur in medium and small arteries, resulting in diminished pulses, cold extremities, renovascular hypertension, angina, and cerebrovascular accidents.[120]

The degeneration and calcification of elastic fibers in the intima and media of peripheral arteries can progress to discrete plaques, causing severe luminal narrowing. Similar changes occur in the elastic fibers in the deeper layers of the endocardium, particularly those of the atria.[123]

Coronary involvement may lead to sudden death, although myocardial infarction is rare. Involvement of the aorta is infrequent, but changes in the mitral, aortic, and tricuspid valves have been described. As is the case with other disorders of connective tissue, mitral valve prolapse occurs with increased frequency in pseudoxanthoma elasticum.[124]

The typical skin manifestations of pseudoxanthoma elasticum are yellowish papular lesions in the flexures associated with mild skin redundancy. Gastrointestinal bleeding, although infrequent, is most probably the result of structural weakness in the submucosal vessels of the stomach.[125] The ocular lesions, although not pathognomonic, are characterized by angioid streaks or breaks of the retina associated with neovascularization, hemorrhage, and eventual fibrosis that leads to visual deterioration.[126]

Cutis laxa

This is a dermatologic term, and therefore not a strict disease entity. The term is used to describe abnormally loose, poorly elastic skin that hangs from the patient in loose folds, giving an appearance of premature aging.[127]

Acquired forms of cutis laxa may be associated with other diseases, whereas congenital forms of both autosomal recessive and autosomal dominant types have been described.[128]

Decreased lysyl oxidase activity has been found in a rare X-linked form of cutis laxa.[129] The defect appears to be one of elastin synthesis and/or cross-linking (decreased lysyl oxidase).

Cardiovascular findings in cutis laxa. The autosomal recessive form is characterized by cardiovascular and pulmonary manifestations, either of which (but especially pulmonary) can cause death in childhood. Vascular involvement is manifested as dilatation, tortuosity, and occasional rupture of the aorta and its branches.[130]

Histologic changes consist of decreased, coarse, and irregular elastic fibers and accumulation of extracellular acid mucopolysaccharides. In contrast to pseudoxanthoma elasticum, calcification is not seen. Ultrastructural abnormalities, such as separation between the amorphous and fibrillary components of elastic fibers, have been described.[127]

Right ventricular enlargement may represent cor pulmonale secondary to either severe emphysema or pulmonary vascular disease.

Combined Marfan syndrome and Ehlers-Danlos syndrome

A condition with features of both Marfan syndrome and Ehlers-Danlos syndrome has been described.[131] Biochemical studies of this combined connective tissue disorder are lacking.

The patients usually present with the typical skeletal findings of Marfan syndrome, along with marked hyperextensibility of the joints and extreme skin fragility. Mitral and tricuspid valve prolapse and aortic valvular regurgitation are the usual cardiovascular manifestations.[132]

Adult polycystic kidney disease

Such an association has recently been recognized.[133] Enlargement of the aortic root and mitral valvular regurgitation have been the main manifestations of this disorder. The usual histologic findings from the aortic and mitral valves is myxomatous degeneration with loss and disruption of collagen fibers (see chapter 3).

Annuloaortic ectasia

The term *annuloaortic ectasia* is used to describe aneurysmal dilatation of the aortic annulus and ascending aorta in patients without evidence of connective tissue abnormalities in other organ systems.[132] This condition has significant morbidity and mortality because of its propensity for aortic dissection, rupture, or regurgitation.[134]

Controversy exists about the specificity of the histologic features in this entity, although it appears that the degree of elastic lamellae fragmentation correlates better and more consistently with the presence of dissection than does the accumulation of mucopolysaccharides in the aortic media.[135]

The question whether this condition represents a variant of Marfan syndrome remains unanswered. Some investigators point out that cystic medial necrosis, elastic fragmentations, and fibrosis are common and nonspecific findings in the normal aging aorta, and therefore their role in the pathogenesis of the aortic dissection may be incidental.[136]

About 94% of the known causes of death in these patients were related to the cardiovascular system, with 65% being the result of aortic dissection, rupture, or sudden death.[135] These patients are usually at an older age, and have hypertension, coronary artery disease, and left ventricular dysfunction.

ENDOCRINE DISORDERS

Several endocrine disorders may directly or indirectly effect the cardiovascular system. Conditions characterized by hyperfunction or hypofunction of the thyroid gland, adrenals (both cortex and medulla), and pituitary gland are well recognized causes of both structural and functional alterations in the heart and vessels. However, the most frequent and by far the most grave effects on the cardiovascular system are those inflicted by diabetes mellitus.

The thyroid and the cardiovascular system

The effects of the thyroid hormone on the heart are multiple and may be direct or indirect. The biologic hallmark of increased thyroid function is a change in the basal metabolic rate, which is reflected by an increased total body oxygen consumption. This increased metabolic activity demands the heart to deliver more blood to all tissues. Although the exact mechanisms of action are not clear, it is accepted that T4 and T3 act primarily to stimulate cellular oxygen consumption and substrate utilization.[137]

Thyrotoxicosis

Cardiovascular manifestations in thyrotoxicosis. The cardiovascular manifestations in thyrotoxicosis include tachycardia, hyperdynamic circulation, warm skin, and bounding pulses. In the early stages, these findings may be subtle; in advanced stages they are dramatic, with explosive arrhythmias that are relatively resistant to treatment. Atrial fibrillation with a rapid ventricular response is the classic arrhythmia that may introduce this syndrome. Less frequent are high grade AV block, congestive heart failure, mitral valve abnormalities, and dyspnea. The latter, in patients with no underlying cardiovascular abnormality, has been attributed to weakness and fatigue of respiratory and other skeletal muscles.[138] Mitral valve prolapse appears to be more prevalent in patients with hyperthyroidism, particularly women with Grave's disease or autoimmune thyroiditis.[139]

Approximately one third of patients with diffuse toxic goiter have systolic hypertension caused by thyrotoxicosis-mediated increases in cardiac output, blood volume, and pulse pressure. Furthermore, a reversible cardiomyopathy has been described in a subset of patients with abnormal left ventricular function.[140]

Hyperthyroidism

Pathophysiologic cardiovascular manifestations in hyperthyroidism. Many of the clinical symptoms of hyperthyroidism suggest excessive sympathoadrenal stimulation and show quite striking similarities with the clinical presentation of pheochromocytoma. However, in spite of the clinical impression of increased adrenergic stimulation, studies have revealed normal or low levels of serum norepinephrine and epinephrine in thyrotoxicosis.[141]

The increased sensitivity of the heart to beta-adrenergic stimuli by the thyroid hormone, perhaps indicates that both the total numbers of cardiac adrenoreceptors and their distribution between the plasma membrane and vesicular fraction are influenced by the status of the thyroid activity.[142] It is also believed that the thyroid hormone has direct inotropic and chronotropic effect on the cardiac muscle; there-

fore the hyperkinesia of hyperthyroidism is caused by augmented contractility.[143]

Studies have addressed the effects of preload, afterload, contractility, and heart rate on the overall left ventricular performance and myocardial oxygen requirements in hyperthyroid patients. These studies have shown that preload is not an important determinant of the augmented ventricular performance in hyperthyroidism, that afterload reduction is not responsible for the hyperdynamic state, and that chronotropic factors (e.g., heart rate) do not contribute significantly to the increased contractility.[143] However, there was strong positive correlation between thyroid hormone levels and myocardial contractility, consistent with a shift in the force velocity curve upward and to the right.[144]

Similar to exercise, thyroid hormone administration produces a decline in systemic vascular resistance and an increase in cardiac output and contractility. It has been speculated that increased cellular respiration leads to the release of local vasodilators, and therefore to changes in vascular tone.[145] The rise in stroke volume and cardiac work reflect changes in systemic hemodynamics (e.g., decline in systemic vascular resistance) as the result of decreased smooth muscle contractility by T3 altering sodium and potassium flux in smooth muscle cells.[145]

Hyperthyroidism exerts a positive cardiac inotropism as the rate of ventricular pressure development or velocity of contraction are increased.[146] Moreover, changes in serum T4 and T3 may directly increase muscle fiber shortening as a consequence of increased myosin ATPase activity.[147]

Cardiac hypertrophy in hyperthyroidism. Excess thyroid hormone induces cardiac hypertrophy and structural remodeling at the cellular level. There is an increased myocyte cross-sectional area in both ventricles, but it is greater in the right ventricle in experimental animals.[148] Factors such as hypertrophy of myocyte mitochondria may contribute to cell enlargement. Cell length also increases in the thyroid hormone treated animals. This increase is again twice as great in the right ventricle than in the left ventricle. These cellular changes in cross-diameter and length indicate that, at least in the experimental model, thyroid hormone induces combined eccentric and concentric cardiac hypertrophy that is more pronounced in the right ventricle.[148] Furthermore, the cellular hypertrophy within the left ventricle is not uniform because there is a preferential epimyocardial hypertrophy.

Reversal of the hyperthyroid state in experimental animals brings about a rapid regression of the cardiac hypertrophy during the first 10 days and a more gradual reduction in heart size over several months.[148] For regression to occur, the rate of proteolytic mechanisms in the cardiac myocyte must be greater than the rate of protein synthesis.

Hyperthyroid-induced cardiac hypertrophy has been associated with an increase of membrane-bound β-adrenoreceptors and consequently enhanced β-agonist effects.[149]

The increase of cardiac β-adrenoceptors is found in both the membrane-bound and the intracellular receptor pools. However, receptor cycling depends on the presence of intact microtubules. Microtubules may influence the transduction of signals to the nucleus that initiate cardiac hypertrophy or β-receptor synthesis and may also be involved in the insertion of newly synthesized β-receptors from the Golgi apparatus to the plasma membrane.[150] Although the perinuclear microtubular system undergoes striking proliferation and rearrangement during induction of cardiac hypertrophy, no data are available on microtubular involvement in cardiac gene expression.[150]

This thyroid-induced modulation of β-adrenoceptors has not explained adequately the mechanisms involved in the development and regression of cardiac hypertrophy. For example, it has not been clarified whether receptor shifts from intracellular pools to membrane-bound β-adrenoceptors follows administration of thyroid hormone. The existence of such intracellular pools has been identified for several receptors.[151]

Experimental thyroid hormone-induced cardiac hypertrophy. Studies using a heterotopic cardiac transplantation experimental model and administration of excess T4 led to hypertrophy of the situ working heart, but not of the transplanted heart.[138] These studies also revealed the lack of direct effect of T4 on protein synthesis and provided strong support for the concept that thyroxine-induced cardiac hypertrophy is mediated by increased workload.[138] Furthermore, in experimental hyperthyroidism, isolated cardiac muscle reveals increased rate of contraction and relaxation with an abbreviation of contraction independently of catecholamines. In thyroid hormone-treated animals, the increased contractility and heart rate are not completely removed by β-adrenergic blockade.[152]

Receptor studies in hyperthyroidism. Studies have shown that hyperthyroidism changes the distribution of β-receptors by preferentially increasing the membrane pool, and that synthesis of β-receptors is regulated by thyroid hormones.[142] Cardiac α1-adrenoceptors show a different pattern of response to hyperthyroidism from that of the β-adrenoceptors. Perhaps, the regulation of β-adrenoceptors and α1-adrenoceptors in the heart involves different mechanisms.[142]

Studies on the thyroid hormone interaction with cellular receptors have shown that high affinity (but low capacity) nuclear receptors are probably the sites of the initiation of thyroid hormone action.[153] The receptors are identified as nonhistone proteins of molecular weight 50,500 with a sedimentation constant of 3.55.[154] The nuclear sites are found in all thyroid hormone-responsive tissues. Occupancy of these nuclear sites appears to be the physiologic constraint to the biologic response elicited by thyroid hormone.[155] It is believed that the thyroid hormone effect is determined by the number of nuclear sites occupied and

the duration of such occupancy. Furthermore, the biologic response to variations of T3-nuclear receptor complex concentration is thought to be mediated by altered levels of specific messenger RNAs.[155] Because it is similarly structured, investigators believe that a nuclear receptor for T3 is related to the glucocorticoid receptor and the c-erb-A oncogene.[156] Although complete characterization of the transport of T3 from plasma to cytoplasm and the reverse direction has not been completely accomplished, it has been suggested that it involves specific transport units.[157] Extranuclear sites for T3 binding have not been recognized.

Molecular phenomena in thyroid hormone excess. Metabolic and physiologic functions of the heart and other tissues are controlled by thyroid hormone. However, cellular mechanisms involved in the action of thyroid hormone excess still remain unclear. Augmented rate of cardiac protein synthesis, which provides sufficient components to deal with an increased cardiac output, is an example of structural and functional adaptation of the heart in hyperthyroidism. In addition, thyroid hormone increases the number of $Na+/K\pm ATPase$ pump sites, consistent with an elevation in protein synthesis.[158] Recent studies have shown that glycogenolysis is stimulated in the hyperthyroid state. It is believed that the increased glycolytic aerobic capacity is essential or even critical to the survival of the heart in dealing with the increase in $Na+/K\pm ATPase$ activity.[159] However, our present understanding of the effects of hyperthyroidism on fuel selection by the heart is rather limited.

Hypothyroidism (myxedema)

Cardiovascular impairment in advanced hypothyroidism with myxedema has been well recognized for almost a century. Signs and symptoms of the hypothyroid state include bradycardia, diminished peripheral pulses, low voltage ECG, and nonpitting edema. Symptoms such as dyspnea, orthopnea, and nocturia may suggest congestive heart failure. However, the low plasma volume in the hypothyroid patient, and the response to thyroid hormone (but not to digitalis), support the view that this constellation of symptoms is related to deficiency of thyroid hormone rather than to heart failure.

Contrary to the high cardiac output and the hyperdynamic state that characterize hyperthyroidism, the hypothyroid state is recognized by a low cardiac index, decreased stroke volume, decreased vascular volume and increased systemic vascular resistance. In spite of all these changes, however, the hemodynamic response of the hypothyroid patient to exercise is quite normal.

Both symptoms and signs in hypothyroidism suggest a decreased sympathetic tone exhibited by bradycardia, decreased metabolic rate, cool dry skin, and decreased gastrointestinal motility. Plasma levels of norepinephrine in hypothyroid patients are elevated, suggesting either increased transmitter release or decreased clearance.[160] The explanation for this apparent contradiction of elevated norepinephrine in hypothyroidism may reflect increased "spillover" at the level of the synapse.[161]

Myxedema is also characterized by effusion of serous cavities such as the pericardium, pleura, and peritoneum. The pericardial effusion is slow to accumulate and is probably the reason for the enlarged cardiac silhouette and low voltage ECG. The pericardial fluid is high in protein and cholesterol content.

Hypotension is relatively common in hypothyroid patients, and probably results from a direct effect of thyroid hormone deficiency on the heart.

Recent echocardiographic studies have suggested that a reversible cardiomyopathy is associated with the hypothyroid state. Global decrease in left ventricular function, increased septal thickness, and thickening of the free wall of the right ventricle were noted, all of which reversed after treatment with thyroxine.[162]

The relation of hypothyroidism to ischemic heart disease is controversial. Most investigators, however, accept the idea that there is an increased risk of atherosclerosis in overtly hypothyroid patients. Clinical manifestations of ischemic heart disease are relatively uncommon in these patients, probably because the reduced myocardial consumption prevents or lessens the risk of ischemia.

Laboratory findings in hypothyroidism. Besides the hypercholesterolemia and elevated LDL levels in hypothyroidism, effects on triglyceride transport lead to hypertriglyceridemia. LDL clearance and catabolism are impaired in the hypothyroid state. This impaired LDL removal from plasma is thought to be associated with decreased receptor-mediated LDL degradation.

The normal removal of chylomicron and very low density lipoprotein (VLDL) remnants also appears to be affected by hypothyroidism.[163] The hyperlipidemia, which resolves with thyroxine therapy, may be secondary to decreased lipoprotein lipase activity or cholesterol esterase activity.[164]

Morphologic features of the heart in myxedema. The usual gross finding from the heart in myxedema is four-chamber dilatation without significant hypertrophy. Histologic studies of the myocardium usually reveal pale, swollen fibers, some of which contain vacuoles distorting the myofibrils and staining positive with PAS (basophilic mucoid degeneration) (Fig. 11-13). Interstitial edema and fatty infiltration also occur. However, none of these histopathologic changes are specific for myxedema, and their functional significance is not clear.

ADRENAL DISORDERS

The normal products of the adrenal cortex are glucocorticoids (cortisol), mineralocorticoids (aldosterone), and the androgen precursors. The production of glucocorti-

coids is regulated by pituitary adrenocorticotropic hormone (ACTH), whereas the production of aldosterone is under the regulation of the renin-angiotensin system. Although it is well established that glucocorticoids affect the cardiovascular system, the mechanisms of such influence are not entirely clear.

Cushing syndrome

This syndrome is caused by increased glucocorticoids either synthesized in the adrenal cortex—as a result of primary hyperplasia, pituitary-dependent adrenocortical hyperplasia (Cushing syndrome), ectopic ACTH secretion, adrenal cortical adenoma, or carcinoma—or induced iatrogenically by glucocorticoid therapy. The latter is the most common cause of Cushing syndrome.

Clinical manifestations in Cushing syndrome. Truncal obesity, abdominal striae, "moon faces," amenorrhea, and glucose intolerance are some of the multiple and complex effects of glucocorticoids. Systemic arterial hypertension and accelerated atherosclerosis are the most common cardiovascular complications in Cushing syndrome. It has been estimated that approximately 80% of patients with Cushing syndrome have mild to moderate and occasionally severe hypertension, although the pathogenesis of this complication is not well understood.[165]

Pathogenesis of hypertension in Cushing syndrome. Hypertension in Cushing syndrome is characterized by increases in both cardiac output and total peripheral resistance. Because cardiac sensitivity to both the chronotropic and the inotropic effects of catecholamines result in increased cardiac output, such an effect may be one of the factors involved in the hypertension in this syndrome.[166]

In Cushing syndrome caused by ACTH excess, there is overproduction of cortisol and a variable excess of the mineralocorticoids II-deoxycorticosterone (DOC) and corticosterone.[167]

Considerable evidence exists that mineralocorticoids and glucocorticoids have opposite effects on one possible pathogenetic factor: sodium retention. Mineralocorticoids promote renal sodium and water retention, and kaliuresis, whereas glucocorticoids increase glomerular filtration rate, and therefore promote sodium and water loss.[168]

In a recent study of patients with Cushing syndrome, plasma II-DOC and corticosterone (B) levels were high, although still in the normal range, but total exchangeable sodium (NaE) and serum potassium were normal, and there was no correlation between blood pressure and NaE.[169] In these patients, no evidence of mineralocorticoid excess was found, nor was there any evidence of sodium retention by any mechanisms independent of mineralocorticoids. However, the possibility that steroids such as cortisol may alter blood pressure directly without altering electrolyte metabolism still remains open.[170]

Studies have shown that patients with Cushing syndrome have normal catecholamine levels and receptors,

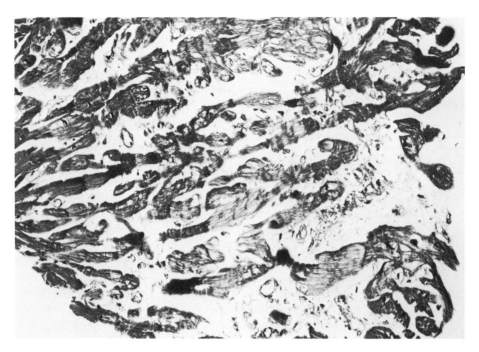

Fig. 11-13. Focally swollen myocytes and marked interstitial edema in endomyocardial biopsy from a patient with myxedema.

but reveal an increased β-adrenoceptor sensitivity. Except for elevation of plasma renin substrate, most reports indicate that the renin-angiotensin system is normal in Cushing syndrome.[171] In a study by Ritchie et al,[169] plasma renin was normal and at a level appropriate for the sodium status. Although this finding rules out a vascular role, it does not exclude a tissue angiotensin II-mediated mechanism for blood pressure elevation in Cushing syndrome.

Other investigators that studied patients with cortisol-secreting adrenal adenomas found an increased pressor responsiveness to noradrenaline and angiotensin II, possibly as a result of inhibition of their extraneuronal uptake and degradation. These findings were thought to indicate that increased vascular sensitivity to vasopressors was a likely cause of the elevated blood pressure in Cushing syndrome.[171]

An association of Cushing syndrome with Sertoli's cell tumors of the testes and cutaneous labial letiginosis was reported to occur in one fifth of patients with familial cardiac myxoma.[172] Cushing syndrome, cardiac myxoma, other myxoid tumors, and spotty skin pigmentation probably present a heritable syndrome.[173]

Addison disease

Addison disease features are the opposite of those of Cushing syndrome. They include hypotension, hyperkalemia, and weight loss. The heart is small and disproportionate to systemic weight loss, and the myocytes are thin and atrophic.

Addison disease also includes a deficiency of both cor-

tisol and aldosterone. Because of the deficiency of the latter, sodium reabsorption and potassium secretion in the renal distal tubule are impaired. Such patients, because of their inability to conserve sodium, have a propensity for volume depletion, and therefore are prone to vascular collapse when stressed.[174]

Pheochromocytoma

The adrenal medulla contains enterochromaffin cells derived from the neural crest. Similar cells are also found in the organs of Zuckerkandl and along the paraaortic sympathetic chain. A neoplasm arising from enterochromaffin cells in the adrenal medulla is called a pheochromocytoma, whereas a similar neoplastic growth in other locations is designated as an extraadrenal paraganglioma. Although it is the epinephrine-secreting pheochromocytoma that has a profound effect on the cardiovascular system, a norepinephrine-secreting extraadrenal paraganglioma may also produce hypertension, palpitations, and facial flushing. Pheochromocytoma is a rare tumor with an estimated incidence of 0.8 per 100,000 population.[175]

Clinical manifestations. Pheochromocytoma may mimic numerous clinical syndromes, thus presenting a significant diagnostic challenge, although cardiac manifestations dominate the overall clinical picture in the great majority of cases. When the tumor is symptomatic, hypertension, palpitations, headache, chest pain, and sudden death have been observed. Although symptoms and ECG changes may suggest angina pectoris, coronary angiographic findings are usually normal, and blood pressure measurement reveals cyclic changes. ECG abnormalities in pheochromocytoma include ST-T change and arrhythmias. The cause of ST-T change may be either a relative ischemia resulting from increased oxygen demands or a catecholamine effect that shortens depolarization time and produces ST-T depression.[176] Echocardiograms have revealed wall motion abnormalities and in some cases a hypokinetic basal portion, but a hyperkinetic apex attributed to different catecholamine sensitivity at the two sites.[176]

On rare occasions, an acute, severe myocardial event may be the initial clinical presentation of the pheochromocytoma. Such an event may occur without any provocation or may be manifested during an unrelated operation. Usually, the event is life-threatening and may only be recognized at autopsy. Although association of pheochromocytoma with myocardial infarction is rare, at least 28 cases of such association have been reported.[177] In some pheochromocytoma cases inappropriate for the patient's age, coronary atherosclerosis was noted. It is not clear whether the known activation of lipoprotein lipase by catecholamines, and subsequent degradation of triglycerides to free fatty acids and glycerol play any role in this premature atherosclerosis.[178]

Systemic hypertension occurs in most cases of pheochromocytoma and may be either intermittent or sustained. The fluctuation (cyclic) of blood pressure and heart rate often recorded in patients with pheochromocytoma may be related to episodic secretion of catecholamines by the tumor, or a change in vascular resistance. Even though they are hypertensive, many patients exhibit a drop in blood pressure on standing (orthostatic hypotension). The hypertension is almost certainly a direct effect of catecholamines. Most pheochromocytomas secrete primarily norepinephrine, which has a dominant effect on α-adrenergic receptors in the peripheral vasculature and β-adrenergic receptors in the heart, thus causing peripheral vasoconstriction, increased heart rate, and contractility.[179] Epinephrine, which is secreted with norepinephrine by some tumors but rarely alone, may cause hypertension by means of a β 2-agonist effect on the peripheral vasculature. However, ectopic arrhythmias occur after infusion of both epinephrine and norepinephrine. Moreover, with greater stretching of cardiac muscle caused by hypertension, there is an increased cardiac automaticity. Catecholamines also facilitate ectopic rhythms by changing ionic transport mechanisms across the cell membrane that increase the speed of diastolic depolarization.[177]

In addition to the direct effect of catecholamines, an indirect effect on renin secretion may exacerbate the hypertension. Data show high nonsuppressable renin levels in some patients with pheochromocytoma.[180] Catecholamines can mediate renin release by stimulating β-adrenergic receptors, whereas α-adrenergic stimulation appears to suppress renin release.

Laboratory findings. Laboratory documentation of pheochromocytoma relies on the presence of urinary catecholamine metabolites (particularly metanephrines and vanillylmandelic acid) in increased amounts. Although increased plasma epinephrine and nonepinephrine concentrations have been observed parallel to the elevation of blood pressure, the reliability of plasma measurements in the diagnosis of this condition is controversial.[181]

Morphologic manifestations in pheochromocytoma. Infusions of *l*-norepinephrine in experimental animals can cause subepicardial and subendocardial hemorrhages, focal myocyte necrosis in some instances, and biochemical and morphologic changes in the arterial walls, such as intimal hyperplasia and diffuse proliferative endarteritis.[177] Similar myocardial lesions have been described in patients dying of pheochromocytoma. Foci of myocardial necrosis of the contraction band type are seen. The cytoplasm of the myocytes between the bands appears fine granular, and basophilic because of aggregates of mitochondria, containing calcific deposits, a sign of irreversible cell injury. Lysis of damaged muscle (myocytolysis) is followed by stromal collapse and focal scarring. Neutrophilic inflammation is characteristically scant or absent in this process, although some investigators have described histiocytes, plasma cells, and some eosinophils around the necrotic myocytes, referring to this condition as *acute catecholamine myocarditis* (Fig. 11-14).

An acute catecholamine crisis can be precipitated by foods high in tyramine, positional pressure on the tumor, induction of anesthesia, and labor and delivery.[179] In a study of 10 patients dying suddenly of acute cardiovascular complications (out of a total of 34 with pheochromocytoma found during a 20-year period), the cause of death was myocardial infarction in 5, left ventricular failure in 2, cerebral hemorrhage (hypertensive bleed) in 2, and circulatory collapse in 1.[182]

Mediastinal paragangliomas. Mediastinal paragangliomas (intrathoracic pheochromocytomas) are rare, estimated to be about 2% of all pheochromocytomas. Even more rare are pericardial and cardiac paragangliomas, which are usually located on the posterior wall of the left atrium, but can occur in other locations in the heart. Twelve of the sixteen resected cardiac paragangliomas were located in the atria, and four involved the ventricle.[183]

PITUITARY DISORDERS
Hypopituitarism

Studies have shown that life expectancy in hypopituitarism is shortened because of cardiovascular and cerebrovascular disorders. Such disorders include myocardial infarction, cardiac failure, cerebrovascular events, and arterial and pulmonary emboli.[184]

Although it is believed that growth hormone deficiency is responsible for premature death from vascular disorders,

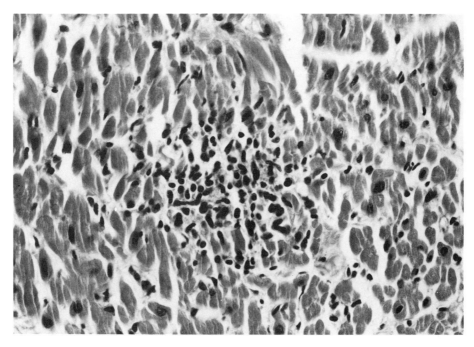

Fig. 11-14. Focal myocyte necrosis and mononuclear cell infiltrate from a patient with pheochromocytoma.

no correlation was found between the estimated duration of the disease before diagnosis of hypopituitarism and risk of vascular death.

Acromegaly

Hypersecretion of growth hormone by a pituitary adenoma results in the clinical syndrome of acromegaly. This syndrome is characterized by hypertrophy of soft tissues, muscles, and bones, and enlargement of internal organs, particularly the heart, liver, and kidneys. The documented effect of growth hormone (GH) production is an increase in insulin growth factor 1 (IGFI) or somatomedin C. Although increased morbidity and mortality from heart disease in acromegalics is well established, a controversy continues regarding whether these individuals suffer from a specific cardiomyopathy or cardiac dysfunction secondary to diabetes, coronary atherosclerosis, or hypertension.[185] However, several authors continue to suggest that acromegaly may induce a specific cardiomyopathy in the absence of hypertension, atherosclerosis, or severe valvular disease. Whether coronary atherosclerosis and diabetes play a major role in the cardiac hypertrophy of acromegaly is still controversial.

Clinical manifestations in acromegaly. Cardiac hypertrophy (often disproportional to that of other organs), increased cardiac output, and decreased systemic vascular resistance are all characteristic of the acromegalic patient. While echocardiographic studies in acromegalic patients have stressed the disproportional increased thickness of the interventricular septum,[186] postmortem studies failed to demonstrate asymmetric septal hypertrophy.[187]

Cardiac dilatation and congestive heart failure may be the end result and is often the major cause of death in acromegalics. However, the pathophysiologic mechanisms responsible for the cardiac dysfunction remain unclear, although it is recognized that the associated hypertension contributes to left ventricular hypertrophy and dysfunction. Other proposed etiologic factors for the acromegalic symptoms include coronary atherosclerosis, valvular abnormalities, compensatory hypertrophy caused by increased work load (splanchnomegaly and somatomegaly), and direct effects of the growth hormone. Although valvular disease in acromegaly may be present in approximately one fifth of the patients, its role in the cardiac hypertrophy appears to be limited.[187] Abnormal diastolic indices have been recorded even in acromegalic patients without hypertension and/or coronary atherosclerotic heart disease. A reduced diastolic compliance in acromegaly may be the result of the reported increased interstitial fibrosis or the mononuclear cell infiltrates within the myocardium.[187]

Cardiac morphologic findings in acromegaly. The usual microscopic findings in the hearts of acromegalics are myocyte hypertrophy, interstitial fibrosis, focal myofiber disarray, wall thickening of small intramyocardial arteries, and focal interstitial infiltrates of mononuclear cells. The latter are rarely diffuse and may occasionally simulate lesions seen in the hearts of patients with pheochromocytoma (norepinephrine lesions).

Increased number of mitochondria, vacuolization of the sacrotubular system, myofibrillar loss, z-band remnants, and crenation of nuclear membranes are the usual electron microscopic (EM) findings.[188] However, none of these EM alterations are specific for the entity.

Pathogenesis of cardiomegaly in acromegaly. Although cardiomegaly is a common phenomenon in acromegalic patients, the correlation between the plasma levels of GH or duration of GH hyperproduction and the degree of left ventricular hypertrophy is generally weak. Furthermore, the underlying mechanism by which elevated GH induces cardiac hypertrophy is not completely clear. Volume work overloading due to increased blood supply and water retention under the influence of excessive GH may be an important factor in the induction process.[189]

Echocardiographic studies on a limited number of patients with acromegaly at our institution have shown increased left ventricular mass, marked septal thickness, and a lesser degree of hypertrophy of the posterior left ventricular wall. These patients were noted to have abnormal ventricular diastolic function and decreased ejection fraction. These morphologic findings in the absence of coronary atherosclerosis, hypertension, and diabetes strongly suggest that a specific cardiomyopathy in acromegaly may be present.

EFFECTS OF PARATHYROID HORMONE ON THE CARDIOVASCULAR SYSTEM
Hyperparathyroidism

The classic effects of the parathyroid hormone (PTH) are encountered in the kidneys and skeletal system. A peptide called PTH-related protein (PTHrp), or humoral hypercalcemia of malignancy factor, has recently been reported. This factor mimics the biologic actions of PTH, thus stimulating bone resorption and elevating blood calcium concentration. Both PTH and PTHrp are specifically bound to the same receptor protein.[190]

PTH has been shown to elicit a hypotensive response resulting from peripheral vasodilation of small resistance vessels. This action of PTH is thought to be manifested at the vascular smooth muscle site. It is independent of endothelial cell regulation.[191]

The effects of both PTH and PTHrp on the heart are less well known; the suggested chronotropic and inotropic activity remains controversial. However, it is possible that such activity may result from increased oxygen delivery secondary to coronary artery vasodilatation.[190] Moreover, the PTHrp may be a regulatory or modulatory factor of cardiovascular function in an autocrine or paracrine fashion.[192]

Calcific deposits in hyperparathyroidism, hypervitaminosis D, renal failure, sarcoidosis, and metastatic carcinoma are most often found in the mitral valve annulus. Less often calcium deposition is seen on individual myocardial fibers and coronary arteries (medial calcinosis).

The hemodynamic derangement of such depositions is rarely significant except when massive.

Hypocalcemia

Severe acute hypocalcemia can adversely effect ventricular function because calcium ions are of integral importance in translating the depolarization impulse into muscle contraction (excitation contraction coupling). However, chronic hypocalcemia has not been known to cause ventricular dysfunction.

DIABETES MELLITUS

Despite significant clinical and laboratory research on the etiology and pathogenesis of cardiovascular disease associated with diabetes mellitus, considerable controversies exist about the link between the two conditions. There is, however, general agreement about the epidemiologic evidence of increased morbidity and mortality from heart disease in diabetics. The Framingham study revealed that mortality from cardiovascular causes was 4.5 times greater in diabetic women than in control group patients, and two times greater in diabetic men.[193] The study also disclosed that obese diabetic women with low high-density lipoprotein (HDL) cholesterol levels had a specially high risk for cardiovascular disease. Furthermore, data from the Framingham study indicate that congestive heart failure is twice as common in diabetic men, and five times more common in diabetic women in the age range of 45 to 74 than in age-matched control group patients.

Other studies have revealed that diabetic patients more often have multivessel coronary disease, left anterior descending lesions, higher left ventricular end-diastolic pressure, more distal coronary artery disease, and higher incidence of left ventricular aneurysms.[194] Comparative studies of patients with insulin-dependent diabetes and nondiabetic control subjects of comparable age have shown that diabetics are more likely to have severe coronary stenoses, three-vessel disease, and significant narrowings of distal epicardial coronary arteries, rendering them unsuitable for bypass surgery.[195] Diabetics with coronary artery disease have left main atherosclerotic occlusive lesions more often than nondiabetics with CAD. Although the severity of diabetes does not appear to correlate with the severity of coronary artery disease, diabetics treated with insulin have a higher risk of coronary disease than those treated with oral hypoglycemic agents or diet alone.[196]

The inpatient mortality is higher among diabetics with myocardial infarction, particularly those with poor control of diabetes. Diabetics more frequently experience atrioventricular and interventricular conduction defects post-MI than do control patients with MI. Furthermore, congestive heart failure is more common after an MI in diabetics than in control group patients. It remains unclear whether an underlying cardiac dysfunction in diabetes, in addition to coronary artery disease, predisposes to the development of congestive heart failure.[197] The long-term survival rates of diabetics who have undergone coronary bypass are worse, particularly those with insulin-dependent diabetes.[198]

Morphology of epicardial coronary arteries in diabetes. Histopathologic differences in the epicardial coronary arteries between diabetic and nondiabetics have been reported. The media of epicardial coronary arteries in diabetics reveal reduced thickness, decreased amounts of acid mucopolysaccharides, and increased periodic acid-Schiff-positive material compared with controls.[199] Moreover, an increase in connective tissue at the nonatheromatous segment of the arterial wall has been noted in diabetics.

Diabetic cardiomyopathy. Because some diabetics may present with congestive heart failure in the absence of occlusive coronary artery disease, it has been suggested that perhaps a primary diabetic cardiomyopathy may exist with diabetes alone or in association with hypertension.[200] Although the often-recorded clinical deterioration of left ventricular performance in diabetics is suggestive of specific heart muscle disease, the pathogenesis for the cardiac dysfunction is not clear. Some reports have indicated that the pathogenesis of diabetic cardiomyopathy is secondary to metabolic alterations in the diabetic heart. Those metabolic alterations include impaired glucose transport and decreased phosphorylation, increased lipid metabolism, altered protein synthesis and degradation, and decreased calcium transport by the sarcoplasmic reticulum.[201]

Morphologic features in diabetic cardiomyopathy. Recent studies have reported significant differences in heart weight, interstitial fibrosis, replacement fibrosis, and perivascular fibrosis between patients with hypertension, diabetes mellitus, or both. The heart weight is higher in the hypertensive-diabetic patients, and the amount of microscopic fibrosis is greater than in patients with either hypertension or diabetes.[202] The above study suggested that the myocardial fibrosis seen in the hypertensive-diabetic cardiomyopathy may contribute to the diastolic dysfunction of the heart because the function of connective tissue is to ensure proper diastolic alignment of the myocytes. Furthermore, the degree of myocardial fibrosis appears to be greater in patients with congestive heart failure. Similar diminished ventricular compliance has been recorded in diabetics without hypertension.[203]

The microscopic findings in the hearts of patients with diabetic cardiomyopathy are not considered pathognomonic. The pathogenesis of fibrosis remains unknown, although it has been postulated to result from diabetic microangiopathy. Whether an additional microangiopathy caused by hypertension may also be contributory remains speculative.

Diabetic microangiopathy. Microangiopathic lesions of diabetic patients may include microaneurysms and thickening of the basement membrane of small coronary arteries and arterioles. It is unlikely, however, that the microangiopathic lesions can cause clinical cardiomyopathy.

It is entirely possible, however, that other microvascular changes not specific for diabetes, such as thickening of the arterial wall caused by myointimal proliferation, may produce critical reduction of the arterial lumen and lead to focal fibrosis.

Whether these microvascular myocardial changes are more frequent and more pronounced in diabetics and may lead to diabetic cardiomyopathy is vigorously debated in the literature. Studies based on endomyocardial biopsies of diabetic patients have concluded that there is no correlation between diabetes and small vessel disease.[204] Although association between diabetes and myocardial small vessel disease has been reported by some investigators,[205] others have been unable to identify significant morphologic or functional abnormalities in the microvasculature of diabetics in the absence of hypertension.[206]

It is believed, however, that adequate control of blood glucose levels in type I diabetes may prevent the microangiopathic changes. In this regard, a hemorheologic hypothesis has been advanced. This hypothesis proposes that the combination of reduced erythrocyte deformability specific to diabetes, and increased erythrocyte aggregation caused by nonspecific plasma protein changes, gradually induces the diabetic microangiopathy.[207] Both increased blood and erythrocyte viscosity and reduced erythrocyte deformability are linked to the degree of hyperglycemia.[208] Furthermore, increased erythrocyte aggregation in diabetes is associated with fibrinogen and haptoglobin elevations present with glucose intolerance.

The erythrocyte aggregates pass into the microcirculation, where they must ultimately be disrupted to be accommodated within the marrow lumina. Their disruption (aggregates) necessitates unusually high short-lived local pressure gradients because of reduced erythrocyte deformability in diabetics. At the sites of erythrocyte aggregate disruption, the peak shearing force exerted on local endothelial cells is as much as 12 times the normal. The response of the endothelial cells to such an increased force is to generate thicker basement membranes.[207]

Pathophysiology of the diabetic heart. Currently, there is general agreement about the role of the autonomic nervous system in controlling the cardiovascular response to exercise. The interaction of the parasympathetic and sympathetic components is involved in the adjustment of the heart rate during exercise. Defects in parasympathetic innervation, clinically presented as an increased resting heart rate and decreased respiratory variation in heart rate, are common and occur fairly early in diabetics.[209] Sympathetic innervation defects (decrease in heart rate rise on standing) are not as common and occur only in long-standing diabetes. However, during exercise, regional increases in vascular resistance (e.g., splanchnic, renal beds) are mediated by the sympathetic nervous system. Thus degeneration of sympathetic fibers in the splanchnic beds of diabetics could result in a blunted rise of blood pressure during exercise.[210] Orthostatic dysfunction, characterized by excessive drop in blood pressure and protracted and diminished heart rate rise on standing has been observed in diabetics with vagal dysfunction.

The most well-known phenomenon of neurologic dysfunction in the hearts of diabetics is silent ischemia and/or infarction. The clinical assessment of individuals with diabetes is made very difficult because of the phenomenon of silent ischemia. Exercise may produce no symptoms yet S-T segments may become depressed.[211] Recognition of this phenomenon by the physician should lead to additional diagnostic evaluation of the underlying coronary status. In the Framingham study, almost half of the diabetic patients with coronary disease were asymptomatic. Autopsy studies of diabetic patients often reveal decreased numbers of autonomic nerve fibers in the heart. These fibers are often fragmented with focal spindle-shaped and beaded thickenings.[212] Data from several studies indicate that sudden cardiac death is increased among diabetics with autonomic neuropathy.[213]

Atherogenesis in diabetes. It remains unclear whether hyperglycemia plays a role in the induction of vascular changes and vascular complications commonly seen in diabetes. However, accumulated evidence in recent years indicates that hyperglycemia may induce pathologic alterations in a number of plasma proteins through the process of nonenzymatic glycation.[214] This multistep process occurs when the carbonyl group of glucose undergoes a nucleophilic attack by an amino group and produces an unstable, nonenzymatic glycation adduct (an aldimine) in rapid fashion. A second, slower step is the formation of a relatively stable ketoamine, which after long periods (months to years) rearranges itself to form advanced irreversible structures.[215]

An increased nonenzymatic glycation in a protein sequence may have a profound effect on enzyme activity, the binding of regulatory molecules, the cross-linking of proteins, proteolysis,[214] and immunogenicity.[216] Increased nonenzymatic glycation could alter endothelial functions and affect its interactions with monocytes,[215] which are well-known participants in the early steps of atherogenesis.

Assays of cultured monocytes in high glucose/low NaCl media have shown a 75% increase in monocyte adherence to endothelial cells.[215] These experimental data suggest that relatively small but long-lasting alterations of monocyte-endothelial cell interactions could be an important event in the pathogenesis of slowly progressive vascular disease in diabetes.

Alterations in the composition of arterial glucosaminoglycans in diabetes may also influence the progress of the atherosclerotic process. Such an observation is based on the belief that LDL entering into the neointima may be bound and retained by the glycosaminoglycan (GAG) portion of the proteoglycan molecule. At present, there is ample documentation of the binding of chondroitin sulfate/dermatan sulfate proteoglycans to LDL, both in vivo and in vitro. Both of these glycosaminoglycans form soluble and insoluble complexes with LDL. Desulfation of the glycosaminoglycans abolishes the interaction, an indication that sulfate ester groups are important in the binding.[217]

Proteoglycans are macromolecules present in plasma membranes and extracellular matrix. Certain properties of GAG are recognized as potential important factors in atherogenesis. For example, GAG heparan sulfate has antiproliferative properties, antithrombogenic, and antilipemic effects and influences the permeability of basement membranes.[218]

There are a number of additional ways by which the responses of the vessel wall to injury are modified by diabetes. Several of the molecular alterations observed in diabetes tend to increase the proliferative response of the vessel wall and facilitate the deposition of lipid. Features of the diabetic state that may facilitate the development of atherosclerotic lesions include increased synthesis of thromboxane by platelets and decreased production of prostacyclin (PGI2). Reduced production of the latter may have an effect on lipid metabolism in the vessel wall. Prostacyclin enhances the production of lysosomal (acid) cholesteryl ester hydrolase by smooth muscle cells and increases their cyclic adenosine monophosphate (cAMP) levels.[219] Furthermore, the effects of glycosylation of connective tissue proteins in the atherosclerotic plaque may be important. For example, the nonenzymatic glycosylation of collagen may provide a strong stimulus for platelet aggregation in diabetes.[220]

In humans both type I and type II diabetes are considered risk factors for atherosclerosis, although these two types reveal different lipoprotein profiles. Endothelial dysfunction has been described in both type I and type II diabetes as determined by an increased loss of von Willebrand factor and decreased production of prostacyclin and plasminogen activator.[221]

Experimental studies in diabetic atherogenesis. The endothelium of alloxan-induced diabetes in rabbits reveals altered function indicated by increased thromboxane A2 synthesis and reduced synthesis of endothelium-derived relaxing factor.[222] Furthermore, alloxan diabetic rabbits develop more extensive atherosclerosis when fed a mild atherogenic diet than nondiabetic animals fed the same diet.

At 2 weeks after alloxan-induced diabetes, the animals reveal histopathologic evidence of endothelial injury, endothelial replication, and intimal hyperplasia without lipid accumulation.[223] Although there was no endothelial denudation, ultrastructural evidence of endothelial injury was present in the form of blebs, craters, raised cell margins, and microvillus formation. Focal adhesion of mononuclear cells on the endothelial surface was observed, some of which was found within the intima, but did not contain lipid.

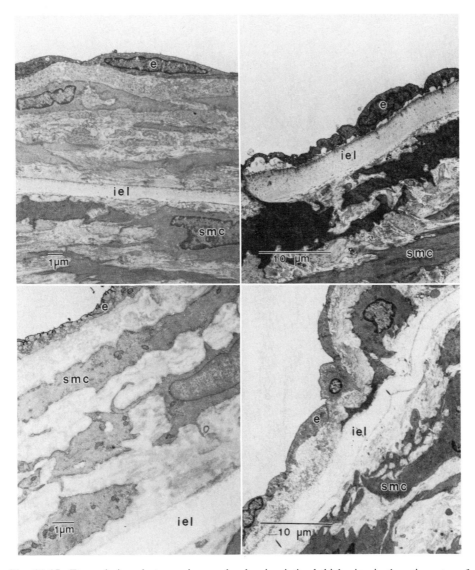

Fig. 11-15. Transmission electron micrographs showing intimal thickening in thoracic aortas of diabetic rabbits and age-matched controls. *Upper left panel:* 2 weeks after alloxan treatment. Upper right panel: 2-week control. *Lower left panel:* 3 months after alloxan treatment. Lower right panel: age-matched 3-month control. There is no intimal thickening in the control vessel at 2 weeks, but two layers of myointimal cells are evident in diabetic aortas. At 3 months, control vessel contains one layer of cells in contrast to the diabetic vessel, which shows three layers of myointimal cells. (*iel* = internal elastic lamina; *smc* = smooth muscle cell; *e* = endothelium.) (Reprinted by permission of Mary Richardson, MD and *Arteriosclerosis Thrombosis* 11 (3):517, 1991.)

At 3 months, platelets, increased numbers of RBCs, and fibrin-like material were present on the endothelial surface of all the diabetic animals, but there was no evidence of thrombus formation. The aortic endothelial basement membrane increased its thickness and reached its maximum at about 1 week after alloxan injection.[223]

All vessels examined at 6 months revealed increased numbers of intimal smooth muscles and deposition of connective tissue. The intimal thickening was more marked in the diabetic aortas than in those of nondiabetic age-matched animals. The smooth muscle cells in the intima expressed the secretory phenotype that is capable of migration and proliferation.[224]

The above experimental study in rabbits indicates that alloxan-induced diabetes is associated with nondenuding endothelial injury and intimal hypertrophy, changes that are considered consistent with atherogenesis[223] (Fig. 11-15).

From the discussion above, it is apparent that diabetes is associated with a spectrum of cardiovascular disorders. The association with coronary heart disease, myocardial infarction, and congestive heart failure is well established. However, whether diabetes induces a specific type of cardiomyopathy or whether there is a condition such as hypertensive-diabetic cardiomyopathy is not entirely clear.

CARCINOID HEART DISEASE

Carcinoid tumors are neoplasms of neuroendocrine cells of amine precursor uptake and decarboxylation type (APUD). The great majority of carcinoids arise from the small intestine (44%) and bronchus (32%). Less often encountered locations are the ovary, stomach, appendix, colon, pancreas, rectum, gallbladder, and other sites.[225]

Clinical manifestations. The most frequent clinical manifestation of the carcinoid syndrome is attacks of flushing. Repeated attacks of flushing over many months or years may lead to skin telangiectasia or leonine facies. Although the cause of flushing remains elusive, it has been postulated that kinins, prostaglandins, dopamine, various gut peptides (particularly the substance P-related peptides), and the tachykinins are probably involved. Because of the diversion of tryptophan to 5-hydroxytryptamine (5HT) in the carcinoid syndrome, there are reduced amounts of the former for protein and nicotinamide synthesis. 5-Hydroxytryptamine is believed to be responsible for the diarrhea and bronchospasm in this syndrome.[225]

The frequency of heart lesions in patients with the carcinoid syndrome ranges from 19% to 53% of cases.[226]

Pathogenesis of carcinoid heart disease. The pathogenesis of carcinoid heart disease has not been elucidated. Agents released by the tumor, such as serotonin, kallikrein, bradykinin, histamine, gastrin, ACTH, and prostaglandins have been incriminated, but they have not been proved responsible for the lesions.[227]

Recent studies have indicated that patients with severe carcinoid heart disease had higher urinary 5-hydroxyindoleacetic acid (5-HIAA) excretion than patients without or with lesser degree of heart involvement. Furthermore, these studies have demonstrated high plasma concentrations of the tachykinins neuropeptide K (NPK) and substance P (SP) in patients with established cardiac lesions.[228] In vitro fibroblast stimulation by tachykinins such as SP and neurokinin A is known to occur.[229]

The severity of cardiac involvement does not seem to be related to the duration of carcinoid disease or to the extent of liver involvement but rather to the higher plasma levels of serotonin and tachykinins.[228] Interestingly, carcinoids proximal to the right heart without liver metastasis rarely produce lesions of right heart valves, whereas carcinoids proximal to the left heart (bronchial carcinoids) may cause left-sided valvular lesions.[230] The diagnosis of carcinoid heart disease should be considered in cases of isolated right heart failure, even though the classic signs of the syndrome are absent.

Morphologic findings in carcinoid heart disease. The morphologic appearance of carcinoid lesions is that of diffuse elevated fibrotic endocardial plaques primarily seen in the tricuspid and pulmonic valves. The plaques are most frequently seen on the ventricular surface of the posterior and septal leaflets of the tricuspid valve, causing adherence to the underlying ventricular endocardium and thus

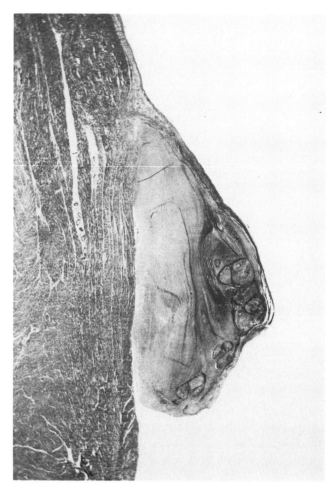

Fig. 11-16. Tricuspid valve with carcinoid plaque on the undersurface of a completely immobilized leaflet. Note that in contrast to the leaflet, the plaque contains no elastic fibers.

tricuspid regurgitation (Fig. 11-16). Involvement of the pulmonic valve causes cuspal thickening and contraction, often resulting in significant stenosis. The edges of the leaflets of both valves are often curled and embedded in the fibrous plaque that immobilizes them. Left-sided lesions occur but rarely are hemodynamically significant.[231] Carcinoid plaques are rarely seen on the intima of great veins, the coronary veins, and the proximal ascending aorta.[227]

The main components of the carcinoid plaques are an extracellular matrix rich in mucopolysaccharides and collagen intermingled with a moderate number of cells. The more superficial cells are elongated, slender, and are parallel to the endothelial surface. Deeper layers of cells are more irregular, stellate, and randomly oriented. The lesions are devoid of elastic components and are usually sharply demarcated from the normal underlying tissues. However, in some instances the acid mucopolysaccharide stroma appears to extend into the underlying leaflet tissues.

The cells within the plaque are immunoreactive with the antiactin and antidesmin antibodies, suggesting the presence of muscle characteristics (e.g., smooth muscle and myofibroblasts). Specific lectin (UEAI) binding to endothelial cells has shown that carcinoid lesions are covered by a layer of such cells. It appears, however, that the proliferative activity of the carcinoid plaque cells is very low; the cells were negative to Ki67 antibody.[232]

Although the connective tissue within or adjacent to the primary site of carcinoid tumors, or the liver metastases, reveals an increased number of PDGF-B receptors, this is not the case with carcinoid plaques in the heart. Such diversity argues against PDGF as a common pathogenetic mechanism for the fibromuscular proliferation.[232]

The hemodynamic derangements of both tricuspid regurgitation and pulmonic stenosis secondary to carcinoid heart disease are discussed in Chapter 3.

INFILTRATIVE SYSTEMIC DISORDERS AND DEPOSITIONS

Amyloidosis and sarcoidosis are two entities that may significantly affect the heart and, to a lesser degree, the vascular system.

Amyloidosis

Amyloidosis comprises a group of diseases characterized by the deposition of abnormal fibrillar proteins in the extracellular spaces. The accumulation of these deposits leads to cellular dysfunction and disease states.

All amyloid fibrils (deposits), regardless of their biochemical composition, share similar properties: (1) a serum precursor; (2) a high degree of antiparallel beta-pleated sheet conformation; (3) green birefringence under polarized light after Congo Red staining; and (4) a fibrillar quaternary structure with a typical electron microscopic appearance.[233] Amyloid proteins are also known to be highly insoluble; therefore they resist complete degradation in vivo by cellular proteases.

It appears that tissue-specific factors are also involved in amyloidogenesis since amyloid fibrils may be deposited in several organs in the systemic forms, or to one organ in the localized forms.[233]

The amyloid fibrils are organized as rigid, nonbranching rods with a slight twist longitudinally. They are of indeterminate length, with a constant diameter of 75 to 100 Å. Each fibril contains two or more filamentous subunits (25 to 35 Å diameter).[234] Amyloid deposits are consistently associated with a glycoprotein known as amyloid P-component of normal basement membrane, a finding that adds additional weight to the possibility that a basement membrane disturbance is involved in amyloid deposition.[235]

AL amyloidosis. AL amyloidosis, the most common form of amyloidosis, occurs in primary amyloidosis and in multiple myeloma. The proliferating plasma cells in these two disorders produce either whole immunoglobulin light chains or fragments of it. The immunoglobulins are present in the plasma, urine or both, and are the source of the amyloid deposits.[236]

In AL amyloidosis, excessive amounts of either kappa or lambda chains are synthesized (occasionally with fragments of heavy chains). However, lambda light chains are more frequently associated with AL amyloidosis than are kappa light chains.[237] There is also significant preponderance of lambda VI (and Kappa I) proteins in AL fibrils. It has been suggested that these two subtypes may be inherently amyloidogenic as a result of certain key amino acid sequences present in each.[238]

Recent reports indicate that at least some amyloid fibrils are unequivocally created in the rough endoplasmic reticulum (RER) of plasma cells. Such production is accomplished by polymerization or degradation of the precursor proteins, which are subsequently deposited in the extracellular space.[239]

A certain ethnic predisposition for AL amyloidosis has been reported recently in individuals of Hispanic extraction.[240]

Secondary amyloidosis. Secondary or reactive amyloidosis (AA) is a rare complication of common chronic inflammatory disorders such as tuberculosis, osteomyelitis, rheumatoid arthritis, and of some malignancies (Hodgkin's lymphoma and renal cell carcinoma).[233] AA amyloidosis is also a common feature and cause of early death resulting from renal failure in the autosomal recessive familial Mediterranean fever.

The amyloid fibrils in secondary amyloidosis are made up of non-immunoglobulin natural protein called AA. This is the amino terminal fragment of 76 residues of a serum precursor protein SAA.[241] SAA, an acute-phase reactant with a molecular weight of 12 kd, is produced in the liver and circulates as part of the HDL3 complex. This precursor protein increases in inflammatory states, and its production by the hepatocytes is enhanced by interleukin-1.[242]

A group of systemic amyloidoses that includes the familial amyloidotic polyneuropathies, senile cardiac or systemic amyloidosis, and familial cardiomyopathy of Danish origin, shares the same serum precursor prealbumin as the amyloid subunit. Familial amyloid polyneuropathy (FAP) is an autosomal dominant disease and has been described in several kinships throughout the world (Portuguese, Japanese, Swedish, Jewish, Swiss-German, and Appalachian types).[233]

A new type of AA amyloidosis has been described in long-term subcutaneous heroin abusers. These individuals develop typical renal and other systemic organ AA disease.[243] It is of considerable interest that most cases of systemic amyloidosis in Europe are AA disease, whereas in the United States most cases are AL disease.[244]

Another recently described type of amyloidosis has

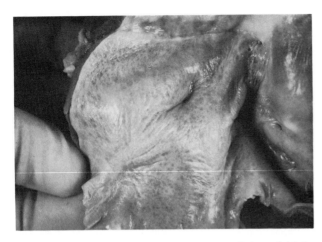

Fig. 11-17. Left atrium with multiple endocardial amyloid deposits (dark spots).

been seen in patients receiving long-term hemodialysis, in whom the amyloid fibril is composed of beta-2 microglobulin.[245] These individuals have carpal tunnel syndrome and cystic bone lesions. It is believed that this condition is caused by an accumulation of beta-2 microglobulin, which does not cross the dialysis membrane.

Cardiac amyloidosis. Cardiac involvement by amyloidosis may occur in any form of systemic amyloidosis, although it is most common in primary immunocyte-derived disease (AL). Clinical cardiac dysfunction may manifest as heart failure, restrictive cardiomyopathy, dysrhythmias, conduction abnormalities, valvular dysfunction, myocardial ischemia caused by involvement of intramyocardial arteries, and/or sudden death.[246] ECG abnormalities are particularly common and include low QRS voltage, myocardial infarct pattern, abnormal QRS axis, and heart block. Sinoatrial node dysfunction and ventricular ectopy may also occur, and the latter may be a marker for patients prone to sudden death.[247]

Morphologic features of cardiac amyloidosis. The heart in amyloidosis is glossy, enlarged, and maintains its shape. The myocardium is rather pale and waxy, but firm in consistency. Dilatation of the atria is often present. Amyloid deposits in the endocardium, particularly in the atria, may appear as pink or gray nodular elevations (Fig. 11-17). Amyloid deposits may also involve the valvular apparatus, imparting a firmness to the leaflets or cusps. Histologically, amyloid fibrils are seen on the myocyte sarcolemma membrane, in the perivascular and interstitial spaces, and within the walls of intramyocardial vessels, producing luminal narrowing (Fig. 11-18). Amyloid deposits are rare in the major epicardial coronary arteries. Amyloid in the heart may be deposited in a linear or nodular fashion (Fig. 11-19). When these deposits are extensive, atrophy or necrosis of myocytes may be detected.

It is of significant interest that although abnormal ECG

and various dysrhythmias are frequent, actual amyloid infiltration of the conduction system is rare. However, damage of the conduction system may be the result of subendocardial amyloid deposits and may account for the electrocardiographic abnormalities noted in these patients.

Cardiac involvement in AA amyloidosis appears to be less extensive and of lesser clinical importance than that associated with AL amyloidosis. Rare cases of nonimmunoglobulin nature, isolated, severe, cardiac amyloidosis with sudden death have been reported. In such cases, amyloid deposition in the conduction system was the cause of first degree heart block.[248]

Light chain deposition disease. Recently, evidence from a number of reported cases has indicated that nonfibrillar deposits of immunoglobulin light chains may be deposited in the heart as a complication of myeloma or other proliferative disorders of plasma cells. Although these nonfibrillatory deposits can induce clinical manifestations of amyloid heart disease, they differ morphologically from fibrillary deposits, and therefore are not evident unless histochemical and ultrastructural studies are carried out.[249] Thus Congo Red stains under polarized light fail to reveal these nonfibrillar amyloid deposits because they are noncongophilic and nonbirefringent. The nonfibrillar amyloid appears as a linear deposit on the surface of myocytes (basement membrane), arteriolar walls, and neural elements. On electron microscopy, the deposits are identified as electron-dense amorphous clumps that measure up to 2000 nm in diameter. Direct immunofluorescent studies of the myocardium reveal the presence of either kappa or lambda light chains. The clinical presentation may be that of restrictive cardiomyopathy[249] or ischemic heart disease caused by amyloid deposits in the small intramyocardial coronary arteries.[250]

These patients are often referred to as having "light chain deposition disease." In this disorder, synthesis of structurally abnormal immunoglobulin chains occurs. Abnormal chain glycosylation, aberrations in chain length, and defects in the "variable" region of the chain (critical for the formation of fibrils) are some of the spectrum of biochemical abnormalities that favor the deposition of amorphous material instead of the accumulation of fibrillar material.[251]

The deposits in light chain deposition disease (LCDD) lack the amyloid P component, a glycoprotein that has been found in all amyloid deposits.[252] Conceptually, an autologous light chain with excessive amino groups that impart a positive charge could bind to anionic sulphated proteoglycans that are present in basement membranes.[253]

It remains unclear why only some patients with gammopathy develop LCDD.

Senile cardiac amyloidosis. Three distinct forms of senile cardiac amyloidosis are recognized with the use of immunohistochemical techniques: (1) isolated atrial amyloidosis, which is characterized by focal deposits only in

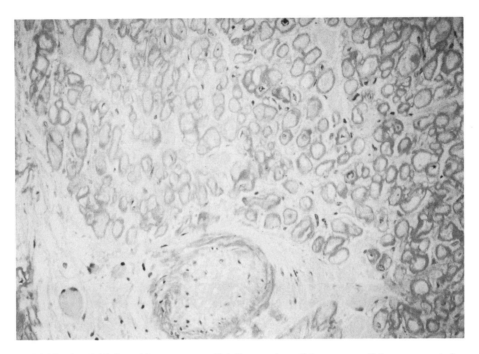

Fig. 11-18. Amyloid deposition on myocardial fibers and small intramyocardial coronary arteries. Note the atrophic changes (reduced size) in many myocardial cells.

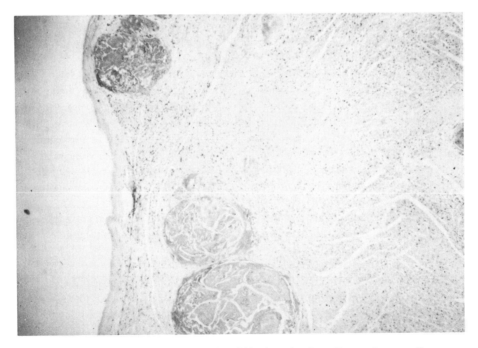

Fig. 11-19. Nodular amyloid deposits within the subendocardium and myocardium.

the atria; (2) senile aortic amyloidosis, which commonly affects the aortas of elderly individuals; and (3) senile systemic amyloidosis, in which, in addition to the heart, the lungs, liver, and kidneys are also involved.[254] The primary structure of the amyloid protein in senile systemic amyloidosis has been partly characterized and appears similar to human prealbumin.[255] Senile systemic amyloidosis produces diffuse amyloid infiltration of the heart, and therefore is an important, although uncommon, cause of cardiovascular morbidity. However, patients with senile systemic amyloidosis with cardiac involvement appear to have a better prognosis than patients with immunoglobulin-derived amyloidosis with comparable degree of cardiac involvement (echocardiography).

Heart transplantation for severe cardiac amyloidosis. In recent years, patients with severe heart disease secondary to amyloidosis have been accepted in many programs as heart recipients. Reports have begun to appear indicating recurrence of cardiac amyloidosis in the donor heart. In one recent report, endomyocardial biopsy obtained 4 months posttransplantation showed amyloid infiltration on electron microscopy, although the deposits were not detected by light microscopy.[256] The early recurrence and progression of cardiac infiltration by amyloid, as demonstrated in the above case, may suggest that heart transplantation in patients with severe compromise of cardiac function secondary to amyloidosis may only offer short-term palliation at best.

Cardiac sarcoidosis

Sarcoidosis is a granulomatous disorder of unknown cause characterized by bilateral hilar adenopathy, interstitial pulmonary infiltrates, and varying involvement of systemic organs. Clinical recognition of cardiac involvement by sarcoid is uncommon, although autopsy studies of consecutive autopsies in patients with sarcoidosis have shown up to 27% of the cases to have myocardial sarcoid.[257]

Approximately one third of patients with myocardial lesions confirmed at autopsy did not reveal evidence of cardiac sarcoidosis during life. However, cardiac abnormalities, detectable when patients were stressed by exercise, manifested as chronotropic and/or inotropic changes.[258]

In a series of 300 cases of cardiac sarcoid, supraventricular arrhythmias were present in 75%, complete heart block was demonstrated in 26%, and cardiomyopathy was confirmed in 24%. Only a small minority of patients (15%) exhibited chest pain simulating myocardial infarction. Of 138 fatal cases in this series, 77 patients died suddenly.[259] Ventricular tachycardia and VF may also be manifestations of cardiac sarcoidosis.

Echocardiography and radionuclide angiography in patients with cardiac sarcoidosis have disclosed left ventricular dysfunction and a pattern of fibrosis quite dissimilar from that encountered in coronary artery disease. Cardiac sarcoidosis patients reveal abnormal regional wall motion in the basal portion of the ventricular septum and free wall with sparing of the apex. This pattern is distinctly different from that seen in ischemic heart disease, in which the wall motion abnormality is primarily localized at the apical region.[260]

Progressive congestive heart failure may be the cause of death in one fourth of patients with cardiac sarcoidosis. In general terms, cardiac sarcoidosis should be suspected in a patient with acute onset cardiac symptomatology, or rapidly progressive or unexplained congestive heart failure.[261] Rarely, patients may present with mitral stenosis caused by leaflet granulomas or mitral regurgitation resulting from granulomatous infiltration of the papillary muscles.[260]

Morphologic manifestations in cardiac sarcoidosis. Cardiac sarcoidosis can be detected by endomyocardial biopsy, although granulomas are often deeply seated, and therefore inaccessible to the bioptome. Sarcoid granulomas tend to involve the basal half of the heart more than the apical region, which is usually favored in cardiac biopsies.[262]

The heart in cardiac sarcoidosis appears enlarged because of dilatation of both ventricles and atria. Rarely, a left ventricular aneurysm may be present adjacent to the mitral annulus.[263] Nonnecrotizing granulomas may be found throughout the ventricular myocardium and the atria, but pericardial involvement is less common. Granulomas consist of nodular aggregates of epithelioid histiocytes, multinucleated giant cells often containing "asteroid" bodies, and a scanty admixture of lymphocytes. Central necrosis is conspicuously absent. However, the acute phase of myocardial sarcoidosis may resolve to a diffuse interstitial fibrosis with no recognizable granulomas and only occasional giant cells. At this stage, its distinction from a dilated cardiomyopathy may be difficult.

Some controversy exists regarding the terms *giant cell myocarditis* and *granulomatous (sarcoid) myocarditis*. We believe that the two entities are different, with the former being either infectious or idiopathic.

Pathogenesis of sarcoidosis. The pathogenesis of sarcoidosis remains unknown. Currently, the sarcoid granuloma is felt to represent an immunologic phenomenon in which T-lymphocytes interact with macrophages in the presence of an unknown antigenic stimulus, leading to mutual activation and proliferation.[264]

Gout

The major cardiovascular clinical manifestations in patients with gout are arrhythmias and conduction abnormalities. Patients may reveal urate deposits in the myocardial interstitium, aortic and mitral valves, conduction system, vascular walls, and pericardium.[265] Depending on their location and size, these urate deposits may induce structural dysfunction of the heart and blood vessels. Although the association between gout and atherosclerosis has been suspected for more than a century, some studies of large populations have reported contradictory results of such a relationship.[266] Data from the Framingham study indicated that men with gout experienced a 60% excess of coronary heart disease compared with those without gout (95% confidence limits). There was no significant association between gout and coronary heart disease in women. The association between gout and coronary heart disease in men remained significant after control of age, systolic blood pressure, total cholesterol, alcohol intake, body mass index, and diabetes.[267] Furthermore, this study showed that men with gout experienced angina pectoris twice as often than those without gout. However, hyperuricemia may be a secondary finding without any independent pathogenic significance.

Although it has not been conclusively demonstrated that uric acid per se can cause vascular damage, in vitro studies suggest the possibility that urate crystals may have a role in atherogenesis. For example, incubation of monosodium urate crystals with platelets results in rapid release of serotonin, adenosine triphosphate, and adenosine diphosphate. The latter is a potent stimulator of platelet aggregation, which results in endothelial cell damage and possibly atherosclerosis.[268] It is possible, however, that gouty patients have a greater risk for coronary atherosclerosis chiefly because they often have other risk factors such as hypertension, hyperlipidemia, and obesity.

The data above indicate that it is difficult to draw conclusions about the independent relationship between gout and coronary heart disease from epidemiologic studies alone. However, gout is still considered a marker for susceptibility to coronary artery disease.

IMMUNE DEFICIENCY DISEASES
Human immunodeficiency virus infection

Morbidity and mortality associated with HIV disease in the United States is primarily caused by the pulmonary, lymphoreticular, central nervous, and alimentary systems. Cardiac morbidity and mortality, which has remained constant since the epidemic began, is estimated to be 6% to 7% and 1% to 6%, respectively.[269] However, the clinical and pathologic cardiovascular findings of AIDS are still being elucidated.

Cardiac manifestations. Overall, pathologic changes are seen in the myocardium, pericardium, endocardium, and vasculature in a descending rate of frequency. Recognized clinical syndromes in patients with HIV infection include pericardial effusion or hemorrhage with or without cardiac tamponade, myocardial disease as evidenced by dilated cardiomyopathy, ventricular tachycardia, sudden death, cardiac failure, and infectious or noninfectious thrombotic endocarditis with or without thromboembolic phenomena.

Pericardial involvement in AIDS. Pericardial effusion is usually seen in about one third of AIDS patients with cardiovascular involvement. Infection or neoplasia (Kaposi sarcoma) causes the effusion. Nonspecific pericardial effusion unassociated with either infection or neoplasia is thought to be multifactorial. Chronic pulmonary disease with right ventricular dilatation has been reported to correlate positively with nonspecific pericardial effusion.[270] A variety of infectious agents have been identified in pericardial fluid, although in asymptomatic effusions pericardial fluid cultures are often unrevealing. Statistics from echocardiographic studies indicate that pericardial effusion occurs in 30% of infected children and in 23% of adults, with tamponade developing in 8%.[271]

Myocardial involvement in AIDS. Fatal dilated cardiomyopathy has been clinically observed in patients with AIDS. Left ventricular dilatation with diffuse wall motion abnormalities (with or without mitral regurgitation) have been detected in these patients.

The gross and microscopic findings are similar to dilated cardiomyopathy in non-AIDS patients, although evidence of myocarditis is present in almost half of the cases[270] with AIDS. The myocarditis may play an etiologic role in the development of dilated cardiomyopathy, although nutritional deficiencies and wasting may also contribute to the cardiac dilatation.

The usual histologic finding in AIDS-associated myocarditis is that of nonspecific inflammatory infiltrates without myocyte necrosis (Fig. 11-20). Lack of myocyte damage may reflect long-term stress, cytomegalovirus infection, or an autoimmune process (Fig. 11-21). Viral etiology is likely, although biologic evidence for an opportunistic viral agent has not been described. The possibility of HIV inflicting myocyte damage either by direct cytolytic effect or via the mechanism of "innocent bystander destruction" has been raised.[270] According to this hypothesis, the myocyte injury is inflicted by the toxic enzymes released by replicating HIV in the interstitial lymphocytes and macrophages. Although recent reports have confirmed the presence of HIV in cardiac tissue, a cause-effect relationship has not been established.[271] Endomyocardial biopsies from HIV-positive patients with and without cardiovascular symptoms, prepared by individual cell microdissection, have shown that myocytes are often infected by HIV in both groups of patients, although a direct lethal effect of the HIV on the myocytes is unlikely.[272] Dendritic cells also harbor HIV.

Dilated cardiomyopathy in children with AIDS. Fatal cases of dilated cardiomyopathy have been reported also in children with AIDS.[273] Their clinical features consisted of signs and symptoms of cardiovascular compromise or congestive heart failure with cardiomegaly. The microscopic findings in the myocardium (myocyte hypertrophy, fatty change, focal interstitial fibrosis, and endocardial thickening) did not provide definitive clues to the pathogenesis of dilated cardiomyopathy in those children, except perhaps the sparse lymphocytic inflammatory infiltrates with or without myocyte necrosis. Bacteria, fungi,

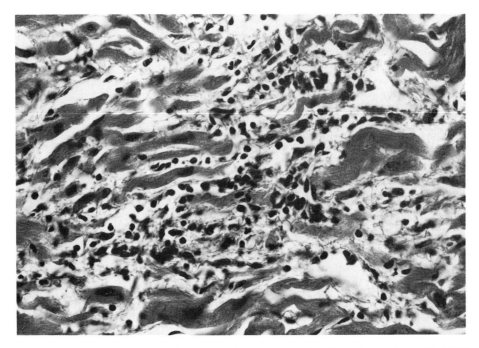

Fig. 11-20. Focal myocyte necrosis surrounded by a round cell infiltrate in a patient with AIDS.

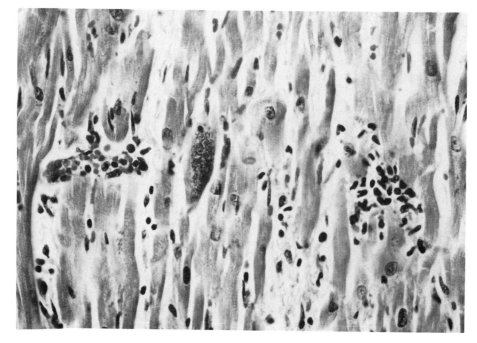

Fig. 11-21. Intracytoplasmic (myocyte) *Toxoplasma* cysts in a patient with AIDS. Note the complete absence of inflammatory reaction in the immediate vicinity of the infected myocyte.

or acid-fast bacilli were demonstrated in none of the cases.

Congestive heart failure in AIDS patients. Cardiac failure in AIDS patients may occur in nondilated hearts and in the absence of septic shock, apparently indicating severe myocardial dysfunction. Extensive neoplastic infiltration by either Kaposi sarcoma or malignant lymphoma may produce a low cardiac output syndrome or a restrictive cardiomyopathy.[274]

Refractory ventricular tachycardia and ventricular fibrillation have been recorded in patients with AIDS. An etiologic association between myocarditis and dysrhythmias has been suggested.[275]

Nonbacterial thrombotic endocarditis, which can involve all valves (most commonly the left-sided ones), is usually asymptomatic in most patients with HIV disease.[269] It is rarely the cause of death in these patients, although systemic or pulmonary embolization may occur. However, infectious endocarditis has not been found to be more frequent in patients with AIDS.

Cardiac neoplasms in AIDS patients. Kaposi sarcoma in AIDS patients has been reported in the visceral and parietal pericardium and less often within the myocardium.[276] Extension of the neoplastic growth to the adventitia of the coronary arteries and the great vessels has been observed. Rare cases of malignant lymphoma involving the hearts of AIDS patients have also been recorded. In one of our patients, the heart appeared to be the primary site of the malignant lymphoma.

REFERENCES

1. Tan EM, Cohen HS, Fries JF, et al: The 1982 revised criteria for the classification of SLE, *Arthritis Rheum* 75:1271, 1982.
2. Chang RW: Cardiac manifestations of SLE, *Clin Rheum Dis* 8:197, 1982.
3. Wallace DJ, Dubois EL, eds: *Lupus erythematosus,* ed 3, Philadelphia, 1987, Lea & Febiger.
4. Ansari A, Larson PH, Bates HD: Cardiovascular manifestations of systemic lupus erythematosus: current perspective, *Prog Cardiovasc Dis* 27:421, 1985.
5. Kelly TA: Cardiac tamponade in systemic lupus erythematosus: an unusual initial manifestation, *South Med J* 80:514, 1987.
6. Browning CA, Bishop RL, Heilpern RJ, et al: Accelerated constrictive pericarditis in procainamide-induced systemic lupus erythematosus, *Am J Cardiol* 53:376, 1984.
7. Bulkley BH, Roberts WC: The heart in systemic lupus erythematosus and the changes induced in it by corticosteroid therapy: a study of 36 necropsy patients, *Am J Med* 58:243, 1975.
8. Mandell BF: Cardiovascular involvement in systemic lupus erythematosus, *Semin Arthritis Rheum* 17:126, 1987.
9. James TN, Rupe CE, Monto RW: Pathology of the cardiac conduction system in systemic lupus erythematosus, *Ann Intern Med* 63:402, 1985.
10. Moffitt GR: Complete atrioventricular dissociation with Stokes-Adams attacks due to disseminated lupus erythematosus, *Ann Intern Med* 63:402, 1985.
11. Litsey SE, Noonan JA, O'Connor WN, et al: Maternal connective tissue disease and congenital heart block: demonstration of immunoglobulin in cardiac tissue, *N Engl J Med* 312:98, 1985.
12. Singson BH, Akhter JE, Weinstein MM, et al: Congenital complete

13. Deng J, Bair LW, Shen-Schwarz S, et al: Localization of Ro (SS-A) antigen in the cardiac conduction system, *Arthritis Rheum* 30:1232, 1987.
14. Bidani AK, Roberts JL, Schwartz MM, et al: Immunopathology of cardiac lesions in total systemic lupus erythematosus, *Am J Med* 69:849, 1980.
15. Fukumoto S, Tsumagari T, Kinso M, et al: Coronary atherosclerosis in patients with systemic lupus erythematosus at autopsy, *Acta Pathol Jpn* 37:1, 1987.
16. Elias M, Eldor A: Thromboembolism in patients with the "lupus"-type circulating anticoagulant, *Arch Intern Med* 144:510, 1984.
17. Asherson RA, Gibson DG, Evans DW, et al: Diagnostic and therapeutic problems in two patients with antiphospholipid antibodies, heart valve lesions and transient ischemic attacks, *Ann Rheum Dis* 47:947, 1988.
18. Galve E, Candell-Riera J, Pigrau C, et al: Prevalence, morphologic types, and evolution of cardiac valvular disease in systemic lupus erythematosus, *N Engl J Med* 319:817, 1988.
19. Kinkhoff AV, Thompson CR, Reid GD, et al: M-mode and two-dimensional echocardiographic abnormalities in systemic lupus erythematosus, *JAMA* 253:3273, 1985.
20. Senignen RP, Borer JS, Redwood DR, et al: Libman-Sacks endocardoma: diagnosis during life, *Radiology* 113:597, 1974.
21. Straaton KV, Chatham WW, Reveille JD, et al: Clinically significant valvular heart disease in systemic lupus erythematosus, *Am J Med* 85:645, 1988.
22. Ford SE, Lillicrap D, Brunet D, et al: Thrombotic endocarditis and lupus anticoagulant, *Arch Pathol Lab Med* 113:350, 1989.
23. Chartash EK, Lans DM, Paget SA, et al: Aortic insufficiency and mitral regurgitation in patients with systemic lupus erythematosus and the antiphospholipid syndrome, *Am J Med* 86:407, 1989.
24. Asherson RA, Oakley CM: Pulmonary hypertension and systemic lupus erythematosus, *J Rheumatol* 13:1, 1986.
25. Quismorio FP, Sharma O, Koss M, et al: Immunopathologic and clinical studies in pulmonary hypertension associated with systemic lupus erythematosus, *Semin Arthritis Rheum* 13:349, 1984.
26. Alpert MA, Goldberg SH, Singsen BH: Cardiovascular manifestations of mixed connective tissue disease in adults, *Circulation* 68:1182, 1983.
27. Tan EM, Chan EKL, Sullivan KF, et al: Antinuclear antibodies (ANAs) diagnostically specific immune markers and clues towards understanding systemic autoimmunity, *Clin Immunol Immunopathol* 47:121, 1988.
28. Miller MH, Littlejohn GO, Davidson A, et al: The clinical significance of the anticentromere antibody, *Br J Rheumatol* 26:71, 1987.
29. McGregor AR, Watson A, Yunis E, et al: Familial clustering of scleroderma spectrum disease, *Am J Med* 84:1023, 1988.
30. Botstein GR, Leroy EC: Primary heart disease in systemic sclerosis (scleroderma): advances in clinical and pathological features, pathogenesis and new therapeutic approaches, *Am Heart J* 102:913, 1981.
31. Goldman AP, Kotler MN: Heart disease in scleroderma, *Am Heart J* 110:1043, 1985.
32. Bulkley BH, Ridolfi RL, Salyer WR, et al: Myocardial lesions of progressive systemic sclerosis: a cause of cardiac dysfunction, *Circulation* 53:483, 1976.
33. Reimer KA, Murry CE, Jennings RB: Cardiac adaptation to ischemia: ischemic preconditioning increases myocardial tolerance to subsequent ischemic episodes, *Circulation* 82:2266, 1990.
34. Kahan A, Nitenberg A, Foult JM, et al: Decreased coronary reserve in primary scleroderma myocardial disease, *Arthritis Rheum* 28:637, 1985.
35. Follansbee WP, Curtiss EI, Medsger TA, et al: Physiologic abnormalities of cardiac function in progressive systemic sclerosis with diffuse scleroderma, *N Engl J Med* 310:142, 1984.

heart block and SSA antibodies: obstetrical implications, *Am J Obstet Gynecol* 152:655, 1985.

36. Alexander EL, Firestein GS, Weiss JL, et al: Reversible cold-induced abnormalities in myocardial perfusion and function in systemic sclerosis, *Ann Intern Med* 105:661, 1986.

37. Goldman AP, Kotler MN: Heart disease in scleroderma, *Am Heart J* 110:1043, 1985.

38. Comens SM, Alpert MA, Sharp GC, et al: Frequency of mitral valve prolapse in systemic lupus erythematosus, progressive systemic sclerosis, and mixed connective tissue disease, *Am J Cardiol* 63:369, 1989.

39. Ferri C, Bermini L, Bongiorni MG, et al: Noninvasive evaluation of cardiac dysrhythmias and their relationship with multisystemic symptoms in PSS patients, *Arthritis Rheum* 28:1259, 1985.

40. Janosik HL, Osborn TG, Moore TL, et al: Heart disease in systemic sclerosis, *Semin Arthritis Rheum* 19:191, 1989.

41. Davies MJ: *Disorders of the conduction system.* In Ansell BM, Simkin PA, eds: *The heart and rheumatic disease,* London, 1984, Butterworths.

42. Ridolfi RL, Bulkley BH, Hutchins GM: The cardiac conduction system in progressive systemic sclerosis, *Am J Med* 61:361, 1976.

43. Stastny P: Association of the B cell alloantigen HLA-DRW4 with rheumatoid arthritis, *N Engl J Med* 298:869, 1978.

44. McDermott M, Molloy M, Cahin P, et al: A multicase family study of rheumatoid arthritis in SW Ireland, *Dis Markers* 4:103, 1986.

45. Sigal LH and Friedman HD: Rheumatoid pericarditis in a patient with well controlled rheumatoid arthritis, *J Rheumatol* 16:368, 1989.

46. Mody GM, Stephens JE, Meyers OL: The heart in rheumatoid arthritis—a clinical and echocardiography study, *Q J Med* 65:921, 1987.

47. Thould AIC: Constrictive pericarditis in rheumatoid arthritis, *Ann Rheum Dis* 45:89, 1986.

48. Siegel LH, Johnson JL, Phillips PE: Peripheral blood mononuclear cell responses to cartilage components in rheumatoid arthritis and osteoarthritis, *Clin Exp Rheumatol* 6:59, 1988.

49. Villecco AS, DeLiberali E, Bianchi FB, et al: Antibodies to cardiac conducting tissue and abnormalities of cardiac conduction in rheumatoid arthritis, *Clin Exp Immunol* 53:536, 1983.

50. Krane SM, Simon LS: Rheumatoid arthritis: clinical features and pathogenetic mechanisms, *Med Clin North Am* 70:263, 1986.

51. Slack JD, Waller B: Acute congestive heart failure due to the arteritis of rheumatoid arthritis: early diagnosis of endocardial biopsy, a case report, *Angiology* 37(6):477, 1986.

52. Gravallese EM, Corson JM, Coblyn JS, et al: Rheumatoid arthritis: a rarely recognized, but clinically significant entity, *Medicine* 68:95, 1989.

53. Askari AD: The heart in polymyositis and dermatomyositis, *Mt Sinai J Med* 55:479, 1988.

54. Tamir R, Pick AJ, Theodor E: Constrictive pericarditis complicating dermatomyositis, *Ann Rheum Dis* 47:961, 1988.

55. Strongwater SL, Annesley T, Schnitzer TJ: Myocardial involvement in polymyositis, *J Rheumatol* 10:459, 1983.

56. Behan WMH, Behan PD, Gairns J: Cardiac damage in polymyositis associated antibodies to tissue ribonucleoproteins, *Br Heart J* 57:176, 1987.

57. Dalakas MC: Polymyositis, dermatomyositis, and inclusion-body myositis, *N Engl J Med* 21:1487, 1991.

58. Kissel JT, Halterman RK, Rammohan KW, et al: The relationship of complement-mediated microvasculopathy to the histologic features and clinical duration of disease in dermatomyositis, *Arch Neurol* 48:26, 1991.

59. Condemi JJ: The autoimmune diseases, *JAMA* 258:2920, 1987.

60. Arahata K, Engel AG: Monoclonal antibody analysis of mononuclear cells in myopathies: III immunoelectron microscopic aspects of cell-mediated muscle fiber injury, *Ann Neurol* 19:112, 1986.

61. Karpati G, Pouliot Y, Carpenter S: Expression of immunoreactive major histocompatability complex products in human skeletal muscle, *Ann Neurol* 23:64, 1988.

62. Isenberg DA, Rowe DJ, Shearer M, et al: Localization of IFN and interleukin-2 in polymyositis and muscular dystrophy, *Clin Exp Immunol* 63:450, 1986.

63. Emslie-Smith AM, Arahata K, Engel AG: Major histocompatibility complex class I antigen expression, immunolocalization of interferon subtypes, and T-cell mediated cytotoxicity in myopathies, *Hum Pathol* 20:224, 1989.

64. Brenner MB, Strominger JL, Krangel MS: The gamma delta T-cell receptor, *Adv Immunol* 43:133, 1988.

65. Born W, Happ MP, Dallas A, et al: Recognition of heat-shock proteins and γ/δ cell function, *Immunol Today* 11:40, 1990.

66. Hohlfeld R, Engel AG, Ii K, et al: Polymyositis mediated by T lymphocytes that express the γ/δ receptor, *N Engl J Med* 324:877, 1991.

67. Fauci AS, Wolff SM: Wegener's granulomatosis and related diseases, *Dis Mon* 23:(7)1, 1977.

68. Boudes P, Andre C, Belghiti D, et al: Microscopic Wegener's disease: a particular form of Wegener's granulomatosis, *J Rheumatol* 17:1412, 1990.

69. Parrillo JE, Fauci AS: Necrotizing vasculitis, coronary arteritis and the cardiologist, *Am Heart J* 99:547, 1980.

70. Van der Woude FJ, Rasmusen N, Lobatto S, et al: Autoantibodies against neutrophils and monocytes: tool for diagnosis and marker of disease activity in Wegener's granulomatosis, *Lancet* 1:425, 1985.

71. Ewert BH, Jennette JC, Falk RJ: The pathogenic role of antineutrophil cytoplasmic autoantibodies, *Am J Kidney Dis* 18:188, 1991.

72. Feldman M: Whipple's disease, *Am J Med Sci* 291:56, 1986.

73. Sossai P, DeBoni M, Cielo R: The heart and Whipple's disease, *Int J Cardiol* 23:275, 1989.

74. Southern JF, Moscicki RA, Margo C, et al: Lymphedema, lymphocytic myocarditis, and sarcoid-like granulomatosis, *JAMA* 261:1467, 1989.

75. Pelech T, Fric P, Huslarova A, et al: Interstitial lymphocytic myocarditis in Whipple's disease, *Lancet* 237:553, 1991.

76. Ho K, Crowell WT, Herrera GA: Whipple's disease: pathogenetic considerations, *South Med J* 76:284, 1983.

77. Weiner SR, Utsinger P: Whipple's disease, *Semin Arthritis Rheum* 15:157, 1986.

78. Dobbins WO: HLA antigens in Whipple's disease, *Arthritis Rheum* 30:102, 1987.

79. Remuzzi G: HUS and TTP: variable expression of a single entity, *Kidney Int* 32:292, 1987.

80. Kwaan HC: Miscellaneous secondary thrombotic microangiopathy, *Semin Hematol* 24:141, 1987.

81. Bell W: Thrombotic thrombocytopenic purpura, *JAMA* 265:91, 1991.

82. Lian EC-Y: Thrombotic thrombocytopenic purpura, *Annu Rev Med* 39:203, 1988.

83. Van der Linden S, Valkenburg H, Cats A: The risk of developing ankylosing spondylitis in HLA-B27 positive individuals: a family and population study, *Br J Rheumatol* 22 (suppl 2):18, 1983.

84. Archer JR, Winrow VR: HLA-B27 and the course of arthritis: does molecular biology help? *Ann Rheum Dis* 46:713, 1987.

85. Alves MG, Espirito-Santo J, Queirez MV, et al: Cardiac alterations in ankylosing spondylitis, *Angiology* 39 (7 pt 1):567, 1988.

86. Sukenik S, Pras A, Buskila D, et al: Cardiovascular manifestations of ankylosing spondylitis, *Clin Rheumatol* 6:588, 1987.

87. Hull RG, Asherson RA, Rennie JAN: Ankylosing spondylitis and aortic arch syndrome, *Br Heart J* 51:663, 1984.

88. Roberts WC, Hollingsworth JF, Bulkley BH, et al: Combined mitral and aortic regurgitation in ankylosing spondylitis: angiographic and anatomic features, *Am J Med* 56:237, 1974.

89. Brewerton DA, Gibson DG, Goddard DH, et al: The myocardium in ankylosing spondylitis: a clinical, echocardiographic and histopathological study, *Lancet* 1:995, 1987.

90. Nagyhegyi G, Nades I, Banyai F, et al: Cardiac and cardiopulmo-

nary disorders in patients with ankylosing spondylitis and rheumatoid arthritis, *Clin Exp Rheumatol* 6:17, 1988.

91. Pyeritz RE, McKusick VA: The Marfan syndrome: diagnosis and management, *N Engl J Med* 300:722, 1979.

92. Beighton P, Paepe A de, Danks A, et al: International nosology of heritable disorders of connective tissue, Berlin 1986, *Am J Med Genet* 29:581, 1988.

93. Pyeritz R: The Marfan syndrome, *Am Fam Physician* 34:83, 1986.

94. Geva T, Hegesh J, Frand M: The clinical course and echocardiographic features of Marfan's syndrome in childhood, *Am J Dis Child* 141:1179, 1987.

95. Vetter V, Mayerhofer R, Land D, et al: The Marfan syndrome—analysis of growth and cardiovascular manifestation, *Eur J Pediatr* 149:452, 1990.

96. Gilbert EF: The effects of metabolic diseases on the cardiovascular system, *Am J Cardiovasc Pathol* 1:189, 1987.

97. Roman MJ, Devereux RB, Kramer-Fox R, et al: Comparison of cardiovascular and skeletal features of primary mitral valve prolapse and Marfan syndrome, *Am J Cardiol* 63:317, 1989.

98. Erbel R, Daniel W, Visser C, et al: Echocardiography in diagnostic aortic dissection, *Lancet* 1:457, 1989.

99. Hirata K, Triposkiadis F, Sparks E, et al: The Marfan syndrome: abnormal aortic elastic properties, *J Am Coll Cardiol* 18:57, 1991.

100. Marsalese DL, Moodie DS, Vacante M, et al: Marfan's syndrome: natural history and long term follow-up of cardiovascular involvement, *J Am Coll Cardiol* 14:422, 1989.

101. Ferrans VJ, Boyce SW: *Metabolic and familiar diseases.* In Silver MD, ed: *Cardiovascular pathology,* New York, 1983, Churchill Livingstone.

102. Boucek RJ, Noble NL, Gunja-Smith Z, et al: The Marfan syndrome: a deficiency in chemically stable collagen cross-links, *N Engl J Med* 305:988, 1981.

103. Dalgleish R, Hawkins JR, Keston M: Exclusion of the alpha 2 (I) and alpha 1 (III) collagen genes as the mutant loci in a Marfan syndrome family, *J Med Genet* 24:148, 1987.

104. Abraham PA, Perejda AJ, Carnes WH, et al: Marfan syndrome: demonstration of abnormal elastin in aorta, *J Clin Invest* 70:1245, 1982.

105. Perejda AJ, Abraham PA, Carnes WH, et al: Marfan's syndrome: structural, biochemical, and mechanical studies of the aortic media, *J Lab Clin Med* 106:376, 1985.

106. Kainulainen K, Pulkkinen L, Savolainen A, et al: Location on chromosome 15 of the gene defect causing Marfan syndrome, *N Engl J Med* 323:935, 1990.

107. Pignatelli M, Bodmer WF: Genetics and biochemistry of collagen binding-triggered glandular differentiation in a human colon carcinoma cell line, *Proc Natl Acad Sci USA* 85:5561, 1988.

108. Retting WJ, Real FX, Spengler BA, et al: Human melanoma proteoglycan: expression in hybrids controlled by intrinsic and extrinsic signals, *Science* 231:1281, 1986.

109. Gunning P, Ponte P, Kedes L, et al: Chromosomal location of the co-expressed human skeletal and cardiac actin genes, *Proc Natl Acad Sci USA* 81:1813, 1988.

110. Hollister DW, Godfrey M, Sakai LY, et al: Immunohistologic abnormalities of the microfibrillar-fiber system in the Marfan syndrome, *N Engl J Med* 323:151, 1990.

111. Maslen CL, Corson GM, Maddox BK, et al: Partial sequence of a candidate gene for the Marfan syndrome, *Nature* 352:334, 1991.

112. Dietz HC, Cutting GR, Pyeritz RE, et al: Marfan syndrome caused by a recurrent de novo missense mutation in the fibrillin gene, *Nature* 352:337, 1991.

113. Lee B, Godfrey M, Vitale E, et al: Linkage of Marfan syndrome and a phenotypically related disorder to two different fibrillin genes, *Nature* 352:330, 1991.

114. McKusick VA: The defect in Marfan syndrome, *Nature* 352:279, 1991.

115. Sillence DO: *Osteogenesis imperfecta: clinical variability and classification.* In Akeson WH, Bornstein P, Glimcher MJ, eds: *Symposium on heritable diseases of connective tissue, San Diego, CA, May 1980,* St Louis, 1982, CV Mosby.

116. Kuivaniemi H, Tromp G, Prockop DJ: Mutations in collagen genes: causes of rare and some common diseases in humans, *FASEB J* 5:2052, 1991.

117. Rogerson ME, Buchanan JD, Morgan CM: Left atrial rupture in osteogenesis imperfecta, *Br Heart J* 56:187, 1986.

118. Hortop J, Tsipouras P, Hanley JA, et al: Cardiovascular involvement in osteogenesis imperfecta, *Circulation* 73:54, 1986.

119. McKusick VA: *Mendelian inheritance in man, catalogs of autosomal dominant, autosomal recessive, and X-linked phenotypes,* ed 6, Baltimore, 1983, The Johns Hopkins University Press.

120. Viljoen D: Pseudoanthoma elasticum (Gronbland-Strandberg syndrome), *J Med Genet* 25:488, 1988.

121. Viljoen DL, Pope FM, Breighton P: Heterogeneity in pseudoxanthoma elasticum: delineation of a new form? *Clin Genet* 32:100, 1987.

122. Strobe WE, Margolis RJ: Gastrointestinal bleeding with ocular and cutaneous abnormalities, case records of the Massachusetts General Hospital: weekly clinicopathologic exercises, case #10 1983, *N Engl J Med* 308:579, 1983.

123. Mendelsohn J, Bulkley B, Hutchins G: Cardiovascular manifestations of pseudoxanthoma elasticum, *Arch Pathol Lab Med* 102:298, 1978.

124. Lebwhol MG, Distefano D: Pseudoxanthoma elasticum and mitral valve prolapse, *N Engl J Med* 307:228, 1982.

125. McKusick VA: *Heritable disorders of connective tissue.* ed 4, St Louis, 1973, CV Mosby.

126. Clarkson JG, Altman RD: Angioid streaks, *Surv Ophthalmol* 26:235, 1982.

127. Brown FR III, Holbrook KA, Byers PH, et al: Cutis laxa, *Johns Hopkins Med J* 150:148, 1982.

128. Beighton P: The dominant and recessive forms of cutis laxa, *J Med Genet* 9:216, 1972.

129. Byers P, Narayanan A, Bornstein P, et al: An X-linked form of cutis laxa due to deficiency of lysyl oxidase, *Birth Defects* 12:293, 1976.

130. Muster AJ, Bharati S, Herman JJ, et al: Fatal cardiovascular disease and cutis laxa following acute febrile neutrophilic dermatosis, *J Pediatr* 102:243, 1983.

131. Goodman R, Baba N, Wooley C: Observations on the heart in a case of combined Echlers-Danlos and Marfan syndromes, *Am J Cardiol* 24:734, 1969.

132. Bowen J, Boudoulas H, Wooley CF: Cardiovascular disease of connective tissue origin, *Am J Med* 82:481, 1987.

133. Leier C, Baker P, Kilman J, et al: Cardiovascular abnormalities associated with adult polycystic kidney disease, *Ann Intern Med,* 100:683, 1984.

134. DeSanctis RW, Doroghazi RM, Austen WG: Aortic dissection, *N Engl J Med* 317:1060, 1987.

135. Marsalese DL, Moodie DS, Lytle BW, et al: Cystic medial necrosis of the aorta in patients without Marfan's syndrome: surgical outcome and long-term follow-up, *J Am Coll Cardiol* 16:68, 1990.

136. Schlatmann TJ, Becker AE: Pathogenesis of dissecting aneurysm of aorta: comparative histopathologic study of significance of medial changes, *Am J Cardiol* 39:21, 1977.

137. Oppenheimer JH, Schwartz HL, Mariash CN, et al: Advances in our understanding of thyroid hormone at the cellular level, *Endocr Rev* 8:288, 1987.

138. Klein I: Thyroid hormone and the cardiovascular system, *Am J Med* 88:631, 1990.

139. Marks AD, Chonnick BJ, Allen EV, et al: Chronic thyroiditis and mitral valve prolapse, *Ann Intern Med* 102:479, 1985.

140. Forfar JC, Muir AL, Sawers SA, et al: Abnormal left ventricular

function in hyperthyroidism: evidence for a possible reversible cardiomyopathy, *N Engl J Med* 307:1120, 1982.

141. Coulombe P, Dussault JH, Letarte J, et al: Catecholamine metabolism in thyroid disease. I. Epinephrine secretion rate in hyperthyroidism and hypothyroidism, *J Clin Endocrinol Metab* 42:125, 1976.

142. Limas C, Limas CJ: Influence of thyroid status on intracellular distribution of cardiac adrenoceptors, *Circ Res* 61:824, 1987.

143. Feldman T, Borow KM, Sarne DH, et al: Myocardial mechanics in hyperthyroidism: importance of left ventricular loading conditions, heart rate and contractile state, *J Am Coll Cardiol* 7:967, 1986.

144. Gunning JF, Harrison CE, Coleman NH: Myocardial contractility and energetics following treatment with d-thyroxine, *Am J Physiol* 226:1166, 1979.

145. Klein I: *Thyroid hormone and high blood pressure.* In Laragh JH, Brenner BM, Kaplan NM, eds: *Endocrine mechanisms in hypertension,* vol 2, New York, 1985, Raven Press.

146. Ikram H: The nature and prognosis of thyrotoxic heart disease, *Q J Med* 54:19, 1985.

147. Schwartz K, Lecarpenter Y, Martin JL, et al: Myosin isoenzyme distribution correlates with speed of myocardial contraction, *J Mol Cell Cardiol* 13:1071, 1981.

148. Campbell SE, Gerdes AM: Regional changes in myocyte-size during the reversal of thyroid induced cardiac hypertrophy, *J Mol Cell Cardiol* 20:379, 1988.

149. Gross G, Lues I: Thyroid-dependent alterations of myocardial adrenoceptors and adrenoceptor-mediated responses in the rat, *Arch Pharm* 329:427, 1985.

150. Limas C, Limas CJ: Disparate effects of colchicine on thyroxine-induced cardiac hypertrophy and adrenoceptor changes, *Circ Res* 68:309, 1991.

151. Weiel JE, Hamilton TA: Quiescent lymphocytes express intracellular transferrin receptors, *Biochem Biophys Res Commun* 119:598, 1984.

152. Rutherford JP, Vatner SF, Braunwald E: Adrenergic control of myocardial contractility in conscious hypertrophied dogs. *Am J Physiol* 237:590, 1980.

153. Oppenheimer JH: *The nuclear receptor-triodothyronine complex: relationship to thyroid hormone distribution, metabolism and biological action.* In Oppenheimer JH, Samuels HH, eds: *Molecular basis of thyroid hormone action,* New York, 1983, Academic Press.

154. Latham KR, Ring JC, Baxter JD: Solubilized nuclear receptors for thyroid hormones, *J Biol Chem* 251:7388, 1976.

155. Oppenheimer JH, Schwartz HL, Mariash CN, et al: Advances in our understanding of thyroid hormone action at the cellular level, *Endocr Rev* 8:288, 1987.

156. Weinberger C, Thompson CC, Ong ES, et al: The c-erb-A gene encodes a thyroid hormone receptor, *Nature* 324:641, 1986.

157. Mol JA, Krenning EP, Docter R, et al: Inhibition of iodothyronine transport into rat liver cells by a monoclonal antibody, *J Biol Chem* 264:7640, 1986.

158. Kim D, Smith TW: Effects of thyroid hormone on sodium pump sites, sodium content and contractile responses to cardiac glycosides in cultured chick ventricular cells, *J Clin Invest* 74:1481, 1984.

159. Seymour AML, Eldar H, Radda GK: Hyperthyroidism results in increased glycolytic capacity in the rat heart, a 31P-NMR study. *Biochim Biophys Acta* 1055:107, 1990.

160. Polikar R, Kennedy B, Ziegler M, et al: Norepinephrine plasma kinetics in hypothyroid patients before and following replacement therapy (abstr), *Circ Res* 37:362A, 1989.

161. Levey GS: Catecholamine-thyroid hormone interactions and the cardiovascular manifestations of hyperthyroidism, *Am J Med* 88:642, 1990.

162. Shenoy MM, Goldman JM: Hypothyroid cardiomyopathy, echocardiographic documentation of reversibility, *Am J Med Sci* 294:1, 1987.

163. Bierman EL, Glomset JA: *Disorders of lipid metabolism.* In Wilson JD, Foster DW, eds: *Williams textbook of endocrinology,* Philadelphia, 1985, WB Saunders.

164. De Martino GN, Goldberg AL: A possible explanation of myxedema and hypercholesterolemia in hypothyroidism: control of lysosomal hyaluronidase and cholesterol esterase by thyroid hormones, *Enzyme* 26:1, 1981.

165. Urbanic RC, George JM: Cushing's disease—18 years experience, *Medicine (Baltimore)* 60:14, 1981.

166. Agrest A, Finkilman S, Elijovich F: Haemodinamica de la hipertension arterial en al sindrome de Cushing, *Medicina (Buenos Aires)* 34:457, 1974.

167. Cassar J, Loizou S, Kelly WF, et al: Deoxycorticosterone and aldosterone excretion in Cushing's syndrome, *Metabolism* 29:115, 1980.

168. Gaunt R: *Action of the adrenal cortical steroids on electrolyte and water metabolism.* In Christy NP, ed: *The human adrenal cortex, New York, 1983, Harper and Row.*

169. Ritchie CM, Sheridan B, Froser R, et al: Studies on the pathogenesis of hypertension in Cushing's disease and acromegaly, *Q J Med* 76(280):855, 1990.

170. Frazer R, Davies DL, Connell JMC: Hormones and hypertension, *Clin Endocrinol* 31:701, 1989.

171. Saruta T, Suzuki H, Handa M, et al: Multiple factors contribute to the pathogenesis of hypertension in Cushing's syndrome, *J Clin Endocrinol Metab* 62:275, 1986.

172. Carney JA: Differences between nonfamilial and familial cardiac myxoma, *Am J Surg Pathol* 9:53, 1985.

173. Carney JA, Gordon H, Carpenter PC, et al: The complex of myxomas, spotty pigmentation, and endocrine overactivity, *Medicine* 64:270, 1985.

174. Abrass IB, Scarpace PJ: Glucocorticoid regulation of myocardial beta-receptors, *Endocrinology* 108:977, 1981.

175. Beard CM, Sheps SG, Kurland LT, et al: Occurrence of pheochromocytoma in Rochester, Minnesota, 1950 through 1979, *Mayo Clin Proc* 58:802, 1983.

176. Murai K, Hirota K, Niskikimi T, et al: Pheochromocytoma with electrocardiographic change mimicking angina pectoris, and cyclic change in direct arterial pressure—a case report, *Angiology* 42(2):157, 1991.

177. Nirgiotis JG, Andrassy RJ: Pheochromocytoma and acute myocardial infarction, *South Med J* 83:1478, 1990.

178. Smith U: Adrenergic control of lipid metabolism, *Acta Med Scand* 672(suppl):41, 1983.

179. Harris RB, DelaRoca RR: Pheochromocytoma: a medical review, *Heart Lung* 13:73, 1984.

180. Ganguly A, Weinberger MH, Grim CE: The renin-angiotensin-aldosterone system in Cushing's syndrome and pheochromocytoma, *Horm Res* 17:1, 1983.

181. Bravo EL, Gifford RW Jr: Pheochromocytoma: diagnosis, localization and management, *N Engl J Med* 311:1298, 1984.

182. Cohen CD, Dent DM: Pheochromocytoma and acute cardiovascular death (with special reference to myocardial infarction), *Postgrad Med J* 60:111, 1984.

183. Chang C-H, Lin PJ, Chang J-P, et al: Intrapericardial pheochromocytoma, *Ann Thorac Surg* 51:661, 1991.

184. Rosen T, Bengtsson B-A: Premature mortality due to cardiovascular disease in hypopituitarism, *Lancet* 336:285, 1990.

185. Thuesen L, Christensen SE, Weeke J, et al: A hyperkinetic heart in uncomplicated active acromegaly: explanation of hypertension in acromegalic patients? *Acta Med Scand* 233:338, 1988.

186. Lacka K, Piszczek I, Kowowicz J, et al: Echocardiographic abnormalities in acromegalic patients, *Exp Clin Endocrinol* 91:212, 1988.

187. Lie JT, Grossman SJ: Pathology of the heart in acromegaly: anatomic findings in 27 autopsied patients, *Am Heart J* 100:41, 1980.

188. Van den Heuvel PACMB, Elbers HRJ, Plokker HWM, et al: Myocardial involvement in acromegaly, *Int J Cardiol* 6:550, 1984.

189. Xu X, Best PM: Decreased transient outward K+ current in ventricular myocytes from acromegalic rats, *Am J Physiol* 260:H935, 1991.

190. Nickols GA, Nana AD, Nickols MA, et al: Hypotension and cardiac stimulation due to the parathyroid hormone-related protein, humoral hypercalcemia of malignancy factor, *Endocrinology* 125:834, 1989.

191. Asimakis GK, Dipette DJ, Conti VR, et al: Hemodynamic action of calcitonin gene-related peptide in the isolated rat heart, *Life Sci* 41:597, 1987.

192. Keda K, Weir EC, Mangin M, et al: Expression of messenger ribonucleic acids encoding a parathyroid hormone-like peptide in normal human and animal tissues with abnormal expression in human parathyroid adenomas, *Mod Endocrinol* 2:1230, 1988.

193. Kannel WB, McGee DL: Diabetes and cardiovascular disease: the Framingham study, *JAMA* 241:2035, 1979.

194. Schurtz CI, Lesbre JP, Jarry G, et al: Coronary artery disease in diabetics: an angiographic study of 238 patients, *Arch Mal Coeur Vaiss* 76:872, 1983.

195. Valsania P, Zarich SW, Kowalchuk GK, et al: Severity of coronary artery disease in young patients with insulin-dependent diabetes mellitus, *Am Heart J* 122:695, 1991.

196. Lemp GF, Vander Zwaag R, Hughes JP, et al: Association between the severity of diabetes mellitus and coronary arterial atherosclerosis, *Am J Cardiol* 60:1015, 1987.

197. Jaffe AS, Spadaro JJ, Schechtman K, et al: Increased congestive heart failure after myocardial infarction of modest extent in patients with diabetes mellitus, *Am Heart J* 108:31, 1984.

198. Lawrie GM, Morris GC, Glaeser DH: Influence of diabetes mellitus on the results of coronary bypass surgery: follow-up of 212 diabetic patients ten to fifteen years after surgery, *JAMA* 256:2967, 1986.

199. Dybdahl H, Ledet T: Diabetic macroangiopathy: quantitative histopathological studies of the extramural coronary arteries from Type 2 (non-insulin-dependent) diabetic patients, *Diabetologia* 30:882, 1987).

200. Factor SM, Minase T, Sonnerblick EH: Clinical and morphological features of human hypertensive-diabetic cardiomyopathy, *Am Heart J* 99:446, 1980.

201. Van Hoeven KH, Factor SM: Diabetic heart disease: the clinical and pathological spectrum, Part I, *Clin Cardiol* 12:600, 1989.

202. Van Hoeven KH, Factor SM: A comparison of the pathological spectrum of hypertensive diabetic and hypertensive-diabetic heart disease, *Circulation* 82:848, 1990.

203. Regan TJ, Lyons MM, Ahmed SS, et al: Evidence for cardiomyopathy in familial diabetes mellitus, *J Clin Invest* 60:885, 1977.

204. Peng SK, French WJ: Morphologic changes in small vessels on endomyocardial biopsy, *Ann Clin Lab Sci* 16:180, 1986.

205. Fisher BM, Gillen G, Lindop GBM, et al: Cardiac function and coronary arteriopathy in asymptomatic type I (insulin-dependent) diabetes patients: evidence for a specific diabetic heart disease, *Diabetologia* 29:706, 1986.

206. Van Hoeven KH, Factor SM: Diabetic heart disease, Part II: the clinical and pathological spectrum, *Clin Cardiol* 12:667, 1989.

207. McMillian DE: Relationship of abnormalities in blood viscosity to early vascular changes in diabetic children and adolescents, *Pediatr Adolesc Endocr* 17:1, 1988.

208. McMillian DE: Physical factors important in the development of atherosclerosis in diabetes, *Diabetes* 30:97, 1981.

209. Oikawa N, Umetsu M, Sakurada M, et al: Discrimination between cardiac para-and sympathetic damage in diabetics, *Diabetes Res Clin Pract* 1:203, 1985.

210. Kahn JK, Zola B, Juni JE, et al: Decreased exercise heart rate and blood pressure response in diabetic subjects with cardiac autonomic neuropathy, *Diabetics Care* 9:389, 1986.

211. Charcello M, Indalfi C, Cotecchia MR, et al: Asymptomatic transient ST changes during ambulatory ECG monitoring in diabetic patients, *Am Heart J* 110:529, 1985.

212. Faerman I, Faccio E, Milei J, et al: Autonomic neuropathy and painless myocardial infarction in diabetic patients: histologic evidence of their relationship, *Diabetes* 26:1147, 1977.

213. Page MMcB, Watkins PJ: The heart in diabetes: autonomic neuropathy and cardiomyopathy, *J Clin Endocrinol Metab* 6:377, 1977.

214. Cerami A, Vlassara H, Brownlee M: Protein glycosylation and the pathogenesis of atherosclerosis, *Metabolism* (12 suppl 1):37, 1985.

215. Gilerease MZ, Hoover RL: Examination of monocyte adherence to endothelium under hyperglycemic conditions, *Am J Pathol* 139:1089, 1991.

216. Vlassara H, Brownlee M, Cerami A: Novel macrophage receptor for glucose-modified proteins is distinct from previously described scavenger receptors, *J Exp Med* 164:1301, 1986.

217. Sambandam T, Baker JR, Christner JE, et al: Specificity of the low-density lipoprotein glycosaminoglycan interaction, *Arterioscler Thromb* 11:561, 1991.

218. Deckert T, Horowitz IM, Kofoed-Enevoldsen A, et al: Possible genetic defects in regulation of glycosaminoglycans in patients with diabetic nephropathy, *Diabetes* 40:764, 1991.

219. Moore S: Pathogenesis of atherosclerosis, *Metabolism* 34:13, 1985.

220. Le Pape A, Gutman N, Guitton JD, et al: Nonenzymatic glycosylation increases platelet aggregating potency of collagen from placenta of diabetic human beings, *Biochem Biophys Res Commun* 111:602, 1983.

221. Colwell JA, Lopes-Virella MF, Winocour PD, et al: *New concepts about the pathogenesis of atherosclerosis in diabetes mellitus.* In Levin ME, O'Neal LW, eds: *The diabetic foot,* St Louis, 1988, CV Mosby.

222. Tesfamarian B, Jakubowski JA, Cohen RA: Contraction of diabetic rabbit aorta caused by endothelium-derived PGI2-TxA2, *Am J Physiol* 257:H1327, 1989.

223. Hadcock S, Richardson M, Winocour PD, et al: Intimal alterations in rabbit aortas during the first six months of alloxan-induced diabetes, *Arterioscler Thromb* 11:517, 1991.

224. Campbell GR, Campbell JH, Manderson JA, et al: Arterial smooth muscle: a multifactorial mesenchymal cell, *Arch Pathol Lab Med* 122:977, 1988.

225. Maton PN: The carcinoid syndrome, *JAMA* 260:1602, 1988.

226. Forman MB, Byrd BF, Oates JA, et al: Two-dimensional echocardiography in the diagnosis of carcinoid heart disease, *Am Heart J* 107:492, 1984.

227. Stickman NE, Rossi PA, Massumkhani GA, et al: Carcinoid heart disease: a clinical pathologic and therapeutic update, *Curr Probl Cardiol* 6:1, 1982.

228. Lundin L, Norheim I, Landelius J, et al: Carcinoid heart disease: relationship of circulating vasoactive substances to ultrasound-detectable cardiac abnormalities, *Circulation* 77:264, 1988.

229. Nilson K, Von Euler AM, Dalsgaard CJ: Stimulation of connective tissue cell growth by substance P and substance K, *Nature* 315:61, 1985.

230. Lachter JH, Lavy A, Eidelman S: Right heart failure as the sole presentation of carcinoid syndrome, *Int J Cardiol* 25:129, 1989.

231. Ross EM, Roberts WC: The carcinoid syndrome: comparison of 21 necropsy subjects with carcinoid heart disease to 15 necropsy subjects without carcinoid heart disease, *Am J Med* 79:339, 1985.

232. Lundin L, Fuuna K, Hansson HE, et al: Histochemical and immunohistochemical morphology of carcinoid heart disease, *Pathol Res Pract* 187:73, 1991.

233. Castano EM, Frangione B: Biology of disease: human amyloidosis, Alzheimer disease, and related disorders, *Lab Invest* 58:122, 1988.

234. Cohen AS, Connors LH: The pathogenesis and biochemistry of amyloidosis, *J Pathol* 151:1, 1987.

235. Dyck RF, Lockwood CM, Kershaw M, et al: Amyloid P-component is a constituent of normal glomerular basement membrane, *J Exp Med* 152:1162, 1980.

236. Diebold J: Letters to the case, *Pathol Res Pract* 180:200, 1985.

237. Laurent M, Toulet R, Ramee MP, et al: Maladie des chaines legeres avec myocardiopathie terminale, *Arch Mal Coeur Vaiss* 78:943, 1984.

238. Solomon A, Frangione B, Franklin EC: Bence-Jones proteins and light chains of immunoglobulins: preferential association of the lambda VI group of human light chains with amyloidosis AL (lambda), *J Clin Invest* 70:453, 1982.

239. Ishihara T, Takahashi M, Koga M, et al: Amyloid fibril formation in the rough endoplasmic reticulum of plasma cells from a patient with localized A amyloidosis, *Lab Invest* 64:265, 1991.

240. Buck FS, Koss MN, Sherrod AE, et al: Ethnic distribution of amyloidosis: an autopsy study, *Mod Pathol* 2:372, 1989.

241. Levin M, Pras M, Franklin EC: Immunologic studies of the nonimmunoglobulin protein of amyloid, identification and characterization of a related serum component, *J Exp Med* 138:373, 1973.

242. Ramadori G, Sipe JD, Dinarello CA, et al: Pretranslational modulation of acute phase hepatic protein synthesis by murine recombinant interleukin I (IL1) and purified human IL-1, *J Exp Med* 162:930, 1985.

243. Neugartern J, Gallo GR, Buxbaum J, et al: Amyloidosis in subcutaneous heroin abusers ("skin poppers' amyloidosis"), *Am J Med* 81:635, 1986.

244. Browning MJ, Banks RA, Tribe CR, et al: Ten years' experience of an amyloid clinic: a clinicopathologic survey, *Q J Med* 54:213, 1985.

245. Gejyo F, Yamada T, Odani S, et al: A new form of amyloid protein associated with chronic hemodialysis was identified as B2-microglobulin, *Biochem Biophys Res Commun* 129:701, 1985.

246. Kyle RA, Greipp PR: Amyloidosis (AL): clinical and laboratory features in 229 cases, *Mayo Clin Proc* 58:665, 1983.

247. Falk RH, Rubinow A, Cohen AS: Cardiac arrhythmias in systemic amyloidosis: correlation with echocardiographic abnormalities, *J Am Coll Cardiol* 3:107, 1984.

248. Lindholm PF, Wick MR: Isolated cardiac amyloidosis associated with sudden death, *Arch Pathol Lab Med* 110:243, 1986.

249. McAllister HA, Seger J, Bossart M, et al: Restrictive cardiomyopathy with kappa light chain deposits in myocardium as a complication of multiple myeloma, *Arch Pathol Lab Med* 112:1151, 1988.

250. Peng S-K, French WJ, Cohen AH, et al: Light chain cardiomyopathy associated with small-vessel disease, *Arch Pathol Lab Med* 112:844, 1988.

251. Ganeval D, Mignon F, Peud'home J-L, et al: Depots de Chaines legeres et d'immunoglobulines monoclonales: aspects nephrologiques et hypotheses physiopathologiques, *Actualities Nephrogogiques de l' Hospital Necker, Paris*, Flammarion Medecine, Sciences 179, 1981.

252. Picken MM, Frangione B, Barlogie ML, et al: Light chain deposition disease derived from the K1 light chain subgroup, *Am J Pathol* 134:749, 1989.

253. Gallo G, Picken MM, Frangione B, et al: Deposits in monoclonal immunoglobulin deposition disease lack amyloid P component, *Mod Pathol* 1:453, 1988.

254. Olson LJ, Gertz MA, Edwards WD, et al: Senile cardiac amyloidosis with myocardial dysfunction: diagnosis by endomyocardial biopsy and immunohistochemistry, *N Engl J Med* 317:738, 1987.

255. Sletten K, Westermark P, Natrig JB: Senile cardiac amyloid is related to prealbumin, *Scand J Immunol* 12:503, 1980.

256. Valantine HA, Billingham ME: Recurrence of amyloid in a cardiac allograft four months after transplantation, *J Heart Transplt* 8:337, 1989.

257. Silverman KJ, Hutchins GM, Bulkley BH: Cardiac sarcoid: a clinicopathologic study of 84 unselected patients with systemic sarcoidosis, *Circulation* 58:1204, 1978.

258. Gibbons WJ, Levy RD, Nava S, et al: Subclinical cardiac dysfunction in sarcoidosis, *Chest* 100:44, 1991.

259. Fleming HA: *Death from sarcoid heart disease, United Kingdom series 1871 to 1986, 300 cases with 138 deaths.* In Grassi C, Rizzato G, Pozzi E, eds: *Sarcoidosis and other granulomatous disorders: 11th World Congress, Milan, 1987,* Amsterdam, 1988, Elsevier.

260. Valantine H, McKenna WJ, Nihoyannopoulos P, et al: Sarcoidosis: a pattern of clinical and morphological presentation, *Br Heart J* 57:256, 1987.

261. Stewart RE, Graham DM, Godfrey GW, et al: Rapidly progressive heart failure resulting from cardiac sarcoidosis, *Am Heart J* 115:1324, 1988.

262. Gravanis MB: Endomyocardial biopsy: a pathologist's view, *J Invas Cardiol* 1:191, 1989.

263. Oakley CM: Cardiac sarcoidosis, *Thorax* 44:371, 1989.

264. Lemery R, McGoon MD, Edwards WD: Cardiac sarcoidosis: a potentially treatable form of myocarditis, *Mayo Clin Proc* 60:549, 1985.

265. Jaworski RC, Gibson M: Tophaceous aortic valve: a case report, *Pathology* 15:197, 1983.

266. Viozzi EJ, Bluhm GB, Riddle JM: Gout and arterial thrombosis, *Henry Ford Hosp Med J* 20:119, 1972.

267. Abbott RD, Brand FN, Kannel WB, et al: Gout and coronary heart disease: the Framingham study, *J Clin Epidemiol* 41:237, 1988.

268. Jargensen L, Hevig T, Roswell HC, et al: Adenosine diphosphate induced platelet aggregation and vascular injury in swine and rabbits, *Am J Pathol* 61:161, 1970.

269. Anderson DW, Virmani R: Emerging patterns of heart disease in human immunodeficiency virus infection, *Hum Pathol* 21:253, 1990.

270. Anderson DW, Virmani R, Reilly JM, et al: Prevalent myocarditis at necropsy in the acquired immunodeficiency syndrome, *J Am Coll Cardiol* 11:792, 1988.

271. Kaul S, Fishbein MC, Siegel RJ: Cardiac manifestations of acquired immune-deficiency syndrome: a 1991 update, *Am Heart J* 122:535, 1991.

272. Rodriquez ER, Nasim S, Hsia J, et al: Cardiac myocytes and dendritic cells harbor human immunodeficiency virus in infected patients with and without cardiac dysfunction: detection by multiplex, nested, polymerase chain reaction in individually microdissected cells from right ventricular endomyocardial biopsy tissue, *Am J Cardiol* 68:1511, 1991.

273. Joshi VV, Gadol C, Connor E, et al: Dilated cardiomyopathy in children with acquired immunodeficiency syndrome: a pathologic study of five cases, *Hum Pathol* 19:69, 1988.

274. Corallo S, Mutinelli MR, Moroni M, et al: Echocardiography detects myocardial damage in AIDS: prospective study in 102 patients, *Eur Heart J* 9:887, 1988.

275. Levy WS, Varghese J, Anderson DW, et al: Myocarditis diagnosed by endomyocardial biopsy in human immunodeficiency virus infection with cardiac dysfunction, *Am J Cardiol* 62:658, 1988.

276. Cammarosano C, Lewis W: Cardiac lesions in acquired immune-deficiency syndrome (AIDS), *J Am Coll Cardiol* 5:703, 1985.

Chapter 12

CARDIAC MANIFESTATIONS OF INHERITED METABOLIC AND NUTRITIONAL DISORDERS

Patricia A. O'Shea

Disorders of Carbohydrate Metabolism
   Glycogen Storage Disease (GSD)
   Mucopolysaccharidoses
Disorders of Glycoprotein Metabolism
   Sialidosis
   Free Sialic Acid Storage Diseases
   Mucolipidoses
Sphingolipidoses
   GM_1 Gangliosidosis
   GM_2 Gangliosidosis
   Fabry Disease
   Gaucher Disease
Neuronal Ceroid Lipofuscinosis
Disorders of Amino Acid and Organic Acid Metabolism
   Alcaptonuria
   Homocystinuria
   X-Linked Dilated Cardiomyopathy With 3-Methyl-glutaconic Aciduria
   Phenylketonuria
   Oxalosis
Disorders of Mineral Metabolism
   Iron Overload
   Disorders of Copper Metabolism
Disorders of Lipid Metabolism
   Hyperlipidemias I - V
   Disorders of Fatty Acid Beta Oxidation
Neuromuscular Disorders
   Muscular Dystrophy
   Nemaline Myopathy
   Friedreich Ataxia
   Kugelberg-Welander Disease
   Neuronal Intranuclear Inclusion Disease
   Mitochrondrial Encephalomyopathies

Peroxisomal Disorders
   Zellweger Syndrome
Nutritional Deficiencies
   Kwashiorkor
   Beriberi
   Scurvy
Endocardial Fibroelastosis

Systemic metabolic and nutritional diseases may affect the development, morphology, and function of the cardiovascular system at any stage from earliest embryo to old age. Overall, however, these effects assume disproportionate physiologic and clinical significance in childhood and young adult life. Patterns of cardiovascular involvement in systemic disorders are diverse; most commonly encountered are cardiomyopathies, which pathophysiologically may be hypertrophic, restrictive, or congestive. Although we are not accustomed to thinking of congenital cardiac malformation as a manifestation of systemic disease, there is no doubt that metabolic derangements of the embryonic and fetal milieu by fetal or maternal systemic disease can give rise to cardiovascular malformation. Structural myocardial disease in infants of diabetic or phenylketonuric mothers is a case in point.[1] Moreover, in infants of diabetic mothers cardiomyopathy and structural defect may coexist, illustrating the sometimes complex anatomic and functional relationships seen in this group of disorders. Valvular heart disease, as seen in the mucopolysaccharidoses and in Marfan syndrome, is often a complication of systemic disease. Many conditions (homocystinuria and Ehlers-Danlos syndrome, for example) lead to loss of vascular integrity, producing either obstructive lesions or aneurysmal dilatation.

DISORDERS OF CARBOHYDRATE METABOLISM
Glycogen storage disease (GSD)

The glycogenoses are a group of autosomally inherited recessive conditions characterized by the accumulation of abnormal amounts of glycogen or, in the case of type IV, amylopectin in many tissues. Ten distinct types, each corresponding to a different metabolic defect, are currently recognized.[2] Cardiac involvement may dominate the clinical picture in types II, III, and IV.

Type II glycogen storage disease. Type II GSD (Pompe disease), was the first storage disease to be localized to the lysosome.[3] Several different genetic errors are known, all of which result in generalized deficiency of lysosomal alpha-1,4-glucosidase (acid maltase) activity. In most patients, renal acid maltase activity is normal.[4] Glycogen accumulates within lysosomes in many tissues, most prominently the heart, skeletal muscle, and liver. Profound cardiomegaly, heart failure, hypotonia, and muscle weakness dominate the clinical picture. Three clinical variants of acid maltase deficiency are recognized; the infantile type is most severe and most common. Affected infants develop massive cardiomegaly and hypotonia in the first 6 months of life and are generally dead by 1 year of heart failure or its complications. The heart is massively and usually symmetrically hypertrophied and globular (Fig. 12-1); endocardial fibroelastosis may be prominent.[5] However, several patients have been reported in whom the septum was particularly thickened, causing outflow obstruction of one or both ventricles.[5,6] These patients present with a systolic murmur or with signs or symptoms of ventricular outflow obstruction, mimicking idiopathic hypertrophic subaortic stenosis.

Microscopically, the condition is characterized by striking vacuolization of myocardial cells caused by huge glycogen deposits (Fig. 12-1). Involvement of the conduction system probably explains at least some of the electrocardiographic abnormalities in Pompe disease.[7] Ultrastructurally, cardiac muscle contains abundant cytoplasmic glycogen in addition to the characteristic lysosomal glycogen.[4,8,9] Vascular smooth muscle and endothelium also contain lysosomal glycogen.[10] Definitive diagnosis is accomplished by demonstration of deficient activity of lysosomal alpha-1,4-glucosidase.[2]

The juvenile[10,11] and adult onset[10] forms of Type II GSD are much less common; both are primarily skeletal myopathies, and cardiac involvement is overshadowed by progressive weakness.

Type III glycogen storage disease. In type III GSD, also known as Cori disease or limit dextrinosis, cardiac involvement is much less severe than in cases of type II. A structurally abnormal glycogen with short outer chains accumulates in muscle and liver. Patients with Cori disease present with hepatosplenomegaly and weakness in childhood. An adult onset myopathic form also has been described. Patients with Cori disease clinically resemble a milder form of von Gierke disease, but the renal enlargement and severe hypoglycemia that characterize type I GSD are not seen in type III.[2] The morphologic changes in cardiac muscle are similar to but generally more subtle than those in type II. A small subset of type III patients with massive cardiomegaly and sudden death in infancy has been reported.[12] Despite concerns regarding cardiomyopathy and the occasional development of cirrhosis, Cori disease is amenable to dietary manipulation and is not incompatible with a long and reasonably normal life.[2] Distinction from type I GSD (von Gierke disease or glucose-6-phosphatase deficiency) on clinical or morphologic grounds is not reliable, and diagnosis rests on demonstration of amylo-1,6-glucosidase (debrancher) deficiency.

Type IV glycogen storage disease. Type IV GSD, also known as amylopectinosis or Andersen disease, results from deficient activity of brancher enzyme (alpha-1,4-glucan: alpha-1,4-glucan 6 glycosyl transferase). Tissue glycogen stores are not increased in this disorder, but glycogen is abnormal in structure, with few branches and long inner and outer chains, similar to amylopectins. This structure renders the molecule less water soluble than glycogen and resistant to diastase digestion; the polysaccharide accumulates in the cytoplasm of hepatocytes and skeletal and cardiac myocytes, forming large PAS-positive diastase-resistant inclusions of irregular shape that are highly characteristic of this disease.[13] Affected infants fail to thrive, develop hepatosplenomegaly in the first months of life, and die of hepatic cirrhosis in infancy or early childhood. In exceptional cases, myopathic or neurologic disease is the dominant clinical feature, and cardiomyopathy has been the presentation in a small group of older children.[2,14] Morphologic and enzymatic findings do not distinguish among these clinically variant groups. Greene et al[15] have reviewed a small group of patients with similar clinicopathologic changes but without demonstrable deficiency of brancher enzyme. Patients with Type IV disease and cardiomyopathy develop congestive heart failure during childhood that progresses rapidly to death. They have cardiac hypertrophy and large ragged PAS-positive diastase resistant inclusions (Fig. 12-2). Despite the relative paucity of clinical signs and symptoms related to hepatic or CNS disease, cirrhosis is seen. The characteristic inclusions are present in skeletal muscle, liver, and nervous system, and branching enzyme is deficient in all these tissues.[14] The explanation for variable severity of expression in different organs is not known, nor is it clear how the

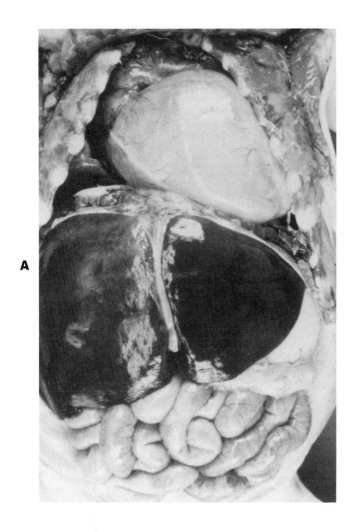

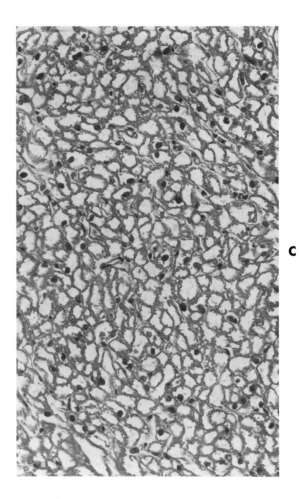

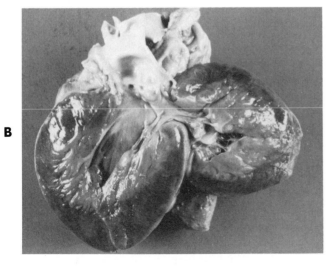

Fig. 12-1. Type II Glycogen storage disease (Pompe disease). **A,** Massive cardiomegaly and hepatomegaly in an infant with generalized GSD. **B,** Symmetrical hypertrophy and pallor of left ventricle are striking. **C,** The cytoplasm of myocardial muscle cells is filled with glycogen, displacing the myofibrils to the periphery and giving the myocardium a lace-like pattern.

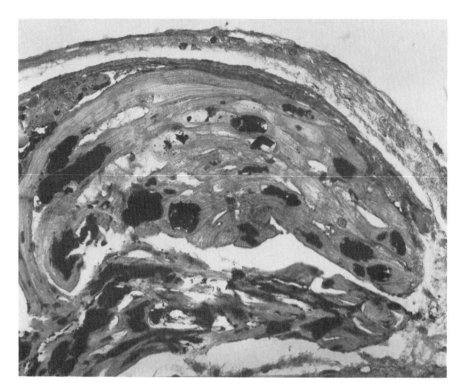

Fig. 12-2. Type IV Glycogen storage disease (Andersen disease). In this form of GSD, brancher enzyme deficiency leads to myocardial cytoplasmic accumulation of deposits of abnormal amylopectin-like molecules, which are insoluble in water and resistant to diastase digestion. (courtesy Dr. Claire Langston, Texas Children's Hospital, Houston, Texas).

presence of the abnormal polysaccharide causes tissue damage. Andersen postulated that the insoluble molecule acts as an irritant. This theory is unproved, but a more satisfactory explanation has not been forthcoming. Recent studies in patients undergoing hepatic transplantation for type IV GSD have demonstrated amylopectin deposits in cardiac muscle of all four patients studied perioperatively; amazingly, the deposits decreased dramatically following transplantation. The children did not die of progressive myopathy, and began to grow and develop normally.[16] The mechanisms by which liver transplantation effects a metabolic cure in distant enzyme deficient tissues are not at present understood; clearly their elucidation would have exciting implications for the treatment of genetic metabolic disease.

Mucopolysaccharidoses (MPS)

The mucopolysaccharidoses are a group of diseases resulting from deficiencies of the lysosomal enzymes that degrade the glycosaminoglycans: dermatan sulfate, heparan sulfate, and keratin sulfate. Chondroitin sulfate is sometimes involved as well. The undegraded mucopolysaccharides accumulate within distended lysosomes, giving rise to the widespread cytoplasmic vacuolation that is the morphologic hallmark of these diseases, and to the

resulting functional disturbances. They are also excreted in the urine, providing a useful diagnostic screening test for the mucopolysaccharidoses.

To date, six different groups of disorders are described, involving 10 different enzyme deficiencies.[17] Type II MPS, or Hunter Syndrome, is an X-linked trait. All the other diseases are transmitted in autosomal recessive fashion. Each shows a wide spectrum of severity, and there is much overlap in clinical and pathologic features. These chronic and progressive disorders are characterized by variable degrees of corneal clouding, abnormal facies (gargoylism), hepatosplenomegaly, and profound, often crippling skeletal abnormalities. The Hurler (MPS I), Hunter (MPS II), and Sanfilippo (MPS III) syndromes may, in addition, produce marked mental impairment. It appears likely that cardiovascular involvement is universal in the mucopolysaccharidoses,[18] but the severity of functional impairment varies greatly and is most severe in MPS I.

Mucopolysaccharidosis I. MPS I is actually three conditions; Hurler, Scheie, and Hurler-Scheie syndromes all result from alpha-L-iduronidase deficiency. Hurler phenotype is the most severe, and a prototype for the group. Myocardial storage of glycosaminoglycans leads to some degree of enlargement of the heart, but valvular and vascular deposition account for most of the functional impair-

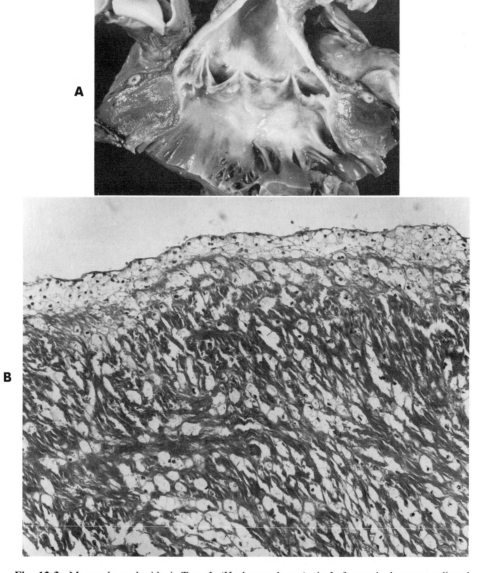

Fig. 12-3. Mucopolysaccharidosis Type I, (Hurler syndrome). **A,** Left ventricular myocardium is hypertrophied, and there is thickening of aortic and mitral valves and coronary arteries. Chordae are thickened and shortened. **B,** Mitral valve with vacuolated "gargoyle" cells and marked fibrosis. (Case contributed by Dr Carlos Abramowsky, Emory University School of Medicine, Atlanta GA)

Continued.

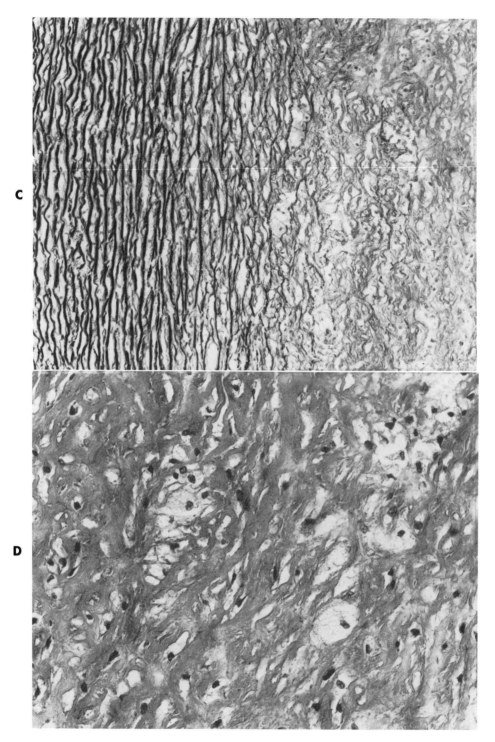

Fig. 12-3, cont'd. C, Aortic plaque in Hurler syndrome; intima is thickened and medial elastic fibers separated by large collections of mucopolysaccharide-laden cells. **D,** Detail of **C** with large vacuolated myointimal cells in a mucinous matrix.

ment and lead to childhood death in most patients.[19,20,21] Endocardium, mitral and aortic valves, and uncommonly the pulmonic and tricuspid valves, are thickened, pale, and opaque (Fig. 12-3). Stenosis and regurgitation result in rolled or nodular and short thick chordae. There is intimal thickening of the muscular arteries, including the coronary arteries, leading to luminal obliteration and rarely, myocardial infarction. Large elastic arteries show plaque-like lesions similar to arteriosclerotic plaques (Fig. 12-3). In all sites, the microscopic feature is the accumulation in connective tissue and smooth muscle cells of granular and vacuolar PAS-positive and Alcian blue–positive substances. Accompanying the deposition of abnormal metabolites is fibroblastic proliferation, resulting in collagenization, stiffness, and insufficiency of valves and stiffness and concentric intimal thickening of muscular arteries. The latter is accompanied by sometimes striking reduplication of elastic laminae. Vacuolated "gargoyle" cells and fibrosis have been described in the conduction system. Death from valvular and/or ischemic heart disease in childhood is to be expected in Hurler syndrome.

Lipid accumulation also can be demonstrated in some tissues, notably in the brain. A possible explanation for the lipid deposition is contained in the observation that in some patients with MPS, secondary reductions in activity of other lysosomal enzymes have been identified.[22] Scheie syndrome is a much less severe form of MPS I characterized by corneal clouding and stiff joints. Mental retardation is not a feature, and most patients have a normal lifespan. Cardiac involvement is also much less severe than in Hurler syndrome, though similar pathologically. Aortic or less commonly, mitral valve dysfunction may necessitate valve replacement.[23] The Hurler-Scheie type of MPS I is intermediate in phenotype between the Hurler and Scheie types.

Mucopolysaccharidosis II. Hunter syndrome (MPS II, iduronate sulfatase deficiency) shares many phenotypic features with Hurler syndrome, including coarse facies, dysostosis multiplex, and mental retardation. A severe and a mild form are described, and both may have cardiac disease in proportion to other organ system involvement. The changes are not distinguishable from those in Hurler syndrome.

Mucopolysaccharidosis III. The Sanfilippo syndromes A, B, C, and D (MPS III) are a group of four phenotypically indistinguishable conditions, each of which is caused by a different enzyme deficiency. They are characterized by profound neurologic impairment with relatively little somatic involvement, although isolated cases of valvular disease have been described in types A and B. Mitral and occasionally tricuspid insufficiency result in nodular leaflets and thick, short chordae.[24,25,26]

Mucopolysaccharidosis IV. Morquio syndrome (MPS IV) is caused by deficiency of either galactose-6-sulfatase or beta-galactosidase; skeletal changes are distinctive.[18]

Aortic regurgitation and childhood coronary artery disease are recognized in some patients with the severe form of the disease.[27]

Mucopolysaccharidosis V. MPS V is now referred to as *MPS I-Scheie*.

Mucopolysaccharidosis VI. MPS VI, or Maroteux-Lamy syndrome (arylsulfatase B deficiency), is primarily a skeletal disorder sometimes complicated by valvar heart disease.[28,29] Aortic and mitral stenosis and insufficiency may require valve replacement. The valves are thickened, the chordae are short, and there is sometimes fusion of aortic cusps. Tricuspid involvement is rare. Endocardial fibroelastosis has been reported in siblings.[30]

Mucopolysaccharidosis VII. A single patient with MPS VII (Sly syndrome, or beta-glucuronidase deficiency) has been reported with obstructive large vessel disease resembling fibromuscular dysplasia, which required an aortic graft.[31]

DISORDERS OF GLYCOPROTEIN METABOLISM

Derangement of glycoprotein degradation and transport accounts for a group of disorders clinically resembling the mucopolysaccharidoses but lacking urinary mucopolysaccharide excretion. Mannosidosis, fucosidosis, sialidosis, and aspartylglycosaminuria result from defective degradation of N-glycosidically linked oligosaccharides that are stored within lysosomes and overflow into the urine. As in MPS, there are infantile, juvenile, and adult forms of each, with a wide range of severity. Common features include dysostosis multiplex, coarse facial features, visceromegaly, and psychomotor disturbances. Intracellular storage is demonstrable in most tissues, including the heart, but seldom causes clinically significant cardiac dysfunction.[32] Patients with the severe infantile type of fucosidosis have cardiac hypertrophy.[33]

Sialidosis

In type II infantile sialidosis (alpha-neuraminidase deficiency), membrane-bound vacuoles in endothelial and smooth muscle cells are described, and one patient has had clinically significant mitral regurgitation; details of cardiac pathology are not given.[34] A severe congenital form of type II sialidosis is characterized by fetal hydrops and ascites; patients with this condition also have pericardial effusions. Extensive renal involvement is a feature of congenital type II sialidosis. This involvement may account for effusions and edema. Cardiac involvement has not been documented in this condition.[35] Galactosialidosis is a near phenocopy of Type II sialidosis, with secondary deficiencies of both beta galactosidase and neuraminidase caused by a defective 34-kDa protein that is necessary for stabilization of both enzymes.[36] Details of cardiovascular pathology are not well studied; because these patients are also beta-galactosidase deficient, cardiomyopathy as seen in cases of GM_1 gangliosidosis would not be unexpected.

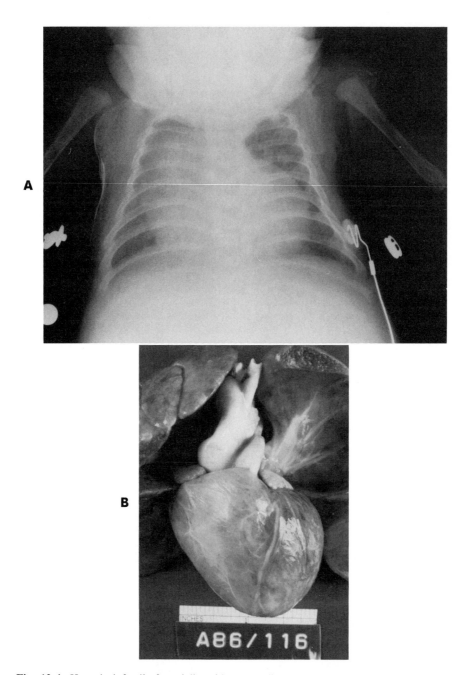

Fig. 12-4. Heart in infantile free sialic acid storage disease. This hydropic newborn male infant had ascites, hepatosplenomegaly, and coarse facial features. **A,** Chest roentgenograph showed cardiomegaly. **B,** At autopsy the heart was symmetrically hypertrophied, globular, and pale.

Free sialic acid storage diseases

The sialic acid storage disorders, infantile free sialic acid storage disease (IFSSD) and Salla disease, are distinct from sialidosis. Alpha neuraminidase activity is normal. Degradation of sialoglycoconjugates proceeds unimpeded within the lysosome, but liberated free sialic acid cannot be removed from the lysosome. The defect presumably lies in a dysfunction in transport of free sialic acid across the lysosomal membrane, and free sialic acid is stored within lysosomes and is excreted in the urine.[37,38] IFSSD is characterized by fetal or neonatal onset, growth retardation, developmental delay, hypotonia, visceromegaly, coarse dysmorphic facial features, blond hair, and a rapidly lethal course.[39,40,41] Fetal hydrops and ascites are frequent findings. Lysosomal and cytoplasmic storage of sialic acid is demonstrable in all viscera and in the central nervous system. Hypertrophic cardiomyopathy has been documented in half of affected patients. The heart is huge, often twice normal weight, globular, and pale (Fig. 12-4). Myocardial cells are swollen and vacuolated; the stored substance can be confirmed as sialic acid by lectin staining.[39]

Patients with hydrops or ascites have also shown pronounced glomerular involvement; at least one has had hepatic fibrosis as well. The relative contributions of hepatic, renal, and myocardial disease to hydrops are not easily determined. Placental involvement by storage is quite prominent and may provide a presumptive diagnosis. The precise enzyme defect is not known at present. In the late onset form of free sialic acid storage disease (Salla disease) and in sialuria, cardiac involvement has not been described.[40]

Mucolipidoses

I-cell disease (mucolipidosis II) and pseudo-Hurler polydystrophy (mucolipidosis III) are the result of defective transport of lysosomal enzymes.[42] In I-cell disease synthesis of enzymes is normal, but targeting to the lysosome is faulty. The enzymes are excreted into the blood, where they are ineffective, while intralysosomal enzyme deficiency leads to the accumulation in mesenchymal cells of large membrane-bound inclusions containing electron lucent and fibrillogranular materials. Clinically, the condition resembles Hurler syndrome. Infants with I-cell disease present at birth or in early infancy with growth retardation and facial and skeletal manifestations resembling MPS I. They are profoundly retarded and die of cardiorespiratory disease in childhood. Well-documented cardiac changes include thickening and nodularity of the endocardium and aortic, mitral, and tricuspid valves by large clear cells in an Alcian blue positive matrix.[43,44] Aortic insufficiency is a frequent manifestation.[45] Similar large clear cells and dense matrix cause marked arterial intimal thickening in the aorta and coronary arteries. Myocardial cells are variably involved.[44] Mucolipidosis III patients also have aortic insufficiency, but pathologic changes are not documented.[42]

SPHINGOLIPIDOSES

Sphingolipids are large molecules made up of sphingosine (an organic base) esterified with a fatty acid to form ceramide. The latter is in turn esterified to either phosphoryl-choline (yielding sphingomyelins), sialyoligosaccharides (to form gangliosides), or unsubstituted monosaccharides or disaccharides (to form neutral glycolipids).[46] Catabolic derangements in the complex metabolic pathways of these molecules result in a family of neurovisceral lysosomal storage diseases of widely variant clinicopathologic manifestations. Cardiovascular disease is described in four: GM_1 and GM_2 gangliosidosis, Fabry disease, and Gaucher disease.

GM_1 Gangliosidosis

GM_1 gangliosidosis results from a number of different structural mutations that produce deficient activity of acid beta-galactosidase.[36] Infantile, juvenile, and adult-onset types are recognized; only infantile (type I, or Landing disease) and juvenile (type II) forms cause cardiovascular disease.[47,48,49]

In infantile GM_1 gangliosidosis, mental and motor retardation, dysostosis multiplex, coarse facies, and hepatosplenomegaly dominate the clinical picture. Most patients have cardiomegaly and nodularity of the atrioventricular valves, which contain deposits of PAS and Alcian blue positive cytoplasmic storage material. Arrhythmia is a frequent cause of death, and a cardiomyopathic variant is described.[49]

In type II (juvenile) GM_1 gangliosidosis, cardiomegaly and valvar disease also occur. Gilbert et al[50] have described vacuolated cells with both lamellar and reticulogranular inclusions in valve leaflets.

GM_2 gangliosidosis

GM_2 Gangliosidosis consists of a group of three nonallelic mutations, all of which result in hexosaminidase deficiency.[51] A defective alpha subunit of hexosaminidase A leads to Tay-Sachs disease. Defective beta subunits are responsible for Sandhoff disease, and a deficient activator protein causes the AB variant, phenotypically identical to Tay-Sachs disease. Of these, Sandhoff disease is the only form with symptomatic heart disease, although myocardial ganglioside storage can be demonstrated in Tay-Sachs disease.[52] Infants with Sandhoff disease have cardiac hypertrophy, endocardial fibrosis, and mitral insufficiency. Storage of concentric lamellar lipids can be demonstrated in myocardium, valvar and endocardial fibrocytes, endothelium, and vascular smooth muscle.[53,54]

Fabry disease

Fabry disease is an X-linked recessive disorder with onset in childhood or adolescence. The condition results from defective lysosomal alpha-galactosidase deficiency, leading to deposition of glycosphingolipids with terminal galactosyl groups in endothelium, perithelium, vascular smooth muscle, myocardium, glomerular epithelium, renal tubular epithelium, perineurium, and multiple ocular tissues. Pain and paresthesia in the extremities, cutaneous and mucous membrane angiokeratomas (vascular ectasia), hypohidrosis, and corneal and lenticular opacity are characteristic early clinical manifestations. Eventually renal or cardiac failure leads to death. An unusual variant of Fabry disease apparently confined to myocardium has been recognized.[55]

Cardiovascular involvement in Fabry disease is global and progressive; globotriaosylceramide is deposited in myocardium, leading to hypertrophic or dilated cardiomyopathy. Vascular endothelial deposits lead to angina and infarction, and valvar connective tissue involvement accompanies mitral insufficiency.[56,57,58] An obstructive hypertrophic cardiomyopathy is also recognized.[59] The heart is markedly enlarged; myocardial cells contain perinuclear vacuoles that are birefringent, sudanophilic, and PAS positive. Endothelial and fibroblastic cells are filled with similar material. Ultrastructurally, the material consists of intralysosomal densely packed parallel or concentric lamellae. A peculiar sunburst pattern is occasionally encountered in lysosomes of endothelium.[60]

Gaucher disease

Gaucher disease results from glucocerebrocidase deficiency. It is the most prevalent of the sphingolipidoses, but rarely leads to cardiovascular disease.[46] There is a great deal of clinical diversity in Gaucher disease. Type I, the nonneuronopathic form, is a chronic skeletal disease of adults. Type II, acute neuronopathic Gaucher disease, is characterized by opisthotonus and spasticity in the first months of life, with death ensuing within a year. Type III (juvenile or subacute neuronopathic) patients have seizures and retardation beginning in the first year and die in the second decade. In all types, glucosylcerebroside accumulates within cells of the reticuloendothelial system. The resulting "wrinkled tissue paper" appearance of the Gaucher cell cytoplasm is very close to pathognomonic. Cardiac disease is seen occasionally in types I and III, mainly resulting from cor pulmonale secondary to pulmonary hypertension.[61] Myocardial involvement has been reported in only one case.[62] Pericarditis is also infrequent and results from bleeding.[63,64] Gaucher cells and intimal and medial fibrosis of coronary arteries led to cardiac hypertrophy, myocardial infarction, and death in a 6-year-old.[65]

NEURONAL CEROID LIPOFUSCINOSIS (NCL)

The neuronal ceroid lipofuscinoses are a group of familial neurodegenerative disorders characterized clinically by psychomotor retardation, visual impairment, seizures, and cerebellar and extrapyramidal dysfunction. They are distinguished morphologically by the accumulation of autofluorescent lipofuscin-like pigments in neurons and a wide variety of other cells. Four groups are recognized, based on the age of onset: infantile (Santavuori), late infantile (Jansky-Bielschowsky), juvenile (Batten or Spielmeyer-Vogt), and adult (Kufs) diseases.[66] Because the stored material is intralysosomal, classification of NCL with the lysosomal storage disorders is conceptually attractive, but in fact no lysosomal enzyme defect has been established, and the metabolic basis for the condition is unknown. Diagnosis is at present established by the demonstration of characteristic curvilinear and fingerprint profiles by electron microscopic examination of the skin, conjunctiva, rectal mucosa, or lymphocytes.[67] Myocardial fibers also accumulate storage material in vacuoles. Cardiac hypertrophy and valve thickening are reported.[68]

DISORDERS OF AMINO ACID AND ORGANIC ACID METABOLISM

Alcaptonuria

Alcaptonuria is a systemic disorder caused by homogentisic acid oxidase deficiency; the classical triad of features is homogentisic aciduria, ochronosis, and arthritis. Ochronotic pigment is a polymer of homogentisic acid. Onset of symptoms ordinarily does not begin until adult years; major clinical problems are related to pigment deposition in skin, eyes, and joints, and to ochronotic renal calculi.[69] In the cardiovascular system, sites of involvement include endocardium, valves, and walls of arteries and veins. The endocardium is diffusely or focally stained gray or black, and pigmentation is most prominent in valve rings and at the base of valves.[70] Symptomatic disease usually results from aortic stenosis; the ochronotic pigment is associated with extensive dystrophic calcification, and a causal relationship has been suggested. The myocardium is not involved except in areas of scarring. All layers of the arterial wall contain pigment, but the intima of large arteries is most prominently affected. Atherosclerotic plaques are heavily pigmented, but it is not clear whether the atherosclerotic process is accelerated. Microscopically, pigment can be identified in macrophages, fibroblasts, and smooth muscle cells, and in the extracellular space. Intracellular deposits are electron dense and membrane-bound.[70]

Homocystinuria

The homocystinurias are a group of inherited and acquired metabolic disorders; the most common, and the only one with cardiovascular consequences, is caused by cystathione-beta-synthetase deficiency.[71,72] Acquired ectopia lentis, osteoporosis, lengthened tubular bones, and thromboembolism are cardinal clinical features. The correct diagnosis is frequently first suspected by an ophthalmologist, but catastrophic vascular occlusion may be the initial presentation[72] and is usually the cause of death. Pulmonary embolism, stroke, and myocardial infarction are common; any vessel may be affected regardless of the patient's age.[71] Arteries show the most striking changes.[73,74] There is marked fibrous intimal thickening, which may be concentric or patchy. Both elastic fibers and smooth muscle cells are fragmented and frayed, and the media is fibrotic. Atherosclerosis is accelerated, and thrombosis is superimposed. Aneurysmal dilation has been noted, but does not seem to be as common as in cases of Marfan syndrome.[75] Abnormalities of collagen cross-linking, increased endothelial fragility, and a variety of platelet function and survival abnormalities have been described. The relative contribution of each of these changes to the pathogenesis of vascular disease is not clearly delineated.[71] The disease is transmitted as an autosomal recessive condition. Heterozygote detection and prenatal diagnosis are feasible.

X-Linked dilated cardiomyopathy with 3-methylglutaconic aciduria

This recently described organic aciduria is characterized by growth retardation, neutropenia, and dilated cardiomyopathy of infantile or early childhood onset.[76] Most patients have died of sepsis or heart failure in infancy. Early in the course of disease, cardiac dilatation predominates; hypertrophy occurs late if at all. Some patients have had endocardial fibroelastosis. Details of cardiac morphology are not described. The condition may be closely related to the x-linked cardiomyopathy with endocardial fibroelastosis and abnormal mitochondria reported by Neustein et al.[77] The metabolic defect leading to methylglutaconic aciduria has not been established.

Phenylketonuria (PKU)

Phenylketonuria is one of a group of autosomal recessive conditions that cause hyperphenylalaninemia.[78] In PKU, phenylalanine hydroxylase activity is deficient; very high levels of phenylalanine lead, by mechanisms not well understood, to profound disturbances of nervous system growth and development and mental retardation. There is recent evidence that infants with PKU have more congenital heart disease than non-PKU subjects.[79] As widespread neonatal screening and low phenylalanine diet have permitted survival of a large number of women of normal intelligence to childbearing age, it has become apparent that maternal PKU, like maternal diabetes mellitus, is a potent teratogen, producing growth retardation, microcephaly, mental retardation, and a variety of congenital malformations, most of which are cardiac.[80,81,82] These include but are not limited to heterotaxy, single atrium, single ventricle, hypoplastic left heart syndromes, pulmonary and aortic stenosis and atresia, septal defects, anomalies of pulmonary venous return, and arrhythmias.[1] The teratogenic effect is dose related, operates throughout pregnancy and is not organ specific. It is thought to be due to growth inhibition by elevated phenylalanine levels.[1] In further analogy to maternal diabetes, it is apparent that the deleterious effects of maternal PKU can be averted by meticulous dietary management prior to and throughout pregnancy.[78]

Oxalosis

Oxalosis includes two rare autosomal recessive disorders that both lead to primary hyperoxaluria.[83] The more common type I, or glycolic aciduria, results from deficiency of peroxisomal alanine-glyoxalase transferase. Large amounts of glyoxylic and glycolic acids appear in the urine. Type II, or L-glyceric aciduria, results from a hitherto incompletely defined defect in hydroxypyruvate metabolism; excess hydroxypyruvate is converted to excess L-glyceric acid. Both oxalic and L-glyceric acids are excreted in the urine. In both diseases, nephrocalcinosis and nephrolithiasis are the overriding concern, but calcium oxalate crystals are deposited in many tissues, including myocardium, conducting system, and vascular smooth muscle.[84,85,86] The crystalline deposits are accompanied by muscle cell necrosis and inflammation, including foreign body giant cells. Arrythmias, including complete heart block, are encountered.[87] Vascular occlusive disease may result from crystal deposition.[88] In all locations the crystals are yellow to brown, strongly birefrin-gent, and insoluble in acetic acid.[68] Secondary forms of oxalosis result from pyridoxine deficiency, ethylene glycol ingestion, excessive intake of oxalate (in, for example, spinach and rhubarb), and inflammatory bowel disease.[68,83]

DISORDERS OF MINERAL METABOLISM
Iron overload

Diseases of iron overload include primary idiopathic hemochromatosis, neonatal hemochromatosis, and secondary or transfusional hemochromatosis. The last condition is the most common of the three. Exogenous iron overload is manifest first in the reticuloendothelial system, and later in various epithelia, liver, and many mesenchymal organs, including myocardium. In chronic iron overload states such as the thallassemias, cardiac iron deposition may become a major clinical problem limiting survival. Iron is deposited in conducting and contractile elements, conferring a dark brown color and leading to marked cardiac hypertrophy, fibrosis, and eventually cardiac failure.[89]

Primary (idiopathic) hemochromatosis. This condition is an autosomal recessive disorder, closely linked to the HLA locus. Excessive iron is absorbed from the intestinal tract[90]; iron accumulates first in the liver and subsequently in other parenchymal organs, with relative sparing of the reticuloendothelial system until late into the disease.[91] Myocardial involvement usually is not manifested until adulthood, but childhood presentation with congestive cardiomyopathy is described.[92] Arrhythmia (especially tachyarrhythmias and ventricular premature contractions) and dilated cardiomyopathy are the most common cardiac complications of primary hemochromatosis. Less common is restrictive cardiomyopathy with impaired ventricular filling.[93]

Morphologically, primary hemochromatosis may be indistinguishable from transfusional hemochromatosis. The heart is large, brown, and usually dilated; iron pigmentation is greater in the ventricles than in the atria, with relative sparing of conducting fibers, valves, and coronary arteries.[68] Iron is stored in hemosiderin granules in the cytoplasm of myocytes. Early in the disease, cytoplasmic pigmentation may be limited to the perinuclear area; eventually pigmentation becomes widespread. Ultrastructural examination shows most of the hemosiderin to be contained in membrane-limited granules. Fibrosis is a relatively late occurrence. Endomyocardial biopsy is extremely useful in making the diagnosis of hemochromatosis.[94] The mechanisms by which iron causes cellular damage are incompletely understood; hydroxyl free radical toxicity and derangements of mitochondrial energy production have been implicated.[95,96]

Neonatal hemochromatosis (NH). This condition is an uncommon but increasingly recognized disorder of intrauterine onset characterized by severe liver disease, hepatic iron storage, and widespread extrahepatic siderosis

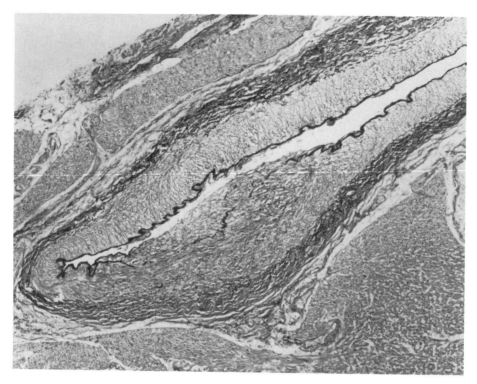

Fig. 12-5. Menkes disease. A section of the left anterior descending coronary artery from 7-month old male infant shows a plaque-like focus of intimal thickening with splitting, fraying, and disruption of the internal elastic membrane. Such lesions lead to dilatation and tortuosity of the vessel. (Courtesy Dr. Jennifer Ahearn, Rhode Island Hospital, Providence, RI).

that spares the reticuloendothelial system. A primary disorder of iron metabolism has not been established, and there is evolving consensus that NH may be a final common pathway for intrauterine liver disease.[97] Myocardial iron deposition is uniformly present in NH, and endomyocardial biopsy has been useful in documenting extrahepatic siderosis in the condition, but infants with NH have not to date had myocardial dysfunction attributable to iron storage.

Disorders of copper metabolism

Wilson disease. Impaired biliary copper excretion and impaired copper incorporation into ceruloplasmin lead to hepatotoxic copper accumulation and liver disease of protean clinicopathologic manifestations. The ocular and neuropsychiatric extrahepatic manifestations of this autosomal recessive disease are the sequela of overflow of copper from the liver.[98] Myocardial involvement (hypertrophic cardiomyopathy) is very uncommon.[99]

Menkes kinky hair syndrome. This extremely rare x-linked condition is a copper deficiency state related to defective intestinal copper absorption. Affected infants seldom live beyond 2 years. The heart is normal, but large vessels show striking degenerative changes: fragmentation,

disruption, and duplication of elastic lamellae, intimal proliferation, thrombosis, aneurysmal dilation, and tortuosity (Fig. 12-5).[98]

DISORDERS OF LIPID METABOLISM

The hyperlipoproteinemias are a complex and heterogeneous family of genetically determined and acquired disorders characterized by elevated levels of plasma lipids. Current classification recognizes five types of hyperlipoproteinemias; most are associated with precocious onset or accelerated development of systemic and coronary atherosclerosis.

Hyperlipidemias I-V

The primary hyperlipidemias are summarized in Table 12-1. Secondary (acquired) forms result from many metabolic derangements; the most common include diabetes mellitus, alcoholism, chronic renal disease, dysglobulinemias, and a variety of endocrine disorders.[104]

Disorders of fatty acid beta oxidation

Inherited defects of fatty acid oxidation are increasingly recognized as causes of hepatic disease, cardiac and skeletal myopathy, and encephalopathy. They are characterized

Table 12-1. The hyperlipidemias

Type	Name	Elevated lipopopratien	Primary disorder	ASCVD
I	Exogenous Hyperlipemia	Chylomicrons	Familial lipoprotein lipase deficiency CII Apolipoprotein deficiency	No predisposition
II-A	Hypercholesterolemia	LDL	Familial hypercholesterolemia	Accelerated especially in homozygous individuals
II-B	Combined Hyperlipidemia	LDL + VLDL	Familial multiple lipoprotein-type hyperlipidemia	Most common cause of premature AS-CVD
III	Remnant Hyperlipidemia	beta VLDL	Familial dyslipoproteinemia	Precocious coronary and peripheral ASCVD
IV	Endogenous Hyperlipidemia	VLDL	Familial hypertriglyceridemia (mild form) Tangier Disease	Accelerated CAD
V	Mixed Hyperlipidemia	VLDL Chylomicrons	Familial hypertriglyceridemia (severe form) Familial lipoprotein lipase deficiency	Unknown

Data modified from Brunzell,[100] Goldstein,[101] Kane,[102] Mahley,[103] and Havel.[104]
ASCVD   Arteriosclerotic Cardiovascular Disease
CAD   Coronary Artery Disease

by fasting hypoglycemia, vomiting, coma, increased urinary dicarboxylic acids, and reduced levels of plasma or tissue carnitine.[105] Known disorders include deficiencies of long, medium, and short chain acyl-CoA dehydrogenases (LCAD, MCAD, and SCAD respectively), long chain L-3-lydroxyacyl-CoA dehydrogenase (LCHAD), electron transfer flavoprotein (ETF) and ETF dehydrogenase, carnitine transporter, and carnitine palmitoyl-transferase. These are disorders of fasting adaptation and therefore may remain clinically silent in the absence of significant stress. Onset of illness may be abrupt; a Reye syndrome-like picture, sudden infant death, and encephalomyopathy are well-recognized modes of presentation. Cardiac involvement may consist only of myocardial neutral lipid accumulation, which is clinically silent and frequently inconspicuous unless lipid stains are employed.[106] MCAD should be suspected in cases of unexpected sudden death, particularly in families with recurring disease. It is now possible by mutational analysis to demonstrate the MCAD mutation in paraffin-embedded tissues.[107] In LCAD, hypertrophic cardiomyopathy has been a consistent finding.[108] Endocardial fibroelastosis is a feature of both primary and secondary alterations in carnitine metabolism.[109]

Glutaric acidemia type II, or multiple acyl-CoA deficiency, results from ETF deficiency or ETF: ubiquinone oxidoreductase deficiency. It is characterized by acidosis, hypoglycemia, hyperammonemia, organic aciduria, and early death.[110] Affected infants are said to smell like sweat socks. A unique feature is the association of multiple congenital anomalies with the metabolic defect in a subset of patients; these include dysmorphic facies, renal medullary dysplasia and glomerular cysts, pachygyria, lung hypoplasia, and anomalies of external genitalia. Cardiomyopathy

leads to heart failure in early infancy; autopsies have shown myocardial lipid accumulation with or without hypertrophy.[111,112]

NEUROMUSCULAR DISORDERS
Muscular dystrophy

Cardiomyopathy is a recognized component of many of the muscular dystrophies; in Duchenne muscular dystrophy, dilated cardiomyopathy is a common cause of death. The left ventricle and septum show fiber size variation, fragmentation, fatty infiltration, and epimyocardial fibrosis. The right side is rarely affected. Mitral valve prolapse occurs in some patients with papillary muscle dysfunction.[113,114] In patients with Becker muscular dystrophy, cardiomyopathy is less common than in Duchenne dystrophy.[115] The conducting system may be involved, giving rise to arrhythmia. In myotonic dystrophy, arrhythmia is related to fibrosis and fatty infiltration of the conducting system; these patients also have myxoid changes of the mitral valve associated with prolapse, and myofiber disarray.[68]

Nemaline myopathy

Nemaline myopathy is a congenital nonprogressive and usually relatively benign myopathy characterized morphologically by rod-shaped cytoplasmic inclusions that stain dark red with modified Gomori trichrome stain. Dilated cardiomyopathy of childhood or adult onset is a rarely reported complication; in most cases the characteristic rod structures are demonstrable in cardiac muscle.[116]

Friedreich ataxia

Patients with autosomal recessive Friedreich ataxia uniformly have cardiac hypertrophy and fibrosis at autop-

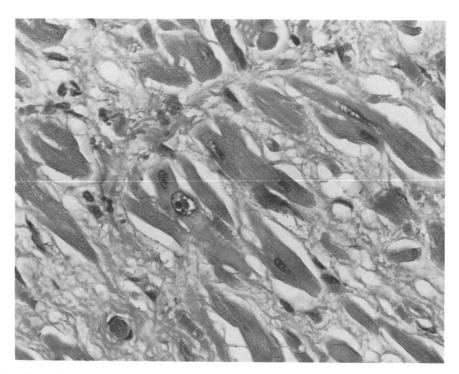

Fig. 12-6. Myocardial involvement in neuronal intranuclear inclusion disease. This 9-year-old boy with a 6-year history of progressive neurologic deterioration had dilated cardiomyopathy with hypertrophied myocytes, fibrosis, and eosinophilic intranuclear inclusions, which are Feulgin and methyl green pyronine negative.

sy,[68,117] though only a third have clinical difficulties. In symptomatic patients, cardiac involvement may take the form of asymmetric hypertrophic cardiomyopathy, with or without obstruction. Myocardial fibrosis is widespread, and coronary artery occlusion has resulted from intimal thickening of intramyocardial arteries.[68] The conducting system is seldom involved.

Kugelberg-Welander disease

Kugelberg-Welander disease is the juvenile form of progressive spinal muscular atrophy. Both cardiomyopathy and arrhythmia are reported; endomyocardial biopsies have shown myocardial fibrosis. The heart is usually enlarged.[68,118]

Neuronal intranuclear inclusion disease (NIID)

NIID is a rare progressive neurodegenerative disorder of unknown etiology defined morphologically by large eosinophilic intranuclear inclusions in neurons and occasionally in adrenal medulla and skeletal muscle (Fig. 12-6). Congestive cardiomyopathy with fibrosis and the characteristic inclusions in cardiac myocytes has been noted in a juvenile case.[119]

Mitochondrial encephalomyopathies

This is a diverse group of neuromuscular diseases associated with defective function of one or more components of the mitochondrial respiratory chain. Common features include dementia, short stature, hearing loss, lactic acidemia, weakness, ragged red fibers on muscle biopsy, and both quantitative and qualitative structural abnormalities of mitochondria. Several of these diseases are known to be encoded by mitochondrial DNA and are therefore maternally inherited; these include Leber optic neuropathy, *m*yoclonic *e*pilepsy with *r*agged *r*ed *f*ibers (MERRF), a syndrome of mitochondrial *m*yopathy with *e*ncephalopathy, *l*actic *a*cidosis, and *s*troke-like episodes (MELAS), Alper progressive infantile poliodystrophy, Leigh subacute necrotizing encephalopathy, and Kearns-Sayre syndrome.[120,121,122] Of these, Kearns-Sayre syndrome, MELAS, and MERRF have shown fairly consistent cardiac involvement that is variable in onset and clinical manifestations. Heart block, supraventricular tachycardia, sudden death, and hypertrophic nonobstructive cardiomyopathy have been described. MELAS patients have an obstructive microangiopathy with endothelial swelling and thickened basal lamina, which is thought to contribute an ischemic component to their disease.

Another group of mitochondrial disorders consists of infantile onset myopathies, some of which are rapidly lethal. Some of those disorders are severe at birth and show gradual improvement during the first year, suggesting developmental modulation of the oxidative phosphorylation sequence.[120] There is not a consistent correlation between

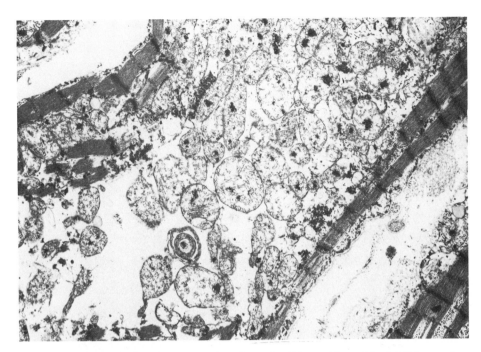

Fig. 12-7. Mitochondrial cardiomyopathy in a 4-month-old boy with combined deficiency of respiratory complexes I and IV. His course was characterized by hypotonia, seizures, hepatic dysfunction, lactic acidosis, and hypertrophic cardiomyopathy. Electron micrograph of cardiac muscle with increased numbers of abnormal mitochondria displacing myofibrils to the periphery of the fiber. (courtesy Dr. Kevin Winn, Emory University School of Medicine, Atlanta, GA).

the oxidative defect and phenotype. Several infants with the lethal form have had progressive hypertrophic nonobstructive cardiomyopathy. Increased numbers of deformed mitochondria and cytoplasmic vacuolation of myocardial cells are described (Fig. 12-7).[123]

PEROXISOMAL DISORDERS

Peroxisomes are membrane-bound cytoplasmic organelles that carry out a wide variety of anabolic and catabolic functions including biosynthesis of plasmalogens, cholesterol, and bile acids, breakdown of polyamines, purines, and pipecolic acid, and beta oxidation of fatty acids.[124] Defects in either peroxisomal biogenesis or peroxisomal enzyme function lead to Zellweger cerebrohepatorenal syndrome, rhizomelic chondrodysplasia punctata, neonatal adrenal leukodystrophy, and infantile Refsum disease.

Zellweger syndrome

This condition is a lethal constellation of characteristic dysmorphic features, renal cystic disease, and hepatic fibrosis and cirrhosis. Absence of hepatic peroxisomes is a constant finding. Like glutaric acidemia type II and hyperphenylalaninemia, the Zellweger syndrome is an example of *metabolic dysplasia,* a term coined by Opitz to refer to a group of metabolic disorders resulting in defects of cellular differentiation. Zellweger patients also have an in-

creased prevalence of congenital heart disease, particularly ventricular septal defects and various aortic abnormalities.[125]

Cardiac disease has not been widely recognized in rhizomelic chondrodysplasia punctata. However, ventricular septal defect, myxoid dysplasia of atrioventricular valves, and advanced pulmonary hypertensive vascular disease have been seen in an affected infant.

NUTRITIONAL DEFICIENCIES

Cardiovascular involvement is a component of many nutritional disorders, most importantly kwashiorkor, scurvy (vitamin C deficiency), and beriberi (thiamine deficiency).

Kwashiorkor

Kwashiorkor is caused by inadequate protein intake in the presence of adequate carbohydrate intake. It occurs mainly in infants and young children; affected individuals are edematous, apathetic, and withdrawn. Diarrhea, hair and skin depigmentation, anemia, and fatty change in the liver are characteristic findings. There is a profound loss of skeletal muscle mass in patients who have kwashiorkor. Myocardial changes are difficult to assess in the presence of coexisting vitamin deficiencies. Thinning of myocardium, dilatation of the heart, interstitial edema, and myocardial vacuolation have been described.[126] In marasmus

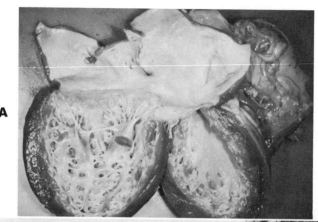

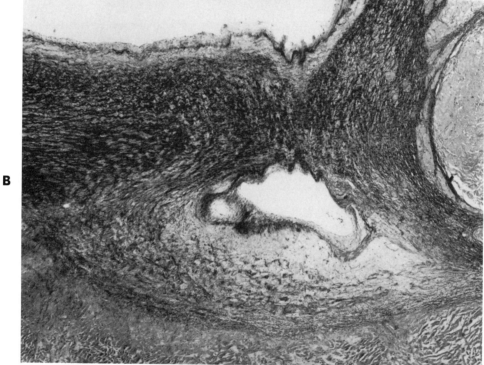

Fig. 12-8. Idiopathic endocardial fibroelastosis. **A,** The heart is both hypertrophied and dilated. Left atrium and ventricle are lined by a thick white opaque layer of fibroelastic tissue. The mitral valve and chordae are short and thick, probably the result of cardiac dilatation and relative mitral insufficiency. **B,** Left atrial and ventricular endocardium in a 17-year-old boy who underwent cardiac transplantation for familial EFE. The endocardium is thickened by layers of elastic fibers that partially surround the left circumflex coronary artery.

and adult starvation syndromes, cardiac atrophy is proportional to decreased cardiac output in response to reduced body mass.

Beriberi

Vitamin B_1, or thiamine, functions as an important cofactor in decarboxylation of alpha-ketoacids and transketolation in the pentose phosphate pathway; it is required for acetylcholine synthesis. Deficiency results in defective energy production, impaired carbohydrate metabolism, and altered nerve conduction. In large parts of the world, dietary deficiency of thiamine results from diets consisting largely of polished rice; in developed countries chronic alcoholism is the main associated condition.

Clinically, beriberi heart disease, or "wet" beriberi, is characterized by tachycardia, peripheral vasodilatation, arteriovenous shunting, and high output cardiac failure. Edema results from cardiac and renal failure. An acute form, Shoshin beriberi, consists of profound predominantly right-sided failure, and rare cases of low output failure have been ascribed to derangements of cardiac pyruvate metabolism.[127]

The heart in beriberi heart disease is enlarged, flabby, pale, and globular. The right ventricle is particularly dilated, and mural thrombi are often present. Microscopic findings include interstitial edema, cytoplasmic hydropic change, and nonspecific degenerative changes with loss of striation and myocyte necrosis. Fibrosis and inflammation are occasionally reported but inconspicuous.[128,129]

Scurvy

Right ventricular hypertrophy and sudden death have been attributed to infant scurvy.[130]

ENDOCARDIAL FIBROELASTOSIS (EFE)

EFE is a cardiac lesion characterized morphologically by increased thickness of the endocardium caused by proliferation of elastic and collagen fibers. Left ventricular involvement is most frequent and most severe, but any cardiac chamber may be involved. Although it may be encountered, albeit infrequently, in adolescents and adults, EFE is overwhelmingly a condition of prenatal or perinatal onset. More than 80% of patients are infants under 1 year of age who present with respiratory distress or rapidly progressive cardiac failure.[131] Abrupt onset and death in ostensibly normal infants leads in some cases to initial misdiagnosis as sudden infant death syndrome. The association of EFE with nonimmune fetal hydrops, and the diagnostic utility of prenatal ultrasound and fetal echocardiography are well documented.[132]

Historically, classification schemes have recognized primary and secondary forms of EFE. Primary EFE is by definition idiopathic and has no recognized underlying structural or cardiomyopathic abnormality. Cardiac hypertrophy and an incompetent mitral valve are consistent features of so-called primary EFE. Secondary EFE is associated with and presumably a consequence of any of a variety of structural, ischemic, inflammatory, and metabolic diseases. These include congenital obstruction to left ventricular outflow (aortic stenosis, coarctation of the aorta, and hypoplastic left heart syndrome), anomalous origin of coronary arteries, interstitial myocarditis, myocardial infarction, disorders of carnitine metabolism, Pompe disease, mucopolysaccharidoses I (Hunter) and IV (Maroteux-Lamy), and mitochondrial cardiomyopathy.* Increasing utilization of endomyocardial biopsy in the diagnosis of EFE during life, coupled with greater sophistication in the diagnosis of metabolic disorders, has caused many cases of primary EFE to be reclassified as secondary. We regard EFE as a non-specific reactive and proliferative response of young endocardium to increased tension, and concur with Lurie's view that "there is no primary EFE. All EFE is secondary".[135] The etiology may or may not be known in an individual case, but the use of the term *idiopathic* rather than the term *primary* at least serves as reminder that further inquiry may be fruitful and of more than academic interest. A significant minority (about 10%) of index cases have been shown to have at least one affected sibling.[136]

The heart in EFE is invariably large, frequently two or three times the expected weight, and usually dilated. In a small minority of cases, especially those with hypoplastic left heart syndromes, the heart is contracted and small. The endocardium of the left ventricle is diffusely thickened, white, and opaque (Fig. 12-8). Left atrium and right atrium and ventricle may be affected. Papillary muscles and trabeculae are encased in a dense rubbery tissue, which has the effect of smoothing out the contours of the chamber. In idiopathic cases, the mitral valve is thickened and the chordae are short as a result of mitral regurgitation. Microscopically, the normal, transparently thin endocardium is replaced by many layers of relatively acellular collagen and elastic fibers. They may reach several millimeters in thickness and extend around vessels and into the myocardium for a short distance (Fig. 12-8).[137] The mechanisms evocative of this proliferative response are beginning to be understood; it has been shown that increased intraluminal tension in pulmonary arteries stimulates elastin production by vascular smooth muscle via humoral intermediates.[138]

REFERENCES

1. Fisch RO, Burke B, Bass J et al: Maternal phenylketonuria–chronology of the detrimental effects in embryogenesis and fetal development: pathological report, survey, clinical application, *Pediatr Pathol* 5:449-461, 1986.
2. Hers HG, VanHoof F, DeBarsy T: *Glycogen storage diseases.* In Scriver CR, Beaudet Al, Sly WS et al eds: *The Metabolic Basis of Inherited Disease,* ed 6, vol 1, New York, 1989, McGraw-Hill.

*References 5, 30, 77, 113, 132, 133, 134.

3. Hers HG: Alpha glucosidase deficiency in generalized glycogen storage disease (Pompe's disease), *Biochem J* 86:11-16, 1963.

4. Hug G: *The glyocgen storage diseases.* In Behrman RE, Vaughn VC III, eds: *Nelson's textbook of pediatrics,* ed 13, Philadelphia, 1987, *WB Saunders.*

5. Rees A, Elbl F,Minhaus K et al: Echocardiographic evidence of outflow tract obstruction in Pompe's disease (glycogen storage disease of the heart), *Am J Cardiol* 36:1103-1106, 1976.

6. Cottrill CM, Johnson GL, Noonan JA: Parental genetic contributions to mode of presentation in Pompe disease, *Pediatrics* 79:379-381, 1989.

7. Gillette PC, Nihill MR, Singer DB: Electrophysiological mechanism for the short PR interval in Pompe disease, *Am J Dis Child* 128:622-626, 1974.

8. Dincsoy, MY, Dincsoy HP, Kessler AD et al: Generalized glycogenesis and associated endocardial fibroelastosis. Report of three cases with biochemical studies, *J Pediatr 67:728-740, 1965.*

9. Bruni CD, Paluello FM: A biochemical and ultrastructural study of liver, muscle, heart, and kidney in type II glycogenosis, *Virchows Archiv B Cell Pathol* 4:196, 1970.

10. Engel AG, Gomez MR, Seybold ME et al: The spectrum and diagnosis of acid maltase deficiency, *Neurology* 23:95-106, 1973.

11. Tanaka K, Shimazu S, Oya M et al: Muscular form of glycogenosis type II (Pompe's disease), *Pediatrics* 63:124-129, 1979.

12. Miller CG, Alleyne GA, Brooks SEH: Gross cardiac involvement in glycogen storage disease type III, *Br Heart J* 34:862-864, 1972.

13. Bannayan GB, Dean WJ, Howell RR: Type IV glycogen storage disease. Light microscopic, electron microscopic, and enzymatic study, *Am J Clin Pathol* 66:702-209, 1976.

14. Servidei S, Riepe RE, Langston C et al: Severe cardiopathy in branching enzyme deficiency, *J Pediatr* 111:51-56, 1987.

15. Greene GM, Weldon DC, Ferrans VJ et al: Juvenile polysaccharidosis with cardioskeletalmyopathy, *Arch Pathol Lab Med* 111:977-982, 1987.

16. Selby R, Starzl TE, Yunis E et al: Liver transplantation for type IV glycogen storage disease, *N Engl J Med* 324:39-42, 1991.

17. Neufeld EF, Muenzer J: *The mucopolysaccharidoses.* In Scriver CR, Beaudet AL, Sly WS et al eds: *The metabolic basis of inherited disease,* ed 6, New York, 1989, McGraw-Hill.

18. McKusick VA, Neufeld EF: *The mucopolysaccharide storage diseases.* In Stanbury JB, Wyngaarden JB, Fredrickson DS et al eds: *The metabolic basis of inherited disease,* New York, 1983, McGraw-Hill.

19. Renteria VG, Ferrans VJ, Roberts WC: The heart in Hurler syndrome. Gross, histologic, and ultrastructural observations in five necropsy cases, *Am J Cardiol* 38:487, 1976.

20. Goldfischer S, Coltoff-Schiller B, Biempica L et al: Lysosomes and the sclerotic arterial lesion in Hurler's disease, *Hum Pathol* 6:633-637, 1975.

21. Krovetz LJ, Lorinca AE, Scheibler GL: Cardiovascular manifestation of the Hurler syndrome. Hemodynamic and angiographic observations in 15 patients, *Circulation* 31:132, 1965.

22. Baumkotter J, Cantz M: Decreased ganglioside neuraminidase activity in fibroblasts from mucopolysaccharidosis patients, *Biochem Biophys Acta* 761:163, 1983.

23. Peyritz RE: *Cardiovascular manifestations of heritable disorders of connective tissue.* In Steinberg AG, Bearn AG, Motulsky AG, et al eds: *Progress in medical genetics, vol 5,* Philadelphia, 1983, Saunders.

24. Herd JK, Subramanian S, Robinson H: Type III mucopolysaccharidosis: report of a case with severe mitral valve involvement, *J Pediatr* 82:101, 1973.

25. Cain H, Enger E, Kresse H: Mucopolysaccharidosis III A (Sanfilippo disease type A). Histochemical, electron microscopical, and biochemical findings, *Beitr Pathol* 160:58, 1977.

26. Witting C, Muller KM, Kresse H et al: Morphological and bio-

chemical Findings in a case of mucopolysaccharidosis type III A (Sanfilippo's disease type A), *Beitr Pathol* 154:324, 1975.

27. Factor SM, Biempica L, Goldfischer S: Coronary intimal sclerosis in Morquio's syndrome, *Virchows Arch (A) Pathol Anat Histopathol* 379:1, 1978.

28. Tan CTT, Schaff HV, Miller FA et al: Valvular heart disease in four patients with Maroteux-Lamy syndrome, *Circulation* 85:188-195, 1992.

29. Wilson CS, Mankin HT, Pluth JR: Aortic stenosis and mucopolysaccharidosis, *Ann Intern Med* 92:496, 1980.

30. Fong LV, Menahem S, Wraith JE et al: Endocardial fibroelastosis in mucopolysaccharidosis type VI, *Clin Cardiol* 10:362-364, 1987.

31. Lee, JES, Falk RE, Ng WG et al: Beta-glucuronidase deficiency: a heterogeneous mucopolysaccharidosis, *Am J Dis Child* 139:57, 1985.

32. Beaudet AL, Thomas GH: *Disorders of glycoprotein degradation: mannosidosis, fucosidosis, sialidosis, and aspartylglycosaminuria,* In Scriver CR, Beaudet AL, Sly WS et al, eds: *The metabolic basis of inherited disease,* New York, 1989; McGraw-Hill.

33. Duran P, Borrone CY, DellaCella G: Fucosidosis, *J Pediatr* 75:665, 1969.

34. Roth KS, Chan JC, Ghatak NR et al.: Acid alpha-neuraminidase deficiency: a nephropathic phenotype?, *Clin Genet* 34:185-194, 1988.

35. Aylsworth AS, Thomas, GH, Hood JL et al: A severe infantile sialidosis: clinical, biochemical, and microscopic features, *J Pediatr* 96:662-668, 1980.

36. O'Brien JS: *B-galactosidase deficiency (GM$_1$ gangliosidosis, galactosialidosis, and Morquio syndrome type B); ganglioside sialidase deficiency (Mucolipidosis IV).* In Scriver CS, Beaudet AL, Sly WS, et al, eds: *The metabolic basis of inherited disease* ed 6, New York: 1989, McGraw-Hill.

37. Mancini GMS, Verheijen FW, Galjaard H: Free n-acetylneuraminic acid (NANA) storage disorders: evidence for defective NANA transport across the lysosomal membrane, *Hum Genet* 73:214-217, 1986.

38. Paschke E, Hofler G, Roscher A: Infantile sialic acid storage disease: the fate of biosynthetically labeled n-acetyl-(^{3}H)-neuraminic acid in cultured human fibroblasts, *Pediatr Res* 20:773-777, 1986.

39. Pueschel SM, O'Shea PA, Alroy J et al: Infantile sialic acid storage disease associated with renal disease, *Pediatr Neurol* 4:207-212, 1988.

40. Gahl WA, Renlund M, Thoene J: *Lysosomal transport disorders: cystinosis and sialic acid storage disorders.* In Scriver CR, Beaudet AL, Sly WS et al, eds: *The metabolic basis of inherited disease,* ed 6, New York, 1989, McGraw-Hill.

41. O'Shea PA, Alroy J, Ambler M et al: Pathologic features of a severe form of infantile free sialic acid storage disease, *Lab Invest* 58:7P, 1988.

42. Nolan CM, Sly WS: *I-cell disease and pseudo-Hurler polydystrophy: disorder of lysosomal enzyme phosphorylation and localization.* In Scriver CR, Beaudet AL, Sly WS et al, eds: *The metabolic basis of inherited disease* ed 6, New York, 1989, McGraw-Hill.

43. Martin JJ, Leroy JG, Van Eygen M et al: I-cell disease: a further report on its pathology, *Acta Neuropathol* (Berl) 64:234, 1984.

44. Gilbert EF, Dawson G, ZuRhein GM et al: I-cell Disease, mucolipidosis II. Pathological, histochemical, ultrastructural, and biochemical observations in four cases, *Z Kinderheilk* 114:259, 1973.

45. Okada S, Owada M, Sakiyama T et al: I-cell disease: clinical studies of 21 Japanese cases, *Clin Genet* 28:207, 1985.

46. Barranger JH, Ginns EI: *Glucosylceramide lipidoses: Gaucher disease.* In Scriver CS, Beaudet AL, Sly WS et al, eds: *The metabolic basis of inherited disease,* New York: 1989, McGraw-Hill.

47. Landing BH, Silverman FN, Craig JM et al: Familial neurovisceral lipidosis, *Am J Dis Child* 108:503, 1964.

48. Hadley RN, Hagstrom JWC: Cardiac lesions in a patient with fa-

milial neurovisceral lipidosis (generalized gangliosidosis), *Am J Clin Pathol* 55:237-240, 1971.

49. Kohlschuetter A, Sieg K, Schulte FJ et al: Infantile cardiomyopathy and neuromyopathy with beta-galactosidase deficiency, *Eur J Pediatr* 139:75-81, 1982.

50. Gilbert EF, Varakis J, Opitz JM et al: Generalized gangliosidosis type II (juvenile GM gangliosidosis). A pathological, histochemical and ultrastructural study, *Z Kinderheilk* 120:151-180, 1975.

51. Sandhoff K, Counzelmann E, Neufeld EF et al: *The GM₂ gangliosidoses*. In Scriver CS, Beaudet AL, Sly WS et al, eds: *The metabolic basis of inherited disease,* New York, 1989, McGraw-Hill, 1807-1839.

52. Rodriguez-Torres R, Schneck L, Kleinberg W: Electrocardiographic and biochemical abnormalities in Tay-Sachs disease, *Bull N Y Acad Med* 47:717, 1971.

53. Dolman CL, Chang E, Duke RJ: Pathologic findings in Sandhoff disease, *Arch Pathol Lab Med* 96:272-275, 1973.

54. Hadfield MG, Mamunes P, David PB: The pathology of Sandhoff's disease, *J Pathol* 123:137-144, 1977.

55. von Scheidt W, Eng CM, Fitzmaurice TF et al: An atypical variant of Fabry's disease with manifestations confined to the myocardium, *N Engl J Med* 324:395-399, 1991.

56. Ferrans VJ, Hibbs RG, Burda CD: The heart in Fabry's disease: A histochemical and electron microscopic study, *Am J Cardiol* 24:95-110, 1969.

57. Desnick RL, Bleiden LC, Sharp HL et al: Cardiac valvular anomalies in Fabry's disease: Clinical, morphologic, and biochemical studies, *Circulation* 54:818-825, 1976.

58. Desnick RL, Bishop DF: *Fabry's disease. Alpha galctosidase deficiency; Schindler disease: alpha-N-acetyl-galactosaminidase deficiency*. In Scriver CS, Beaudet AL, Sly WS et al, eds: *The metabolic basis of inherited disease,* New York, 1989, McGraw-Hill.

59. Colucci WS, Lorell BH, Schoen FJ et al: Hypertrophic obstructive cardiomyopathy due to Fabry's disease, *N Engl J Med* 307:926-928, 1982.

60. Elleder M, Ledvinova J, Vosmik F et al: An atypical ultrastructural pattern in Fabry's disease: a study on its nature and incidence in seven cases, *Ultrastruct Pathol* 14:467-474, 1990.

61. Roberts WC, Fredrickson DS: Gaucher's disease of the lung causing severe pulmonary hypertension with associated acute recurrent pericarditis, *Circulation* 35:783-789, 1967.

62. Smith RRL, Hutchins, GCM, Sack GH et al: Unusual cardiac, renal, and pulmonary involvement in Gaucher's disease. Interstitial glucocerebroside accumulation, pulmonary hypertension, and fatal bone marrow embolization, *Am J Med* 65:352, 1978.

63. Benbassat J, Bassan H, Milwidski H et al: Constrictive pericarditis in Gaucher's disease, *Am J Med* 44:647, 1968.

64. Harvey PKP, Jones MC, Anderson EG: Pericardial abnormalities in Gaucher's disease, *Br Heart J* 31:603, 1969.

65. Wilson ER, Barton MW, Barranger JA: Vascular involvement in type 3 neuronopathic Gaucher's disease, *Arch Pathol Lab Med* 109:82-84, 1984.

66. Rapola J, Järvelä T, Peltonen L: The neuronal ceroid lipofuscinoses: Unfolding the genetic defect, *Pediatr Pathol* 11:799-806, 1991.

67. Vogler C, Rosenberg H, Williams J et al: *Electron microscopy in the diagnosis of lysosomal storage disease*. In Opitz JM, Bernstein J, Spano LM, eds: *Topics in pediatric genetic pathology: the Enid Gilbert-Barness festschrift, New York, 1987, Alan R Liss*.

68. Gilbert, EF: The effects of metabolic diseases on the cardiovascular system, *Am J Cardiovasc Pathol* 1:189-213, 1987.

69. LaDu BM: *Alcaptonuria*. In Scriver CS, Beaudet AL, Sly WS et al, ed: *The metabolic basis of inherited disease,* New York: 1989, McGraw-Hill.

70. Gaines JL: The pathology of alkaptonuric ochronosis, *Hum Pathol* 20:40-46, 1989.

71. Mudd SH, Levy H, Flemming S: *Disorders of transsulfuration*. In Scriver CS, Beaudet AL, Sly WS et al, eds: *The metabolic basis of inherited disease,* New York, 1989, McGraw-Hill.

72. Valle D, Pai GS, Thomas Gh et al: Homocystinuria due to cystathione beta-synthetase deficiency: clinical manifestation and therapy, *Johns Hopkins Med J* 146:110-117, 1980.

73. McCully KS: Homocystein theory of arteriosclerosis: development and current status, *Atherosclerosis Rev* 11:157-246, 1983.

74. Gibson JB, Carson, NAJ, Neill DW: Pathological findings in homocystinuria, *J Clin Pathol* 17:427-437, 1964.

75. Almgren B, Eriksson I, Hemmingsson A et al: Abdominal aortic aneurysm in homocystinuria, *Acta Chir Scand* 144:545-548, 1978.

76. Kelley RI, Cheatham JP, Clark BJ, et al: X-Linked cardiomyopathy with neutropenia, growth retardation, and 3-methylglutaconic aciduria, *J Pediatr* 119:738-747, 1991.

77. Neustein HB, Lurie PR, Dahms B, et al: An x-linked cardiomyopathy with abnormal mitochondria, *Pediatrics* 64:24-29, 1979.

78. Scriver CR, Kaufman S, Woo SLC: *The hyperphenylalaninemias*. In Scriver CS, Beaudet AL, Sly WS et al, eds: *The metabolic basis of inherited disease,* New York: 1989, McGraw-Hill.

79. Verkerk PH, van Spronsen FJ, Smit GPA et al: Prevalence of congenital heart disease in patients with phenylketonuria, *J Pediatr* 119:282-283, 1991.

80. Mabry CC, Denniston JC, Nelson TL et al: Maternal phenylketonuria, *N Engl J Med* 269:1404-1408, 1963.

81. Stevenson RE, Huntley CC: Congenital malformations in offspring of phenylketonuric mothers, *Pediatrics* 40:33-45, 1967.

82. Lenke RR, Levy HL: Maternal phenylketonuria and hyperphenylalaninemia. An international survey of the outcome of untreated and treated pregnancies, *N Engl J Med* 303:1202-1208, 1980.

83. Hillman RE: *Primary hyperoxalurias*. In Scriver CS, Beaudet AL, Sly WS, et al, eds: *The metabolic basis of inherited disease,* New York: 1989, McGraw-Hill.

84. Coltart DJ, Hudson REB: Primary oxalosis of the heart: a cause of heart block, *Br Heart J* 33:315-319, 1971.

85. Pikula B, Plamenac P, Curfcic B, Nikulin A: Myocarditis caused by primary oxalosis in a four year old child, *Virchows Arch (A) Anat Histopathol* 358:99, 1973.

86. Tonkin AM, Mond HG, Matthew TH et al: Primary oxalosis with myocardial involvement and heart block, *Med J Aust* 1:873-874, 1976.

87. West RR, Salyer WR, Hutchins GM: Adult-onset Primary Oxalosis with Complete Heart Block, *JohnsHopkins Med J* 133:195-200, 1973.

88. Arbus GS, Sniderman S: Oxalosis with peripheral gangrene, *Arch Pathol Lab Med* 97:107, 1974.

89. Buja LM, Roberts WC: Iron in the heart. Etiology and clinical significance, *Am J Med* 51:209, 1971.

90. McLaren GD, Nathanson MH, Jacobs A et al: Regulation of intestinal iron absorption and mucosa iron kinetics in hemochromatosis, *J Lab Clin Med* 117:390-401, 1991.

91. Edwards GQ, Dodone MM, Skolnick MH et al: Hereditary hemochromatosis, *Clin Lab Haematol* 11:411-435, 1982.

92. Menahem S, Salmon AP, Dennett V: Hemochromatosis presenting as severe cardiac failure in a young adolescent, *Int J Cardiol* 29:86-89, 1990.

93. Dabestani A, Child JS, Perloff JK et al: Cardiac abnormalities in primary hemochromatosis, *Ann NY Acad Sci* 526:234, 1988.

94. Olson LJ, Edwards WD, Holmes DR et al: Endomyocardial biopsy in hemochromatosis: clinicopathologic correlation in six cases, *J Am Coll Cardiol* 13:116, 1989.

95. Link G, Pinson A, Hershko C: Heart cells in culture: a model of myocardial iron overload and chelation, *J Lab Clin Med* 106:147, 1985.

96. Hanstein WG, Sacks, PV, Muller-Eberhard V: Properties of liver mitochondria from iron loaded rats, *Biochem Biophys Res Commun* 67:1175, 1975.

97. Knisely AS: Neonatal Hemochromatosis, *Adv Pediatr* 39:383-403, 1992.

98. Danks DM: *Disorders of copper transport.* In Scriver CS, Beaudet AL, Sly WS et al, eds: *The metabolic basis of inherited disease,* New York: 1989, McGraw-Hill.

99. Azevedo EM, Scaff M, Barbosa ER et al: Heart involvement in hepatolenticular degeneration, *Acta Neurol Scand* 58:296, 1978.

100. Brunzell JD: *Familial lipoprotein lipase deficiency and other causes of the chylomicronemia syndrome.* In Scriver CS, Beaudet AL, Sly WS et al, eds: *The metabolic basis of inherited disease,* New York: 1989, McGraw-Hill.

101. Goldstein JL, Brown MS: *Familial hypercholesterolemia.* In Scriver CS, Beaudet AL, Sly WS et al, eds: *The metabolic basis of inherited disease,* New York: 1989, McGraw-Hill.

102. Kane JP, Havell RJ: *Disorders of the biogenesis and secretion of lipoproteins containing the B apolipoproteins.* In Scriver CS, Beaudet AL, Sly WS et al, eds: *The metabolic basis of inherited disease,* New York: 1989, McGraw-Hill.

103. Mahley RW, Rall SC: *Type III hyperlipoproteinemia (dysbetalipoproteinemia): the role of apolipoprotein E in normal and abnormal lipoprotein metabolism.* In Scriver CS, Beaudet AL, Sly WS et al, eds: *The metabolic basis of inherited disease,* New York: 1989, McGraw-Hill.

104. Havel RJ, Kane JP: *Introduction: structure and metabolism of plasma lipoproteins.* In Scriver CS, Beaudet AL, Sly WS et al, eds: *The metabolic basis of inherited disease,* New York: 1989, McGraw-Hill.

105. Roe CR, Coates PM: *Acyl-CoA dehydrogenase deficiencies.* In Scriver CS, Beaudet AL, Sly WS et al, eds: *The metabolic basis of inherited disease,* New York, 1989, McGraw-Hill.

106. Bennett MJ, Hale DE, Coates PM et al: Postmortem recognition of fatty acid oxidation disorders, *Pediatr Pathol* 11:365-370, 1991.

107. Ding JH, Roe CR, Iafolla AK: Medium chain acyl coenzyme A dehydrogenase deficiency and sudden infant death, *N Engl J Med* 325:61-62, 1991.

108. Treem WR, Stanley CA, Hale DE et al: Hypoglycemia, hypotonia, and cardiomyopathy: the evolving clinical picture of long-chain Acyl-CoA dehydrogenase deficiency, *Pediatrics* 87:328-333, 1991.

109. Ino T, Sherwood WG, Benson LN et al: Cardiac manifestations in disorders of carnitine metabolism, *J Am Coll Cardiol* 11:1301-1308, 1988.

110. Frerman FE, Goodman SI: *Glutaric acidemia type II and defects of the mitochondrial respiratory chain.* In Scriver CS, Beaudet AL, Sly WS et al, eds: *The metabolic basis of inherited disease,* New York: 1989, McGraw-Hill.

111. Colevas AD, Edwards JL, Hruban RH et al: Glutaric acidemia type II: comparison of pathologic feature in two infants, *Arch Pathol Lab Med* 112:1133-1139, 1988.

112. Kamiya M, Eimoto T, Kishimoto H et al: Glutaric aciduria type II: autopsy study of a case with electron-transferring flavoprotein dehydrogenase defiency, *Pediatr Pathol* 10:1007-1019, 1990.

113. Patterson K, Donnelly WH, Dehner LP: *The cardiovascular system.* In Stocker JT, Dehner LP, eds: *Pediatric pathology,* Philadelphia, 1992, JB Lippincott.

114. Frankel KA, Rosser RJ: The pathology of the heart in progressive muscular dystrophy: epimyocardial fibrosis, *Hum Pathol* 7:375-386, 1976.

115. Lazzeroni E, Favaro L, Botti G: Dilated cardiomyopathy with regional myocardial hypoperfusion in Becker's muscular dystrophy, *Int J Cardiol* 22:126, 1989.

116. Ishibashi-Ueda H, Imakita M, Yutani C et al: Congenital nemaline myopathy with dilated cardiomyopathy: an autopsy study, *Hum Pathol* 21:77-82, 1990.

117. Smith ER, Sangaland VE, Hoffernan LP et al: Hypertrophic cardiomyopathy: the heart disease of Friedreich's ataxia, *Am Heart J* 94:428, 1977.

118. Tanaka H, Uemura N, Toyama Y et al: Cardiac involvement in the Kugelberg-Welander syndrome, *Am J Cardiol* 38:588, 1976.

119. Oyer CE, Cortez S, O'Shea PA et al: Cardiomyopathy and myocyte intranuclear inclusions in neuronal intranuclear inclusion disease, *Hum Pathol* 22:722-724, 1991.

120. Robinson BH: *Lactic acidemia.* In Scriver CS, Beaudet AL, Sly WS, et al, eds: *The metabolic basis of inherited disease,* New York: 1989, McGraw-Hill.

121. Tulinius MH, Holme E, Kristiansson B et al: Mitochondrial encephalomyopathies in childhood. I. Biochemical and morphologic investigations, *J Pediatr* 119:242-250, 1991.

122. Tulinius MH, Holme E, Kristiansson B et al: Mitochondrial encephalomyopathies in childhood II. Clinical manifestations and syndromes, *J Pediatr* 119:251-259, 1991.

123. Zheng X, Shoffner JM, Lott MA et al: Evidence in a lethal infantile mitochondrial disease for a nuclear mutation affecting respiratory complexes I and IV, *Neurology* 39:1203-1209, 1989.

124. Lazarow PB, Moser PB: *Disorders of peroxisome biogenesis.* In Scriver CS, Beaudet AL, Sly WS et al, eds: *The metabolic basis of inherited disease,* New York: 1989, McGraw-Hill.

125. Heymans HSA: Cerebro-hepato-renal (Zellweger) syndrome: clinical and biochemical consequences of peroxisomal dysfunction. Thesis, University of Amsterdam, 1984.

126. Piza J, Troper L, Cespedes R et al: Myocardial lesions and heart failure in infant malnutrition, *Am J Trop Med Hyg* 20:343, 1971.

127. Standstead HH: *Clinical manifestations of certain classical deficiency diseases.* In Goodhardt RS, Shil S, eds: *Modern nutrition in health and disease,* ed 6, Philadelphia, 1980, Lea & Febiger.

128. Benchimol AB, Schlesinger P: Beriberi heart disease, *Am Heart J* 46:245, 1953.

129. Vedder EB: The pathology of beriberi, *JAMA* 110:893, 1978.

130. Follis RH Jr: Sudden death in infants with scurvy, *J Pediatr* 20:347, 1942.

131. Ino T, Benson LN, Freedom RM: Natural history and prognostic risk factors in endocardial fibroelastosis, *Am J Cardiol* 62:431-434, 1988.

132. Wolfson DJ, Pepkowitz SH, Van de Velde R, et al: Primary endocardial fibroelastosis associated with hydrops fetalis in a premature infant, *Am Heart J* 120:708-711, 1990.

133. Hutchins GM, Vie SA: The progression of interstitial myocarditis to idiopathic endocardial fibroelastosis, *Am J Pathol* 66:483-496, 1972.

134. Stephan MJ, Stevens EL, Wenstrup RJ et al: Mucopolysaccharidosis I presenting with endocardial fibroelastosis of infancy, *Am J Dis Child* 143:782-784, 1989.

135. Lurie PR: Endocardial fibroelastosis is not a disease, *Am J Cardiol* 62:468-470, 1988.

136. Chen S, Thompson MW, Rose V: Endocardial fibroelastosis: family studies with special reference to counseling, *J Pediatr* 79:385-392, 1971.

137. Fishbein MC, Ferrans VJ, Roberts WC: Histologic and ultrastructural features of primary and secondary endocardial fibroelastosis, *Arch Pathol Lab Med* 101:49-54, 1977.

138. Rabinovitch M, Bothwell T: An inhibitor of pulmonary artery smooth muscle growth is released by cells pulsated at high pressure, *Fed Proc* 46:730, 1987.

Chapter 13

PATHOGENESIS AND PATHOPHYSIOLOGY OF STRUCTURAL CONGENITAL HEART DISEASE

George C. Emmanouilides
Michael B. Gravanis

Single ventricle (univentricular heart)
    Group I: double inlet to a left ventricular chamber
    Group II: double inlet to a right ventricular chamber
    (DIRV)
    Group III: double inlet to an indeterminate ventricular
    chamber
Malpositions of the heart
    Dextrocardia
    Levocardia
    Left atrial isomerism
    Right atrial isomerism
Anomalous left coronary artery arising from the pulmonary artery

---

ETIOLOGY AND PATHOGENESIS

Despite extensive research during the past 20 years regarding cardiac morphogenesis, the exact mechanisms by which genetic and environmental factors may influence normal early development of the cardiovascular system are not completely understood.[1]

The cardiovascular system is the first functioning organ in the early development of the embryo. As soon as the "cardiac tube" is formed, this primitive heart begins to pump blood, supplying the swiftly growing and metabolically active embryo. The transition of the muscle-bound "cardiac tube" to four distinct cardiac chambers involves a complex and still incompletely understood developmental process. It has been well accepted that pathogenetic influences that result in congenital cardiovascular malformations most likely occur during the period of primary morphogenesis.[2] It should be realized, however, that aberrations and anomalies in the developing fetal heart do not occur in a haphazard way. The same congenital malformations, with only a few minor variations, are seen predictably over and over again. It appears that in the interplay between genetic and environmental factors, either or both affect the looping and septation of the developing heart in a way that suggests a certain embryologic timetable.[3]

Based on recent embryologic and clinical advances, the following classification of cardiovascular malformations has been proposed:

(1) *looping anomalies* (malpositions of the heart with or without situs inversus); (2) *conotruncal anomalies,* or disorders of the mesenchymal tissue migration (Tetralogy of Fallot, truncus arteriosus, transposition of the great arteries); (3) *anomalies involving extracardiac matrix* (atrioventricular septal defects); and (4) *defects of hemodynamic molding or flow defects* (left-sided defects, atrial and ventricular defects, pulmonic stenosis).[3,4]

Our knowledge is quite limited as far as etiology of congenital cardiac malformations is concerned. No more than 10% of such malformations can be attributed to genetic factors with very little if any contribution from the environment, whereas 90% are best explained by a genetic-environmental interaction *(multifactorial inheritance),* in which both genetic and environmental contributions are of comparable importance.[5,6]

Primarily genetic causes

These include the gross *chromosomal anomalies* such as trisomies 13, 18, and 21, and Turner syndrome, which account for 5% to 7% of all congenital cardiac malformations. It should be pointed out that some of the familial or nonfamilial cases of congenital heart disease, without being part of a recognized syndrome, may be associated with chromosomal aberrations that are nondetectable by current diagnostic techniques. Moreover, even a minor anomaly of a chromosome may affect many gene loci and is likely to cause abnormalities of other structures besides the heart. This is well demonstrated to be true in gross chromosomal disorders in which the addition or subtraction of hundreds of genes causes a developmental aberration in many cell lines and systems and produces a syndrome. With the exception of 45X Turner syndrome, the most common defect in the general population—ventricular septal defect—is also the most common defect in the various chromosomal syndromes. In trisomy 21 (Down syndrome), however, where approximately 50% of individuals have congenital heart disease, endocardial cushion defects (atrioventricular defects) are the most common cardiac malformations (at least 50%).

Single mutant gene causes of congenital cardiac malformations, as in chromosomal ones, constitute a part of a syndrome. There may be some exceptions such as familial hypertrophic cardiomyopathy, with or without asymmetric septal hypertrophy (a dominantly inherited disorder), which may not constitute a cardiac "maldevelopment" in its strict sense, but a progressive myocardial disease manifesting in very rare instances in newborns and young infants. Another example may be an atrial septal defect (secundum) occurring in three consecutive generations, suggesting a dominant inheritance.

Because many genes are required for normal cardiogenesis, a mutant gene must be of large effect to produce a cardiac maldevelopment. Genes of large effect, in general, may influence the development of more than one structure, thus producing a syndrome rather than an isolated cardiac defect. Sometimes on closer scrutiny, minor anomalies of the hands, in cases of familial atrial septal defect, may lead to the diagnosis of Holt-Oram syndrome, which is dominantly inherited. The question of cytoplasmic inheritance has been also raised in families in which there is maternal transmission to almost all offspring.[7] It is essential to recognize families in which the congenital heart defects are transmitted by Mendelian inheritance because the risks of recurrence are greater than in the usual families demonstrating multifactorial inheritance. Typically a congenital heart anomaly caused by a single mutant gene will be found as part of a syndrome. The recurrence risk of the syndrome, if the gene is recessive, will be 25%, and 50%

if the gene is dominant. Congenital heart disease may not be present in every subject affected by the syndrome.

Some examples of autosomal recessive syndromes associated with cardiovascular abnormalities are: Ellis-van Creveld, mucopolysaccharidoses, glycogenosis, and cutis laxa. Examples of autosomal dominant syndromes associated with cardiovascular abnormalities are: Holt-Oram, Ehlers-Danlos, Marfan, Noonan, Treacher-Collins; idiopathic hypertrophic cardiomyopathy, and tuberous sclerosis.[5]

Multifactorial inheritance (genetic-environmental interaction)

The great majority of congenital heart diseases fall in this category. As mentioned earlier, the situations in which the factors are primarily genetic or primarily environmental are uncommon.

It appears that the etiologic basis for most congenital cardiac anomalies is a hereditary predisposition to cardiovascular maldevelopment interacting with an environmental trigger (e.g., drug or virus) at the vulnerable period of cardiogenesis. This specific mode of inheritance presupposes the existence of three important ingredients. The individual must be genetically predisposed to cardiovascular maldevelopment; there must exist also a genetic predisposition to react adversely to the environmental teratogen; and the environmental insult must occur at the vulnerable period of cardiac development very early in pregnancy. According to this theory, there is a precarious balance of the many genes that determine the formation of an organ. These genes may be individually normal, but their collective balance may be influenced by environmental triggers producing acceleration or delay of primary gene products, thus disturbing the schedule of the orderly development of the specific organ or tissue.[5,8]

The overall risk of significant congenital cardiovascular malformations is approximately 8 per 1000 live births. This number is much greater if one takes into account the prenatal detection of cardiac malformations using current echocardiographic Doppler techniques.[9] Moreover, bicuspid aortic valve, a very common malformation, and mitral valve prolapse are not included in these statistics. If there is one first-degree relative with congenital cardiac malformation, the recurrence risk may range from 1% to 4%, depending upon how common the heart defect is, i.e., the more common the heart defect, the more likely it is to recur. The risk in multifactorial inheritance increases rapidly with the number of affected first-degree relatives. With two affected first-degree relatives, the risk is approximately tripled. In the rare instances where the genetic balance is so precarious that the majority of first-degree relatives will have cardiac maldevelopment, probably with minimal or without much environmental insult, the risk of recurrence exceeds that of Mendelian inheritance.

The risk to the offspring of an affected parent varies again with the mode of inheritance. For example, an adult with pulmonic stenosis who has no recognizable syndrome and no affected children, has a risk of only 3% recurrence in the next child. If the adult has Noonan syndrome, the risk is 50% that the next child will have the syndrome and 25% that there will be an associated heart disease.

From the data available, it appears that the risk is much higher to the children of mothers with congenital cardiovascular malformation than to children of affected fathers. The risk differences between parents in transmitting their cardiac defects to their offspring may be explained by the influence of teratogenic triggers during pregnancy in the genetically predisposed mother or the possibility of cytoplasmic inheritance (mitochondrial) from the mother.[7]

Environmental factors

According to some authors, careful inquiry may identify potentially teratogenic exposures in more than 50% of pregnant mothers giving birth to a child with congenital cardiovascular malformations. However, for obvious reasons, it is difficult to prove with certainty a cause-and-effect relationship between these potential teratogenic triggers and organ malformation.

Drugs such as anticonvulsants, alcohol, lithium, thalidomide, and retinoic acid have been found to be associated with cardiovascular malformations. Infections such as rubella during the early part of pregnancy have been definitely implicated as a cause of peripheral pulmonary artery stenosis and patent ductus arteriosus along with deafness, microcephaly, and cataracts. Maternal conditions such as diabetes and lupus erythematosus have been also associated with specific cardiac conditions.

The dangerous period for exposure to cardiac teratogens is early in pregnancy, just at the time a woman is not yet certain she is pregnant. It appears that an effective teratogenic insult must occur between 1 and 2 weeks before the completion of the embryologic event during the development of the heart. For example, in order to implicate a teratogen in the etiology of transposition of the great arteries, its effect should have occurred before the 34th day of gestation (completion of conotruncal septation) but not before the 22nd day. In contrast, the vulnerable period for persistent ductus arteriosus, atrial septal defect, or semilunar valve abnormalities (defects of hemodynamic molding) is much later (6 to 8 weeks of gestation).[3]

That the genetic makeup of an individual plays an important role in the incidence of congenital cardiovascular defects is supported by the fact that differences exist between sexes not only in the overall incidence but also in certain types of defects. Males seem to be more often affected with congenital heart disease than females. Moreover, males are more prone to have transposition of the great arteries, tetralogy of Fallot, aortic valve stenosis, and coarctation of the aorta. Conversely, females are prone to have patent ductus arteriosus and secundum atrial septal defect.

There is a wide variation of statistics regarding the prevalence of various cardiac defects, depending upon the reporting center and the mode of collection of the data. However, the true frequency of congenital cardiac defects will not be known until the effect of the new diagnostic modalities (echocardiographic Doppler technology, magnetic resonance imaging, and prenatal diagnosis) is shown in the next few years.

FETAL AND NEONATAL (TRANSITIONAL) CIRCULATION

Knowledge of the anatomic and physiologic features of fetal and transitional-neonatal circulation is essential for understanding the pathophysiology of congenital heart disease both prenatally and postnatally. Most of the available information is derived from anatomic observations, whereas physiologic studies of human fetal circulation have been, for obvious reasons, very rare. Thus our current concepts regarding human fetal circulation have been extrapolated from investigations in other mammals, particularly in sheep. It is only recently, with the increasing application of two-dimensional echocardiographic Doppler technology, that direct observations of fetal cardiac structure and function in the intact human fetus during the last half of gestation are appearing in the literature. Moreover, using the same technology, prenatal diagnosis of congenital malformations of the heart is being widely applied in many specialized centers. The pathophysiology of cardiac malformations can be studied now in the developing human fetus, and for the first time we are able to observe directly anatomic and physiologic adaptations of the fetal circulation to morphologic derangements of cardiac and vascular structures.

Fetal circulation

The major characteristics of mammalian fetal circulation are summarized as follows:

1. Intracardiac and extracardiac vascular shunts are present, i.e., foramen ovale, ductus arteriosus, and ductus venosus.
2. The right and left ventricle work in parallel rather than in series.
3. The right ventricle is pumping blood against higher-than-systemic pulmonary vascular resistance, resulting in pulmonary blood flow that is a fraction of its output. The blood bypasses the lung via the ductus arteriosus, enters the descending aorta, and is directed toward the low-vascular resistance placenta.
4. The lung secretes fluid continually into the respiratory passages and extracts oxygen from the blood rather than providing oxygen for it.
5. The placenta is the major site for exchange of gases and nutrients.
6. The liver is the first organ to receive oxygen and nutrients provided by the mother via the placenta.

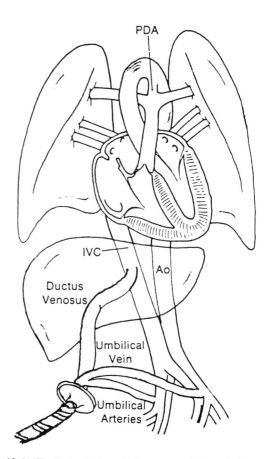

Fig. 13-1. Fetal circulation. (*AO* = aorta, *IVC* = inferior vena cava, *PDA* = patent ductus arteriosus.)

7. The upper part of the fetal body receives blood that has slightly higher oxygen saturation.

The course of the fetal circulation (Fig. 13-1)

In the placenta, the most important "fetal" organ, fetal metabolic end-products are exchanged for oxygen and other nutrients such as glucose, amino acids, fatty acids, water, and electrolytes. Moreover, the placenta is an active "endocrine" organ secreting a number of "hormones" essential for fetal development and maintenance of gestation. The enriched blood from the placenta via the umbilical vein enters the portal sinus of the liver. Approximately 50% of the umbilical venous blood under normal conditions bypasses the liver via the *ductus venosus,* wherein the remainder joins the small amount of blood coming from the portal vein and passes through the liver. The left lobe of the liver, because of its location and the proportionally large umbilical blood flow, is supplied exclusively by the placenta. The physiologic significance and the exact mechanisms controlling the function of the ductus venosus are not completely understood. Although in some mammalian species the ductus venosus is absent at term, it appears that this fetal structure may play an important role in the regulation of the preload of the fetal heart and the oxygenation of the fetus under adverse conditions. For example, it is conceivable that under optimal fetal conditions, i.e., sleep, the ductus venosus may become partially constricted, allowing more blood to enter the liver, whereas it relaxes in situations in which high fetal output is needed.

The oxygenated umbilical venous blood, via the ductus venosus, joins the blood returning from the lower part of the body at the level of the inferior vena cava and from there, without significant mixing in the right atrium, enters the left atrium via the patent foramen ovale. In the fetal lamb, about a third of the inferior vena cava blood flow normally enters the left side of the heart, where it mixes with the relatively small amount of less-oxygenated blood returning from the pulmonary circulation. Thus the slightly higher oxygenated blood from the left ventricle is being ejected to the upper part of the body. Only a small portion of the fetal left ventricular output passes the aortic isthmus (15% to 20%) and enters the descending thoracic aorta. For this reason, the narrowest segment of the normal fetal and newborn aorta is located at the distal transverse aortic arch, just before the junction of the ductus arteriosus. The blood from the superior vena cava coming from the upper part of the body joins the two thirds of the inferior vena cava flow in the right atrium, and from there the blood enters the right ventricle and pulmonary artery.

Because of the high pulmonary vascular resistance (the lung is full of fluid), only a small portion of the right ventricular output enters the pulmonary circulation. The rest bypasses the lung via the ductus arteriosus and is directed toward the low vascular resistance placental circulation. A small portion of this blood perfuses the lower part of the body, including the kidneys and the abdominal viscera.[10,11]

Fetal cardiac output

Fetal cardiac output and its distribution have been extensively studied in animal models and particularly in the sheep. The best available data are those obtained with the use of radiolabeled microspheres in chronically instrumented *fetal lambs*. In the near-term lamb fetus, approximately 70% of the combined ventricular output is directed toward the lower part of the body and the placenta, 20% to the upper body, 7% to the lungs, and 3% to the coronary circulation. The superior vena cava flow, together with close to two thirds of the inferior vena cava and coronary sinus flow, enters the right ventricle. Thus at least 65% of the combined ventricular output in the fetal lamb is ejected by the right ventricle and only 35% by the left.[12,13]

The combined ventricular output increases with fetal growth. However, the proportions distributed to the various organs change as gestation progresses. The proportion of flow perfusing the placenta gradually decreases, whereas there is an increase in the percentage of blood flow supplying the brain, lungs, and gastrointestinal tract. In the human fetus, because the brain is larger, the relative distribution between right and left ventricular output may be closer to 55% and 45%, respectively.

Fetal pulmonary circulation

The fetal pulmonary circulation is characterized by increased pulmonary vascular resistance (higher than that of the systemic circulation), which incorporates the low resistance placental circulation. The factors determining the high pulmonary vascular resistance and its location have been the subject of many investigations and are not completely understood.

The structure and distribution of the pulmonary arterial tree, including the precapillary small arteries, as well as histologic changes that take place during lung development, have been intensively studied in recent years.[14,15] Toward the end of any arterial pathway, a complete smooth muscular coat can be seen (muscular artery) giving way to a region where the muscle is incomplete (partially muscular artery) before the muscle disappears from arteries that are still larger than the capillaries (nonmuscular artery). Moreover, the size of the artery at which the transition from one structural type to another takes place is not always the same. Thus the structure of the artery cannot always be predicted from the external diameter. For this reason, to characterize the peripheral pulmonary circulation, the "population" distribution of the various types of arteries needs to be known. The adult pattern of pulmonary arterial branching is generally complete by about the 20th week of fetal life. In the fetus and newborn infant the precapillary arterial unit is at the level of the terminal, or respiratory, bronchiole.[15] On the venous side, the structural arrangement of a postcapillary unit is similar to the precapillary unit. The alveolar capillaries drain into thin-wall venules which, in turn, lead to the pulmonary veins.

At birth half of the arteries running with respiratory bronchioles are virtually free of muscle. The bronchial arteries arise from the thoracic aorta and the intercostal arteries and supply the airway structures. Anastomoses exist between the bronchial and pulmonary arteries at the precapillary level and are more commonly seen in the fetus than in the newborn. The intrapulmonary bronchial veins join the pulmonary venous drainage, whereas the true bronchial veins connect with the azygos or hemiazygos system. The true bronchial veins drain only the region of the hilus. The veins that drain the bronchial walls may be considered tributaries of the pulmonary veins. Thus elevation of the left atrial pressure is transmitted to airways as well as to alveolar walls.

In reviewing the development of the lung, the preacinar airways are apparently complete in the human fetus by the 16th week of intrauterine life. The alveolar, or respiratory, region is represented by primitive saccules. The true alveolar region develops mainly after birth. As bronchi branch, the pulmonary artery gives off supernumerary and conventional arteries appropriate for each generation. As alveoli multiply, so do arteries. Arterial multiplication, however, usually precedes alveolar multiplication so that the arterial-to-alveolar ratio (per unit) increases. Muscularization of the new arteries is slow, thus quite large arteries may be found without significant muscle layer. In the premature lung, there are fewer alveoli than at term. The 28-week-old fetus has about half as many alveoli as the term infant (per unit area).

Although at birth the alveolar surface is relatively free of muscularized arteries, indicating that the fetal pulmonary circulation is less muscular, the fetal lung appears to be more muscular in one respect. The fetal and newborn arteries of all sizes have a thicker wall when related to external diameter than they do in the child and adult. The smallest muscular arteries are the most muscular, i.e., they have the thickest coat when expressed as a percentage of external diameter. It is in this vascular compartment that the greatest portion of pulmonary vascular resistance resides. The same arteries undergo considerable thinning postnatally, corresponding to the decrease in pulmonary vascular resistance after birth.[14,15,16]

Contrary to what was believed in the past, the amount of smooth muscle in the small pulmonary arteries (30 to 50 μ in diameter) does not change during the last trimester of pregnancy. After birth, the amount of smooth muscle in the media of the pulmonary arteries regresses toward normal adult values. The amount of muscle in the larger arteries generally reaches adult levels only after a child is 2 to 3 years of age. The smaller (less than 200 μ) diameter vessels generally reach adult values of medial smooth muscle when a child is 3 to 4 months of age.

Fetal pulmonary flow gradually increases with fetal growth. At term approximately 7% to 8% of combined ventricular output reaches the lung.[13] The fetal pulmonary blood flow appears to be partially regulated by the autonomic nervous system and humoral factors that are not yet completely understood.[16] Norepinephrine and epinephrine cause pulmonary vasoconstriction, whereas agents such as bradykinin, oxygen, acetylcholine, isoproterenol, histamine, and E-type prostaglandins produce pulmonary vasodilation. The exact contribution of such humoral agents upon the maintenance of high pulmonary vascular resistance in the fetus is not known. The relative hypoxemia in the fetus appears to have a major influence in the maintenance of pulmonary vasoconstriction. The role of ductus arteriosus in the human fetus in regulating pulmonary blood flow, as gestation progresses, is being studied directly by several investigators. It appears that the velocity of blood crossing the ductus arteriosus, as determined by Doppler echocardiography, is higher than that of the pulmonary artery and thoracic aorta, suggesting that the lumen of the ductus is narrower. The fact that the wall of the fetal ductus arteriosus contains a large amount of smooth

muscle that responds not only to intravascular pressure changes but also to humoral or autonomic nervous stimuli, suggests that this structure may play an important role in the regulation of the right ventricular afterload and pulmonary blood flow, a necessary element in the development of the fetal pulmonary vascular bed. Factors that may increase the pulmonary arterial pressure during fetal life, such as premature constriction of the ductus arteriosus or chronic hypoxemia, appear to cause hypertrophy of the smooth muscle layers of the muscular arteries and further muscularization of the nonmuscular arteries. Thus it has been postulated that this abnormal muscularization of the fetal pulmonary vessels may be causally related to the development of persistent pulmonary hypertension of the newborn (persistent fetal circulation syndrome).[10,15] The role of the stretch-induced reflex pulmonary hypertension in the maintenance of high pulmonary vascular resistance in the fetus has not been elucidated. The fetal lung is a metabolically active organ despite the fact that it is not actively involved in gas exchange. It produces fluid that, as gestation progresses, contains increasing amounts of surfactant. The fluid produced by the fetal lung distends the developing potential air spaces and is periodically discharged into the pharynx and amniotic cavity. This fluid is rapidly removed from the potential air spaces within the first few breaths after birth, allowing normal gas exchange.

Fetal arterial blood pressure

Fetal arterial pressure increases gradually as pregnancy progresses. Studies in several animal species have shown that fetal cardiovascular autonomic reflex responses appear to be intact during the last part of gestation.[12] Stimulation of the carotid sinus or the peripheral end of the vagus nerve causes profound bradycardia. Acute, artificially induced elevation of fetal blood pressure causes bradycardia, a characteristic postnatal barostatic response.

Fetal heart

The fetal heart ultrastructurally differs considerably from that of the adult. In addition, its mechanical properties and autonomic innervation are also different. Although there are differences between species, depending upon the relative maturity of the animal at term, the unique cardiac properties of the fetus may render it less efficient in adapting to cardiocirculatory stress.[17] The fetal myocardial cells are fewer and smaller in diameter, and the young heart contains less contractile mass per gram of tissue and more noncontractile elements, such as mitochondria, nuclei, and surface membranes, than does the adult heart. Consequently, force generation and the extent and velocity of shortening are decreased. The fetal myocardium develops greater tension at rest and less active tension with contraction, i.e., it is less compliant than that of the adult.[17,18] Although acute studies of left ventricular performance in the fetal lamb heart suggested that the Frank-Starling mechanism is operative to a large extent, more recent observations made in chronic preparations indicate that fetal cardiac output is controlled primarily by heart rate rather than the classic Frank-Starling mechanism. The fetal heart apparently has a limited ability to increase its output in the presence of either volume overload (preload) or pressure overload (afterload). Moreover, the fetal myocardium lacks complete development of sympathetic but not parasympathetic innervation.[17,18]

Neonatal (transitional) circulation

At birth two major events take place: First, the infant initiates breathing, and, second, he or she is separated from the placenta. These two events result in profound changes in the infant's circulation, which does not immediately acquire the adult pattern.[10]

The characteristics of the transitional or neonatal circulation can be summarized as follows:

1. With establishment of normal respiration, pulmonary blood flow increases because of a reduction of pulmonary vascular resistance.
2. Systemic vascular resistance increases as a result of elimination of placental circulation.
3. The right and left ventricle now work in series rather than in parallel.
4. Within a few minutes after birth, blood flow through the ductus arteriosus is directed from left to right, i.e., from the aorta to the pulmonary artery; this may last as long as the ductus remains functionally open (usually 24 to 48 hours).
5. The ductus venosus blood flow ceases, and the portal and inferior vena cava blood flow decreases (because of cessation of the fetal umbilical flood flow).
6. The foramen ovale functionally closes.

The exact stimulus that causes the first breath is not known. The progressive hypoxia, hypercarbia, and acidosis that ensue at birth, in conjunction with the sudden increase of sensory input that stimulates the central nervous system, have been considered as important stimuli for the initiation of breathing.

The separation of the placenta at birth results in an increase in systemic arterial pressure (increased afterload) caused by the elimination of the low resistance placental circulation. Concurrently, with initiation of breathing and removal of the lung fluid, pulmonary flow increases mainly because of reduction of the pulmonary vascular resistance. A fivefold or more increase in pulmonary blood flow takes place. Besides the mechanical expansion of the lung, oxygen diffusion from the alveoli to the capillaries and precapillary arterioles appears to be the major cause of the reduction of pulmonary vascular resistance. It has been suggested that increases in Pao_2 or simple distension of the alveoli activate the synthesis and/or release of vasoactive substances such as bradykinin or prostaglandins, which may contribute to the initial decrease in pulmonary vascular resistance on ventilation, as well as to the subsequent maintenance of a low pulmonary vascular resistance (PVR).[10,11,16]

During the first few hours after birth, the left-to-right shunt via the ductus may be as high as 30% to 50% of the left ventricular output, depending on the relative size of the lumen of the ductus and the degree of reduction of the PVR. Consequently, the amount of blood returning from the lungs into the left side of the heart is greater than that during fetal life. This greater volume leads to distension of the left atrium and helps in the functional closure of the foramen ovale. Moreover, a temporary left ventricular volume overloading occurs during the first few hours of postnatal circulatory adaptation.

Foramen ovale

In the normal newborn soon after birth, the foramen ovale flap apposes to the left surface of the atrial septum. This apposition is partly caused by the marked reduction of the inferior vena cava blood flow following the occlusion of the umbilical cord. Moreover, with the increase in pulmonary venous return the left atrial pressure increases and aids in the closure of the foramen. However, the factors that control the closure of the foramen ovale may change during the first week of life. For example, if there is a substantial left-to-right shunt through the ductus arteriosus for a longer time than normal (such as that frequently seen in very small preterm infants), the left atrial dimensions may increase the flap deficiency and allow a left-to-right shunt at the atrial level. Such shunts have been documented during the first few hours of life in normal term infants. Conversely, right-to-left shunts through the foramen ovale also can exist for variable periods, especially when the pulmonary blood flow is decreased because of persistence of high pulmonary vascular resistance. During hypoxic pulmonary vasoconstriction, whether associated with right ventricular dysfunction or not, such venoarterial shunts at the atrial level are present quite frequently.[19] Anatomic closure of the foramen ovale eventually occurs within a few months, but a probe patent foramen may persist in up to 15% to 20% of normal adult individuals.

Closure of the ductus arteriosus

Within the first 24 hours in the majority of term neonates, the ductus closes functionally. A right-to-left, bidirectional, or left-to-right shunt may occur during the first few hours of life, depending on many factors. A left-to-right shunt, however, persists for 15 to 20 hours and may last for several days in some instances.[20] Right-to-left shunt is usually present immediately after birth. Moreover, hypoxemia, by promoting the patency of the ductus arteriosus and inducing pulmonary vasoconstriction, may cause persistence of the right-to-left ductal shunt. Administration of 100% oxygen to term infants younger than 15 hours of age will constrict the ductus arteriosus, whereas 13% oxygen will cause its dilation.[21] These responses were found to be more pronounced in term infants under 3 hours of age. The various factors that control the patency of the ductus arteriosus have been extensively studied. The most important physiologic factor contributing to its closure is the constrictive effect of oxygen tension in the arterial blood. This constriction response appears to be stronger with increasing fetal age and occurs at lower oxygen tensions as the fetus approaches term.[11] It has been suggested that intermediate transmitter substances released by oxygen may help control the patency of the ductus. There is ample evidence now that prostaglandins play a major role in maintaining patency of the ductus during fetal life.[11,16] Infusion of the prostaglandin of the E type in human neonates has been shown to dilate a previously constricted ductus arteriosus, whereas prostaglandin synthetase inhibitors may close a persistent patent ductus arteriosus during the first few days or weeks of life. The role of the autonomic nervous system on the patency of the ductus has not been completely elucidated. Both sympathetic and parasympathetic nerve fibers are known to be present in the ductus in humans and other animal species. Their chemical mediators are known to be capable of constricting the ductus, and the effects of these mediators plus oxygen have been shown to be additive.[11,16] Anatomic closure of the ductus arteriosus begins soon after birth and is completed after several weeks or months.

Cardiac output

Following birth and after the closure of the ductus arteriosus and foramen ovale, the combined cardiac output, i.e., right and left ventricular output, in the newborn lamb increases significantly in comparison with that of the fetus.[11,13] Delayed clamping of the umbilical cord may result in higher systemic and pulmonary arterial pressures and higher respiratory rates for the first 24 hours of life.

Pulmonary arterial pressure

Following the establishment of respiration, the pulmonary artery pressure does not fall abruptly in spite of the marked reduction of the pulmonary vascular resistance. Pulmonary arterial systolic pressure is near systemic levels during the first hour of life, and thereafter it decreases slowly to reach 50% of systemic levels by 24 hours of age.[22] Normal adult values are not reached until several days or weeks. The various factors that contribute to the persistence of elevated pulmonary arterial pressure and vascular resistance are summarized as follows:

1. Pulmonary vasoconstriction caused by hypoxemia and acidosis.
2. Increased pulmonary blood flow caused by left-to-right ductal shunt.
3. Reduction of the pulmonary vascular capacitance be-

cause of medial hypertrophy of the small pulmonary arteries.
4. Delayed clamping of the umbilical cord.

Pulmonary arterial pressure and vascular resistance gradually decrease over the next few weeks of life, most likely because of lung growth and the involution of the thickened smooth muscle of the media of the small pulmonary arteries.[15] A number of infants born at high altitudes tend to maintain some degree of pulmonary hypertension, and histologic examination of their pulmonary arterioles shows changes resembling the persistence of fetal pattern.

ATRIAL SEPTAL DEFECTS

Atrial septal defects (ASD) are relatively common malformations and frequently are isolated. They are located in various parts of the interatrial septum and lead to free communication between the atria (Fig. 13-2). Their hemodynamic and clinical significance depends primarily upon their size and the compliance of the right ventricle.

During early cardiac development the embryonic single atrium is partially divided by the growth of the septa. The separation of the two atria is accomplished by 6 to 8 weeks of gestation except for the persistence of the *patent foramen ovale* (through which blood flows from the right atrium to the left atrium) which occurs throughout fetal life. The *septum primum* provides an incomplete separation of the two atria. Its anteroinferior free edge lies above the atrioventricular canal and becomes lined by tissue derived from the superior and inferior endocardial cushions. Subsequently the resultant *ostium primum* is completely obliterated by growth of endocardial cushion tissue. This takes place only after the simultaneous development of fenestrations of the septum primum, which coalesce to form the ostium secundum. Concurrently, to the right of the septum primum from the anterior-superior area of the atrial roof, an infolding of atrial tissue develops and forms the *septum secundum*. The posteroinferior deficiency of the septum secundum is the *fossa ovalis*.

In the normal-term fetus postnatally, when left atrial pressure exceeds right atrial pressure, the valve of fossa ovalis (septum primum) is forced against the limbus (septum secundum), resulting in functional closure of the foramen (valve-competent foramen ovale). This communication potentially remains patent in a large number of otherwise normal adults (up to 20%). The most common location of atrial septal defects involves the fossa ovalis. They are caused by a deficiency or fenestrations of the valve with or without deficiency of the limbus of the fossa ovalis, resulting in enlargement of the ostium secundum. For this reason, these defects involving the central part of the septum are commonly called *ostium secundum* or *secundum atrial septal defects* (Fig. 13-2). They may be present in association with other more serious cardiac malformations, such as tricuspid atresia, or pulmonary atresia or stenosis with intact ventricular septum. In addition, secundum atrial septal defects may be associated with prolapsed mitral valve with or without mitral valve insufficiency. Rarely, the typical gross and microscopic features of the floppy mitral valve syndrome have been associated with secundum atrial septal defects.

The second most common atrial septal defect is the *ostium primum defect,* which involves the inferior portion of the atrial septum (persistence of the ostium primum) and embryologically belongs to the *spectrum of the endocardial cushion defects.* It can be associated with cleft in the mitral or tricuspid valve with varying degrees of mitral or tricuspid regurgitation.

Another less frequent atrial septal defect is the so-called *sinus venosus type.* It is located high in the atrial septum posterior to the fossa ovalis. The defect is usually rimmed by atrial septal tissue only antero-inferiorly. Its posterior aspect is bordered by the atrial wall and superiorly in many instances there is no actual border because of an overriding large superior vena cava. Rarely the defect may be located directly posterior or posteroinferior to the fossa ovalis, allowing the inferior vena cava to join both atria. The sinus venosus defect is usually associated with partial anomalous pulmonary venous connection of the right lung. The superior right pulmonary vein or occasionally both veins connect directly with the right atrium or the superior vena cava near its atrial junction. A very rare type of atrial septal defect called *coronary sinus type* is located inferior and slightly anterior to the fossa ovalis near the anticipated location of the ostium of the coronary sinus. In most instances, it is a part of a developmental complex that includes absent coronary sinus and a persistent left superior vena cava that enters the roof of the left atrium. This malformation may be associated with complete atrioventricular canal and is often seen in the *asplenia* syndrome. In such cases, the coronary sinus ASD is usually merged with the ostium primum ASD (a component of the A-V canal). Secundum atrial septal defects are twice as common in females than in males. A number of familial cases also have been reported.[23]

According to their hemodynamic significance, atrial septal defects, regardless of their type, can be classified as small, medium and large. With the exception of very small defects, the size of the ASD has less effect on the flow of blood from the left to right atrium than does the relative filling resistance (compliance) of the right and left ventricle. The direction of the blood flow across the defect throughout the cardiac cycle is primarily related to differences in pressure between the left and right atria. The pressures in the atria are mainly determined by the relative compliances of the respective ventricles. Thus soon after birth, even in the presence of a large atrial septal defect, the left-to-right shunt through it will be minimal because of the low right ventricular compliance (thick wall), which is at least equal to that of the left ventricle. As pulmonary vascular resistance normally decreases, due to the gradual

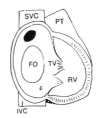 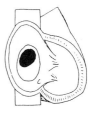

Sinus Venosus Defect   Ostium Secundum Defect

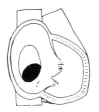 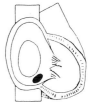

Ostium Primum Defect   Coronary Sinus Defect

Fig. 13-2. Diagrammatic illustration of four types of atrial septal defects viewed from the right atrium. (*SVC* = superior vena cava, *PT* = pulmonary trunk, *FO* = foramen ovale, *RV* = right ventricle, *IVC* = inferior vena cava, *TV* = tricuspid valve.)

reduction in right ventricular afterload, the compliance of the right ventricle improves (via thinning of its wall), resulting in decrease in its filling pressure and preferential flow during diastole from the left atrium to the right ventricle. The left ventricle, because of its high afterload (systemic circulation) maintains its low compliance (thick wall); consequently the major portion of the blood returning from the lungs preferentially enters the right ventricle through the large ASD.

Atrial septal defects of similar size in preterm or near-term infants may present with signs of heart failure earlier than the majority of term infants.[24] It appears that the right ventricular compliance improves faster in preterm infants than in term infants because of the lesser thickness of the right ventricular wall at birth and the more accelerated reduction of pulmonary vascular resistance, caused by the presence of less smooth muscle in the pulmonary arterioles and the faster growth of the lung.

As mentioned earlier, the shunt is left-to-right because the left atrial pressure exceeds that of the right during most of the duration of the cardiac cycle. A very small right-to-left shunt of blood returning from the inferior vena cava is usually present and occurs at the onset of ventricular contraction or during early diastole. It is obvious that because of the proximity of the ostia of the right pulmonary veins to the ASD, the right lung preferentially contributes the major portion of the left-to-right shunt.

With large atrial septal defects, the resultant left-to-right shunt leads to a progressive volume overload of the right ventricle. Thus the right atrium and right ventricle enlarge, whereas the pulmonary artery pressure remains

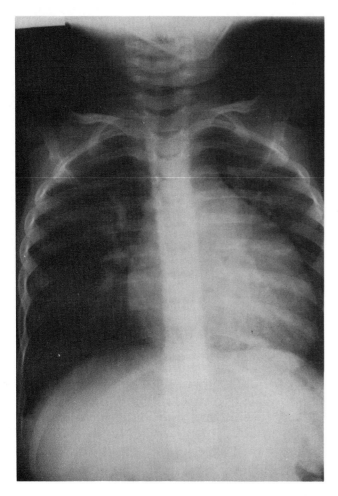

Fig. 13-3. Chest roentgenogram in a 3-year-old boy with large ostium secundum atrial septal defect. Note the considerable cardiomegaly and the increase in pulmonary vascular markings. (Courtesy of Kenneth Dooley, M.D., Egleston Children's Hospital, Atlanta, Ga.)

normal or increases only slightly. This results from the high capacitance of the pulmonary vasculature caused by vascular recruitment and dilation of perfused vessels. The pulmonary flow may increase to three times normal with only minimal increase, if any, of pulmonary arterial pressure. Thus the calculated pulmonary vascular resistance remains quite low (lower than normal). Structural changes in the pulmonary arteries may occur only late in adult life and only in a few selected cases.

Because of the large volume overload of the right ventricle, its stroke volume increases considerably, causing small systolic pressure gradients across the pulmonary valve (10 mm to 15 mm). This pressure gradient is reflected by the typical grade 2-3/6 ejection systolic murmur, heard best at the upper left sternal border. A mid-diastolic rumble can also be heard at the lower left sternal border, and it is caused by the increase in blood flow across the tricuspid valve (prolongation and accentuation of the filling sound of the right ventricle). However, the most char-

acteristic auscultatory finding of an ASD is the widely split second sound, which remains fixed with inspiration and expiration. This splitting is attributed to delay in pulmonary valve closure secondary to the large stroke volume, and it remains fixed because of the fact that the right ventricle is always filled to capacity, i.e., during both inspiration and expiration.

The chest roentgenogram shows cardiomegaly and increased pulmonary vascularity, depending upon the magnitude of the left-to-right shunt. The main pulmonary arterial segment as well as the right atrium and right ventricle are prominent (Fig. 13-3).

The electrocardiogram shows right atrial and right ventricular hypertrophy with normal or right QRS frontal axis, except in ostium primum ASD, where a left-axis deviation with counter-clockwise frontal vector is usually present (left anterior hemiblock).[25] Two-dimensional echocardiography reveals both right atrial and right ventricular enlargement, and paradoxic systolic anterior ventricular septal motion (i.e., the ventricular septum contracts with the right ventricle rather than with the left).[26] Color Doppler echocardiography in conjunction with esophageal echocardiographic techniques has become the most valuable noninvasive diagnostic method in detecting atrial septal defects. Only rarely is cardiac catheterization indicated, especially when the presence of pulmonary hypertension is suspected.[27]

Ostium secundum ASD

Ostium secundum ASD is the most common congenital malformation of the heart in adults.[27] The reason is that young patients with this defect are notoriously asymptomatic. Unless a careful physical examination by an experienced physician is performed, the defect may go undetected for many years. Very often, a secundum ASD may be suspected in an otherwise healthy adult from a chest roentgenogram.

Although life expectancy is not normal, a number of patients may reach advanced age. Natural survival (without surgery) beyond 40 to 50 years is less than 50%, with an attrition rate after 40 years of 6% per year. Older patients with ASD usually deteriorate because of atrial arrhythmias (fibrillation, flutter, paroxysmal tachycardia); age-related decreased compliance of the left ventricle (coronary artery disease, hypertension) resulting in increase in left-to-right shunt; and development of pulmonary hypertension usually of moderate degree, so the right ventricle is subjected not only to volume overload but also increasing amounts of afterload. Major pulmonary hypertension seldom ensues before the third decade. Some of these patients may reach the fourth decade, showing evidence of varying degrees of right-to-left shunt (Eisenmenger reaction) and become inoperable.[27,28]

Complications following surgical repair of secundum ASD are apparently related to the age at which the repair had occurred. In general, children and young adults operated on before 25 years of age can expect a normal life expectancy. In one study, late survival of patients with systolic pulmonary arterial pressure more than 40 mm has been reported to be half of the control subjects.[29] In general, symptomatic adults following surgical repair do not do as well as asymptomatic individuals. In patients with preoperative right heart failure and tricuspid regurgitation, late postoperative right atrial and right ventricular dilatation may persist, and right ventricular ejection fraction seldom returns to normal. Although there is some improvement in their clinical status, in general they remain symptomatic.[30,31] In patients with high pulmonary vascular resistance, there is progressive deterioration of their clinical status, with continued rise of pulmonary artery pressure and right ventricular failure.

A small number of children undergoing ASD repair may experience late onset of premature atrial extrasystoles, supraventricular tachycardias, atrial flutter, and atrial fibrillation. The exact cause of these arrhythmias is not known. It has been suggested that they may be related to atrial fibrosis and/or sinus node dysfunction. Late-onset junctional rhythm or second-degree atrioventricular block occur infrequently.[32] Nonsurgical closure of secundum atrial septal defects using a transcatheter technique has been reported recently with very good short-term results. A *double umbrella* device with a clamshell configuration that uses spring tension to attach the umbrella to the atrial septum is inserted under fluoroscopic guidance.[33] A number of selected older patients with a small secundum ASD or a patent foramen ovale have been treated successfully with this technique to prevent paradoxic emboli. In spite of the preliminary results, it has been suggested that a transcatheter approach may, in the future, supplant surgery as the procedure of choice for closure of an isolated ostium secundum ASD or patent foramen ovale.[34]

VENTRICULAR SEPTAL DEFECTS

Ventricular septal defect (VSD) as a solitary lesion is the most frequent congenital malformation of the heart, if one excludes bicuspid aortic valve and ductus arteriosus associated with extreme prematurity. According to several studies, it constitutes approximately 20% of all congenital cardiac defects. A slight female prevalence has been reported.[35]

In the developing heart, the single ventricular cavity is divided into two by a septum between the fourth and eighth week of gestation. Final closure of the interventricular foramen is dependent upon three components: continued growth of connective tissue located on the "free" edge at the muscular ventricular septum; inferior growth at the ridges dividing the conus and truncus arteriosus; and the projections into the atrioventricular canal of the endocardial cushions. A faulty development in any of these factors may result in a ventricular septal defect.

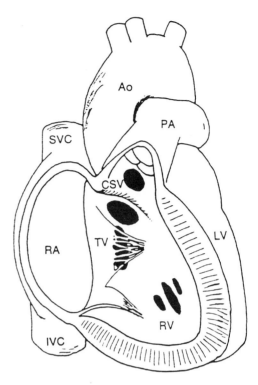

Fig. 13-4. Diagrammatic illustration of different types of ventricular septal defects viewed from the right ventricle. (*AO* = aorta, *PA* = pulmonary artery, *SVC* = superior vena cava, *RA* = right atrium, *LV* = left ventricle, *TV* = tricuspid valve, *CSV* = crista supraventricularis, *RV* = right ventricle, *IVC* = inferior vena cava.)

The ventricular septum is considered to have four components: the inlet septum separating the mitral and tricuspid valves; the trabecular septum, which extends from attachments at the tricuspid leaflet distally to the apical region of the ventricle and superiorly to the crista supraventricularis; the infundibular septum extending from the crista to the pulmonary valve; and the membranous septum, which is relatively small and is covered in part by the septal leaflet of the tricuspid valve.

Classification according to location

There are several different classifications of ventricular septal defects depending upon their anatomic location.[36] There are at least four morphologically distinct varieties of ventricular septal defects (Fig. 13-4).

Perimembranous VSD. The most common (80%) variety, this type is located in the outflow of the left ventricle immediately beneath the aortic valve. When seen from the right ventricle, it is clearly located below the crista supraventricularis and posterior to the papillary muscle of the conus. The defects may involve only the membranous septum or additionally various amounts of muscular tissue adjacent to it. They may be associated with minor anomalies of the tricuspid valve, which in part may be acquired from the impact of the shunted blood. Tricuspid valve anomalies may resemble *membranous septal aneurysms,* and they actually constitute "extra" separate leaflet tissue or pouches that can partially or completely occlude the defect. An anterior malalignment between the infundibular septum and the anterior ventricular septum may produce varying degrees of overriding at the aortic root. Posterior or leftward malalignment of the septum may produce subaortic stenosis. Moreover, a deficiency of the attachment of septal commissure of the tricuspid valve to the membranous septum may result in a direct obligatory *left ventricular-right atrial shunt.* These defects may be located both above and below the tricuspid annulus and result in both left ventricular-right ventricular and left ventricular-right atrial shunts. Very rarely an isolated left ventricular-right atrial defect is found.

Supracristal or subpulmonic VSD. This type of defect is located in the outflow tract (infundibulum) of the right ventricle and beneath the pulmonary valve. Such defects contribute 5% to 7% of all VSDs except for Oriental subjects, in whom the percentage is much higher (up to 30%).[37]

Defects of the muscular septum. These frequently are multiple and comprise 5% to 20% of defects found at surgery or autopsy. They may be associated with other VSDs and are difficult to visualize from the right ventricle because of the overlying muscular trabeculae and the presence of tortuous channels. They may be quite large, involving the apical portion or midportion of the muscular septum. Very rarely the "Swiss cheese" type of multiple muscular ventricular septal defects may be present, involving the entire muscular septum (primitive myocardium).

Isolated inlet defects. Located posterior and inferior to the membranous defects lying beneath the septal cusp of the tricuspid valve and inferior to the papillary muscle of the conus, these defects have been previously called VSDs of the atrioventricular canal type. However, because of the frequent absence of associated mitral or tricuspid abnormalities and the absence of left axis deviation (left anterior hemiblock in the ECG), some authors do not consider them as part of the spectrum of endocardial cushion defects. Prolapse (herniation) of the right or noncoronary aortic cusp, with varying degrees of aortic valve regurgitation, has been found to be associated with supracristal and some large perimembranous VSDs. The prolapsed leaflet may produce moderate right ventricular outflow pressure gradients or partially obliterate the moderate to large ventricular septal defect.[37]

Location and conduction pathways. Knowledge of the course of the atrioventricular conduction pathways and its relationship to the position of the VSD is very important to the operating surgeon. In *perimembranous defects,* the bundle of His is located in a subendocardial position as it courses the posterior-inferior margin of the defect. Surgical damage to the bundle of His can produce occasionally complete heart block.

In *inlet defects* (A-V canal type), the bundle of His passes anterosuperiorly to the defect. In *muscular defects* and *outlet defects* the conduction tissue is far removed from the area of the defect, and the risk for complete heart block is minimal unless the defect extends toward the perimembranous area. Right bundle branch block (RBBB) occurs frequently after repair of ventricular septal defects. This may result from damage of the right bundle branch, which can course along the posterior-inferior margin of infracristal defects. However, right vertical ventriculotomy alone may cause postoperative RBBB in up to 80% of cases of repaired ventricular septal defects, suggesting that the block is caused by disruption of a distal branch or branches of the right bundle.[38]

Classification according to size

Another useful clinical classification of VSDs is based upon their size. Therefore, VSDs have been classified as *small, medium,* and *large.* In small and medium VSDs, the limiting factor determining the magnitude of the left-to-right shunt is the actual size of the defect. However, in large defects with sizes approximately the size of the aortic orifice, there is no resistance to blood flow across the opening of the defect. Therefore in such cases the relative systemic and pulmonary vascular resistances will determine the flow across the defect. Accordingly, defect size and the respective circulatory resistances determine the magnitude of the systemic and pulmonary flow, the pressures in the two circulations, the work characteristics of the atria and ventricles, and the clinical features.

As discussed earlier, after birth the rate of decline of the pulmonary vascular resistance (PVR) determines the magnitude of right ventricular pressure. In the absence of pulmonary disease and hypoxemia, the right ventricular pressure may reach near normal adult levels within 7 to 10 days after birth.

Small VSD. With this type, where the resistance to flow resides in the defect itself, left-to-right shunt producing a loud systolic murmur (turbulence) may appear within the first few hours after birth and continue to be audible as long as the defect is present. Children with small VSDs are generally asymptomatic and have a normal chest roentgenogram and electrocardiogram.

Large defects. However, in the presence of a large VSD, the rate of maturational changes of the pulmonary vascular bed (reduction of PVR) is delayed and the resultant maintenance of a relatively high PVR acts as a protective mechanism against massive left-to-right shunting of blood through the VSD and flooding of the lungs. In addition, increases of left atrial pressures and left ventricular overloading secondary to the large left-to-right shunt may play an important role in maintaining peripheral pulmonary arterial constriction. When the pulmonary vessels are stretched to the limit of their surrounding fibrous tissues, further increases in blood flow result in directly proportional increases in pressure. Thus the markedly stretched vessels may undergo injury that results eventually in thickening of the adventitia, medial wall smooth muscle hypertrophy, and even intimal injury. These progressive vascular changes in the pulmonary circulation have been repeatedly documented, but the exact basic mechanisms involved in the development of end-stage pulmonary vascular disease have not been completely understood. The contribution of humoral vasoactive substances, produced locally with or without the influence of the autonomic nervous system, triggered by the stretch of the wall of the pulmonary arterial vessels, has not been elucidated as yet.

Medium VSD. With this type of defect (and large ones as well), as the pulmonary vascular resistance gradually declines within the first few weeks of life, the left-to-right shunt increases, progressively resulting in pulmonary blood flow that is three to four times larger than systemic flow. The increase in pulmonary flow in the absence of a patent foramen ovale or an ASD leads to elevation of pulmonary venous and left atrial pressures. This increase in pulmonary venous return leads to left atrial and left ventricular dilatation, as well as an increase in left ventricular mass. This increase in volume overloading of the left ventricle may lead to left ventricular failure in infants during the first 4 to 12 weeks of life. Symptoms of left ventricular failure are respiratory difficulties such as tachypnea or dyspnea, feeding difficulties, and failure to thrive. The mechanisms by which such infants adapt to the volume load include the Frank-Starling effect, increased sympathetic cardiac stimulation, and myocardial hypertrophy.[39] The rate of development of myocardial hypertrophy determines the ability to adapt and compensate adequately to the load imposed on the heart by the large left-to-right shunt.[40] An overactive precordium with loud heart sounds and loud systolic murmur are usually present. Cardiomegaly and increased pulmonary vascular markings are seen in the chest roentgenogram and left or combined ventricular hypertrophy is shown by electrocardiogram. Doppler echocardiographic examination usually confirms the diagnosis.

In the presence of some elevation of PVR and a large left-to-right shunt, the pulmonary and aortic peak systolic pressures may be about equal. The continued pulmonary vascular response in such instances may be variable. In some cases there is little change in PVR, and the amount of left-to-right shunt remains stable. However, in certain patients under similar conditions, the dilatation and stretch of the pulmonary arteries and the increase in vascular tone is followed by hypertrophy of the smooth muscle of the vascular media, continued pulmonary hypertension, and gradual development of intimal sclerotic changes. Usually such changes occur in patients with large VSD, in which there is a common ejectile force from both ventricles. With progressive increase of PVR there is a diminution of the pulmonary flow and reduction in the left atrial and left

ventricular size. These changes are usually associated with improvement in the clinical status of the infant and reduction of the length and intensity of the systolic murmur. As the PVR exceeds the SVR, the pressure between the two ventricles will equalize, and the direction of the blood flow will be predominantly right-to-left (Eisenmenger complex).[41] Although this sequence of events is the most common, there is a group of infants who seem to maintain high PVR throughout infancy, balanced shunting via the VSD, and normal or near-normal left ventricular size and muscle mass. These infants do not show clinical signs of left ventricular decompensation either in infancy or childhood. Thus the *end-stage Eisenmenger complex* is indistinguishable between these two groups.[41] Severe degrees of polycythemia and right ventricular decompensation will eventually ensue early in adulthood.

Right ventricular workload. In patients with small VSD right ventricular workload remains normal, as does the right ventricular systolic pressure and wall thickness. In a medium defect, where some pulmonary hypertension may be present, the right ventricle may be called upon to perform some extra work. Thus mild to moderate hypertrophy may develop as a result of this increase in pressure. In the presence of large VSD with a common ejectile impulse, the right ventricle is called upon to perform considerable work to overcome the increased resistance during the ejection. Thus the right ventricle, hypertrophies to a greater extent. Moreover, with moderate or large left-to-right shunts, the right ventricle may also enlarge in volume depending upon the degree of diastolic left-to-right shunting from the left ventricle. However, because the major shunting occurs during systole, the right ventricle does not enlarge to the same extent as the left ventricle, i.e., during ventricular systole the right ventricle acts as a "contracting tube" that accepts the blood shunted from the left ventricle.

Spontaneous closure

It has been well documented that a large number of ventricular septal defects, especially muscular defects, spontaneously close within the first 2 years of life (30%).[42] Spontaneous closure may also occur later in life, especially during adolescence. The smaller the size of the VSD, the more likely is its spontaneous closure (up to 80%) whereas large VSDs close spontaneously less frequently (10%).[35,43] Spontaneous closure is the reason why ventricular septal defects are not seen commonly during adulthood. Defects located in the inlet and the infundibular septum do not usually decrease in size, unlike perimembranous and muscular defects.

Survival

Patients with VSD who survive into adulthood without surgical intervention comprise two groups: those with small or moderately restrictive defects that have closed spontaneously or decreased in size enough to become clinically not apparent or hemodynamically insignificant; and patients with nonrestrictive VSD who belong to the Eisenmenger complex, i.e., with suprasystemic pulmonary hypertension caused by an increase in PVR and right-to-left shunt. They usually develop right ventricular failure during the third or fourth decade, although occasionally patients may survive longer.[44] Heart and lung transplantation has been offered in some of these older patients with not very satisfactory results. The patient with a small restrictive VSD is apparently prone to development of bacterial endocarditis following potentially bacteremic conditions such as dental procedures.

In general, perimembranous defects are repaired from the right atrium via the tricuspid valve. Right ventriculotomy is usually reserved for supra-cristal defects, whereas left ventriculotomy has been utilized for multiple muscular defects. Transatrial repair of VSD reduces the risk of late postoperative occurrence of right ventricular ectopic rhythms by avoiding right ventriculotomy. However, it may induce proximal right bundle branch block. When the operation is performed during the first 2 years of life, the results are usually excellent. Patients can be expected to reach adulthood and to be asymptomatic with normal ventricular size and function. However, when surgical repair is performed in older children, a late postoperative increase in left ventricular chamber size and mass may persist together with reduced incidence of left ventricular systolic function. A residual ventricular septal defect with small left-to-right shunt may persist postoperatively. This is caused by incomplete closure of the defect (10% to 25%) or a loosening of one or two superficially placed sutures during the closure of VSD.

In older children operated with borderline increase in pulmonary vascular resistance, progressive increase in PVR, despite elimination of the left-to-right shunt, leading to right ventricular failure has been reported. The attrition rate for individuals with VSD and PVR exceeding 10 Wood units per square meter, is approximately 25% within 5 years. A small number of adults with relatively stable, moderate postoperative pulmonary vascular disease apparently have survived 20 years following the operation.[44]

ENDOCARDIAL CUSHION DEFECTS (ATRIOVENTRICULAR CANAL DEFECTS)

Endocardial cushion defects are caused by faulty development of the endocardial cushions and the atrioventricular septum. There are three general types of endocardial cushion (atrioventricular canal) defects: the *partial type,* consisting most frequently of an *ostium primum atrial septal defect* (ASD) with or without a cleft in the anterior leaflet at the mitral valve; the *complete type,* which is commonly seen in patients with Down syndrome; the *transitional type,* a rare defect in which the anterior and posterior bridging leaflets of the common A-V valve are fused in the midline.

Less common forms of the partial type include common atrium, ventricular septal defect of the inlet type, isolated cleft of the anterior leaflet of the mitral valve, and a widened medial tricuspid commissure.[23,45]

The development of the tubular heart into a four-chambered functioning pump is usually complete by 8 to 10 weeks gestation. This transition is accomplished by a number of processes involving the proliferation of the endocardial cushions, which are responsible for the formation of the atrioventricular valves, the septum primum separating the two atria, the ventricular septum, and the development of dextrodorsal conus. Thus developmental errors in the formation of these components may result in the persistence of a centrally located atrioventricular communication (atrioventricular foramen) and variable anatomic abnormalities of the atrioventricular valves (Fig. 13-5). In such cases the anterior leaflet of the mitral valve is almost always deformed, and occasionally the anteroseptal commissure of the tricuspid valve is involved.

Pathophysiology of these defects varies with the nature and severity of the defect.

Ostium primum atrial septal defect

This is the most common type of partial A-V canal defect and is usually associated with a cleft in the anterior leaflet of the mitral valve. The defect is located anteroinferiorly to the fossa ovalis and is bordered by a crescentic rim of atrial septal tissue posterosuperiorly and by mitral-tricuspid valvular continuity anteroposteriorly. This defect is less common than the secundum ASD, and sex distribution is equal.[23]

The resultant left-to-right shunt may be large depending upon the size of the defect and the compliance of the right ventricle, and almost invariably there is mitral valve insufficiency of varying degree. The left-to-right shunt from the ASD and the obligatory left ventricular-right atrial shunt via the mitral valve insufficiency may cause significant right ventricular volume overloading. Occasionally, in patients with ostium primum ASD, left ventricular obstruction may be present (subaortic stenosis), which may become progressively more severe after surgical closure of the ASD.[46] Hypoplasia of the left ventricle, as well as hypoplasia of the aortic isthmus or coarctation of the aorta, also has been rarely seen in association with partial A-V canal.[47]

Infants with primum ASD may become symptomatic earlier and more frequently than those with secundum ASD. Besides the typical ejection systolic murmur at the upper left sternal border and the tricuspid mid-diastolic murmur, a holosystolic murmur of mitral insufficiency may be present. The electrocardiogram has a characteristic superior frontal QRS axis ($-30°$ to $-120°$) with counterclockwise frontal QRS vector, with evidence of right ventricular hypertrophy. The *left axis deviation* persists even after surgical repair of the defect, and results from the ab-

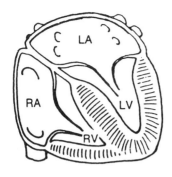

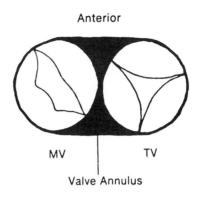

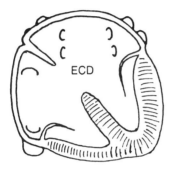

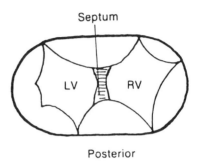

Fig. 13-5. Diagrammatic illustration of normal relation of the atrioventricular valves (upper) and their relation in endocardial cushion defect *(ECD)* (atrioventricular canal). (*MV* = mitral valve, *TV* = tricuspid valve.)

normal course of the branches of the left bundle of His (left anterior hemiblock pattern).[48] Two-dimensional and Doppler echocardiography are considered the most useful tools for the diagnosis of both partial and complete A-V canal defects.

The complete form of endocardial cushion defect

This type is characterized by a large atrioventricular septal defect, a common atrioventricular valve originating from both atria, and variable deficiency of the superior edge of the muscular ventricular septum. Thus the septal defect extends to the level of the membranous septum, which is usually markedly deficient or absent. The length from the crux to apex is foreshortened. The left ventricular outflow tract is long and narrow and has been referred to angiocardiographically as the *goose neck* deformity. After surgical repair of either partial or complete A-V canal defects, subaortic stenosis may develop in some patients.[46,49] The stenosis may be caused by either mitral valve or left ventricular abnormalities. The common atrioventricular valve usually has five major leaflets and commissures. The interventricular defect lies between the two bridging leaflets and in the majority of cases is located beneath these

two leaflets. The posterior bridging leaflet overhangs the ventricular septum and has extensive chordal attachments to it that frequently obliterate completely the potential interventricular communication.

The morphologic relationship between the anterior bridging leaflet and the underlying ventricular septum varies considerably and has been utilized in the subclassification of the complete form of the A-V canal defect. Three subtypes have been proposed.

In *Type A,* the anterior bridging leaflet is committed almost completely to the left ventricle, and its commissure with the anterior tricuspid leaflet lies along the right anteroposterior rim of the ventricular septum. Beneath this commissure there is either a distinct medial papillary muscle or, more frequently, multiple direct chordal insertions into the septum. This type of defect is most common.

Type B is characterized by a larger anterior bridging leaflet that overhangs the ventricular septum more than in Type A. The medial papillary muscle attaches on the septomarginal trabecula or on the moderator band. Because of the absence of chordal connection to the underlying ventricular septum, a free interventricular communication exists. This type is relatively rare.

Type C has a much larger anterior bridging leaflet that overhangs the ventricular septum more than that of types A and B. The anterior tricuspid leaflet is very small, and the medial papillary muscle attaches to the anterior tricuspid papillary muscle. Thus the large anterior bridging leaflet is "free floating," leaving a free unimpeded interventricular communication.[23,45]

Endocardial cushion defects may be associated with other congenital malformations of the heart. Type A defects are commonly associated with Down syndrome.[23] Type C defects are often associated with other complex cardiac anomalies such as tetralogy of Fallot, double outlet right ventricle, D-transposition of the great arteries, and polysplenia-asplenia syndromes (situs ambiguous). The common A-V valve of the complete form of the A-V canal defect often shows gross and microscopic features of a "floppy valve." The intermediate form of the A-V canal defect resembles the complete form except for the fusion of the anterior bridging leaflets on top of the ventricular septum. These leaflets often have insufficient tissue from which a competent anterior mitral valve leaflet could be reconstructed by the operating surgeon.

Infants with complete A-V canal defect may present with signs of congestive heart failure associated with frequent lower respiratory infections and failure to grow. They are small and undernourished, and virtually all become symptomatic during the first year of life. In the absence of severe pulmonary vascular obstruction, they do not show arterial desaturation. They may have both abnormal right and left ventricular precordial impulse and loud heart sounds. A holosystolic apical murmur of mitral insufficiency may be present, as well as an ejection systolic murmur over the left upper sternal border (increased blood flow across the pulmonary valve). A mid-diastolic murmur may be also audible at the lower left sternal border and the apex. This is caused by the increase in diastolic flow across the common A-V valve. These findings may be indistinguishable from those of an isolated VSD or partial A-V canal. The electrocardiogram shows the typical left frontal QRS axis deviation seen in endocardial cushion defects and usually more right ventricular hypertrophy covering the left ventricular forces (hypertrophy) that may be present.

Two-dimensional echocardiography and Doppler echocardiography are the most reliable and informative examinations for the diagnosis and anatomic classification of the complete A-V canal. Moreover, anatomic subgroups can be recognized by the characteristic chordal insertions and the size and special features of the anterior bridging leaflet of the common A-V valve. Cardiac catheterization and angiocardiography are recommended preoperatively for the assessment of pulmonary vascular resistance, the size of the left ventricle and its outflow tract, and associated other defects.

The clinical course of patients with the complete form

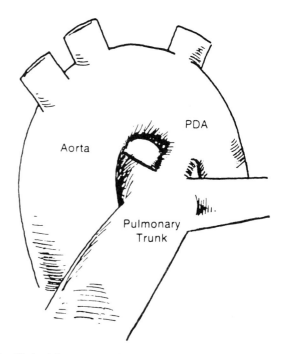

Fig. 13-6. A large patent ductus arteriosus. The shunt through it will depend on the differences in vascular resistance between the pulmonary and systemic circulation.

of A-V canal defect depends upon several underlying factors: the size of the defect, the magnitude of the atrioventricular valve insufficiency, the magnitude of the pulmonary vascular resistance, the size of the left ventricle, and the extent of the A-V valve malformation.

Postoperatively, complete heart block as well as atrial and ventricular dysrhythmias may complicate the long-term survival of these patients.[48] In many instances, postoperative residual mitral stenosis and/or insufficiency requires further surgical intervention. A number of children with Down syndrome and very high pulmonary vascular resistance, prohibitive for surgical correction, may survive for 2 or 3 decades in spite of the development of Eisenmenger syndrome.

PATENT DUCTUS ARTERIOSUS

The ductus arteriosus is a large vascular channel connecting the main pulmonary arterial trunk with the descending thoracic aorta, just distal to the left subclavian artery (Fig. 13-6). Its role in fetal circulation has been discussed earlier.[11]

At approximately the sixth week of gestation, the ductus arteriosus (DA) is sufficiently developed to carry the major portion of right ventricular output. This large vascular channel is derived from the distal portion of the left sixth aortic arch. In the presence of a right aortic arch the DA may be on the right side, joining the right pulmonary artery. However, more commonly it is found on the left side, connecting the left pulmonary artery and the proximal portion of the left subclavian artery. The DA is rarely bilateral. In the normal-term fetus its diameter is similar to that of the descending aorta.

The histologic structure of the wall of the DA is quite different from that of the pulmonary artery and aorta. In contrast to the aorta and pulmonary artery, the media of which are composed by circumferentially arranged layers of elastic fibers, the media of a DA contains dense layers of smooth muscle arranged spirally in both directions (right and left). Moreover, the intimal layer of the DA is thicker than the adjoining arteries and contains increased amounts of mucoid substance.[50]

The process of postnatal closure of the DA in the normal-term newborn involves two stages: functional closure produced by contraction of the smooth muscle of its wall, which thickens, and the protrusion into the lumen of intimal cushions (thickened intima). This process generally occurs within 10 to 15 hours after birth. The second stage of closure is usually completed by 2 to 3 weeks and involves disruption and proliferation of the subintimal layers, resulting in connective tissue formation and permanent closure (ligamentum arteriosum).

Although the exact mechanisms of postnatal closure of DA are not well understood, factors such as length of gestation, oxygen, and vasoactive substances such as prostaglandins and catecholamines seem to play an important role in this process.[11,50] For example, a large number of preterm infants with respiratory distress syndrome (RDS), kept alive by respiratory assistance and more recently with the use of pulmonary surfactant therapy, were found to have patent ductus arteriosus (PDA) with large left-to-right shunts, complicating the course of their disease.[51] Moreover, in term infants with systemic hypoxemia caused by pulmonary disease, delay in the closing process of the DA has been observed with clinically detrimental results ("persistent fetal circulation syndrome").[10] Histologic changes in the wall of the DA resulting in its partial anatomic closure, even before birth, have been described in some stillborn infants and neonates dying within a few hours after birth.[52]

Whereas the incidence of PDA in preterm infants, depending upon their gestational age and the presence of RDS, ranges from 30% to 80%, the incidence of isolated PDA in the term infant beyond the neonatal period is considerably less (1 in 2000 live births). It accounts for 5% to 10% of all types of congenital heart disease. Unlike the PDA in premature infants, in whom failure to close is caused by physiologic developmental causes, the PDA in full-term infants is abnormal and related to a significant structural abnormality. As mentioned earlier, exposure to rubella in the first trimester of pregnancy may cause multiple congenital abnormalities in various systems, including the cardiovascular system.[5] The rubella virus apparently interferes with the normal formation of arterial elastic tissue, resulting in patency of the ductus arteriosus and

peripheral pulmonary and systemic arterial stenoses. PDA has been observed in more than one member of certain families, suggesting the existence of genetic factors in its pathogenesis. Arterial hypoxemia induced by nonpulmonary causes, such as living in high altitudes, has been also shown to be associated with delayed closure of the DA. It has been reported that the incidence of PDA is 30 times greater at high altitude (4500 m. to 5000 m.) than at sea level.

The initial constriction of the DA starts at its pulmonary arterial end and progresses toward the aorta. Such constriction results in the typical cone shape of the small PDA in which the diameter of its lumen at the aortic end is much larger than that of the lumen at the pulmonary end. Even after spontaneous complete closure of a small DA, the dilated aortic end may persist for several weeks, months, or years as "ductus diverticulum," a site from which a dissecting aneurysm may originate later on in adult life.

Control of the magnitude of shunt across the DA, as with other types of shunts, depends primarily upon three factors: the diameter of its lumen; the pressure difference between the aorta and pulmonary artery; and the respective pulmonary (PVR) and systemic vascular resistances (SVR). With a small PDA, because of the high resistance offered by the constricted ductus, the left-to-right shunt will be small despite the presence of large pressure differences between the aorta and pulmonary artery. In contrast, with a large PDA, the pressures between the two circulations may become almost equal, and the magnitude of the shunt is primarily determined by the relationship between pulmonary and systemic vascular resistances. Thus the left-to-right ductal shunting through the DA has been called *dependent shunting;* in the presence of relatively high and stable SVR, change in PVR after birth is the major determinant of the amounts of shunted blood.

The amount of blood shunted from the aorta to the pulmonary artery will cause an increase in left atrial and ventricular preload. Although with small shunts this volume load can be easily handled by the left atrium and ventricle, large volumes of pulmonary venous blood will result in increase of left ventricular diastolic volume and consequently in increased left ventricle stroke volume (Frank-Starling mechanism). Left ventricular dilatation will result in increase of left ventricular end-diastolic pressure and left atrial pressure, and may lead to heart failure and pulmonary edema. Right ventricular failure may only occur in the presence of a large PDA associated with pulmonary hypertension and/or pulmonary edema.

Compensatory physiologic mechanisms aimed at maintaining a normal effective systemic output include the following: Frank-Starling mechanism, myocardial hypertrophy, and stimulation of the sympathetic adrenal system. The latter will result in increases of the force of contraction, as well as increases in heart rate. These mechanisms are most likely responsible for the rapid heart rate and the sweating usually seen in infants with heart failure. With continued persistence of the volume overload, compensatory myocardial hypertrophy ensues. In general, these compensatory mechanisms are well developed in older children and adults but are not as well developed in newborn infants and even less developed in preterm infants. Thus it is very important to pay attention to the degree of maturity of the infant, i.e., the gestational age at the time of birth of an infant who has clinical evidence of PDA. Sympathetic innervation of the left ventricular myocardium may only be completed at term, so the premature infant is likely to have incomplete responses to sympathetic stimulation.[18] Moreover, the myocardial response to stretch of the premature animal (Frank-Starling mechanism) appears to be less vigorous than that of the more mature animal.[17,18] Another important factor in the cardiovascular adaptation of the infant with large DA and left-to-right shunt is the maintenance of coronary perfusion of the myocardium. The low aortic diastolic pressure, a consequence of the diastolic runoff, in conjunction with the elevated left ventricular end-diastolic pressure, may adversely influence myocardial perfusion.

With large communications between the aorta and pulmonary artery, the normal postnatal involution of the medial smooth muscle of small pulmonary arteries will be delayed, resulting in slower-than-normal rates in the postnatal reduction of PVR.[50]

Progressive development of pulmonary vascular disease leading to right-to-left shunting (Eisenmenger complex) may develop in certain cases with large DA and persistence of high PVR.

Older patients with small ductus arteriosus are usually asymptomatic. They have normal heart sounds and precordial activity. The only significant finding in these patients is the presence of a loud continuous murmur. In preterm infants initially the heart murmur is crescendo systolic, and only later does it become continuous. Jet lesions in the pulmonary artery may result from longstanding untreated PDA (caused by the shunting of blood). Such lesions always carry the risk of becoming the site of infectious endocarditis.

Infants and older children with moderate or large PDA become symptomatic in a manner similar to those with large ventricular septal defects: with signs of left ventricular failure (i.e., tachypnea, feeding problems, irritability, and failure to thrive). There is usually a hyperactive precordium, bounding pulses, loud heart sounds, and a loud continuous murmur over the upper left sternal border. However, in preterm infants recovering from RDS, the heart murmur is usually only systolic, and in many instances no murmur is audible (silent DA).[51]

In the chest roentgenogram cardiomegaly is usually present (left atrial and left ventricular enlargement), as well as increase in pulmonary vascularity. In older chil-

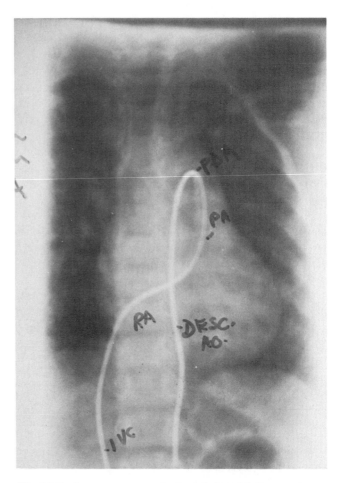

Fig. 13-7. A roentgenogram obtained during right heart catheterization showing the course of the catheter through the patent ductus arteriosus from the pulmonary artery to the descending aorta. (Courtesy of Kenneth Dooley, M.D., Egleston Children's Hospital, Atlanta, Ga.)

dren with large PDA, the electrocardiogram may show left ventricular or combined ventricular hypertrophy and left atrial dilatation.

At the present time, the most useful diagnostic aid is provided by Doppler echocardiography. The DA can be visualized as can the systolic and diastolic flow through it. In addition, assessment of left atrial and ventricular chamber size and function can be easily obtained. Cardiac catheterization is indicated only to accurately assess the pulmonary hemodynamics and the presence of other associated lesions (Fig. 13-7).

Occasionally with the progressive development of pulmonary vascular disease (Eisenmenger complex), the heart murmur becomes shorter and may disappear. A loud pulmonary closure sound is present and differential cyanosis may be detected, i.e., cyanosis and clubbing of the lower extremities with pink upper body caused by the right-to-left shunt across the ductus.

Surgical ligation of the DA is usually recommended for symptomatic infants and children. Asymptomatic children

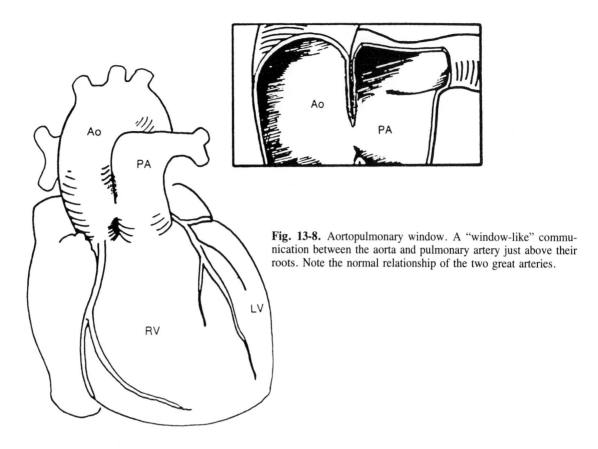

Fig. 13-8. Aortopulmonary window. A "window-like" communication between the aorta and pulmonary artery just above their roots. Note the normal relationship of the two great arteries.

over 1 year of age with small DA also undergo ductus ligation on an elective basis. The long-term results of surgery are excellent. The use of indomethacin in the treatment of preterm infants with PDA has practically eliminated the need for surgical ligation of the DA.

Patent ductus arteriosus associated with other cardiac malformations

Persistent patency of the DA may be associated with other shunting lesions such as ventricular septal defect, atrial septal defect, and endocardial cushion defects. Clinical recognition may be difficult because of the similarity of symptoms and the masking of clinical signs by the dominant associated lesion. It is prudent to always seek subtle signs such as prominent pulses in infants with heart failure, and other findings suggestive of ventricular septal defect. In many instances, careful two dimensional Doppler echocardiographic studies may uncover an associated PDA complicating a VSD or endocardial cushion defect.[50]

However, PDA is essential for survival in certain complex congenital malformations of the heart such as pulmonary atresia with or without a VSD, hypoplastic left heart syndrome, infantile coarctation of the aorta, or interrupted aortic arch. In cases of pulmonary atresia, the DA may be the only source of pulmonary blood flow, and its spontaneous closure is incompatible with extrauterine survival. The intravenous administration of prostaglandin E_1, by relaxing

the constricted DA, results in marked improvement in oxygenation and stabilization of these infants, prior to palliative surgical intervention necessary for long survival.

Ductus dependency for survival is of a different nature in cases of coarctation of the aorta, interrupted aortic arch, or hypoplastic left heart syndrome. In such instances, the blood crossing the usually large DA is the only source of supply to the lower part of the body in cases of coarctation of the aorta or the entire body in cases of hypoplastic left heart syndrome. Prostaglandin E_1 infusion, again by relaxing the constricted ductus arteriosus, results in reestablishment of systemic perfusion and improvement of the clinical status and renal function prior to palliative or definitive surgical intervention.

Aortopulmonary window

The pathophysiology of this cardiac malformation is similar to a patent ductus arteriosus. It consists of a direct communication ("window") between the left side of the aorta and the right side of the main pulmonary trunk (Fig. 13-8). It is frequently associated with a ventricular septal defect. The defect is located just above the roots of the great vessels, and its opening may vary from a few millimeters to more than 20 mm. It is obvious that spontaneous closure of such a defect is not expected and, depending upon its size, left-to-right shunting will occur soon after birth, producing murmurs similar to those of PDA heard in

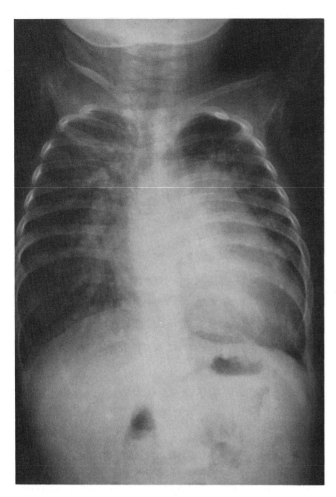

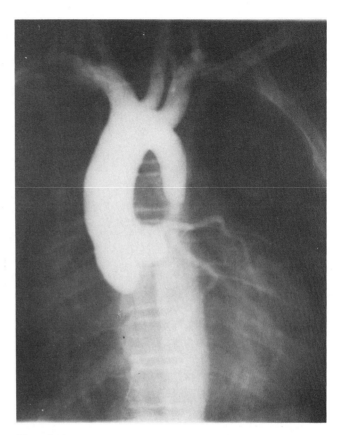

Fig. 13-10. Aortogram from a child showing typical (adult-type) coarctation of the aorta (see text). There is a bicuspid aortic valve and normally arising aortic arch branches. (Courtesy of Kenneth Dooley, M.D., Egleston Children's Hospital, Atlanta, Ga.)

Fig. 13-9. Chest roentgenogram obtained from a 5-month-old infant with aortopulmonary window. Note the massive cardiomegaly, prominence of the main pulmonary artery segment, and markedly increased pulmonary vascularity. (Courtesy of Kenneth Dooley, M.D., Egleston Children's Hospital, Atlanta, Ga.)

a lower location at the left sternal border. Larger defects may lead to equalization of systemic and pulmonary arterial pressures where shunting through the defect is controlled by the respective differences between pulmonary and systemic vascular resistances (Fig. 13-9). Reversal of the shunt, (right-to-left) will eventually ensue in cases of large defects and increases in PVR (Eisenmenger complex).

Embryologically the defect is apparently caused by incomplete spiral separation of the primitive fetal truncus arteriosus into the two great arteries. This defect occurs less than 2% of all cases of DA. The differentiation of this rare lesion from an isolated DA is absolutely necessary before surgical treatment is contemplated because the operative approach is different.

COARCTATION OF THE AORTA

Coarctation of the aorta is a relatively common vascular malformation, consisting of a narrowing of the aortic lu-

men, located usually opposite the insertion of the ductus arteriosus and distal to the left subclavian artery. The narrowing can be discrete or may involve a long segment. Rarely, its location may be lower down in the thoracic or abdominal aorta (Figs. 13-10 and 13-11).[53,54]

Coarctation of the aorta (CA), isolated or in combination with other cardiac anomalies, is a frequent cause of heart failure in infancy. In one large study among infants under 1 year of age with cardiac malformations, CA was found to be the fifth most common defect, occurring for 7.5% of all malformations.[55] The true incidence of this lesion, however, is much higher because a large number of affected individuals remain undiagnosed during the first year of life.

The exact *pathogenesis* of this anomaly has not been completely elucidated but most likely it involves a disturbance in the formation of the left fourth aortic arch during the sixth to eighth week of gestation. It has long been postulated that coarctation may develop because of the presence of aberrant fibromuscular-ductal tissue in the aortic wall.[56,57] However, this theory cannot explain the association of a widely patent ductus arteriosus with severe coarctation frequently involving a long segment of the distal aortic arch. It appears that certain prenatal hemodynamic

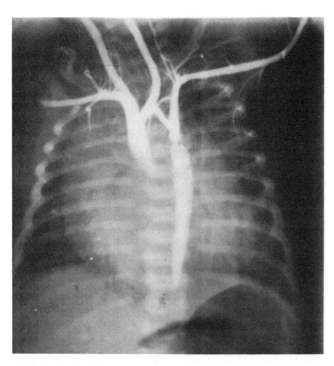

Fig. 13-11. Aortogram in a very young infant with heart failure demonstrating discrete coarctation of the aorta associated with marked hypoplasia of the transverse aortic arch. Note the marked cardiomegaly and prominent pulmonary vasculature. (Courtesy of Kenneth Dooley, M.D., Egleston Children's Hospital, Atlanta, Ga.)

factors may also play a significant role in the development of this lesion.[58] In the normal fetus the aortic isthmus receives a relatively small fraction of the left ventricular output, normally causing an anatomic narrowing of the isthmus in comparison with the descending aorta distal to the insertion of the ductus.[13] Any interference with the normal fetal left ventricular output, caused by either a large ventricular septal defect, or mitral valve abnormalities and/or significant narrowing of the left ventricular outflow tract, may lead to further decrease in blood flow through the aortic isthmus and thus promote the development of coarctation.[58]

There is definite male preponderance of CA, an observation that is concordant with the sex distribution of other left-sided obstructive lesions. Like most other congenital aortic malformations, the sporadic occurrence of CA is most likely determined by multifactoral inheritance. However, specific genetic factors occasionally may have a major influence on the development of coarctation, such as the XO Turner syndrome, in which CA is commonly associated with other cardiac malformations. Moreover, there are certain families where more than one member was found to have CA, and it was reported to affect two sets of monozygotic twins.[56,57]

A typical CA consists of a localized narrowing of the aortic lumen distal to the origin of the left subclavian artery and opposite of the insertion of the ductus arteriosus,

patent or obliterated. For this reason, the term *juxtaductal coarctation* is currently used instead of *preductal* or *postductal* CA, terms commonly used in the past. There is usually a ridge-like posterior infolding of the aortic wall (shelf), which could be an isolated lesion or associated with varying degrees of tubular hypoplasia of the aortic isthmus and distal transverse arch. Occasionally, the left subclavian artery may arise distal to the stenotic transverse arch, or rarely the right subclavian artery may aberrantly arise distal to the coarctation. For this reason blood pressure measurements always should be obtained from both upper extremities to avoid missing the presence of hypertension secondary to coarctation of the aorta. Rarely, there is *complete interruption of the aortic arch* and in such cases the term *preductal* coarctation is an appropriate one.[57] The lower part of the body is perfused exclusively by blood from the right ventricle via the ductus arteriosus. In such cases invariably there is an associated ventricular septal defect.

The terms *simple coarctation* and *complex coarctation* also have been used to describe, respectively, isolated coarctation and coarctation associated with other significant intracardiac defects. Simple CA in infancy is frequently associated with a patent ductus arteriosus. In some infants the aortic end of the unconstricted ductus arteriosus opposite of the "self" of coarctation allows for the blood to flow freely through the coarctation to the descending aorta. The coarctation may become clinically detectable only after constriction and closure of the ductus.

Complex coarctation in infancy occurs more frequently than isolated coarctation. Ventricular septal defect, subvalvular or valvular aortic stenosis, and mitral valve anomalies are the most common coexisting intracardiac malformations. The VSD may be single or multiple, of the membranous, muscular, or malalignment type. A malalignment VSD with a posterior displacement of the conal septum may impinge on the left ventricular outflow tract, leading to subaortic stenosis. Bicuspid aortic valve is the most frequently associated lesion in CA (50% to 80%). Mitral stenosis may be caused by a supravalvular ring, dysplasia of the leaflets and chordae tendineae, or papillary muscle abnormalities, including the "parachute" deformity, in which the chordae tendineae insert into a single papillary muscle. The complex anomaly of coarctation of the aorta with subaortic and mitral stenosis constitutes what has been called a *Shone* syndrome. Less frequently, endocardial cushion defect, double outlet right ventricle, D-transposition with tricuspid atresia, L-transposition, and endocardial fibroelastosis, have been also found to be associated with CA.[56,57]

Arterial collateral circulation between the upper and lower part of the body is usually developed in patients surviving infancy without surgical intervention. An anterior collateral system develops between the internal thoracic arteries and the superior and inferior epigastric arteries, which connect to the external iliac arteries. A posterior arterial collateral system also develops between branches of the thyrocervical trunk that connect to intercostal arteries and the descending thoracic aorta. Thus blood flows in a retrograde fashion through the intercostal arteries in the descending aorta. These dilated and tortuous arteries may erode the lower margins of the ribs in older children, causing the frequently seen "rib notching" in the chest roentgenograms.

A localized area of intimal thickening and distortion of the media is often seen distal to the contraductal shelf. This is apparently caused by the jet of blood across the coarctation, which erodes the intima over a small area of distal aorta. If there is marked disruption of the elastic tissue, a saccular aneurysm may develop later in life. Moreover, intimal dissection also can develop from this site. Other vascular anomalies such as intracranial "berry" aneurysms of the circle of Willis have been associated with longstanding CA. Abnormalities of other organ systems such as the musculoskeletal, gastrointestinal, genitourinary, and respiratory frequently may be present in infants with CA (up to 25%).

Coarctation of the aorta in infancy (infantile coarctation) may present acutely with signs of left ventricular failure with tachypnea or dyspnea and occasionally with circulatory collapse with low cardiac output. Unless it is recognized promptly and treated appropriately, it may be fatal, especially during the newborn period. The reason for the acuteness of presentation is the sudden constriction of the ductus arteriosus, which was supplying the lower part of the body, and the resultant significant decrease of blood flow distal to the coarctation. In such very sick neonates intravenous administration of prostaglandin E_1 has been proven to be indeed life-saving. Relieving the constriction of the ductus arteriosus provides prompt amelioration of the symptoms and adequate stabilization of the infant so further diagnostic studies, such as cardiac catheterization and aortography, can be safely performed before surgical repair.[57] As long as the ductus arteriosus is widely patent, there is no difference in the quality of pulses between the upper and lower extremities, and the arterial pressures are equal. However, determination of arterial Po_2 or percent hemoglobin saturation obtained by pulse oximeter will reveal varying degrees of hypoxemia in the lower part of the body. Cyanosis may not be visually apparent, especially in the presence of VSD. If the constriction of the ductus is gradual, collateral circulation will develop as a result of development of systemic hypertension in the upper body and relative hypotension of the lower body. The femoral pulses under these circumstances will be absent or barely palpable, whereas the pulses in the upper extremities will be prominent. A short ejection systolic murmur can be heard over the upper left and right sternal borders and over the left interscapular area. The heart murmur and the difference in the quality of pulses, as well as the pressure differences between upper and lower extremities, may not be apparent in the acutely symptomatic infant because of the concomitant reduction of the left ventricular output.

In infants with isolated coarctation of the aorta, and gradual constriction of the ductus arteriosus, the clinical presentation is different because of the development of collateral circulation. The infants may show only mild signs of left ventricular failure manifested with varying degrees of failure to thrive. In such infants, careful examination will suggest the diagnosis, and surgical intervention may be deferred for a later time as long as the infant responds appropriately to the anticongestive measures and does not develop severe hypertension.

The electrocardiogram in infants with symptomatic CA invariably shows right ventricular hypertrophy. This is probably caused by the prenatal overloading of the right ventricle, which continues to be present postnatally by maintaining pulmonary arterial pressures at systemic levels and perfusing the lower part of the body via the ductus arteriosus. Cardiomegaly and increased pulmonary vascularity in the chest roentgenogram are usually present. The diagnosis is usually made by two-D-echocardiography and Doppler interrogation across the coarctation. Cardiac catheterization and angiocardiography are now utilized only when preoperative hemodynamic measurements are needed and better delineation of other associated intracardiac anomalies is desired.

Coarctation of the aorta in older children is rarely symptomatic. It appears that the reason for this is the gradual development of collaterals that provide adequate flow distal to the coarctation. An occasional patient may complain of weakness and/or pain in the lower extremities, especially following exercise. The pathognomonic features include differential blood pressure between upper and lower extremities with systolic hypertension at least in one arm (usually the right) or both upper extremities. Absent or decreased femoral or pedal pulses are characteristic. Ejection systolic murmur, at the mid-left sternal border transmitted to the neck, is usually present even in the absence of significant aortic valvular stenosis. Because of the high frequency of associated bicuspid aortic valve, an ejection sound (click) may be present along with the systolic murmur. A characteristic blowing late ejection systolic murmur is usually present in the left interscapular area. In older patients, systolic and/or continuous murmur may be heard in the back because of well-developed collateral blood flow.[56]

In asymptomatic patients, the ECG is usually normal. Occasionally it may show evidence of left ventricular hypertrophy. Chest roentgenograms usually show normal heart size and prominent ascending and descending aorta (distal to the coarctation) with a localized indentation at the area of coarctation (3 sign). "Rib notching" may be present, usually in children older than 5 years of age. Magnetic resonance imaging produces excellent pictures depicting the severity and the extent of the coarctation.

However, aortography provides additional information regarding the size and extent of collateral coarctation (Figs. 13-10 and 13-11).

The majority of patients that survive infancy may reach adulthood if they remain undiscovered in between (a not uncommon occurrence). They may become symptomatic and die of complications, although sporadic examples of exceptional longevity have been reported in the literature; on the average, death occurs in the mid 30s. More than three quarters die by age 50. Rupture of the aorta or dissecting aneurysm is a dramatic complication of CA, with the peak incidence occurring in the third or fourth decade. The rupture originates usually in the proximal ascending aorta but it may occur in the area of postcoarctation aneurysm.[27]

The malformation most commonly associated with CA, as mentioned earlier, is a bicuspid aortic valve. The development of progressive aortic valve insufficiency, accelerated by the long-standing systemic hypertension in patients with CA and bicuspid aortic valve, is not a rare occurrence. Less common but potentially lethal are the congenital "berry" aneurysms located usually in the circle of Willis, which may rupture at any time. The majority of patients who succumb to cerebral hemorrhage do so during the second or third decade of life. However, the presence of hypertension is not always a prerequisite for cerebral hemorrhage; it may also occur in the absence of hypertension many years after successful surgical repair in childhood. It should be noted that pregnancy increases the risk for aortic rupture and intracranial hemorrhage. Left ventricular failure in unoperated patients with CA, besides infancy, may occur in older patients surviving beyond 40 years of age.[27]

Long-term postoperative residua, sequelae, and complications in patients with CA are quite frequent and require follow-up for life.[29,59,60] Residual systolic hypertension despite adequate relief of the coarctation, has been reported to occur, especially during exercise. Progressive aortic valve disease resulting from fibrosis and calcification of the bicuspid aortic valve may occur many years later. However, recoarctation of the aorta requiring additional surgical repair or therapeutic catheterization (balloon angioplasty) is quite commonly seen, especially in children operated before 1 year of age. Exercise testing may be needed to uncover significant systolic pressure gradients across the recoarctation. Aneurysm formation, many years after repair of coarctation using a plastic patch, have been reported (Fig. 13-12).[61] These late complications, i.e., restenosis or aneurysm formation, can be easily detected by Doppler echocardiography or magnetic resonance imaging (MRI). Assessment of the function and morphology of aortic valve can be also accomplished by echocardiography, Doppler interrogation, and color flow imaging.[29,59] It has been suggested (and partially substantiated so far) that longevity following surgical repair is influenced by the pa-

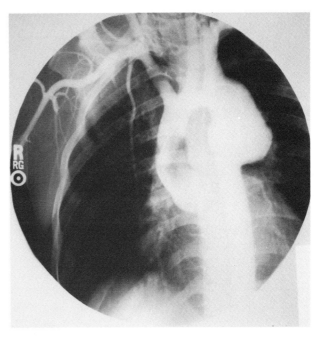

Fig. 13-12. Retrograde aortogram from a 16-year-old adolescent boy, 10 years post patch-surgical repair of coarctation of the aorta, showing a giant "aneurysm" of the thoracic aorta originating from site of the repair. A semi-emergency surgical repair of the aorta using a graft has been carried out successfully, and the young man is doing well.

tient's age at operation. After repair of isolated coarctation of the aorta in infancy, late survival is approximately 92%. It is obvious that coexisting cardiac malformations significantly modify the outcome. Repair of CA in childhood results in 89% survival in 15 years and 83% in 25 years. When surgery is performed on patients after 40 years of age, only 50% survive 15 years after the operation. Correction of CA in women patients reduces the risk of complications during pregnancy.[29]

AORTIC STENOSIS

There is a spectrum of cardiovascular malformations that can be considered obstructive to the ejection of blood from the left ventricle. These include: bicuspid aortic valve with or without valvar stenosis, discrete subaortic stenosis, supravalvar aortic stenosis, coarctation of the aorta, and hypoplastic left heart syndrome with aortic and/or mitral atresia. In this section, valvar, discrete subvalvar, and supravalvar aortic stenoses will be discussed separately (Fig. 13-13).

The division of truncus arteriosus into the two great arteries (pulmonary artery and aorta) is accomplished between the fourth and sixth weeks of gestation. The semilunar valves develop somewhat later (sixth week) at the interface of the truncal cushions and the aorticopulmonary septum, initially as small tubercles that subsequently undergo differentiation through a process of proliferation, re-

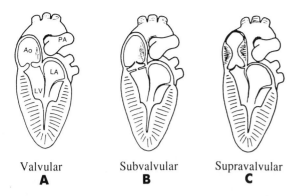

Valvular   Subvalvular   Supravalvular
A   **B**   **C**

Fig. 13-13. Diagrammatic illustration of three types of aortic stenosis: valvar (**A**), subvalvar (**B**), and supravalvar (**C**). The left ventricular myocardium is equally hypertrophied regardless of the location of stenosis.

sorption, and hollowing of their margins. The coronary arteries develop a week later. Presumably any interference with the process of cusp formation will result in maldevelopment of either aortic or pulmonary valve. However, the effects of early intracardiac and extracardial blood flow patterns, secondary to what appears to be a rather insignificant deviation from normal blood flow patterns, may have a profound influence on the final development and evolution of the various cardiovascular malformations.

Valvar aortic stenosis

This maldevelopment of the aortic valve has been considered to occur in approximately 3% to 6% of patients with congenital heart disease. However, if one includes *bicuspid aortic valve,* which is often undetected early in life and becomes stenotic with time, the prevalence of congenital aortic stenosis is much greater. It has been estimated that the prevalence of bicuspid aortic valve is between 0.7% and 2% in the population of the United States, i.e., a prevalence larger than that of all other congenital cardiac malformations put together. Valvar aortic stenosis (AS) appears to occur more frequently in men than women (up to 3:1 sex ratio), and the prevalence of other associated cardiovascular anomalies may be as high as 20%. Patent ductus arteriosus and coarctation of the aorta are the most frequently associated defects with valvar AS, and all three may coexist in the same patient. Particularly, bicuspid aortic valve, usually without appreciable obstruction, is commonly a part of the coarctation syndrome.

Morphologically, the maldeveloped valve appears to be thickened and rigid with varying degrees of commissural fusion. Quite often the aortic valve is bicuspid and has a single fused commissure with an eccentric orifice. In some cases, a third hypoplastic or incomplete commissure is present. The aortic valve may be unicuspid and dome-shaped and sometimes attached to the wall of the aorta at the level of its stenotic orifice. Less frequently, the valve may be tricuspid with symmetrically fused commissures and a central opening of variable size. In very severe

forms of valvar AS (infantile critical AS), the root of the aorta may be relatively hypoplastic. This form of AS could be considered as the mildest form of the spectrum of *hypoplastic left heart syndrome,* which extends to hypoplasia of the ascending aorta and aortic valve atresia. It has been well documented that malformed aortic valves, because of physical stresses of high velocity of blood flow passing through them, undergo progressive fibrosis and calcification late in life.[62]

Concentric left ventricular hypertrophy is invariably present with hemodynamically significant obstruction, regardless of its location. Poststenotic dilatation of the ascending aorta is also a frequent finding only with valvar stenosis. Myocardial fibrosis (located usually in the subendocardial areas) and even endocardial fibroelastosis (in neonates with critical AS) has been associated with longstanding cases of severe aortic stenosis.[63]

Left ventricular obstruction, in general, regardless of its location and depending upon its severity, poses varying degrees of afterload to the ventricular myocardium, which compensates with development of hypertrophy. Consequently, the main hemodynamic abnormality produced by the obstruction is the systolic pressure gradient between the left ventricle and aorta. This gradient may be mild or very large (up to 200 mm Hg) and is usually measured by cardiac catheterization or estimated by Doppler interrogation.[64,65] The magnitude of the transvalvar gradient is directly proportional to the square of blood flow velocity across the stenotic valve and inversely proportional to the square root of the diameter of the orifice. The systolic pressure gradient across the stenosis varies with changes in the contractile state of the left ventricle and peripheral vascular resistance. Thus the gradient may increase with positive inotropic stimuli, or decrease with increases of distal systemic vascular resistance. It is obvious that the severity of valvar stenosis is reflected by the magnitude of the systolic pressure gradient. Therefore it is necessary to measure blood flow rates across the valve and pressure gradient simultaneously in order to assess hemodynamic severity of stenosis. A peak systolic pressure gradient exceeding 75 mm Hg in the presence of normal cardiac output or an effective aortic orifice less than 0.5 cm^2/m^2 of body surface area is considered as evidence of critical obstruction to the left ventricular outflow.

The effective systolic orifice area of the valve is calculated using the Gorlin formula. The normal outflow orifice is approximately 2.0 cm^2/m^2 BSA; areas of 0.5 cm^2/m^2 to 0.8 cm^2/m^2 reflect moderate obstruction, and areas larger than 0.8 cm^2/m^2 indicate mild obstruction. The left atrial and left ventricular end-diastolic pressure are usually elevated with severe stenosis, reflecting the low compliance of the hypertrophied left ventricle or impaired ventricular function. The resting cardiac output and stroke volume in well-compensated aortic stenosis are normal. With exercise, because of increases in cardiac output, the transvalvar pressure gradient increases.[65] In contrast, with left ventricular failure and decreases in cardiac output, the pressure gradient across the valve decreases, and the left ventricular end-diastolic, left atrial, and pulmonary vascular pressures increase. Studies in children with compensated AS have frequently shown the presence of supernormal pump function as indicated by increases in ejection fraction and circumferential fiber shortening. Moreover, in spite of elevated left ventricular systolic pressures, left ventricular systolic stress appears to be lower than normal during systole, because of possible overcompensation for the pressure overload provided by the increases in wall thickness.

The myocardial blood supply may be compromised in severe AS, in spite of widely patent coronary arteries. This is particularly true for the areas of subendocardium where the flow of blood is entirely diastolic because of the very high left ventricular systolic pressure. In patients with severe AS, despite coronary autoregulation, any additional increase in myocardial oxygen demand (i.e., with exercise) will not be adequately met. Under these circumstances, the major determinants of the magnitude of the subendocardial myocardial flow will be the coronary artery driving pressure and the duration of diastole. Diastole is shortened, especially at high heart rates, when systolic ejection time lengthens across the stenosis. Thus coronary driving pressure is decreased if left ventricular end-diastolic pressure is high or aortic diastolic pressure is low.[63]

The great majority of children with aortic stenosis are asymptomatic and grow and develop normally. The presence of an ejection systolic murmur localized at the right upper sternal border and radiating to the neck and apex is usually the first sign that brings attention to these children. An ejection sound (click) may be present in the apex and may extend to the left and right upper sternal border. A "click" signifies usually the presence of mild-to-moderate stenosis. This sound is produced by the sudden opening of the thickened but still mobile aortic valve.

The usual symptoms, when they occur, include fatigability, dyspnea on exertion, chest pain, and syncope. Sudden death is another potential threat in patients with severe AS and usually occurs in association with strenuous exercise in previously asymptomatic patients. Death most likely is the result of ventricular arrhythmias secondary to reduced myocardial blood supply in the presence of increased demand and increase in the intracavitary pressure. Left ventricular lift is usually present only in cases of severe aortic stenosis. There is usually a slow upstroke and decrease in pulse pressure in older patients with severe aortic stenosis. With nonobstructive bicuspid aortic valve, the only auscultatory finding may be an ejection sound (click).[64]

The chest roentgenogram shows normal or only minimally increased heart size. The concentric left ventricular hypertrophy seen in severe stenosis may manifest with rounding of the apex in the frontal view and some posterior displacement in the lateral projection. Poststenotic dilatation of the ascending aorta is a common finding in patients with valvar aortic stenosis. Calcification of the aortic valve, a relatively common finding in adults, is rarely seen in children.

A normal electrocardiogram does not always correlate with the severity of stenosis. Severe obstruction, besides voltage criteria for left ventricular hypertrophy, may be associated with T-wave inversion in the left precordial leads (discordant T waves), suggesting subendocardial ischemia ("strain").

Two-dimensional echocardiography and continuous wave Doppler flow analysis are presently the most useful noninvasive techniques in establishing the diagnosis and severity of the stenosis. Aortic valve thickness and mobility, ventricular wall thickness, and estimates of pressure gradients across the stenosis have been obtained quite accurately with these techniques. A simple estimate of the transvalvular pressure gradient can be calculated as four times the square of the peak Doppler velocity (m/sec.).[65,66]

Cardiac catheterization is necessary to confirm exact site and severity of the obstruction, rather than its presence, which is usually diagnosed by clinical and echocardiographic examination. In addition, therapeutic transcatheter balloon aortic valvoplasty can be tried at the time of cardiac catheterization.[67] Angiocardiographic studies usually complement the echocardiographic and Doppler studies by confirming the site of stenosis, the appearance of the malformed valve, presence or absence of mitral or aortic valve insufficiency, ventricular size, and contractility parameters.

It has been demonstrated in several studies that aortic valvar stenosis is frequently a progressive disorder, even in young patients, presenting initially with relatively mild-to-moderate obstruction. In individuals with bicuspid aortic valves without initial obstruction, progressive fibrocalcific thickening of the valve may ensue, producing severe aortic stenosis during the course of many years. It has been estimated that more than half of the cases of surgically important, pure calcific aortic stenosis in adults result from progressive calcification of a fibrotic bicuspid valve.[68] Mild-to-moderate aortic valve insufficiency may develop progressively in patients with bicuspid aortic valve, in the absence of episodes of bacterial endocarditis. Moreover, varying degrees of aortic regurgitation or restenosis may also develop postoperatively. It has been said that aortic valve surgery or valvoplasty at best is a palliative procedure in childhood and that the great majority of these patients eventually will need aortic valve replacement later on in life.

Subvalvar or discrete subaortic stenosis

Discrete subaortic stenosis consists of a fibrous ring or diaphragm located just below the aortic valve. It accounts for approximately 8% to 10% of all cases of aortic stenosis and occurs more frequently in men than women (2:1). Its differentiation from valvular stenosis is very difficult to establish from clinical findings alone.[64,69] The ejection systolic murmur is similar to that heard in valvar stenosis, but the ejection sound (click) is usually absent. An early diastolic murmur of mild aortic valvar insufficiency is caused by the thickening and retraction of the cusps of the adjacent aortic valve, which frequently may be biscupid. Dilatation of the ascending aorta may be present, but calcification of the aortic valve is uncommon.

Two-dimensional echocardiography and Doppler interrogation of the stenotic subaortic area will invariably establish the diagnosis and determine the severity of the lesion, including estimates of systolic pressure gradients across the stenosis.[70] In addition, associated coexisting hypertrophic subaortic stenosis can be easily differentiated from fixed subvalvar stenosis.

Cardiac catheterization will definitively differentiate between valvar and subvalvar stenosis by obtaining careful withdrawal pressure recordings across the left ventricular outflow tract, whereas left ventriculography will localize the stenotic membrane or the fibrous ring. It is generally believed that early surgical correction of the discrete subaortic stenosis may prevent the likelihood of progressive development of valvar stenosis and insufficiency. However, in spite of careful removal of the fibromuscular obstructive tissue, pressure gradients across the left ventricular outflow tract persist and may progressively increase, requiring reoperation.[71]

In rare instances, valvar and subvalvar stenosis may coexist, producing a tunnel-like narrowing of the left ventricular outflow tract. Hypoplasia of the aortic valve ring and ascending aorta as well as very thickened valve leaflets may be associated with this form of *tunnel stenosis*. These complex forms of stenosis often require extensive surgical reconstruction of the left ventricular outflow tract.

Supravalvar aortic stenosis

This form of left ventricular outflow obstruction is quite rare. It consists of localized or diffuse narrowing of the aorta, usually originating at the superior margin of the sinuses of Valsalva, just above the level of the coronary arteries. It has been found to be associated with *idiopathic infantile hypercalcemia,* a disease probably related to a disturbance of vitamin D metabolism.[64] Supravalvar aortic stenosis syndrome, or Williams syndrome, has been applied to describe a distinct clinical entity produced by coexistence of cardiac and multiple system anomalies.[72] Mental retardation, friendly and happy demeanor, elfin facies, multiple stenoses of pulmonary and systemic arteries, and abnormalities of dental development are some of the features associated with the syndrome. Aortic valve thickening and pulmonary valvar stenosis may occasionally be present along with the peripheral pulmonary stenoses.

Supravalvar stenosis associated with multiple peripheral pulmonary arterial stenoses have been observed in familial and sporadic cases not associated with Williams syndrome. When the anomaly is familial, it is transmitted as an autosomal-dominant trait with variable expression. There is no sex predilection in the various forms of familial and nonfamilial forms of supravalvular aortic stenosis.

There are three anatomic types of this malformation: the hourglass type, the membranous type, and the hypoplastic type. In the *hourglass type* the constricting annular ridge located at the superior margins of the sinuses of Valsalva is produced by extreme thickening and disorganization of the aortic media. The *membranous type* is produced by a fibrous or fibromuscular semicircular diaphragm with a small central opening. The *hypoplastic type* is characterized by a uniform hypoplasia of the ascending aorta. The coronary arteries are usually dilated and tortuous because they are subjected to high systolic pressures, being located proximal to the stenosis. Premature coronary atherosclerosis has been observed, as well as medial thickening of the walls of the coronary vessels.

Patients with supravalvar aortic stenosis are subject to the same risks of unexpected sudden death and endocarditis as those with valvar and subvalvar stenosis. The ejection systolic murmur and systolic thrill are transmitted more extensively to the neck, and usually there is no ejection sound. Coexisting heart murmur of peripheral pulmonary stenosis widely transmitted over the entire anterior chest and back may be present. A disparity of pulses and pressures between the upper extremities may exist because the right brachial pulse is more prominent and the arterial pressure is higher. This disparity in pulses may relate to the tendency of a jet stream to adhere to a vessel wall (Coanda effect) and selective streaming of blood into the innominate artery.

The diagnosis of this lesion is easily made by two-dimensional echocardiography, angiography, and cardiac catheterization (Fig. 13-14, *A* and *B*). The electrocardiogram invariably reveals varying degrees of left ventricular hypertrophy. Except for cases with relatively discrete supravalvar stenosis, surgical repair of these lesions is difficult and carries a higher risk.

HYPOPLASTIC LEFT HEART SYNDROME

Hypoplastic left heart syndrome (HLHS) is a continuum of congenital cardiac anomalies characterized by varying degrees of underdevelopment of the left-sided cardiac structures, including the aorta, aortic valve, and mitral valve, as well as the left atrium and left ventricle (Fig. 13-15). Although aortic valve atresia alone has been referred to synonymously as hypoplastic left heart syndrome, occasionally a normal-size left ventricle has been found with normal mitral valve and an associated ventricular septal defect. The frequency of this malformation has been cited to be 7% to 9% of all congenital malformations of the heart during the neonatal period.[73] It has been reported to occur in several sets of siblings. However, there is no

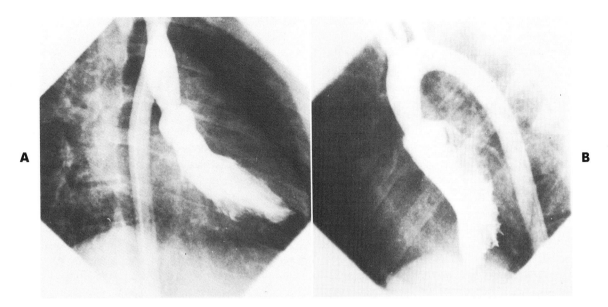

Fig. 13-14. Left ventriculogram in a 15-year-old adolescent with moderate supravalvular aortic stenosis. A = RAO view, B = long axial LAO view. Note constriction of ascending aorta above the sinuses of Valsalva, and large left coronary artery supplying the hypertrophied left ventricular myocardial wall (LAO view). (Courtesy of Kenneth Dooley, M.D., Egleston Children's Hospital, Atlanta, Ga.)

agreement regarding whether the mode of transmission is autosomal, recessive, or multifactorial.

The pathogenesis of this syndrome may be attributed to a number of developmental errors in combination with fetal hemodynamics. Premature closure of the foramen ovale has been suggested as a cause of the milder forms of this syndrome, resulting in a generalized hypoplasia of the left atrium, left ventricle, and mitral and aortic valves. A diminished inflow because of mitral atresia (failure of endocardial cushions, interventricular septum, and ventricular muscle), a diminished outflow because of aortic atresia (failure of proliferation and hollowing of aortic lumen tubercles), and a hypoplastic ascending aorta and aortic arch caused by profound changes in blood flow patterns), may individually or in combination lead to varying degrees of hypoplasia of the left ventricular chamber. The syndrome appears to be more prevalent in males than in females. Extracardiac malformations have been reported to occur in at least 10% of cases. The most severe form of the syndrome is associated with aortic valve atresia, which may or may not be associated with mitral atresia or severe stenosis (hypoplasia). With aortic valve atresia, the ascending aorta is very hypoplastic and constitutes the vessel that exclusively provides the coronary circulation. The left atrium is also hypoplastic, and there is a patent foramen ovale of variable size.[73]

In fetal life, this malformation apparently does not pose significant embarrassment to the fetus. The right ventricle adapts itself as the fetus grows, assuming the role of a "functional" single ventricle (univentricular heart), which, through a large pulmonary artery and ductus arteriosus,

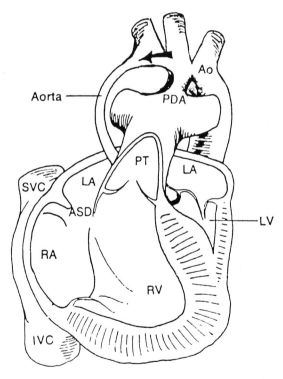

Fig. 13-15. Diagrammatic illustration of hypoplastic left heart syndrome with aortic valve atresia. Note the markedly hypoplastic proximal aorta with retrograde perfusion, functioning as a feeding artery to the coronary circulation. (ASD = atrial septal defect, PT = pulmonary trunk.)

supplies both the entire body and placental circulation. The upper part of the body is perfused in a retrograde fashion from blood entering the systemic circulation via the ductus arteriosus. The pulmonary blood flow is provided by the two normal branches of the main pulmonary arterial trunk. Depending on the presence and the degree of obstruction to the pulmonary flow (i.e., mitral atresia with small restrictive foramen ovale), the small pulmonary arteries may show excessive smooth muscle hypertrophy of their media, a very important adaptation of the pulmonary circulation that has important postnatal implications.[74] In the presence of mitral atresia, the blood flow through the foramen ovale is left-to-right and remains so postnatally. Frequently, because of very high left atrial pressure in the presence of restrictive intraatrial communication, there is bulging of the atrial septum to the right.

Postnatally, as long as the large ductus arteriosus remains widely patent and the pulmonary hypertension persists, adequate systemic flow is maintained, and these infants initially appear relatively asymptomatic. However, they may suddenly deteriorate and present with respiratory distress, grunting, and signs of *cardiogenic shock* with poor peripheral perfusion and severe metabolic acidosis. The clinical deterioration of these infants is caused by partial postnatal constriction of the ductus arteriosus, resulting in inadequate supply of blood flow to the body. The birth weight is usually normal. Approximately two thirds of babies with HLHS become symptomatic during the first 3 days of life, and by 2 weeks 90% of them will require medical attention. Almost 90% of affected infants are dead within the first month of life.[73]

Although there is complete mixing of the arterialized blood with the venous blood, initially the infants are not cyanotic. When they become symptomatic, they present with mild-to-moderate cyanosis (duskiness) and poor peripheral perfusion. They have poor pulses and hypotension in spite of prominent right ventricular impulse on palpation and loud heart sounds. Short nonspecific systolic heart murmur and occasionally loud tricuspid insufficiency murmur may be audible. In most instances, however, there is no heart murmur. Moderate-to-marked cardiomegaly with prominent lung vessels and pulmonary congestion are usually seen in the chest roentgenogram. The ECG invariably shows right ventricular hypertrophy, more than is expected for an infant of that age.

The systemic arterial oxygen saturation depends upon the magnitude of pulmonary blood flow and the relative pulmonary to systemic blood flow ratio. The arterial Pao_2 with oxygen breathing may reach 90 mm Hg to 100 mm Hg or more in an infant with profound circulatory collapse and markedly diminished systemic flow. This results from the continuous recirculation of large amounts of super-oxygenated blood through the lungs, which mixes via the patent foramen ovale with a relatively small amount of unsaturated blood returning from the systemic circulation.

The diagnosis of HLHS is made by two-dimensional echocardiographic and Doppler studies, which usually demonstrate the very small left ventricle and the aortic and/or mitral atresia or stenosis, the hypoplastic ascending aorta, and the large right ventricle and pulmonary artery. Right-to-left shunt is demonstrated at the ductal level and a retrograde blood flow in the small ascending aorta, which feeds the coronary arteries. Infants with *generalized moderate hypoplasia* of the left-sided structures and mitral and aortic stenosis may be recognized clinically a little later and certainly require cardiac catheterization and angiocardiography for definitive diagnosis (Fig. 13-16).

Continuous infusion of prostaglandin E_1 dramatically improves the very ill infant with circulatory collapse. This is accomplished by relaxation of the constricted ductus arteriosus and consequent increase in the systemic blood flow. This improvement in peripheral circulation is similar to that seen in infants with preductal coarctation of the aorta and closing ductus arteriosus who present with profound cardiac failure and hypoperfusion of the lower part of the body. Treatment with prostaglandin E_1 is continued until a decision is reached regarding palliative surgical intervention (Norwood procedure) or cardiac transplantation.[75] In recent years a number of neonates with HLHS have survived this lethal cardiac malformation by undergoing a series of palliative procedures that eventually transform their hearts into "two-chambered" organs containing a single large vessel that supports the systemic circulation. The final stage of this palliative procedure is a modified Fontan procedure, in which the systemic venous return is diverted directly to the pulmonary artery, whereas the two-chambered heart supports only the systemic circulation.[76]

Cardiac transplantation has been successfully performed in a few medical centers with gratifying results.[77] The long-term prognosis in these infants with successful palliative surgery or cardiac transplantation is not known.[78]

RIGHT VENTRICULAR OUTFLOW OBSTRUCTIONS

Obstructive lesions to the right ventricular outflow can be classified as valvar, subvalvar, or supravalvar, involving the main pulmonary trunk and pulmonary arterial branches (Fig. 13-17). These obstructions can be associated with a variety of other congenital heart defects and, together with the isolated ones, occur in 25% to 30% of all patients with congenital heart disease.[79]

Pulmonary valvar stenosis (isolated)

The development of the pulmonary valve occurs after the division of the common truncus arteriosus into the aorta and pulmonary artery. Similar to the development of the aortic valve, there is a proliferation of tubercles that undergo resorption and hollowing of the tissues, thus forming the cusps of the valve. The right ventricular infundibulum originates from the proximal part of the bulbus

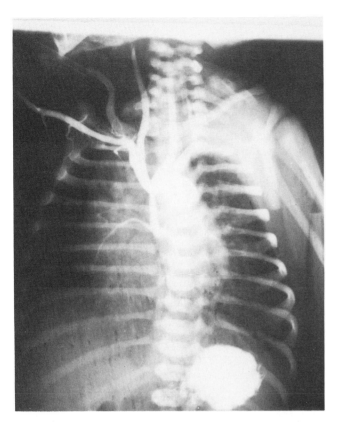

Fig. 13-16. Aortogram taken from a 5-day-old newborn with hypoplastic left heart syndrome with aortic valve atresia. Note the marked hypoplasia of the ascending aorta, which fills in a retrograde fashion and supplies the coronary arteries. (Courtesy of Kenneth Dooley, M.D., Egleston Children's Hospital, Atlanta, Ga.)

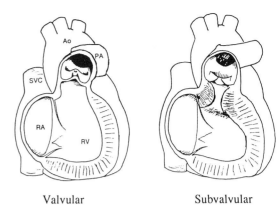

Valvular   Subvalvular

Fig. 13-17. Diagrammatic illustration of valvar and subvalvar pulmonary stenosis.

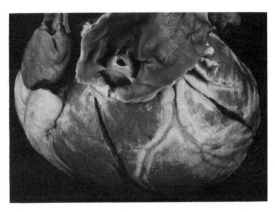

Fig. 13-18. Anatomic specimen showing severe congenital pulmonary valvar stenosis and poststenotic dilatation of the pulmonary arterial trunk. Note the narrow opening of the thickened pulmonary valve and the fusion of the commissures. (Courtesy of William D. Edwards, M.D., Mayo Clinic.)

cordis and precedes the development of the pulmonary valve. Errors of resorption or hollowing of the tissues (tubercles) at the period of normal development of the valve may result in different types of maldevelopment. The appearance of the malformed valve depends on the severity of stenosis. In mild-to-moderate cases, there is some thickening of the valves, which can be bicuspid or tricuspid, and minimal fusion at the base of the commissures. In severe forms of stenosis the pulmonary valve is conical or dome-shaped, projecting superiorly into the pulmonary trunk, and is formed by the fusion of the valve leaflets. The fused leaflets can be recognized from the arterial side as three equidistant raphes radiating to the pulmonary arterial wall (Fig. 13-18). The actual opening of the valve is influenced by the degree of thickness and rigidity of the fused cusps. In a small number of patients with valvar obstruction, the valve appears to be "dysplastic," i.e., the cusps are exceptionally thick and immobile with little or no fusion. They are composed of disorganized myxomatous tissue. There is usually an associated narrowing (hypoplasia) of the pulmonary annulus, which accentuates the severity of the obstruction. Such dysplastic pulmonary valves frequently are present in patients with Noonan syndrome or in some familial cases.[80]

As a consequence of the stenosis, varying degrees of right ventricular hypertrophy are present, especially in the infundibular area, where a dynamic narrowing occurs during ventricular systole. The endocardium and the tricuspid valve may be thickened, and in some severe cases of stenosis endocardial fibroelastosis may be present. The right atrium is frequently dilated and its walls may be thickened. A patent foramen ovale is present in the majority of patients and, less commonly, a true atrial septal defect. The ventricular septum is intact, and there is usually poststenotic dilatation of the main pulmonary trunk, except in patients with dysplastic valves, infundibular stenosis, and valvar stenosis associated with bilateral pulmonary arterial stenosis. Right aortic arch is extremely rare with isolated pulmonary stenosis, and when it is present, infundibular stenosis should be suspected.

The main functional consequence in valvar pulmonic stenosis (PS) is obstruction to the ejection of blood from the right ventricle, leading to an increase in right ventricular pressure proportional to the degree of obstruction. As the stenosis develops in fetal life, it is accompanied by an increase in right ventricular muscle mass. The latter is accomplished both by hyperplasia and hypertrophy of the right ventricular muscle fibers. In contrast, in older children and adults, the myocardium responds to the obstruction primarily by hypertrophy of the muscle fibers with minimal or no hyperplasia. With hypertrophy alone, there is usually no increase in capillary density; thus, the diffusion distance between the capillaries and the distal portion of the myocardial cells is increased. In the fetus and newborn, however, the myocardial response to the obstruction is primarily hyperplasia of the muscle cells with an associated increase in the number of capillaries. Thus the relationship between cells and capillaries remains normal in the newborn. This developmental property of the fetal and neonatal myocardium is very important because it provides the newborn the capacity to generate the high ventricular pressures needed to maintain normal blood flow across the obstruction.

Because the ventricular septum is intact, the pressure generated by the right ventricle may exceed that of the left ventricle. This constitutes a distinct hemodynamic difference from other types of right ventricular obstruction such as tetralogy of Fallot. The compensatory hypertrophy of the right ventricle tends to maintain a normal stroke volume. However, if the PS remains fixed, as the child grows the right ventricle eventually dilates, and heart failure ensues. In the presence of a patent foramen ovale or atrial septal defect, with marked ventricular hypertrophy and consequent decrease in ventricular compliance, right-to-left shunt across the interatrial communication will occur with varying degrees of systemic hypoxemia.

There is a syndrome of pulmonary valvar stenosis with a relatively small (hypoplastic) right ventricle associated with a large patent foramen ovale or ASD, in which significant degrees of systemic hypoxemia and cyanosis may occur caused by a right-to-left interatrial shunt. This syndrome simulates pulmonary valve atresia with intact ventricular septum.

The prevalence of pulmonary valvar stenosis with intact ventricular septum has been estimated to be between 8% and 10% of all congenital cardiac malformations. Familial occurrence also has been reported. The estimated recurrence risk ranges from 2% to 3%.

The majority of patients with valvar stenosis are asymptomatic and are discovered only during routine examination by the presence of a loud systolic ejection murmur. When symptoms are present, they may vary from mild exertional dyspnea and mild cyanosis to signs and symptoms of heart failure, depending on the severity of obstruction and the level of myocardial compensation.

With increasing age, subjective complaints may increase, but there are reports in the literature describing asymptomatic adults well into their 50s or 60s with moderately severe PS.[27] Occasionally, however, in patients with severe PS, strenuous exercise may provoke syncope and even sudden death. Growth and development in children is usually normal, even with severe stenosis. A right ventricular impulse and systolic thrill at the upper left sternal border are usually present in moderate-to-severe PS. Depending upon the degree of stenosis, a harsh ejection systolic murmur of variable duration is usually present over the upper precordium. This murmur is widely transmitted to the anterior and posterior chest. The severity of the stenosis is proportionally related to the length of the heart murmur. An "ejection click" is usually present in cases of mild or moderate valvar stenosis. The second sound is diminished over the pulmonary area and may even be absent with severe PS. In mild stenosis the ejection systolic murmur is short, and its peak never passes mid systole. When tricuspid insufficiency is present, a holosystolic murmur also may be heard at the lower left sternal border.[79]

The electrocardiogram may show varying degrees of right ventricular hypertrophy in cases of moderately severe or severe stenosis. The chest roentgenogram usually shows normal or slightly increased heart size, and in the majority of cases, prominence of the main pulmonary arterial segment caused by poststenotic dilatation. When cardiac failure develops, cardiomegaly is seen resulting from right ventricular and right atrial dilatation. The pulmonary vascularity is usually normal unless there is significant right-to-left atrial shunt (cyanosis) or right ventricular failure and decrease in right ventricular stroke volume.

Two-dimensional echocardiography will confirm the clinical diagnosis by demonstrating the stenotic valve, poststenotic dilatation of the pulmonary trunk, ventricular hypertrophy, and associated anomalies, whereas Doppler interrogation of the stenotic pulmonary valve gives accurate estimates of pressure gradients across the valve.

Diagnostic cardiac catheterization and angiocardiography are not necessary unless they are combined with therapeutic balloon valvoplasty. In the last decade or so, therapeutic transvenous balloon valvoplasty has almost completely replaced surgical repair of pulmonary valvar stenosis.[81,82]

The long-term prognosis of patients with surgical repair or relief of stenosis by balloon valvoplasty is very good to excellent. In contrast to aortic stenosis, pulmonary restenosis following surgical relief or valvoplasty seldom occurs. However, in infants with critical PS and hypoplasia of the annulus, progressive residual stenosis has been frequently observed. It should be pointed out that the creation of pulmonary valve insufficiency, by generous relief of the stenosis, can be tolerated fairly well because of low diastolic pulmonary arterial pressure.[81,82]

Pulmonary valvar stenosis due to *dysplastic* pulmonary cusps is frequently seen in patients with Noonan syndrome.[80] Moreover, hypertrophic cardiomyopathy affecting the left ventricle, isolated or in association with dysplastic pulmonary stenosis, has been seen in up to 25% of cases of this syndrome. In cases of PS with dysplastic valve, besides the stenotic pulmonary valvar annulus, there is usually hypoplasia of the proximal main pulmonary artery, immobility of the thickened pulmonary valve leaflets, and absence of an ejection click on auscultation.[79]

Infundibular stenosis

Primary infundibular stenosis, isolated, is a very rare malformation, and may be considered as part of the spectrum of *double-chambered right ventricle*. The prevalence of this entity has been reported to range from 2% to 10% of all cases of right ventricular outflow obstructions.

There are two types of isolated primary infundibular stenosis: the most common type, in which a *fibrous band,* located at the junction of the main right ventricular cavity and the infundibulum, produces a stenosis of the proximal portion of the infundibulum and divides the cavity into two chambers; and the type in which the infundibulum is relatively *"hypoplastic,"* with a thickened muscular wall forming a narrow outlet to the right ventricle. The narrow area of the infundibulum may be short or long, and located either immediately below the pulmonary valve or lower.

The physiologic and clinical manifestations of the entity are indistinguishable from those seen in right ventricular obstruction caused by anomalous muscle bundles of the right ventricle.

Right ventricular obstruction caused by anomalous muscle bundles (two-chambered right ventricle)

This cardiac malformation is characterized by aberrant hypertrophied muscular bands that divide the right ventricular cavity into a proximal high-pressure chamber and a low-pressure chamber located distal to the anomalous muscle bands.[83] Ventricular septal defect and/or pulmonary valve stenosis are frequently associated with this lesion.

The anomalous hypertrophied muscle bundles are muscle masses that run from the ventricular septum to the anterior wall of the right ventricle. There are usually two types of bundles: the ventral bundle, which attaches to the wall of the right ventricle adjacent to the septum; and the dorsal bundle, which is usually larger and has its attachments at the base of the anterior papillary muscle of the tricuspid valve. Thus the right ventricular cavity is divided into two compartments: a proximal chamber consisting of the sinus portion of the right ventricle and a distal chamber, the infundibulum. The obstruction of right ventricular outflow in this entity is completely different from that seen in tetralogy of Fallot. In the latter, the anatomic obstruction is located in the infundibulum itself, and the hypertrophied muscle bundles present protrude from the walls of the infundibulum into its cavity, without crossing the cavity from one wall to another. The anomalous muscle bundles, however, because their septal attachments are near the base of the tricuspid ring, cross the main channel of the right ventricle, and with progressive hypertrophy cause obstruction.[79]

The origin of these bundles is unknown. It has been postulated that they may be caused by a localized growth of the trabeculated myocardium very early in development. For the blood to pass from the right ventricular inflow to the outflow, it must course either between the muscle bundles and the tricuspid valve, above the muscle bundles, or through the narrow channel between the bundles and septal wall. Particularly during ventricular contraction, the size of these channels is markedly reduced; frequently the lumen of the channel adjacent to the septum may be completely obliterated.

Clinically, patients with anomalous muscle bundles and intact ventricular septum closely resemble patients with isolated PS. In the presence of ventricular septal defect (VSD), the clinical features may be dominated by the VSD. A very loud systolic murmur, which resembles that of a VSD and PS, is usually heard along the left sternal border. A prominent systolic thrill also is present.

The electrocardiogram may show right ventricular hypertrophy of moderate degree. The diagnosis may be suspected by Doppler echocardiography and confirmed by cardiac catheterization and angiocardiography.

The results of surgical repair of this malformation are very gratifying, resulting in complete relief of the obstruction and disappearance of the loud systolic murmur. However, in some instances, mild residua such as mild right ventricular obstruction, residual VSD, and tricuspid insufficiency have been observed.[84] In time, spontaneous closure of the associated VSD may occur, leaving the right ventricular obstruction caused by anomalous muscle bundles as an isolated lesion.

Peripheral pulmonary artery stenosis with intact ventricular septum

Stenosis of the pulmonary arteries, isolated or in association with other defects, is quite common. The frequency of pulmonary arterial stenosis is between 2% to 3% of all patients with congenital heart disease.[79] The stenosis may be single, involving the main pulmonary arterial trunk or either of its branches, or multiple, involving both main and several branches.[85] In about two thirds of the cases, other associated cardiac defects may be present, such as valvar PS or VSD. Patent ductus arteriosus and atrial septal defects are also frequent, perhaps more so in cases associated with the rubella syndrome.[86] Peripheral pulmonary arterial stenoses are also frequently seen with tetralogy of Fallot. Supravalvar aortic stenosis in association with multiple peripheral pulmonary arterial stenoses, mental retardation, and peculiar facies has been described as a separate syndrome (Williams syndrome). Peripheral pulmonary arterial stenoses have been associated with

Noonan syndrome, Alagille syndrome, cutis laxa, and Ehlers-Danlos syndrome.

The pathogenesis of peripheral pulmonary arterial stenosis is unknown. It appears that many types of pathologic changes produce the same result: narrowing of the lumen of the main pulmonary artery and its branches. The high frequency of associated intracardiac anomalies suggests that the pathogenesis of these lesions must be developmental in origin. Any teratogenic insult on the components of the developing pulmonary arteries may arrest their normal development and lead to atresia, hypoplasia, or stenosis. At least one teratogenic agent, the rubella virus, has been implicated in the pathogenesis of peripheral pulmonary arterial stenoses. With the rubella syndrome, interference with normal formation of the elastic tissues may be the principal mechanism in the development of the lesion.[86]

Depending upon the severity of the obstruction, varying degrees of right ventricular hypertrophy may be present. Elevations of right ventricular systolic pressure and, proximal to the stenosis, pulmonary arterial systolic pressure are usually present.

Clinically these patients are often asymptomatic. Symptoms of right ventricular failure may be present, but only in severe forms of stenosis. Loud ejection systolic murmur, widely transmitted over the chest, is usually present with severe stenosis. In multiple peripheral pulmonary arterial stenoses, soft continuous murmurs may be heard over both lung fields.[79]

In the chest roentgenogram, the main pulmonary artery segment is not prominent. With cardiac failure, cardiomegaly and decrease in pulmonary vascularity may be seen. Cardiac catheterization and angiocardiography are necessary to determine the location and severity of the stenoses.[85,86]

Surgical relief of severe stenosis at the bifurcation has been attempted with not completely satisfactory results. Similarly, balloon angioplasty has been applied in certain cases of proximal pulmonary arterial stenosis with variable results.[87]

Progressive increases of the degree of obstruction of peripheral pulmonary arterial stenosis may occur. However, in many instances, pressure gradients recorded early in life disappear with growth. Patients with multiple peripheral pulmonary arterial stenosis of severe degree have similar prognosis to those with primary pulmonary hypertension. Death in early infancy or later in life has been reported to occur with severe pulmonary artery stenosis. Severe peripheral pulmonary artery stenosis in late adult life is apparently very rare.

Pulmonary atresia with intact ventricular septum

In this cardiac malformation there is no outlet to the right ventricle. There is *pulmonary valve atresia,* and the ventricular septum is intact, i.e., there is no ventricular septal defect, and the right ventricle usually is not developed normally, showing varying degrees of hypoplasia. Tricuspid valve abnormalities and rarely right ventricular-coronary artery fistulae may be present. This combination of lesions is referred to as *hypoplastic right heart syndrome.* In 20% of cases an infundibular atresia may be associated with valve atresia. Although in the majority of cases the right ventricle is hypoplastic, a normal or near-normal size, (or even dilated) right ventricle (in the presence of Ebstein anomaly of the tricuspid valve) may be seen. The pulmonary arteries are usually moderately hypoplastic, and there is always a ductus arteriosus supplying the pulmonary circulation. The right atrium is enlarged, and invariably there is a larger-than-usual foramen ovale or atrial septal defect providing an outlet for the right atrium. The tricuspid annulus is frequently small, and the valve leaflets may be dysplastic or hypoplastic.[88]

Ebstein anomaly of the tricuspid valve is present in 20% to 25% of cases of pulmonary atresia with intact ventricular septum. In such cases, because of severe tricuspid insufficiency, massive right atrial dilatation and frequently intrauterine heart failure is seen. Thus there is a continuum of right ventricular dimensions ranging from extremely diminutive to massively enlarged, in decreasing order of frequency. The former division of the right ventricle into sinus and outlet portions has been more recently modified to a tripartite right ventricle with *inlet, trabecular,* and *outlet* portions. Based on this anatomic division, cases of pulmonary atresia with intact ventricular septum, regardless of ventricular size, are divided into those with neither trabecular nor outflow portions. This classification has very important implications regarding the potential for ventricular growth and prognosis following surgical relief of the valvar atresia.

In some cases with competent tricuspid valve, fistulous communications may exist between the right ventricular cavity and the right, left, and rarely both coronary arteries. These *intramyocardial sinusoids* apparently represent persistent fetal trabecular myocardial communications in the small right ventricle that may generate systemic or suprasystemic pressures. Retrograde coronary blood flow from the right ventricle into the aorta (right-sided circular shunt) has been implicated as causing both right and left ventricular ischemia, necrosis, and fibrosis.

The atretic pulmonary valve is usually represented as an imperforate, diaphragm-like membrane with a hypoplastic ring. There may be complete atresia of the infundibulum with no identifiable valvular structure, and the main pulmonary arterial trunk is replaced by a cordlike structure connecting with the bifurcation of the pulmonary artery.[88]

The exact pathogenesis is not known. It must involve a specific insult to the developing, already formed right ventricle, certainly an etiologic mechanism quite different from that of conotruncal abnormalities, such as pulmonary atresia with a ventricular septal defect (severe tetralogy of Fallot).

In the absence of severe tricuspid insufficiency, the fetus with pulmonary atresia and intact ventricular septum apparently tolerates the malformation quite well as long as there is adequate interatrial communication. The left atrium and ventricle receive two to three times more blood than in the normal fetus. The ductus arteriosus is always patent at birth, but survival of the infant depends upon its continuous patency. These infants present with hypoxemia and cyanosis soon after birth; time of presentation depends upon the size and patency of the ductus arteriosus. Moderate tachypnea and a soft crescendo systolic ductal murmur may be present. This murmur may or may not spill into diastole. A single second sound and relatively quiet precordium are usually present. In cases with cardiomegaly and tricuspid insufficiency, a systolic murmur at the lower left sternal border and hepatomegaly are invariably present. Rapid deterioration of the hypoxemia and cyanosis may ensue any time after birth because of the constriction and closure of the ductus arteriosus. Unless the condition is recognized early and the patient is given intravenous prostaglandin E$_1$ followed by palliative surgery (modified Blalock-Taussig shunt with or without pulmonary valvotomy), the infant will invariably die.[89] During the last decade or so a number of such infants with very small ventricles survived the initial palliative surgery and have undergone definitive surgery (such as Fontan or modified Fontan or Glenn procedures) with very good results.[89] In such procedures, the systemic venous return is diverted to the pulmonary artery either totally (Fontan) or partially (Glenn). Moreover, in cases where the right ventricle is normal or near-normal size, surgical valvotomy resulted in complete normalization of the circulation.

TETRALOGY OF FALLOT

Tetralogy of Fallot (TOF) is the most common cyanotic congenital heart anomaly in children and accounts for the largest proportion of adults with cyanotic congenital heart disease. In its classic description it consists of a *large nonrestrictive ventricular septal defect* (VSD), pulmonary stenosis (PS), right ventricular hypertrophy, and overriding of the aorta (Fig. 13-19). Because right ventricular hypertrophy and overriding of the aorta appear to be consequences of the combination of severe right ventricular outflow obstruction and equalization of the pressures between the two ventricles, the most important anomalies in the TOF are the pulmonic stenosis and the ventricular septal defect. The aortic override is considered to be caused by a normally positioned aorta with an enlarged root. The PS should be sufficiently severe so as to result in normal or decreased pulmonary arterial pressures and predominantly right-to-left shunt through the VSD. Although there may be some disagreement about the location of the VSD and the site of right ventricular outflow obstruction, factors that may have important pathogenetic implications, in the typical TOF there is a large perimembranous VSD of the

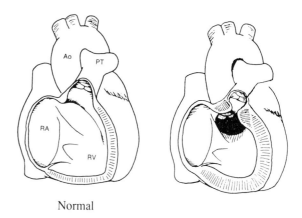

Fig. 13-19. Diagrammatic illustration of tetralogy of Fallot. Note the large high ventricular septal defect, infundibular stenosis, overriding of the aorta, and right ventricular hypertrophy. (See text.)

malalignment variety, and infundibular stenosis with or without valvar or supravalvar components.[90,91]

Pathogenesis

It has been postulated that TOF results from truncal malseptation at the expense of the pulmonary artery. However, malseptation does not readily explain the development of the malalignment VSD and the infundibular abnormality seen in this malformation.[90] It appears that the infundibular stenosis is at least in part caused by anterior deviation of the infundibular septum, and the malalignment VSD is clearly related to this septal deviation. It has been suggested that both the malalignment VSD and the deviation of the infundibular septum result from the underdevelopment of the infundibulum of the right ventricle, and that this *hypoplasia* is the primary pathogenetic event responsible for the development of all other components of TOF.[92] However, there are some patients with similar clinical picture and hemodynamics who do not have the "typical" anatomic features of TOF, requiring similar palliative and corrective surgical procedures. For example, the large VSD may just be perimembranous and the right ventricular obstruction may be in a different location, valvular or supravalvular. Moreover, there are also patients with TOF who are initially acyanotic because of the less severe infundibular stenosis but become cyanotic with growth. Therefore, in the broader definition of TOF, cyanosis may not always be a necessary requirement.

As mentioned earlier, the large perimembranous VSD results from malalignment of the infundibular septum with the remainder of the muscular septum. The defect is roofed superiorly by the aortic valve and is bordered posteroinferiorly by the area of fibrous continuity between tricuspid, mitral, and aortic valves. Often a remnant of ventricular membranous septum may be present in this area of "confluence" of the three valves. The border of the defect anteriorly and anteroinferiorly is always muscle. In some cases there is a muscular rim between the inferior margin of the defect and the tricuspid valve. In very few cases, the VSD is associated with straddling of the tricuspid valve and malalignment of the atrial and ventricular septa. A second VSD may also occasionally be present.

The infundibulum is always narrow in typical cases of TOF. This narrowing is caused by varying degrees of generalized hypoplasia with or without associated hypertrophy and fibrosis of the endocardium. Obstruction caused by anomalous muscle bundles, as described elsewhere, is another form of intraventricular obstruction proximal to the infundibulum.[83]

The pulmonary valve is abnormal in the majority of cases. It is found to be bicuspid in half and unicuspid in one sixth of autopsied cases. In most cases, the valve is stenotic and occasionally it may be the only site of stenosis. The annulus of the valve may be hypoplastic, resulting in severe stenosis that cannot be relieved at surgery by valvoplasty alone and requires placement of a transannular patch. Pulmonary valve atresia with ventricular septal defect is considered to be a severe form of TOF.[91] The infundibulum is usually very hypoplastic, but it can be completely atretic as well. Pulmonary flow is provided by the ductus arteriosus, bronchial arteries, or large aberrant arteries originating from the thoracic aorta or from large branches of the aortic arch.

Supravalvular pulmonary artery stenoses are most commonly found near the origin of the right or left pulmonary arteries from the main pulmonary arterial trunk. In the great majority of cases of "typical" TOF, there are varying degrees of generalized hypoplasia of the pulmonary arterial tree. Absent left pulmonary artery may occasionally be detected by angiography. In such cases, there is a hypoplastic left pulmonary artery that is not connected with the main pulmonary trunk, having been originally supplied by a patent ductus arteriosus. There is frequently a right aortic arch (20% to 25%). The overriding of the aortic root is variable. Even in extreme degree of override, there is always aortic-mitral valve continuity, a distinguishing feature of TOF from *double outlet right ventricle,* in which there is always a muscular ridge separating the mitral from the aortic valve. Other morphologic features associated with TOF include abnormalities in the course of the bundle of His and its branches because of the position and extent of the VSD; anomalies of the coronary arteries, such as anomalous origin of the anterior descending artery from the right coronary artery crossing anteriorly over the infundibulum; and single right or left coronary artery with major branches crossing similarly over the right ventricular outflow area. For this reason, preoperative identification of the coronary arteries and their branching is necessary to avoid intraoperative coronary vascular injury.

Associated cardiac abnormalities

The lungs of patients with TOF may be somewhat smaller than normal. The number of alveoli may be decreased, and the hilar and proximal intrapulmonary arteries are smaller than normal. These pulmonary and vascular changes were attributed to decreased pulmonary blood flow, and it has been suggested that early surgical repair or palliation may give a better chance of normalization because most lung and arterial growth takes place during the first 2 years of life. Other associated cardiac abnormalities include: patent foramen ovale or true atrial septal defect; absent pulmonary valve with massive dilatation of the proximal pulmonary arteries and pulmonary valve insufficiency; arterioventricular canal defects (usually in patients with Down's syndrome); and systemic and pulmonary venous anomalies, such as left superior vena cava connection with the coronary sinus, or directly into the left atrium, intrahepatic interruption of the IVC with azygous continuation to the superior vena cava, and partial or total pulmonary venous return.[90,91]

TOF has been estimated to occur in approximately 10% of all congenital cardiac malformations. The etiology is unknown, and it is slightly more prevalent in men than in women. The recurrence risks have been estimated to be at least 3% in siblings. A morphologic anomaly similar to TOF has been produced in chick embryos by temporarily placing a fine silk thread about the developing conus. Approximately half of the embryos that survived had PS, VSD, and overriding aorta. It was postulated that insult caused by the ligature resulted in abnormal septation of the conus, thus producing the PS and the malalignment VSD.[93]

Because the VSD in TOF is, by definition, nonrestrictive, i.e., equal or larger than the aortic root, the systolic pressure is equal in both ventricles. Thus the direction and amount of blood flow across the defect will depend upon the degree of obstruction of the right ventricular outflow. Early in systole there may be a small left-to-right shunt, even in patients with severe pulmonary stenosis, because the pressure rise in the left ventricle slightly precedes that of the right ventricle. With mild or moderate stenosis, there will be a net left-to-right shunt at the ventricular level, and pulmonary flow will exceed systemic (acyanotic TOF). With increasing severity of obstruction, resistance to blood flow into the pulmonary and systemic circuits may be nearly equal, resulting in bidirectional shunt across the defect. More severe degrees of obstruction will lead to large right-to-left shunt and decrease in pulmonary flow (cyanotic TOF). Because pulmonary flow under these circumstances is much less than systemic, most of the blood entering the aorta comes from the right ventricle and therefore is highly undersaturated. Systemic blood flow is usually normal or slightly increased.

In spite of the severity of pulmonary stenosis in cyanotic TOF, the pulmonary artery pressure is usually normal or low normal. As long as the VSD is nonrestrictive and the obstruction is severe, the location of the VSD, the site of stenosis, and even the degree of overriding at the aorta seem to be of little hemodynamic importance. In contrast to pulmonic stenosis with intact ventricular septum, right ventricular hypertrophy in TOF is not extreme. This is related to the fact that right ventricular pressure never exceeds left ventricular pressure, and its hypertrophy is commensurate to systemic vascular resistance. Thus, the right ventricular compliance is not impaired, as is reflected in the right ventricular end-diastolic pressure, which is not higher than left ventricular end-diastolic pressure.

With exercise, however, arterial oxygen saturation usually falls and sometimes quite dramatically. This reduction in arterial saturation is primarily caused by the exercise-induced decrease in systemic vascular resistance, which promotes larger amounts of right-to-left shunt across the VSD. Another factor that may play a significant role in the production of systemic hypoxemia during exercise is tachycardia, which results in relative reduction to pulmonary flow (at a time when it is needed most) secondary to a decrease in diastolic filling time of the right ventricle in the presence of fixed pulmonary stenosis. Similarly, during the "hypercyanotic ("blue") spells" seen frequently in infants with severe TOF, marked reduction in systemic arterial saturation occurs, leading to metabolic acidosis and fainting.[90,91]

The hemoglobin and hematocrit levels in cyanotic patients with TOF are usually elevated. They depend directly upon the degree of systemic hypoxemia and the availability of iron to the body, especially in milk-fed infants during the first 2 years of life. Microcytic, hypochromic anemia may be present, despite what appears to be "normal" hemoglobin and hematocrit values. Marked polycythemia (small hypochromic red cells) may be present even though the patient is anemic. Decreased exercise tolerance and frequent hypercyanotic spells may be caused by this relative anemia. For this reason, adequate supply of iron should be provided to those infants. As the "anemia" improves, the patients become more cyanotic but they are less symptomatic. In contrast, very high levels of hemoglobin may have serious consequences, especially in older individuals. Exercise intolerance and headaches may be caused by the hyperviscosity of the blood. However, both very high hematocrit (greater than 70%) or polycythemia with iron-deficient red blood cells may place individuals with cyanotic heart disease at risk for cerebrovascular accidents.

Clinical presentation

The clinical presentation of patients with TOF may range from the distressed, cyanotic, hypoxemic newborn to the young adult with no cyanosis and only a few, if any, symptoms. The range of symptoms is directly related to the broad spectrum of severity of the pulmonary stenosis. Cyanosis may be present at birth (in cases of pulmonary atresia), or it may occur with passage of time. Occasionally, with mild or moderate outflow obstruction, the patient presents with clinical picture of a large VSD with excessive pulmonary flow and even heart failure. As the ob-

struction becomes progressively more severe, a more typical picture of TOF emerges with disappearance of the heart failure and eventually appearance of hypoxemia and cyanosis. Patients with TOF and absent pulmonary valve may present with minimal symptoms or may be severely distressed early in infancy because of airway obstruction secondary to massive aneurysmal dilatation of the proximal pulmonary arteries.[94] They may not have severe hypoxemia and may show signs of heart failure caused by a large left-to-right shunt.

Infants with TOF may develop "hypercyanotic" spells characterized by labored respirations and altered levels of consciousness. These spells occur more frequently in patients with TOF, but also may be seen in patients with other cyanotic congenital cardiac malformations. They usually occur during morning hours, and when the episodes are severe the infant may become lethargic or unconscious. Their occurrence is considered an indication for surgical intervention. The characteristic systolic murmur of TOF usually becomes shorter or even disappears during the spell, suggesting infundibular "spasm," leading to further obstruction of the right ventricular outflow. Hyperpnea itself, by increasing the systemic venous return, has been suggested as the initiating event of a "blue spell" in the presence of fixed pulmonary blood flow. Consequently, the systemic arterial blood contains a larger proportion of unsaturated systemic venous blood, leading to more severe hypoxemia. The decrease in arterial oxygen saturation further stimulates the respiratory center, leading to more hyperpnea, and the cycle continues.[90,91]

In older patients, easy fatigability and dyspnea on exertion is usually present. Squatting is another common symptom in children with TOF beyond infancy, especially following a physical effort. The improvement in oxygenation with squatting has been attributed to a decrease in venous return of the highly unsaturated blood coming from the lower extremities. Slowing of the heart rate, together with the associated increase in peripheral vascular resistance (angulation and compression of the femoral arteries) during squatting, by increasing the pulmonary blood flow through the fixed pulmonary stenosis, appears to be a more important hemodynamic factor responsible for the improvement in systemic oxygenation.

Heart failure is not part of the clinical picture of TOF. There is usually generalized cyanosis, but when it is mild-to-moderate the cyanosis may be evident only in the lips, nailbeds, and mucous membranes. "Clubbing" of the fingers and toes is commonly seen in patients with long-standing cyanosis. The precordium is usually quiet without abnormal ventricular heaves. This is because of the fact that the combined ventricular volume work in TOF is less than "normal." The first heart sound is usually normal, and the second sound is loud and single (aortic valve closure sound). Aortic ejection sounds (clicks) may be present at the apex in cases with severe TOF and are caused by the dilated aortic root. A harsh ejection systolic murmur is in-

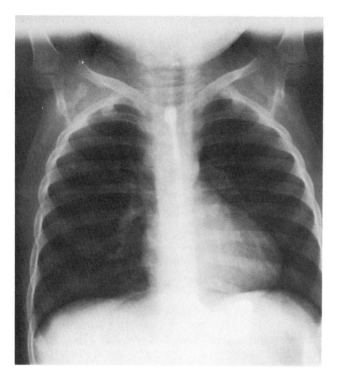

Fig. 13-20. Chest roentgenogram from a 3-year-old child with tetralogy of Fallot. Note the normal heart size, uplifted apex of the heart, absence of the main pulmonary arterial segment, and decrease in pulmonary vascularity. There is a right aortic arch. (Courtesy of Kenneth Dooley, M.D., Egleston Children's Hospital, Atlanta, Ga.)

variably heard over the mid and high left sternal border and is caused by the pulmonic stenosis. The more severe the obstruction in TOF, the shorter and softer is the systolic murmur, in contrast with pulmonic valvular stenosis and intact ventricular septum, in which the opposite occurs, i.e., the more severe the stenosis the louder and longer is the heart murmur. In pulmonary atresia, there is no pulmonary ejection systolic murmur. A much louder and longer systolic murmur is present with moderate PS and VSD with left-to-right shunt. In TOF with absent pulmonary valve, a "to and fro" systolic and diastolic murmur is usually present because of stenosis and insufficiency of the pulmonary valve (narrow pulmonary valve ring and absent or rudimentary pulmonary valve cusps).[94] A continuous murmur suggests the presence of either a patent ductus arteriosus and/or aberrant aortopulmonary collaterals.[91]

The physical findings described above are different following surgical repair of TOF.[29] The cyanosis disappears, and the clubbing usually regresses with time. In cases with significant residual pulmonary valve insufficiency, produced by a transannular patch, a diastolic murmur is usually present. A systolic ejection murmur of varying intensity resulting from residual relative pulmonary stenosis is heard together with the diastolic murmur. A holosystolic murmur at the lower left sternal border, when present,

may be caused by either a small residual VSD or rarely, postoperative tricuspid insufficiency.[95]

The electrocardiogram in TOF shows usually right ventricular hypertrophy and rightward QRS frontal axis. In older individuals unoperated beyond 16 years of age, premature ventricular contractions have been detected in more than 50% of patients.[27] Right bundle branch block (RBBB) is almost invariably observed following complete repair of TOF. This ECG abnormality has been attributed to damage of conduction tissue in at least three levels: in the proximal bundle that runs along the rim of the VSD; in the area of the moderator band; and more distally in the parietal wall of the right ventricle. Left anterior hemiblock is also seen postoperatively in a small number of patients.[96] By reducing the length of right ventriculotomy, the incidence of RBBB was reduced by 40%, according to one report.[97] However, RBBB is common even after transatrial repair.

The chest roentgenogram usually shows a normal or smaller-than-normal heart size and decreased pulmonary vascularity. The apex of the heart is often upturned, and there is absence of the normal main pulmonary artery segment (concave border). These findings cause the typical "boot-shaped" heart seen in most patients with TOF (Fig. 13-20). The heart in TOF with absent pulmonary valve may be enlarged, showing massive dilatation of the proximal pulmonary arteries that compress the large bronchi. Varying degrees of partial or generalized overinflation of the lungs is also present in this syndrome.[94]

The Doppler echocardiographic studies are essential in confirming the diagnosis noninvasively. All the components of this malformation as well as other associated anomalies can be visualized.[91] However, cardiac catheterization and angiocardiography is usually recommended prior to surgical repair. This is done to delineate more accurately the level and severity of stenosis, the presence of coronary arterial abnormalities, the size of the pulmonary arteries and their branches, as well as the aberrant aortopulmonary collaterals, particularly in cases of severe TOF with pulmonary atresia (Fig. 13-21).

Residua and sequelae

The long-term results of surgical repair of TOF are quite satisfactory. It has been reported that patients who had their intracardiac repair at about 2 years of age, following an initial palliative shunt, had a 96% 10-year survival, and 87% survival 10 to 22 years after the operation.[29,95] The great majority were free of significant symptoms and led practically normal lives. Significant postoperative problems usually manifest within the first 2 years after the operation. The most common problems are failure to relieve the obstruction of the right ventricular outflow and residual ventricular septal defects. Reoperation rates have been reported to range from 5% to 15%. Primary intracardiac repair in infancy has been found to be associated

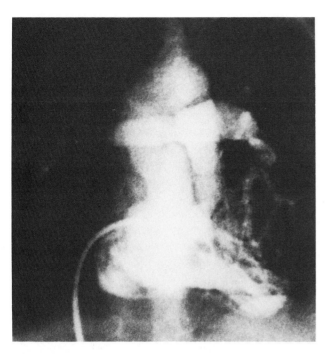

Fig. 13-21. Right ventriculogram (AP view) taken from a 1-year-old child with tetralogy of Fallot. Note the marked infundibular stenosis and the moderately hypoplastic pulmonary valve annulus and proximal pulmonary artery. The majority of contrast media enters the overriding dilated aorta via the ventricular septal defect. There appears to be marked hypoplasia of the distal pulmonary arterial branches. (Courtesy of Kenneth Dooley, M.D., Egleston Children's Hospital, Atlanta, Ga.)

with higher reoperation rate for residual outflow obstruction and/or VSD. Patients who have reached adulthood, after palliative shunts during childhood, fall into two groups: those who had Potts anastomosis (descending thoracic aorta to left pulmonary artery) and may present with inoperable pulmonary vascular disease; and those who had Blalock-Taussig shunts (subclavian artery to pulmonary artery anastomosis) and maintained symptomatic improvement and could benefit from intracardiac repair as adults.[29] However, such patients operated on after 40 years of age have significant mortality (17%). Late postoperative right ventricular function in patients operated before 5 years of age apparently remains good, with normal ejection fraction and diastolic volume as long as their residual pulmonary valve insufficiency is mild-to-moderate and there is no significant residual obstruction. Ventricular arrhythmias and sudden death have been reported in postoperative patients who had significant residual obstruction and/or pulmonary valve regurgitation.[98] Right ventricular aneurysms have been observed when pericardial patches were utilized for relief of the infundibular and/or transannular stenosis. The response to exercise is normal or near-normal in those patients operated on during early childhood. In contrast, there is general agreement that the response to exercise is generally decreased in those patients operated on in late

childhood or adulthood. A recent study reported serial follow-up of a cohort of 151 patients with repaired tetralgy of Fallot. The patients were prospectively studied regarding their clinical outcome and factors that could potentially affect their survival. Fifty-six percent of the patients had a palliative procedure (Blalock, Potts, Waterston) performed before repair. The study showed that 94% of patients have remained in New York Heart Association functional class I, and that adults with repaired tetralogy of Fallot have a very good prognosis and a low risk for sudden death.[98a]

The results of reparative surgery in patients with pulmonary atresia and VSD (severe TOF) are not as good as in those with pulmonic stenosis and VSD (usual TOF). There are multiple reasons for this difference: hypoplasia or peripheral stenoses of the pulmonary arteries with resultant postoperative right ventricular hypertension; severity of residual obstruction of the right ventricular outflow; the size of the aortopulmonary collateral arterial communications; and the durability of prosthetic conduits utilized to establish the necessary continuity between the right ventricle and pulmonary artery.[97]

TRICUSPID ATRESIA

The principal abnormality in tricuspid atresia (TA) is "agenesis" of the tricuspid valve, resulting in no direct communication between the right atrium and right ventricle. A patent foramen ovale or an atrial septal defect is always present along with a hypoplastic right ventricle and a ventricular septal defect (VSD). The prevalence of TA ranges from 1% to 3% of all congenital cardiac malformations, according to various clinical or autopsy series.

The exact etiology of TA is not known. The formation of the tricuspid valve occurs about the fifth week of gestation and involves several tissue components: the anterior and posterior endocardial cushions, a portion of the intraventricular septum, and the ventricular muscle. An error in balance of the contributions of these tissues may result in an anomaly such as TA. It appears that the development of tricuspid valve is intimately related to the development of the right ventricular sinus. It has been postulated that TA is the result of malalignment between the ventricular loop and the atria. Underdevelopment of the right ventricle may cause this malalignment in such a way that the ventricular septum completely blocks the tricuspid orifice.[99,100]

In tricuspid atresia and intact ventricular septum the right ventricle is markedly hypoplastic or absent, and there is usually pulmonary valve and trunk atresia. Under these circumstances, the pulmonary flow in the fetus and neonate is provided exclusively by the PDA and the bronchial circulation. In the presence of VSD, however, depending on its size, the pulmonary circulation is primarily supplied from the left ventricle via the VSD.

In 25% of the cases TA is associated with *D-transposition of the great arteries* (D-TGA), and usually there is no impedance of the pulmonary circulation (Fig. 13-22). The

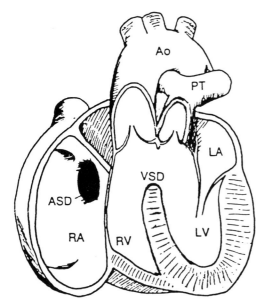

Fig. 13-22. Diagrammatic illustration of tricuspid atresia with D-transposition of the great arteries, ventricular septal defect, and atrial septal defect, Type II. (See text.)

ductus arteriosus is large in the fetus, whereas the anteriorly placed aorta arises from a hypoplastic right ventricle and its blood flow is supplied by the left ventricle through the VSD. Tubular hypoplasia of the aorta is present, resulting from the intrauterine preference of the blood flow to the placenta via the pulmonary artery and ductus arteriosus.

In TA the right ventricle is composed largely of the conus and the incompletely developed sinus portion of the cavity. When a large VSD is present, the sinus portion of the right ventricular cavity is better developed; consequently, the pulmonary arteries may be normal or near normal size. The atretic tricuspid valve is usually muscular, and its location becomes visible by the presence of a "dimple" in the floor of the right atrium. Less frequently, the atresia is fibrous or membranous, most likely when it is associated with Ebstein anomaly of the tricuspid valve.[100]

In 80% of cases, the intraatrial mode of communication is a large patent foramen ovale. In the remaining cases, it is a true secundum-type ASD and only rarely an ostium primum ASD. The VSD is usually located at the basal or muscular portion of the septum. Obstruction of the pulmonary flow may be located at several levels: the site of the restrictive small VSD; the long and narrow hypoplastic right ventricular cavity; the infundibular area; or at the stenotic pulmonary valve. In patients with associated D-TGA, if there is an obstruction to pulmonary blood flow, it is usually subpulmonary or valvular.[99,100]

Tricuspid atresia is associated with a number of other cardiac defects that generally determine the magnitude of pulmonary blood flow and, consequently, the pathophysiology, clinical picture, and type of medical or surgical treatment.

A number of classifications of TA have been proposed. Two types of TA should be recognized: one with normally related great arteries (type I), and type II, which is associated with D-TGA (Fig. 13-22). Each type is further subdivided according to the presence of pulmonary stenosis or atresia and the absence and size of the VSD. A smaller group of patients, comprising 3% to 7% of all cases of tricuspid atresia, is associated with "corrected" transposition of the great arteries (L-TGA) (type III). Coarctation of the aorta, hypoplasia of the aortic arch, PDA, and juxtaposition of the atrial appendages are more commonly seen in type II (D-TGA) tricuspid atresia.

There are two distinct types of clinical presentation of individuals with TA. Although varying degrees of hypoxemia are always present (the entire systemic venous return enters the left atrium from the right atrium), the presence of true cyanosis depends upon the amount of blood entering the pulmonary circulation. Thus infants with TA and pulmonary atresia or with a very small restrictive VSD will present with cyanosis soon after birth. Conversely, the infant with TA and D-TGA without pulmonic stenosis will present with signs of congestive heart failure and without clinical cyanosis.[99]

Central cyanosis or *harsh systolic murmur* are present at birth in at least 50% of cases with TA. Cyanosis is caused by the obligatory right-to-left shunt via the intraatrial communication, and its intensity is inversely related to the amount of pulmonary blood flow. In older patients, chronic hypoxemia leads to polycythemia and its related consequences. Exertional dyspnea and easy fatigability are common, and squatting may be present. "Hypoxic" ("blue") spells are frequently seen in infants under 6 months of age. These spells are usually related to either spontaneous diminution in size or closure of VSD, or progressive infundibular or valvular stenosis. The pathogenesis of the blue spells is similar to that described in tetralogy of Fallot. The occurrence of such spells is an ominous sign indicating critical reduction in pulmonary blood flow and urgent need for surgery.

Heart failure caused by increased pulmonary blood flow is usually seen in patients with TA with D-TGA (type II) and occasionally in patients with normally related great arteries who have a large VSD and/or a PDA. Cyanosis is minimal or even absent, but there is always mild-to-moderate arterial hypoxemia. Tachypnea or dyspnea, frequent respiratory infections, feeding difficulties, and failure to gain weight are common in such patients. Infants with severe cyanosis and relative iron deficiency anemia and older children with marked polycythemia are prone to develop cerebrovascular accidents. In older children, hemiplegia may result from brain abscess, emboli from endocarditis, or complications of a systemic-to-pulmonary artery shunt.

Because of the obligatory right-to-left intracardiac shunt, transient bacteremia may colonize particularly the brain, which has been damaged by severe hypoxemia and hypoperfusion, resulting in abscess formation. Endocarditis occurs quite frequently in patients with TA with surgical arteriopulmonary shunts.

Patients who have TA and D-TGA with large pulmonary flows and pulmonary hypertension may develop early pulmonary vascular obstructive disease. Such a course of events is very unusual in patients with normally related great vessels and decreased pulmonary flow in the absence of large systemic-to-pulmonary arterial shunts (Potts or Waterston).

There is invariably a harsh systolic murmur at the left sternal border in patients with a restrictive VSD and decreased pulmonary flow. The precordium is usually quiet, and occasionally a systolic thrill may be present. The first heart sound is single and accentuated, and the second sound is single in patients with severe pulmonic stenosis. Decreasing intensity of the murmur suggests either more severe pulmonary stenosis or spontaneously closing VSD. A continuous murmur is usually present in patients with functioning surgical shunts.[100]

The electrocardiogram is specific for this malformation. It shows almost invariably left axis deviation in the frontal plane with right atrial enlargement and prominent left ventricular forces. Right ventricular forces are usually absent or decreased. The radiologic features of TA with normally related arteries are decreased pulmonary vascular markings; normal or slightly increased cardiac size; and decreased prominence of the main pulmonary arterial segment. In contrast, patients with TA and a large VSD with increased pulmonary blood flow show gross cardiomegaly and increase in pulmonary vascular markings. A transition from increased to decreased pulmonary vascularity may be caused by a spontaneously closing VSD.

Echocardiographic and Doppler studies are most useful in the noninvasive diagnosis of the various forms of TA. The atretic tricuspid valve, the right atrium, and the size of interatrial communication, as well as the large left ventricle, hypoplastic right ventricle, VSD, and semilunar valves, can be easily delineated. Moreover, pressure gradients across the VSD and pulmonary valve, as well as blood flow and pressure gradients across the ductus arteriosus or across surgically created shunts, can be estimated with fairly good accuracy. Of course, cardiac catheterization and angiocardiography are still "gold standards" for definitive diagnosis.

With the wide application of the Fontan procedure and its modifications in recent years, a large number of individuals, following initial palliative procedures, survive to adulthood and have a fairly reasonable quality of life.[101] Exercise performance improves postoperatively, but it remains abnormal. At best, no more than a twofold increase in cardiac output is achieved with exercise.[102] The results

of the Fontan procedure depend upon the size of the pulmonary arteries (pulmonary vascular resistance) and the function of the left ventricle. Successful operation results in reduction of left ventricular size, regression to a normal mass-to-volume ratio, and an increase in contractility. Operations performed earlier without adequate myocardial protection have occasionally resulted in marked ventricular dilatation and decreased function.[103] Patients who are properly selected for operation have done quite well with minimal symptoms up to 15 years postoperatively. The 5-year survival is 87%, with most deaths occurring within a year after surgery. The right atrial pressure following the Fontan operation increases to levels slightly higher than mean pulmonary arterial pressure and increases more with exercise.[102] Arrhythmias, such as atrial fibrillation or flutter, may lead to further elevation in the right atrial mean pressure. The latter is partially caused by the effect of the atrial arrhythmias upon the left ventricular filling pressure. Fluid accumulation (pleural effusion, ascites, and generalized edema) can be severe and last for weeks and months after the Fontan repair. The majority of patients gradually adapt to increased systemic venous pressure and improve clinically, achieving a state of functional stability. As mentioned above, atrial arrhythmias are caused by markedly increased right atrial pressures.[104] Recent modifications of the Fontan procedure involving total caval-to-pulmonary arterial connection, by obviating right atrial distension, seem to reduce the frequency of the atrial arrhythmias.[105]

Following a Fontan procedure, isotonic exercise was found to be associated with an elevated physiologic dead space and a ventilation-perfusion mismatch, reflecting maldistribution of pulmonary blood flow. The pulmonary arterial blood flow postoperatively is not pulsatile and results in abnormal distribution of blood in both lungs, similar to that observed in the right lung after a classic Glenn procedure.[106] The acquired right lower lobe *pulmonary arteriovenous fistula* seen after the Glenn anastomosis (superior vena cava-to-right pulmonary artery end-to-end anastomosis) has been attributed to the nonpulsatile flow, which causes a decreased ratio of upper lobe-to-lower lobe blood flow distribution. Because similar patterns of pulmonary blood flow occur following the Fontan operation, it is conceivable that such pulmonary arteriovenous fistulae may further complicate the long-term prognosis of these patients.[106]

EBSTEIN ANOMALY OF THE TRICUSPID VALVE

Congenital malformations involving the tricuspid valve leading to stenosis or insufficiency of the valve are relatively infrequent. The most common is Ebstein anomaly. Other types of isolated dysplasia of the tricuspid valve producing insufficiency or stenosis are quite rare. In his original report, Ebstein described the marked redundancy of the valve and its abnormal origin from the right ventricular

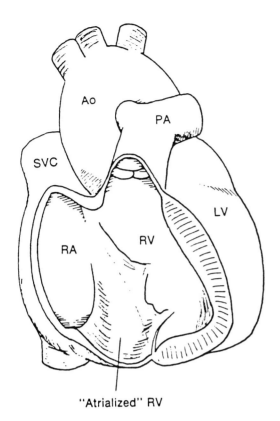

"Atrialized" RV

Fig. 13-23. Diagrammatic illustration of Ebstein anomaly of the tricuspid valve. Note the downward displacement of the tricuspid opening and the "atrialized" portion of the right ventricular inflow area. (See text.)

wall well below the tricuspid valve annulus. Only the anterior cusp of the tricuspid valve originated from the normal position.[107] The prevalence of Ebstein anomaly among patients with congenital heart disease is 0.5% to 0.7%. There is no clear dominance between either sex. However, familial occurrence of the malformation has been reported. There is no particular association of the anomaly with any genetic syndrome, but there is unusually high frequency among infants born to mothers who were treated with lithium preparations during pregnancy.[108]

The morphologic appearance of the tricuspid valve is extremely variable. The characteristic features are redundancy of the valve tissue, and adherence of a variable portion of the septal (medial) and posterior cusps to the right ventricular wall so that the origin of the free wall of the right ventricle is located some distance away from the atrioventricular junction. The redundancy of the valve may be less apparent if most of the valve tissue is adherent to the right ventricular wall. In some instances the posterior and medial leaflet of the valve are so completely plastered to the wall that there is no free portion of the valve left, and the valve opening appears to be unguarded. The anterior cusp arises normally from the atrioventricular annulus and appears to be elongated and redundant. The portion of

the right ventricle between the atrioventricular junction and the origin of the dominant displaced valve forms a common chamber with the right atrium and is usually referred to as an *atrialized* ventricle (functionally it has become part of the right atrium) (Fig. 13-23). The degree of right ventricular malfunction depends primarily on the extent to which its right ventricular inflow portion is atrialized and how intimately the valve tissue is adherent to the ventricular wall. In some instances the cusp tissue is only superficially adherent to the "atrialized" wall of the ventricle, which is muscular, whereas at the other extreme end of the spectrum, the adherence is so intimate that the corresponding ventricular wall is reduced to a very thin fibrous sac that has lost its ability to contract. In rare instances the membrane formed by the redundant valve tissue is imperforate and cannot be distinguished from the classic form of tricuspid atresia. However, there is usually one opening located near the crista supraventricularis, substituting the normal tricuspid valve.[107]

The leaflets of the tricuspid valve, embryologically, are almost exclusively derived from the inner layers of the embryonic right ventricular myocardium by a process of resorption "undermining" the right ventricular wall (the same process that forms the trabeculations of the ventricular cavity). Thus the inner layer of ventricular myocardium is freed from the rest of the ventricular wall and forms a muscular "skirt." At the same time, the atrial side of this separated inner wall is partially covered by endocardial cushion tissue. Perforations appear in the apical portion of the skirt, which enlarges until papillary muscle and chordae tendineae remain. The cusps and the chordae initially are muscular structures and become fibrous later. The anterior cusp is apparently formed much earlier than the posterior and medial cusps. The latter is not fully formed even in a fetus of 3 months gestational age. Thus the pathogenesis of Ebstein anomaly may be explained by an abnormality of the process of undermining the inner muscular layers of the embryonic right ventricular wall, which remained incomplete and did not reach the atrioventricular annulus. The formation of chordae and papillary muscles by the perforating process of the primitive "muscular" skirt does not take place at all or is aborted altogether. The latter may explain the redundancy of the valve. The normal origin of the anterior cusp is apparently related to the earlier formation.

The most common intracardiac anomalies are interatrial communications, i.e., patent foramen ovale or true secundum atrial septal defect. Less frequent are pulmonary valve stenosis or atresia, ventricular septal defect alone or in combination with other defects, and occasionally tricuspid valve atresia.

The hemodynamic consequences of Ebstein anomaly are quite variable and depend upon the corresponding pathologic anatomy of the tricuspid valve and the associated defects. The anomaly may be so mild that it is completely unnoticed until adult life or incidentally found at autopsy. On the other hand, because of the severity of the valve dysfunction, cyanosis may be present as a result of right-to-left shunt at the atrial level. The mean right atrial pressure is usually higher than the left atrial pressure and is primarily caused by the stenosis and/or insufficiency of the malformed tricuspid valve opening. In cases where large areas of "atrialized" right ventricular muscular wall is present, atrial systole may result in bulging of the atrialized wall (which is depolarized later) by the blood propelled into it. With ventricular systole, the "contracting" atrialized ventricle will send the blood contained in it back to the right atrium. This "back and forth" effect is particularly pronounced in cases where the "atrialized" ventricle has a well-developed muscular wall.[107]

In the fetus and newborn infant immediately after birth, the insufficiency of the malformed tricuspid valve is accentuated because of the right ventricular hypertension resulting from the high pulmonary vascular resistance. The newborn infant may present initially with intense cyanosis that gradually diminishes as the pulmonary vascular resistance (PVR) drops postnatally. This fall in PVR leads to significant reduction of the magnitude of the tricuspid regurgitation. Recurrent episodes of cyanosis may be precipitated by *paroxysmal supraventricular tachycardia,* which further impairs right ventricular function and may lead to increase in the right-to-left interatrial shunt. Cyanosis tends to decrease and even disappear early in life but almost invariably returns later on. It appears that in time the function of the abnormal valve deteriorates along with its associated myocardial structure. The tricuspid insufficiency results in dilatation of the right ventricular outflow tract and the proximal right heart structures, including the incompetent tricuspid valve ostium. Thus a vicious cycle sets in whereby insufficiency begets more insufficiency, resulting in further increases in right atrial pressure and right-to-left shunt across the interatrial communication. Bidirectional atrial shunt or only left-to-right shunt may occur if an ASD is present, especially associated with milder forms of the malformation.

As might be expected, clinical manifestations of the anomaly vary tremendously. In some cases, diagnosis of Ebstein anomaly is not made until adult life; on the other end of the spectrum are fetuses in whom the anomaly is so severe as to lead to intrauterine demise. In the neonatal period, moderate-to-severe cyanosis and a heart murmur may be present. The cyanosis improves with time and may reappear again in a few years. If symptoms appear after infancy, their onset may be insidious. Dyspnea on exertion, fatigability, and cyanosis are usually the presenting symptoms. The degree of hypoxemia may have little relationship to the ability of the individual to perform physical work.

Arrhythmias are common and occur in more than 50% of patients. Paroxysmal supraventricular tachycardia (SVT) including atrial flutter and fibrillation is very common. Ventricular extrasystoles or varying degrees of atrioventricular block are less common.[109] Syncope associated with tachyarrythmias may also occur. Transient vision loss, dizzy spells, and thromboembolic phenomena are occasionally seen, most likely caused by small "paradoxic" emboli. Symptoms of cardiac failure in older children and adults are present only in terminal stages of the disease, although they may be seen frequently during bouts of SVT. The cardiac impulse may be normal, and a systolic thrill may be present. The majority of patients, however, have a systolic murmur of varying intensity at the lower left sternal border. The murmur results from either tricuspid insufficiency or right ventricular outflow obstruction. A split second sound and loud third and fourth heart sounds are frequently audible, giving the impression of a *triple* or *quadruple rhythm.* A prominent mid or late diastolic murmur may be present and occasionally resemble precordial friction rub.

The electrocardiogram is always abnormal. Right bundle branch block pattern is the most common abnormality. A Wolf-Parkinson-White (WPW) syndrome is also seen in 5% to 20% of cases and typically is of the type B pattern, i.e., resembling the LBBB. The PR interval is prolonged, and the P waves are prominent, reflecting right atrial hypertrophy and dilatation. Supraventricular tachycardia is more commonly seen in infants and children, whereas in adults arrhythmias such as PVCs, atrial flutter and fibrillation, and junctional rhythm are more frequent.

Two-dimensional echocardiography with Doppler interrogation is the best noninvasive diagnostic technique in confirming the clinically suspected diagnosis. It demonstrates very well the distally displaced tricuspid valve, its opening, the atrial septal defect, and the presence of stenosis and insufficiency of the malformed valve.[110]

Chest roentgenograms rarely show a normal heart size. In infancy there may be slight-to-massive cardiomegaly with decreased pulmonary vascular markings. The right atrial segment is usually prominent (Fig. 13-24). Cardiac catheterization and angiocardiography very rarely are necessary for the diagnosis of this disorder and always carry the risk of inducing cardiac arrhythmias; for this reason they are rarely recommended, even preoperatively.[111]

Surgical intervention has been recommended for patients in functional class III and IV (New York Heart Association classification), signs of increasing cyanosis and polycythemia, paradoxic emboli, or tachyarrhythmias secondary to accessory conduction pathway. The aims of surgical "repair" are relief of the regurgitation, improvement of right ventricular function, closure of the interatrial communication, and ablation of the atrioventricular bypass track. Artificial valve replacement is currently avoided, and efforts are made to reconstruct the abnormal valve. Tissue valves are preferred instead of mechanical valves.[112] Tricuspid valve replacement carries 10% to 15% late mortality.

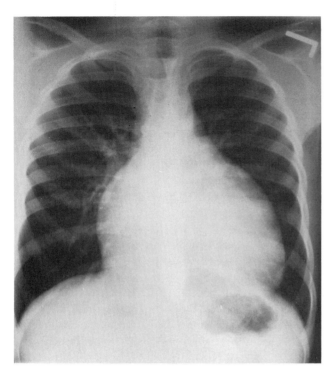

Fig. 13-24. Chest roentgenogram from a 6-year-old child with Ebstein anomaly of the tricuspid valve. There is cardiomegaly with prominent right atrium and normal pulmonary vascular markings. (Courtesy of Kenneth Dooley, M.D., Egleston Children's Hospital, Atlanta, Ga.)

Approximately one third of patients die before the age of 10 years, most in early infancy. There are many reports of survival beyond the sixth decade. The majority of patients surviving early infancy apparently have a relatively good prognosis. Pregnancy is tolerated very well in those patients with the milder forms of the anomaly.[29]

TRANSPOSITION OF THE GREAT ARTERIES

In transposition of the great arteries (TGA), there is complete reversal of the position of the great arteries, i.e., the aorta arises from the right ventricle and the pulmonary artery arises from the left ventricle. Consequently, the undersaturated systemic venous blood is misdirected back to the transposed aorta, whereas the highly oxygenated pulmonary venous blood is misdirected into the pulmonary circulation.

In its simple form with intact ventricular septum, this malformation is incompatible with extrauterine survival unless there is an associated interatrial communication and/or an extracardiac connection between the two circulations, such as a patent ductus arteriosus. Whereas in fetal life the hemodynamic derangements caused by TGA do not greatly influence fetal well-being and development, infants born with this defect become severely hypoxemic soon after birth, and without treatment may survive only a few days because of the persistence of the foramen ovale and the ductus arteriosus. In contrast, infants with TGA and a ventricular septal defect with or without associated pulmonic stenosis usually survive for months or years because of the mixing of blood from the two circulations.[113]

TGA is a relatively frequent malformation and accounts for 5% to 7% of all congenital cardiac malformations. The incidence of TGA varies from 19 to 34 per 100,000 live births, and there is a strong male preponderance (60% to 70%). Extracardiac anomalies are relatively infrequent (9%) in comparison with other more common cardiac malformations, such as VSD and tetralogy of Fallot.

In spite of much controversy among morphologists concerning the exact description and anatomic classification of TGA and other malpositions of the great arteries, there appears to be a general consensus in describing the various cardiac and great artery segments in terms of *connections* (or *alignments*), *spatial relationships,* and *internal morphology.*[114] The great arteries may be related normally or abnormally to each other, to the ventricles, to the ventricular septum, and to the atrioventricular valves. Thus normally and abnormally related great arteries are designated in terms of their ventriculoarterial connections or alignments: normal, transposed, and double outlet right ventricle or left ventricle. The term *TGA* implies the presence of discordant ventriculoarterial connection, so that the aorta arises entirely or in large part from the right ventricle, and the pulmonary artery arises entirely or in large part from the left ventricle.[115,116]

The terms *partial* or *incomplete* transposition used in the past have been replaced by *double outlet* right ventricle or left ventricle. The term *complete TGA* is now used to indicate that the transposed arteries are *physiologically uncorrected,* i.e., because of normal atrioventricular connections (concordance), the systemic venous blood flows predominantly to the aorta and the pulmonary venous blood flows to the pulmonary artery. In contrast, the term *corrected transposition of the great arteries,* i.e., *physiologically corrected,* is used when, together with the ventriculoarterial discordance (TGA), there is atrioventricular discordance that provides the physiologic correction, i.e., systemic venous blood enters the pulmonary artery and pulmonary venous blood enters the aorta.

The term *simple* has been used to exclude those cases of TGA associated with complex malformations such as *tricuspid atresia, mitral atresia, common atrioventricular canal,* or *univentricular heart.* Simple TGA comprises 80% of all transposition malformations and includes those with intact ventricular septum, ventricular septal defect (VSD), patent ductus arteriosus (Fig. 13-25) (PDA), and left ventricular outflow obstruction (pulmonic stenosis). Very commonly, clinicians and surgeons use the term simple for the largest group of TGA with intact ventricular septum (or very small VSD) but without any other significant associated lesions (large VSD, PDA, or PS).

The exact developmental aspects of abnormal ventricu-

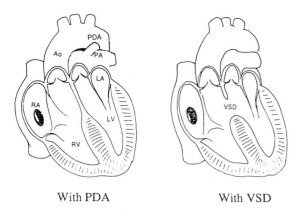

With PDA   With VSD

Fig. 13-25. Diagrammatic illustration of complete transposition of the great arteries with an associated PDA (left) and VSD (right). Note the patent foramen ovale present in both drawings.

loarterial relationships are largely unknown. A number of hypotheses regarding the pathogenesis of TGA have been advanced, including abnormal (straight) truncoconal separation; abnormal fibrous skeleton; abnormal embryonic hemodynamics; phylogenetic regression; and inverted development of the truncal cushions. Abnormal development, i.e., growth and absorption, of the distal infundibulum (conus) plays an important role in the morphogenesis of this malformation. The normal conus is subpulmonary, left-sided and anterior, preventing fibrous continuity between the pulmonary and tricuspid valve rings. In typical TGA, the infundibulum is subaortic, right-sided, and anterior, and prevents fibrous continuity between the aortic and tricuspid valve rings. In human embryos, the pulmonary valve normally moves posteroanteriorly and towards the left side after 30 to 34 days of gestation, and its movement is related to normal development of the subpulmonary infundibulum. During the same time, the aortic valve remains stationary, apparently because of normally occurring resorption of the subaortic infundibulum. It has been postulated that the pathogenesis of TGA may be the result of abnormal growth and development of the subaortic infundibulum and the absence of growth (resorption) of the subpulmonary infundibulum. The aortic valve is displaced superiorly and anteriorly by the development of subaortic infundibulum above the anterior right ventricle. Failure of development of the subpulmonic conus prevents the normal posterior-anterior movement of the pulmonary valve and results in abnormal pulmonary artery-to-mitral valve ring fibrous continuity.[117]

A fundamental pathogenetic mechanism for development of complex segmental cardiac malformations may be related to genetic decontrol events that result in cardiac segmental discordance. Thus the etiology of TGA and other conotruncal malformations may be related to an abnormality of normally dominant genetic material for situs solitus, allowing deviations from normal anatomic organization of various cardiac segments.[117]

The atria are usually normal, and there is almost always a patent foramen ovale. Only rarely is there a true secundum atrial septal defect. The right ventricle is hypertrophied and remains so as long as it supports the systemic circuit. When the ventricular septum is intact, there is always a subaortic conus that separates the aortic valve from the tricuspid valve. The left ventricle is connected to the pulmonary circuit, and its wall thickness and shape of its cavity depend upon the age and associated defects such as VSD, PDA, and pulmonic stenosis. The status of the left ventricle is of major importance in deciding about the arterial switch operation. In the majority of cases, the position of the aorta is anterior and slightly to the right of the pulmonary trunk, but it may be anterior to the left as well. The coronary arteries in TGA, in general, arise from the aortic sinuses facing the pulmonary artery. Thus in the normal heart, the noncoronary sinus is located posteriorly, whereas in TGA it is located anteriorly.[118] This origin of the coronary arteries facilitates the transfer of the coronary ostia and vessels posteriorly to the root of the pulmonary artery (neoaorta) during the arterial switch operation. There is also considerable variability in the origin and course of the three major coronary arteries from the sinuses. The course of the *sinus node artery* has been given much attention because of its possible implication in the development of supraventricular arrhythmias ("sick sinus syndrome") following the Mustard or Senning intraatrial switch operations. It has been postulated that the sinus node artery, partially embedded in the anterosuperior area of the interatrial septum, can be easily damaged during the intraatrial surgery.[113]

Ventricular septal defect is the most frequent (35%) coexisting anomaly in TGA. It may be small, large, or multiple and can be located in any part of the septum. In 10% of cases the VSD may be associated with left ventricular outflow obstruction (LVOO). Isolated LVOO, i.e., with intact ventricular septum, is quite rare (5%). The great majority of VSDs are perimembranous or malalignment defects. A large outlet VSD, depending upon the degree of malalignment of the conal septum and its displacement, may lead to either LVOO (posterior) or pulmonary annulus overriding (anterior) of the right ventricle. Extreme degrees of pulmonary overriding may culminate in what is referred to as *double outlet right ventricle with subpulmonic VSD* (Taussig-Bing anomaly). Left ventricular outflow tract obstruction is a common coexisting anomaly in TGA, and it is located mainly in the subpulmonic area (subpulmonary stenosis).

Valvar or annular pulmonary stenosis is very rare. With intact ventricular septum, a dynamic type of "obstruction" is quite common. It is usually mild and is caused by leftward bulging of the basal muscular ventricular septum during systole into the low-pressure left ventricle.[113] This systolic narrowing of the LVO tract is demonstrated by angiocardiography or echocardiography, and it is not readily apparent on autopsy specimens. This dynamic septal bulge "obstruction" is not present in the newborn or infant with an associated VSD who underwent pulmonary arterial banding.[119] It is usually seen following intraatrial surgical repair, in which the pressure in the left ventricle remains relatively low in contrast to that of the right ventricle. The dynamic obstruction is produced by the closing anterior mitral leaflet and the posterior displacement of the ventricular septum during systole (a dynamic mechanism similar to that of hypertrophic obstructive cardiomyopathy but without asymmetric septal hypertrophy). A fixed subpulmonic obstruction may develop in some infants. Initially this may appear as an area of endocardial thickening on the septal bulge, later evolving into a fibrous ridge.

Left ventricular outflow obstruction may coexist in up to 30% of patients with TGA and VSD. The stenosis may be more severe and more complex than in TGA and intact ventricular septum. It is again mostly subvalvar, and it can be produced by a localized fibrous ring, a tunnel line of fibromuscular narrowing, or a muscular obstruction related to malposition of the outlet septum. Very rarely, stenosis may be produced by redundant tricuspid valve tissue protruding like a pouch through the VSD.

Patent ductus arteriosus is invariably present at birth and may remain open up to a month. Presently with the introduction of prostaglandin E_1 treatment, the ductus may be kept open beyond its natural time of closure until palliative or surgical repair is accomplished.

Other less frequent anomalies associated with TGA include tricuspid and mitral valve defects that may produce varying degrees of valvular dysfunction. Coarctation of the aorta can also coexist with TGA (5%) and is frequently seen with an associated large VSD. Coarctation syndrome most commonly exists (20%) in patients with double outlet right ventricle and subpulmonary defect (Taussig-Bing anomaly).

In patients with TGA and particularly in those with intact ventricular septum, the dominant physiologic abnormalities are a deficiency in oxygen supply to the body and excessive overloading of both ventricles. The systemic and pulmonary circulations function in parallel rather than in series, i.e., the great majority of blood ejected from each ventricle to the respective circuit returns to the same ventricle. Only a relatively small amount of blood is exchanged between the two circuits via intercirculatory shunts and reaches the appropriate vascular bed. Consequently, oxygen saturations in the aorta and pulmonary artery depend exclusively on the amount of blood exchanged through the following anatomic paths: intracardiac (PFO, ASD, VSD) and extracardiac (PDA and bronchopulmonary collateral circulation).

The net volume of blood passing from the pulmonary circulation to the systemic circulation via their interconnections represents the *anatomic left-to-right shunt* and is actually the *effective systemic blood flow,* i.e., fully oxygenated blood from the pulmonary veins enters the systemic circulation and perfuses its capillary bed). On the other hand, the net amount of blood passing from the systemic circulation to the pulmonary circulation is the *true anatomic* right-to-left shunt and actually constitutes the *effective pulmonary blood flow,* i.e., underoxygenated blood returning from the systemic veins enters the pulmonary circulation and perfuses its pulmonary capillary bed. At any given interval of time, volumes of these net anatomic shunts (right-to-left and left-to-right) are equal and comprise the *intercirculatory mixing shunt,* i.e., the blood flow in TGA on which survival depends. The "effective blood flows" are relatively small in comparison to the total amount of blood that circulates via the systemic and pulmonary circuit, which includes the large amount of recirculating blood (physiologic left-to-right and right-to-left shunts). Physiologic left-to-right shunt is the volume of pulmonary venous blood that recirculates through the lungs without having perfused the body, whereas physiologic right-to-left shunt is the volume of systemic venous blood that reenters the systemic circulation without having perfused the lungs. The magnitude of the mixing between the two circulations depends directly on the number, size, and location of the anatomic communications, and on the total blood flow through the pulmonary circuit.[113] In the newborn with intact ventricular septum and a closed or closing ductus arteriosus, severe hypoxemia caused by inadequate mixing at the foramen ovale level is usually present. Prostaglandin E_1 infusion reestablishes ductal flow, i.e., undersaturated blood enters the pulmonary circulation, and increases the volume of blood in the pulmonary circulation. Consequently, left atrial blood flow and pressure increase will result in more *effective left-to-right shunt* and ameliorate the systemic hypoxemia. Thus when the intracardiac shunt sites are of adequate size, the degree of arterial saturation is influenced primarily by the pulmonary-to-systemic flow ratio. As long as the left ventricle can adequately maintain the high output state, the higher the pulmonary flow, the higher the systemic blood saturation will be. Conversely, if pulmonary blood flow is decreased either from pulmonary stenosis or increased pulmonary vascular resistance, arterial oxygen saturation will decrease in spite of the large anatomic shunt sites. The exact mechanisms that quantitatively control the interchange between the two circulations are not completely elucidated. The location and size of the anatomic communication, along with respirations and respective ventricular and atrial compliances, as well as the level of pulmonary and systemic vascular resistances, play a role in this process of intercirculatory mixing.

It has been postulated that bronchopulmonary collateral circulation plays a major role in the pathophysiology of TGA. Bronchopulmonary anastomotic channels have been visualized by angiography in more than 30% of infants with TGA under 2 years of age. These anastomotic channels apparently communicate freely with the pulmonary vascular bed proximal to the pulmonary capillary bed. They may provide substantial amounts of unsaturated blood to the pulmonary circulation, contributing significantly to the intermixing of the two circuits. It also has been postulated that these precapillary bronchopulmonary anastomoses may play a role in the accelerated and more widespread pulmonary vascular disease observed in some patients with TGA.[120] For this reason, estimates of pulmonary blood flow based on the Fick principle are notoriously unreliable because the contribution of the bronchopulmonary anastomoses to the pulmonary blood flow cannot be assessed with this method.

In neonates with intact ventricular septum, the systemic arterial pO_2 may be as low as 25 mm Hg to 30 mm Hg, with resultant anaerobic glycolysis and severe metabolic acidosis. Unless intracardiac mixing is improved by either enlargement of the interatrial communication or administration of prostaglandin E_1, severe systemic hypoxemia will result in advanced metabolic acidosis, hypoglycemia, hypothermia, and death.

In the fetus with TGA, the physiologic derangement of the circulation appears to be tolerated very well. The fetus survives without apparent difficulty and develops normally. The average birth weight of infants with TGA is slightly greater than normal. Because the aorta arises from the right ventricle, the relatively more hypoxemic blood from the superior vena cava preferentially enters the right ventricle, and instead of being directed to the pulmonary artery, ductus arteriosus, and descending aorta, is ejected back into the ascending aorta. Thus the coronary circulation, cerebral circulation, and the rest of the upper body receives blood with somewhat lower pO_2. In contrast, the blood entering the left ventricle and the pulmonary circulation and descending aorta and placenta is derived from the inferior vena cava via the foramen ovale and has somewhat higher pO_2 than is expected in normal fetuses. Postnatally, as pulmonary vascular resistance drops, and in the presence of a PDA, unsaturated systemic arterial blood enters the pulmonary circulation and provides a much needed mixing.

Right ventricular dysfunction has been repeatedly documented before and after intraatrial repair.[121,122] Some of the causes considered responsible for depressed preoperative right ventricular function include intense cyanosis with prolonged myocardial hypoxemia, hypertension, and perhaps some intrinsic anatomic-geometric properties of the right ventricle.[113] Postoperatively, numerous studies have shown right and left ventricular dysfunction in a large percentage of patients, both at rest and with exercise. Several years postoperatively, more than 50% of patients have shown right ventricular ejection fraction at rest significantly below normal.[113] Abnormal exercise responses were also documented for both the right and left ventricle. These objective findings of mild to moderately depressed

right ventricular function may not be significant because most of these patients appear to be asymptomatic with minimal, if any, subjective complaints.[123]

With successful application of the *arterial switch operation* for anatomic correction of TGA, some of the postoperative residua involving the right ventricle will be completely avoided.[124] To date, long-term postoperative observations of left ventricular function have been quite encouraging regarding this type of definitive repair.[125]

The relatively early development of pulmonary vascular obstruction in patients with TGA has been fairly well documented by autopsy findings, lung biopsies, and hemodynamic data.[126,127] Compared with other forms of congenital heart disease, TGA has an apparent accelerated rate and an increased occurrence of this complication. In patients with associated large VSD and increased pulmonary flow, development of pulmonary vascular disease is more frequent than in those with intact ventricular septum. Pulmonary vascular changes grade III or greater (Heath-Edwards classification) are almost always present in infants older than 1 year of age. In patients over 1 year of age with TGA and intact ventricular septum, only a third will have similar pulmonary vascular obstructive changes.[127]

Even after intraatrial repair, progressive pulmonary vascular disease has been reported by several authors. It appears that hypoxemia, both systemic (chemoreceptor reflexes) and pulmonary (local effects), can induce pulmonary arteriolar constriction. Increased pulmonary blood flow and pressure, as well as the presence of hyperviscosity caused by polycythemia and development of microthrombi within the pulmonary microcirculation, may contribute to accelerated pulmonary vascular obstructive disease.[126,127]

Clinical features

Cyanosis, progressively severe hypoxemia or heart failure, and early death are the clinical manifestations of an infant with untreated TGA. As previously noted, the clinical manifestations will depend upon several anatomic and functional factors influencing the volume of intercirculatory mixing. The following is a useful clinical classification:

Transposition of the great arteries with intact ventricular septum. Patients with small VSD may be included in this group. Because of inadequate intermixing, these patients present with progressive cyanosis in the newborn period, requiring prostaglandin E_1 administration for stabilization, and early surgical correction (arterial switch operation) with or without balloon atrial septostomy (Rashkind procedure) prior to surgery.[128] Heart murmur may not be present in half of these patients, and the heart sounds may be only slightly accentuated. There is mild tachypnea or dyspnea in 50%. When a small VSD or persistent ductus arteriosus is present the cyanosis may not be as severe, and systolic or continuous murmur may be audible. The diagnosis is made easily now by a Doppler echocardiographic examination. Cardiac catheterization is not absolutely necessary unless there is a question about the origin of coronary arteries or a need for atrial septostomy. Chest roentgenogram shows mild-to-moderate cardiomegaly with increased pulmonary arterial markings and an "egg-shaped" cardiac silhouette.

Transposition of the great arteries with ventricular septal defect. These infants may not show symptoms of heart disease initially. Mild cyanosis may be noted only with crying. Signs of heart failure resembling those seen with large VSD may develop within 2 to 6 weeks of age. Tachypnea and tachycardia with moderate cyanosis are the usual presenting symptoms. Overactive precordium with loud heart sounds and loud systolic murmur, associated with a diastolic rumble at the apex, are usually present. These patients will show cardiomegaly and increased pulmonary vascularity in chest roentgenograms and combined left and right ventricular hypertrophy in the electrocardiogram. Echocardiographic and Doppler studies will establish the diagnosis adequately, and cardiac catheterization may be indicated to assess cardiopulmonary hemodynamics. Spontaneous decreases in the size of the VSD occurs in a small number of patients.

Corrective cardiac surgery [arterial switch operation, or palliative surgery (pulmonary arterial banding)] is recommended by 3 months of age when multiple VSDs or other complicating valve defects are present.

Patients who develop progressive pulmonary vascular obstructive disease become more cyanotic and symptomatic. The heart murmur from the VSD previously present diminishes in intensity and length, and there may be an ejection sound and a loud pulmonary closure sound. These patients follow a course similar to those with isolated large VSD and pulmonary hypertension (Eisenmenger complex). Palliative Mustard or Senning procedure has been successfully offered to some of these patients, resulting in marked improvement of their oxygenation.[121,122]

Transposition of the great arteries with ventricular septal defect and left ventricular outflow obstruction. These patients present with cyanosis and a loud systolic murmur caused by pulmonary or subpulmonary stenosis. Clinical findings are similar to those of tetralogy of Fallot. Diagnosis is usually made now by Doppler echocardiography. Cardiac catheterization and angiocardiography are usually performed prior to palliative or definitive surgical repair. Modified Blalock-Taussig shunting procedures are usually offered (prior to definitive repair) to such patients who may have relatively hypoplastic pulmonary arteries.

For more than 2 decades, the definitive corrective repair of patients with TGA has been the intraatrial switch of the systemic and pulmonary venous return (Senning and Mustard procedures).[121,122] These procedures were usually performed during the first or second year of life, following

life-saving balloon atrial septostomy (Rashkind procedure) performed soon after birth. More recently, these surgical procedures have given way to anatomic repair—the *arterial switch operation*—with apparently very promising results.[124,129]

It should be pointed out, however, that there are large numbers of patients who have undergone intraatrial repair in whom a variety of persistent abnormalities and complications have been recognized.[123] These conditions include superior or inferior vena cava obstruction, pulmonary venous obstructions, residual intraatrial baffle shunts, tricuspid valve insufficiency, and right ventricular dysfunction. Moreover, long-term follow-up studies have shown high prevalence of postoperative arrhythmias secondary to extensive intraatrial surgery.[130,131] Indeed, the high frequency of these atrial electrophysiologic disturbances constitutes one of the major arguments for embracing the arterial switch operation. The most frequent arrhythmias include bradycardia, ectopic atrial rhythm, junctional rhythm, and supraventricular tachycardia, particularly atrial flutter. Atrioventricular conduction disturbances, surgical complete heart block, and premature ventricular extra systoles have been also noted, especially in patients with repair of an associated ventricular septal defect.

A very disturbing late complication has been sudden unexplained death, probably caused by dysrhythmias, reported with a frequency of 2% to 9%. Sinus node dysfunction or rapid atrial tachycardias, either alone or in combination, have been frequently observed in such patients and could be the cause of sudden death. The term *sick sinus syndrome* has been applied to the arrhythmias characterized by periods of marked bradycardia, sinoatrial arrest or block with atrioventricular junctional escape, and slow junctional rhythms. Origin of the various arrhythmias has been attributed to intraoperative damage to sinus node or sinus node artery, damage to internodal pathways, or damage to AV node conduction tissue. A number of patients with extreme degrees of bradycardia even in the absence of symptoms have undergone placement of permanent pacemakers.[113] As expected, postoperative arrhythmias after arterial switch operations have been extremely rare. Some of the potential problems following the arterial switch operation are primarily related to translocation of the coronary arteries. Mild degrees of aortic insufficiency and supravalvular pulmonary stenosis at the site of repair have been reported.[132]

CORRECTED TRANSPOSITION OF THE GREAT ARTERIES (L-TRANSPOSITION)

Congenitally corrected transposition of the great arteries (CTGA) is a rare cardiac malformation in which there is transposition of the great arteries with anatomic inversion of the ventricles and situs solitus atria. Because of the arrangement of the cardiac segments, the normal hemodynamic pathways are not altered by the malformation, i.e., the systemic venous return enters the right atrium normally and via the right-sided A-V valve (mitral), then is directed into the anatomic left ventricle, and from there is ejected into the transposed pulmonary artery. The pulmonary venous return enters the normal left atrium, which is connected via a tricuspid valve to the left-sided anatomic right ventricle, and from there the blood is ejected into the transposed anterior aorta. In this malformation, the presence of atrioventricular discordance physiologically corrects the transposition of the great arteries (ventriculoarterial discordance), and there is no cyanosis.

The frequency of this malformation is probably less than 2% of all congenital malformations of the heart; in the absence of associated cardiac defects individuals with this malformation may have normal life expectancy. Corrected transposition of the great arteries is frequently associated with malpositions of the heart, especially those without atrial inversion ("dextroversion"). It is frequently associated with other congenital cardiac defects such as ventricular septal defect, pulmonary valve or subpulmonary stenosis, and left-sided atrioventricular valve insufficiency (Ebstein anomaly).[133]

The embryologic defect leading to this malformation is abnormal rotation of the bulboventricular loop and septation. In the presence of normal visceral-atrial situs solitus, the primitive heart tube loops to the left instead of to the right. Consequently, the anatomic right ventricle (arterial ventricle) is displaced posteriorly and leftward, and the anatomic left ventricle (venous ventricle) is displaced anterior and rightward. In addition, there is a lack of spiral rotation of the truncoconal septum.[134] The result of all these developmental errors is that the pulmonary artery is connected to the anatomic left ventricle, which receives systemic venous blood, and the aorta is connected to the anatomic right ventricle, which receives pulmonary venous (oxygenated) blood. The anatomic inversion of the two ventricles is followed by inversion of the conduction system, whereby the ventricular septal depolarization is directed from right to left.[135] As mentioned earlier, there is always inversion of the atrioventricular valves, and consequently there is no aorta-left sided (tricuspid) valve continuity, but such continuity exists between the pulmonary valve and the anterior leaflet of the right-sided (mitral) valve. The left-sided ventricle has an outflow chamber (infundibulum) below the aortic valve, whereas no infundibulum is present on the right side. The aorta is located anteriorly and to the left of the pulmonary artery, which is located posteriorly and medially to the aorta (Fig. 13-26).[133]

The left-sided ventricle has the architectural characteristics of the right ventricle, with heavy trabeculations and triangular shape and is hypertrophied in comparison with the right-sided ventricle, which has the anatomic characteristics of the left ventricle with a smooth wall without trabeculations. The coronary arteries are also inverted,

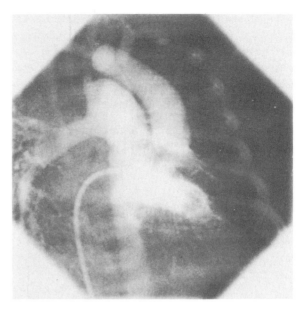

Fig. 13-26. Cineangiocardiogram from a 3-year-old child with corrected transposition of the great arteries and a large VSD. The injection of contrast material is made in the smooth-walled right sided ventricle (anatomic left ventricle). The aorta opacifies via a large VSD and is located anteriorly and to the left of the pulmonary artery. The dilated pulmonary artery is positioned medially and posteriorly to the aorta. Pulmonary hypertension caused by high pulmonary vascular resistance was present in this patient. (Courtesy of Kenneth Dooley, M.D., Egleston Children's Hospital, Atlanta, Ga.)

arising from the posterior sinuses. The anterior sinus is usually the noncoronary. The right coronary artery arises above the right aortic sinus and gives off the anterior descending; the left coronary artery arises above the left sinus, continues around posteriorly, and gives off the conal branch and the posterior descending artery, i.e., the coronary arteries supply their respective inverted ventricles. The most common associated malformation is ventricular septal defect (VSD). Its frequency has been reported as high as 80%. The VSD is usually large, and it is located beneath the crista supraventricularis in the membranous septum near the pulmonary valve. Supracristal, muscular, or multiple defects are much less common. Pulmonary outflow obstruction is also frequent and may involve the valve or the subvalvar area. Subpulmonary stenosis (like subaortic stenosis in hearts with normally related vessels) may be produced by either a fibrous ring, accumulation of fibrous or myxomatous tissue, or a fibromuscular tunnel.

Systemic A-V valve insufficiency has been reported to occur in one third of cases of CTGA. The posterior leaflet of the left-sided tricuspid valve is malformed and morphologically resembles that seen in cases of Ebstein anomaly. In contrast to Ebstein anomaly of the right-sided tricuspid valve, the circumference of the valve and the ventricle are not enlarged, the anterior leaflet is frequently cleft, and the malformed valve may interfere with the ventricular outflow tract.

The clinical manifestations are related to the associated lesions. As mentioned earlier, it is well documented that individuals with CTGA and without associated cardiac malformation may live normal lives. However, in such cases there is a possibility that symptoms may appear later in life because of arrhythmias.

The majority of patients with CTGA present with serious cardiac symptoms during the first few months of life. In all cases there is a large VSD or an associated lesion with or without pulmonary stenosis. Signs of heart failure with large left-to-right shunts or cyanosis and "blue" spells with associated severe pulmonary outflow obstruction are commonly the presenting symptoms. A loud single second heart sound over the upper sternal border, even in the absence of associated malformations, may suggest the presence of CTGA to the astute observer. It is caused by the closure of the anterior positioned aortic valve.

Systolic heart murmur at the lower left sternal border could represent either a small restrictive VSD or left A-V valve insufficiency. A harsh ejection systolic murmur is usually heard at the middle or lower left sternal border when pulmonary stenosis is present.

The electrocardiogram shows left axis deviation with evidence of Q wave inversion in the precordial leads caused by the inversion of the septum and the ventricles, i.e., QS and QR pattern in V_1 and R/S (no Q wave) in V_5 and V_6. Rhythm and conduction disturbances occur in over 50% of symptomatic cases.[136] This high frequency of arrhythmias has been attributed to the "abnormal" course of the conduction system. The ventricular inversion (A-V discordance) produces malalignment of the ventricular and atrial septa so that the bundle of His is elongated. The posterior A-V node is usually not connected with the bundle of His. An "accessory" anterior A-V node is connected with the bundle of His that passes anteriorly to the pulmonary valve annulus and branches in a mirror image of normal. It appears that the dual A-V modes and the long and tortuous course of the bundle of His are responsible for the high frequency of arrhythmias and A-V dissociation that occur naturally and quite frequently following cardiac surgery for associated defects. First degree A-V block may be present up to 50% of cases; complete A-V block may be present in up to 10%.

The diagnosis of CTGA and associated lesions can be made by a careful Doppler echocardiographic study. Cardiac catheterization and angiocardiography are indicated prior to surgical interventions and when associated malposition of the heart is present (Fig. 13-26).

Incompetence of the left A-V valve may not be present early in life and may manifest later. In such cases, it may be misdiagnosed as acquired mitral regurgitation rather than the congenital type. With increasing age, the risk of complete atrioventricular block in patients with CTGA continues to be present at a rate of 2% per year. Thus the complete heart block may manifest as an Adams-Stokes attack or sudden death.[136,137]

PERSISTENT TRUNCUS ARTERIOSUS

Persistent truncus arteriosus (PTA) is a rare cardiovascular malformation accounting for 2% to 3% of all the cardiac anomalies found at autopsy. It is characterized by the presence of a single arterial trunk arising from the base of the heart that gives origin to the coronary, pulmonary, and systemic arteries. In addition, there is a single semilunar valve without a remnant of a second atretic valve, a feature that differentiates PTA from pulmonary or aortic valve atresia, in both of which a single arterial vessel also receives the entire cardiac output.[138,139] A large ventricular septal defect is almost invariably present. There appears to be a slight male preponderance.

In the majority of cases truncus arteriosus occurs as an isolated cardiovascular malformation, but on occasion it has been reported in association with anomalies of other systems, particularly the DiGeorge syndrome.[140] As with other congenital cardiac malformations, an ever-increasing number of patients are reaching adolescence and adulthood because of successful reparative surgery.[141] These patients are in need of long-term follow-up, and for this reason this lesion is of some interest not only for the pediatric cardiologist but also for the cardiologist who treats adults.

The truncus arteriosus in the early embryo lies between the conus cordis proximally and the aortic sac and aortic arch system distally. The truncal lumen is divided in two channels by the appearance of truncal swellings, the proximal ascending aorta, and the pulmonary trunk. During the process of fusion between the truncal septum and the developing conal septum, the right ventricular origin of the pulmonary trunk and the left ventricular origin of the aorta are being established. The respective semilunar valves are being formed from tissue swellings at the sites of conotruncal fusion. Meanwhile, the paired sixth aortic arches (the primitive pulmonary arteries), along the aortic sac, migrate leftward, and the paired fourth aortic arches move rightward. Concurrently, invagination of the roof of the aortic sac forms an aortopulmonary septum that eventually fuses with the distal truncal septum. Consequently, the right and left pulmonary arteries originate from the pulmonary trunk, and the aortic arch is a continuation of the ascending aorta. The spiral course of the truncoaortic partition leads to the normal intertwinement of the great arteries.

Abnormal development of the conotruncal and truncoaortic septation may result in a number of congenital ventriculoarterial anomalies, one of which is PTA. Deficiency or absence of the conal (infundibulum) septum may result in a large ventricular septal defect. The single truncal valve may be deformed, leading to insufficiency or very rarely to stenosis. If remnants of distal truncoaortic septation develop, the pulmonary arteries may arise together from a short pulmonary trunk; otherwise, they may arise directly and separately from the root of the common trunk.[142]

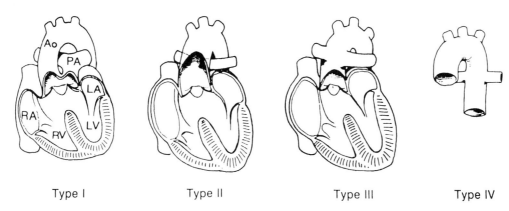

Type I Type II Type III Type IV

Fig. 13-27. Diagrammatic illustration of four types of persistent truncus arteriosus. Type IV is no longered considered as true truncus arteriosus (pseudotruncus). It is classified as severe tetralogy of Fallot with pulmonary atresia. (See text.)

Based upon the anatomic origin of the pulmonary arteries, four types of PTA have been recognized (Fig. 13-27).[143]

Type I—There is a short pulmonary trunk that originates from the left side of the common trunk and gives off both pulmonary arteries.

Type II—The pulmonary arteries arise separately from a common opening, usually located in the posterior wall of the common trunk, with no remnant of a pulmonary trunk.

Type III—The pulmonary arteries arise separately at some distance from each other.

Type IV—There is a common arterial trunk with two arteries ("bronchial") arising from the descending thoracic aorta and supplying the lung. This type is now considered to represent a variant of pulmonary atresia with ventricular septal defect.

The VSD is usually large and is located below the truncal root. Very rarely the VSD is small and even absent. In 70% of cases the truncal valve is tricuspid and 20% quadricuspid. Bicuspid valve is less common, and very rarely a pentacuspid valve is present. The truncal valve is always in continuity with the mitral valve. There is overriding of the VSD by the truncal root in more than 70% of cases. In 20% the truncus may arise entirely from the right ventricle; it originates from the left ventricle in only 5% of cases.[138]

Truncal valvar insufficiency is not uncommon and results from cusp abnormalities and dilatation of the root of the common trunk. Right aortic arch is present in at least one third of cases. In at least 50% of cases the ductus arteriosus is absent. Very rarely, hypoplasia of the aortic arch with or without coarctation of the aorta is seen. A distinct category of PTA has been described showing interruption of the aortic arch with ductal continuity to the descending thoracic aorta.

Type I is the most commonly encountered PTA (60%),

with Type II being the second most common (35%). Occasionally stenosis of the ostium of one or both pulmonary arteries may be present. In some cases of PTA one pulmonary artery may be absent, usually on the same side of the aortic arch. This is in contrast with tetralogy of Fallot with a single pulmonary artery, in which the absence of the artery occurs on the opposite side of the aortic arch.

There are several abnormalities of the origin and distribution of the coronary arteries. The left anterior descending artery is frequently very small, and frequently the conus branch of the right coronary artery is more prominent, with several large branches supplying the right ventricular outflow area. The posterior descending coronary artery arises from the left circumflex in at least 30% of cases, a variation that is three times as frequent as normal. Single coronary artery or one hypoplastic coronary artery with marked dominance of the other arising from the same sinus also has been observed. Rarely, a coronary artery may arise from a pulmonary artery trunk. Other cardiovascular anomalies of less hemodynamic significance also have been found in association with PTA, including secundum ASD, partial anomalous pulmonary venous connection, aberrant left subclavian artery, and persistent left SVC draining into the coronary sinus.[138,139]

There is always biventricular hypertrophy because both ventricles work in parallel to support the common circulation. Biventricular dilatation may be present in cases with severe truncal valve insufficiency. As a consequence of chronic exposure of the pulmonary vascular bed to systemic arterial pressure, pulmonary vascular disease often develops more rapidly and to a more severe extent in PTA than in isolated VSD.[138]

The clinical features of PTA depend largely upon the volume of pulmonary blood flow and the competence of the truncal valve. Symptoms such as mild cyanosis or signs of heart failure may appear in the neonatal period, and the great majority of patients will be recognized early

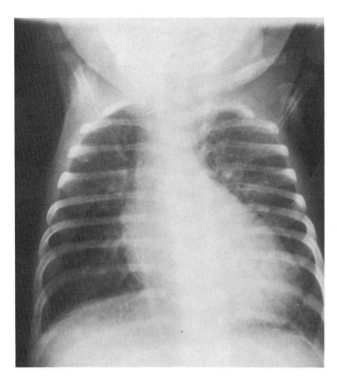

Fig. 13-28. A chest roentgenogram from a 1-month-old infant with persistent truncus arteriosus. Note the marked cardiomegaly, the increase in pulmonary vascularity, and the "straight" pulmonary artery segment. (Courtesy of Kenneth Dooley, M.D., Egleston Children's Hospital, Atlanta, Ga.)

in infancy. As the pulmonary vascular resistance drops postnatally, the pulmonary blood flow increases proportionally and leads to heart failure caused by volume overloading. The mild cyanosis present early after birth may diminish or disappear as the pulmonary flow increases with time. However, there is always moderate arterial hypoxemia caused by the mixing of the systemic and pulmonary venous return. Respiratory and feeding difficulties with failure to thrive and other signs of heart failure will appear within a few weeks, in a way similar to that seen in infants with large VSD or PDA. An overactive precordium with loud and single second sound and an ejection click may be present. A systolic murmur at the left sternal border and a diastolic apical rumble are usually audible in cases with markedly increased pulmonary blood flow. The pulses are usually prominent (bounding) because of the diastolic runoff into the pulmonary circulation. The combined ventricular output, after passing the truncal valve, is distributed according to the relative regional vascular resistances.[139] Mild-to-moderate arterial hypoxemia will easily differentiate a patient with PTA and heart failure from one with large patent ductus arteriosus in failure. The electrocardiogram usually shows combined right and left ventricular hypertrophy, and the chest roentgenogram shows cardiomegaly with increased pulmonary vascularity (Fig. 13-28).

In patients who develop early pulmonary vascular dis-

ease, the cyanosis becomes progressively more pronounced, and the clinical signs of heart failure recede. The heart murmur diminishes in intensity and even disappears, whereas the second sound remains single and loud. Two-dimensional and Doppler echocardiography are most helpful in establishing the diagnosis of PTA and detecting pressure gradients or truncal valve insufficiency.

Cardiac catheterization and angiocardiography are still recommended for some cases in which the precise diagnosis is not clear. Aortography and even selective coronary angiography is indicated for detection of coronary arterial abnormalities, as well as for establishing the exact location of the origin of the pulmonary arteries and the degree of truncal regurgitation (Fig. 13-29).

Without palliative or reparative surgery the majority of symptomatic infants die within the first year of life. However, patients who survive infancy are usually those who develop pulmonary vascular disease. There are a few isolated cases of patients with PTA who survived to the third and fourth decades of life. Complications resulting from polycythemia and paradoxic emboli such as cerebrovascular accidents and brain abscesses are as common as with other cyanotic cardiac defects.

Because of the dismal prognosis of infants with PTA and heart failure unresponsive to medical treatment, surgical treatment has been the only hope for them. Presently, primary repair of the malformation is offered to infants before 1 year of age with excellent results (Rastelli procedure).[144] This repair includes closure of the VSD and interposition of a conduit (valved plastic tube or aortic homograft) between the right ventricle and the pulmonary arteries, which have been separated from the common trunk. However, late development of "aortic" valve insufficiency requiring valve replacement has been frequently observed. In addition, replacement of the conduit becomes necessary with the growth of the child. Late survival has been compromised when the repair occurred in patients older than 2 years of age and in those with a single pulmonary artery or moderate truncal valve insufficiency. In older children with borderline increase in PVR who had definitive repair, the pulmonary vascular changes may continue to progress in spite of the decrease of the pulmonary blood flow.[145]

TOTAL ANOMALOUS PULMONARY VENOUS RETURN

In total anomalous pulmonary venous return (TAPVR), all pulmonary veins connect anomalously either directly to the right atrium or to one of its venous tributaries. When one or more but not all of the veins connect anomalously, the condition is called partial anomalous pulmonary venous return (PAPVR).

Embryologically, in the early stages of development, the lungs are connected by the vascular plexus of the foregut, the splanchnic plexus. As pulmonary differentiation progresses, a portion of the splanchnic plexus forms the

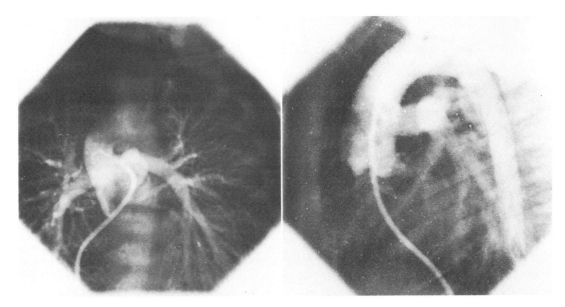

Fig. 13-29. A, Aortogram from a 3-year-old girl with Type I persistent truncus arteriosus. Note the large truncal root and the immediate take-off at the pulmonary artery. **B,** A lateral aortogram from a 1-year-old boy with persistent truncus arteriosus, Type II. Note the high and posterior origin of the pulmonary artery. (Courtesy of Kenneth Dooley, M.D.)

pulmonary vascular bed. At this stage of development there is no direct connection of the pulmonary vessels to the heart. The blood drainage of this primitive pulmonary vascular bed is carried via the splanchnic plexus (umbilicovitelline and cardinal vein system). The connection of the pulmonary vascular bed to the heart proper occurs later and depends upon the junction of an outpouching of the sinoatrial area of the heart with the pulmonary portion of the splanchnic plexus. This bulge ("common pulmonary vein") originates leftwards from the developing septum primum. As the direct connection with the heart proceeds, the initial communication of the pulmonary portion of the splanchnic plexus to the umbilicovitelline and cardinal venous systems gradually disappears. The drainage of the pulmonary vascular bed is carried out by four major veins and a common pulmonary vein that empties into the left atrium. The common pulmonary vein is apparently a transient structure and rapidly becomes incorporated into the left atrium, resulting in the final normal anatomic arrangement, i.e., direct and separate connections of the pulmonary veins with the left atrium. An interference with the development of the common pulmonary vein may result in TAPVR, as well as other pulmonary venous anomalies. If atresia of the common pulmonary vein occurs early in the development, the collateral channels draining the developing primitive lung will persist and enlarge, resulting in one of the types of TAPVR.[146] When the atresia of the common pulmonary vein is incomplete, i.e., it involves only the right or left side of it, partial anomalous pulmonary venous drainage will result. When the atresia of the common pulmonary vein occurs after the obliteration of the collat-

eral venous channels, a rare lethal malformation will result, whereby all four pulmonary veins empty into an isolated cul-de-sac, that does not have any connection either to the left atrium nor to systemic venous system (atresia of the common pulmonary vein).[146]

The frequency of TAPVR was reported to be 2% of a large number of autopsied cases with congenital heart disease. There is a definite male preponderance (3:1) in TAPVR connecting infradiaphragmatically to the portal vein. However, there is no sex prevalence in the other types of supradiaphragmatic connections. By definition, all pulmonary veins from both lungs connect anomalously to the right atrium or to systemic veins that in turn empty directly or indirectly into it. TAPVR is associated with additional major cardiac defects in 30% of cases.

There are several classifications of this malformation depending upon the location of the abnormal anatomic connections or the presence or absence of pulmonary venous obstruction, i.e., supracardiac, cardiac, infracardiac, or mixed type. An embryologic and anatomic classification taking into consideration the presence of venous obstruction has been well accepted and seems to be more appropriate. Based upon this classification, the following four types of anomalous pulmonary connections have been described (Fig. 13-30):

Type I—Common pulmonary vein → vertical vein → innominate vein → → superior vena cava → right atrium

Type II—Common pulmonary vein → coronary sinus → right atrium

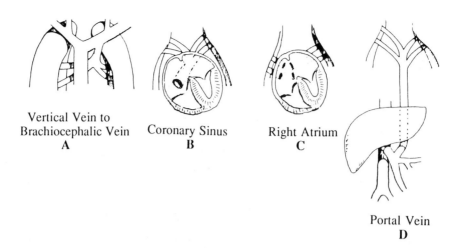

Vertical Vein to
Brachiocephalic Vein
A

Coronary Sinus
B

Right Atrium
C

Portal Vein
D

Fig. 13-30. Diagrammatic illustration of four types of total anomalous pulmonary venous return. (See text.)

Type III—All pulmonary veins enter the right atrium

Type IV—Common pulmonary veins → portal vein → ductus venosus → inferior vena cava → right atrium

In types I and II, the pulmonary veins form a confluence posterior to the left atrium and connect via a vertical vein to the innominate vein or to the coronary sinus, respectively. In type III, the pulmonary veins may enter the right atrium separately or via a common pulmonary vein. In type IV, the pulmonary veins join together in a confluence behind the left atrium and via an elongated common vein join the portal vein (below the diaphragm). In this type of TAPVR, there is always obstruction of the pulmonary venus return. The obstruction is offered by the hepatic sinusoids, i.e., the oxygenated blood from the lung passes through the liver to reach the right atrium. Other sites of obstruction of venous return may be at the interatrial septum (small patent foramen ovale), or at any site of the anomalous channel because of intrinsic causes (stenosis), or as a result of compression from an external structure (bronchus, pulmonary artery, diaphragm).[147]

Associated serious cardiac malformations may be present with TAPVR and include cor biloculare, single ventricle, truncus arteriosus, TGA, pulmonary atresia, and anomalies of the systemic veins. Frequently TAPVR is seen in asplenia. In TAPVR with pulmonary venous obstruction, severe degrees of arteriolar thickening and intimal vascular changes have been observed in the lungs.

The physiologic characteristics of TAPVR are determined by several factors: the degree of blood mixing of the pulmonary and systemic venous return in the right atrium and its distribution between the two circuits; the size of the interarterial communication; and the presence or absence of pulmonary venous obstruction. If the intraarterial communication is small, the amount of blood reaching the left atrium is decreased, leading to reduced left ventricular output.[147] The right atrial pressure increases to secure adequate systemic blood flow; consequently the ve-

nous pressures in both circuits also increase. In the presence of a widely patent foramen ovale or ASD, there is free communication between the two atria, and the distribution of mixed venous blood will depend upon the relative compliance of the atria and ventricles and the relative vascular resistances of both circuits.

TAPVR without pulmonary venous obstruction

In the presence of an adequate patent foramen ovale, the distribution of blood between the pulmonary and systemic circulation, at birth, is approximately equal because of almost equal vascular resistances. Postnatally, as the PVR gradually decreases, proportionally larger amounts of the mixed venous blood will enter the pulmonary circulation. Pulmonary blood flow three to four times systemic blood flow may be present. The systemic blood flow is usually normal. Because of the marked increase of pulmonary flow, the resultant arterial hypoxemia caused by the blood mixing is relatively mild. Blood entering all four chambers of the heart and both great vessels has practically the same oxygen saturation. Infants with TAPVR are usually asymptomatic at birth. However, within a few weeks they will develop symptoms such as tachypnea, feeding difficulties, and failure to thrive. They are subject to repeated respiratory infections and develop heart failure within a few months. Cyanosis is usually very mild and clinically inapparent. However, pulse oximetry or arterial blood gases invariably show moderate arterial hypoxemia. Cyanosis may be present in infants with heart failure or in older children who survived infancy and are acquiring secondary pulmonary vascular changes. There is always a prominent right ventricular heave. The first sound is loud and may be followed by an ejection click. The second sound is widely split and the splitting is fixed, i.e., does not change with respiration. A loud third and fourth heart sound in older patients may be present. A grade 2/6 ejection systolic murmur is usually heard at the upper left sternal border and results from turbulence produced by the

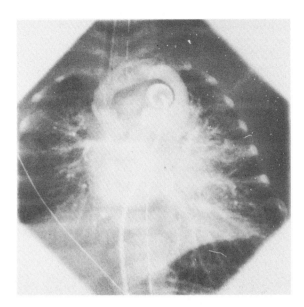

Fig. 13-31. Pulmonary angiogram from a 3-year-old girl with total anomalous pulmonary venous return into the superior vena cava via left vertical vein ("snowman" appearance). (See text.) (Courtesy of Kenneth Dooley, M.D., Egleston Children's Hospital, Atlanta, Ga.)

large right ventricular stroke volume across the pulmonary valve. A mid-diastolic murmur at the lower left sternal border also can be heard in at least 50% of cases and is caused by increased tricuspid flow. Hepatomegaly is always present and less frequently, so is peripheral edema.

The electrocardiogram shows right atrial enlargement and right ventricular hypertrophy. The chest roentgenogram shows always cardiomegaly with right atrial and right ventricular enlargement, prominent pulmonary arterial segment, and increased vascularity. A "snowman" appearance of the cardiac shadow is usually seen in older patients with TAPVR to the innominate vein. The two-dimensional echocardiogram shows volume-overloading of the right-sided chambers, with a leftward bulging of the atrial septum and paradoxic movement of the ventricular septum. Right-to-left direction of blood flow across the foramen ovale can be easily demonstrated by Doppler interrogation, and the absence of pulmonary venous connection to the small left atrium are both diagnostic signs for TAPVR. The exact location of the anomalous venous connections, especially when the connections are mixed, is difficult to determine and requires special expertise. Cardiac catheterization and angiocardiography are indicated preoperatively (Fig. 13-31).

TAPVR with pulmonary venous obstruction

Pulmonary venous obstruction is always present in cases of infradiaphragmatic TAPVR, and in at least 50% of those with supradiaphragmatic connections. Pulmonary venous obstruction is less common in patients with connection to the coronary sinus or directly to the right

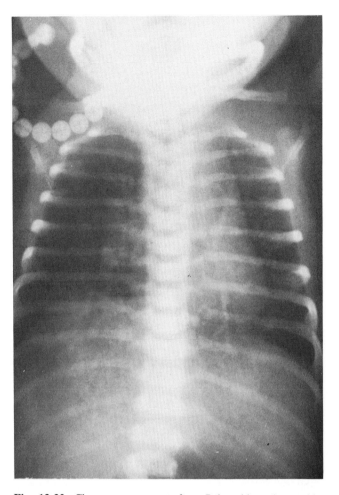

Fig. 13-32. Chest roentgenogram for a 7-day-old newborn with infradiaphragmatic total anomalous pulmonary venous return. Note the *normal heart size* and prominent pulmonary venous pattern. (See text.) (Courtesy of Kenneth Dooley, M.D., Egleston Children's Hospital, Atlanta, Ga.)

atrium. The clinical profile of these patients is similar regardless of the site of the obstruction. Infants with TAPVR below the diaphragm present with cyanosis and respiratory distress within the first few hours of life, and resemble those with respiratory distress syndrome (RDS). Infants with TAPVR are born usually at term, whereas typical RDS involves preterm infants. In spite of the severity of the symptoms, the cardiac findings may be minimal. The heart does not appear to be enlarged, and there is no significant right ventricular heave. There is usually no cardiac murmur, and the second sound may be split with an accentuated second component. There is always hepatomegaly.

The chest roentgenogram shows normal heart size and abnormal pulmonary vascular markings characterized by diffuse, reticular, stippled densities that fan out from the hilar regions. Kerley B lines may be present, and the cardiac borders are often obscured (Fig. 13-32). Two-dimensional echocardiography and Doppler echocardiography are again very valuable at arriving at the

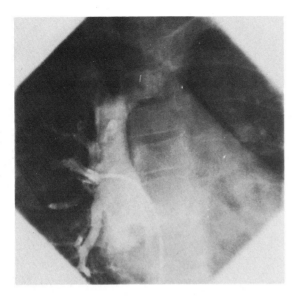

Fig. 13-33. Pulmonary venous angiogram in a 13-year-old girl with partial anomalous venous return. The catheter entered the anomalous vein from the right atrium. An ASD of the sinus venosus type was present in this patient. (Courtesy of Kenneth Dooley, M.D., Egleston Children's Hospital, Atlanta, Ga.)

diagnosis. However, in neonates, obtaining a blood sample from the umbilical vein will invariably suggest the diagnosis by finding highly saturated blood in the presence of peripheral cyanosis and systemic hypoxemia. Cardiac catheterization and angiocardiography will confirm the diagnosis.

The long-term results of corrective cardiac surgery in TAPVR without venous obstruction are very gratifying. Occasionally, isolated pulmonary venous obstruction secondary to scarring at the site of repair have been observed, necessitating revision of the anastomosis. Otherwise, the great majority of these patients are expected to live normal lives. Atrial dysrhythmias and rarely, atrioventricular block have been observed as postoperative sequelae.[146]

Partial anomalous pulmonary venous return (PAPVR)

In this type of pulmonary venous malformation, one or more (but not all) pulmonary veins are connected to the right atrium or its feeding veins (Fig. 13-33). There is frequent association of PAPVR with an atrial septal defect. Embryologically, it has been suggested that PAPVR may be the result of partial early obliteration of the common pulmonary vein and persistence of the still-present pulmonary-systemic venous channels that drain portions of the lung.

Left-sided pulmonary veins may connect anomalously to derivatives of the left cardinal system such as the coronary sinus or the left innominate vein. Abnormal connections of the right pulmonary veins are usually derivatives of the right cardinal system, i.e., superior vena cava, right

atrium, and inferior vena cava.[148] Occasionally, there is crossover of anomalous connections to the contralateral derivatives of the cardinal venous system. Anomalous right-sided pulmonary veins are more frequent than left-sided ones.

Right pulmonary veins to superior vena cava. This is the most common PAPVR. It involves the veins draining the upper and midlobe of the right lung. In the majority of cases, an ASD of the sinus venosus type is present. Occasionally, a secundum ASD may be present and very rarely, an ostium primum ASD. The signs and symptoms in such cases are difficult to differentiate from those of an ASD.

Right pulmonary veins to inferior vena cava (Scimitar Syndrome). All the right pulmonary veins, or only the veins draining the middle and lower lobe, enter the IVC just above or below the diaphragm. The atrial septum is usually intact. There is usually hypoplasia of the right lung and abnormalities of the bronchial system, dextroposition of the heart, hypoplasia of the right pulmonary artery, and anomalous arterial connection to the right lung from the aorta.[149]

Left pulmonary veins to the left innominate vein (LIV). The veins from the left upper lobe or of the entire left lung connect to the LIV via a derivative of the left cardinal system. The connecting vein has been called a persistent vertical vein. The atrial septum may be intact.

Stenosis of the common pulmonary vein (Cor triatriatum). This is a very rare abnormality whereby the pulmonary vein enters an accessory chamber, which in turn connects to the left atrium via a narrow opening. Failure of the common pulmonary vein to incorporate into the left atrium is considered the most plausible theory regarding the embryogenesis of cor triatriatum. There are a number of variants of this malformation, and the clinical manifestations are variable depending on the degree of narrowing at the connecting site. It presents with signs of pulmonary hypertension, sometimes later in life. Usually the patients present with respiratory symptoms that are persistent and resemble primary pulmonary disease. There is usually a loud second sound, ejection click, and signs of right ventricular failure. The electrocardiogram shows right ventricular hypertrophy (systolic overloading) and right atrial enlargement. The chest roentgenogram reflects pulmonary venous obstruction. Two-dimensional echocardiography is very helpful in suspecting diagnosis, but cardiac catheterization and angiocardiography are usually recommended for establishing the diagnosis preoperatively.[150]

SINGLE VENTRICLE (UNIVENTRICULAR HEART)

Single ventricle (SV) or univentricular heart, as the name indicates, is a serious form of cyanotic congenital heart disease characterized by the presence of two atrioventricular valves (or a common A-V valve) connected with one ventricular chamber (double inlet ventricle), which anatomically could be either the left ventricle or right ventricle. The most common variety of single ventricle is one in which the two atria are connected to a morphologic left ventricular chamber in the presence of a rudimentary right ventricular chamber.[151]

The ventricular morphology in hearts with absent atrioventricular connection (tricuspid or mitral valve atresia) is comparable to that of the true double inlet ventricle, i.e., the presence of a dominant left or right ventricle and hypoplastic contralateral ventricle ("functionally single ventricle"). However, such hearts are not considered true cases of SV and will not be included in this section. Classification of the various types of SV depends upon the morphology of the dominant ventricle, the nature of the ventricular connections, and the presence of other associated lesions. Single or univentricular hearts may be associated with any of the four possible atrial arrangements: normally related atria (situs solitus); mirror image atria (situs inversus); right atrial isomerism; and left atrial isomerism. Double inlet connection of the atria to the ventricle may occur via two separate A-V valves or a common valve. In many instances it is very difficult (when there are two valves) to distinguish, morphologically, a tricuspid from a mitral valve. For this reason, they are referred to as right-sided or left-sided A-V valve, irrespective of the atrial situs or ventricular morphology. Overriding or straddling of the A-V valve may also be present. The ventricular chambers are usually differentiated according to their trabecular characteristics. Whenever there are two ventricular chambers, they usually possess their different trabecular patterns.[152] In contrast, when there is only one chamber (common chamber), it is almost always neither anatomically right nor left, but of indeterminate ventricular pattern ("primitive ventricle").

The chamber lacking the A-V connection is always the nondominant or rudimentary one. Thus the septum separating the two ventricles, out of necessity, cannot be an inlet septum. It is always a trabecular septum. According to ventricular morphology, the ventricular arterial connections are *concordant* or *discordant*. Double outlet or single outlet (truncus arteriosus) may also occur from either the dominant or "rudimentary" chamber.

Based on the morphology of the double inlet dominant ventricle, three groups of single ventricles have been recognized: those with double inlet to a left ventricular chamber (DILV), to a right ventricular chamber (DIRV), and to an indeterminate ventricular chamber.

Group I: double inlet to a left ventricular chamber

In this type of SV, both A-V valves or a common valve are connected with the morphologically left ventricle posterior to the trabecular septum. The septum never extends to the crux of the heart. The rudimentary right ventricle is located anteriorly and to the right or anteriorly and to the

left. The dominant chamber has the characteristics of the left ventricle, with a relatively smooth wall, in contrast to the rudimentary anterior chamber, which has a trabecular component of the right ventricular pattern. It is usually hypoplastic, but in cases in which there is straddling or overriding of one of the A-V valves, this chamber may attain a larger size. Subpulmonary obstruction may be present within the left ventricular chamber, primarily caused by a posterior deviation of the infundibular septum. Valvar stenosis also may be present. Subaortic obstruction also occurs, frequently from a restrictive ventricular septal defect. More than 90% of the ventricular arterial connections in DILV are discordant, i.e., there is transposition. Significant subaortic obstruction is almost always associated with coarctation of the aorta. Ventriculoarterial concordance is rare.

Group II: double inlet to a right ventricular chamber (DIRV)

In this group both A-V valves (or a common valve) are connected with a ventricle that morphologically resembles the right ventricle (trabeculated). The location of the valves are anterior to the trabecular septum, which extends to the crux. The location of the rudimentary left ventricular chamber may be on the left and posterior aspect of the heart (normally related); on the anterior-inferior aspect (inverted); or at a midline posterior position. It may be of variable size, from a well-defined hypoplastic chamber to a very small slit-like structure resembling a trabeculation. This type of SV is found more often with atrial isomerism. Straddling and overriding of the valves is commonly seen, and it is usually found on the same side as the rudimentary left ventricular chamber. The ventriculoarterial connection is the double outlet type, usually occurring via a bilateral infundibulum. The rudimentary left ventricular chamber may have the appearance of a small smooth wall pouch connected with the dominant RV.

Group III: double inlet to an indeterminate ventricular chamber

The two A-V valves or the common valve connect to a common ventricle without outflow chamber, which does not resemble either the left or the right ventricle. It has the appearance of a more primitive ventricle with loose apical trabeculations, large criss-crossing trabeculae, and wall that appears much smoother in the inflow and outflow areas. The atrial situs is solitus but atrial isomerism is not infrequent. With atrial isomerism, there is usually a common A-V valve. Because there is only one chamber, both great vessels and occasionally one vessel arise from it, and the relationship between the two great arteries is variable. The aorta is usually anterior to the pulmonary trunk.

In cases with a very large VSD, there is always an apical rim of ventricular septum separating the two anatomic ventricles. This rim extends up the crux and carries the regular conduction system. This entity has been referred to in the literature as *common ventricle.*

Embryologically, the formation of the ventricular mass in hearts with double inlet ventricles depends upon the development of their trabecular components. Normally, the left ventricular trabecular component is formed from the inlet segment of the primary heart tube ("primitive ventricle"), whereas the right ventricular trabecular component is derived from the outlet segment ("bulbus"). Failure of development of both ventricular trabecular components will result in a sole chamber without a septum and indeterminate morphology that has a double A-V valve connection. This sequence of abnormal developmental events may be the possible mode of development of the double inlet univentricular heart with indeterminate ventricular morphology.[151]

Usually during the development of the ventricular mass, the inlet portions (A-V junction) of the trabecular components are shared by both ventricles. Failure of this normal sharing explains the other forms of the double inlet, as well as the different types of straddling A-V valves. Thus if the A-V junction retains its initial connection to the left ventricular trabecular zone, the result will be the development of DILV, with the trabecular component of right ventricular type forming the basis for the rudimentary chamber. Conversely, if there is an exaggeration of the connection of the A-V junction to the right ventricular component, a DIRV will be formed, and the trabecular component of the left ventricle will form the rudimentary ventricular chamber.[152]

The clinical features of patients without obstruction of the pulmonary blood flow are typical of large left-to-right shunts. Signs of heart failure with tachypnea, feeding difficulties, and failure to thrive are the common symptoms. Minimal cyanosis, overactive precordium, systolic thrill, and a loud systolic murmur at the left sternal border are common. In the presence of mild-to-moderate pulmonary obstruction, cyanosis is the dominant clinical symptom. The electrocardiogram, echocardiogram, and magnetic resonance studies may aid in the diagnosis of SV.[152,153] Biplane angiocardiography, however, obtained in special long axial oblique views as well as four-chamber views, is essential for establishing accurate diagnosis prior to palliative or definitive surgical procedures.[151] Palliative surgical procedures, such as *pulmonary arterial banding,* in patients with markedly increased pulmonary blood flow, or systemic-to-pulmonary arterial shunting for cyanotic patients with decreased pulmonary flow, are indicated and successfully performed. Definitive surgical reparative operations requiring cardiopulmonary bypass, such as Fontan-type repairs or even high risk *septation* operations, have been attempted with variable results in a selective group of patients.[151]

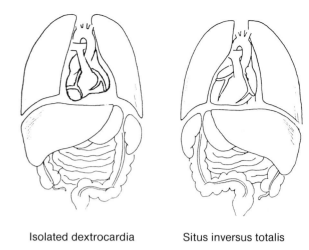

Isolated dextrocardia   Situs inversus totalis

Fig. 13-34. Diagrammatic illustration of isolated and mirror image dextrocardia. (See text.)

MALPOSITIONS OF THE HEART

The phrase *malposition of the heart* is used to describe abnormalities of the position of the heart either within or outside the thorax. The heart may be located in either side of the thorax or reside outside the thorax, as in *ectopia cordis,* or be shared in thoracopagus twins. Cardiac anomalies are frequently present in such cases and can be quite complex. Because of the malposition of the heart and the associated intracardiac and extracardiac malformations, the interpretation of clinical echocardiographic and angiocardiographic data is frequently difficult. Moreover, the various classifications and terms used to describe cardiac malpositions and their associated anomalies have contributed to the difficulties in understanding the complex nature of the defects in a given patient.

Several excellent reviews of the subject are available.[154,155] In this section, an attempt will be made to present a rather simplified description of the more common malpositions of the heart. Familiarity with various concepts used to describe developmental phenomena of the cardiovascular system (such as the types of *visceroatrial situs;* situs solitus, situs inversus, and situs ambiguous; the anatomic features of cardiac chambers; the connections between atria and ventricles, and ventricles and great arteries) is necessary to understand the various malpositions discussed.[154] In general, the terms *dextrocardia* and *levocardia* denote that the heart is located in the right side of the chest or the left side of the chest, respectively.

Dextrocardia

The heart is located in the right hemithorax (Fig. 13-34). There are five types of dextrocardia: two with situs solitus, one with situs inversus, and two with situs ambiguous with either right or left atrial isomerism. In the two forms of dextrocardia with situs solitus, the visceroatrial connection is normal, and concordance is present. The liver, inferior vena cava, and right atrium are right-sided, and the stomach, descending aorta, and left atrium are left-sided. The heart, though, is located in the right hemithorax. The two forms of dextrocardia with situs solitus are: *dextroposition of the heart,* in which the heart is displaced to the right chest by an extrinsic cause, such as hypoplasia of the right lung; and *dextroversion of the heart,* which results from rotational developmental abnormalities of the cardiac loop.[154]

Dextroposition. In this form of dextrocardia (with normally related atria, ventricles, and great arteries) the heart is displaced into the right hemithorax, but the cardiac apex points medially and to the left. It results, usually, from hypoplasia, dysplasia, or agenesis of the right lung. The pulmonary arterial branches of the right lung are smaller and have less arborization than those of the left lung. However, any abnormally occupying space in the left hemithorax (diaphragmatic hernia or a large pulmonary cyst) may also result in dextroposition of the heart. The term *scimitar* has been used to describe a condition in which there is dextroposition of the heart associated with varying degrees of hypoplasia of the right lung, partial anomalous pulmonary venous connection of the right pulmonary veins to the inferior vena cava, and anomalous arterial vessels originating from the descending aorta and supplying the right lower lobe of the lung.[149] The bronchial system of the right lung is hypoplastic and may show cystic changes. The condition derives its name from the curvilinear shadow produced by the anomalous venous connection in the right lung, which appears like a scimitar, or curved Turkish sword. Atrial septal defect, ventricular septal defect, and tetralogy of Fallot have been occasionally found to coexist with dextroposition of the heart.

Dextroversion (isolated dextrocardia). In this type of dextrocardia there is situs solitus, and the cardiac apex points to the right. There is usually atrioventricular concordance, but A-V discordance or a single ventricle may be associated with dextroversion. A faulty rotation of the primitive bulboventricular loop has been implicated as the pathogenetic mechanism of this malposition of the heart. Consequently, corrected transposition of the great arteries is a frequently associated anomaly, together with other common defects such as VSD, pulmonary stenosis, or atresia.

Dextrocardia associated with situs inversus (mirror image dextrocardia). There is always concordance because of the situs inversus. The liver, inferior vena cava, and the right atrium are located on the left side of the body. The descending aorta, stomach, and left atrium are found on the right side. The lungs and gastrointestinal tract are positioned in direct opposition to their normal positioning. The incidence of this form of dextrocardia is 1:10,000

live births. The frequency of cardiac malformations in this type of dextrocardia is not known. The distribution of various cardiac defects is similar to that found in cases of situs solitus and normal cardiac position. A subset of patients with dextrocardia and situs inversus have sinusitis and bronchiectasis, associated with infertility in males. This multisystem association of lesions comprise *Kartagener syndrome*. Study of the cilia of these patients revealed functional abnormalities believed to be responsible for the sinusitis, bronchiectasis, and infertility. It appears that ciliar function is important during normal embryogenesis. Absence of ciliar function in the embryo may result in a randomly determined situs. Moreover, abnormal ciliar function has been described in patients with polysplenia syndrome. Accordingly, individuals with the "immotile cilia syndrome" may have situs solitus, situs inversus, or situs ambiguous.[155]

Levocardia

The types of situs resulting in levocardia resemble those of dextrocardia: two with situs solitus, one with situs inversus, and two with situs ambiguous.

Situs solitus heart. This is the normal heart with visceroatrial concordance. In almost all individuals there is atrioventricular and ventriculoarterial concordance as a result of the normal rotation of the bulboventricular loop. In a very small proportion, there is an atrioventricular and ventriculoarterial discordance resulting in the anomaly known as congenitally corrected transposition of the great arteries.

Levoposition of the situs solitus. The heart is displaced further to the left from extrinsic causes, such as hypoplasia of the left lung. Absent left pulmonary artery may also result in hypoplasia of the left lung and further levoposition of the heart.

Levoversion of situs inversus. This condition is the opposite of dextroversion with situs solitus, i.e., there is situs inversus totalis, but the heart is in the left hemithorax with visceroatrial concordance. This malposition is extremely rare and may be associated with atrioventricular and ventriculoarterial discordance (corrected TGA).

Situs ambiguous. As mentioned in earlier discussion, visceroatrial situs refers to the relationship between the atria and the major viscera. There are three types of situs: situs solitus, situs inversus, and situs ambiguous. In the first two types there is always a concordant relationship between the viscera and right atrium. In situs ambiguous, the concordant relationship between organs does not exist, and there is no clear-cut laterality of the organs. The atria frequently show anatomic symmetry and appear to be either right atria (right atrial isomerism) or left atria (left-sided isomerism), and the lungs appear to be either trilobed and bilobed (epiarterial or hypoarterial bronchi). There is also abnormal morphology and position of the abdominal organs (liver, spleen, and intestine). Cases of situs ambiguous, very often, have been classified not according to their visceroatrial relationships, but according to the splenic status (asplenia or polysplenia). In most instances, asplenia is associated with right atrial isomerism and polysplenia with left atrial isomerism. However, there are cases where the status of the spleen does not correlate well with the cardiac anatomic features.

Regardless of the atrial isomerism (right or left), in 60% of the cases the heart is located in the left hemithorax (levocardia). There is no definite pattern of visceroatrial concordance, and for this reason they are referred to as ambiguous or indeterminate situs. The presence of situs ambiguous may be suspected frequently by the radiographic appearance of the chest and upper abdomen, which shows a relationship between the heart and the abdominal viscera that is neither situs solitus or situs inversus.[156]

Left atrial isomerism

This entity is synonymous with polysplenia syndrome. Right-sided organs tend to be absent in this condition, and bilaterally placed organs tend to have anatomic characteristics of the normal left-sided organ. Patients with left atrial isomerism have less complex cardiac defects and apparently longer survival than those with right atrial isomerism.

The lungs are bilobed and symmetric and show a relationship between the main stem bronchus and pulmonary artery similar to that seen in the normal left lung; the bronchus of each lung is hypoarterial, i.e., the respective pulmonary arteries course over and finally behind the bronchus. On heavily penetrated roentgenograms of the thorax, one can identify the symmetry of the bronchi. The liver is abnormal in shape and lobulation and may be symmetric. The gallbladder may be hypoplastic or absent. Rarely, extrahepatic biliary atresia has been observed. There may be two or more splenic masses present, located along the great curvature of the stomach. Absence of rotation or reverse rotation of the midgut loop may cause intestinal obstruction.

Cardiac anomalies are quite frequent and may include: bilateral superior venae cavae each entering the ipsilateral atrium; absent coronary sinus; azygous continuation of the inferior vena cava, with the hepatic veins connecting directly to the floor of the atrium; and partial anomalous pulmonary venous connection, with the pulmonary veins from each lung connecting separately with the posterior wall of the ipsilateral atrium. The atria show certain anatomic features of a left atrium. Their appendages are long and narrow, and the septum secundum and the crista terminalis are absent. In 65% of cases there is an ostium primum ASD. A ventricular septal defect is present in two thirds of cases, and in a few instances a univentricular heart may be present. The atrioventricular connection is usually ambiguous, either with two valves or a common valve. In 70% of cases there is ventriculoarterial concordance. The pulmonary valve may be stenotic or atretic in 30% of cases. The clinical features of these patients depend upon the underlying cardiac anomalies. The presence of dextrocardia with a midline (horizontal) liver may suggest left atrial isomerism.[155,156]

The electrocardiogram may show an ectopic atrial pacemaker with left and superior QRS frontal axis (because of frequent association of endocardial cushion defect). Thoracic and abdominal roentgenograms may be helpful in suspecting the diagnosis by demonstrating possible discordance between cardiac structures, the stomach, and the liver. Echocardiography is most useful in the diagnosis; angiocardiography is best utilized in demonstrating the long and narrow atrial appendages bilaterally.

Right atrial isomerism

Although this condition is practically synonymous with asplenia syndrome, there are a few cases described with normal spleen present. In right atrial isomerism, there is a tendency for bilaterally placed organs each to show characteristics of the right-sided organ. The left-sided organs are absent. Patients with this condition present themselves early in life because of associated serious and complex cardiac malformations. In the past, 90% of patients with asplenia syndrome could not survive the first year of life. With the use of prostaglandin E_1, echocardiographic diagnosis, and surgical interventions, survival has improved considerably. The lungs are trilobed and have eparterial bronchi bilaterally. However, because of the frequent presence of pulmonary atresia and hypoplastic pulmonary arteries, the relationship of the bronchi to the pulmonary arterial tree is difficult to establish. The major portion of the pulmonary arterial flow is derived from systemic collateral circulation. The liver is symmetric and occupies a transverse position across the upper abdomen. Malrotation of the bowel is usually present. The stomach is relatively small and is located in the midline. Renal and adrenal anomalies also may be present.

Cardiac anomalies include bilateral superior vena cava (50%); absence of coronary sinus; azygous continuation of the IVC (less frequently seen than in polysplenia); total anomalous pulmonary venous connection (80%) with frequent obstruction; pyramidal atrial appendages (right atrial–like); absence of the atrial septum; common atrioventricular valve with double inlet ventricle; pulmonary atresia and stenosis (75%); double outlet ventricle (right or univentricular); discordant ventriculoarterial connection (25%); and anterior position of the aorta.[156]

Patients with right atrial isomerism, because of the frequent association of pulmonary atresia, present with intense cyanosis during the neonatal period. No murmur is heard unless there is pulmonic stenosis. The QRS frontal axis of the electrocardiogram is superior, as it is in endocardial cushion defects. The thoracic roentgenograms show normal heart size with decreased pulmonary vascular markings, with the heart in the left or right hemithorax. Pulmonary venous obstruction may become evident only following increases in pulmonary blood flow, by either prostaglandin E$_1$ infusion or surgically created arteriopulmonary shunt.

ANOMALOUS LEFT CORONARY ARTERY ARISING FROM THE PULMONARY ARTERY

In this rare vascular anomaly, the left coronary artery arises from the left sinus of Valsalva of the pulmonary arterial trunk and assumes the course and branching of the normally arising coronary artery. Although a quite rare lesion, it has important physiologic and clinical features. It usually produces symptoms early in life but can be found occasionally in older patients with relatively few or no symptoms. It is often referred to as Bland-White-Garland syndrome.[157]

The development of coronary arteries in the normal human fetus occurs after the seventh week of gestation and follows the partition of the primitive arterial trunk to aorta and pulmonary artery. At this time small buds appear at the base of the aorta that rapidly mature and evolve as coronary arteries. The development of similar buds at the base of the pulmonary artery also has been observed in a number of embryos studied. These buds usually involute, but their persistence may lead to anomalies of the origin of the coronary arteries from the pulmonary artery. The anomalous origin of the left coronary artery (ALCA) from the pulmonary artery can be easily attributed to such embryologic aberration.[158]

Accessory coronary arteries arising from the pulmonary artery are usually small and supply a limited area of the right ventricle without ill effect. Anomalous origin of a single coronary artery from the pulmonary artery has not been reported. However, both coronary arteries arising from the pulmonary artery, although very rare, has been reported and is compatible with survival beyond early infancy as long as there is associated pulmonary hypertension.[159]

The myocardium is a specialized muscle with an unusual avidity for oxygen, which permits it to extract all the available oxygen in the blood in the coronary arteries. As long as there is adequate coronary perfusion pressure, low tension of oxygen in the blood perfusing the myocardium can be tolerated within a rather broad range. For example, patients with uncorrected cyanotic cardiac malformations and severe degrees of hypoxemia may develop myocardial dysfunction or damage only over a period of years.

In fetal and neonatal life, anomalous origin of the left coronary artery does not interfere with coronary perfusion because of the presence of pulmonary hypertension. Thus there is no need for development of intercoronary collateral circulation because both coronary arteries are perfused

with equal pressures. However, as pulmonary arterial pressure falls postnatally, a gradual decrease in left coronary arterial perfusion pressure ensues, leading to global underperfusion of the left ventricular myocardium. The left ventricle, in spite of the decrease in myocardial perfusion, is forced to develop systemic pressures to support the peripheral circulation. Decrease in coronary perfusion, however, will result in reduction of cardiac output and consequently to elevation of left atrial pressure and secondary pulmonary hypertension. It appears that this reactive pulmonary hypertension, to which the young infant is especially prone, prevents the pulmonary arterial and coronary pressure from falling precipitously and provides time for development of collateral circulation from the right coronary artery to the ischemic left coronary arterial bed. Therefore the extent and magnitude of this collateral circulation determines the severity of the clinical signs and symptoms and survival of the infant. If the collateral circulation is adequate, it may be life-saving. If not, it may lead to myocardial infarction and death. If large, the collateral circulation may cause a left-to-right shunt at the pulmonary arterial level and LV volume overloading, i.e., forward blood flow via the collaterals from the RCA to LCA and, from there, retrograde to the pulmonary artery (Fig. 13-35). Only in such cases has surgical ligation of the left coronary artery near its origin apparently resulted in marked improvement in left ventricular function. However, in the majority of cases, progressive left ventricular myocardial ischemia, especially in the subendocardial regions, as well as the development of small infarctions, may lead to permanent changes such as secondary endocardial fibroelastosis, papillary muscle scarring, and shortening of the chordae tendineae, resulting in varying degrees of mitral valve insufficiency.[158]

A very small number of patients with ALCA who apparently develop a generous pattern of collateral circulation may never present with appreciable symptoms.[160] In such cases, the malformation is discovered only at autopsy. The majority of patients become symptomatic within the first few weeks of life and progressively deteriorate with manifestations of myocardial ischemia and heart failure, which usually lead to death if the lesion is left unrecognized and not treated.

The adult heart with ALCA usually has a very large, thick-walled right coronary artery with large branches that gradually taper over the course normally occupied by distal branches of the left coronary artery (very similar distribution to that seen normally with dominant right coronary artery). The proximal branches of the anomalous left coronary artery are smaller than normal, have thin walls, and have the gross appearance of veins. These branches become larger peripherally as they merge with the distal branches of the right coronary artery. The heart is normal in size or only slightly enlarged, and there is only minimal myocardial fibrosis.

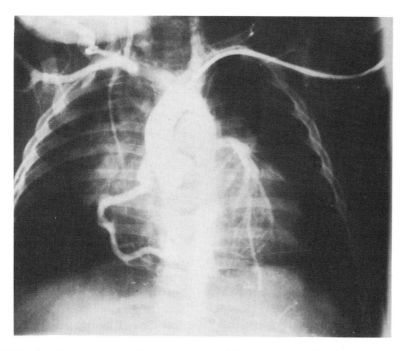

Fig. 13-35. Selective aortogram from a 4-month-old boy with anomalous left coronary artery arising from the pulmonary artery. Note the large right coronary artery. The anomalous left coronary artery opacifies via collaterals from the right coronary artery. The main pulmonary artery is visualized from the left-to-right shunt via the coronary circulation.

The hearts of infants who die are large because of dilated left ventricles. Evidence of multiple infarcts, old and recent ones, are usually present. Scars and thinning of the apical region, septum, and papillary muscles, as well as evidence of endocardial fibroelastosis involving the adjacent areas of the mitral valve, are invariably seen. The size of the collateral coronary arterial branches may vary considerably. In some infants, there is no gross evidence of intercoronary collaterization, and in others large localized collaterals may be present.

The clinical manifestations vary considerably, depending upon the development of adequate intercoronary communications. Episodes of paroxysmal attacks of acute discomfort precipitated by the exertion of nursing have been repeatedly described in very young infants. Grunting, pallor, cold sweat, and occasionally transient loss of consciousness are associated with such attacks. Chronic dyspnea and signs of heart failure may appear soon, and a number of these infants succumb within a few weeks if not recognized and appropriately treated. Some infants improve gradually because of the development of collateral circulation, and their acute painful episodes decrease in frequency and eventually disappear. Some of the older children who survive may have an occasional anginal attack with exertion or under the influence of emotion, or may present with signs of mitral valve insufficiency. There is invariably cardiomegaly caused by thin-walled underperfused left ventricle. An apical systolic murmur of mitral

valve insufficiency is usually audible. In the presence of large collaterals and aortopulmonary shunting through the coronary arteries, a continuous murmur, similar to that heard in coronary arteriovenous fistulae, may be heard over the precordium.

In the presence of infarction, the electrocardiogram resembles that of an adult with atherosclerotic coronary artery disease. Various stages of myocardial necrosis, scarring, and fibrosis may be reflected in the ECG with profound ST-T wave changes and "coving." Electrocardiographic changes compatible with anterior or anteroseptal myocardial infarction may be present, as well as deep q waves and inverted T waves in the left precordial leads. In older children with better myocardial perfusion, signs of infarction or ischemia are usually absent, but there is evidence of left ventricular hypertrophy.[158,161]

The chest roentgenogram may show varying degrees of cardiomegaly with dilated left ventricle and left atrium. Thallium-201 myocardial perfusion imaging may show abnormalities of perfusion.

Echocardiography (both M-mode and two-dimensional) is quite helpful in detecting left ventricular size and contractility, as well as the abnormal origin of the left coronary artery. Localized hypokinesis and dyskinesis, and thinning of the anterior and lateral and anterior ventricular wall and septum can be readily assessed. Doppler interrogation of the mitral valve will reveal valve regurgitation.

The extent and magnitude of the intercoronary collaterals can be easily assessed by selective aortography. The normal origin of the left coronary artery from the aorta will not be found, and only late opacification of the vessel through right coronary collaterals will be visualized. The right coronary artery is large, and its size is determined by the extent of collateral flow and the presence of left-to-right aortopulmonary shunt through the coronary circulation (Fig. 13-35).

Because the risk of sudden death in symptomatic patients is high, early diagnosis and surgical treatment is recommended. Ligation of the anomalous artery at its origin from the pulmonary trunk has been tried in the past and met with variable results.[158] It appears that it is beneficial only in those symptomatic patients with large intercoronary collaterals and left-to-right aortopulmonary shunt. Ligation of the left coronary artery and grafting of the left subclavian artery to it has been tried successfully in older infants and children with very good results.[161] More recently, direct connection of the anomalous left coronary artery to the aortic root via a transpulmonary baffle and creation of an aortopulmonary window also has been successfully applied.

At present, it appears that the creation of a two-coronary arterial system by applying various surgical methods as early as possible, is preferable to the originally proposed simple ligation of the anomalous coronary artery at its origin.[158]

REFERENCES

1. Clark EB, Takao A, eds: *Developmental cardiology: morphogenesis and function.* Mount Kisco, NY, 1990, Futura.
2. Van Mierop LSH: *Morphological development of the heart.* In Bern RM, ed: *Handbook of physiology,* sec 2, vol 1, Bethesda, 1979, American Physiological Society.
3. Clark EB, Van Mierop LHS: *Development of the cardiovascular system.* In Adams FH, Emmanouilides GC, Riemenschneider TA, eds: *Moss' heart disease in infants, children and adolescents,* ed 4, Baltimore, 1989, Williams & Wilkins.
4. Manasek FJ, Nakamura A: *Forces and deformations: their origins and regulation in early development.* In Ferrans VJ, Rosenquist GC, Weinstein C, eds: *Cardiac morphogenesis,* New York, 1985, Elsevier.
5. Nora JJ: *Etiologic aspects of heart diseases.* In Adams FH, Emmanouilides GC, Riemenschneider TA, eds: *Moss' heart disease in infants, children and adolescents,* ed 4, Baltimore, 1989, Williams & Wilkins.
6. Ferencz C, Villasenor AC: Epidemiology of cardiovascular malformations: the state of the art, *Cardiol Young* 1:264, 1991.
7. Nora JJ, Nora AH: Maternal transmission of congenital heart diseases: new recurrence risk figures and the question of cytoplasmic inheritance and vulnerability to teratogens, *Am J Cardiol* 59:459, 1987.
8. Kirby ML: Cardiac morphogenesis: recent research advances, *Pediatr Res* 21:219, 1987.
9. Devore GR, Siassi B: *Prenatal diagnosis and fetal monitoring.* In Adams FH, Emmanouilides GC, Riemenschneider TA, eds: *Moss' heart disease in infants, children and adolescents,* ed 4, Baltimore, 1989, Williams & Wilkins.
10. Emmanouilides GC, Baylen BG: *Neonatal cardiopulmonary distress.* Chicago, 1988, Yearbook Medical Publishers.
11. Heymann MA: *Fetal and neonatal circulations.* In Adams FH, Em-
manouilides GC, Riemenschneider TA, eds: *Moss' heart disease in infants, children and adolescents,* ed 4, Baltimore, 1989, Williams & Wilkins.
12. Rudolph AM, Heymann MA: Cardiac output in the fetal lamb: the effects of spontaneous and induced changes of heart rate on right and left ventricular output, *Am J Obstet Gynecol* 124:183, 1976.
13. Rudolph AM: Distribution and regulation of bloodflow in the fetal and neonatal lamb, *Circ Res* 57:811, 1985.
14. Hislop A, Reid L: Intrapulmonary arterial development during fetal life: branching pattern and structure, *J Anat* 113:35-48, 1972.
15. Kulik TJ, Reid LM: *Neonatal pulmonary vasculature.* In Moller JH, Neal WA, eds: *Fetal, neonatal and infant cardiac disease,* Norwalk, 1990, Appleton & Lange.
16. Cassin S: *Physiological changes in the circulation after birth.* In Moller JH, Neal WA, eds: *Fetal, neonatal and infant cardiac disease,* Norwalk, 1990, Appleton & Lange.
17. Friedman WF: The intrinsic physiologic properties of the developing heart. In Friedman WF, Lesch M, Sonnenblick EH, eds: *Neonatal Heart Disease,* New York, 1973, Grume & Stratton.
18. Anderson PAW: *The immature myocardium.* In Moller JH, Neal WA, eds: *Fetal, neonatal and infant cardiac disease,* Norwalk, 1990, Appleton & Lange.
19. Emmanouilides GC: *Persistent pulmonary hypertension in the neonate.* In Moller JH, Neal WA, eds: *Fetal, neonatal and infant cardiac disease,* Norwalk, 1990, Appleton & Lange.
20. Moss AJ, Emmanouilides GC, Duffie ER, Jr: Closure of the ductus arteriosus in the newborn infant, *Pediatrics* 32:35, 1963.
21. Moss AJ, Emmanouilides GC, Adams FH et al: The effect of hypoxia and status of ductus arteriosus on acid-base balance in newborn infants, *J Pediatr* 65:819, 1964.
22. Emmanouilides GC, Moss AJ, Duffie, E et al: Pulmonary arterial pressure changes in human newborn infants from birth to 3 days of age, *J Pediatr* 65:327, 1964.
23. Feldt RH, Porter CJ, Edwards WD et al: *Defects of the atrial septum and the atrioventricular canal.* In Adams FH, Emmanouilides GC, Riemenschneider TA, eds: *Moss' heart disease in infants, children and adolescents,* ed 4, Baltimore, 1989, Williams & Wilkins.
24. Mahoney LT, Truesdell SC, Krzmarzick TR et al: Atrial septal defects that present in infancy, *Am J Dis Child* 140:1115, 1986.
25. Ruschhaupt DG, Khoury L, Thilenius OG et al: Electrophysiologic abnormalities of children with ostium secundum atrial septal defect, *Am J Cardiol* 53:1643, 1984.
26. Shub C, Dimopoulos IN, Seward JB et al: Sensitivity of two-dimensional echocardiography in the direct visualization of atrial septal defect utilizing the subcostal approach: experience with 154 patients, *J Am Coll Cardiol* 2:127, 1983.
27. Child JS, Perloff JK: *Natural survival patterns.* In Perloff JK, Child JS, eds: *Congenital heart disease in adults,* Philadelphia, 1991, WB Saunders.
28. Craig RJ, Selzer A: Natural history and prognosis of atrial septal defect, *Circulation* 37:805, 1968.
29. Kaplan S, Perloff JK: *Survival patterns after surgery or interventional catheterization.* In Perloff JK, Child JS, ed: *Congenital heart disease in adults,* Philadelphia, 1991, WB Saunders.
30. St. John Sutton MG, Tajik AJ, McGoon DC: Atrial septal defect in patients 60 years or older: operative results and long term postoperative follow-up, *Circulation* 64:403, 1981.
31. Murphy JG, Gersh BJ, McGoon DC et al.: Long term outcome of patients undergoing surgical repair of isolated atrial septal defect: follow-up at 28-32 years, *N Engl J Med* 323:1645, 1990.
32. Bolens M, Fredli B: Sinus node function and conduction system before and and after surgery for secundum atrial septal defect: An electrophysiologic study, *Am J Cardiol* 53:1415, 1984.
33. Rome JJ, Keane JF, Perry SB et al: Double-umbrella closure of atrial septal defects: initial applications, *Circulation* 82:751, 1990.
34. Borow KM, Karp R: Atrial septal defects; lessons from the past, directions for the future, *N Engl J Med* 323:1698, 1990.

35. Graham TP Jr, Bender HW, Spach MS: *Ventricular septal defects.* In Adams FH, Emmanouilides GC, Riemenschneider TA, eds: *Moss' Heart disease in infants, children and adolescents,* ed 4, Baltimore, 1989, Williams & Wilkins.

36. Van Praagh R, Geva T, Kreutzer J: Ventricular septal defects: how shall we describe, name and classify them, *J Am Coll Cardiol* 14:1298, 1989.

37. Momma K, Toyama K, Takao A et al.: Natural history of subarterial infundibular ventricular septal defect, *Am Heart J* 108:1312, 1988.

38. Krongard E, Heffler SE, Bowman FO Jr et al: Further observations on the etiology of the right bundle branch block pattern following right ventriculotomy, *Circulation* 50:1105, 1974.

39. Jarmakani MM, Graham TP Jr, Canent RV Jr et al: Effect of site of shunt on left heart volume characteristics with ventricular septal defect and patent ductus arteriosus, *Circulation* 40:411, 1969.

40. Rosenthal A, Bank ER: *Ventricular septal defect.* In Moller JH, Neal WA, eds: *Fetal, neonatal and infant cardiac disease,* Norwalk, 1990, Appleton & Lange.

41. Graham, TP Jr: In Roberts WC, ed: *Adult congenital heart disease,* Philadelphia, 1987, FA Davis.

42. Hoffman JLE, Rudolph AM: The natural history of ventricular septal defects in infancy, *Am J Cardiol* 16:634, 1965.

43. Moe DG, Guntheroth WG: Spontaneous closure of uncomplicated ventricular septal defect, *Am J Cardiol* 60:674, 1987.

44. Perloff JK, Child JS, eds: *Congenital heart disease in adults,* ed 1, Philadelphia, 1991, WB Saunders.

45. Titus JL, Rastelli GC: *Anatomic features of persistent common atrioventricular canal.* In Feldt RH, McGoon DC, Ongley PA eds: et al, *Atrioventricular canal defects,* Philadelphia, 1976, WB Saunders.

46. Lappen RS, Muster AJ, Idriss FS et al: Masked subaortic stenosis in ostium primum atrial septal defect; recognition and treatment, *Am J Cardiol* 52:336, 1983.

47. Piccoli GP, Ho SY, Wilkinson JL et al: Left-sided obstructive lesions in atrioventricular septal defects: an anatomic study, *J Thorac Cardiovasc Surg* 83:453, 1982.

48. Portman MA, Beder SD, Cohen MH et al: Conduction abnormalities detected by electrophysiologic testing following repair of ostium primum atrioventricular septal defect, *Int J Cardiol* 11:111, 1986.

49. Studer M, Blackstone EH, Kirklin JW et al: Determinants of early and late results of repair of atrioventricular septal (canal) defects, *J Thor Cardiovasc Surg* 84:523, 1982.

50. Heymann MA: *Patent ductus arteriosus.* In Adams FH, Emmanouilides GC, Riemenschneider TA, ed: *Moss' heart disease in infants, children and adolescents,* ed 4, Baltimore, 1989, Williams & Wilkins.

51. Thibeault DW, Emmanouilides GC, Nelson RJ et al: Patent ductus arteriosus complicating the respiratory distress syndrome in preterm infants, *J Pediatr* 86:120-1975.

52. King DT, Emmanouilides GC, Andrews JC et al: Morphologic evidence of accelerated closure of the ductus arteriosus in preterm infants, *Pediatrics* 65:872, 1980.

53. Edwards JE: *Congenital malformations of the heart and great vessels.* In Could SE, ed: *Pathology of the heart,* ed 2, Springfield, IL, 1960, Charles C Thomas.

54. Riemenschneider TA, Emmanouilides GC, Hirose F et al: Coarctation of the abdominal aorta in children; report of three cases and review of the literature, *Pediatrics* 44:716, 1969.

55. Fyler DC, Buckley LP, Hellenbrand WE et al: Report of the New England Regional Infant Cardiac Program, *Pediatrics* 65(suppl):2, 1980.

56. Gersony WM: *Coarctation of the aorta.* In Adams FH, Emmanouilides GC, Riemenschneider TA, eds: *Moss' heart disease in infants, children and adolescents,* ed 4, Baltimore, 1989, Williams & Wilkins.

57. Beekman RH, Rocchini AP: *Coarctation of the aorta and interruption of the aortic arch.* In Moller JH, Neal WA, eds: *Fetal, neonatal and infant cardiac disease,* Norwalk, 1990, Appleton & Lange.

58. Rudolph AM, Heymann MA, Spitznas U: Hemodynamic considerations in the development of narrowing of the aorta, *Am J Cardiol* 30:514, 1972.

59. Koller M, Rothlin M, Senning A: Coarctation of the aorta; review of 362 operated patients. Long-term follow-up and assessment of prognostic variables, *Eur Heart J* 8:670, 1987.

60. Cohen M, Fuster V, Steele DM et al: Coarctation of the aorta: long-term follow-up and prediction of outcome after surgical correction, *Circulation* 80:840, 1989.

61. Bromberg EI, Beekman RH, Rocchini AP et al: Aortic aneurysm after patch aortoplasty repair of coarctation: a prospective analysis of prevalence, screening tests and risks, *J Am Coll Cardiol* 14:734, 1989.

62. Roberts WC: Valvular, subvalvular and supravalvular aortic stenosis; morphologic features. *Cardiovasc Clin* 5:97, 1973.

63. Hoffman JIE: Determinants and prediction of transmural myocardial perfusion, *Circulation* 58:381, 1978.

64. Friedman WF: *Aortic stenosis.* In Adams FH, Emmanouilides GC, Riemenschneider TA, ed: *Moss' heart disease in infants, children and adolescents,* ed 4, Baltimore, 1989, Williams & Wilkins.

65. Seitz WS, McIlroy MB, Kline H et al: Echocardiographic application of the Gorlin formula for assessment of aortic stenosis: correlation with cardiac catheterization in pediatric patients, *Am Heart J* 111:1118, 1986.

66. Cyran SE, James FW, Daniels S et al: Comparison of the cardiac output and stroke volume response to upright exercise in children with valvular and subvalvular aortic stenosis, *J Am Coll Cardiol* 11:651, 1988.

67. Rocchini AP, Beekman RH, Shachar GB et al: Balloon aortic valvoplasty; results of the valvoplasty and angioplasty of congenital anomalies registry, *Am J Cardiol* 65:784, 1990.

68. Roberts WC: The congenitally bicuspid aortic valve; a study of 85 autopsy cases, *Am J Cardiol* 26:72, 1970.

69. Newfeld EA, Muster AJ, Paul MH et al: Discrete subvalvular aortic stenosis in childhood, *Am J Cardiol* 38:53, 1976.

70. Berry TE, Aziz KU, Paul MH: Echocardiographic assessment of discreet subaortic stenosis, *Am J Cardiol* 43:951, 1979.

71. Leichter DA, Sullivan I, Gersony WM: "Acquired" discrete subvalvular aortic stenosis; natural history and hemodynamics, *J Am Coll Cardiol* 14:1539, 1989.

72. Williams JCP, Barrat-Boyce BG, Lowe JB: Supravalvular aortic stenosis, *Circulation* 24:1311, 1961.

73. Freedom RM: *Hypoplastic left heart syndrome.* In Adams FH, Emmanouilides GC, Riemenschneider TA, eds: *Moss' heart disease in infants, children and adolescents,* ed 4, Baltimore, 1989, Williams & Wilkins.

74. Newman MP, Heidelberger KP, Dick MH et al: Pulmonary vascular changes associated with hypoplastic left heart syndrome, *Pediatr Cardiol* 1:301, 1980.

75. Norwood WJ: Hypoplastic left heart syndrome: experience with palliative surgery, *Am J Cardiol* 45:87, 1980.

76. Chang AC, Farrell PE Jr, Murdison KA: Hypoplastic left heart syndrome: hemodynamic and angiographic assessment after initial reconstructive surgery and relevance to modified Fontan procedure, *J Am Coll Cardiol* 17:1143, 1991.

77. Bailey LL, Nehlsen-Cannarella SL, Doroshow RW et al: Cardiac allotransplantation in newborns as therapy for hypoplastic left heart syndrome, *N Engl J Med* 315:949, 1986.

78. Puga FJ: Modified Fontan procedure for hypoplastic left heart syndrome after palliation with Norwood operation, *J Am Coll Cardiol* 17:1150, 1991.

79. Rocchini AP, Emmanouilides GC: *Pulmonary stenosis.* In Adams FH, Emmanouilides GC, Riemenschneider TA, eds: *Moss' heart*

disease in infants, children and adolescents, ed 4, Baltimore, 1989, Williams & Wilkins.

80. Noonan JA: Hypertension with Turner's phenotype; a new syndrome with associated congenital heart disease, *Am J Dis Child* 116:373, 1968.

81. Stanger P, Cassidy SC, Girod DA et al: Balloon angioplasty, pulmonary valvuloplasty; results of the valvuloplasty and angioplasty of congenital anomalies registry, *Am J Cardiol* 65:775, 1990.

82. McCrindle BW, Kan JS: Long-term results after balloon pulmonary valvuloplasty, *Circulation* 83:1915, 1991.

83. Lucas RV Jr, Marshall RJ, Morgan DZ et al: Anomalous muscle bundle of the right ventricle with intact ventricular septum; a newly recognized cause of right ventricular obstruction, *Circulation* 28:759, 1963.

84. Kveselis D, Rosenthal A, Ferguson P et al: Long-term prognosis after repair of double-chamber right ventricle with ventricular septal defect, *Am J Cardiol* 54:1292, 1984.

85. Gay BB, Franch RH, Shufford WH et al: Roentgenologic features of simple and multiple coarctations of the pulmonary artery and branches, *Am J Roentgenol* 90:599, 1963.

86. Emmanouilides GC, Linde LM, Crittenden IH: Pulmonary artery stenosis associated with ductus arteriosus following maternal rubella, *Circulation* 29:514, 1964.

87. Kan JS, Marvin WJ, Bass JL et al: Balloon angioplasty-branch pulmonary artery stenosis: results from valvuloplasty and angioplasty congenital anomalies registry, *Am J Cardiol* 65:798, 1990.

88. Marvin WJ, Mahoney LT: *Pulmonary atresia with intact ventricular septum.* In Adams FH, Emmanouilides GC, Riemenschneider TA, eds: *Moss' heart disease in infants, children and adolescents,* ed 4, Baltimore, 1989, Williams & Wilkins.

89. Foker JE, Braunlin EA, Cyr JAS et al: Management of pulmonary atresia with intact ventricular septum, *J Thorac Cardiovasc Surg* 92:706, 1986.

90. Zuberbuhler JR: *Tetralogy of Fallot.* In Adams FH, Emmanouilides GC, Riemenschneider TA, eds: *Moss' heart disease in infants, children and adolescents,* ed 4, Baltimore, 1989, Williams & Wilkins.

91. Mair DD, Edwards WD, Hagler DJ et al: *Tetralogy of Fallot and pulmonary atresia with ventricular septal defect.* In Moller JH, Neal WA, eds: *Fetal, neonatal and infant cardiac disease,* Norwalk, 1990, Appleton & Lange.

92. Van Praagh R, Van Praagh S, Nebesar RA, et al: Tetralogy of Fallot; underdevelopment of the pulmonary infundibulum and its sequelae, *Am J Cardiol* 26:25, 1970.

93. Arenega A, Egea J, Alvarez L et al: Tetralogy of Fallot produced in chick embryos by mechanical interference with cardiogenesis, *Anat Rec* 213:560, 1985.

94. Emmanouilides GC, Thanopoulos B, Siassi B et al: "Agenesis" of ductus arteriosus associated with the syndrome of tetralogy of Fallot and absent pulmonary valve, *Am J Cardiol* 37:403, 1976.

95. Kirklin JW, Blackstone EH, Kirklin JK et al: Surgical results and protocols in the spectrum of tetralogy of Fallot, *Ann Surg* 198:251, 1983.

96. Steeg CN, Krongrad E, Davachi F et al: Postoperative left anterior hemiblock and right bundle branch block following repair of tetralogy of Fallot. *Circulation* 51:1026, 1975.

97. Kirklin JW, Blackstone EH, Shimazaki Y et al: Survival, functional status and reoperations after repair of Tetralogy of Fallot with pulmonary atresia, *J Thorac Cardiov Surg* 96:102, 1988.

98. Gillette PC, Yeoman MA, Mullins CE et al: Sudden death after repair of tetralogy of Fallot, *Circulation* 56:566, 1977.

98a. Waien SA, Liu PP, Ross BL et al: Serial follow-up of adults with repaired tetralogy of Fallot, *J Am Coll Cardiol* 20:295, 1992.

99. Rosenthal A, Dick M: *Tricuspid atresia.* In Adams FH, Emmanouilides GC, Riemenschneider TA, eds: *Moss' heart disease in infants, children and adolescents,* ed 4, Baltimore, 1989, Williams & Wilkins.

100. Rao PS: *Tricuspid atresia.* Mount Kisco, NY, 1982, Futura Publishing.

101. Fontan F, Bandet E: Surgical repair of tricuspid atresia, *Thorax* 26:240, 1971.

102. Driscoll DJ, Danielson GK, Puga FJ et al: Exercise tolerance and cardiorespiratory response to exercise after the Fontan operation for tricuspid atresia or functional single ventricle, *J Am Coll Cardiol* 7:1087, 1986.

103. Girod DA, Fontan F, Deville C et al: Long-term results after Fontan operation for tricuspid atresia, *Circulation* 75:605, 1987.

104. Kürer CC, Tanner CS, Norwood WI et al: Perioperative arrhythmias after Fontan repair, *Circulation* 82:Suppl IV:190, 1990.

105. de Leval MR, Kilner P, Gewillig M et al: Total cavopulmonary connection; a logical alternative to atriopulmonary connection for complex Fontan operations. Experimental studies and early clinical experience, *J Thorac Cardiovasc Surg* 96:682, 1988.

106. Cloutier A, Ash JM, Smallhorn JF et al: Abnormal distribution of pulmonary blood flow after the Glenn shunt or Fontan procedure; risk of development of arteriovenous fistulae, *Circulation* 72:471, 1985.

107. Van Mierop LHS, Kutsche LM, Victorica BE: *Ebstein anomaly.* In Adams FH, Emmanouilides GC, Riemenschneider TA, eds: *Moss' heart disease in infants, children and adolescents,* ed 4, Baltimore, 1989, Williams & Wilkins.

108. Park JM, Sridaromont S, Ledbetter ED et al: Ebstein's anomaly of the tricuspid valve associated with prenatal exposure to lithium carbonate, *Am J Dis Child* 134:703, 1980.

109. Oh JK, Holmes DR Jr, Hayes DL et al: Cardiac arrhythmias in patients with surgical repair of Ebstein's anomaly, *J Am Coll Cardiol* 6:1351, 1985.

110. Shiina A, Seward JB, Edwards WD et al: Two-dimensional echocardiographic spectrum of Ebstein's anomaly; detailed anatomic assessment, *J Am Coll Cardiol* 3:356, 1984.

111. Leung MP, Baker EJ, Anderson RH et al: Cineangiographic spectrum of Ebstein's malformation; its relevance to clinical presentation and outcome. *J Am Coll Cardiol* 11:154, 1988.

112. Quagebeur JM, Sreeram N, Fraser AG et al: Surgery for Ebstein's anomaly; the clinical and echocardiographic evaluation of a new technique, *J Am Coll Cardiol* 17:722, 1991.

113. Paul MH: *Complete transposition of the great arteries.* In Adams FH, Emmanouilides GC, Riemenschneider TA, eds: *Moss' heart disease in infants, children and adolescents,* ed 4, Baltimore, 1989, Williams & Wilkins.

114. McCartney FJ, Shinebourne EA, Anderson RH: Connections, relations, discordance and distortions, *Br Heart J* 38:323, 1976.

115. Van Mierop LH: Diagnostic code for congenital heart disease. *Pediatr Cardiol* 5:331, 1984.

116. Van Praagh R: The importance of segmental situs in the diagnosis of congenital heart disease. *Semin Roentgenol* 29:254, 1985.

117. Van Praagh R, Layton WM, Van Praagh S: *The morphogenesis of normal and abnormal relationships between the great arteries and the ventricles; pathologic and experimental data.* In Van Praagh R, Takao A, eds: *Etiology and morphogenesis of congenital heart disease,* Mount Kisco, NY, 1980, Futura Publishing.

118. Gittenberger-de Groot AC, Sauer U, Oppenheimer-Dekker A et al: Coronary arterial anatomy in transposition of the great arteries. A morphological study. *Pediatr Cardiol* 4(suppl):15-24, 1983.

119. Yacoub MH, Arensman FW, Keck E, et al: Fate of dynamic left ventricular outflow obstruction after anatomic correction of transposition of the great arteries, *Circulation* 68:1153, 1983.

120. Aziz KU, Paul MH, Rowe RD: Bronchopulmonary circulation in D-transposition of the great arteries: possible role in genesis of accelerated pulmonary vascular disease, *Am J Cardiol* 39:432, 1977.

121. Senning A: Surgical correction of transposition of the great vessels, *Surgery* 45:966, 1959.

122. Mustard WT: Successful two-stage correction of transposition of the great vessels, *Surgery* 55:469, 1964.

123. Torino MI, Siebeumann R, Nussbaumer P et al: A long-term outlook after atrial correction for transposition of great arteries; cautious optimism. *J Thorac Cardiovasc Surgery* 95:828, 1988.

124. Jatene AD, Fontes VF, Paulista PP et al: Anatomic correction of transposition of the great vessels, *J Thorac Cardiovasc Surg* 72:364, 1976.

125. Castaneda AR, Norwood WI, Jonas RA et al: Transposition of the great arteries and intact ventricular septum: anatomical correction in the neonate, *Ann Thorac Surg* 38:438, 1984.

126. Rosengart R, Fishbein M, Emmanouilides GC: Progressive pulmonary vascular disease after surgical correction (Mustard procedure) of transposition of the great arteries with intact ventricular septum, *Am J Cardiol* 35:107, 1975.

127. Newfeld EA, Paul MH, Muster AJ et al: Pulmonary vascular disease in transposition of the great vessels and intact ventricular septum, *Circulation* 59:529, 1979.

128. Rashkind WJ, Miller WW: Creation of an atrial septal defect without thoracotomy, *JAMA* 196:991, 1966.

129. Casteneda AR, Trusler GA, Paul MH et al: The early results of simple transposition in the current era, *J Thorac Cardiovasc Surg* 95:14, 1988.

130. Flinn CJ, Wolff GS, Dick M II, et al: Cardiac rhythm after Mustard operation for complete transposition of the great arteries, *N Engl J Med* 310:1635, 1984.

131. Vetter VL, Tanner CS, Horowitz LN: Electrophysiologic consequences of the Mustard repair of D-transposition of the great arteries, *J Am Coll Cardiol* 10:1265, 1987.

132. Martin RP, Ladusans EG, Parsons JM et al: Incidence and site of pulmonary stenosis after anatomical correction of transposition of great arteries, *Br Heart J* 59:122, 1988.

133. Ruttenberg HD: *Corrected transposition of the great arteries and splenic syndromes.* In Adams FH, Emmanouilides GC, Riemenschneider TA, eds: *Moss' heart disease in infants, children and adolescents,* ed 4, Baltimore, 1989, Williams & Wilkins.

134. Grant RP: Morphogenesis of corrected transposition and other anomalies of cardiac polarity, *Circulation* 29:71, 1964.

135. Anderson RH, Becker AG, Arnold R et al: The conduction tissues in congenitally corrected transposition, *Circulation* 50:911, 1974.

136. Daliento L, Corrado D, Buja G et al: Rhythm and conduction disturbances in isolated, congenitally corrected transposition of the great arteries, *Am J Cardiol* 58:314, 1986.

137. Lundstrom U, Bull C, Wyse RKH et al: The natural and "unnatural" history of congenitally corrected transposition, *Am J Cardiol* 66:1222, 1990.

138. Mair DD, Edwards WD, Julsrud PR et al: *Truncus arteriosus.* In Adams FH, Emmanouilides GC, Riemenschneider TA, eds: *Moss' heart disease in infants, children and adolescents,* ed 4, Baltimore, 1989, Williams & Wilkins.

139. Stanger P: *Truncus arteriosus.* In Moller JH, Neal WA, eds: *Fetal, neonatal and infant cardiac disease,* Norwalk, 1990, Appleton & Lange.

140. Van Mierop LH, Kutsche LM: Cardiovascular anomalies in DiGeorge syndrome and importance of neural crest as a possible pathogenetic factor, *Am J Cardiol* 58:133, 1986.

141. Ebert PA, Turley K, Stanger P et al: Surgical treatment of truncus arteriosus in the first six months of life, *Ann Surg* 200:451, 1984.

142. Van Praagh R, Van Praagh S: The anatomy of common aorticopulmonary trunk (truncus arteriosus communis) and its embryologic implications. A study of 57 necropsy cases, *Am J Cardiol* 16:406, 1965.

143. Collett RW, Edwards JE: Persistent truncus arteriosus; a classification according to anatomic types, *Surg Clin North Am* 29:1245, 1949.

144. Rastelli GC, Titus JL, McGoon DC: Honograft of ascending aorta and aortic valve as a right ventricular outflow. An experimental approach to the repair of truncus arteriosus, *Arch Surg* 95:698, 1967.

145. DiDonato RM, Fyfe DA, Puga FJ et al: Fifteen-year experience with surgical repair of truncus arteriosus, *J Thorac Cardiovasc Surg* 89:414, 1985.

146. Lucas RV, Krabill KA: *Anomalous venous connections, pulmonary and systemic.* In Adams FH, Emmanouilides GC, Riemenschneider TA, eds: *Moss' heart disease in infants, children and adolescents,* ed 4, Baltimore, 1989, Williams & Wilkins.

147. Ward, KE, Mullins CH, Huhta JC et al: Restrictive interatrial communication in total anomalous pulmonary venous connection, *Am J Cardiol* 57:1131, 1986.

148. Van Meter C Jr, LeBlanc JC, Culpepper WS et al: Partial anomalous pulmonary venous return, *Circulation* (82(suppl IV):IV-195, 1990.

149. Canter CE, Martin TC, Spray TL et al: Scimitar syndrome in childhood, *Am J Cardiol* 56:653, 1986.

150. Marin-Garcia J, Tandon R, Lucas RV Jr et al: Cor triatriatum: study of 20 cases, *Am J Cardiol* 35:59, 1975.

151. Elliott LP, Anderson RH, Bargeron LM: *Single ventricle or univentricular heart.* In Adams FH, Emmanouilides, Riemenschneider TA, eds: *Moss' heart disease in infants, children and adolescents,* ed 4, Baltimore, 1989, Williams & Wilkins.

152. Van Praagh R, Ongley PA, Swan HJC: Anatomic types of single or common ventricle in men; morphologic and geometric aspects of sixty necropsied cases, *Am J Cardiol* 13:367, 1964.

153. Bevilacqua M, Sanders SP, Van Praagh S et al: Double-inlet single ventricle: echocardiographic anatomy with emphasis on the morphology of the atrioventricular valves and ventricular septal defect, *J Am Coll Cardiol* 18:559, 1991.

154. Van Praagh R, Weinberg PM, Smith SD et al: *Malpositions of the heart.* In Adams FH, Emmanouilides GC, Riemenschneider TA, eds: *Moss' heart disease in infants, children and adolescents,* ed 4, Baltimore, 1989, Williams & Wilkins.

155. Moller JH: *Malposition of the heart.* In Moller JH, Neal WA, eds: *Fetal, neonatal and infant cardiac disease,* Norwalk, 1990, Appleton & Lange.

156. Van Praagh S, Kreutzer J, Alday L et al: *Systemic and pulmonary venous connections in visceral heterotaxy, with emphasis on the diagnosis of atrial situs: a study of 109 postmortem cases.* In Clark EB, Takao A, eds: *Developmental cardiology: morphogenesis and function,* Mount Kisco, NY, 1990, Futura.

157. Bland EF, White PD, Garland J: Congenital anomalies of the coronary arteries, *Am Heart J* 8:787, 1933.

158. Takahashi M, Lurie PR: *Abnormalities and diseases of the coronary vessels.* In Adams FH, Emmanouilides GC, Riemenschneider TA, eds: *Moss' heart disease in infants, children and adolescents,* ed 4, Baltimore, 1989, Williams & Wilkins.

159. Roberts WC: Anomalous origin of both coronary arteries from the pulmonary artery, *Am J Cardiol* 10:595, 1962.

160. Gouley BA: Anomalies of left coronory artery arising from the pulmonary artery (adult type), *Am Heart J* 40:630, 1950.

161. Yoshida Y, Emmanouilides GC, Nelson RJ et al: Anomalous origin of the left coronary artery from the pulmonary artery; a case report with remarkable improvement of myocardial function following subclavian artery-coronary artery anastomosis, *Cathet Cardiovasc Diagn* 6:293, 1980.

Chapter 14

PATHOGENESIS AND PATHOPHYSIOLOGY OF ARRHYTHMIAS AND CONDUCTION DISORDERS

Conduction Abnormalities
Angel R. Leon
Ventricular Tachycardias
Sina Zaim

Congenital or acquired abnormalities of the cardiac conduction system provide the substrate for rhythm disorders that result in a spectrum of clinical syndromes ranging from asymptomatic dysrhythmia and benign dysrhythmia to sudden death. This chapter reviews normal conduction system anatomy and the anatomic variations and conduction system abnormalities that disrupt the orderly genesis and propagation of the heartbeat and its rhythm.

ANATOMY OF THE CONDUCTION SYSTEM IN THE HEART

Correlations between clinical syndromes and pathologic findings are not very strong. Examination of the conduction system in patients with arrhythmias, sick sinus syndrome, and conduction blocks often fails to determine a specific anatomic abnormality responsible for the clinical diagnosis. However, knowledge of the normal conduction system anatomy is important to understanding the genesis of heart rhythm disorders.

The major structures of the cardiac conduction system appear in Figure 14-1. The sinoatrial (SA) node is a spindle-shaped collection of cells located in the sulcus terminale at the junction of the anterior superior vena cava and the right atrial appendage. Its location is more epicardial than endocardial. The most common anatomic variation is the horseshoe-shaped SA node (10% of autopsy cases),

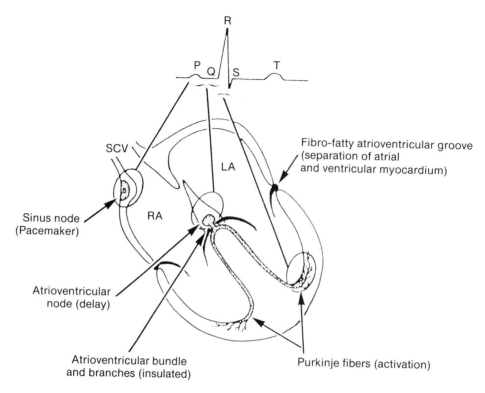

Fig. 14-1. The normal anatomy of the cardiac conduction system appears on the left panel. The sinus node occupies an area near the junction of the right atrial terminal sulcus and the superior vena cava. The AV node lies at the floor of the intraatrial septum. It is the most proximal component of the atrioventricular conduction axis, which consists of the AV node, the bundle of His, and the bundle branches. (From Becker AE, Anderson RH, et al[6]).

which straddles the sulcus terminalis. SA node cells are fusiform, narrower than contractile atrial cells, and contain few myofibrils. Electron microscopy shows gap junctions and intercalated discs present between SA node cells. At birth, cells are the primary constituent of the SA node, and they are separated by thin fibrous tissue. With aging, the fibrous material, composed of collagen and fine elastic fibers, infiltrates the intracellular space and total cell count decreases, suggesting that SA node cells are gradually replaced by fibrous tissue. The blood supply to the SA node arrives via the SA node artery, which is usually the first major branch of either the right (55%) or the left circumflex coronary artery (45%). Postganglionic fibers of the vagus nerve innervate the SA node and surrounding atrial tissue.[1,2]

Cells of the SA node spontaneously depolarize due to influx of calcium during phase 4 of the SA node cell action potential. Sodium channels are either lacking or insignificant in sinoatrial cell membranes. Beta agonist agents exert a positive chronotropic effect on SA node firing via adenyl cyclase by increasing the rate of phase 4 depolarization. Vagal stimulation of SA node cells inhibits adenyl cyclase activity and slows the inward calcium current.[3]

The wave of depolarization travels out of the SA node and across the right atrium. Specialized conduction pathways referred to as Bachmann's bundles transport the current across the intraatrial septum to the left atrium. The atrial activation sequence has been studied in experimental models and in patients undergoing surgery. The SA node communicates with multiple centers of impulse origination in the atria, forming the pacemaker complex, from which dissemination of conduction occurs. The earliest impulse origin corresponds to the junction of the superior vena cava and right atrium, near the SA node itself. Autonomic manipulations reveal the presence of numerous pacemaker centers throughout the atria driven by the SA node. Removal of the SA node causes a disorganized firing of the different foci of this pacemaker complex, suggesting the existence of a hierarchy dominated by the SA node.[4]

The SA node communicates with the atrioventricular (AV) node by three internodal pathways. Controversy exists regarding whether the internodal tracts contain specialized cells, or are simply composed of typical atrial myocytes. Internodal conduction may proceed preferentially along the internodal tracts simply because anatomic barriers producing physical or functional block in the atrium create the three conduits of relatively less resistance between the SA and AV nodes.[5]

Atrial impulses travel down to the ventricles across the atrioventricular node, which arises in the posteromedial aspect of the floor of the right atrium within what is surgically described as the triangle of Koch. The boundaries of the triangle are, posteriorly, the anterior border of the coronary sinus os, superiorly, the tendon of Todaro, and inferoanteriorly, the attachment of the septal leaflet of the tricuspid valve. Like the SA node, the AV node is an epicardial structure, lying on a tissue plane posterior to the intraatrial septum. Three cell types define the layers of the AV node: the transitional zone, the compact node, and the penetrating atrioventricular bundle. Cells of the transitional zone interdigitate among left and right atrial myocytes and proceed distally into the compact node. The transitional cells attach to atrial myocytes from the area of the coronary sinus os to the intraatrial septum. The transitional zone and the compact node lie above the fibrous atrioventricular ring. As the compact node crosses the atrioventricular ring, it becomes the penetrating bundle of His.[6]

Cells of the AV node are small, and there is no sharp demarcation between the three zones. Below the AV ring, the cells become larger and elongated.

Proximal septal perforators from the left anterior descending artery, as well as the first branch of the posterior descending artery arising at the crux of the heart from the right coronary or the circumflex artery, provide the AV node with a dual blood supply. Autonomic innervation of the AV node comes from the vagus nerve, and it ends immediately above the penetrating bundle. Therefore, components of the conduction system proximal to the penetrating bundle, such as the SA node or the proximal AV node, are under vagal influence, whereas the conduction system below the penetrating bundle is not.

The AV node is capable of both antegrade and retrograde conduction. AV node cells also depolarize after the slow influx of calcium. AV node cells have decremental conduction properties; they become increasingly refractory to successive stimuli as the frequency of stimulation increases. The phenomenon of decremental conduction permits the AV node to limit the rate at which atrial impulses are transmitted to the ventricles. Mobitz type I atrioventricular block results from the decremental properties of the AV node (Fig. 14-2). Fibers of the vagus nerve innervate the AV node, decrease the rate of phase 4 depolarization, and prolong refractoriness. Therefore conduction block at this level is attributed to autonomic influences rather than to anatomic factors. Sympathetic input to the AV node cells is similar to the effect on the SA node; the rate of phase 4 depolarization increases, and refractoriness shortens.[7]

The most distal region of the AV node, the penetrating bundle, extends below the tricuspid annulus and bifurcates

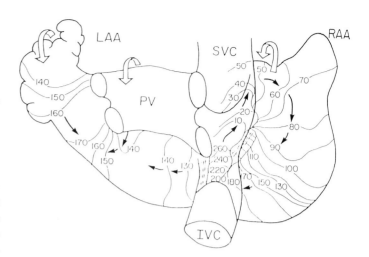

Fig. 14-2. The atrial activation sequence during atrial flutter shows a reentrant circuit in the right atrium that passively depolarizes the left atrium. The numbers indicate activation times, with the higher numbers indicating the atrial regions that are activated last. (From Boineau JP, Schuessler RB, Cain PB et al: *Activation mapping during normal atrial rhythm and atrial flutter.* In Zipes DP, Jalife J: *Cardiac electrophysiology: from cell to bedside,* Philadelphia, 1990, WB Saunders.)

at the crest of the muscular septum into the right and left bundle branches. The penetrating bundle may lie more superficially to the left ventricular surface of membranous septum, a finding of importance during transcatheter ablation of the bundle of His. Depolarization of the His bundle produces a discrete, recordable electrical potential (Fig. 14-2). His bundle recordings during atrial pacing distinguish between block at the AV node caused by extrinsic autonomic influences, and infrahisian block caused by intrinsic conduction system disease.

The short penetrating bundle divides into the left and right bundle branches at varying distances after crossing the tricuspid annulus. The right bundle branch is a long, discrete tract extending distally within the septum to the apex of the right ventricle, toward the base of the medial papillary muscle of the triscuspid valve, across the septal base, and toward the right ventricular apex. The left bundle quickly divides into two or three fascicles. The left bundle branches into various patterns.[8] A fibrous sheath encases the penetrating bundle, the bundle branches, and the Purkinje network until it divides and intermingles with ventricular myocytes. Ventricular myocytes are therefore insulated from receiving electrical impulses from the proximal components of the conduction system. Dissemination of conduction occurs after the fascicles divide into the Purkinje network. The mechanism of interaction between Purkinje fibers and ventricular muscle cells has not been determined.[9]

The blood supply to the right bundle branch comes from the left anterior descending coronary artery. The proximal left bundle branch and the anterior fascicle also receive blood exclusively from the left anterior descending artery and its branches; the posterior fascicle receives a dual blood supply from marginal branches of the left circumflex artery and from the distal right coronary. A single occlusion proximal to the first septal branch of the LAD can produce right bundle branch block. However, because the left bundle divides early, and because the left posterior fascicle has a dual blood supply, complete left bundle branch block occurs only after massive myocardial infarction.[10]

The Purkinje cell system is the final ramification of the specialized conduction system of the heart. These glycogen-rich cells have little contractile function; they serve mainly to propogate the wave of depolarization to the ventricular myocytes. The Purkinje cell network lies along the endocardial surface of the heart. These cells directly absorb oxygen and nutrients from intracavitary blood, and therefore, unlike endocardial myocytes, are protected from ischemia caused by coronary occlusion.

The metabolic needs of the specialized conduction cells are approximately one-fifth of those of contractile myocardial cells. Therefore the former are more resistant to ischemic injury. The viability of Purkinje cells in the vicinity of infarcted myocytes is an important factor in the genesis of a substrate for ventricular arrhythmias in patients with coronary artery disease.

CLINICAL MANIFESTATIONS OF CONDUCTION SYSTEM DISEASE
Sinus node dysfunction

Sinus node dysfunction results from infarction, fibrosis, inflammation, or surgical trauma. Replacement of sinus node cells by fibrotic tissue is a component of the aging process. It is unclear whether excessive fibrosis produces sinus node dysfunction, but it is the most common pathologic finding in patients with clinical sinus node dysfunction.[11] Direct injury to the SA node cells during canalization for cardiopulmonary bypass, or resulting from other instrumentation during surgery for congenital heart disease (such as the Mustard procedure and atrial septal defect closure) is another common cause of sinus node dysfunction.[12,13] Coronary artery disease producing occlusion of the SA node artery is an uncommon pathologic association with sinus node dysfunction. Inflammation from pericarditis, rheumatic heart disease, or collagen vascular diseases also produces sinus node dysfunction.[14] Infiltrative cardiomyopathic processes, such as amyloidosis, sarcoidosis, and thyrotoxicosis may also damage SA node cells. The common clinical manifestations of sinus node dysfunction are chronotropic incompetence, sinus exit block, sinus arrest, the tachycardia-bradycardia syndrome, and atrial fibrillation.

Chronotropic incompetence. The failure of the sinus node to increase its rate of depolarization when challenged with appropriate autonomic stimuli reflects the presence of intrinsic sinus node dysfunction. Chronotropic incompetence is present when either atropine or isoproterenol infusion fails to increase the heart rate by 15% to 20%.[15]

Sinoatrial exit block (SAEB). The delay or failure of SA cell depolarizations to appropriately depolarize the atria results in apparent sinus pauses on the surface electrocardiogram. First degree SAEB, which involves a delay in the transmission of each SA depolarization, can only be detected during invasive electrophysiologic studies by direct recordings of SA node firing, or by estimation of the sinoatrial conduction time. Otherwise first degree SAEB is invisible on the surface ECG.[16]

Two types of second degree SAEB exist. Mobitz type I SAEB occurs with the same periodicity as Mobitz I atrioventricular block. Following a pause, the P-P interval progressively shortens leading to another pause. Mobitz type II SAEB occurs when the length of a pause between P waves is an exact multiple of the normal P wave cycle length.[17]

Third degree SAEB produces long pauses between P waves that are indistinguishable on the surface electrocardiogram from sinus arrest.

Sinus arrest. Failure of the SA node to depolarize will cause asystole in the surface electrocardiogram when secondary pacemakers fail to fire. Pauses are considered abnormal when they are longer or equal to 3 seconds. Shorter pauses may be caused by autonomic suppression of SA node firing. Longer pauses are associated with intrinsic sinus node dysfunction.[18]

ATRIOVENTRICULAR BLOCK

Atrial depolarizations fail to stimulate the ventricles when conduction block occurs at any level of the AV node, the bundle of His, or in both bundle branches.

First degree AV block consists of a conduction time greater than 200 msec from the onset of the P wave to the onset of the QRS. This delay represents conduction slowing through the atria and AV node proximal to the bundle of His. Mobitz I second degree AV block results from the decremental conduction properties of the AV node; the conduction time and refractoriness of the AV node to successive rapid stimuli progressively increase, until complete block of one impulse ends one cycle and allows the AV node cells to recover excitability, starting a new cycle. Increasing parasympathetic stimulation further slows the rate of AV node cell depolarization and increases refractoriness, producing block at slower atrial rates. Direct recordings of atrial and bundle of His depolarizations show progressively longer atrium to His intervals until block of an atrial depolarization occurs without a bundle of His depolarization (Fig 14-2); the His-to-ventricle interval remains constant. Reversal of block by atropine at the same pacing rate confirms that vagal input proximal to the penetrating bundle contributes to the block. Mobitz II block occurs when an atrial stimulus depolarizes the His bundle but fails to depolarize the ventricles. Prolongation of the atrium-to-His interval prior to the block may be absent, and atropine does not reverse the block.[19]

Mobitz I block can occur simultaneously at more than one level of the AV node, resulting in the variable AV conduction ratios seen in atrial flutter. Mobitz II block occurs anywhere along the penetrating bundle. Third degree block can occur in the AV node as a result of increased vagal tone or nodal ischemia, or distal to the node as a result of damage to the infranodal structures. Atropine infusion may distinguish between the two forms of third degree AV block[20]

The pathophysiology of AV block is divided into congenital, acquired intrinsic disease, and acquired extrinsic damage to the conduction system. Components of the AV conduction system (AV node, penetrating bundle, or bundle branches) may be absent at birth, resulting in third degree AV block. Absence of the AV node itself is most common. The distal interatrial structures are replaced by fatty tissue. Less commonly, the penetrating bundle is discontinuous, or the bundle branches are disrupted. Also, congenital structural anomalies may displace the AV conduction system. Infants of mothers with systemic lupus erythematosus may be born with high grade AV block. The presence of circulating maternal anti-Rho antibodies has some correlation with the presence of AV block in the infants.[21]

Intrinsic degeneration of the components of the conduction axis can cause AV block. Lev[22] described degeneration, disappearance, and fibrosis of the proximal left bundle branch, the distal penetrating bundle, and less commonly, the proximal right bundle branch as a cause of conduction block. Accelerated aging processes worsened by high intracavitary pressures or other traumata may produce the changes. Lenegre disease consists of diffuse fibrosis throughout the ventricular conduction system. It is not a focal process, and it also differs from Lev disease in that fibrosis is a major component of the damage to the conduction system.[23]

The most common source of extrinsic damage to the conduction system producing atrioventricular block is coronary artery disease. Acute myocardial infarction causes AV block either by direct ischemia or necrosis of the infrahisian conduction structures during anterior infarcts, or by vagally mediated AV node block, more commonly during inferoposterior infarcts. AV block during inferoposterior infarction also results from ischemia to the AV node. The node has a dual blood supply, therefore, AV block in the setting of an inferoposterior infarct has been attributed to the presence of multivessel coronary disease.[24] AV block during inferoposterior infarction is almost always transient, and permanent pacing is rarely needed. AV block during an anteroseptal infarct results from an occlusion in the left anterior descending artery proximal to its first septal branch, signalling extensive infarction. Damage to the

conduction system during anteroseptal infarcts occurs at the distal penetrating bundle or at the proximal segments of both bundle branches.[25]

Valvular heart disease or senile calcification of the valvular annuli may penetrate the infranodal conduction system, producing AV block.[25] Calcific aortic stenosis and mitral annulus calcification may extend into the penetrating bundle, producing conduction abnormalities. AV block also occurs from direct trauma during aortic or mitral valve replacement or repair, because the proximal segment of the penetrating bundle lies adjacent to the noncoronary aortic cusp and the septal attachment of the anterior mitral leaflet. Pressure and edema from prosthetic valve sewing rings, or direct trauma by sutures damages the penetrating bundle and bundle branches. Surgical resection of septal hypertrophy commonly results in bundle branch block or AV block.

Burrowing valve ring abcesses complicate infectious endocarditis in native and prosthetic valves, causing AV block of varying degrees and bundle branch block.[26]

Malignancies, either primary or metastatic, can produce high grade AV block. Primary tumors of the heart, including rhabdomyosarcoma and mesothelioma can destroy and replace the AV node and upper ventricular septum. Metastatic tumors such as melanoma, and infiltration by lymphoma into the AV node also produce AV block. Sarcoidosis, amyloidosis, myocarditis, collagen vascular diseases, and trypanosomysis can produce AV block by destroying the AV node, penetrating bundle, or bundle branches.[7,28,29,30]

Fascicular block

Destruction of the left anterior fascicle (LAF) produces left axis deviation on the surface electrocardiogram. The most common causes of LAF block are coronary artery disease and Chagas disease.[31] The posterior fascicle is a more diffuse structure, and it has a dual blood supply. Therefore, isolated left posterior fascicular block (LPFB) is uncommon. When present it creates right axis deviation on the surface electrogram. However, other causes of right axis deviation, including right ventricular hypertrophy, must be excluded before inferring the presence of LPFB.

Bundle branch block

The pathologic processes described above that produce AV block or fascicular block may also selectively damage either of the bundle branches. Acute anterior myocardial infarction produces right bundle branch block more often than left bundle branch block. Because the left bundle is a more diffuse structure, the presence of new left bundle branch block in the setting of an acute infarct is an ominous sign, indicating extensive destruction of the left ventricle and an extremely poor prognosis. Right bundle branch block can result from a discrete septal infarction. However, because a proximal occlusion of the left anterior descending artery must be involved, the prognosis associated with a new right bundle branch block in the setting of infarction is worse than in anterior infarcts without right bundle branch block. The indication for temporary pacing with a new right bundle branch block in the setting of an acute myocardial infarction is controversial. The progression to complete AV block with a new right bundle occurs when evidence of other conduction abnormalities is present.[32]

TACHYARRHYTHMIAS
Sinus tachycardia

Sinus tachycardia is an appropriate physiologic response to physical or emotional stress that produces increased sympathetic tone. The heart rate increases and decreases gradually; the PR interval may shorten, and the P-wave axis may become more inferior, with peaking of P-waves in the inferior limb leads. Because of increased sympathetic tone, the pacemaker focus becomes an area in the superior right atrium[5] producing the P-wave changes described above. Persistent sinus tachycardia is abnormal, and may be caused by disease (thyrotoxicosis); it also occurs in the denervated hearts of heart transplant recipients.

Sinus node reentry tachycardia (SNRT)

An abrupt increase in the sinus rate without a change in the P-wave morphology has been attributed to a reentrant circuit within and around the sinus node. The sudden rate increase is often triggered by atrial ectopy. SNRT can only be inferred; the direct diagnosis has not been clinically demonstrated by electrophysiologic studies, and few experimental models of it exist. Persistent, symptomatic sinus tachycardia, in the absence of an extrinsic cause, and attributed to SNRT, has been treated by surgical ablation of the SA node.[32]

Atrial tachycardia

Atrial fibrillation, atrial flutter, and automatic and reentrant atrial tachycardias are confined to atrial muscle tissue, and do not require the participation of ventricular or AV node components for their initiation and maintenance. All atrial tachycardias result from either atrial myocyte automaticity or from reentry circuits. Disparities in conduction velocities and refractoriness in the atrium facilitating reentry result from physical barriers created by the various atrial structures, scar from previous procedures in the atrium, or by the asymmetric orientation of atrial myocytes, producing what is referred to as anisotropic reentry (Fig. 14-2). Atrial automaticity may be caused by calcium channel-mediated afterdepolarizations.[34]

The designation of atrial tachycardia refers to atrial rhythms with rates less than 250. These arrhythmias are often regular, chronic, and sometimes incessant.[35] Distinguishing whether automaticity or reentry produces an atrial tachycardia may be difficult. Reentrant rhythms are usu-

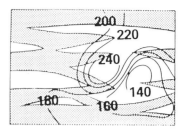

Fig. 14-3. Geometric irregularities in atrial fibers create microrentrant circuits by creating areas of functional block (relatively slow conduction). The numbers indicate activation in milliseconds, with the higher numbers representing areas activated last due to physical or functional block. (From Boineau JP, Schuessler RB, Cain PB et al: *Activation mapping during normal atrial rhythm and atrial flutter*. In Zipes DP, Jalife J: *Cardiac electrophysiology: from cell to bedside*. Philadelphia, 1990, WB Saunders.)

ally induced and terminated by premature stimuli or by electrical cardioversion; automatic tachycardias are not. Reentrant atrial tachycardias occur commonly in patients who have had atrial surgery; automatic tachycardias are more common in children, but can occur in all age groups without structural heart disease.[36] Disruption of the sinus node-dominated pacemaker complex may result in irregular and chaotic atrial ectopy, such as multifocal atrial tachycardia in patients with chronic lung disease.

Incessant atrial tachycardia may produce congestive heart failure if the rhythm continues for years. Surgical removal of the tachycardia focus, or disruption of AV conduction can prevent or reverse the cardiomyopathy.[37]

Atrial flutter

Atrial rhythms with rates 250 or greater (producing a "saw-tooth"-shaped baseline on the surface electrocardiogram) are referred to as atrial flutter. Two types of atrial flutter have been described; type I flutter with rates from 250 to 340, and type II flutter with rates from 340 to 440.[38]

Atrial automaticity was once thought to be the mechanism of type I atrial flutter. The ability to entrain the tachycardia by atrial pacing proved that a single reentry circuit confined within the atria is the pathophysiologic mechanism for atrial flutter.[39] The arrhythmia originates in the reentry circuit and the remainder of the atria are passively depolarized. A disparity in the refractoriness of different areas of the atria leads to unidirectional block in a relatively fast conduction pathway that recovers excitability in time to receive retrograde activation from slower conducting zones, thus completing the reentry loop. Macroscopic anatomic barriers in the atria, such as vein orifices, valvular annuli, and the coronary sinus os, combine with microscopic anisotropy to create unidirectional block and reentry circuits. The conduction sequence in a patient with previous atrial surgery was found to consist of a cir-

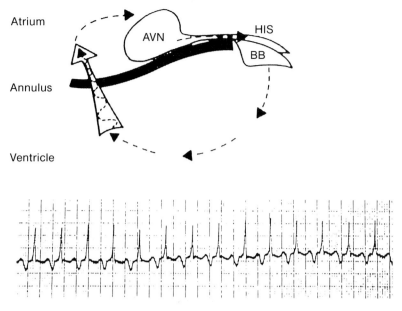

Fig. 14-4. The paranodal pathway responsible for the permanent form of junctional reciprocating tachycardia creates a reentrant circuit, producing a tachycardia similar to the uncommon variety of atrioventricular node reentry tachycardia. Retrograde conduction is relatively slower than antegrade conduction down the atrioventricular node, as reflected in the long R to P time on the surface ECG. Note the negative P waves indicating a low atrial activation site. (From Gallagher JJ, Selle JG, Sealy WC, et al: *Variants of pre-excitation.* In Zipes DA, Jalife J, eds: *Cardiac electrophysiology: from cell to bedside,* Philadelphia, 1990, WB Saunders.)

cular pattern of reentry in the right atrium around the surgical scar, with passive stimulation of the left atrium.[35] Atrial activation during atrial flutter mapped during surgical resection of the arrhythmia occurs earliest in the inferolateral atrial wall near the coronary sinus os (Fig. 14-3). The area of slow conduction critical to reentry lies in the posteroseptal area between the coronary sinus os and the tricuspid annulus.[36] Ablation of the slow zone cures the arrhythmia and proves that atrial flutter occurs from a reentry in a single circuit.

The etiology of type II atrial flutter remains unclear.

Atrial fibrillation

Unlike atrial flutter, atrial fibrillation is caused by the competition and fusion between multiple reentry circuits within the atria. Atrial fibrillation could be experimentally induced by application of aconitine to animal atria or by rapid atrial pacing. When atrial fibrillation occurred from a single focus, isolating that focus terminated the arrhythmia.[40] However, rapid pacing of the atrial appendage activates a large enough atrial mass, producing stable atrial fibrillation; isolating the atrial appendage does not terminate fibrillation. Theoretically, pacing activates various reentry circuits in the atria that conduct and fire throughout areas of different refractoriness, perpetuating the fibrillation.[41]

The sequence of atrial activation during atrial fibrillation in humans has been studied by intraoperative mapping. Multiple waves of depolarizations occur in the right atrium, each dividing into smaller wavelets at areas of functional conduction block that fuse with each other as they travel across the atria. These wavelets confirm previous experimental models of the "multiple wavelet" theory for the etiology of atrial fibrillation.[42] The presence of multiple wavefronts of depolarization throughout the atria explains why overdrive pacing does not terminate atrial fibrillation, and why ablating a single zone of slow conduction does not cure it. Surgery designed to redirect sinus node and atrial depolarization wavefronts terminates atrial fibrillation by preventing the interaction of the multiple wavelets that perpetuate the arrhythmia.

Atrial flutter and atrial fibrillation occur most commonly in patients with structurally abnormal hearts. Atrial scarring and enlargement caused by valvular heart disease, hypertension (systemic and pulmonary), and cardiomyopathy often results in macroscopic atrial abnormalities, producing fibrillation and flutter. Metabolic processes such as hyperthyroidism, and infiltrative processes such as amyloidosis have direct injurious effects on the heart that produce microscopic disruption in atrial tissue, creating the substrate for these arrhythmias.

Atrioventricular junctional tachycardia

Tachyarrhythmias originating in the atrioventricular junction result from automaticity or reentry. The vast ma-

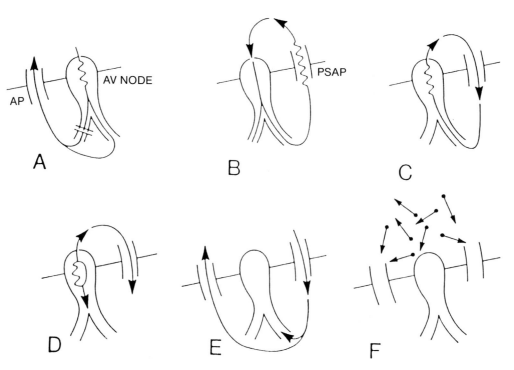

Fig. 14-5. Six different tachycardias associated with accessory pathways are diagrammed: **A,** Orthodromic atrioventricular reciprocating tachycardia with bundle branch block; **B,** The permanent form of junctional reciprocating tachycardia with a posteroseptal paranodal pathway with decremental properties; **C,** Antidromic atrioventricular reciprocating tachycardia; **D,** Atrioventricular node reentry tachycardia with antegrade conduction down an accessory pathway; **E,** Atrioventricular reciprocating tachycardia and antegrade and retrograde conduction occurring over two different accessory pathways; and **F,** atrial tachycardia or flutter or fibrillation with antegrade conduction down an accessory pathway. (From Yee R, Klein GJ, Sharma AD, et al: *Tachycardia associated with accessory autoventricular pathways.* In Zipes DP, Jalife J, eds: *Cardiac electrophysiology: from cell to bedside,* Philadelphia, 1990, WB Saunders.)

jority of AV junctional tachycardias are caused by atrioventricular node reentry.[43] Automatic junctional tachycardias occur rarely; automaticity should be considered as a tachycardia mechanism only after reentry has been excluded. Automatic junctional tachycardia is often associated with increased automaticity caused by digoxin toxicity.

The substrate for atrioventricular node reentry tachycardia (AVNRT) consists of two longitudinally distinct pathways of atrioventricular conduction within or in the vicinity of the AV node. Each pathway has distinct electrophysiologic properties. One pathway courses anteriorly along the intraatrial septum superior to the penetrating bundle; the other pathway courses posteriorly along the floor of the right atrium between the septal tricuspid ring and the os of the coronary sinus. It appears that more than one posterior pathway or multiple posterior pathways are present. In the common form of AVNRT, antegrade conduction during tachycardia occurs down the posterior pathway, which has relatively slower conduction than the anterior pathway (which conducts retrograde to the atria). In the uncommon form of AVNRT, antegrade conduction occurs down the

anterior pathway, with retrograde activation travelling up the posterior pathway. It is unclear whether both pathways are confined within the AV node, or whether atrial tissue participates in the reentrant circuit.

For reentry to occur, the two pathways must have different conduction properties. Unidirectional block occurs in a refractory pathway at a time when the second pathway is able to conduct antegrade. The once-refractory pathway then recovers, and is activated retrograde as the two pathways fuse distally. In the common form of AVNRT, retrograde activation of the atria by the anterior pathway occurs relatively faster (less than 60 msec) than during the uncommon form of AVNRT, where retrograde conduction over the posterior pathway takes longer. The diagnosis of a longitudinally dissociated atrioventricular node, or dual nodal physiology, can be made during programmed atrial stimulation in which two distinct refractory periods for antegrade AV node conduction are uncovered. Dual retrograde nodal physiology can be detected in the same manner by programmed ventricular stimulation.[44]

AVNRT can be cured by modification of AV node conduction. The anterior or pathways can be located and one

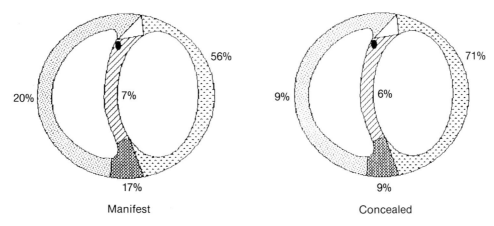

Fig. 14-6. The anatomic locations of concealed and manifest pathways are compared. The only difference is that concealed right free wall pathways are rare; also note that 15% of concealed pathways lie in the septum.

can be ablated by administration of radiofrequency current, thereby eliminating the reentrant loop.

Permanent form of junctional reciprocating tachycardia (PJRT)

PJRT is an often incessant reentrant tachycardia confined to the vicinity of the AV node. Normal AV node conduction serves as the antegrade limb of the reentrant loop. Retrograde activation proceeds along a paranodal tract that connects the penetrating bundle to the proximal compact node (Fig. 14-5). The extranodal tract has decremental properties, and the tachycardia associated with it may be clinically indistinguishable from the uncommon variety of AVNRT.[45]

Nodofascicular and atriofascicular connections

Reciprocating tachycardia with a left-bundle branch block morphology, long atrioventricular conduction times, and ventriculoatrial dissociation may result from an anomalous connection between the AV node and the right bundle branch. During sinus rhythm, preexcitation is present with the same left bundle branch pattern. When an atriofascicular pathway is present, the atria participate in the tachycardia, and there is no ventriculoatrial dissociation.[40]

Tachycardias associated with accessory pathways

Anomalous atrioventricular connections that bypass the insulating atrioventricular ring are associated actively and passively with a number of clinically important tachyarrhythmias. Accessory pathways are generally classified by the presence (manifest) or absence (concealed) of antegrade conduction and preexcitation on the surface electrocardiogram.

Manifest preexcitation across an accessory pathway associated with clinical tachycardia forms the basis of the Wolff-Parkinson-White syndrome.[46] Atrioventricular re-

ciprocating tachycardia (AVRT) occurs over a macrorentrant circuit involving the atria, ventricles, the normal atrioventricular conduction system, and the accessory pathway. Concealed accessory pathways become clinically significant when involved with atrioventricular reciprocating tachycardias. Because they are usually incapable of antegrade conduction they do not participate in other tachycardias. Atrial fibrillation, atrial flutter, and atrial tachycardias may preexcite the ventricles by conducting exclusively down the bypass tract at high rates, during which the atrioventricular node is refractory. The pattern of preexcitation in that case is similar to the pattern of preexcitation seen in sinus rhythm. The accessory pathway may be a bystander during another reentrant tachycardia such as AVNRT and conduct the atrial activation to the ventricles with a preexcited pattern (Fig. 14-6).

AVRT is divided into two types based on the location of antegrade conduction during the tachycardia. Orthodromic tachycardias involve antegrade conduction down the atrioventricular node and retrograde conduction up the accessory pathway. The tachycardia is not preexcited. Antidromic tachycardias involve antegrade conduction the bypass tract and retrograde conduction up the atrioventricular node. Preexcitation is present during the tachycardia, and as occurs during atrial fibrillation, flutter, and tachycardia with manifest accessory pathways, the pattern of preexcitation during tachycardia is similar to the pattern of preexcitation during sinus rhythm.

In patients with multiple accessory pathways, a reciprocating tachycardia may involve two accessory pathways without participation of the atrioventricular node. The pattern of preexcitation during tachycardia depends on which accessory pathway forms the antegrade limb of the tachycardia.

Manifest accessory pathways are distributed throughout the atrioventricular ring. Concealed accessory pathways are more common along the left ventricular free wall, and in the right posteroseptal area. Right free wall pathways are rare. Studies of conduction along concealed accessory pathways reveal that conduction block occurs at the ventricular insertion site of the pathway.[47] The distribution and conduction properties of accessory pathways has become more important since the introduction of techniques for transcatheter ablation of accessory pathway-mediated tachycardias.

VENTRICULAR ARRHYTHMIAS

Ventricular arrhythmias vary greatly in complexity and clinical importance. The spectrum of this rhythm disorder encompasses isolated ventricular premature beats, nonsustained and sustained ventricular tachycardia as well as ventricular fibrillation. It may occur in the presence or absence of underlying structural cardiac disease. Clinically its expression ranges from benign palpitations to syncope to sudden death.

Sudden cardiac death, the most devastating and feared presentation of ventricular arrhythmias, is operationally defined as unexpected death within 1 hour of onset of symptoms in a previously healthy person. It accounts for over 300,000 deaths per year in the United states, the overall incidence being 0.1% to 0.2% per year in the general population.[42] The terminal arrhythmia is most often ventricular fibrillation; less commonly it is rapid sustained ventricular tachycardia. Twenty-four hour ambulatory electrocardiographic recordings fortuitously obtained from patients at time of sudden cardiac death show that ventricular fibrillation is usually preceded by an initial period of ventricular tachycardia.[47,48] Severe bradycardia or asystole may also result in sudden cardiac death in a minority of patients.[49]

VENTRICULAR TACHYCARDIA

Ventricular tachycardia may be classified, for clinical convenience, by its association with coronary artery disease, other structural disease, or with absence of structural disease. In addition to the entities described in the text, an idiopathic ventricular tachycardia is known to occur in those patients with no structural disease.

Ventricular tachycardia associated with coronary artery disease

Very commonly, significant coronary artery disease and a left ventricular scar resulting from a remote myocardial infarction is found in patients with ventricular tachycardia. In such a setting of chronic ischemic heart disease the mechanism of ventricular tachycardia appears to be reentry, a disorder of impulse conduction. Reentry may occur in one or more ways. The possibilities include classic "circus movement" arrhythmias over a defined anatomic pathway, "anisotropic" and "leading edge" reentry, both of which do not require a fixed anatomic pathway.

Reentrant activity occurs only if a specific sequence of steps develops in the cardiac tissues. First, conduction of the antegrade impulse must be blocked in an "arrhythmogenic" zone (Fig. 14-7), which is usually composed of abnormal tissues because of damage by ischemia or stretch. The antegrade impulse consequently reaches the distal margin of this arrhythmogenic zone by another route and then conducts slowly in a retrograde direction through a "protected" pathway also located in the arrhythmogenic zone. This "protected" pathway is the same one that had earlier blocked the antegrade impulse. The pathway is thus capable of "unidirectional block." The retrograde impulse next travels through the normal tissues proximal to the site of antegrade block to reactivate the normal zones of the heart and complete the circuit. If the retrograde impulse conducts too rapidly through the arrhythmogenic zone it will arrive at a critical site in the reentrant circuit (i.e., at, or proximal to, the site of antegrade block) while that site is still refractory. Such an event will produce bi-directional conduction block, and reentry will not occur. Reentry is therefore possible only if both antegrade unidirectional block and retrograde slow conduction occur in the same arrhythmogenic zone and the timing is appropriate.

The endocardial surface of the chronic ischemic heart seems to be the site of reentry in most instances[43] but intramyocardial or epicardial sites may also participate.[50]

Anisotropy, another form of reentry, has also been proposed as a mechanism for ventricular tachycardia. In this type of reentry, there is no fixed anatomic circuit with the requisite electrophysiologic abnormalities just described.

In normal ventricular myocardium, impulse conduction along the long axis of the ventricular fiber bundles is faster than conduction in the transverse direction across the bundles. This directional difference in conduction is attributed to variations in the distribution of gap junctions and consequent cell-to-cell coupling in the longitudinal direction along the fibers, as compared to the transverse direction, and is referred to as uniform anisotropic conduction.[51,52] If functional changes develop that alter the coupling between the ventricular muscle fibers, the wavefront will no longer advance smoothly, but will instead become irregular and fractionated, as slow conduction and blocks occur at some sites but not others, and nonuniform anisotropy will be said to occur. These changes in the uniformity of conduction lead to the initiation and perpetuation of reentrant tachycardias involving variable anatomic circuits.[52]

The "figure of eight" ventricular tachycardia (Fig. 14-8) is such an example. This model was proposed by El Sherif and workers[53] based on studies of the activation sequence of premature ventricular beats in canine hearts with 3 to 5-day-old anteroseptal myocardial infarcts.[53]

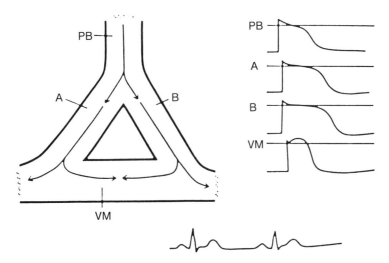

Fig. 14-7. Top panel: Normal conduction through a branch of the His-Purkinje system. Schmitt-Erlanger diagram at the left shows one of the branches of the Purkinje network. (*PB,* proximal bundle; *A* and *B,* two distal branches; and *VM,* ventricular muscle.) Action potential duration and refractory periods are longest in distal Purkinje fibers of A and B. The impulses normally conduct through A and B and activate ventricular muscle. The wavefronts of activation then collide in ventricular wall and terminate. Action potentials at right are from point indicated in drawing at left. Action potential show activation sequence in the ventricle, producing normal ECG as shown below. **Bottom panel:** Reentry depicted in the Schmitt-Erlanger diagram. Same format as top panel. Antegrade impulse conducts normally through proximal bundle (PB) and distal bundle A but slowly and decrementally through B *(wavy line)* and blocks in the damaged zone. The impulse conducts through the ventricle from insertion sites of branch and enters the damaged zone from the distal margin. It conducts slowly in the retrograde direction through B and reenters the proximal bundle. This can cause premature coupled ventricular depolarizations as depicted by action potentials at right and ECG below. (From Dangman KH, Boyden PA: *Cellular mechanisms of cardiac arrhythmias.* In Fox PR, ed: *Canine and feline cardiology,* New York, 1988, Churchill Livingstone.)

Reentry beats were found to occur in the thin surviving layer of epicardial muscle overlying the myocardial infarct. When the wavefront of an antegrade impulse encountered a long zone of functional conduction block (an "arc of block"). The presence and location of this zone of conduction block is determined by the ischemia induced spatially nonuniform distribution of refractoriness in epicardial muscle layer. Premature impulses tend to block along the long axis of the muscle bundles because of abrupt increases in refractoriness between adjacent fibers, or poor coupling. When the advancing antegrade impulse blocks along this arc, the wavefront splits into two wavefronts of activation that then slowly conduct around both ends of the arc of block and meet on the distal side of the arc. They may either collide and extinguish each other there or they may merge, summate, and lead to a reentrant beat. The reentrant beat occurs only if the impulse breaks through in the retrograde direction across the central portion of the arc of block. The impulse then reactivates the proximal area and the reentrant wavefront subsequently propagates laterally in the opposite directions, along the two remnant segments of the zone of block, resulting in a stable reentrant tachycardia. Figure of eight tachycardias may occur in the subepicardial, intramural, or subendocardial muscle layers.[53]

Allessie and colleagues[54] have described yet another reentry tachycardia mechanism in small pieces of rabbit atrial myocardium, the "leading circle" model.[56] This tachycardia also has no need for a permanent fixed anatomic obstacle. The impulse of the reentrant tachycardia travels in the smallest possible circular pathway, such that the head of the wavefront "continuously biting" its own tail of refractoriness.[46] The central region inside the circle remains functionally refractory because of continuous convergence of multiple centripetal wavelets emanating from the circulating wavefront. According to one report,[55] sustained ventricular tachycardia caused by the leading circle mechanism has been shown to occur in canine ventricular tissue.

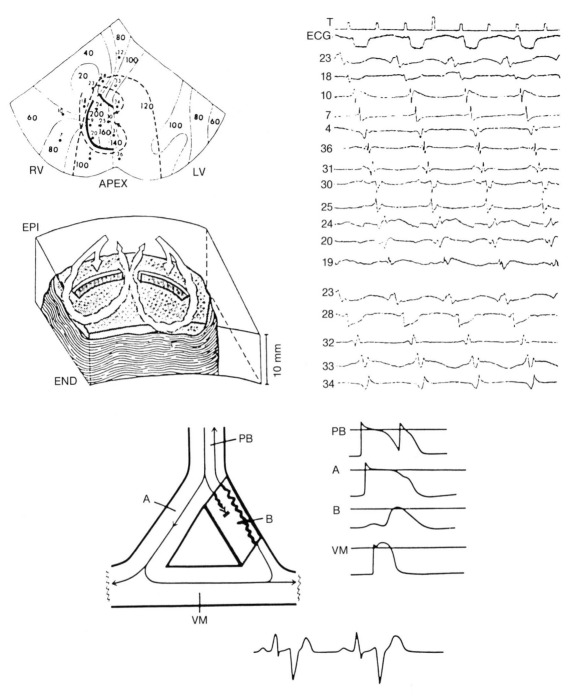

Fig. 14-8. Figure eight model of reentry. Isochronal activation map during monomorphic reentrant ventricular tachycardia occurring in the surviving epicardial layer overlying an infarct. Recordings were obtained from the epicardial surface of a canine heart 4 days after ligation of the left anterior descending coronary artery. Activation isochrones are drawn at 20 msec intervals *(upper left)*. The reentrant circuit has a characteristic figure eight pattern. Two circulating wavefronts advance in clockwise and counterclockwise directions, respectively, around two zones (arcs) of conduction block *(represented by heavy solid lines)*. The epicardial surface is depicted as if the ventricles were unfolded following a cut from the crux to the apex. The right panel shows selected simultaneous electrograms recorded along the two arcs of functional conduction block and the common reentrant wavefront. A three-dimensional diagrammatic illustration of the ventricular activation pattern during the reentrant tachycardia is shown at the lower left corner. RV = right ventricle, LV = left ventricle, EPI = epicardium, END = endocardium, T = time lines at 100 msec intervals. (From EL Sherif N: Reentry revisited, *PACE Pacing Clin Electrophysiol* 11:1358, 1988).

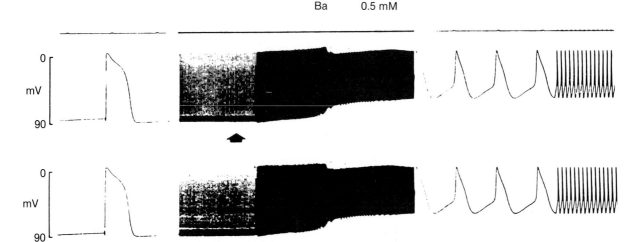

Fig. 14-9. Example of abnormal automaticity: effects of 500 μM barium on normal canine Purkinje fiber. Within a minute the maximum diastolic potential begins to decrease, and soon abnormal automaticity occurs *(right)*. In a healthy Purkinje fiber this abnormal automaticity persists unchanged for hours. (From Dangman KH, Hoffman BF: In vivo and in vitro antiarrhythmic and arrhythmogenic effects of N-acetyl procainamide, *J Pharmacol Exp Ther* 217:851, 1981).

Correlation of histologic findings in patients with chronic ischemic heart disease and reentrant ventricular tachycardia has been investigated by De Bakker et al.[56] The apparently focal origin of reentrant tachycardias, as determined by mapping, was actually found in some cases to be the site of impulse exit, via small isolated bundles of surviving muscle fibers, of a reentrant circuit actually located in a larger subendocardial muscle mass.

Ventricular tachycardias may arise not only in the setting of chronic ischemic heart disease as described above but also during the course of an acute coronary artery occlusion, as well as during the subsequent subacute phase.

The acute phase arrhythmias may be initiated by abnormal impulse formation, in contrast to abnormal impulse conduction, in the tissues (Purkinje or ventricular muscle cells) on the periphery of the ischemic zone. It is thought that a "current of injury" develops between the highly depolarized cells in the center of the ischemic zone and the more normal cells in the periphery and leads to abrupt depolarization of these peripheral, or border zone, cells to produce "depolarization induced automaticity" (Fig. 14-9) (i.e., abnormal automaticity[57]). A more likely possibility is that the same current gives rise to early afterdepolarizations and triggered activity (explained below). Nevertheless, reentrant ventricular tachycardia may be the most frequent mechanism at this stage because of the likelihood of the formation of a suitable arrhythmogenic zone resulting from ischemia-induced slowed conduction and nonhomogeneous refractoriness.[58]

Arrhythmias during the subacute phase, (i.e., the first 24 hours) may also be caused by a variety of mechanisms.

It has been shown in dog studies that enhanced or abnormal automaticity occurs in partially depolarized Purkinje fibers or ventricular muscle cells in the periphery of the infarct between 18 and 40 hours after coronary occlusion.[59] It is also known that reentry occurs in the Purkinje fiber network on the border of the 24-hour infarct zone.[45] Additionally, delayed afterdepolarizations and resultant triggered activity have also been shown to occur in the border zone of Purkinje fibers[60] and subepicardial ventricular muscle[61] in canine hearts with subacute infarcts.

Triggered activity is another type of mechanism of ventricular tachycardia.[62] This abnormal rhythm is thought to result from oscillations in the membrane potential. These oscillations are of two types: early afterdepolarizations and delayed afterdepolarizations. Early afterdepolarizations arise during phase 2 and 3 of the action potential and result in further depolarization and thus another action potential after the depolarization threshold is reached (Fig. 14-10). Delayed afterdepolarizations, on the other hand, arise during phase 4 of the action potential duration and result in a subsequent depolarization once the depolarization threshold of the fiber is reached (Fig. 14-11). The oscillations described do not arise de novo, i.e., there is no pacemaker current; they are dependent on the presence of an appropriate preceding (triggering) action potential.[62] The mechanism responsible for early afterdepolarizations has not been fully clarified. It may be the result of both a decrease in the outward potassium current and an increase in the inward calcium current.[62] Delayed afterdepolarizations seem to be secondary to intracellular calcium overload, which then leads to an increased inward sodium current and depolarization.[62]

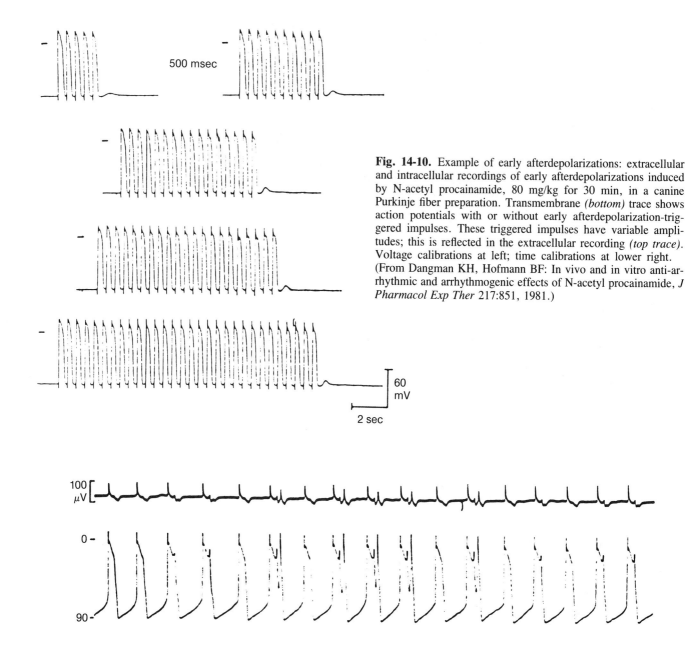

Fig. 14-10. Example of early afterdepolarizations: extracellular and intracellular recordings of early afterdepolarizations induced by N-acetyl procainamide, 80 mg/kg for 30 min, in a canine Purkinje fiber preparation. Transmembrane *(bottom)* trace shows action potentials with or without early afterdepolarization-triggered impulses. These triggered impulses have variable amplitudes; this is reflected in the extracellular recording *(top trace).* Voltage calibrations at left; time calibrations at lower right. (From Dangman KH, Hofmann BF: In vivo and in vitro anti-arrhythmic and arrhythmogenic effects of N-acetyl procainamide, *J Pharmacol Exp Ther* 217:851, 1981.)

Figure 14-11. Example of delayed afterdepolarizations: delayed afterdepolarizations in a goat Purkinje fiber induced by 1 μM isoproterenol. The preparation was stimulated at a cycle length of 500 msec for trains of 5 to 30 beats. Note that the amplitude of the delayed afterdepolarizations increases between 5 and 15-20 beats; minimal increases occur with longer stimulus trains. Reference potential marked to the left of each panel, time and voltage calibrations at lower right. (From Dangman KH: *Electrophysiology of the Purkinje fiber.* In Dangman KH, Miura DS, eds: *Electrophysiology and pharmacology of the heart. A clinical guide,* New York, 1991, Dekker.)

Ventricular tachycardia associated with abnormal cardiac structure

Idiopathic dilated cardiomyopathy. Ventricular arrhythmias become more frequent and more significant as the left ventricular function deteriorates. Nonsustained ventricular tachycardia has been documented, by 24-hour ambulatory electrocardiographic monitoring, in up to 60% of patients with idiopathic dilated cardiomyopathy.[63,64] The risk of sudden cardiac death has been found to increase at least fivefold in patients with congestive heart failure secondary to idiopathic dilated cardiomyopathy when compared to the general population.[65]

Reentry is believed to be the most common mechanism of ventricular tachycardia in this group of patients.[66] However, one may occasionally find bundle branch reentry as the mechanism of ventricular tachycardia.[67] The reentry circuit in this tachycardia is large and consists of the bundle of His, the right bundle branch, the interventricular septum, and the left bundle branch. The impulse travels down the right bundle across the interventricular septum, up the left bundle to the bundle of His before going back down the right bundle. The preexisting differences in refractoriness between the right and left bundle branches may be a predisposing factor for this tachycardia. Ventricular tachycardia/ventricular fibrillation may not be the sole mechanism of death. In these patients, severe bradycardia and asystole also have been documented as immediate cause of demise.[49]

Hypertrophic cardiomyopathy. Hypertrophic cardiomyopathy is a disorder in which the primary finding is marked left ventricular hypertrophy with concomitant reduction of left ventricular cavity size.

There is a high incidence of complex ventricular arrhythmias in these patients, with the occurrence of sudden cardiac death being more common in those with asymptomatic nonsustained ventricular tachycardia as detected by 24-hour ambulatory electrocardiographic monitoring[68,69,70,71] The annual incidence of sudden death is estimated at 2% to 4%.[70]

The mechanisms responsible for ventricular tachycardia/ventricular fibrillation resulting in sudden cardiac death are not fully known.[72] Aronson[73,74] has shown in animal models, in which left ventricular hypertrophy was induced by pressure overload, that there is a consistent prolongation of the duration of repolarization. This finding has also been reported in the human heart.[75] The prolonged duration of repolarization has additionally been found to be more marked on the endocardial (as compared to the epicardial surface). Such a disparity in recovery of excitability had been previously proposed as a suitable condition for reentry.[76] Aronson, however, has shown that both early and delayed afterdepolarizations and ensuing triggered activity can be observed in papillary muscles isolated from hypertrophied hearts. The tendency to develop early afterdepolarizations is thought to be caused by the prolonged phase of repolarization. The early afterdepolarizations may thus lead to triggered activity or may even result in the formation of delayed afterdepolarizations and subsequent triggered activity. Of interest is that monophasic action potential catheters have recorded early and delayed afterdepolarizations in dogs and humans respectively with left ventricular hypertrophy.[77,78]

Arrhythmogenic right ventricular dysplasia. Right ventricular dysplasia is a pathologic entity in which there is fatty infiltration of the right ventricle that usually leads to a large dilated ventricle, although only localized areas of dysfunction may be present in some cases. The infiltration seems to have a propensity for the inferior wall, the apex, and the infundibulum of the right ventricle—the "triangle of dysplasia."[79]

The 12 lead surface electrocardiogram during sinus rhythm usually shows precordial T wave inversions and sometimes a uniquely characteristic "epsilon" wave that occurs after the QRS complex and is thought to represent the late activation of the right ventricle.[80]

The natural history of this entity seems to be very variable. Patients who did not have syncopal episodes had a lower incidence of mortality in one study.[81]

Ventricular tachycardia in these patients appears as a left bundle branch pattern on the 12 lead surface electrocardiogram because the origin of the tachycardia is the right ventricle. Isolated ventricular premature complexes also have a left bundle branch block pattern. However, it should be noted that this feature alone does not distinguish this entity from others because ventricular tachycardia originating from the interventricular septum of other etiologies may also appear as a left bundle branch tachycardia on the electrocardiogram.

The exact mechanism of the ventricular tachycardia is not known. The fact that programmed stimulation can elicit this arrhythmia in a reproducible fashion is suggestive of reentry, but the possibility of a triggered mechanism can not be ruled out.

Mitral valve prolapse. Patients with mitral valve prolapse—a common disorder that can be found in 5% to 10% of the population[84]—seem to have a higher prevalence of ventricular premature complexes than the normal population. However, this relationship has not been unequivocally established.[85] It has been further suggested that patients with mitral valve prolapse and mitral regurgitation have more complex ventricular ectopy than those with prolapse alone, but some studies have not confirmed this.[83]

The relationship between mitral valve prolapse and sudden cardiac death is also not clearly established. The incidence of sudden cardiac death in this group of patients is very low.[83] Interestingly, there is no preponderance of mitral regurgitation in those mitral valve prolapse patients with sudden cardiac death.[83]

Nevertheless, several mechanisms have been proposed as the cause of ventricular arrhythmias. Wit et al,[84] have shown that the anterior leaflet of a normal human mitral valve contains atrial muscle and that delayed afterpolarizations could be elicited from the fiber with stimulation in the presence of catecholamines. Nondriven spontaneous automatic activity was also noted during catecholamine infusion. Cobbs and King[85] have proposed that excessive traction of the papillary muscle, resulting in local pacemaker activity, may be the cause. Chessler et al[86] have reported the presence of aggregates of platelets and fibrin at the level of the left atrial wall and posterior mitral valve leaflet in 5 of 14 patients with mitral valve prolapse who had died suddenly. It was then conjectured that microembolization to the coronary arteries may occur and result in ischemia and ventricular fibrillation.

Ventricular tachycardia associated with normal cardiac structure

Congenital long QT syndrome. Patients with primary long QT syndrome have structurally normal hearts but show a prolonged duration of repolarization (QT interval) on their surface electrocardiograms, as well as abnormal appearance of the T waves. The prolongation is present in the absence of any abnormal metabolic conditions.

These patients have a propensity for sudden death secondary to sustained ventricular tachycardia or ventricular fibrillation. A recent prospective study of 328 patients with an average follow-up period of 54 months reported the rate of sudden cardiac death to be 0.9% per year and noted that the majority of the patients had died by the age of 20.[87]

The type of ventricular tachycardia associated with the long QT syndrome is known as torsades de pointes ("twisting of the points"). It is a tachycardia in which the axis of the QRS complexes of the surface electrocardiogram rotates in a relatively regular fashion so that the QRS complexes appear to twist about the isoelectric baseline.

The mechanism for torsades de pointes is postulated to be an intrinsic abnormality of ventricular repolarization. The effect of increased adrenergic tone in such cardiac tissue is thought to lead to triggered activity associated with early afterpolarizations and subsequently to torsades.[88]

The long QT syndrome may also present as an acquired entity. The acquired form can occur with any type of structural heart disease in settings such as severe hypokalemia and hypomagnesemia. It may, quite paradoxically, also occur during antiarrhythmic drug therapy.[89] The resulting ventricular tachycardia is then referred to as a "proarrhythmic" effect of the antiarrhythmic medication.

Catecholamine dependent ventricular tachycardia. This type of ventricular tachycardia is usually found in the young, is usually well tolerated, and is usually associated with a benign prognosis.[90,91] Exercise frequently precipitates the arrhythmia. Infusion of isoproterenol, during the course of electrophysiologic testing, can also frequently initiate the tachycardia. The mechanism is thought to be triggered activity involving delayed afterpolarizations. Catecholamines give rise to delayed afterpolarizations in Purkinje fibers and ventricular muscle by ultimately causing an increase in the intracellular calcium by effecting an increase in intracellular cyclic AMP. In support of this hypothesis has been the finding that the substance adenosine, an endogenous nucleotide with no direct effect on Purkinje fiber or ventricular muscle, membrane can terminate these tachycardias when administered intravenously.[90,91] Adenosine is believed to act by suppressing the catecholamine mediated intracellular production of cyclic AMP and thereby inhibit the formation of delayed afterpolarizations. These tachycardias often are found to have the focus localized to the right ventricular outflow tract as determined during mapping studies in the electrophysiology laboratory and thus characteristically show left bundle branch morphology on the surface.

REFERENCES

1. Becker AE: *General comments.* In Bonke FIM ed: *The sinus node structure, function and chemical relevance,* The Hague, 1978, Martinus Nijhoff.
2. Anderson KR, Ho SY, Anderson RH: The location and vascular supply of the SA node in the human heart, *Br Heart J* 41:28, 1979.
3. Loffelholz K, Pappano AJ: The parasympathetic neuroeffector junction of the heart, *Pharmacol Rev* 37:1, 1985.
4. Boineau JP, Canavan TE, Schuessler RB, et al: Demonstration of a widely distributed atrial pacemaker complex in the human heart, *Circulation* 77:1221, 1988.
5. Janse MJ, Anderson RH: Internodal atrial specialized pathways - fact or fiction? EUR Cardiol 2:117, 1974.
6. Becker AE, Anderson RH: *Morphology of the human atrioventricular junctional area.* In Wellens HJJ, Lie KI, Janse MJ, eds: *The conduction system of the heart. Structure, function and clinical implications,* Leiden, 1976, Stenfest Kroese BV.
7. Zipes DP, Miyazaki T: *The autonomic nervous system and the heart: basis for understanding interactions and effects on arrhythmia development.* In Zipes DP, Jalye J, eds: *Cardiac electrophysiology: from cell to bedside.* Philadelphia 1990, WB Saunders.
8. Rosenbaum MB, Elizari MV, Lazzari JO: *The hemiblocks: new concepts of intraventricular conduction based on human anatomical, physiological and clinical studies.* Oldsmar, Fla, 1970, Tampa Tracings.
9. Toshimori H, Toshimori K, Oura C, et al: Immunohistochemical identification of purkinje fibers and transitional cells in a terminal portion of the impulse conducting system of porcine hearts, *Cell Tissue Res* 253:47, 1988.
10. Davies MJ, Anderson RH, Becker AE: *The conduction system of the heart.* London, 1983, Butterworth & Co.
11. Lev M: Ageing changes in the human sinoatrial node, *J Gerontol* 9:1, 1954.
12. Sasaki R, Theilen EO, et al: Cardiac arrhythmia associated with the repair of atrial and ventricular septal defects, *Circulation* 18:909, 1958.
13. Greenwood RO, Rosenthal A, Sloss LJ, et al: Sick sinus syndrome after surgery for congenital heart disease, *Circulation* 52:208, 1975.
14. Evans R, Shaw DB: Pathologic studies in sinoatrial disorder (sick sinus syndrome), *Br Heart J* 39:778, 1977.
15. Mandel WJ, Laks MM, Obayashi K: Sinus node function evaluation in patients with and without sinus node disease, *Arch Intern Med* 135:388, 1975.

16. Dauchot P, Esravenstein JS: Effects of atropine on the electrocardiogram in different age groups, *Clin Pharmacol Ther* 12:274, 1971.

17. Engel TR, Bond RC, Schaul SF: First degree sinoatrial heart block in the sick sinus syndrome, *Am Heart J* 91:303, 1976.

18. Asseman P, Berzin B, Desry D, et al: Persistent sinus nodal electrograms during post pacing atrial pauses in sick sinus syndrome in humans: sinoatrial block versus, overdrive suppression, *Circulation* 68:33, 1983.

19. Ector H, Robies L, DeGeest H: Dynamic electrocardiography and ventricular pauses of 3 seconds or more: etiology and therapeutic implications, *PACE Pacing Clin Electrophysiol* 6:548, 1983.

20. Slama R, LeClerq JF, Rosengarten M, et al: Multilevel block in the atrioventricular node during atrial tachycardia and flutter alternating with Wenkeback phenomenon, *Br Heart J* 42:463, 1979.

21. McCue CM, Mantakas ME, Tingelstad JB, et al: Congenital heart block in newborns of mothers with connective tissue disease, *Circulation* 56:82, 1977.

22. Lev M: The pathology of complete atrioventricular block. *Prog Cardiovasc Dis* 6:317, 1964.

23. Lenegre J: Etiology of bilateral branch fibrosis in relation to complete heart block, *Prog Cardiovasc Dis* 6:317, 1964.

24. Bassan R, Maia IG, Bozza A, et al: Atrioventricular block in acute inferior wall myocardial infarction: harbinger of associated obstruction of the left anterior descending coronary artery, *J Am Coll Cardiol* 8:773, 1986.

25. Davies MJ: *Pathology of conducting tissue of the heart*. London, 1971, Butterworth & Co.

26. Nair CK, Runco V, Everson GT, et al: Conduction defects and mitrial annular calcification, *Br Heart J* 44:162, 1980.

27. Arnett EN, Roberts WC: Active infective endocarditis. A clinicopathologic analysis of 137 necropsy patients, *Curr Probl Cardiol* 7:1, 1976.

28. Weed CL, Kulander BG, Mazzarella JA, et al: Heart Block in ankylosing spondylitis, *Arch Intern Med* 177:800, 1966.

29. Ahern M, Lever J, Cosh J: Complete heart block in rheumatoid arthritis, *Ann Rheum Dis* 41:319, 1982.

30. Roberts WC, Waller BF: Cardiac amyloidosis, causing cardiac dysfunction: analysis of 54 necropsy patients, *Am J Cardiol* 52:137, 1983.

31. Morales AR, Levy S, Davis J, et al: *Sarcoidosis and the heart*. In Sommers SC ed: *Pathology Annual*, New York, 1974, Appleton-Century-Crofts.

32. Hindman MC, Wagner, GS, JaRo M, et al: The clinical significance of bundle branch block complicating acute myocardial infarction II. Indicators for temporary and permanent therapy, *Circulation* 58:689, 1978.

33. Bonke FIM, Kirchof CJH Allessie MA: *Sinus Node Re-entry*. In Zipes DP, Jalife J, eds: *Cardiac electrophysiology: from cell to bedside*, Philadelphia, 1990, WB Saunders.

34. Gillette PC: The mechanisms of supraventricular arrhythmia in children, *Circulation* 54:133, 1976.

35. Boineau JP, Schuessler RB, Cain ME, et al: *Activation mapping during normal atrial rhythm and atrial flutter*. In Zipes DP, Jalife J, eds: *Cardiac electrophysiology: from cell to bedside*, Philadelphia, 1990, Saunders WB.

36. Guiraudon, Klein GJ, Sharma AD, et al: *Surgery for atrial flutter, atrial fibrillation, and atrial tachycardia*. In Zipes DP, Jalife J, eds: *Cardiac electrophysiology: from cell to bedside*, Philadelphia, 1990, Saunders WB.

37. Giorgi LV, Hartzler GO, Hamaker WR: Incessant atrial tachycardia: a surgically remediable cause of cardiomyopathy, *J Thorac Cardiovasc Surg* 87:466, 1984.

38. Wells JL Jr, McLean WAH, James TN, et al: Characterization of atrial flutter. Studies in man after open heart surgery using fixed atrial electrodes, *Circulation* 60:665, 1979.

39. Waldo AL, McLean WAH, Karp RB, et al: Entertainment and interruption of atrial flutter with atrial pacing: studies in man following open heart surgery, *Circulation* 56:737, 1977.

40. Myerburg RJ, Kessler KM, Castellanos A: Sudden cardiac death. Structure, function and time-dependence of risk, *Circulation* 85 [suppl I]:I-1, 1992.

41. Moe GK, Abildskov, JA: Atrial fibrillation as a self-sustaining arrhythmia independent of focal discharge, *Am Heart J* 58:59, 1959.

42. Moe GK: On the multiple wavelet hypothesis of atrial fibrillation, *Arch Int Pharmacodyn Ther* 140:183, 1962.

43. Friedman PL, Stewart JR, Wit A: Spontaneous and induced cardiac arrhythmias in subendocardial Purkinje fibers surviving extensive myocardial infarction, *Circ Res* 33:612, 1973.

44. Sung RJ, Styperek JL, Myerburg RJ, Et al: Initiation of two distinct forms of atrioventricular node re-entry in man, *Am J Cardiol* 42:404, 1978.

45. Critelli G, Gallagher JJ, Monda V, et al: Anatomic and electrophysiologic substrate of the permanent form of junctional reciprocating tachycardia. *J Am Cardiol* 4:601, 1984.

46. Allessie MA, Bonke FIM, Schopman FJG: Circus movement in rabbit atrial muscle as a mechanism of tachycardia, *Circ Res* 41:9, 1977.

47. Panidis JP, Morganroth J: Sudden death in hospitalized patients: cardiac rhythm disturbances detected by ambulatory electrocardiographic monitoring, *J Am Coll Cardiol* 2:798, 1983.

48. Pratt CM, Francis AJ, Luck CJ et al: Analysis of ambulatory electrocardiograms in 15 patients during spontaneous ventricular fibrillation with special reference to preceding arrhythmia events, *J Am Coll Cardiol* 2:789, 1983.

49. Luu M, Stevenson WG, Stevenson LW et al: Diverse mechanism of unexpected cardiac arrest in advanced heart failure, *Circulation* 80:1675, 1989.

50. Kaltenbrunner W, Cardinal R, Dubuc M et al: Epicardial and endocardial mapping of ventricular tachycardia in patients with myocardial infarction. Is the origin of the tachycardia always subendocardially localized? *Circulation* 84:1058, 1991.

51. Wasserstrom JA, TenEick RE. *Electrophysiology of mammalian ventricular muscle*. In Dangman KH, Miura DS, eds: *Electrophysiology and pharmacology of the heart, a clinical guide*, New York, 1991, Dekker.

52. Sorota S, Boyden P: *Electrophysiology of the atrial myocardium*. In Dangman KH, Miura DS, eds: *Electrophysiology and pharmacology of the heart, a clinical guide*, New York, 1991, Dekker.

53. El Sherif N, Gough WB, Zeiler RH et al: Re-entrant ventricular arrhythmias in the late myocardial infarction period. 12. Spontaneous vs. induced re-entry and intramural vs. epicardial circuits, *J Am Coll Cardiol* 6;124, 1985.

54. Allessie MA, Schalij MJ, Kirchof CJHJ et al: Experimental electrophysiology and arrhythmogenicity. Anisotropy and ventricular tachycardia, *Eur Heart J* 10:(Suppl E)2-8, 1989.

55. Kamiyama A, Eguchi K, Shibayama R: Circus movement tachycardia induced by a single premature stimulus on the ventricular sheet-evaluation of the leading circle hypothesis in the canine ventricular muscle, *Circ J* 50:65, 1986.

56. De Bakker JMT, Van Capelle FJL, Janse MJ et al: Re-entry as a cause of ventricular tachycardia in patients with chronic ischemic heart disease: electrophysiologic and anatomic correlation, *Circulation* 77:589, 1988.

57. Janse M, VanCappelle FJL, Morsink H: Flow of "injury" current and pattern of excitation during early ventricular arrhythmias in acute regional myocardial ischemia in isolated porcine and canine hearts: evidence for two different arrhythmogenic mechanisms, *Circ Res* 47:151, 1980.

58. Wit AL, Janse MJ: Experimental models of ventricular tachycardia and fibrillation caused by ischemia and infarction, *Circulation* 85 [suppl I]:I-32, 1992.

59. Lazzara R, El Sherif N, Scherlag BJ: Electrophysiological prperties

of canine Purkinje cells in one-day-old myocardial infarction, *Circ Res* 33:722, 1973.

60. Dangman KH, Hofmann BF: In vivo and in vitro anti-arrhythmic and arrhythmogenic effects of N-acetyl procainamide, *J Pharmacol Exp Ther* 217:851, 1981.

61. Dangman KH, Dresdner KP, Zaim S: Automatic and triggered impulse initiation in canine subepicardial ventricular muscle cells from border zones of 24 hr transmural infarcts. New Mechanisms for malignant cardiac arrhythmias? *Circulation* 78:1020, 1988.

62. Binah O, Rosen MR: Mechanisms of ventricular arrhythmias, *Circulation* 85 [suppl I]:I-25, 1992.

63. Huang SK, Messer JV, Denes P: Significance of ventricular tachycardia in idiopathic dilated cardiomyopathy: Observations in 35 patients, *Am J Cardiol* 51:507, 1983.

64. Meinerz T, Hofmann T, Kasper W et al: Significance of ventricular arrhythmias in idiopathic dilated cardiomyopathy, *Am J Cardiol* 53:902, 1984.

65. Kannel WB, Pleher JF, Cupples LA: Cardiac failure and sudden death in the Framingham study, *Am Heart J* 115:869, 1988.

66. Miller JM, Josephson MA: *Ventricular arrhythmias.* In Parmley WW, Chatterjee K, eds: *Cardiology,* Philadelphia, 1990, JP Lippincott.

67. Caceres J, Jazayeri M, Mckinnie J et al: Sustained bundle branch reentry as a mechanism of clinical tachycardia, *Circulation* 79:256, 1989.

68. Maron BJ, Savage DD, Wolfson JK, et al: Prognostic significance of 24 hour ambulatory electrocardiographic monitoring in patients with hypertrophic cardiomyopathy: a prospective study, *Am J Cardiol* 48:252, 1981.

69. McKenna W, Deanfield J, Farnqui A et al: Prognosis in hypertrophic cardiomyopathy: role of age and clinical, electrocardiographic and hemodynamic features, *Am J Cardiol* 47:532, 1981.

70. Stewart JT, McKenna WJ: Arrhythmias in hypertrophic cardiomyopathy, *J Cardiovasc Electrophysiol* 2:516, 1991.

71. Fananapazir L, Epstein SE, Epstein ND: Investigation and clinical significance of arrhythmias in patients with hypertrophic cardiomyopathy, *J Cardiovasc Electrophysiol* 2:525, 1991.

72. Maron BJ, Fananapazir L: Sudden death in hypertrophic cardiomyopathy, *Circulation* 85 [suppl]:I-57, 1992.

73. Aronson RS: Mechanisms of arrhythmias in ventricular hypertrophy, *J Cardiovasc Electrophysiol* 2:249, 1991.

74. Aronson RS: *Cellular basis for arrhythmias in cardiac hypertrophy and cardiomyopathy.* In Dangman KH, Miura DS, eds: *Electrophysiology and pharmacology of the heart,* New York, 1991, Dekker.

75. Coltart DJ, Meldrum SJ: Hypertrophic cardiomyopathy. An electrophysiology study, *Br Med J* 218:217, 1970.

76. Han J, Moe GK: Nonuniform recovery of excitability in ventricular muscle, *Circ Res* 14:44, 1964.

77. Ben-David J, Ayers GM, Pride HP et al: Left ventricular hypertrophy predisposes to development of early afterdepolarizations that cause ventricular tachycardia in dogs, *Circulation* 82:III-99, 1990.

78. Goethals MA, Sys SU, Stroobandt R et al: Delayed afterpotentials elicit diastolic aftercontractions in the hypertrophied ventricle of human aortic stenosis, *Circulation* 82:III-581, 1990.

79. Marcus FI, Fontaine GH, Guiradon G et al: Right ventricular dysplasia: a report of 24 adult cases, *Circulation* 65:384, 1982.

80. Fontaine G, Frank R, Fontaliran F et al: *Right ventricular dysplasia.* In Parmley WW, Chatterjee K eds: *Cardiology,* Philadelphia, 1991, JP Lippincott.

81. Marcus FI, Fontaine GH, Frank R et al. Long-term follow-up in patients with arrhythmogenic right ventricular disease, *Eur Heart J* 10:(Suppl D) 68, 1989.

82. Braunwald E: *Valvular heart disease.* In Braunwald E, ed: *Heart disease,* Philadelphia, 1991, WB Saunders.

83. Schaal SF: *Mitral valve prolapse: cardiac arrhythmias and electrophysiological correlates.* In Boudoulas H, Wooley CF, eds: *Mitral valve prolapse and the mitral valve syndrome,* Mount Kisco, 1988, Futura.

84. Wit AL, Fenoglio JJ, Hordof AJ et al: Ultrastructure and transmembrane potentials of cardiac muscle in the human anterior mitral valve leaflet, *Circulation* 59:1284, 1979.

85. Cobbs BW, King SB: Ventricular buckling: a factor in the abnormal ventriculogram and peculiar hemodynamics associated with mitral valve prolapse, *Am Heart J* 93:741, 1977.

86. Chesler E, King R, Edwards JE: The myxomatous mitral valve and sudden death, *Circulation* 67:632, 1983.

87. Moss AJ, Schwartz PJ, Crampton RS et al: The long QT syndrome. Prospective longitudinal study of 328 families, *Circulation* 84:1136, 1991.

88. Zipes DP: The long QT syndrome. A Rosetta stone for sympathetic related ventricular tachyarrhythmias, *Circulation* 84:1414, 1991.

89. Jackman WM, Friday KJ, Anderson JL et al: The long QT syndromes: a critical review, new clinical observations and a unifying hypothesis, *Prog Cardiovasc Dis* 31:115, 1988.

90. Lerman BB. *Ventricular tachycardia unassociated with coronary artery disease.* In Zipes DP, Rowlands DJ, eds: *Progress in cardiol,* Philadelphia, 1988, Lea & Febiger.

91. Lerman BB, Belardinelli L, West A et al: Adenosine-sensitive ventricular tachycardia: evidence suggesting cyclic AMP-mediated triggered activity, *Circulation* 74:270, 1986.

Chapter 15

CARDIAC TRANSPLANTATION

Kirk R. Kanter
Gary L. Hertzler
Michael B. Gravanis

Et Toi Mon Coeur?
. . . .
Alas, new times arrived mon coeur
and you became a pump
just another mortal
with tarnished halo, the wings clipped.
Your queenship has ended as
the royal chambers were probed and intruded.
The inspiring figure was altered and distorted
with devices and euphemistic assists
and then the dreadful nightmare
you were declared replaceable.
Oh gods, where to place the feelings,
where to house the internal turmoil,
a state of wrath,
an inner ebullition, an impulse of love.

              Michael B. Gravanis, M.D.

(reprinted from Clin. Cardiol. 13.305 (1990))

INDICATIONS AND CONTRAINDICATIONS

Clinical cardiac transplantation has progressed significantly since the first human-to-human heart transplantation was performed by Barnard[1] in Cape Town, South Africa in 1967. Since the introduction of the immunosuppressive drug cyslosporine in the early 1980s, cardiac transplantation has become an accepted and generally successful treatment for end-stage cardiac disease. The most recent report of the Registry of the International Society for Heart and Lung Transplantation reveals that cardiac transplantation has matured from a bold headline-grabbing event in the late 1960s to a near-everyday procedure in the 1990s, with 16,687 heart transplants performed up to January 1, 1991.[2]

In general, candidates for cardiac transplantation are individuals with end-stage heart disease with an expected survival of less than 1 year in whom standard medical and surgical options have been exhausted. The vast majority of these patients are New York Heart Association functional class IV, with a large percentage of recipients in an intensive care unit on inotropic support or mechanical circulatory assistance such as an intraaortic balloon pump, a ventricular assist device, or a totally artificial heart at time of transplantation. Dilated cardiomyopathy is the most common indication for heart transplantation in adults and children, accounting for roughly 50% of transplants in both age groups. Ischemic heart disease accounts for another 40% of cases in adults, whereas congenital heart disease has been until recently the second most common indication for transplantation in children (36%). Since 1988, however, congenital heart disease has surpassed cardiomyopathy as the most common indication for transplantation in children. Conditions accounting for small numbers of heart transplants include valvular heart disease (4%) and cardiac retransplantation (2.5%). Refractory arrhythmias, doxorubicin-induced cardiomyopathy, amyloidosis, Chagas disease, and cardiac tumors each account for less than 1%.[2]

In the past, contraindications for potential cardiac transplant recipients have been fairly rigorous, with strict age constraints (less than 55 years old) and exclusion of patients with diabetes, cancer, active infection, pulmonary emboli, other serious irreversible organ dysfunction, irreversible pulmonary hypertension, and presence of another disease process that might significantly decrease life expectancy after transplantation.[3] As experience has been gained, many of the old absolute contraindications to transplantation have been relaxed to serve a larger percentage of the population. Most transplant centers now set the upper age limit for recipients at 60, with some groups performing transplants in patients up to age 70.[4,5] With the use of cyclosporine as the mainstay of immunosuppression, the need for high-dose steroids in the posttransplant period is less, thus allowing transplantation in diabetics.[6] Cardiac transplantation has been performed successfully in patients with a history of cancer who appear disease-free.[7] Even patients with recent pulmonary emboli have been successfully transplanted.[8] Patients with concomitant severe irreversible hepatic or renal failure have undergone successful combined heart and liver[9] or combined heart and kidney transplantation.[10,11]

Although most candidates for cardiac transplantation have elevated pulmonary artery pressures caused by congestive heart failure and elevated left-sided pressures, most of them have an acceptable pulmonary vascular resistance and thus presumably reversible pulmonary arterial hypertension. A certain percentage of potential transplant recipients have irreversible pulmonary hypertension. The donor heart comes from an otherwise normal brain-dead individual, and when faced with an irreversibly elevated pulmonary vascular resistance, will develop right ventricular failure, resulting in subsequent graft loss and patient death.[12] This problem can be averted by performing a heterotopic ("piggyback") heart transplant where the native diseased heart is left *in situ* at time of transplantation. If necessary, concomitant coronary revascularization or valvular reparative procedures are performed on the native heart and the donor heart is placed in the right chest in parallel fashion with essentially a common left atrium.[13] Because the native right ventricle in these patients often has gradually hypertrophied over time as pulmonary hypertension developed, the native right ventricle can cope with the elevated

pulmonary vascular resistance workload.[14] The heterotopic heart transplant accounts for 2% of heart transplants recorded by the Registry of the International Society for Heart Transplantation[2] and 6.25% of transplants done at our institution since 1988.

DONOR/RECIPIENT MATCHING

The paucity of suitable cardiac donors still remains the major factor limiting the more widespread application of cardiac transplantation.[15] It is estimated that annually between 14,000 and 20,000 patients with severe heart disease in the United States could benefit from heart transplantation. Although some authors have proposed that as many as 12,000 to 14,000 brain-dead individuals in the United States meet the criteria for cardiac donation annually,[16] only a small percentage of this potential pool is used, with 2108 heart transplants performed in the United States in 1991.[17]

Donor-recipient pairs are selected on the basis of size (generally no greater than 20% weight difference between donor and recipient), ABO blood group compatibility, clinical urgency, and length of time on the transplant waiting list. In general, a prospective lymphocyte crossmatch is not performed unless the potential recipient on preoperative screening shows greater than 10% to 20% sensitization to a panel of random donors. Although there is now no systematic mechanism to preoperatively match donor and recipient on the basis of HLA histocompatibility, there is compelling evidence that HLA histocompatibility improves long-term survival and reduces rejection episodes.[18,19,20] With current techniques for protection of the donor heart, it would be impractical to perform routine prospective crossmatches and HLA typing because the accepted safe donor ischemia time is generally set at 4 hours. However, if safe donor ischemia time can be significantly extended, as has been done successfully in liver transplantation with the use of University of Wisconsin solution, then HLA matching between donor and recipient may become a clinical reality.[21]

PHYSIOLOGY OF THE TRANSPLANTED HEART

Many of the changes in cardiac physiology seen in the nonrejecting transplanted heart can be directly attributed to the effects of cardiac denervation. As early as 1933, Mann and coworkers[22] demonstrated that a heart could be routinely transplanted from one animal to another with excellent cardiac function. Early in the postoperative period there is an immediate depression of left ventricular function both in autotransplanted animals[23] as well as in allotransplanted humans.[24,25] This transient depression of function is generally attributed to ischemic myocardial injury related to the transplant procedure itself[26,27] and resolves over time.

Small foci of confluent necrosis of the subendocardial myocardium may be seen in biopsy specimens obtained

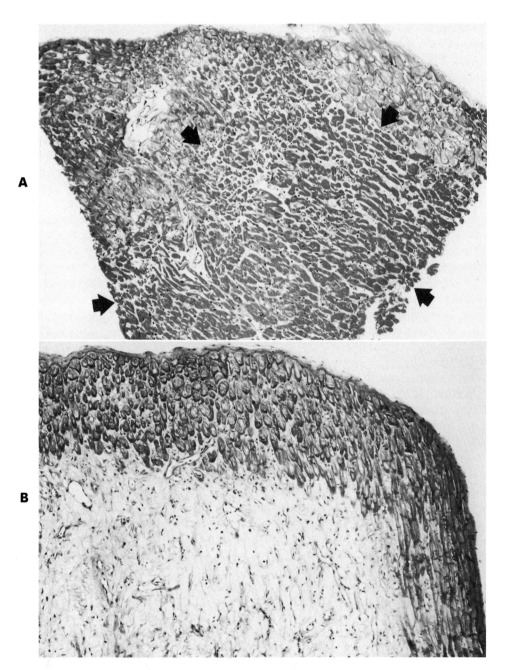

Fig. 15-1. Microinfarct. **A,** Posttransplant day 7. A confluent area of coagulative necrosis is denoted by arrows. The necrotic myocytes are shrunken, wavy, and hypereosinophilic as compared to the surrounding paler viable cells. **B,** A pale area of loose connective tissue and neovascularity denotes a healed microinfarct. A thin layer of myocardium beneath the endocardium remains viable.

within the first 2 weeks post-transplant. Discrete areas of coagulative necrosis of myocytes are accompanied with little or no inflammation. The five to ten layers of myocytes immediately subjacent to the endocardium are spared and remain viable (Fig. 15-1, *A*). Over a period of weeks to months, the necrotic myocytes are gradually removed by macrophages and are replaced by a loosely fibrous scar (Fig. 15-1, *B*). These lesions may be secondary to pressor agents or to localized ischemia.[28] They are readily distin-

guished from rejection by their relative lack of inflammation and their confluent rather than individual myocytic necrosis. These necrotic foci are limited in scope and seldom can be related to allograft dysfunction.

Although myocardial catecholamine levels are not measurable within a week of transplantation because of cardiac denervation,[29] this does not appear to affect intrinsic myocardial function. After the early postoperative period, resting hemodynamics are normal in patients treated with prednisone and azathioprine.[24,30] There is an increase in resting heart rate caused by the vagolytic effect of cardiac denervation.[31] In patients treated with cyclosporine, there appears to be elevation in left ventricular filling pressures, as well as slightly decreased left ventricular ejection fraction and reduced compliance.[30,32,33] An echocardiographic study has shown an increase in left ventricular end-systolic volume without a change in left ventricular mass within 1 year of transplantation.[34] These changes are attributed to the effects of systemic arterial hypertension seen in cyclosporine-treated patients.

The response to exercise in heart transplant recipients is different from normal controls. In normal subjects, moderate exercise results in a sharp increase in cardiac output and blood pressure, mediated mostly though an increase in heart rate with little change in left ventricular end-diastolic volume and stroke volume.[35] By contrast, in heart transplant recipients, the initial rise in heart rate with exercise is severely blunted by cardiac denervation. Instead, the heart responds to demands for increased workload by an early increase in left ventricular end-diastolic volume and stroke volume,[36,37] thus using the Frank-Starling mechanism. In time, there is a steady increase in heart rate of the denervated allograft, presumably related to circulating catecholamines.[36] After about 15 minutes of exercise, heart transplant recipients will achieve peak heart rates almost as high as normal controls.[36,37]

Because of the denervated state of the cardiac allograft, drugs that normally affect the heart may have no effect or different effects on the transplanted heart. For example, because the electrical effects of digoxin on the atrioventricular node are mediated through vagal pathways, there are minimal electrical effects of digoxin on the transplanted heart,[38,39] although the inotropic effects are preserved. As one would expect, atropine, which acts as a parasympathetic blocker, has no effect on the sinus rate of the transplanted heart.[40] Similarly, the normal vagolytic effects of quinidine and disopyramide are not seen in the transplanted heart. Instead of the normal increase in sinus rate and minimal effect on atrioventricular conduction, one sees the direct effect of these two drugs in the transplanted heart with slowing of the sinus node and increased atrioventricular conduction time.[41,42]

Several studies have shown reinnervation of autotransplanted canine hearts after 1 year.[43,44,45] It is widely accepted that reinnervation does not occur in human heart transplant recipients. This belief is based mostly on the lack of appropriate neural reflex-mediated changes in heart rate.[36,46] However, there have been isolated case reports suggestive of reinnervation in humans[47,48] as well as some recent sophisticated neurohumoral studies strongly presumptive of at least partial reinnervation in humans.[49,50]

REJECTION

Allograft injury by a specific immune response of the recipient directed against the graft is termed *rejection*, which if unchecked results in progressive graft dysfunction and loss. Like other solid organ allografts, the cardiac allograft is potentially subject to injury by both major arms of the recipient's immune system: humoral (antibody-mediated) immunity and cellular immunity. Based upon mechanism and duration, rejection of the allograft may be categorized as *hyperacute, acute humoral, acute cellular,* or *chronic*. Hyperacute rejection occurs in the setting of preformed cytotoxic antibodies reactive against graft antigens, with rapid onset at the time of transplantation. Acute humoral rejection occurs following the development of donor-specific antibodies subsequent to transplantation. Rapid onset cytotoxic cell-mediated graft injury is termed acute cellular rejection. Chronic rejection refers to the usually insidious development of occlusive arterial disease and resultant ischemia. In common parlance, cardiac allograft rejection is termed either *acute* or *chronic; acute rejection* is synonymous with *cellular rejection*. As cellular rejection is by far the most common form of acute rejection in the cardiac allograft, this abbreviated terminology has served in everyday practice. However, the occurrence of humoral rejection, either alone or in conjunction with cellular rejection, is increasingly well documented and has important prognostic significance. Terms such as "acute rejection," "vascular rejection," or even "acute vascular rejection" relate time course or site of injury but not mechanism of injury. Therefore discussion of the pathogenesis of rejection requires the use of precise terminology.

Hyperacute rejection

Preformed cytotoxic antibodies present in the recipient at the time of transplantation can result in rapid destruction of the allograft by hyperacute rejection. The antibodies may be directed against a variety of donor antigens, including ABO blood group antigens,[51] major histocompatibility (MHC) antigens,[52] or vascular endothelial antigens.[53] Binding of the antibodies to antigens expressed by the vascular endothelium initiates complement fixation and a cascade of events leading to irreversible tissue injury. Complement-mediated endothelial damage and disruption promotes platelet aggregation, initiation of the clotting cascade, and thrombosis. Inflammatory cells, predominantly neutrophils, are recruited and infiltrate the vascular walls and surrounding interstitium. The combination of small blood vessel occlusion and loss of vascular integrity results in cellular extravasation with diffuse hemorrhage, pronounced edema, and tissue ischemia with frank necrosis.

Hyperacute rejection has been described in different solid organ allografts[51,54] including hearts.[55,56,57] To avoid hyperacute rejection as much as possible, hearts are transplanted only into ABO-compatible recipients. Potential recipients are screened pretransplant for cytotoxic antibodies directed against MHC antigens to identify those with a high level of sensitization. If there is an unacceptably high level of preformed antibodies, a recipient-donor lymphocytotoxicity crossmatch is performed pretransplant to detect performed antibodies directed specifically against potential donor antigens. Fortunately, hyperacute rejection of ABO-compatible cardiac allografts with a negative crossmatch is a rare event.[56,58]

The mainstay of treatment of hyperacute rejection is prevention in the form of identifying potential recipients at risk with preoperative antibody screens and performing prospective crossmatches on sensitized individuals. When hyperacute rejection occurs, it usually is manifested in the operating room at time of transplantation as severe and progressive allograft dysfunction. Immediate treatment consists of aggressive inotropic support with early consideration for mechanical circulatory support. In the most severe forms of hyperacute rejection, immediate retransplantation may be the only viable therapy. In less aggressive forms, consideration can be given to plasmapheresis to remove preformed antibodies[59] or the substitution of cyclophosphamide for azathioprine. Cyclophosphamide theoretically is more active against B lymphocytes.[60] In general, however, in true hyperacute cardiac rejection, these treatment modalities are usually ineffective. Graft loss and patient death are often inevitable unless immediate retransplantation is performed.

Hearts rejected hyperacutely are heavy with visible epicardial, endocardial, and intramural hemorrhages. Microscopically, interstitial edema and extravasated erythrocytes are present throughout the myocardium. Infiltration by segmented neutrophils is patchy. Mononuclear inflammatory cells are few. Many arterioles, capillaries, and venules are occluded by platelet-fibrin microthrombi. Their endothelium is discontinuous with alterations ranging from partial detachment to complete denudation. Scattered segmented neutrophils lie on luminal surfaces and within vessel walls. Frank disruption of some vessels is associated with extensive perivascular and interstitial hemorrhage. Individual and small groups of cardiomyocytes show early acute degenerative and ischemic features with hypereosinophilic coagulated cytoplasm, contraction bands, and nuclear pyknosis. Immunofluorescence or immunohistochemical studies demonstrate finely granular deposits of IgM, IgG, and complement in vascular walls and interstitial deposition of fibrin.

Acute humoral rejection

Rejection of the cardiac allograft mediated by antibodies formed subsequent to transplantation is uncommon in most heart transplantation centers and is a component of only a small minority of acute rejection episodes. Nevertheless, acute humoral rejection is now well documented in heart transplantation.[61,62] It develops early in the posttransplantation period, usually within the first month. The initial and predominant injury is to the intramyocardial blood vessels following deposition of antibody and the activation of complement. Loss of vascular integrity results

in massive allograft edema. The specificities of the antibodies involved remains unknown. Antibodies may be directed against specific vascular and myocytic antigens including major histocompatibility complex (MHC) antigens,[63] or possibly may be deposited as preformed immune complexes. An increased incidence of acute humoral rejection has been reported with OKT3 sensitization and the development of human antimouse antibodies during OKT3 rejection prophylaxis.[64]

Acute humoral rejection is associated with an adverse clinical outcome and high mortality.[62,64] Clinically, this form of rejection should be suspected in the face of significant cardiac dysfunction within the first month of transplantation. Immunofluorescence stains of endomyocardial biopsies will confirm the diagnosis. Once diagnosed, treatment consists of intensified immunosuppression with high-dose steroids, OKT3 monoclonal antibodies and possible plasmapheresis, and cyclophosphamide as is used for hyperacute rejection.

Hammond and her coworkers[62] report the earliest manifestation of acute humoral rejection in biopsy specimens to be deposition of IgG or IgM and complement (C3 and/or C1q) in the microvasculature of the heart demonstrated by immunofluorescence microscopy (Fig. 15-2, *A*). Subsequent biopsies reveal extravasation of fibrin into the interstitium. Schuurman et al[61] describe fine linear perimyocytic deposition of immunoglobulin and complement. We have observed the combination of these two patterns with predominantly vascular deposition of IgG and C3 but with focally linear perimyocytic deposition as well. Immunofluorescence detection of humoral rejection may precede any changes visible by routine light microscopy. The initial changes seen in routine sections include profound swelling and partial detachment of endothelial cells of arterioles, capillaries, and venules (Fig. 15-2, *B*). Segmented neutrophils and mononuclear inflammatory cells adhere to and infiltrate the endothelium. Endothelial cells are enlarged, clumped, and often partially detached (Fig. 15-2, *C*). Sequential biopsies of ongoing vascular rejection reveal frank inflammation of vascular walls and pronounced edema but little inflammatory cell infiltration in the myocardial interstitium (Fig. 15-2, *D*). Serial biopsies of successfully treated humoral rejection document cessation of the vasculitis, reconstitution of the vascular endothelium, and gradual reduction of the interstitial edema.

Humoral and cellular rejection may occur concurrently in a pattern that has been termed *mixed rejection*.[62] The histologic appearance is a combination of the vascular injury and diffuse edema of humoral rejection and the lymphocytic infiltrates and myocytic injury of cellular rejection described below.

Acute cellular rejection

Cellular rejection is characterized by the accumulation of inflammatory cells (predominantly lymphocytes) specifically directed against donor antigens of the allograft with

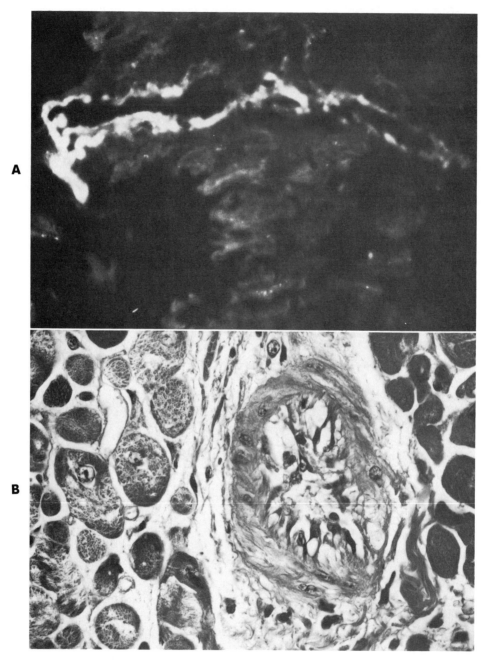

Fig. 15-2. Acute humoral rejection. **A,** Immunofluorescence microscopy demonstrates complement (C3) deposition in a vascular wall. **B,** Endothelial cells of an arteriole are markedly swollen and partially detached.

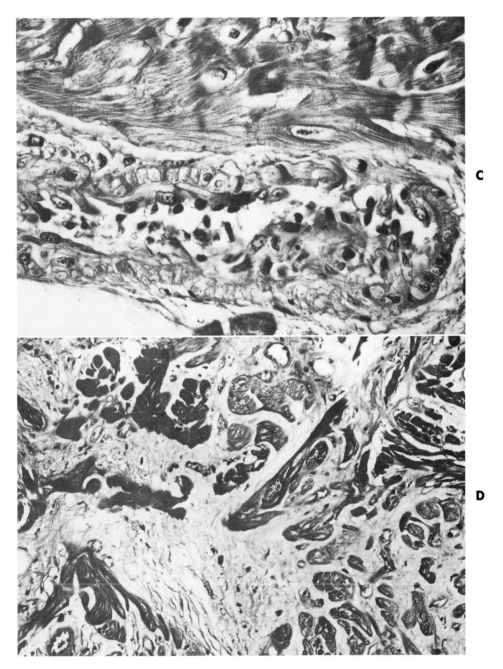

Fig. 15-2, cont'd. C, Inflammatory cells are intermixed with clumped and detached endothelial cells of an arteriole. **D,** The pale edematous interstitium is greatly expanded, widely separating the dark staining myocytes.

demonstrable tissue injury. In the cardiac allograft, cellular rejection is most commonly directed against the myocytes. However, in a minority of episodes vascular injury, particularly to arterioles and arteries, may be a component of or the predominant manifestation of cellular rejection. The complex sequence of events initiating and promoting cellular rejection is incompletely understood. Antigen processing and presentation by tissue dendritic cells and possibly other specialized cells of the macrophage system are important early events.[65] Augmented expression of major histocompatibility (MHC) antigens by vascular endothelium and myocytes may play a role in the development of rejection. High levels of expression of both MHC class I and MHC class II antigens develop prior to the onset of cellular rejection[66] and subside with resolution of rejection. Recognition of foreign MHC class II antigens and other alloantigens by helper/inducer (CD4+) T-lymphocytes initiates a sequence of activation, proliferation, production of lymphokines, and the development of cytotoxic (CD8+) T-lymphocytes specifically directed against graft antigens, including MHC class I antigens.[67] The many lymphokines elaborated include interleukin-2, a potent stimulator of T-cell proliferation, and gamma interferon, an inducer of MHC class II expression. Proliferation of sensitized cells, infiltration of the allograft by those cells, and cytolysis of individual cellular constituents, particularly myocytes, are further important steps.[68] Glucocorticoids act as immunosuppressive agents in inhibiting early T-cell activation. Cyclosporine inhibits helper T-cell (CD4+) production of lymphokines including interleukin-2, which is essential for cytotoxic T-cell proliferation. Cellular infiltrates of rejection in the setting of cyclosporine immunosuppression include natural killer (NK) cells, macrophages, and, at times, eosinophils. The predominant cells, however, are T-lymphocytes, which are most clearly implicated in cellular rejection. Because variable proportions of CD4 and CD8 positive T-cells have been identified in allograft rejection, quantitative analysis of T-cell subtypes in most cases has not been generally useful in predicting or managing rejection.[69,70]

Clinical presentation. In the early days of clinical cardiac transplantation, there were no reliable means to assess the appearance of acute cellular rejection in the cardiac allograft. As a result, fairly nonspecific clinical signs were used to diagnose rejection, including malaise, fever, heart failure, pericardial friction rub, elevated serum LDH, and electrocardiographic abnormalities (including arrhythmias and decreased QRS voltage.[71,72] Although these findings suggest rejection, none could prove its existence unequivocally, occasionally resulting in overimmunosuppression of patients by treating them for rejection when an accurate diagnosis could not be established. Furthermore, by the time these relatively insensitive clinical indicators became apparent, the rejection was fairly advanced, making it more difficult to reverse with intensified immunosuppression therapy and increasing the likelihood of irreparable damage to the graft.

The diagnosis and management of acute cellular rejection was therefore revolutionized with the introduction of routine transvenous endomyocardial biopsy by Caves and

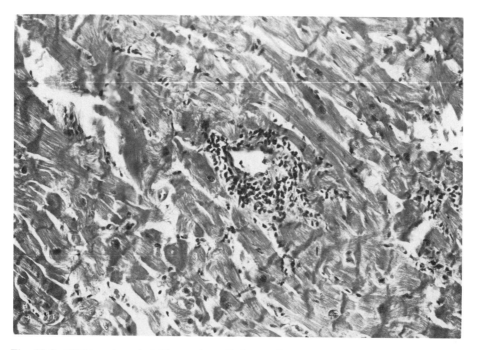

Fig. 15-3. Mild lymphocytic infiltrate. A small cluster of lymphocytes is confined to the perivascular space.

his colleagues[73,74] at Stanford in 1973.[73,74] With this safe and simple technique, it was now possible to perform routine surveillance biopsies to detect acute cellular rejection well before the onset of clinical signs. This development increased the likelihood of reversing rejection and minimizing the possibility of allograft dysfunction. Because the incidence of acute cellular rejection is highest in the first 3 months after transplantation, endomyocardial biopsies are performed at short intervals during that time. As time progresses, biopsies are performed at increasing intervals but are continued indefinitely because the risk of acute cellular rejection exists even years after transplantation. In addition to scheduled surveillance biopsies, endomyocardial biopsies are performed after episodes of rejection to assess response to treatment, after changes in immunosuppression therapy, and at times of clinical suspicion of allograft rejection.

There has been much interest in the development of a reliable non-invasive technique to supplant the endomyocardial biopsy for detection of acute cellular rejection. Various techniques have included serial intramyocardial electrograms,[75] signal-averaged electrocardiograms,[76] echocardiographic measurements of systolic and diastolic function,[77,78] magnetic resonance imaging,[79] cytoimmunologic monitoring of lymphocyte subpopulations,[80] and various measurements of byproducts of lymphocyte activation measured in the serum or urine. Currently, however, endomyocardial biopsy remains the "gold standard" for detection of acute cellular rejection. However, in neonates, where the procedure is somewhat risky, clinical signs, changes in echocardiographic indexes, and evidence of lymphoblast proliferation are used to make the diagnosis of rejection.[81]

Histologic diagnosis. The criteria for rejection on endomyocardial biopsy are usually based upon those initially proposed by Billingham,[82,83] with modifications varying from institution to institution.[84-87] A working formulation has been advanced to standardize the terminology of cardiac rejection.[88] No matter which system is used, the following factors are assessed: (1) the nature, intensity, and distribution of inflammatory cell infiltrates; (2) the presence or absence of edema; and (3) the presence or absence of myocyte injury.

Lymphocytes are the principal effector cell in cellular rejection. However, not all lymphocytic infiltrates are synonymous with rejection. Infections, previous biopsy sites, and microinfarcts must be excluded before the possibility of rejection is considered. Mild lymphocytic infiltrates consisting of sparse perivascular aggregates (Fig. 15-3) are frequently observed in biopsy specimens. These infiltrates approximate mild "rejection" in the original Billingham nomenclature, Emory University Hospital (EUH) grade I, and grade 1A of the International Society for Heart Transplantation (ISHT). In cyclosporine-treated patients, these mild perivascular infiltrates are not associated with tissue injury and do not require augmentation of immunosuppression. Sparse interstitial infiltrates, whether focal or diffuse (EUH grade II), are somewhat more worrisome and require closer follow-up for possible progression to rejection (Fig. 15-4). Herskowitz et al[89] found multifocal interstitial infiltration of lymphocytes between myocytes coupled with the presence of interstitial edema to be highly predictive of

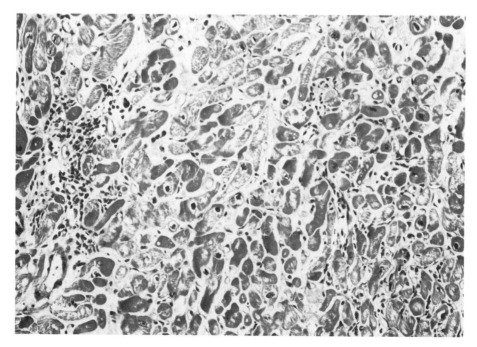

Fig. 15-4. Mild interstitial infiltrate. Lymphocytes lie singly and in small clusters within the interstitium. Edema and myocyte injury are lacking.

myocyte necrosis on subsequent biopsies. Clearly this pattern, even in the absence of frank myocyte necrosis, is an early manifestation of acute cellular rejection that predictably progresses to "moderate" rejection.

Moderate acute cellular rejection is usually a patchy process with dense but localized foci of inflammation lying in expanses of histologically normal myocardium. Occasionally lymphocytes form a large dense aggregate with myocyte damage and necrosis at its periphery (ISHT grade 2) (Fig. 15-5). The more common pattern is that of multiple foci in which enlarged lymphocytes with basophilic cytoplasm accumulate in the interstitium between myocytes (EUH grade III, ISHT grade 3A) (Fig. 15-6, A). These lymphocytes, admixed with variable numbers of macrophages and eosinophils, expand the interstitium. Coupled with localized interstitial edema, the inflammation separates and stretches the myocytes. Lymphocytes lie in close apposition to the myocytes and a few appear to lie within myocytic cytoplasm. Myocyte damage is manifested by stretched, frayed, and often hypereosinophilic cytoplasm (Figure 15-6, B). Frankly necrotic myocytes with disintegrating coagulated cytoplasm may appear, but these are few and widely scattered in a focus of moderate rejection.

With increasing severity, the patches of cellular rejection become larger and more confluent. More intense inflammation is associated with greater frank myocyte necrosis (EUH grade IV). Multinucleated histiocytic giant cells rarely form a prominent component of the process (Fig. 15-7). The most severe form of acute cellular rejection

(EUH grade V, ISHT grade 4) is characterized by intense diffuse inflammation and profound diffuse edema (Fig. 15-8). Numerous segmented neutrophils join the inflammatory infiltrate. Microvascular integrity is compromised so that patchy erythrocyte extravasation becomes prominent. Myocyte injury is apparent throughout the biopsy tissue and small clusters of necrotic myocytes are readily identified.

Endomyocardial biopsies of acute cellular rejection reliably demonstrate the myocardial inflammation and myocyte injury. However, acute cellular rejection may also result in vascular inflammation. Occasionally lymphocytic vasculitis is identified in endomyocardial biopsy specimens, usually with typical cellular rejection elsewhere (Fig. 15-9). Lymphocytes infiltrate vascular walls but are not associated with endothelial disruption or vascular necrosis. In the absence of humoral rejection, these small vessel lesions have resolved with treatment of the cellular rejection. Herskowitz et al[90] associated arteriolar vasculitis with poor outcome but did not distinguish between those with and those without humoral rejection. Lymphocytic vasculitis in the absence of demonstrable humoral rejection has been reported to involve the coronary arteries, resulting in global cardiac ischemia.[91] Because acute lymphocytic coronary arteritis is not detected by endomyocardial biopsy, its true incidence remains unknown, as are the long-term effects upon the vasculature.

Treatment. The backbone of immunosuppression in current clinical cardiac transplantation is the drug cyclosporine, which acts primarily by suppressing the produc-

Text continued on p. 476.

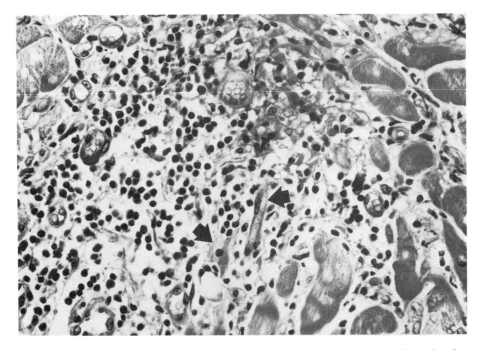

Fig. 15-5. Moderate acute cellular rejection. A relatively dense lymphocytic infiltrate involves the interstitium at its periphery. Injured myocytes *(arrows)* have attenuated cytoplasm with frayed edges.

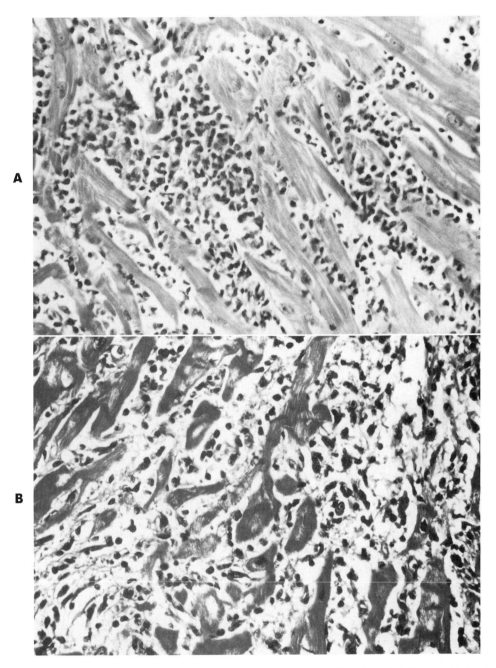

Fig. 15-6. Moderate acute cellular rejection **A,** A focally dense lymphocytic infiltrate with focal edema separates the myocytes. **B,** Damaged myocytes are stretched, hypereosinophilic, and fragmented.

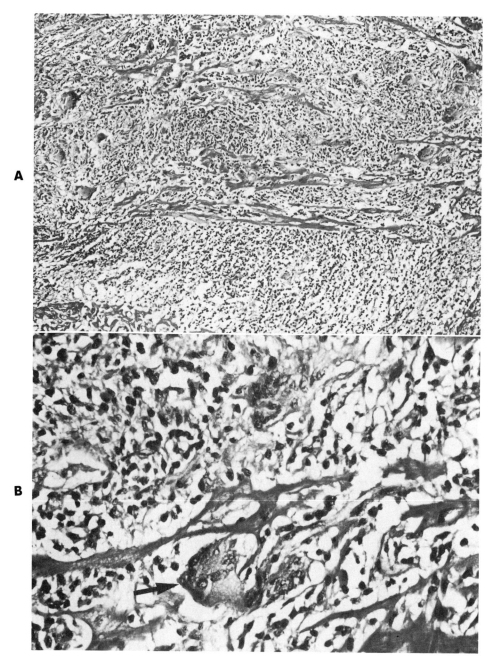

Fig. 15-7. Moderate to severe acute cellular rejection. **A,** A large area of intense lymphocytic inflammation is associated with extensive myocyte necrosis. **B,** Infrequently, multinucleated giant cells *(arrow)* are prominent.

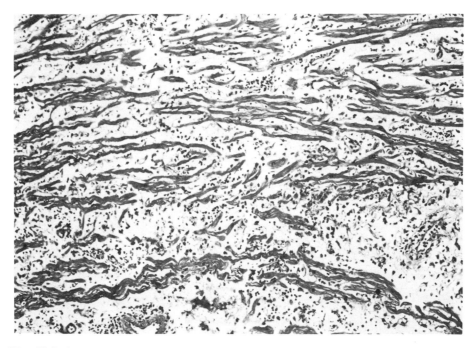

Fig. 15-8. Severe acute cellular rejection. Marked diffuse edema and inflammation separates damaged myocytes.

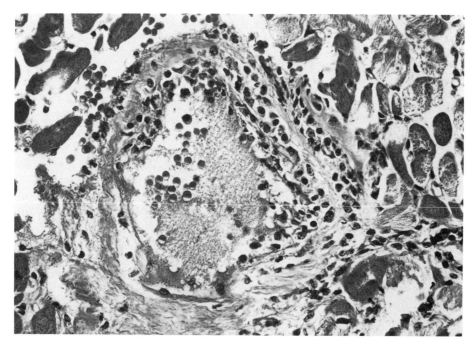

Fig. 15-9. Lymphocytic vasculitis. Lymphocytes infiltrate the endothelium and wall of a small blood vessel in the absence of vascular necrosis.

tion of interleukin-2.[92] The use of cyslosporine has allowed a significant reduction in corticosteroid dosages with a resultant decrease in bacterial and fungal infections. Some centers have even eliminated the use of maintenance corticosteroids[93,94] with very acceptable results. However, most centers use so-called triple therapy, which was first popularized at the University of Minnesota.[95] It consists of cyclosporine, azathioprine, and prednisone. There is controversy concerning the relative risks and benefits of prophylactic cytolytic induction therapy[96] using either a polyclonal antithymocyte/lymphocyte preparation[97] or the murine monoclonal anti-CD3 antibody, OKT3.[98]

At our institution, in 112 heart transplant recipients over 4 years, we have not used induction immunotherapy. Triple-drug immunosuppression is the rule except in infants, in whom maintenance steroids are avoided. Cyclosporine levels, as measured by whole blood monoclonal assays, are maintained between 250 ng/ml to 300 ng/ml for the first 6 months following transplantation, 200 ng/ml to 250 ng/ml from 6 to 12 months, 150 ng/ml to 200 ng/ml for the second posttransplant year, and 100 ng/ml to 150 ng/ml thereafter. Azathioprine is given at 2 mg/kg to 3 mg/kg daily (adjusted to maintain a peripheral white blood cell count above 4000/mm3). After an initial course of high-dose steroids immediately after transplantation (methylprednisolone 125 mg intravenously every 8 hours for six doses in adults), patients are maintained on prednisone at 1 mg/kg/day or less by 3 months after transplantation. Because we believe that steroids greatly increase the incidence of undesirable complications such as infections, hypertension, obesity, hyperlipidemia, and glucose intolerance, we make every effort to lower the maintenance prednisone dose as low as possible. After 6 months, over 90% of our adults are on 5 mg/day or less of prednisone, and 30% of our patients are off steroids completely.

Acute rejection is treated with bolus intravenous methylprednisolone 15 mg/kg for 3 consecutive days, usually on an outpatient basis. For refractory or recurrent rejection or rejection associated with hemodynamic compromise, we add a 10-day course of OKT3. Three of our patients (2.8%) have failed these measures and have been successfully treated with total lymphoid irradiation (800 rad in 10 divided doses)[99] With these immunosuppressive protocols, we have enjoyed a 1-year actuarial survival of 94% in patients ranging from 8 days to 70 years of age at time of transplantation.

Endocardial lymphocytic infiltrates (Quilty effect)

Endomyocardial biopsies occasionally have dense lymphocytic infiltrates forming mounds or plaques in the endocardium. This peculiar phenomenon occurs only in the setting of cyclosporine immunosuppression. Its name derives from the first patient in whom it was observed.[28] Lymphocytes, either predominantly T-lymphocytes with foci of polyclonal B lymphocytes[100] or predominantly B

lymphocytes,[101] form dense infiltrates that expand the endocardium. The infiltrates may be confined to the endocardium, but often extend into the adjacent myocardium and cause marked localized myocyte injury. This aggressive pattern has been termed *Quilty effect with myocyte encroachment*[88] (Fig. 15-10). Nevertheless, in the absence of histologic rejection elsewhere in the biopsy specimen, the Quilty effect, even with myocyte encroachment, does not require treatment. There is no increased incidence or severity of acute rejection associated with the Quilty effect.[100,102] Although the Quilty effect resembles the lymphoproliferation of Epstein-Barr virus (EBV) infection, no EBV has been demonstrated in these lesions.[103] The Quilty effect is presumed to be an incomplete immune response to the cardiac allograft. It may be transient or persist for years in serial biopsies without the development of overt disease.

INFECTIONS

Cardiac allograft recipients are susceptible to a wide variety of bacterial, fungal, protozoal, and viral infections that may involve the allograft itself, giving rise to infectious endocarditis, myocarditis, and pericarditis. Infection remains the leading cause of death in heart transplant recipients in the first year after transplantation,[104] with bacterial infections (particularly pneumonia) the most common. Although an exhaustive discussion on the various types of infections to which a heart transplant recipient is prone is beyond the scope of this chapter, two agents, *Toxoplasma gondii* and cytomegalovirus, are of special interest because they are particularly likely to involve the allograft and may even be first detected on endomyocardial biopsy.[105,106]

Toxoplasmosis

Toxoplasmosis may develop as reactivation of a previous infection in seropositive patients. However, toxoplasma seronegative recipients who receive a graft from a seropositive donor are at much higher risk for developing clinically significant toxoplasmosis. Clinical disease may be limited to the heart, but dissemination and lethal infection is a high risk in these seronegative patients.[107-110] Long-term pyrimethamine prophylaxis is recommended for seronegative recipients of hearts from seropositive donors. We have encountered two heart transplant recipients with toxoplasmosis detected on routine endomyocardial biopsy. Both patients had persistent low-grade fevers and greater than fourfold increase in serologic titers to toxoplasma compared with pretransplant values. Both patients were treated with 6 months of pyrimethamine and sulfadiazine with complete resolution of infection both clinically and on follow-up biopsy.

Toxoplasmosis in the cardiac allograft mimics cellular rejection to a certain extent. Aggregates of inflammatory cells cluster around individual necrotic myocytes. Lym-

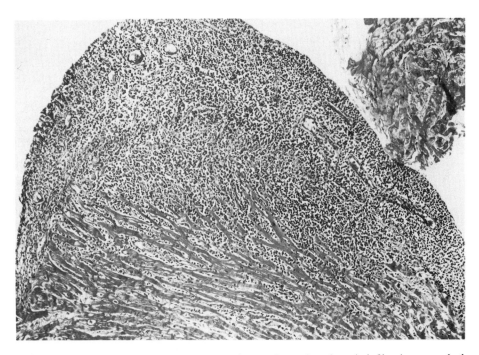

Fig. 15-10. Quilty effect with myocyte encroachment. Dense lymphocytic infiltration expands the endocardium. Lymphocytes also infiltrate the subjacent myocardium.

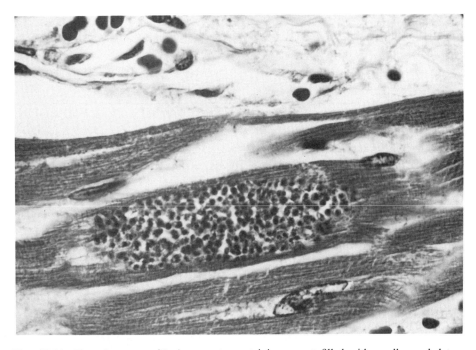

Fig. 15-11. *Toxoplasma gondii.* A myocyte containing a cyst filled with small rounded toxoplasma organisms.

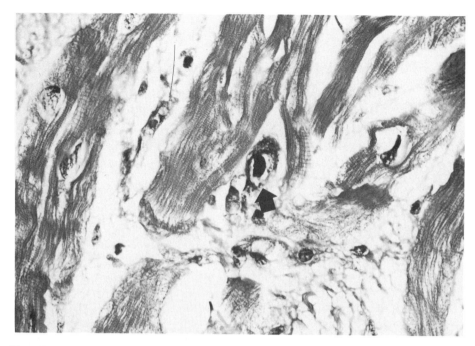

Fig. 15-12. Cytomegalovirus. A cell infected by CMV *(arrow)* has a enlarged nucleus with a characteristic inclusion.

phocytes and macrophages predominate, often with numerous eosinophils. However, eosinophils may be few in some cases of toxoplasmosis and prominent in some cases of cellular rejection. A careful search for the characteristic intramyocytic cysts is required (Fig. 15-11), even in areas lacking inflammation. Cysts that have not ruptured, releasing the trophozoites, usually do not incite an inflammatory reaction.

Cytomegalovirus (CMV)

CMV infection is the most common and important viral infection in heart transplant recipients, with incidences ranging from 73% to 100%.[111,112] Although many of these cases are asymptomatic shedding of virus or increase in serologic titers, 25% to 50% of these patients will develop symptomatic (fevers, malaise, leukopenia) or invasive disease[111,113] which in our experience mandates treatment with ganciclovir. We have seen invasive disease in the lung, urinary tract, colon, duodenum, and bloodstream.

Even in patients with documented invasive or disseminated CMV infections, the virus is detected in only a fraction of endomyocardial biopsy specimens. Involvement of the cardiac allograft is often less severe than that of other organs such as the lungs; and endomyocardial biopsies are insensitive in detecting what is often focal disease. Nevertheless, necrotizing CMV myocarditis is occasionally recognized pathologically.[114,115] Inflammation is usually relatively sparse and focal in these immunosuppressed individuals. A few lymphocytes, histiocytes, and segmented neutrophils cluster around cells showing CMV inclusions or

clumps of necrotic cellular fragments. A variety of cells including endothelial cells, interstitial fibroblasts, and myocytes may be infected. Cells showing diagnostic changes are enlarged and have a large central inclusion surrounded by a pale halo (Fig. 15-12). Less distinct clumped cytoplasmic inclusions may also develop. Immunohistochemistry for CMV early antigens or in situ hybridization for CMV nucleic acids may be required for positive identification in equivocal cases.[116,117]

POSTTRANSPLANT LYMPHOPROLIFERATIVE DISORDERS

Transplant recipients have a markedly increased risk of developing localized or generalized lymphoid proliferations that have morphologically malignant appearances and, if left untreated, have clinically aggressive courses. These lesions fall into a spectrum of polyclonal, oligoclonal, and monoclonal proliferations associated with Epstein-Barr virus (EBV) infection in most instances.[118] Symptomatic EBV infection in transplant recipients may closely resemble mononucleosis with similar constitutional symptoms. On the other hand, EBV infection may induce massive lymphoid proliferations resulting in lymphadenopathy or extranodal tumors of the gastrointestinal tract, brain, or other solid organs. These lesions closely resemble malignant lymphomas arising in nonimmunosuppressed individuals, both clinically and pathologically. The allograft itself may or may not be involved. However, many of these lesions will involute following decreased immunosuppression and are not malignant lymphomas in the conventional sense, giving rise to the less committal term, *posttransplant lymphoproliferative disorders* (PTLD).

The overall incidence of PTLD has been estimated to be about 2%[119] but with longer follow-up and more effective immunosuppressive regimens has been revised upward as high as 4% or 5%[118,120] Increased risk of developing PTLD has been reported with various immunosuppression regimens, including triple drug therapy (cyclosporine, azathioprine, and prednisone)[120] and OKT3 immunotherapy.[121] However, PTLD have developed in patients on FK506 immunosuppression as well.[122] It follows that no single drug, but the overall degree of immunosuppression, determines the risk of PTLD.

In the setting of immunosuppression and lack of normal T-lymphocytic response, B-lymphocytes infected by EBV undergo uncontrolled proliferation. Clinical onset is most commonly in the first year posttransplant, with a peak at 3 to 4 months.[118,119] The B-cell proliferation is presumably polyclonal at the outset, but in some cases a few clones or a single clone proliferate to the exclusion of others. Histologically lesions may be composed of a wide spectrum of sizes and shapes of lymphoid cells (polymorphous) or be monotonous in composition, usually with large cells with plasmacytoid features, including immunoblasts (monomorphous). In either case, the histologic appearance is usually that of a high-grade malignant lymphoma.[123] Polymorphous proliferations may be either nonclonal or monoclonal. Monomorphous lesions are very likely to be monoclonal.

The first line of treatment is reduction or cessation of immunosuppression, often with acyclovir or ganciclovir therapy. Nonclonal PTLD[119] and PTLD arising within the first year[118] are likely to involute; but even some monoclonal PTLD will regress as a result of increased host immune competence. However, monoclonal PTLD and those presenting later than 1 year posttransplant[118] are unlikely to respond and will progress as malignant lymphomas. Radiation and lymphoma chemotherapy are given in such progressive cases, but mortality is high.

We have seen only one presumed PTLD in 112 cardiac transplant recipients. This 63-year-old man presented with abdominal pain 18 months after transplantation. Abdominal CT revealed mesenteric lymphadenopathy presumed to be lymphoproliferative in character. With reduction in immunosuppression, symptoms abated with normalization of the abdominal CT within 3 months.

ALLOGRAFT HEART ACCELERATED ATHEROSCLEROSIS

The problem of accelerated atherosclerosis in the allograft heart continues to adversely effect the long-term survival of transplant patients. It is the third most common cause of death after opportunistic infections and acute allograft rejection. In one center, accelerated atherosclerosis accounted for approximately one fourth of deaths in patients who lived more than 1 year after transplantation.[124] At our institution, accelerated allograft atherosclerosis has been identified in only three patients (severe in one, mild in two) out of a total of 112 transplant recipients, although admittedly the follow-up has been brief (the first heart transplant was conducted in 1988). We attribute our apparently low incidence of accelerated atherosclerosis to our low-dose steroid immunosuppressive protocols, as have others.[94,125]

Clinical presentation

Accelerated coronary atherosclerosis in the early stages is often manifested as a single vessel disease, whereas multivessel disease is more common after the third posttransplantation year. However, intimal proliferative lesions in coronary arteries have been noted as early as 3 months post-cardiac transplantation in patients that died from either infection or acute rejection.

The transplanted patient with allograft coronary atherosclerosis does not present the typical angina pectoris because of the functional denervation of the donor heart. Thus the patient may have silent myocardial infarction detected only by ECG or enzyme studies or succumb to sudden death. Life-threatening ventricular arrhythmias and/or congestive heart failure resulting from ischemia may be the other clinical presentations. A falsely negative thallium exercise test is not unusual in these patients.

Because of distinct morphology and distribution of accelerated atherosclerosis (described below), there is a relative insensitivity of coronary arteriography in detecting the presence of transplant arteriopathy. Qualitative coronary angiography is inadequate,[126] and only systematic use of quantitative angiography provides the means of appreciating subtle changes in luminal diameter over time. Quantitative angiographic studies have indicated that although absolute changes in diameter of small arteries are less than those in larger vessels, there is no significant difference in percent mean reduction between large, medium, and small epicardial vessels.[127]

Morphologic manifestations

Some authors have divided the coronary lesions angiographically into type A lesions, which are discrete, short stenoses in the major coronary arteries or their branches, and type B lesions characterized by diffuse concentric luminal narrowings involving the middle to distal segments of coronary arteries[124] (Figs. 15-13 and 15-14).

There is a morphologic diversity of coronary artery intimal lesions, most of which correlate moderately well with their angiographic appearance. Proximal epicardial vessel lesions may be identical to the naturally occurring atherosclerosis, revealing dense fibrous caps and a central core of lipid containing cells and extracellular lipoproteinaceous debris. In such lesions, similar to the natural occur-

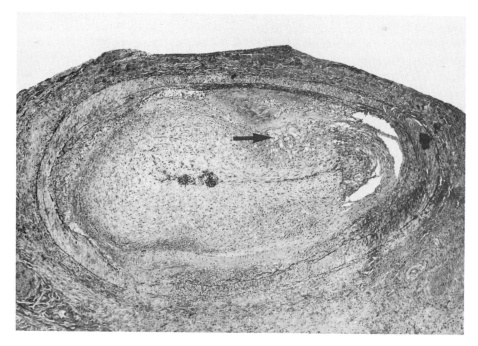

Fig. 15-13. Epicardial coronary artery, allograft heart 14 months posttransplantation, showing severe, occlusive concentric myofibroblastic intimal proliferation. The internal elastica, although reduplicated in areas, is intact. A small focus of foamy cells is present within the intimal lesion *(arrow)*.

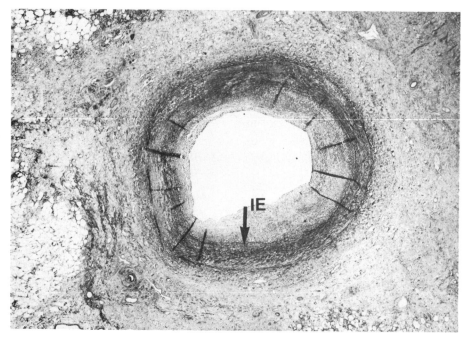

Fig. 15-14. Epicardial coronary artery; allograft heart 6-½ months posttransplantation. Note concentric myofibroblastic intimal proliferation with an intact internal elastica *(arrow 1E)*.

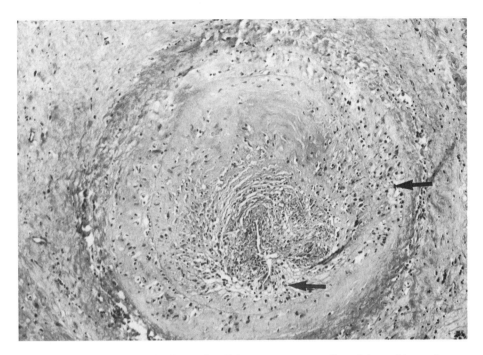

Fig. 15-15. Secondary branch of an epicardial coronary artery, allograft heart 14 months post-transplantation. Note severe concentric intimal myofibroblastic proliferation. Foci of foamy cells are present within the intima and inner media *(arrows)*.

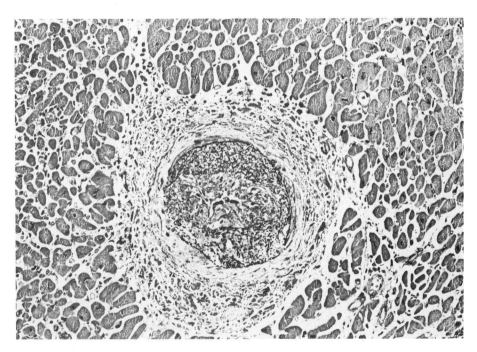

Fig. 15-16. Small intramyocardial coronary artery, allograft heart 5 months posttransplantation, showing complete luminal obliteration by a concentric intimal myofibroblastic reaction.

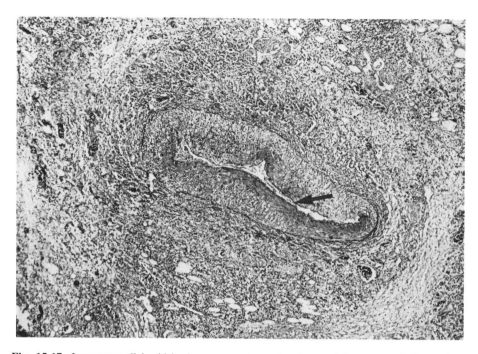

Fig. 15-17. Intramyocardial midsized coronary artery, showing an inflammatory infiltrate (lymphocytes and macrophages) primarily at the outer half of the media and adventitia. Note that there is no intimal proliferation and that the interna elastica is intact *(arrow)*, whereas the external elastica is destroyed in several areas.

ring atheroma, the internal elastic lamina is fragmented and/or completely absent.

Small tributaries of epicardial vessels and penetrating branches reveal concentric lesions (diffuse and tubular) involving the entire length of an artery as well as its branches (Figs. 15-15 and 15-16). These concentric lesions consist of transformed smooth muscle cells, collagen, and varying numbers of macrophages, some of which contain intracytoplasmic lipid. In these lesions the interna elastica is usually intact and the media uninvolved. Furthermore, coronary venous thickening has been noted in the allograft heart, reflecting a more diffuse vasculopathy rather than an exclusively arteriopathic process.[128]

In a significant number of arteries, revealing the above morphologic alterations, lymphocytes may be present primarily in the intima and adventitia, particularly in cases in which a concurrent myocardial rejection is present. It is generally believed that coronary vasculitis is uncommon in patients with accelerated atherosclerosis because the latter usually occurs after the first posttransplantation year. In four of our cases (24 hours to 7 months posttransplantation), vasculitis was observed in primarily medium-sized coronary arteries. The inflammation was segmental, involved primarily the outer two thirds of the media and adventitia, and consisted of round cells. Rarely, the inflammatory infiltrate involved the small intramyocardial arteries and arterioles. The media at the site of inflammatory infiltrate exhibited degenerative changes and contained several foamy macrophages. The external elastica was

fragmented or completely absent, whereas the inner media, interna elastica, intima, and endothelial cells appeared free of morphologic alterations[129] (Fig. 15-17).

Risk factors associated with accelerated atherosclerosis

Several possible causative factors and pathogenetic mechanisms for the development of accelerated atherosclerosis in the allograft heart have been proposed. None of these proposed hypotheses is without controversy.

Traditional risk factors influencing atherogenesis, such as hypercholesterolemia, smoking, hypertension, and diabetes, as well as factors unique to the transplantation milieu, have been considered. The age of the donor heart has been suggested as a possible factor for the atherosclerotic process. Some reports stress that both older donors (more than 40 years) and older recipients (more than 50 years) are significant risk factors.[130]

Somewhat conflicting reports have been published regarding higher rates of accelerated atherosclerosis in patients receiving transplants because of ischemic heart disease. Reports from Europe indicate that patients transplanted for cardiomyopathy had half the incidence of coronary arteriopathy than patients transplanted for ischemic heart disease, although the incidence equalized in 2 years.[131] Others have stressed the possible association of cellular rejection (severity and number of rejection episodes) and obliterative arteriopathy.[132]

Earlier reports from Stanford indicated that elevated plasma triglycerides may be significant predisposing factors for the development of accelerated atherosclerosis.[133] Comparing transplanted patients with and without coronary arteriopathy, no significant differences between the two groups was found, regarding total cholesterol, low density lipoprotein cholesterol, very low density lipoprotein cholesterol, and high density lipoprotein cholesterol.[133]

Others, while recognizing that immune-mediated injury is perhaps the pivotal event, have suggested that a high cholesterol level at 6 months after transplantation is a strong predictor for development of accelerated coronary artery disease.[134] The authors also stressed that early posttransplantation dyslipidemia identifies a subset of patients at high risk for graft failure caused by accelerated atherosclerosis. Some investigators applying multivariate and univariate analysis of several posttransplantation groups have concluded that prednisone administration (not dose-related) and preoperative coronary artery disease are the major contributors to the posttransplant lipid abnormalities.[135]

In a recent study, the luminal coronary narrowing was related to 40 individual risk factors, including demographic, hemodynamic, immune, environmental, and therapeutic factors. Applying multivariate analysis, these investigators concluded the single most predictive risk factor to be posttransplant body mass index.[136] These data strongly indict traditional atherosclerotic risk factors such as obesity and suggest a pervasive role for vascular rejection, which according to the authors begins very early (within 2 weeks) after allograft implantation as a T-cell predominant intimitis.[137] These studies postulate that even minimal myocardial rejection (commonly not treated) may be associated with the insidious development or acceleration of allograft arteriopathy. Independent and additive contributions by serum cholesterol, serum triglycerides, and body mass index with respect to percentage of luminal coronary artery narrowing was observed.[136] Retransplantation for the patient with advanced transplant accelerated atherosclerosis (the only treatment available) is associated with high recurrent rate of coronary arteriopathy in the second graft.[138]

The hypothesis that coronary arteries of heart transplant patients may show endothelial dysfunction before or in the early stages of angiographically evident coronary atherosclerosis has been tested. Acetylcholine was infused into the left anterior descending artery of 13 heart transplant patients at 12 and 24 months after transplantation. In patients with angiographically smooth coronary arteries only few arterial segments showed vasodilator responses, whereas the majority of segments failed to dilate or paradoxically constricted.[139] Similarly, coronary flow reserve and the peak flow response to papaverine are impaired in cardiac transplants with minor proximal coronary occlusive disease.[140] These findings indicate that the endothelium-dependent relaxation is impaired, although endothelial cells may appear morphologically normal.

The role of CMV infections

The idea that cytomegalovirus (CMV) may be etiologically involved in the induction of accelerated atherosclerosis was recently stressed in a retrospective study of 301 heart transplant recipients.[141] One third of the recipients who developed CMV infection following cardiac transplantation had more severe accelerated atherosclerosis than the remaining two-thirds who did not develop CMV infection.

Direct (infection of the graft by CMV) and indirect (activation of the host immune system) mechanisms have been suggested. Heterotopic transplant rat models have shown that CMV infection accelerates the development of vasculitic/proliferative lesions.[142] Endothelial cell infection by herpes simplex has been shown to reduce the anticoagulant properties of these cells, therefore altering the coagulation cascade.[143] Whether CMV infection has similar effect is not clear. It has also been shown that infection by CMV may induce the release of interferon by activated T-lymphocytes and thus upregulate major histocompatability (MHC) antigen expression by endothelial cells. Expression of MHC antigens may by itself be associated with accelerated arteriosclerosis.[144]

Immunologic crossreactivity between human CMV and MHC antigens has been observed as CMV genes may code for proteins that have sequence homology with human proteins (molecular mimicry).[145]

Studies of coronary arteries with accelerated atherosclerosis by in situ DNA hybridization have identified cytomegalovirus nucleic acids in approximately 45% of the vessels examined. Morphologic studies of those arteries failed to reveal intracellular inclusions, indicating a state of latency of the CMV virus.[146] It is of considerable interest that in these studies the strongest hybridization for CMV was found in cells morphologically consistent with smooth muscle cells. Similar localization was observed in our hybridization studies of allograft hearts.[147]

However the presence of CMV nucleic acids in coronary arteries does not prove a causal role of the virus in the development of the coronary arteriopathy of the allograft heart. Critics of the CMV hypothesis point out that if CMV affects endothelial cells, similar changes (intimal proliferation) should be seen throughout the recipient's vascular system rather than solely within the allograft. It is entirely possible, however, that CMV might alter alloantigenicity; therefore only allogeneic endothelial cells (allograft) may become immunologic targets.[148]

Pathogenesis of accelerated atherogenesis

Along with others, we were unable to demonstrate morphologic alterations or damage in the endothelial cells or deposition of platelet thrombi in coronary arteries with accelerated myoproliferative arteriosclerosis. Yet, it seems logical to consider the endothelium the site of initial injury because it is where the donor and the recipient interact directly. Thus our inability to demonstrate structural changes in the endothelium does not exclude the possibility of subtle functional alterations in these pivotal cells.

Recent evidence suggests that accelerated atherosclerosis of the allograft heart may be immunologically mediated. Some investigators consider accelerated atherosclerosis a manifestation of chronic tissue rejection akin to what is seen in the myocardium. Thus coronary artery tissue rejection may provoke in some cases a cellular response that damages the endothelial barrier.

The response to injury hypothesis postulates that death or denudation of endothelial cells is followed by loss of prostacyclin (PGI2) production, increased platelet aggregation, and release of potent smooth muscle mitogens by the platelets.[149] Contrary to naturally occurring atherosclerosis, in which sheer forces are thought to be responsible for the initial endothelial injury, the damage to the endothelium of the allograft is considered immunologic because these cells may express alloantigens and thus become the target of either humoral or cell-mediated immune responses.[148]

Sublethal injury and activation of endothelial cells may result in release of growth factors such as beta fibroblast growth factor (bFGF), transforming growth factor beta (TGF-b) and alpha (TGF-a), and PDGFa and b chains.[148]

Recent evidence indicates that lymphokines and monokines can directly regulate the synthesis of growth factors. Immunohistochemical techniques have shown that although the initial events in accelerated atherosclerosis involve the interaction of macrophages, antibody, and complement, later stages are associated with local production of tumor necrosis factor (TNF) alpha and interleukin-1 (IL-1), which may play an important role in smooth muscle proliferation.[150]

Studies have suggested that accelerated atherosclerosis may be mediated, in part, by a cytotoxic T-lymphocyte-directed endothelialitis; a form of graft rejection.[151] Others, however, have criticized the term endothelialitis because there are no signs of lytic injury in the vascular wall. Such critics stress the consistently high levels of HLA-DR antigen expression of the endothelial cells and the presence of T-lymphocytes and macrophages immediately beneath the class II MHC endothelium.[152] According to this study, the cytokine cascade unleashed by the immunologic activation could stimulate macrophages to produce stimuli for smooth muscle proliferation, such as interleukin-1 (IL-1), tumor necrosis factor (TNF), PDGF, and transforming growth factor a (TGF-a) a chain of events resembling the delayed-type of hypersensitivity.

Although there are strong indications that the initial immunologic injury is directed against the endothelial cells of the allograft heart, other potential target sites, such as the medial smooth muscle cells, may also be involved.[129]

Coronary artery findings in heart and lung transplants

Although the number of episodes of cardiac allograft rejection in combined heart-lung transplants is known to be significantly less than in heart transplants alone, the incidence of accelerated coronary atherosclerosis is similar to cardiac transplants without concomitant lung transplantation. Furthermore, accelerated atherosclerosis is also observed in the pulmonary arteries and veins, although the lesions in those vessels are usually focal or segmental rather than diffuse.[153]

Other types of arteriopathy in the allograft heart

Although accelerated arteriosclerosis is the most critical and most widely recognized complication in the allograft heart, a new subtype of coronary arteriopathy has been reported recently.[154] This new complication, termed *dilated angiopathy,* was observed in about 7% of heart transplants undergoing coronary angiography 1 year or more after transplantation.

The aneurysmal dilatation may involve any of the proximal epicardial coronary arteries and is not accompanied by either diffuse or discrete obliterations of the vascular lumen. Prognosis of this posttransplantation arteriopathy is believed to be better than that of accelerated arteriosclerosis.

Because histologic specimens were not available, it is unclear whether the underlying morphologic alteration in dilated angiopathy is that of active or healed arteritis or some other unspecified medial degenerative process.

FUTURE GOALS

Future developments in the field of cardiac transplantation may include improvements in techniques for cardiac protection, new, less toxic, and more specific immunosuppressive agents, and improved noninvasive techniques for detection of allograft rejection. On the horizon, one solution to the paucity of suitable donors is the development of reliable and effective mechanical devices, such as totally implantable left ventricular assist devices and the totally artificial heart. Another possible solution hinges on improved understanding of the immune system, which may lead to graft tolerance becoming a reality, thus ushering in the promise of xenografting. Finally, accelerated allograft atherosclerosis must be understood and controlled for cardiac transplantation to reach its full potential. Yet, despite the problems of infection, rejection, accelerated atherosclerosis, and escalating costs, cardiac transplantation, in our opinion and that of many others, will remain an excellent therapeutic modality for end-stage heart disease.

REFERENCES

1. Barnard CN: A human cardiac transplant: An interim report of a successful operation performed at Groote Schuur Hospital, Cape Town, *S Afr Med J* 41:1271, 1967.
2. Kriett JM, Kaye MP: The registry of the International Society for Heart and Lung Transplantation: Eighth official report - 1991, *J Heart Lung Transplant* 10:491, 1991.
3. Schroeder JS, Hunt S: Cardiac transplantation: Update 1987, *JAMA* 258:3142, 1987.
4. Kanter KR: Heterotopic heart transplantation, *Emory Univ J Med* 4:77, 1990.

5. Frazier OH, Macris MP, Duncan M, et al: Cardiac transplantation in patients over 60 years of age, *Ann Thorac Surg* 45:129, 1988.

6. Rhenman MJ, Rhenman B, Icenogle T, et al: Diabetes and heart transplantation, *J Heart Transplant* 7:356, 1988.

7. Armitage JM, Kormos RL, Griffith BP, et al: Heart transplantation in patients with malignant disease, *J Heart Transplant* 9:627, 1990.

8. Young JN, Yazbeck J, Esposito G, et al: The influence of acute preoperative pulmonary infarction on the results of heart transplantation, *J Heart Transplant* 5:20, 1986.

9. Shaw BW, Bahnson HT, Hardesty RL, et al: Combined transplantation of the heart and liver, *Ann Surg* 202:667, 1985.

10. Faggian G, Bortolotti V, Stellin G, et al: Combined heart and kidney transplantation: a case report, *J Heart Transplant* 5:480, 1986.

11. Livesey SA, Rolles K, Calne RY: et al: Successful simultaneous heart and kidney transplantation using the same donor, *Clin Transpl* 2:1, 1988.

12. Copeland JG: Cardiac transplantation, *Curr Probl Cardiol* 13:157, 1988.

13. Novitzky D, Cooper DKC, Barnard CN: The surgical technique of heterotopic heart transplantation, *Ann Thorac Surg* 36:476, 1983.

14. Barnard CN, Wolpowitz A: Heterotopic versus orthotopic heart transplantation, *Transplant Proc* 11:309, 1979.

15. Evans RW, Manninen DL, Garrison LP Jr, et al: Donor availability as the primary determinant of the future of heart transplantation, *JAMA* 255:1892, 1986.

16. Robertson JA: Supply and distribution of hearts for transplantation: Legal, ethical and policy issues, *Circulation* 75:77, 1987.

17. Personal communication, United Network for Organ Sharing, Richmond, VA, January 8, 1992.

18. Yacoub M, Festenstein H, Doyle P, et al: The influence of HLA matching in cardiac allograft recipients receiving cyclosporine and azathioprine, *Transplant Proc* 19:2487, 1987.

19. Frist WH, Oyer PE, Baldwin JC, et al: HLA compatibility and cardiac transplant recipient survival, *Ann Thorac Surg* 44:242, 1987.

20. DiSesa VJ, Kuo PC, Horvath KA, et al: HLA histocompatibility affects cardiac transplant rejection and may provide one basis for organ allocation, *Ann Thorac Surg* 49:220, 1990.

21. Terasaki P: Getting the most mileage from donated hearts, *Ann Thorac Surg* 49:177, 1990.

22. Mann FC, Priestley JT, Markowitz J, et al: Transplantation of the intact mammalian heart, *Arch Surg* 26:219, 1933.

23. Stinson EB, Tecklenberg PL, Hollingsworth JF, et al: Changes in left ventricular mechanical and hemodynamic function during acute rejection of the orthotopically transplanted heart in dogs, *J Thorac Cardiovasc Surg* 68:783, 1974.

24. Stinson EB, Caves PK, Griepp RB, et al: Hemodynamic observation in the early period after human heart transplantation, *J Thorac Cardiovasc Surg* 69:264, 1975.

25. Young JB, Leon CA, Short HD, et al: Evolution of hemodynamics after orthotopic heart and heart-lung transplantation: Early restrictive patterns persisting in occult fashion, *J Heart Transplant* 6:34, 1987.

26. Campeau L, Pospisil L, Grondin P, et al: Cardiac catheterization findings at rest and after exercise in patients following cardiac transplantation, *Am J Cardiol* 25:523, 1970.

27. Alyono D, Crumbley AJ, Schneider JR, et al: Early mechanical function in the heterotopic heart transplant, *J Surg Res* 37:55, 1984.

28. Billingham ME: The postsurgical heart: the pathology of cardiac transplantation, *Am J Cardiovasc Pathol* 1:319, 1988.

29. Cooper T, Willman VL, Jellinek M, et al: Heart transplantation: effect on myocardial catecholamine and histamine, *Science* 138:40, 1962.

30. Gaudiani VA, Stinson EB, Alderman E, et al: Long-term survival and function after cardiac transplantation, *Ann Surg* 194:381, 1981.

31. Beck W, Barnard CN, Schrire V: Heart rate after cardiac transplantation, *Circulation* 40:437, 1969.

32. Greenberg M, Uretsky BF, Reddy PS, et al: Long-term hemodynamic follow-up of cardiac transplant patients treated with cyclosporine and prednisone, *Circulation* 71:487, 1985.

33. Uretsky BF, Bernardi L, Greenberg ML, et al: Diastolic dysfunction in long-term survivors of cardiac transplant, *Circulation* 70 (suppl II):II-46, 1984.

34. Tischler MD, Lee RT, Plappert T, et al: Serial assessment of left ventricular function and mass after orthotopic heart transplantation: a four-year longitudinal study, *J Am Coll Cardiol* 19:60, 1992.

35. Brengelmann GL: Circulatory adjustments to exercise and heat stress, *Ann Rev Physiol* 45:191, 1983.

36. Pope SE, Stinson EB, Daughters GT II, et al: Exercise response of the denervated heart in long-term cardiac transplant recipients, *Am J Cardiol* 46:213, 1980.

37. Pflugfelder PW, Purves PD, McKenzie FN, et al: Cardiac dynamics during supine exercise in cyclosporine-treated orthotopic heart transplant recipients: assessment by radionuclide angiography, *J Am Coll Cardiol,* 10:336, 1987.

38. Goodman DJ, Rossen RM, Cannon DS, et al: Effect of digoxin on atrioventricular conduction: studies in patients with and without cardiac autonomic innervation, *Circulation* 51:251, 1975.

39. Leachman RD, Cokkinos DVP, Cabrera R, et al: Response of the transplanted, denervated human heart to cardiovascular drugs, *Am J Cardiol* 27:272, 1971.

40. Hallman GL, Leatherman LL, Leachman RD, et al: Function of the transplanted human heart, *J Thorac Cardiovasc Surg* 58:318, 1969.

41. Mason JW, Winkle RA, Rider AK, et al: The electrophysiologic effects of quinidine in the transplanted human heart, *J Clin Invest* 59:481, 1977.

42. Bexton RS, Hellestrand KJ, Cory-Pearce R, et al: The direct electrophysiologic effects of disopyramide phosphate in the transplanted human heart, *Circulation* 67:38, 1983.

43. Willman VL, Cooper T, Hanlon CR: Return of neural responses after autotransplantation of the heart, *Am J Physiol* 207:187, 1964.

44. Kontos HA, Thames MD, Lower RR: Responses to electrical and reflex autonomic stimulation in dogs with cardiac transplantation before and after reinnervation, *J Thorac Cardiovasc Surg* 59:382, 1970.

45. Mohanty PK, Thames MD, Capeheart JR, et al: Afferent reinnervation of the autotransplanted heart in dogs, *J Am Coll Cardiol* 7:414, 1986.

46. Stinson EB, Griepp RB, Schroeder JS, et al: Hemodynamic observations one and two years after cardiac transplantation in man, *Circulation* 45:1183, 1972.

47. Bexton RS, Hellestrand KJ, Cory-Pearce R, et al: Unusual atrial potentials in a cardiac transplant recipient: possible synchronization between donor and recipient atria, *J Electrocardiol* 16:313, 1983.

48. Mitchell AG, Yacoub M: Efferent autonomic reinnervation after heterotopic cardiac transplantation in humans, *Br Heart J* 57:87, 1987.

49. Wilson RF, Christensen BV, Olivari MT, et al: Evidence for structural sympathetic reinnervation after orthotopic cardiac transplantation in humans, *Circulation* 83:1210, 1991.

50. Stark RP, McGinn AL, Wilson RF: Chest pain in cardiac transplant recipients—evidence of sensory reinnervation after cardiac transplantation, *N Engl J Med* 324:1791, 1991.

51. Gugenheim J, Samuel D, Reynes M, et al: Liver transplantation across ABO blood group barriers, *Lancet* 336:519, 1990.

52. Mason DW, Morris PJ: Effector mechanisms in allograft rejection, *Ann Rev Immunol* 4:119, 1986.

53. Trento A, Hardesty RL, Griffith BP, et al: Role of the antibody to vascular endothelial cells in hyperacute rejection in patients undergoing cardiac transplantation, *J Thorac Cardiovasc Surg* 95:37, 1988.

54. Kissmeyer-Nielsen F, Olsen S, Peterson VP, et al: Hyperacute rejection of kidney allografts associated with pre-existing humoral antibodies to donor cells, *Lancet* 2:662, 1966.

55. Weil R, Clarke DR, Iwaki Y, et al: Hyperacute rejection of a transplanted human heart, *Transplantation* 32:71, 1981.

56. Kemnitz J, Cremer J, Restrepo-Specht I, et al: Hyperacute rejection in heart allografts, *Pathol Res Pract* 187:23, 1991.

57. Rose AG, Cooper DKC, Human PA, et al: Histopathology of hyperacute rejection of the heart: experimental and clinical observations in allografts and xenografts, *J Heart Lung Transplant* 10:223, 1991.

58. Singh G, Thompson M, Griffith B, et al: Histocompatibility in cardiac transplantation with particular reference to immunopathology of positive serologic crossmatch, *Clin Immunol Immunopathol* 28:56, 1983.

59. Minakuchi J, Takahashi K, Toma H, et al: Removal of preformed antibodies by plasmapheresis prior to kidney transplantation, *Transplant Proc* 18:1803, 1986.

60. Zhu LP, Cupps TR, Whalen G, et al: Selective effects of cyclophosphamide therapy on activation, proliferation, and differentiation of human B cells, *J Clin Invest* 79:1082, 1987.

61. Schuurman HJ: Acute humoral rejection after heart transplantation, *Transplantation* 46:603, 1988.

62. Hammond EH, Yowell RL, Nunoda S, et al: Vascular (humoral) rejection in heart transplantation: pathologic observations and clinical implications, *J Heart Transplant* 8:430, 1989.

63. Cherry R, Nielsen H, Reed E, et al: Vascular (humoral) rejection in human cardiac allograft biopsies: relation to circulating anti-HLA antibodies, *J Heart Lung Transplant* 11:24, 1992.

64. Hammond EH, Wittwer CT, Greenwood J, et al: Relationship of OKT3 sensitization and vascular rejection in cardiac transplant patients receiving OKT3 rejection prophylaxis, *Transplantation* 50:776, 1990.

65. Larsen CP, Barker H, Morris PJ, et al: Failure of mature dendritic cells of the host to migrate from the blood into cardiac or skin allografts, *Transplantation* 50:294, 1990.

66. Ahmed-Ansari A, Tadros TS, Knopf WD, et al: MHC-class I and class II expression by myocytes in cardiac biopsies post transplantation, *Transplantation* 45:972, 1988.

67. Krensky AM, Weiss A, Crabtree G, et al: T-lymphocyte-antigen interactions in transplant rejection, *N Engl J Med* 332:510, 1990.

68. Hayry P: Intragraft events in allograft destruction, *Transplantation* 38:1, 1984.

69. Weintraub D, Masek M, Billingham M: The lymphocytic subpopulations in cyclosporine-treated human heart rejection, *J Heart Transplant* 4:213, 1985.

70. Higuchi ML, de Assis RVC, Sambiase NV, et al: Usefulness of T-cell phenotype characterization in endomyocardial biopsy fragments from human cardiac allografts, *J Heart Lung Transplant* 10:235, 1991.

71. Stinson EB, Dong E, Bieber CP, et al: Cardiac transplantation in man, I: early rejection, *JAMA* 207:2233, 1979.

72. Nora JJ, Cooley DA, Fernbach DJ, et al: Rejection of the transplanted human heart: indexes of recognition and problems in prevention, *N Engl J Med* 280:1080, 1969.

73. Caves PK, Stinson EB, Billingham ME, et al: Diagnosis of human cardiac allograft rejection by serial cardiac biopsy, *J Thorac Cardiovasc Surg* 66:461, 1973.

74. Caves PK, Stinson EB, Billingham ME, et al: Serial transvenous biopsy of the transplanted human heart: improved management of acute rejection episodes, *Lancet* 2:821, 1974.

75. Warnecke H, Schuelar S, Goetz HJ, et al:Noninvasive monitoring of cardiac allograft rejection by intramyocardial electrogram recordings, *Circulation* 74 (suppl III):III-72, 1986.

76. Keren A, Gillis AM, Freedman RA, et al:Heart transplant rejection monitored by signal-averaged electrocardiography in patients receiving cyclosporine, *Circulation* 70 (suppl I):I-24, 1984.

77. Dawkins KD, Oldershaw PJ, Billingham ME, et al: Noninvasive assessment of cardiac allograft rejection, *Transplant Proc* 17:215, 1985.

78. Valantine HA, Fowler MB, Hunt SA, et al: Changes in Doppler echocardiographic indexes of left ventricular function as potential markers of acute cardiac rejection, *Circulation* 76 (suppl V):V-86, 1987.

79. Aherne T, Tscholakoff D, Finkbeiner W, et al: Magnetic resonance imaging of cardiac transplants: the evaluation of rejection of cardiac allografts with and without immunosuppression, *Circulation* 74:145, 1986.

80. Ertel W, Reichenspurner H, Hammar C, et al: Cytoimmunologic monitoring: a method to reduce biopsy frequency after cardiac transplantation, *Transplant Proc* 17:204, 1985.

81. Bailey LL, Wood M, Razzouk A, et al: Heart transplantation during the first 12 years of life, *Arch Surg* 124:1221, 1989.

82. Billingham ME: Some recent advances in cardiac pathology, *Human Pathol* 10:367, 1979.

83. Billingham ME: Diagnosis of cardiac rejection by endomyocardial biopsy, *J Heart Transplant* 1:25, 1981.

84. Kemnitz J, Cohnert T, Schafers HJ, et al: A classification of cardiac allograft rejection: a modification of the classification by Billingham, *Am J Surg Pathol* 11:503, 1987.

85. McAllister HA Jr: Histologic grading of cardiac allograft rejection: a quantitative approach, *J Heart Transplant* 9:277, 1990.

86. Zerbe TR, Arena V: Diagnostic reliability of endomyocardial biopsy for assessment of cardiac allograft rejection, *Human Pathol* 19:1307, 1988.

87. Knopf WD, Murphy DA, Sell KW, et al: Cardiac transplantation, *Emory Univ J Med* 1:11, 1987.

88. Billingham ME, Cary NRB, Hammond ME, et al: A working formulation for the standardization of nomenclature in the diagnosis of heart and lung rejection: heart rejection study group, *J Heart Transplant* 9:587, 1990.

89. Herskowitz A, Soule LM, Mellits ED, et al: Histologic predictors of acute cardiac rejection in human endomyocardial biopsies: a multivariate analysis, *J Am Coll Cardiol* 9:802, 1987.

90. Herskowitz A, Soule LM, Ueda K, et al: Arteriolar vasculitis on endomyocardial biopsy: a histologic predictor of poor outcome in cyclosporine treated heart transplant recipients, *J Heart Transplant* 6:127, 1987.

91. Normann SJ, Salomon DR, Leelachaikul P, et al: Acute vascular rejection of the coronary arteries in human heart transplantation: pathology and correlations with immunosuppression and cytomegalovirus infection, *J Heart Lung Transplant* 10:674, 1991.

92. Kahan BD: Immunosuppressive therapy with cyclosporine for cardiac transplantation, *Circulation* 75:40, 1987.

93. Yacoub M, Alivizatos P, Khagani A, et al: The use of cyclosporine, azathioprine, and antithymocyte globulin with or without low-dose steroids for immunosuppression of cardiac transplant patients, *Transplant Proc* 17:221, 1985.

94. Ratkovec RM, Wray RB, Renlund DG, et al: Influence of corticosteroid-free maintenance immunosuppression on allograft coronary artery disease after cardiac transplantation, *J Thorac Cardiovasc Surg* 100:6, 1990.

95. Bolman RM III, Elick B, Olivari MT, et al: Improved immunosuppression for heart transplantation, *Heart Transplant* 4:315, 1985.

96. Menkis AH, McKenzie FN, Thompson D, et al: Benefits of avoidance of induction immunosuppression in heart transplantation, *J Heart Transplant* 8:311, 1989.

97. Szentpetery S, Mohanakumar T, Barnhart G, et al: Beneficial effects of prophylactic use of rabbit antihuman thymocyte globulin in heart transplant recipients immunosuppressed with cyclosporine, *J Heart Transplant* 5:365, 1986.

98. Bristow MR, Gilbert EM, O'Connell JB, et al: OKT3 monoclonal antibody in heart transplantation, *Am J Kidney Dis* 11:135, 1988.

99. Frist WH, Winterland AW, Gerhardt EB, et al: Total lymphoid irradiation in heart transplantation: adjunctive treatment for recurrent rejection, *Ann Thorac Surg* 48:863, 1989.

100. Kottke-Marchant K, Ratliff NB: Endomyocardial lymphocytic infiltrates in cardiac transplant recipients, *Arch Pathol Lab Med* 113:690, 1989.

101. Radio SJ, McManus BM, Winters GL, et al: Preferential endocardial residence of B-cells in the "Quilty effect" of human heart allografts: immunohistochemical distinction from rejection, *Modern Pathol* 4:654, 1991.

102. Forbes RDC, Rowan RA, Billingham ME: Endocardial infiltrates in human heart transplants: a serial biopsy analysis comparing four immunosuppression protocols, *Human Pathol* 21:850, 1990.

103. Nakhleh RE, Copenhaver CM, Werdin K, et al: Lack of evidence for involvement of Epstein-Barr virus in the development of the "Quilty" lesion of transplanted hearts: an in situ hybridization study, *J Heart Lung Transplant* 10:504, 1991.

104. Hofflin JM, Potasman I, Baldwin JC, et al: Infectious complications in heart transplant recipients receiving cyclosporine and corticosteroids, *Ann Intern Med* 106:209, 1987.

105. Ryning FW, McLeod R, Maddox JC, et al: Probable transmission of *Toxoplasmosis gondii* by organ transplantation, *Ann Intern Med* 90:47, 1979.

106. Wreghitt TG, Hakim M, Cory-Pearce R, et al: The impact of donor transmitted CMV and *Toxoplasma gondii* disease in cardiac transplantation, *Transplant Proc* 18:1375, 1988.

107. McGregor CGA, Fleck DG, Nagington J, et al: Disseminated toxoplasmosis in cardiac transplantation, *J Clin Pathol* 37:74, 1984.

108. Hakim M, Esmore D, Wallwork J, et al: Toxoplasmosis in cardiac transplantation, *Br Med J* 292:1106, 1986.

109. Wreghitt TG, Hakim M, Gray JJ, et al: Toxoplasmosis in heart and heart and lung transplant recipients, *J Clin Pathol* 42:194, 1989.

110. Holliman RE, Johnson JD, Adams S, et al: Toxoplasmosis and heart transplantation, *J Heart Lung Transplant* 10:608, 1991.

111. Dummer JS, Gardy A, Poorsattar A, et al: Early infections in kidney, heart, and liver transplant recipients on cyclosporine, *Transplantation* 36:259, 1983.

112. Rubin RH, Russell PS, Levin M, et al: Summary of a workshop on cytomegalovirus infections during organ transplantation, *J Infect Dis* 139:728, 1979.

113. Pollard RB, Arvin AM, Gamberg P, et al: Specific cell-mediated immunity and infections with herpes viruses in cardiac transplant recipients, *Am J Med* 73:679, 1982.

114. Partanen J, Nieminen MS, Krogerus L, et al: Cytomegalovirus myocarditis in transplanted heart verified by endomyocardial biopsy, *Clin Cardiol* 14:847, 1991.

115. Millet R, Tomita T, Marshall HE, et al: Cytomegalovirus endomyocarditis in a transplanted heart: a case report with in situ hybridization, *Arch Pathol Lab Med* 115:511, 1991.

116. Unger ER, Budgeon LR, Myerson D, et al: Viral diagnosis by in situ hybridization, *Am J Surg Pathol* 10:1, 1986.

117. Weiss LM, Movahed LA, Berry GJ, et al: In situ hybridization studies for viral nuclei acids in heart and lung allograft biopsies, *Am J Clin Pathol* 93:675, 1990.

118. Armitage JM, Kormos RL, Stuart S, et al: Posttransplant lymphoproliferative disease in thoracic organ transplant patients: ten years of cyclosporine-based immunosuppression, *J Heart Lung Transplant* 10:877, 1991.

119. Nalesnik MA, Jaffe R, Starzl TE, et al: The pathology of posttransplant lymphoproliferative disorders occurring in the setting of cyclosporine A-prednisone immunosuppression, *Am J Pathol* 133:173, 1988.

120. Wilkinson AH, Smith JL, Hunsicker LG, et al: Increased frequency of posttransplant lymphomas in patients treated with cyclosporine, azathioprine, and prednisone, *Transplantation* 47:293, 1989.

121. Swinnen LJ, Costanzo-Nordin MR, Fisher SG, et al: Increased incidence of lymphoproliferative disorder after immunosuppression with the monoclonal antibody OKT3 in cardiac transplant recipients, *N Engl J Med* 323:1723, 1990.

122. Frayha HH, Nazer H, Kalloghlian A, et al: Lymphoproliferative disorder in a liver transplant patient on FK506, *Lancet* 337:296, 1991.

123. Weintraub J, Warnke RA: Lymphoma in cardiac allotransplant recipients, *Transplantation* 33:347, 1982.

124. Johnson DE, Alderman EL, Schroeder JS, et al: Transplant coronary artery disease: histopathologic correlations with angiographic morphology, *J Am Coll Cardiol* 17:449, 1991.

125. Renlund DG, Brutow MR, Crandall BG, et al: Hypercholesterolemia after cardiac transplantation: amelioration by corticosteroid-free maintenance immunosuppression, *J Heart Transplant* 8:214, 1989.

126. Everett JP, Hershberger RE, Ratkovec RM, et al: The specificity of normal qualitative coronary angiography (QCA) in excluding cardiac allograft vasculopathy (CAV), *J Heart Lung Transplant* 11:193, 1992 (abstract).

127. Gao SZ, Alderman EL, Schroeder JS, et al: Progressive luminal narrowing after cardiac transplantation, *Circulation* 82 (suppl IV):IV-269, 1990.

128. Oni AA, Ray JA, Norman DJ, et al: Cardiac allograft venopathy: a correlate to "accelerated transplant atherosclerosis," *J Heart Lung Transplant* 10:190, 1991 (abstract).

129. Gravanis MB: Allograft heart accelerated atherosclerosis: evidence of cell-mediated immunity in pathogenesis, *Modern Pathol* 1:495, 1989.

130. Sharples LD, Caine N, Mullins P, et al: Risk factor analysis for the major hazards following heart transplantation-rejection, infection, and coronary occlusive disease, *Transplantation* 52:244, 1991.

131. Simon R: Reported at the Tenth European Congress of Cardiology, Vienna, Austria, August 28 - September 1, 1988.

132. Zerbe TR, Kormos RL, Uretsky B, et al: Cardiac obliterative arteriopathy: impact of cellular rejection and donor factors, *J Heart Lung Transplant* 11:193, 1992 (abstract).

133. Gao SZ, Schroeder JS, Alderman EL, et al: Clinical laboratory correlates of accelerated coronary artery disease in the cardiac transplant patient, *Circulation* 76 (suppl V), V-56; 1987.

134. Eich D, Thompson JA, Ko D, et al: Hypercholesterolemia in long-term survivors of heart transplantation: an early marker of accelerated coronary artery disease, *J Heart Lung Transplant* 10:45, 1991.

135. Taylor DO, Thompson JA, Hastillo A, et al: Hyperlipidemia after clinical heart transplantation, *J Heart Transplant* 8:209, 1989.

136. Winters GL, Kendall TJ, Radio SJ, et al: Post-transplant obesity and hyperlipidemia: major predictors of severity of coronary arteriopathy in failed human heart allografts, *J Heart Transplant* 9:364, 1990.

137. McManus BM, Winters GL, Radio SJ, et al: Ubiquity and centrifugal intensification of T-cell mediated coronary arteritis in failed human heart allografts, *Lab Invest* 58:62, 1988 (abstract).

138. Gao SZ, Shroeder JS, Hunt S, et al: Retransplantation for severe accelerated coronary artery disease in heart transplant recipients, *Am J Cardiol* 62:876, 1988.

139. Fish RD, Nabel EG, Selwyn AP, et al: Response of coronary arteries of cardiac transplant patients to acetylcholine, *J Clin Invest* 81:21, 1988.

140. Mullins PA, Chauhan A, Graham TR, et al: Microvascular function is impaired in patients with coronary occlusive disease after cardiac transplantation, *J Heart Lung Transplant* 11:227, 1992 (abstract).

141. Grattan MT, Moreno-Cabral CE, Starnes VA, et al: Cytomegalovirus infection is associated with cardiac allograft rejection and atherosclerosis, *JAMA* 261:3561, 1989.

142. Hatanaka M, Esa AH, Tamura F, et al: Cytomegalovirus and accelerated coronary graft disease, *J Heart Lung Transplant* 10:170, 1991 (abstract).

143. Etingin OR, Silverstein RL, Friedman HM, et al: Viral activation of the coagulation cascade: molecular interactions at the surface of infected endothelial cells, *Cell* 61:657, 1990.

144. von Willebrand E, Patterson E, Ahomen J, et al: CMV infection,

class II antigen expression, and human kidney allograft rejection, *Transplantation* 42:364, 1986.

145. Fujinami RS, Nelson JA, Walker L, et al: Sequence homology and immunologic cross-reactivity of human cytomegalovirus with HLA-DR b-chain: a means for graft rejection and immunosuppression, *J Virol* 62:100, 1988.

146. Hruban RH, Wu TC, Beschorner WE, et al: Cytomegalovirus nucleic acids in allografted hearts, *Hum Pathol* 21:981, 1990.

147. Gravanis MB, Ansari AA, Neckleman N, et al: Evidence of cell-mediated immunity in the pathogenesis of allograft heart arteriosclerosis, *J Am Coll Cardiol* 15:(2), 1990 (abstract).

148. Hosenpud JD, Shipley GD, Wanger CR: Cardiac allograft vasculopathy: current concepts, recent developments, and future directions, *J Heart Lung Transplant* 11:9, 1992.

149. Ross R: The pathogenesis of atherosclerosis-an update, *N Engl J Med* 314:488, 1986.

150. Herskowitz A, Handa N, Lafond-Walker A, et al: The role of cytokines in the immunopathogenesis of coronary graft disease, *J Heart Lung Transplant* 11:193, 1992 (abstract).

151. Hruban RH, Beschorner WE, Baumgartner WA, et al: Accelerated arteriosclerosis in heart transplant recipients is associated with a T-lymphocyte-mediated endothelialitis, *Am J Pathol* 137:87, 1990.

152. Salomon RN, Hughes CCW, Schoen FJ, et al: Human coronary transplantation-associated arteriosclerosis: evidence for a chronic immune reaction to activated graft endothelial cells, *Am J Pathol* 138:791, 1991.

153. Yousem SA, Paradis IL, Dauber JH, et al: Pulmonary arteriosclerosis in longterm human heart-lung transplant recipients, *Transplantation* 47:564, 1989.

154. von Scheidt W, Erdmann E: Dilated angiopathy: a specific subtype of allograft coronary artery disease, *J Heart Lung Transplant* 10:698, 1991.

Chapter 16

HEART FAILURE

Neal A. Scott
Michael B. Gravanis

The concept of heart failure, in addition to its symptoms, signs, and treatments have origins that preceded modern medicine by centuries. A few of the major developments are listed below:[1,2]

460 B.C.—Hippocrates described the importance and prognostic significance of dyspnea and dropsy.

1628—Harvey published *De Cortu Mordis* on the circulatory system.

1707—Lancisi published a work on sudden death, emphasizing the importance of cardiac dilatation and calcified coronary arteries.

1785—Withering described the use of digitalis for the treatment of dropsy.

1832—Ilope, in a treatise on the heart and great vessels, described left ventricular failure with pulmonary vascular congestion and cardiac asthma.

1861—Chauveau and Marey measured intracardiac and pulmonary artery pressures.

1866—Karell introduced a restricted diet for heart failure.

1882—Fick published studies on the determination of cardiac output.

1898—Tigerstedt and Bergman discovered renin.

1905—Carrel and Guthrie performed the first heterotopic heart transplant in a dog.

1914—Starling published observations on the relationship between length of muscle and force of contraction.

1920—Saxl introduced mercurial diuretic injections.

Heart failure is not a specific disease but rather a pathophysiologic state in which the heart is unable to pump enough blood to adequately supply the metabolic demands of the tissues. Failure of the heart as a pump is most commonly associated with primary myocardial dysfunction, a condition that refers to a problem intrinsic to the myocardial or valvular structures and frequently results in an impairment of ventricular contraction.[3] It should be noted that other causes of heart failure, although infrequent, exist; some of these causes are associated with normal ventricular function. Examples are: heart failure resulting from inadequate blood volume (hemorrhage), heart failure caused by inadequate venous return to the heart (tricuspid stenosis or constrictive pericarditis), increased capacity of the vascular bed (profound vasodilation), inadequate oxygen delivery (anemia), and peripheral vascular abnormalities (arteriovenous shunts). Because the vast majority of patients with heart failure have an intrinsic myocardial abnormality, this chapter will focus on heart failure resulting from myocardial causes.

HEMODYNAMICS OF HEART FAILURE

Conceptually, heart failure has usually been approached as failure of the heart as a pump. The hemodynamic abnormalities that result from this condition have been explained as *backward heart failure* caused by inadequate emptying of the venous reservoirs, and *forward heart failure*, which results when the amount of blood ejected from the heart into the aorta is insufficient to meet the metabolic needs. Because the circulatory circuit is closed, forward and backward heart failure frequently coexist. The compensatory adjustments that occur in response to the impaired pump performance are responsible for the clinical findings seen in each condition. Patients who experience left ventricular dysfunction have elevated left ventricular end-diastolic pressures. The elevated end-diastolic pressure is transmitted to the atrium and pulmonary vessels (backward failure). As a result there is increased blood in the pulmonary bed. A transudation of fluid occurs and causes dyspnea, pulmonary congestion, and, if severe, pulmonary edema. When right ventricular function is also compromised, right atrial and systemic venous pressures rise with a resultant transudation of fluid in the liver, abdominal cavity, and lower limbs producing hepatic enlargement, ascites, and pedal edema, respectively. If cardiac output is reduced to a point where adequate tissue

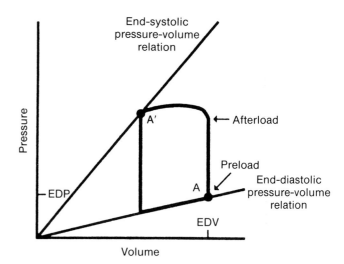

Fig. 16-1. A schematic pressure-volume loop showing its constraint between the end-diastolic pressure-volume relation (lower line) and the end-systolic pressure-volume relation (upper line). Systole begins at the end-diastolic point (A) with isovolumic contraction, followed by ejection. Diastole begins at the end-systolic point (A'). After isovolumic relaxation the ventricle fills and diastolic pressures and volumes increase. The ventricle encounters preload when the mitral valve opens. Afterload is encountered when the aortic valve opens. (Reproduced with permission from Katz, AM: JACC 11:438-445, 1988).

perfusion does not occur, a profound vasoconstriction is induced because the body tends to protect blood pressure at the expense of cardiac output.

In rare situations, the heart is required to pump an abnormally large quantity of blood to meet the metabolic demands of the tissues. These conditions are usually associated with decreased afterload or an elevated metabolic rate (e.g., arteriovenous fistula, hyperthyroidism, anemia, beriberi, on Paget disease). The subsequent development of heart failure ("high output failure") is usually related to the specific underlying disease process and its effect on the myocardium.

Pressure-volume loop

The discovery that the end-diastolic pressure and volume are critical in determining the work of the heart has proved to be one of the historic cornerstones of cardiovascular physiology.[4] A single graphical depiction has been developed to display changes in preload, afterload, and contractility during both systole and diastole. The pressure-volume loop describes the working conditions of the heart by simultaneously plotting pressures and volumes.[5] The pressure-volume loop (Fig. 16-1) begins at the end-diastolic point of the pressure-volume curve (point A) and is inscribed in a counterclockwise direction. Systole begins with isovolumic contraction, during which pressure increases at constant volume; hence, the pressure-volume loop begins with an upward deflection. During ejection,

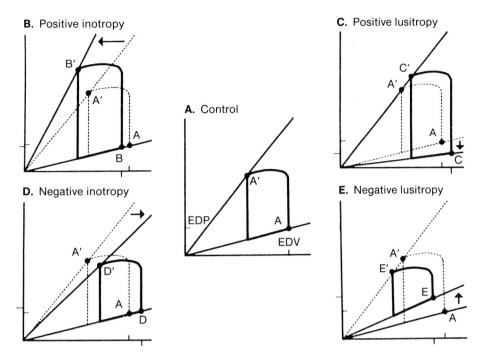

Fig. 16-2. Schematic pressure-volume loops showing responses to interventions that alter inotropy and lusitropy. All examples assume a constant stroke volume. Panel A is a control pressure-volume loop as depicted in Fig. 16-1. Panel B displays the effect of a positive inotropic intervention. The end-systolic pressure-volume relation is shifted upward and to the left. In Panel C, a positive lusitropic intervention shifts the end-diastolic pressure-volume relation downward and to the right. Panel D shows the effect of a negative inotropic intervention. The end-systolic pressure relation is shifted downward and to the right. Note that there is an increase in end-diastolic pressure if stroke volume remains constant. In Panel E, a negative lusitropic intervention is displayed. There is a shift in the end-diastolic pressure-volume relation upward and to the left, causing an increase in end-diastolic pressure. (Reproduced with permission from Katz, AM: JACC 11:438-445, 1988).

after aortic valve opening, the pressure-volume loop turns to the left. Systole ends at a point (point A′) that lies on the end-systolic pressure-volume relation, a key determinant in ventricular function. As diastole begins and the aortic valve closes, the pressure-volume loop first falls during isovolumic relaxation. After the mitral valve opens and the filling phase begins, the pressure-volume loop rises gradually to end at a point along the end-diastolic pressure-volume relation. As in the end-systolic pressure-volume relation, this gradual rise is an important determinant of ventricular performance.[5]

The end-diastolic pressure and volume that begin the pressure-volume loop (Point A) are determined by an interaction between the diastolic properties of the ventricle and the venous return. The former, which can be expressed as the end-diastolic pressure-volume relation of the ventricle, are a manifestation of the intrinsic relaxation (lusitropic) properties of the ventricle.[4]

When relaxation is enhanced (positive lusitropy), filling is increased and diastolic pressures are reduced. The end-diastolic pressure-volume relation shifts downward and to the right. A negative lusitropic intervention would stiffen the ventricle, thereby reducing its size while increasing the filling pressure. The pressure-volume relation would shift upward and to the left (Fig. 16-2).[5]

Ventricular performance is also influenced by the interplay between the contractile (inotropic) state of the ventricle. A positive inotropic intervention shifts the end-systolic pressure-volume relation upward and to the left, whereas negative inotropic interactions shift this relation downward and to the right.[5]

Heart failure commonly reduces the ability of the heart to do work in a manner that impairs relaxation as well as contraction. Therefore there is a rise in the end-diastolic pressure-volume relation accompanied by a fall in the end-systolic pressure-volume relation (Fig. 16-3).

Factors that modify left ventricular distensibility

The pericardium restrains cardiac filling, limits distension of the heart, and influences the left ventricular pressure-volume relation.[6] Changes in the compliance of the pericardium or any alteration of the pericardial-LV pressure gradient will influence left ventricular diastolic chamber compliance. In chronic constrictive pericarditis, the thickened pericardium limits left and right ventricular filling. In acute pericardial tamponade, the increase in intrapericardial pressure can also impair ventricular filling.[7,8]

Extrinsic compression of the ventricles by elevated pleural pressure or by tumor impairs ventricular filling in a manner similar to constrictive pericarditis. A factor intrinsic to the left ventricular chamber that contributes to diastolic dysfunction is thickness of the left ventricular wall. An increase in left ventricular wall thickness without a corresponding change of left ventricular volume is commonly seen in concentric left ventricular hypertrophy. Patients with pathologic left ventricular hypertrophy (as opposed to athletes) have abnormal diastolic pressure-volume curves. An increase in diastolic stiffness (negative lusitropy) shifts the end-diastolic pressure relation to the left and upward. If, for example, contractility and stroke volume are unchanged, filling pressure increases at a reduced end-diastolic volume (point E) (Fig. 16-3). The resulting shift in the pressure-volume loop to the left decreases heart size but, although filling pressure is higher, the work of the smaller ventricle (the area within the pressure-volume loop) is decreased. Because a constant stroke volume is ejected by the smaller ventricle, the end-systolic point moves down the control end-systolic pressure-volume relation to a smaller volume. As the same stroke volume is ejected by a smaller ventricle, the impaired ability of the heart to relax increases ejection fraction.[5]

Patients with abnormalities in the intrinsic composition of the ventricle (e.g., amyloidosis,[9] hemochromatosis, and edema) also display evidence of diastolic dysfunction. Similarly, the deposition of fibrous tissue is a common sequela of ischemia in patients with coronary artery disease. Additionally, animal studies have shown that during cardiac pressure-overload hypertrophy, the amount of collagen relative to muscle increases, accompanied by changes in collagen structure.[10] The increase in the ratio of collagen to muscle has also been shown to be proportional to the severity of the hypertrophy.[11] Correlative studies of hemodynamic data in patients with coronary artery disease and cardiac hypertrophy caused by aortic stenosis and aortic regurgitation have shown that myocardial fibrosis contributes to the elevation of left ventricular diastolic pressure and closely correlates with indices of myocardial stiffness after the relative amount of fibrous tissue exceeds 20%.

Most patients with heart failure have hemodynamic findings that are consistent with an impairment of both systolic and diastolic function. A pressure-volume loop depicting this situation is presented in Fig. 16-3. The resultant amount of cardiac work (area within the loop) is markedly diminished when compared with normal values. This model assumes that no compensatory mechanisms are operative. If, for example, vasoconstriction occurs in re-

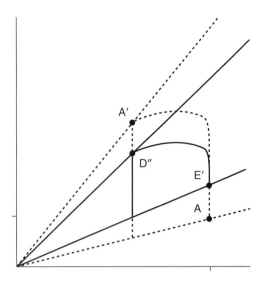

Fig. 16-3. The effect of negative inotropy and lusitropy on the pressure-volume loop. Assuming that stroke volume remains constant, there is a shift of the loop to a higher end-diastolic pressure-volume relation (point E′) in addition to a downward shift in the end-systolic pressure-volume relation that reduces the end-systolic point to D″. (Reproduced with permission from Katz, AM: JACC 11:438-445, 1988).

sponse to decreased pressure, the increase in afterload would move the end-systolic point up and to the right along the depressed end-systolic pressure-volume relation to point D″. This response would decrease stroke volume as well as ejection pressure. On the other hand, the administration of a catecholamine with inotropic and vasodilating properties (e.g., dobutamine) would produce a shift in the end-systolic pressure-volume relation upward and to the left (positive inotropy), in addition to an alteration of the end-diastolic pressure-volume relation so that the pressure-volume loop begins at a lower end-diastolic pressure and a higher end-diastolic volume. As a result, the cardiac work will be greatly increased.[5]

CALCIUM ION AND ITS ROLE IN HEART FAILURE
Cellular regulation of calcium ion concentration

Electromechanical coupling in muscle cells may be broadly defined as the series of reactions initiated by membrane depolarization and culminating in the production of force and movement.[12] The contractile system is sensitive to the concentrations of calcium, magnesium, adenosine triphosphate (ATP), and cyclic nucleotides. There is overwhelming evidence that, physiologically, calcium is the substance that is most important in the acute changes in the state of the myocardial cell, and most other contractile systems. Of the various physiologic ions that have been injected in small amounts into the cell, calcium alone has caused a reversible contraction in the immediate vicinity of the injection.[12] After calcium is removed from the medium

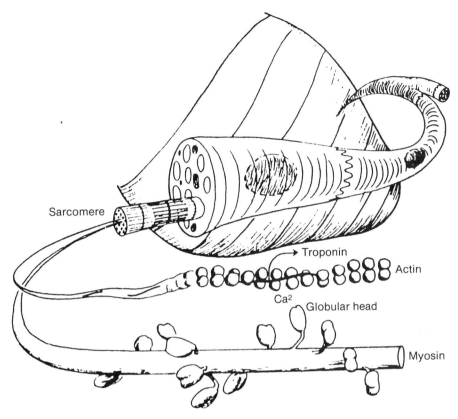

Fig. 16-4. A schematic drawing of a cardiac sarcomere depicting the interaction of the globular head of myosin (thick filament) with actin (thin filament) to form cross-bridging and cause sarcomere shortening (systole or contraction). Contraction occurs when a calcium ion binds to troponin and "depresses" the interaction of actin and myosin. (Reproduced from Coralli RJ, Gravanis MB, *Cardiovascular pathophysiology,* 1987, McGraw-Hill.

bathing an isolated heart, contractions rapidly disappear in spite of maintained electrical activity.[13,14] These experiments proved that extracellular calcium is critical for the steps coupling contraction with membrane depolarization.

The concentration of intracellular calcium ion is regulated by three cellular organelles: the sarcoplasmic reticulum, the mitochondria, and the surface membrane. These structures can transport the ion between the sarcoplasm and another tissue phase, such as the interior of the organelle or the extracellular space.

Calcium ion and muscle contraction

The interaction between actin and myosin is the basis for the generation of force in muscle. Actin and myosin exist in a highly ordered form in the intact muscle cell. Individually, actin molecules are relatively spherical but in the muscle cell they polymerize into double-stranded filaments. The myosin molecules, which consist of an ellipsoid head and a rod-like body, are organized in a highly complex manner to produce a thicker filament. The tail-to-tail arrangement of the rodlike portions of the molecules in the body of the thick filament results in a degree of sym-

metry about the center of the filament, and the heads project from the body of the thick filament at regular intervals in both longitudinal and azimuthal directions. It is generally believed that the myosin heads interact with actin in the thin filament, and during a contraction this interaction occurs cyclically at each head to generate force and produce relative movement of the two sets of filaments. The movement at each zone of overlap of the two sets of filaments is summated along the entire length of the cell to produce a pull and a shortening at its ends (Fig. 16-4). The energy for the work done by the contracting cell is derived from molecules of ATP that are split by an ATPase site on the myosin heads during each cyclic interaction with actin.[15]

The affinity of myosin for actin is so high that in the absence of other proteins and ATP, the two sets of molecules remain bound to each other to produce what has been called *the rigor state.*[16] ATP is responsible for the dissociation of the two molecules, but subsequent cleavage of the terminal phosphate bond on the ATP molecule allows for the recombination of actin and myosin to complete the reaction cycle. Isolated actin and myosin can continuously split ATP and behave as an activated contractile system in an intact muscle cell. Relaxation, or inhibition of the interaction between actin and myosin, is mediated through the action of tropomyosin and troponin, two proteins that exist in the thin filament. These proteins prevent the interaction of actin with myosin in the presence of ATP and the absence of calcium ion.[17] Tropomyosin has a rod-like three-dimensional structure and lies in a groove formed by the two twisted chains of actin monomers. Troponin is bound to tropomyosin in close proximity to actin along the thin filament. The normal state of actin plus myosin is contraction, but the entire protein system in the two sets of contractile proteins is normally relaxed in the presence of the usual cellular concentrations of ATP and calcium. It should be stressed that because calcium ions are actively transported up a concentration gradient during relaxation, whereas they move down a gradient during contraction, the state of myocardial relaxation requires more energy than contraction.

The addition of a small concentration of calcium ions activates the contractile system.[18] At a concentration of Ca^{2+} ions below 10^{-7} M no force is generated by the contractile proteins as long as the concentration of ATP is in the millimolar range; at a concentration of 10^{-5} M, force generation is maximal. Between these two values force is a sigmoidal function of the calcium concentration, with most of the increase in force occurring within a tenfold rise in calcium concentration.[15]

Calcium ions initiate contraction by binding to one of the subunits of troponin and removing the inhibitory effect of the regulatory proteins on the interaction between actin and myosin.[17] Troponin consists of three subunits; one binds calcium ion (troponin C), one is responsible for the inhibition of contraction (troponin I), and a third binds tropomyosin (troponin T).[19] Normal regulation requires the integrated effect of all three subunits on actin, but it is the state of the calcium ion binding sites on troponin C that controls the entire troponin system. Skeletal muscle troponin C has four calcium ion binding sites, two high-affinity sites, and two low-affinity sites. Cardiac troponin has only three calcium ion binding sites,[20] of which two have high affinities and one has a low affinity for calcium ions. Occupation of the low-affinity site is required for activation.[15,21]

Troponin is attached to the thin filaments at two sites; troponin T is attached to tropomyosin, and troponin I is attached to actin. The interaction of troponin C with the other two subunits of troponin depends on the presence or absence of calcium ion. The addition of calcium ion to troponin C promotes the interaction of troponin C with troponin I and dissociates the complex from actin without causing a separation of troponin T from tropomyosin. The resultant movement of tropomyosin relative to the actin chains releases the previously existing inhibition of the actin-myosin interaction.[22] It is not clear whether the movement of tropomyosin removes a steric hindrance or is correlated with a conformational change in actin.[15]

Although the resting contractile system can be converted to an active one by the addition of calcium to troponin, the relationship between the amount of calcium ion bound by contractile proteins is not simple.[23] A sharp rise in the slope of the relation between force generated and free calcium ion concentration suggests that the contractile system is not simply activated by the addition of a calcium ion to a binding site on troponin. Either cooperation or multisite saturation is probably involved in activation.[15]

In general, positive inotropic agents increase the availability of intracellular calcium during systole, whereas negative inotropic agents decrease calcium ion availability.[4] Positive inotropic agents can be divided into two major classes depending on whether their action is mediated by increases in intracellular concentrations of cyclic AMP, which in turn exerts a variety of subcellular actions that increase intracellular calcium ion concentrations and result in positive inotropic and enhanced relaxant effects. Most of the clinically important inotropic agents belong to this category, including the beta adrenergic agonists and phosphodiesterase inhibitors. Drugs in the second class bypass cyclic AMP as an intracellular messenger and activate alternate mechanisms to increase the amount of intracellular calcium available for activation. This class of agents includes digoxin as its most clinically useful member.

Calcium in myopathic muscle

Contraction is initiated when calcium ion enters the cytosol of the heart through channels in the sarcolemmal and sarcoplasmic reticular membranes. These channels are commonly referred to as *slow* or L-type calcium channels. The ability to record the changes in intracellular calcium ion concentrations in actively contracting muscle with the use of calcium indicators has greatly increased the understanding of the influence of calcium in normal and pathological conditions. The signal recorded from the control muscle in Fig. 16-5 consisted of a single component that rose to a peak and declined towards baseline before peak tension was reached. The calcium "transient" peaks and then declines toward the base line before the corresponding mechanical events occur. This relation is consistent with the model of excitation-contraction coupling discussed above and emphasizes the central part played by extracellular calcium ion in modulating systolic and diastolic function.

In contrast, the light signals recorded from myopathic muscle were not only prolonged compared with the controls but consisted of two temporally distinct components (L1 and L2). L2 was diminutive or absent in control preparations but was prominent in all of the myopathic muscles examined. These data suggest that the prolonged contraction of myopathic muscle in vitro as well as the myocardial relaxation abnormalities observed in patients with dilated cardiomyopathy appear to correlate with the intracellular handling of calcium ion.[24]

In myopathic muscles, increasing the concentrations of

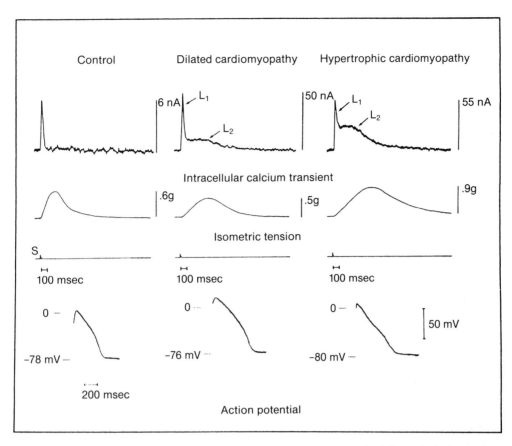

Fig. 16-5. Recordings of the intracellular calcium transient (Aequorin light tracing), isometric tension and stimulus artifact (S) from control group and myopathic human trabeculae maintained in vitro and action potentials in different muscles from the same hearts.
Reproduced from Gwathmey JK et al: *Circ Res* 61:70, 1987 (25), with permission.

extracellular calcium ion produced a progressive increase in the amplitude of L2 relative to L1. This change of calcium transient was associated with a prolongation of isometric contraction. In contrast, the duration of contraction in control muscle was not affected significantly by the concentration of calcium ion in the perfusate. In the myopathic muscles, higher concentrations of extracellular calcium ion were associated with increased end-diastolic levels of intracellular calcium ion and tension, an effect that was not observed in the control muscle.[24] Taken together, these data indicate that muscles from myopathic hearts have a decreased capacity to maintain calcium homeostasis in the presence of normal or increased transsarcolemmal calcium gradients.[25] Additional studies with pharmacologic agents indicated that L2 in myopathic muscle reflects dysfunction of both the sarcolemma and the sarcoplasmic reticulum; the former may cause increased calcium ion entry through voltage-dependent calcium channels, and the latter can cause delayed restoration of low resting tone during diastole because of a decreased rate of calcium ion resequestration by the sarcoplasmic reticulum.[26] The inability of myopathic muscle to maintain calcium homeostasis may be a primary cause of contractile dysfunction in heart failure.[24]

Calcium ion and congestive heart failure

Acute and chronic forms of heart failure involve mechanical dysfunction during systole, diastole, or both phases of the cardiac cycle. Subacute and chronic forms of failure have been associated with a variety of structural and biochemical abnormalities.[24] At the level of the sarcolemma, changes have been reported in the numbers or coupling of adrenergic receptors and voltage-dependent calcium channels. The density of calcium uptake sites on the sarcoplasmic reticulum reportedly is decreased, and the mechanisms that regulate calcium release appear to be impaired. In addition, the structure of the contractile apparatus may change in failing animal and human hearts. The ability of the mitochondria to supply the ATP necessary to fuel the process of excitation-contraction coupling may also be impaired in the failing heart.[27]

A recent study examined the sarcoplasmic reticulum Ca^{2+}-ATPase gene expression in the human ventricle during end-stage heart failure. Ventricular Ca^{2+}-ATPase mRNA levels in patients with heart failure were found to be less than half of the levels seen in myocardial tissue from patients with normal cardiac function.[28] There was no difference in Ca^{2+}-ATPase mRNA content between idiopathic dilated cardiomyopathy and infarct-related cardiac failure, suggesting that the decrease is not related to a specific etiology of heart failure. In rats, the decrease in sarcoplasmic reticulum Ca^{2+}-ATPase mRNA content parallels a decrease in Ca^{2+}-ATPase protein, which suggests a decrease in sarcoplasmic reticulum Ca^{2+}-ATPase pump density.[29]

Both systolic and diastolic dysfunction in the Syrian hamster model of cardiomyopathy, in aged, spontaneously hypertensive rats with clinical heart failure, and in dogs with pacing-induced heart failure are related at least in part to abnormalities in intracellular calcium ion handling. In the whole heart, the increase in end-diastolic pressure that occurs with acute hypoxia is associated with a corresponding increase in end-diastolic levels of intracellular calcium ion, and these increases may be induced by drugs and rapid pacing.[30] In studies of isolated papillary muscle, acute systolic failure induced by drugs with negative inotropic properties (including beta adrenergic blockers and calcium channel antagonists) and hypoxia is associated with corresponding declines in the peak concentration of intracellular calcium ion.[31] Although treatment with calcium channel antagonists has been suggested to be useful in clinical heart failure,[32] the mechanism of the improvement is unclear. When the number of calcium antagonist binding sites are examined, there is no difference between patients with end-stage idiopathic cardiomyopathy and patients with normal hearts.[33]

DIASTOLIC DYSFUNCTION

Classic concepts of heart failure have, in the past, been limited to abnormalities in systolic function. However, studies in patients with left ventricular hypertrophy[34] and coronary artery disease[35] have demonstrated that clinical congestive heart failure may occur in the absence of overtly abnormal systolic performance. In a subgroup of the VA Cooperative study, 83 of the 623 patients with clinically evident heart failure had an ejection fraction greater than 45%. It was postulated that diastolic rather than systolic dysfunction was the most likely etiology for the heart failure seen in this subset of patients. This group had a lower incidence of coronary artery disease, a higher incidence of hypertension, and a better survival than the patients with an ejection fraction less than 45%.[36] However, a recent study has suggested that preserved systolic function in patients with heart failure does not necessarily correlate with a favorable prognosis.[36a] Diastolic dysfunction, defined as increased resistance to filling of one or both ventricles,[37] is frequently seen in structural disorders that increase resistance to ventricular inflow (e.g., constrictive pericarditis and mitral stenosis). Conditions that decrease myocardial relaxation (and subsequent filling) (fibrosis, amyloidosis, hypertrophy) are also associated with diastolic dysfunction. In addition, right-sided heart failure

may itself cause diastolic dysfunction. The elevated right atrial pressure can be transmitted to the coronary sinus, which causes engorgement of the coronary veins, increased myocardial blood volume, and reduced distensibility during diastole.[38]

Calcium and diastolic dysfunction

Recent studies have supported the hypothesis that diastole is an energy-requiring state and that energy is utilized very differently during systole and diastole.[39] Systole is an active, energy-requiring process. However, the activation of muscular contraction occurs via a passive mechanism. Because of the steep concentration gradient favoring the flow of calcium ion into the cell, activation is effected by the very rapid passive diffusion of calcium ion into the cytosol. The inflowing calcium current triggers the release of calcium ion from intracellular stores and, in the presence of ATP, initiates contraction. Thus whereas energy is utilized by the contractile apparatus during contraction, systole is initiated by downhill calcium ion fluxes that do not require the expenditure of energy. During diastole the activator calcium ion must be transported out of the cytosol into the sarcoplasmic reticulum and extracellular space. This transport occurs against a strong concentration gradient and requires energy. The major mechanism involved in the transport of the activator calcium ion out of the cell is a powerful calcium pump, the sarcoplasmic reticular calcium-transporting ATPase, which pumps calcium ions back into the subsarcolemmal cisternae of the sarcoplasmic reticulum. In the normal heart, energy production is not a limiting factor, and the rate of relaxation can increase markedly when needed, as in tachycardia or sympathetic stimulation. However, slowing of relaxation has been observed in conditions where energy resources are limited, such as myocardial ischemia, myocardial hypertrophy, and congestive heart failure.[37]

Hemodynamics of diastole

Diastole can be divided into four phases: isovolumic relaxation, early rapid filling, diastasis, and atrial systole.[40] After left ventricular ejection, the aortic valve closes. During the period between aortic valve closure and mitral valve opening, the left ventricle is a closed chamber. Myocardial relaxation causes a steep, exponential fall in intraventricular pressure. When left ventricular pressure falls below left atrial pressure, the mitral valve opens. Left ventricular pressures continue to fall because of myocardial relaxation and elastic recoil. Because of the large pressure gradient between the left atrium and ventricle, there is a rapid inflow of blood into the ventricle. Approximately 60% to 80% of the stroke volume enters the ventricle during this phase. Much of the inflow occurs early in this period while the left ventricular pressure continues to decrease. The rapid filling phase ends when the left atrial and left ventricular pressures equilibrate. In the absence of tachycardia, rapid filling ends after approximately one third of diastole. During the midportion of diastole, left ventricular filling is slow and consists of a small amount of blood flow into the ventricle (diastasis). Atrial systole increases atrial pressure. The increased atrial pressure augments the left atrial/left ventricular pressure gradient, which causes a further increase in left ventricular volume.

The rapid filling phase of diastole is most sensitive to alterations in diastolic function. The continued fall of the left ventricular pressure after mitral valve opening is, as described above, referred to as "diastolic suction" and is caused by rapid myocardial relaxation. The rapid relaxation is influenced by the lowering of intracellular calcium ion concentration. In the intact heart, if the rapid phase of relaxation slows, the time course of isovolumic pressure decay and the decline of left ventricular pressure just after mitral valve opening also slows. This shifts the early portion of the diastolic pressure-volume relation upward. The mid- and late-diastolic pressure-volume relation is not modified except at fast heart rates with the abbreviation of diastole.

Proposed mechanisms of diastolic dysfunction

The exact mechanism involved in the production of diastolic dysfunction is unknown but is probably multifactorial and related to both hypertrophy and ischemia. Some degree of hypertrophy is present in all chronically failing hearts. Because of an increase in the intercapillary distance seen in hypertrophied myocardial cells,[41] this hypertrophy may lead to a relative imbalance between oxygen supply and demand. This imbalance may be further aggravated in the subendocardium by an increased filling pressure. Thus even in the absence of coronary artery disease, ischemia may alter energy production in the failing heart. Clinical studies have demonstrated that myocardial ischemia causes a slowing of isovolumic relaxation rate, and an upward shift in the left ventricular pressure-volume relation. The severity of the acute change in left ventricular diastolic distensibility appears to relate to the extent of ischemic territory.[42] Although regional dyssynchrony of ischemic and nonischemic regions influences the rise in left ventricular end-diastolic pressure in patients during ischemia, it is not the predominant mechanism responsible for the loss of diastolic distensibility of the ischemic regions. Because upward shifts in the left ventricular diastolic pressure-volume relation can also be seen in a model of global ischemia in isolated, isovolumic rabbit hearts, regional dyssynchrony and pericardial-right ventricular restraint can be excluded as predominant mechanisms.[43] The observation that the upward shift in the pressure-volume relation is present in late as well as in early diastole in response to ischemia is consistent with a mechanism of both a slowed rate of the initial rapid phase of myocardial relaxation and an incom-

plete extent of relaxation.[42] Myocardial ATP depletion has been associated with the changes in relaxation and diastolic distensibility associated with ischemia. It has been suggested that the ATP produced by anaerobic glycolysis in the cytosol is preferentially utilized by the ATP-dependent membrane pumps and is critically important in protecting against depression of myocardial relaxation during ischemia.[44]

Another mechanism likely to occur in end-stage heart failure is mitochondrial dysfunction. The ratio of mitochondria to myofibrils has been shown to decrease with congestive heart failure.[45] In addition, the respiratory function of myocardial mitochondria from patients with heart failure is abnormal.[45] Ultrastructural studies performed in such patients have documented mitochondrial morphologic abnormalities.[46] Dysfunctional mitochondria may contribute to the reduced rate of ATP production in heart failure and therefore reduce the rate that calcium ion is pumped from the cells.

Intracellular concentrations of ionized calcium are often elevated during diastole in myocardial preparations from patients with end-stage heart failure.[25] Depressed function of the sarcoplasmic reticular ion calcium ion pump has been reported in failing myocardium patients.[47] A decrease in gene expression of messenger RNA for the sarcoplasmic reticular calcium ion pump, as well as for its regulatory protein (phospholamban), has been described in ventricular myocardium from failing human hearts.[28,48]

Another important regulator of intracellular calcium ion concentration is cyclic AMP. An increase in cyclic AMP levels mediates the phosphorylation of phospholamban, and increases the activity of the sarcoplasmic reticular calcium ion pump. Downregulation of beta-adrenergic receptors and the resultant decrease in myocardial cyclic AMP has been demonstrated in patients with heart failure.[49]

COMPENSATORY MECHANISMS IN CONGESTIVE HEART FAILURE

In the presence of a defect in myocardial contraction or an excessive hemodynamic burden placed on the ventricle, or both, the heart is dependent on three primary compensatory mechanisms to maintain its necessary function as a pump: (1) the Frank-Starling mechanism, in which an increased preload (i.e., the lengthening of sarcomeres to optimize overlap between thick and thin myofilaments), acts to sustain myocardial pump function; (2) myocardial hypertrophy with or without cardiac chamber dilatation, this alteration causes an increase in the mass of contractile tissue; and (3) increased catecholamine release by noradrenergic cardiac nerves and the adrenal medulla, which increases myocardial contractility and lusitropy. These compensatory mechanisms usually restore a relatively normal level of pumping performance to the heart, although intrinsic myocardial contractility may be substantially reduced.

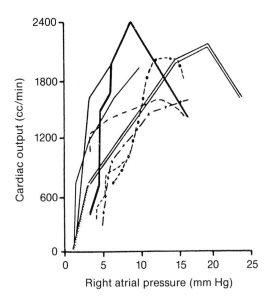

Fig. 16-6. Cardiac function curves obtained in eight heart-lung preparations by Patterson and Starling[52] depicting cardiac output as a function of mean right atrial pressure. Redrawn from Guyton AC: *Circulatory Physiology* et al.[66] C. Guyton, CE Jones, TG Coleman (eds), WB Saunders, Philadelphia, 1973.

Each of these compensatory mechanisms has a limited potential, however, and ultimately fails. The clinical syndrome of heart failure occurs as a consequence of the limitations or the ultimate failure of these compensatory mechanisms or both.[3,50]

Frank-Starling mechanism

In 1915 Starling defined the law of the heart as: "The mechanical energy set free on passage from the resting to the contracted state depends . . . on the length of the muscle fiber, i.e., of the area of chemically active surfaces. This simple formula serves to explain the whole behavior of the isolated mammalian heart."[51,52] Although Starling limited the application of the law of the heart to the isolated organ, this limitation was widely disregarded soon afterward.[53] This capacity of the intact ventricle to vary its force of contraction as a function of its initial end-diastolic size is one of the major principles of cardiac function and is generally referred to as the Frank-Starling phenomenon. The heart is assumed to perform as a static pressure pump: the diastolic filling of the ventricles is a mere passive function depending on venous pressure (vis a tergo), which stretches myocardial ventricular fibers.[54] This concept assumes that the myocardial fiber length determines the stroke volume and that the energy expended during ventricular contraction plays no role in diastolic ventricular filling. Atrial pressure is commonly used as an index of ventricular diastolic stretch (Fig. 16-6). The Frank-Starling law rapidly gained wide acceptance. However, practical and theoretical limitations were later dis-

covered. Robinson et al[55] noted that the Frank-Starling model required diastolic ventricular filling to be determined by a positive diastolic pressure generated by the venous return. In contrast, prior experiments, some performed as early as 1836,[56,57] demonstrated that hearts submerged in saline solution keep ejecting fluid despite the fact that the filling pressure was identical to the external pressure,[58] indicating that active sucking occurs during diastole. Another criticism of the Frank-Starling model was that cardiac output was determined by right ventricular filling pressure, and ultimately, right atrial filling pressure, because right atrial pressure influences the diastolic volume of the right ventricle. Evidence exists to suggest that the wide fluctuations of right atrial pressure during respiration do not cause comparable alterations in stroke volume.[59]

Despite these limitations, the Frank-Starling model has been accepted as a fundamental basis of cardiac function for more than half a century. Several authors have postulated that a major cause for the importance of the law is the experimental model from which the law was derived.[54,55] The original formulation of the law was based on data obtained in the isolated heart. Cardiac function is often depressed in this model, as is suggested by the high filling pressures reported by Starling in his studies. This model therefore is a better model for the failing heart because a normal heart is unlikely to develop pressures of similar magnitude even under severe physiologic stress. At the time when the Frank-Starling model was most widely accepted, invasive cardiac studies were only beginning to be used for the study of clinical heart disease. Most of these patients had impaired cardiac function, usually as a result of valvular heart disease. One can argue that the correlations made between the findings in the isolated heart and clinical studies in patients with impaired myocardial function are appropriate. However, whether the Frank-Starling model is an accurate assessment of normal cardiac function has been the subject of many debates.

The concept of ventricular diastolic suction attracting blood from the atrium into the ventricle during diastole was first advanced by Katz[60] in 1930. This theory (vis a fronte) states that there is a certain ventricular volume, defined as the equilibrium volume. When a freshly excised heart is immersed in a physiologic solution and spontaneous contractions cease, the equilibrium volume is reached when the filling pressure is exactly zero. If there is a further increase in intraventricular volume there will be a positive transmural pressure. Conversely, a reduction in intraventricular volume produces a negative transmural pressure.[61] This observation suggested that in vivo, the ventricles at end-systole would generate a depression of transmural pressure large enough to cause suction. Negative intraventricular diastolic pressures have been documented in experimental animals[62] and in humans[63] with the use of high quality pressure transducers.

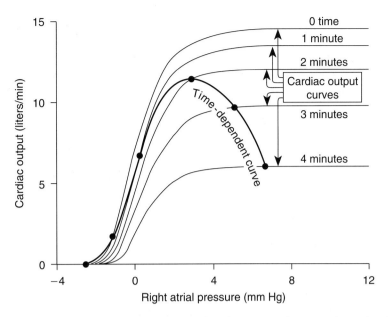

Fig. 16-7. A time-dependent curve recorded during the course of an experiment in which the heart was becoming progressively weaker. The light curves represent the true cardiac output curves, which are changing with time. The dark curve drawn through the points represents the resulting time-dependent curve. (Reproduced with permission from Guyton[66] et al.)

The possible origin of the frontal force creating diastolic suction has been ascribed to two different mechanisms. There is evidence to support the concept that diastole requires much more energy than systole because it requires the active transport of calcium ions up a steep concentration gradient, whereas contraction is mediated by passive movement of calcium ions through membrane channels from the extracellular space and sarcoplasmic reticulum to the cytosol. Although active mechanisms may play a role in the genesis of ventricular diastolic suction by promoting and increasing the rate of muscle relaxation, most data favor the hypothesis that vis a fronte is produced by a passive process, the diastolic elastic recoil of the ventricle. During systole, noncontractile elements (e.g., connective tissue surrounding individual muscle cells) are compressed and elastically deformed beyond their equilibrium state, thus storing potential elastic energy that is released through elastic recoil during diastole. On this basis, the ventricle can be likened to a coil-spring. When the spring is not compressed, it remains at its resting length (resting length in a spring could be analogous to equilibrium volume in a ventricle). When the spring is compressed (systolic contraction) beyond its resting length, its natural tendency is to reexpand. In the ventricle, as in the spring, the level of reexpansion will be proportional to the elastic energy stored during contraction. The more the coil-spring is compressed, the more it will reexpand. If the ventricle loses its elastic properties (e.g., as in the segmental wall motion abnormalities seen with myocardial ischemia and infarction) and/or is excessively stretched because of cardiac dilation (as in congestive heart failure), it

may become unable to determine cardiac elastic reexpansion at end-systole.

Descending limb of Starling's curve

There has been considerable debate concerning the question of whether a descending limb of cardiac function exists in the intact left ventricle.[64] Because a descending limb was not demonstrated in experiments until a left ventricular end-diastolic pressure of 40 mm Hg to 60 mm Hg was reached,[65] it has been postulated that the descending limb of ventricular performance, when observed in the ejecting heart, is not caused by operation of the heart on a descending limb of a sarcomere length-active tension curve; i.e., it is not caused by disengagement of actin and myosin filaments. The descending limb of the Starling curve may be an artifact related to the impaired myocardial function associated with the isolated heart preparation used by the Starling group. Guyton[66] has suggested that the descending limb of the cardiac function curve results from a time-dependent phenomenon that is composed of several plateau curves caused by a progressive decline in the heart's pumping ability (Fig. 16-7).

Left ventricular remodeling

The degree of cardiac enlargement has been shown to be an important predictor of mortality in patients with coronary artery disease.[67,68] In patients with dilated cardiomyopathy, hypertension, and valvular heart disease, increased left ventricular (LV) volume is also an important prognostic factor.[69-71] Indeed, in patients with coronary artery disease, LV volume even more than the extent of coronary artery disease, represents the most potent predictor of subsequent mortality.[67]

When the volume of blood delivered to the systemic vascular bed is chronically reduced, and when one or both of the ventricles fails to expel the normal fraction of its end-diastolic volume, a complex sequence of adjustments occurs that ultimately results in the abnormal accumulation of fluid. Although many of the clinical manifestations of heart failure are secondary to this excessive retention of fluid, hypervolemia also constitutes an important compensatory mechanism that tends to maintain cardiac output by elevating ventricular preload because the myocardium operates on an ascending, albeit depressed, function curve.[3] The augmented ventricular end-diastolic volume must be regarded as aiding the maintenance of cardiac output, except in the terminal stages of heart failure. After heart failure has developed, ventricular remodeling may be accelerated by changes in ventricular load and volume. Renal sodium retention augments diastolic ventricular volume and wall tension. Systemic vasoconstriction may increase the impedance to left ventricular ejection, thereby increasing afterload and wall tension during ejection. The increased wall tension causes progressive hypertrophy and dilatation, with the ventricular shape resembling that of a sphere.

The clinical condition that is best suited for the examination of the temporal relationship between systolic dysfunction and left ventricular dilatation is myocardial infarction. The exact onset of the infarction is usually clinically evident, and the changes can easily be followed with two-dimensional echocardiography. When a subset of patients was examined with echocardiography 2 weeks after infarction, thinning and lengthening of the infarcted segment occured, without evidence of further necrosis.[72] This process is known as infarct expansion. All of the patients with infarct expansion had a transmural anterior wall AMI and on follow-up had a higher incidence of adverse cardiovascular events than patients without infarct expansion. Expansion of the infarct segment with resulting LV dilatation may be detectable within hours of acute myocardial infarction[73] and has been shown to be the major early contributor to LV dilatation within the first 72 hours after infarction of the anterior wall.

Progressive left ventricular remodeling may also occur in the chronic phase after myocardial infarction in the absence of any additional ischemic events or valvular insufficiency. The mechanism of this late left ventricular dilatation has been suggested to be caused by an increase in the length of the contractile segment without any change in noncontractile segment length.[74,75] These results suggest that lengthening or hypertrophy of the contractile segment without additional infarct expansion is the structural change that results in late LV remodeling. In addition, as the left ventricle dilates, it may become more spherical, further adding to the overall LV volume. Results of these

studies and others demonstrate that LV enlargement may be progressive in the first year after myocardial infarction and that both the infarcted and noninfarcted segments participate in the process. Furthermore, as the ventricle dilates, there is further loss of its normal ellipsoidal shape and a subsequent worsening of contractile function[76] and diastolic relaxation.[37]

Hypertrophy

Heart failure, regardless of its precipitating cause, is characterized by an overloading of the active myocardial cells. Compensation at the myocardial level includes cellular hypertrophy, which decreases the rate of mechanical energy expenditure, and dilatation that results in a change of the shape of the heart. However, in time, changes in left ventricular geometry may heighten wall stress and increase myocardial oxygen demand.[50]

Pressure overload stimulates sarcomeres to replicate in parallel fashion, increasing myocardial wall thickness and returning wall stress toward normal according to the Laplace relation. Volume overload stimulates replication of sarcomeres in series, resulting in ventricular dilatation and increased peak systolic wall stress, which in turn stimulate wall hypertrophy in an attempt to normalize this increased systolic wall stress (Fig. 16-8). Although compensatory hypertrophy secondary to chronic pressure or volume overload may be adequate to return systolic wall stress to normal, diastolic wall stress remains elevated in patients with volume overload. Furthermore, uncompensated failure may be associated with elevated systolic wall tension despite compensatory hypertrophy.[77]

Although hypertrophy increases the number of sarcomeres and thus may be beneficial at the early stages of overload states, this compensation usually provides benefit for a limited time. For example, ventricular dilatation initially compensates for the failing heart in states of volume overload by distributing an increased workload over more contractile elements. In a dilated heart much less shortening of myocardial fibers is required to generate a given stroke volume than is needed for a ventricle of smaller dimensions. However, the price paid for this mechanical advantage is an increased myocardial oxygen cost caused by persistently elevated diastolic wall stress that must be sustained by the dilated ventricle. Thus the compensatory mechanism of dilatation eventually fails.[78]

It is widely accepted that cardiac hypertrophy and dilatation are multifactorial and that the sequence of remodeling events may vary depending on the etiology of the heart disease. For example, concentric hypertrophy induced by systemic hypertension precedes dilatation, which is usually a late manifestation. In contrast, in myocarditis or dilated cardiomyopathy, dilatation may precede the hypertrophy. However, after heart failure develops the ventricular remodeling may be accelerated by changes in load and volume.[50] Remodeling of the left ventricle after anterior myo-

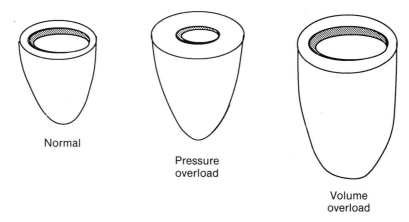

Fig. 16-8. Left ventricular cross-sections depicting anatomic differences in pressure and volume overload.

cardial infarction is considered the most potent predictor of subsequent mortality, although the mechanism whereby postinfarction left ventricular enlargement is linked to congestive heart failure is not entirely clear.[67]

Although it has not been proven, sarcomere slippage in the hypertrophic region of the heart may contribute to the dilation process. Such a concept, however, stresses the importance of the noninfarcted segment of the left ventricle in the pathogenesis of altered ventricular geometry. It also emphasizes that although dyskinetic segments may increase in length, it is the elongation of the contractile region that contributes the most to global left ventricular dilatation. Myocardial hypertrophy is known to increase the distance between capillaries and decrease capillary density, therefore impairing oxygen diffusion. This imbalance is particularly evident in the underperfused subendocardial region of the left ventricle and may be aggravated by a decrease in coronary vasodilator reserve.[79] In addition, reactive hypertrophy is associated with a quantitative increase in collagen fibers. It is not known whether this increase in collagen has any effect on the viscoelastic behavior of the myocardium.

The effect of myocardial hypertrophy on contractility, however, seems to differ depending on the nature of the stimulus and time course of hypertrophy. Structural and metabolic abnormalities that may be associated with depressed contractility in hypertrophy include reduced intracellular volume fraction of myofibrils, massive increase of fiber diameter, increased variability in the thickness of individual fibers, and reduced activity of myofibrilar adenosine triphosphatase (ATPase).[80]

Accumulated evidence supports the concept that there exists an early adaptive or compensatory role for hypertrophy, which in the long-term may be detrimental by contributing to ventricular remodeling and dilation.

The traditional concept that the most important changes occurring in the right ventricle are secondary to left ventricular disease has contributed to the sparsity of studies on chronic hypertrophy and failure of the right ventricle. Furthermore, hypertrophy of the right ventricle may escape detection because it may not be symmetric and occur only in the basal portion.[81] Hypertrophy or dilatation of the right atrium and ventricle are often seen, but most commonly there is a combination of both. The right ventricular trabeculations may be accentuated; this may also involve the right side of the septum. As hypertrophy increases, the right ventricle bulges outward and away from its attachment to the septum, whereas the free wall at the apex may extend beyond the apex of the left ventricle. The atrium and the auricular appendage are enlarged and may contain recent or organized mural thrombi. Although the circumference of both tricuspid and pulmonic valves is increased, this finding is poorly correlated with the degree of hypertrophy. Furthermore, there is a poor correlation between the circumference of the right-sided valves and right ventricular surface area. Thus measurement of valve circumference is an unreliable indicator of right ventricular hypertrophy or dilatation. Finally, in chronic heart disease affecting the right ventricle, increases in surface are proportionate to the increase of ventricular weight.[81]

Although mitotic division of cardiac muscle cells ceases soon after birth, myocyte hypertrophy can be evoked by pathologic states that increase cardiac work. The stimuli for hypertrophy in heart failure are not yet fully elucidated, but there is a growing body of evidence suggesting that protooncogenes may have a critical role in this process. Protooncogenes are genes that are expressed in normal cells and are structurally related to the transforming genes of certain RNA tumor viruses.[82] These protooncogenes are likely to be involved in differentiation and growth regulation of a vast array of cells, including myocytes.[83] Potential stimuli for the initiation of hypertrophy and molecular phenomena involved in the process of cardiac hypertrophy are discussed in detail in Chapter 4.

OTHER ADAPTIVE RESPONSES IN HEART FAILURE

Baroreflex function in congestive heart failure

The distribution of cardiac output is altered in patients with congestive heart failure. Although blood flow to the limb, coronary and cerebral vessels is preserved, skin, splanchnic and renal blood flow is usually decreased. Blood flow to peripheral vascular beds is regulated by complex mechanisms that include inputs from baroreceptors in the heart, lungs, and great vessels.[84] These baroreceptors respond to changes in pressure and volume by altering sympathetic and parasympathetic nervous system activity, pituitary secretion of arginine vasopressin, and renal release of renin. Studies of heart failure in animal models have demonstrated that baroreceptor regulation of regional blood flow is altered.[85] For example, the vasoconstrictor response to carotid artery occlusion and the chronotropic response to phenylephrine response are impaired in animals with low-output heart failure.

A recent study has demonstrated selective regulation of splanchnic and renal vascular resistance but not limb vascular resistance in patients with congestive heart failure. These findings suggest that different sets of receptors can regulate blood flow to specific regions in humans. In patients with heart failure, dysfunction of cardiopulmonary baroreceptors would prevent forearm vasoconstriction, whereas preservation of arterial baroreceptor function could produce renal and splanchnic vasoconstriction.[86]

SYMPATHETIC FUNCTION IN HEART FAILURE

Congestive heart failure is often associated with marked dysfunction of the sympathetic nervous system. The alterations in sympathetic tone are responsible for many of the clinical findings associated with advanced heart failure. The increased sympathetic outflow has also been postulated to contribute to the atrial and ventricular arrhythmias that are often seen in these patients. Plasma levels of norepinephrine have been used as an index of sympathetic activity. Resting plasma norepinephrine levels are approximately two to three times higher in patients with congestive heart failure than in normal volunteers.[87-89] Plasma norepinephrine levels correlate directly with severity of heart failure and subsequent mortality in patients with heart failure.[90] Elevations in plasma dopamine and epinephrine also occur in congestive heart failure. Kinetic studies using tritiated norepinephrine have indicated that these elevated levels of norepinephrine reflect not only an alteration in norepinephrine metabolism, but also an increase in synaptic cleft concentrations, resulting in increased norepinephrine spillover into the circulating blood.[91,92] Recordings of efferent sympathetic nerve traffic in patients with heart failure[93] has correlated with increased norepinephrine secretion. These findings confirm that increased sympathetic activity is present in congestive heart failure. The increased adrenergic drive presumably serves as a compensatory mechanism by stimulating cardiac contractility, redistributing blood flow from nonvital beds, and maintaining arterial pressure in the face of a limited cardiac output.

Under normal circumstances, sympathetic stimulation of the heart improves both contraction and relaxation of the myocardium. The norepinephrine in the heart is synthesized and stored in sympathetic nerve terminals. The effects of released norepinephrine are terminated by two different mechanisms, the first of which involves the reabsorption of 75% of all released norepinephrine into the adrenergic neuron by a process known as reuptake. During the second process, the remaining norepinephrine is enzymatically degraded by catechol-O-methyltransferase and monoamine oxidase.

Even though the circulating levels of norepinephrine are elevated in response to the failing heart, inotropic responsiveness to catecholamines is abnormal. The source of this decreased responsiveness has been examined at several levels. Abnormalities in responsiveness to isoproterenol and several phosphodiesterase inhibitors have been noted in trabeculae carneae from failing hearts of transplant recipients. The response to acetylstrophanthidin and forskolin were normal in these tissues.[94] After a pathologic insult to the myocardium, the remaining viable myocardial tissue adapts and remodels to compensate for diminished pump function. In a rat model, moderate and large infarctions cause progressive ventricular enlargement and death.[95] The same phenomenon has been documented in patients after an acute myocardial infarction.[96,97] Low doses of catecholamines can stimulate myocardial hypertrophy. Alpha-adrenergic stimulation appears to be fundamental to this response.[98-100] Excessive catecholamine stimulation, however, can produce contraction band lesions and myocyte necrosis.[101] The cause of this damage is unclear, but free radical generation, receptor-stimulated myocyte calcium overload, or both are postulated mechanisms.[102] Regardless of the mechanism involved, myocyte loss creates a vicious cycle placing an increased load on the remaining myocardial cells, which stimulates further hypertrophy and a further increase in sympathetic stimulation.[103]

Noradrenergic receptor function

High levels of synaptic cleft norepinephrine are thought to mediate a reduction in beta adrenergic receptor density in the heart through a process of desensitization,[104] causing a reduction in the responsiveness to beta-adrenergic agonists. The cause of the increased spillover of norepinephrine has not yet been determined, but may be due to baroreceptor dysfunction.[105] Examination of cardiac tissue from failing hearts revealed decreased amounts of catecholamines. Animal studies have demonstrated that the depletion of catecholamines is not uniform throughout the myocardium.[106] Histologic analysis revealed that the loss of norepinephrine in the failing myocardium was heterogeneous; some areas remained richly innervated, whereas others sustain a marked loss of norepinephrine and nerve terminals. The pathogenesis of the destruction of sympathetic nerve terminals in the failing myocardium is unknown.

Beta-adrenergic receptors play an important role in the regulation of cardiac function by mediating the positive inotropic, chronotropic, and dromotropic actions of norepinephrine. Exposure to a beta agonist initially causes a functional uncoupling of the beta-adrenergic receptor from adenylate cyclase and makes the tissue less sensitive to the beta receptor-mediated effects. This process occurs within minutes and is not associated with a change in the total number of receptors per cell. This process has also been shown to be reversible upon withdrawal of the increased stimulation. When the exposure to the adrenergic agonist is more prolonged, a decrease in the number of beta-adrenergic receptors occurs (downregulation). The decrease in receptor number is associated with refractoriness to the receptor-mediated effects. Recovery from downregulation requires the synthesis of new receptors and is therefore a slower process.

Myocardial biopsy samples from patients with heart failure have demonstrated that the density of beta-adrenergic receptors is reduced,[107] and the degree of downregulation is inversely related to both the severity of heart failure and the degree of cardiac sympathetic activity, as reflected by the concentration of coronary sinus norepinephrine. The downregulation of beta receptors in patients with heart failure appears to be selective because there was no difference between normal and failing hearts in fluoride-ion and histamine-stimulated muscle contraction. Radioligand studies in myocardial tissue from failing and nonfailing hearts identified a $beta_1$: $beta_2$ ratio of 77:23 in the nonfailing group and 60:38 in the group with heart failure, indicating a decrease in the proportion of $beta_1$ receptors and an increase in the fraction of $beta_2$ myocardial receptors. Thus there may be a selective downregulation of the $beta_1$ subpopulation with little or no change in the $beta_2$ receptor number.[108] As a result, the $beta_2$ receptor may be an important mediator of inotropic support in the failing human heart. In selected patients with heart failure the administration of beta-adrenergic blockers has been shown to produce an increase in myocardial beta-receptor density, improvement in resting cardiac output, and an improved contractile response to catecholamine stimulation.[109]

G proteins

In addition to beta receptor downregulation, evidence now suggests that there are abnormalities in the level and/or functions of one or more of the guanine nucleotide regulatory proteins in the myocardium of patients with heart failure.[49,110] G proteins are a family of guanine nucleotide regulatory proteins that mediate the transduction of receptor activation into modulation of effector molecules in a variety of systems.[111] All G proteins share structural similarities and are composed of three subunits. Beta-adrenergic receptors couple to their second messengers via a GTP-binding protein.[110] The catalytic unit of adenylate cyclase is under the control of two G proteins that mediate the stimulatory and inhibitory actions of various hormones and neurotransmitters that act via adenylate cyclase. Alterations in G protein number have been demonstrated in patients with heart failure.[112] These patients have a diminished number of $beta_1$ receptors and elevated levels of a G protein that mediates the inhibition of adenylate cyclase and probably accounts for the diminished inotropic response to catecholaminergic stimulation. Recent studies of failing human hearts have demonstrated that the alterations existed at the level of transcription and in the posttranslational modification of this G protein.[113]

Vasoconstriction

Activation of the sympathetic nervous system may exert wide range of hemodynamic and metabolic alterations in patients with heart failure. Constriction of the arterial vasculature causes an increase in vascular resistance and a decrease in arterial compliance. These changes eventually increase impedance of left ventricular emptying and further impair ventricular performance. Sympathetic stimulation of renin release may worsen the vasoconstriction.[114] Cardiac sympathetic stimulation may augment heart rate and myocardial contractility, but these effects may be attenuated if the beta-receptors are downregulated.

Altered vagal tone

Inappropriate vagal activation has also been demonstrated in heart failure.

Intravenous injections of phenylephrine cause an enhanced baroreflex-mediated bradycardia in patients with myocardial dysfunction when compared with normal patients.[115] The defective bradycardic response was subsequently shown to be caused by a failure of vagal activation in these patients. Other investigators have also shown that the baroreflex response is attenuated in heart failure. In a canine model of low-output failure, Vatner showed that both the sympathetic and parasympathetic components of the reflex response to hypotension were responsible for the abnormal tachycardia.[116]

NEUROHORMONAL ADAPTATIONS
Atrial natriuretic peptide

The extract derived from the atria of normal rats that produced diuresis and natriuresis is composed of a number of structurally-related small peptides and is collectively defined as atrial natriuretic factor (or peptide) (ANF). Human and rat atria predominantly secrete a peptide of 28 amino acid residues, ANF-(99-126) is a peptide that is composed of the C-terminus of the 126-amino acid precursor.[117] ANF is synthesized and stored in both atrial and ventricular myocardium. ANF reduces blood pressure in normal and hypertensive humans. ANF antagonizes vascular smooth muscle contraction induced by a variety of vasoconstrictors via an endothelium-independent mechanism. ANF also acts as a counterregulatory hormone to the renin-angiotensin-aldosterone system by suppressing renin secretion, inhibiting aldosterone production, and antagonizing the effects of angiotensin II on vascular contraction. ANF also inhibits adrenal cortical steroidogenesis and thirst. ANF influences on body fluid compartmentalization have also been demonstrated. ANF administration causes a shift in fluid from the intravascular bed to the interstitium. Given these actions of this peptide, it is not surprising that the highest serum concentrations of ANF have been recorded in patients with congestive heart failure. Although patients with congestive heart failure are less responsive to ANF infusion than normal subjects, exogenous ANF infusion in patients with CHF does suppress renin and aldosterone secretion. In addition, AF infusion in patients with heart failure can reduce right atrial and pulmonary wedge pressures and increase stroke volume. The major stimulus for ANF release appears to be atrial wall stretch. There also is a correlation between increased atrial or pulmonary arterial pressures and plasma ANF levels.[118] The high plasma ANF levels present in patients with severe heart failure are reduced with successful treatment of cardiac congestion.[119] The finding that angiotensin II has a stimulatory effect on ANF release and that ANF inhibits a number of peripheral effects of angiotensin II suggests that endogenous ANF could be secreted in response to elevated circulating levels of angiotensin II and could antagonize the sodium-retaining and vasoconstrictor actions of angiotensin II.

Arginine vasopressin

Hyponatremia resulting from the retention of water in excess of sodium is often seen in severe congestive heart failure. Although diuretic use is usually a major cause of this finding, an increased concentration of arginine vasopressin (AVP) has been documented in patients with congestive heart failure and hyponatremia who have never received diuretics.[120] AVP is an 8–amino acid peptide that is released from the posterior pituitary. Plasma AVP levels tend to correlate with the degree of heart failure.[121] Although the usual stimulus for AVP release is an increase in serum osmolality, many patients with heart failure have circulating AVP levels that are disproportionately higher than expected for the value of serum osmolality. The stimulus for AVP release in these patients has not yet been identified, but there is evidence to suggest that high-pressure baroreceptors may be a major mediator of nonosmotic stimulation of AVP release in patients with heart failure.[122] There are also data to suggest that there is a "resetting" of the osmotic threshold for AVP release in patients with congestive heart failure.[122] AVP also has potent vaso-

constrictor actions and increases total peripheral resistance. At least two AVP receptors have been described. The V_1 receptor is thought to mediate many of the cardiovascular actions of AVP. These actions include a decrease in cardiac output, bradycardia, increased blood pressure, and increased vascular resistance.[123] Activation of the V_2 receptor is responsible for the antidiuretic response. This action is mediated through the adenylate cyclase system.

Neuropeptide Y

Neuropeptide Y (NPY) is a 36–amino acid peptide that has been found to be co-localized with norepinephrine in many central and peripheral neurons, as well as in the adrenal medulla. NPY exists in high concentrations in sympathetic neurons and is released with nerve depolarization.[124] NPY has been localized in the heart in high concentrations.[125] The major action of this peptide is vasoconstriction.[126] In addition to an independent vasoconstrictor action, NPY has been shown to potentiate the vasoconstriction obtained with norepinephrine.[127] NPY may also possess negative inotropic properties.[126] Patients with heart failure have been shown to possess elevated plasma levels of this peptide.[128]

Calcitonin gene-related peptide

Calcitonin gene-related peptides (CGRP) are alternate products of the calcitonin gene. These peptides have been found to be widely distributed in humans and animals, primarily in the central and peripheral nervous system, the heart, and blood vessels. CGRP is a potent vasodilator and has positive inotropic and chronotropic actions.[129] Endogenous levels of CGRP are elevated in patients with congestive heart failure, and infusion of CGRP to patients with heart failure has been shown to improve hemodynamics and renal blood flow.[130]

Endothelin

Endothelin is a peptide that has been isolated from vascular endothelial cells. Endothelin has potent vasoconstrictor actions, modulates the renin-angiotensin system, and inhibits the release of atrial natriuretic factor.[131] Although endothelin levels were elevated in studies of experimental heart failure,[132] controversy exists regarding whether plasma endothelin levels are elevated in clinical heart failure.

MORPHOLOGIC AND PATHOPHYSIOLOGIC FINDINGS IN HEART FAILURE

Oliguria and azotemia have long been associated with congestive heart failure. Introduction of diuretic agents caused dramatic clinical improvement in patients with this condition. However, the critical importance of the renal response in congestive heart failure was demonstrated when a significant increase in survival was obtained when patients were treated with angiotensin-converting enzyme inhibitors.[133] The presence of heart failure causes the activation of several compensatory mechanisms involving the kidney that are designed for maintaining cardiovascular homeostasis. These mechanisms increase vascular tone and promote sodium retention. Increased systemic vascular resistance maintains systemic blood pressure in the presence of a lowered cardiac output. In addition, an increase in sodium and water retention should increase plasma volume and ventricular filling pressure, thereby augmenting stroke volume. In severe heart failure, excessive vasoconstriction markedly increases afterload on the left ventricle and impairs ejection. An expanded plasma volume can result in transudation of fluid from the capillaries and lead to edema.[134]

Renin

A major discovery that helped to elucidate the importance of the kidney in heart failure was the early observation by Merrill et al[135] that many patients with congestive heart failure had high levels of renin in blood drawn from the renal veins. They postulated that the elevated renin levels were caused by increased secretion of the enzyme by the kidneys, a decrease in blood flow, or a combination of both. They also suggested that the overproduction of renin might contribute to the widespread vasoconstriction seen in heart failure.

Later studies clarified the role of renin and other peptides in the renal response to heart failure. Renin is secreted from the juxtaglomerular apparatus into the lumen of the afferent arteriole. Once in the circulating plasma, renin acts as an enzyme on a specific plasma protein called renin substrate or angiotensinogen. Renin substrate is a protein synthesized by the liver and secreted into the circulation. Under the enzymatic action of renin in the circulating plasma, the ten terminal amino acids are cleaved from renin substrate, leaving the decapeptide angiotensin I. This peptide is physiologically inert. However, it is rapidly altered to angiotensin II, an active form. This alteration consists of an enzymatic removal of two amino acids (histidyl-leucine) from the C-terminal end of the molecule to generate the active octapeptide angiotensin II. This reaction is mediated by converting enzyme. The most abundant source of converting enzyme is the lung, and angiotensin I is largely converted to angiotensin II in a single passage through the pulmonary circulation. Converting enzyme can also be detected in the circulating plasma, although the physiologic significance of this observation is uncertain.[136]

Angiotensin II

Angiotensin II is a peptide containing eight amino acids. The concentration of renin in the circulating plasma is the most important determinant of the plasma concentration of angiotensin II.[136] The actions of angiotensin II are many and varied.[137] It is still uncertain which of these actions are of physiologic importance and which are simple pharmacologic effects demonstrable only on administration of the hormone from exogenous sources. Two of the potential actions of angiotensin II of undoubted physiologic and pathologic importance are the action on vascular smooth muscle, which causes vasoconstriction, and the action on the adrenal cortex, which results in stimulation of the secretion of aldosterone.

Angiotensin II exerts its physiologic effects via specific receptors that are widely distributed throughout the vascular tree. Angiotensin II induces vascular contractions in isolated aortic strips, as well as in vascular rings from femoral, carotid, and coronary vascular beds. Angiotensin II also has an important renal influence. Sodium delivery may be altered solely on the basis of renal artery vasoconstriction.[138] Preferential efferent arteriolar vasoconstriction by angiotensin II may increase transglomerular hydrostatic pressure and the filtration fraction. These physiologic responses may preserve glomerular filtration rate in the setting of decreased renal blood flow.[139] Angiotensin II also causes contraction of glomerular mesangial cells, thereby increasing the ultrafiltration coefficient.[140] Angiotensin II also directly stimulates proximal tubular sodium reabsorption by activating the sodium/hydrogen antiporter.[141] Recently, indirect mechanisms have been identified that allow angiotensin II to influence local vascular responses. Prostacyclin synthesis is increased by angiotensin II.[142] Angiotensin II may also increase the release of endothelium-dependent relaxant factor.[143] Angiotensin II also induces the biosynthesis or release of vasopressin, and atrial natriuretic factor.[144,145]

An important interaction of angiotensin II and the sympathetic nervous system is the angiotensin II-facilitated release of norepinephrine from nerve endings.[146,147] Angiotensin II also enhances the biosynthesis of norepinephrine[148] and has been shown to inhibit the reuptake of norepinephrine from sympathetic nerve endings.[149]

In addition to the classic production of angiotensin II, recent evidence suggests that angiotensin II may be synthesized locally in target tissues and blood vessels. Molecular biologic techniques have confirmed that both renin and angiotensin II genes are expressed in the heart, blood vessels, kidney, and brain.[150,151] The local synthesis of angiotensin II in blood vessels may directly influence regional blood flow regulation.[152]

Aldosterone

The corticosteroid aldosterone is classified as a mineralocorticoid because its action is to enhance sodium and potassium transport across epithelial membranes. It exerts this action on many structures, including the salivary glands and intestinal epithelium, but its most important site of action is the distal segment of the renal tubule. There it increases sodium reabsorption and enhances secretion of potassium and hydrogen ion into the luminal fluid. In performing these functions, aldosterone plays a key role in regulating fluid and electrolyte balance in the body. By increasing sodium reabsorption at the level of the distal tubule, aldosterone tends to increase the osmolality of the extracellular fluid. The rise in osmolality provides a stimulus for secretion of arginine vasopressin, which in turn increases the permeability of the collecting duct to water. As a result, water reabsorption is enhanced and the osmolality of the extracellular fluid is returned to normal. By mediating an increase in tubular reabsorption of water, aldosterone indirectly causes an expansion of extracellular fluid volume.

Acute experimental cardiac decompensation is associated with activation of the renin-angiotensin system, the sympathetic nervous system, and stimulation of vasopressin release. These systems maintain systemic blood pressure and promote renal sodium and water retention. In the chronic "compensated" phase of experimental heart failure, which is associated with expansion of the extracellular fluid volume and restoration of blood pressure, the plasma levels of the hormones generally return to normal.[153] Similar patterns have been observed in humans.[154]

Changes in renal hemodynamics

The primary cause of the renal responses in forward heart failure appears to be a decrease in renal blood flow. Despite this reduction in renal blood flow, both glomerular filtration rate and the capacity to excrete urea are well sustained for a long time in cardiac failure. In animal studies of heart failure secondary to large infarctions, the glomerular plasma flow rate was markedly impaired while the reduction in single-nephron glomerular filtration was proportionately less; these changes resulted in an increase in single-nephron filtration fraction.[155] Measurement of preglomerular, glomerular, and postglomerular pressures and flows revealed that the reduction in the glomerular plasma flow rate and the increase in single-nephron filtration fraction were caused by intense constriction of the efferent arterioles. The increased resistance in the efferent arterioles was responsible for the maintenance of glomerular capillary hydraulic pressure and thus prevented a more marked fall in glomerular filtration rate. It has been suggested that these alterations in glomerular hemodynamics may contribute to the increase in sodium retention in heart failure via a decrease in peritubular hydraulic pressure and an increase in peritubular oncotic pressure, thereby resulting in increased proximal tubular fluid reabsorption.[134,156] In contrast to the experimental models, clinical studies suggest that a mechanism other than proximal tubular reabsorption may be also be involved because the reduced sodium excretion seen in heart failure has been shown to result from a combination of diminished glomerular filtration and enhanced tubular reabsorption beyond the proximal tubule.[157] Treatment with an angiotensin-converting enzyme inhibitor increased renal plasma flow, decreased filtration fraction, and left glomerular filtration rate unchanged, sup-

porting the concept that angiotensin II may play a role in the pathogenesis of abnormal renal hemodynamics in clinical heart failure.

Sympathetic modulation of renal function

Proximal tubules contain both alpha- and beta- adrenergic receptors. Adrenergic agonists have been shown to influence transtubular reabsorption of sodium in microperfused rabbit proximal tubules.[158] Abnormal sympathetic modulation of sodium reabsorption has been demonstrated in experimental heart failure. An infusion of saline to control rats markedly inhibited sympathetic renal nerve activity. However, the inhibitory response was attenuated in rats with heart failure.[159]

In an animal model of congestive heart failure, reversal of sympathetic activity by unilateral denervation produced an increase in single nephron glomerular filtration rate and substantially increased single nephron plasma flow rate. These effects were mainly caused by relief of efferent, i.e., postglomerular, arteriolar vasoconstriction.[160]

These responses consisted primarily of an increased sympathetic neuronal outflow to the kidney and activation of the renin-angiotensin system; a positive feedback mechanism existed because angiotensin II facilitated the release of norepinephrine from nerve endings. Although the renal compensatory mechanisms are aimed at increasing blood volume, these actions may be deleterious in patients with severe heart failure.

Sodium retention resulting from diminished renal excretion of sodium is a hallmark of CHF and is mainly caused by sympathetic overactivity and activation of the renin-angiotensin-aldosterone system. Sympathetic stimulation initiates three mechanisms that ultimately lead to circulatory refilling: an increase in renovascular resistance, activation of the juxtaglomerular cells to release renin, and a direct stimulation of tubular sodium transport.[161]

PULMONARY RESPONSES IN HEART FAILURE

The functional integration of the heart and lungs continues to reveal an interdependency even in altered disease states. A prime example of this association is the occurrence of dyspnea on effort as a result of left ventricular failure. However, the precise stimulus for the respiratory distress of heart failure is not entirely clear. Whether the sensation of dyspnea is caused by an excessive load imposed on the respiratory muscles or an increased drive to breathe is still not clear.[162]

Pulmonary congestion can be defined as an increase of the volume of blood present in the vessels of the lungs. In active pulmonary congestion, there is increased pulmonary flow with or without an arteriocapillary increase of pressure. In passive pulmonary congestion there is increased pulmonary venous capillary pressure. Although active congestion of a moderate degree may be found in a number of conditions (such as anemia or thyrotoxicosis), severe active congestion is observed only in left-to-right shunts.

Passive pulmonary congestion is seen in any condition where there is obstruction to flow at any point from the pulmonary capillary bed to the aortic valve and beyond. A common and important cause of passive pulmonary congestion is chronic left ventricular failure.

As the left ventricle fails, increased ventricular volume moves the ventricle along the passive compliance curve and diastolic intracavitary pressure increases. However, the effects of left ventricular failure on the pulmonary circulation are not compensatory, but passive responses to the increase in pulmonary venous pressure. Such an increase in pulmonary venous pressure has an important effect on pulmonary mechanics, perfusion distribution, and ultimately gas exchange. As in other organs, the lungs are the sites of constant fluid filtration and removal. Filtration is driven by the transvascular hydrostatic pressure while the transvascular protein osmotic pressure acts to retain fluid in the bloodstream. The site of fluid exchange is the pulmonary capillary endothelium.

Under normal conditions, there is an outward force (hydrostatic pressure) of 10 mm Hg and an inward force (protein osmotic pressure) of 6 mm Hg and thus a net outward filtration pressure gradient of 4 mm Hg. An efficient fluid removal system is mandatory to prevent fluid accumulation in the pulmonary interstitial space and flooding of the alveoli. Lymph capillaries are the main vehicles for the fluid removal system, the capacity of which may increase by fivefold to tenfold when necessary. However, at high rates of filtration the capacity of lymphatics is exceeded, and

fluid accumulates in the peribronchovascular cuffs. As the cuffs expand and the tissue pressure within the cuffs rises, fluid begins to flood the alveoli.

Accumulation of fluid in the bronchovascular spaces may reduce the caliber of the airways. Moreover, a reflex constriction of airway smooth muscle may induce an abnormal air flow and manifest clinically as a "cardiac" asthma. While interstitial edema creates minor change in lung volume or the mechanics of breathing, alveolar flooding abolishes gas exchange, the vital capacity decreases, and the lungs become stiffer or less compliant.

In pulmonary edema secondary to congestive heart failure, there is an increase in microvascular hydrostatic pressure. Because the permeability of the endothelial membrane remains normal, the fluid that leaks across contains progressively lower concentrations of protein, resulting in decrease of the perimicrovascular protein osmotic pressure. This important compensatory effect, which depends on a normal microvascular barrier, nullifies approximately 50% of the effect of fluid filtration.[163] Alveolar fluid (edema) has the same composition of the fluid in the interstitial space and a protein concentration that is usually less than 50% of that in blood. However, in pulmonary edema caused by increased permeability, as in seen in adult respiratory distress syndrome, protein concentration within the edema fluid is as high as that in the plasma. In some instances of cardiogenic pulmonary edema fluid may be blood-tinged because of ruptured capillaries resulting from increased hydrostatic pressure in the dependent areas of the lungs.

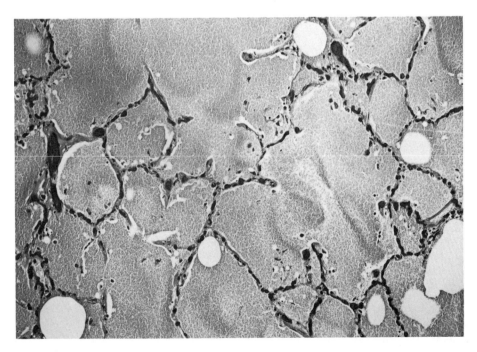

Fig. 16-9. Severe pulmonary edema. Distended alveolar spaces filled with proteinaceous material.

On pathologic analysis, the lungs in pulmonary edema are heavy and wet with no detectable crepitations. The alveolar spaces are filled with proteinaceous material. Hemosiderin-laden macrophages are present in both alveolar spaces and interstitium (Fig. 16-9). In cases of chronic longstanding pulmonary congestion, such as is seen in severe mitral stenosis, besides the abundance of hemosiderin-laden macrophages, there is also widening of the alveolar septa as a result of fibrosis. These morphologic changes of longstanding pulmonary congestion are termed *brown induration* of the lungs.

Pleural effusion

The normal volume of pleural fluid is relatively small and is estimated to be approximately 0.1 to 0.2 ml/kg of body weight. This fluid is filtered through and reabsorbed by the pleural surfaces. Lymphatic stomata (openings) at the diaphragmatic and basilar portions of the parietal pleura may also facilitate the reabsorption of macromolecules and liquid. Current belief is that pleural fluid is an ultrafiltrate of microvessels under the parietal pleural mesothelium. A large portion of this ultrafiltrate is reabsorbed into low pressure microvasculature, whereas the more concentrated protein solution leaks into the pleural space through the mesothelium.

Pleural effusion is a common finding in congestive heart failure. Excessive fluid accumulates in both pleural spaces, although for unknown reasons the effusion is greater on the right hemithorax. Pleural effusions may adversely effect the lungs, which often reveal evidence of collapse. Pleural effusion may also contribute to the sensation of dyspnea and interfere with pulmonary mechanics and gas exchange.

PERIPHERAL CIRCULATION IN HEART FAILURE

The caliber and distensibility of the vasculature is controlled by several factors, including sympathetic activity, endothelial vasoactive substances, circulating hormones, electrolyte and water content, and structural alterations. Moreover, changes in vascular tone may not be homogeneous; thus a response to a stimulus may be different in various vascular beds. Such differences of response may effect individual organ function, but impedance and capacitance depend on the integrated vascular response. The peripheral circulation in patients with heart failure is characterized by an increase in vascular resistance and a decrease in vascular compliance.[164,165] A reduction in distensibility of the aorta and large arteries may impair the storage capacity of the arterial bed during systole. Therefore in the presence of a failing ventricle and a high vascular resistance, the decrease in arterial compliance may cause considerable reduction in left ventricular stroke volume.

GASTROINTESTINAL EFFECTS OF HEART FAILURE

The gastrointestinal phenomena observed in congestive heart failure are mainly passive responses primarily caused by increased venous pressure and decreased perfusion. The right ventricle will respond to the increased pressure in the pulmonary vasculature, secondary to left ventricular failure, with dilatation and hypertrophy. However, as the right ventricle dilates and hypertrophies, it also becomes less compliant. The increased right ventricular stiffness, in addition to an increased blood volume associated with heart failure, will lead to elevation of systemic venous pressure. Furthermore, the catecholamine-induced venous constriction will accentuate the pressures in the systemic venous circulation and cause engorgement of the hepatic and intestinal venous beds.

Hepatic dysfunction in heart failure

The gastrointestinal passive congestion will decrease the arterial perfusion of these organs (enhanced by splanchnic and hepatic arteriolar vasoconstriction), leading to hepatic metabolic dysfunction that impairs the synthesis of hormones, albumin, clotting factors, and other substances. Changes in the absorptive capabilities of the intestines have also been noted. Increased venous pressure can cause hepatic lymphatic and intrasinusoidal pressure to increase, resulting in a postsinusoidal biliary obstruction and jaundice. The elevated lymphatic pressure causes weeping through the hepatic capsule of fluid high in protein and formation of ascites. Hepatic dysfunction is frequently seen in patients with acute circulatory failure, such as shock, prolonged hypotension, and right or left heart failure. The pathogenesis of hepatic dysfunction is thought to be secondary to diminished hepatic blood flow because of the decrease in cardiac output and increased hepatic venous pressure.

An increased central venous pressure is directly transmitted back to the sinusoid because hepatic sinusoidal pressure is very low, and the degree of pressure drop from the sinusoid to the vena cava is very small.[166] The high hepatic venous pressure causes centrilobular cell atrophy and edema of the perisinusoidal area, an evidence of cellular hypoxia. A reduced cardiac output in left heart failure leads to a decrease in the hepatic perfusion via the portal vein and hepatic artery by approximately one third of the normal. This decreased hepatic perfusion is compensated by increased oxygen extraction, leading to further reduction of the hepatic venous oxygen tension. Whereas the periportal hepatocytes continue to receive blood with relatively high oxygen tension, the central area (central vein) is most distant from the portal areas and receives blood of a lower oxygen tension. However, it is doubtful whether the circulatory disturbances stated above are the only cause of significant hepatic dysfunction because hypoxemia

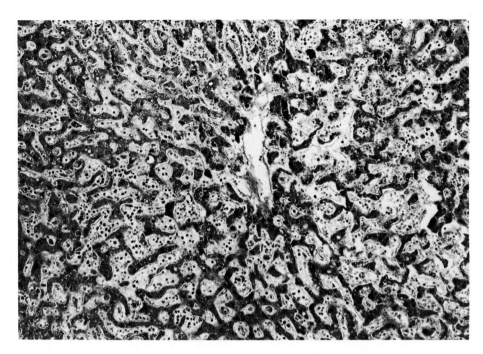

Fig. 16-10. Severe centrilobular congestion of hepatic sinusoids with distortion and atrophy of liver cells.

alone cannot produce centrilobular necrosis. Furthermore, it is known that hepatic necrosis in experimental shock cannot be prevented by hyperbaric oxygen.[167] Thus it has been suggested that factors additional to the hepatic circulatory disturbances may cause fulminant hepatic failure. The alterations in hepatic structure and function are usually mild in most cases of congestive heart failure.

Massive hepatic necrosis and marked elevation of serum transaminase activities were produced in experimental animals when portal endotoxemia was superimposed upon poor hepatic perfusion. In humans, intestinal circulatory disturbances secondary to congestive heart failure may allow an increase in diffusion of endotoxin through the intestinal wall because of the breakdown of the mucosal barrier.[168] In most instances of hepatic dysfunction in congestive heart failure, the GOT values are below 400 units. Occasionally GOT values may reach 1000 to 2000 units and only rarely exceed 3000 units.

Pathologic findings

The classic gross appearance of the liver in chronic passive congestion is that of "nutmeg" (Fig. 16-10). This gross morphology reflects the microscopic alterations occurring primarily in the centrilobular areas. These changes are characterized by centrilobular sinusoidal dilatation with hemorrhage and atrophy and/or necrosis of hepatocytes around the central vein. Light microscopy, electron microscopy, and immunohistochemical studies of hepatocytes from patients with hepatic congestion have shown

the presence of intracellular hyaline globules. Characteristically, these globules are PAS-positive, nonglycogenic (diastase-resistant), and are found within centrilobular hepatocytes and in association with centrilobular congestion. This is not to imply, however, that all patients with passive liver congestion have PAS-positive globules. It is hypothesized that variation in the severity or chronicity of hepatic congestion may play a role in the formation of globules.[169] Some studies have suggested that these nonglycogenic globules are phagocytized plasma proteins produced under conditions of increased intrasinusoidal pressure and/or increased hepatocyte membrane permeability.[170]

In longstanding hepatic congestion, the centrilobular hepatocyte damage may be followed by deposition of collagen and scarring. Severe degrees of hepatic fibrosis secondary to chronic passive congestion are often referred to as cardiac hepatic sclerosis. The intestines in congestive heart failure appear edematous and hyperemic as a result of venous congestion and increased lymphatic pressure. The intestines' absorptive functions may be altered.

SPLENIC FINDINGS IN CONGESTIVE HEART FAILURE

The spleen is significantly enlarged in persistent or chronic venous congestion. This is often referred to as congestive splenomegaly. Systemic or central venous congestion occurs in cardiac decompensation involving the right side of the heart and can be particularly severe in tricuspid or pulmonic valvular disease and in cor pulmonale. Early in chronic passive congestion, the spleen is enlarged (250 g to 300 g), tense, and cyanotic. At this early stage of congestive splenomegaly, there are sinusoidal dilatation, focal hemorrhages, and occasional hemosiderin deposits. In longstanding congestive splenomegaly, the spleen may weigh more than 500 g, is firm, and its capsule may be thick and fibrotic. Depending on the amount of fibrosis the splenic parenchyma may be gray-red to deep red. The malpighian corpuscles are indistinct. Deposition of collagen in the basement membrane of the sinusoids produces dilatation and rigidity of their walls. Focal recent and old hemorrhage is present throughout the splenic parenchyma, and hemosiderin containing histiocytes are plentiful.

PERIPHERAL EDEMA

Although the peripheral edema seen in congestive heart failure may be partially caused by increased hydrostatic pressure in the venular end of the microcirculation, the overall pathogenesis of cardiac edema is multifactorial. Reduction of cardiac output and thus the so-called effective arterial blood volume in congestive heart failure triggers the renin-angiotensin-aldosterone axis in the kidneys, resulting in retention of sodium and water.

The resultant expansion of the intravascular volume constitutes an additional burden on the failing heart, leading to increased venous pressure and edema formation. Although cardiac edema is associated with elevated venous pressure, edema of renal etiology is not. Moreover, cardiac edema is often associated with cyanosis and is typically influenced by gravity, whereas hepatic or renal etiology edema is usually associated with pallor and is more diffuse.

CLINICAL HEART FAILURE
Epidemiology

Prevalence. It has been estimated that more than 2 million Americans have heart failure.[171] It is also estimated that 400,000 new cases occur each year, requiring at least 900,000 hospital admissions annually.[171] The Framingham study provided important information on the evolution of heart failure in a cohort of 5209 men and women who were followed biennially for the development of clinical symptoms and signs of heart failure. It should be noted that the clinical criteria used to identify patients with heart failure were strict by contemporary standards and did not include persons with impaired, subclinical cardiac function who would now be identified because of advancements in modern technology. After more than 30 years of surveillance of the 5209 patients, there were 485 men and women who developed the first clinical evidence of overt heart failure. The annual incidence increased markedly with age, especially beyond 75 years.[172] A recent report of the National Health and Nutrition Examina-

Table 16-1. Etiologies of cardiac failure in the Framingham cohort: 32-year follow-up of the 5209 subjects in the Framingham study

Specified Etiology	Percent of cardiac failures	
	Men	**Women**
Hypertension*	76.4	79.1
Coronary disease[†]	45.8	27.4
Rheumatic heart disease	2.4	3.2
Other[‡]	11.2	16.8

*Blood Pressure greater than 160/95 mm Hg or on antihypertensive therapy.
[†]Any clinical manifestation of coronary disease.
[‡] None of the above, (e.g., cardiomyopathy).
Modified from Kannel WB, Savage D, Castelli WP: *Congestive heart failure: current research and clinical applications.* In Braunwald E, (ed.): *Heart disease,* New York, 1982, Grune and Stratton.

tion Survey showed the prevalence of self-reported congestive heart failure to be 1.1% of the noninstitutionalized U.S. adult population. The prevalence of congestive heart failure based on clinical criteria was 2%.[172a]

Etiology. In the Framingham cohort of patients, systemic arterial hypertension was the most common etiologic factor for the development of congestive heart failure. Of the patients who developed heart failure, 75% had a history of blood pressures of 160/95 mm Hg or greater (Table 16-1). Coronary artery disease was found in 46% of the men and 27% of the women with CHF. Rheumatic heart disease was the etiologic factor in 2.4% of the men and 3.2% of the women. The Framingham Study data suggested a prevalence of less than 11% for other causes of congestive heart failure, including dilated, restrictive, and hypertrophic cardiomyopathy.

Hypertension is thought to be a powerful contributor to the incidence of cardiac failure in the general population mainly because of its high prevalence. Except for stroke, hypertension predisposes as powerfully to cardiac failure as to any other cardiac sequelae[171] (Table 16-2). The risk of cardiac failure increases with the severity of the hypertension and is also increased in patients with isolated systolic hypertension.

Coronary artery disease. Twenty-three percent of the men and thirty-five percent of the women in the Framingham cohort who had symptomatic myocardial infarctions developed cardiac failure. This rate was four to eight times higher than that of patients the same age without coronary disease. There was no difference in the incidence of heart failure between those patients who had silent myocardial infarctions and those who had classic presentations of infarction. The incidence of congestive heart failure in patents with angina was half that of patients with infarction, but two to three times that of the general population of the same age. All but 10% of the patients with coronary dis-

Table 16-2. Risk of heart failure by clinical manifestations of coronary heart disease: subjects 35 to 96 years of age, Framingham study, 30 year follow-up.* Uncomplicated angina

Coronary heart disease status	10-Year per cent probability of congestive heart failure		Age-Adjusted Risk Ratio	
	Men	Women	Men	Women
Angina pectoris*	14.4	14.4	2.1	3.0
Symptomatic myocardial infarction	22.8	34.6	3.7	7.6
Silent or unrecognized myocardial infarction	36.7	27.6	4.6	4.8

Modified from Kannel, WB.[176]

ease who developed CHF in the Framingham cohort had some degree of concomitant hypertension.[171]

Other predisposing factors. Other frequently noted concomitant chronic diseases, such as diabetes mellitus, chronic lung disease, stroke, and claudication, are all probably related to advanced age, but only diabetes mellitus may be uniquely related to CHF. The Framingham study examined this relationship in detail, noting anteced-ent diabetes in 16% of patients who had CHF. A signifi-cant effect of diabetes persisted in multivariate analysis, which also examined the contributions of coronary artery disease risk factors and other possible contributors to the incidence of congestive heart failure. The increased risk of CHF was seen in diabetics of all ages, but was substan-tially limited to those diabetics who were treated with in-sulin. This finding may implicate insulin-dependent, ke-totic, insulinopenic diabetes of early onset as the promoter of cardiac failure, rather than mere duration or severity of the diabetes.[173] Thus rather than simple acceleration of coronary atherosclerosis, it has been suggested that there exists a cardiac microangiopathy related to diabetes that is similar to that seen in the skin, kidney, and retina.[174] This postulated microangiopathy probably could be responsible for the increased risk of CHF in diabetic patients.[175]

Proteinuria, obesity, and cigarette smoking were also examined in the Framingham cohort as possible promoters of heart failure.[176] Proteinuria was associated with an ex-cess risk of cardiac failure, even when other cardiovascu-lar risk factors were taken into account. A modest effect of weight on age-adjusted risk for all ages combined was noted. Cigarette smoking was a weak predictor of cardiac failure in men, but doubled the risk in women.

In another longitudinal study, 973 men were followed for 17 years. The most important predisposing factors for CHF were found to be hypertension, smoking, and obesi-ty.[177]

CLINICAL PRESENTATION OF HEART FAILURE
Dyspnea

The most important mechanism by which cardiac dis-ease can affect lung function is the symptom of dyspnea. Dyspnea is usually the earliest and most important symp-

tom associated with congestive heart failure. The process of accumulation of fluid in the lungs of cardiac patients is driven primarily by increased microvascular pressures. Even compensated patients who display relatively normal hemodynamics at rest can elevate their end-diastolic pres-sures with exercise. The elevation of end-diastolic pres-sures induces compensatory rises in pulmonary venous and pulmonary capillary pressures, causing dyspnea. With chronic passive congestion, pulmonary vessels can un-dergo proliferative changes that further alter the properties of the vessel wall. The work of breathing increases as the transpulmonary airway gradient required for adequate ven-tilation increases. This alters the established length-tension relations of the intercostal muscles. The patient senses an inappropriate relation between the volume of breath achieved and the force required to produce a breath. Spe-cial muscle spindles in the intercostal muscles sense this alteration in length-tension relation and transmit this infor-mation to the central nervous system via afferent impulses. The patient senses this as increased work of breathing, or dyspnea. The development of pleural effusion also may contribute to dyspnea. The classification of heart failure is based to a large extent on the symptom of dyspnea and the amount of physical activity necessary to produce this symptom.

Orthopnea

Orthopnea is the sensation of dyspnea while lying flat that is relieved by elevation of the head. The mechanism of orthopnea is thought to be the pooling of blood into the lower extremities while upright. When assuming a recum-bent position, there is a sudden increase in venous return. The failing left ventricle experiences an increase in left ventricular end-diastolic volume and pressure. The pres-sure is transmitted to the pulmonary circuit, where the rise in pulmonary capillary pressure causes interstitial edema. Recumbency also elevates the diaphragm, which causes a decrease in ventilatory reserve.

Paroxysmal nocturnal dyspnea

Episodes of paroxysmal nocturnal dyspnea usually oc-cur at night when the patient is asleep. The patient awakens, usually quite suddenly, and bolts upright gasping for breath. The mechanism of paroxsymal nocturnal dyspnea appears to be more complex than that of orthopnea. Additional putative etiologies include bronchospasm, caused by congestion of the bronchial mucosa, which increases the work of breathing; reduced adrenergic support of the ventricle during sleep; slow resorption of interstitial fluid from the dependent portion of the body and a resultant increase in blood volume; and normal nocturnal depression of the respiratory center.

Physical findings

The respiratory rate is usually elevated in patients with advanced heart failure. Respiratory distress and tachypnea may worsen when the patient lies flat. Cheyne-Stokes respiration or periodic breathing with periods of hyperpnea alternating regularly with apnea is frequently seen in patients with severe heart failure during sleep.

When the heart failure is uncompensated or the stroke volume is very low, an increase in heart rate develops to maintain cardiac output. The presence of pulsus alternans usually signifies severe myocardial disease, and is usually accompanied by a third heart sound and tachycardia. Pulsus alternans appears to be caused by an alteration in stroke volume of the ventricle. It is probably secondary to incomplete recovery of myocardial cells on alternate beats.

In severe uncompensated heart failure, vasoconstriction of the skin may impair heat loss, causing a low-grade fever.

Persistent elevation of the jugular venous pressure is one of the earlier and most reliable signs of congestive heart failure. The character and type of elevated venous pulsations help to distinguish the underlying pathology in heart failure.

Pulmonary veins become engorged early in the course of heart failure. The transmission of elevated left atrial pressures to the pulmonary veins and capillaries causes transudation of fluid into the alveoli, which then moves into the airways. Rales are usually heard over the lung bases and are often accompanied by dullness to percussion, implying a pleural effusion. In pulmonary edema rales are heard in all lung fields. Wheezing is often noted because of bronchial edema.

Cardiomegaly is usually found in most patients with chronic heart failure, except for those with restrictive cardiomyopathy or constrictive pericarditis. In many acute states, clinical heart failure may appear before cardiomegaly has had a chance to develop. The protodiastolic gallop sound (S3) is caused by the rapid deceleration of blood after rapid ventricular filling. A decrease in ventricular compliance associated with increases in end-diastolic volumes may contribute to the genesis of the S3. This sound characteristically occurs 13 msec to 16 msec after the second heart sound. Although an S3 is frequently heard in healthy children and young adults, it is a rare finding in healthy

patients over age 40. The presystolic gallop sound (S4) is also caused by a rapid deceleration of blood after the rapid ventricular filling that accompanies atrial contraction, and usually signifies atrial hypertrophy without stenosis of the AV valve. The atrial hypertrophy follows the increased resistance to filling that accompanies a decrease in left ventricular compliance.

Hepatomegaly usually occurs before peripheral edema develops but often does not totally reverse, even after compensation of right heart failure and the disappearance of symptoms. If hepatomegaly has occurred rapidly and relatively recently, the liver is usually tender, secondary to stretching of its capsule. Although excessive peritoneal fluid is often found at autopsy in patients who die of heart failure, gross ascites in heart failure is usually associated with chronic venous congestion and very high venous pressures. In patients with severe tricuspid regurgitation or constrictive pericarditis, the ascites may be more prominent than peripheral edema.

Peripheral edema is usually symmetric and generally occurs in the dependent portions of the body. Chronic edema may result in erythema, induration, and pigmentation of the skin of the lower extremities. As a general rule an increase of at least 5 L of extracellular fluid must be present before peripheral edema is detectable in heart failure. The severity of edema does not correlate well with the level of systemic venous pressure in chronic heart failure, in part because the compensatory neurohumoral mechanisms that lead to a decreased excretion of sodium can expand the extracellular volume sufficiently so that edema may result despite normal or only slightly increased systemic venous pressure.

The skin findings associated with heart failure reflect the increased adrenergic tone that accompanies this condition. Not uncommonly, untreated patients display peripheral cyanosis of the digits, pallor of the distal extremities, cool skin, and diaphoresis.

REFERENCES

1. White PD: *Heart disease.* New York, 1937, Macmillan.
2. Callahan JA, Key JD: *Cardiology fundamentals and practice.* Chicago, 1987, Year Book.
3. Braunwald E, Ross J Jr: *Control of cardiac performance.* In Bern RM, eds: *Handbook of physiology,* Baltimore, 1979, Waverly.
4. Winegrad S: *Electromechanical coupling in heart muscle.* In Bern RM, eds: *Handbook of physiology,* Baltimore, 1979, Waverly.
5. Katz AM: Influence of altered inotropy and lusitropy on ventricular pressure-volume loops, *J Am Coll Cardiol* 11:438, 1988.
6. LeWinter MM, Pavelec R: Influence of the pericardium on left ventricular end-diastolic pressure-segment relations during early and later stages of experimental chronic volume overload in dogs, *Circ Res* 50:501, 1982.
7. Janicki JS: Influence of the pericardium and ventricular interdependence on left ventricular diastolic and systolic function in patients with heart failure, *Circulation* 81(Suppl III):III-15, 1990.
8. Grossman W: Diastolic dysfunction and congestive heart failure, *Circulation* 81(Suppl III):III-1, 1990.
9. Klein AL, Hatle LK, Burstow DJ et al: Doppler characterization of left ventricular diastolic function in cardiac amyloidosis, *J Am Coll Cardiol* 13:1017, 1989.

10. Weber KT, Janicki JS, Pick R et al: Collagen in the hypertrophied, pressure-overloaded myocardium, *Circulation* 75(Suppl I):I-40, 1987.

11. Koslovskis PL, Fieber LA, Pruitt DK et al: Myocardial changes during the progression of left ventricular pressure-overloaded myocardium, *J Mol Cell Cardiol* 19:105, 1987.

12. Heilbrunn LJ, Wiercinski FJ: The action of various cations on muscle protoplasm, *J Cellular Comp Physiol* 29:15, 1947.

13. Mines GR: Of functional analysis by the action of electrolytes, *J Physiol* 46:188, 1913.

14. Ringer S: A further contribution regarding the influence of different constituents of the blood on the contraction of the heart, *J Physiol* 4:29, 1883.

15. Reference deleted in galleys.

16. White D: Rigor concentration and the effect of various phosphate compounds on glycerinated insect flight and vertebrate muscle, *J Physiol* 208:583, 1970.

17. Ebashi S, Endo M: Calcium ion and muscle contraction, *Prog Biophys Mol Biol* 18:123, 1968.

18. Weber A: On the mechanism of the relaxing effect of fragmented sarcoplasmic reticulum, *J Gen Physiol* 46:679, 1963.

19. Potter JD, Gergely J: The calcium and magnesium binding sites on troponin and their role in the regulation of myofibrillar adenosine triphosphatase, *J Biochem* 250:4628, 1975.

20. VanErd JP, Takahashi K: Determination of the complete amino acid sequence of bovine cardiac troponin C, *Biochemistry* 15:1171, 1976.

21. Solaro J, Briggs FN: Estimating the functional capabilities of sarcoplasmic reticulum in cardiac muscle, *Circ Res* 34:531, 1974.

22. Haselgrove J: X-ray evidence for conformational changes in the myosin filaments of vertebrate striated muscle, *J Mol Biol* 92:113, 1975.

23. Solaro RJ, Wise RM, Shiner JS et al: Calcium requirements for myofibrillar activation, *Circ Res* 34:525, 1974.

24. Morgan JP: Abnormal intracellular modulation of calcium as a major cause of cardiac contractile dysfunction, *N Engl J Med* 325:625, 1991.

25. Gwathmey JK, Copelas L, MacKinnon R et al: Abnormal intracellular calcium handling in myocardium from patients with end-stage heart failure, *Circ Res* 61:70, 1987.

26. Gwathmey JK, Slawsky MT, Hajjar RJ et al: Role of intracellular calcium handling in force-interval relationships of human ventricular myocardium, *J Clin Invest* 85:1599, 1990.

27. Panagia V, Lee SL, Singh A et al: Impairment of mitochondrial and sarcoplasmic reticular functions during the development of heart failure in cardiomyopathic hamsters, *Can J Cardiol* 2:237, 1986.

28. Mercadier JJ, Lompre AM, Duc P et al: Altered sarcoplasmic reticulum Ca2+−ATPase gene expression in the human ventricle during end-stage heart failure, *J Clin Invest* 85:305, 1990.

29. De la Bastie D, Levitsky D, Rappaport L et al: Function of the sarcoplasmic reticulum and expression of its Ca2+−ATPase gene in pressure overload-induced cardiac hypertrophy in the rat, *Circ Res* 66:554, 1990.

30. Morgan JP, Erny RE, Allen PD et al: Abnormal intracellular calcium handling, a major cause of systolic and diastolic dysfunction in ventricular myocardium from patients with heart failure, *Circulation* 81(suppl III):III-21, 1990.

31. Perrault CL, Meuse AJ, Bentivegna L et al: Abnormal intracellular calcium handling in acute and chronic heart failure: role in systolic and diastolic dysfunction, *Eur Heart Journal* 11(Suppl C):8, 1990.

32. Figulla HR, Rechenberg JV, Wiegand V et al: Beneficial effects of long-term diltiazem treatment in dilated cardiomyopathy, *J Am Coll Cardiol* 13:653, 1989.

33. Rasmussen RP, Minobe W, Bristow MR: Calcium antagonist binding sites in failing and nonfailing human ventricular myocardium, *Biochem Pharmacol* 39:691, 1990.

34. Bonow RO, Rosing DR, Bacharach SL et al: Effects of verapamil on left ventricular systolic function and diastolic filling in patients with hypertrophic cardiomyopathy, *Circulation* 64:787, 1981.

35. Bonow RO, Bacharach SL, Green MV et al: Impaired left ventricular diastolic filling in patients with coronary artery disease: assessment with radionuclide angiography, *Circulation* 64:315, 1981.

36. Cohn JN, Johnson G: Heart failure with normal ejection fraction: the V-HeFT study, *Circulation* 81(Suppl III):III-48, 1990.

36a. Setaro JF, Soufer R, Remetz MS et al: Long-term outcome in patients with congestive heart failure and intact systolic left ventricular performance, *Am J Cardiol* 69:1212, 1992.

37. Grossman W: Diastolic function in congestive heart failure, *N Engl J Med* 325:1557, 1991.

38. Watanabe J, Levine MJ, Bellotto F et al: Effects of coronary venous pressure on left ventricular diastolic distensibility, *Circ Res* 67:923, 1990.

39. Katz AM: Energy requirements of contraction and relaxation: implications for inotropic stimulation of the failing heart, *Basic Res Cardiol* 84(Suppl 1):47, 1989.

40. Little WC, Downes TR: Clinical evaluation of left ventricular diastolic performance, *Prog Cardiovasc Dis* 32:273, 1990.

41. Anversa P, Olivetti G, Melissari M et al: Stereological measurement of cellular and subcellular hypertrophy and hyperplasia in the papillary muscle of adult rat, *J Mol Cell Cardiol* 12:781, 1980.

42. Lorell BH: Significance of diastolic dysfunction of the heart. *Annu Rev Med* 42:411, 1991.

43. Isoyama S, Apstein CS, Wexler L et al: Acute decrease in left ventricular diastolic chamber distensibility during simulated angina in isolated hearts, *Circ Res* 61:925, 1987.

44. Bricknell OL, Daries PS, Opie LH: A relationship between adenosine triphosphate, glycolysis and ischemic contracture in the isolated rat heart, *J Mol Cell Cardiol* 13:941, 1981.

45. Pouleur H: Diastolic dysfunction and myocardial energetics, *Eur Heart J* 11(Suppl):30, 1990.

46. Schaper J, Froede R, Hein S et al: Impairment of the myocardial ultrastructure and changes of the cytoskeleton in dilated cardiomyopathy, *Circulation* 83:504, 1991.

47. Limas CJ, Olivari MT, Goldenberg IF et al: Calcium uptake by sarcoplasmic reticulum in human dilated cardiomyopathy, *Cardiovasc Res* 21:601, 1987.

48. Feldman AM, Ray PE, Silan CM et al: Selective gene expression in failing human heart: quantification of steady-state levels of messenger RNA in endomyocardial biopsies using the polymerase chain reaction, *Circulation* 83:1866, 1991.

49. Maisel AS, Michel MC: Beta-adrenergic receptors in congestive heart failure: present knowledge and future directions, *Cardiology* 76:338, 1989.

50. Francis GS, Cohn JN: Heart failure: mechanisms of cardiac and vascular dysfunction and the rationale for pharmacologic intervention, *FASEB J* 4:3068, 1990.

51. Starling EH: In *The Linacre lecture on the law of the heart, given at Cambridge, 1915,* London, 1918 Longmans, Green.

52. Patterson WW, Starling EH: On mechanical factors which determine output of ventricles, *J Physiol* 48:357, 1914.

53. Harris P: Congestive heart failure: central role of the arterial blood pressure, *Br Heart J* 58:190, 1991.

54. Gioffre PA, Gaspardone A, Crea F: Can the Frank-Starling law be applied to the normal heart? *J Appl Cardiol* 5:275, 1991.

55. Robinson TF, Factor SM, Sonnenblick EH: The heart as a suction pump., *Sci Am* 254:62, 1986.

56. Chassaignac E: Dissertation sur la texture et le development des organes de la circulation sanguine, Paris, June 17, 1836. (quoted in Ebstein E: Die diastole des herzens, *Egreb Physiol* 3:123-194, 1904).

57. Ebstein E: Die diastole des herzens, *Ergeb Physiol* 3:123, 1904.

58. Bloom WL: Diastolic filling of the beating exised heart, *Am J Physiol* 187:H143, 1956.

59. Fragasso G, Davies GJ, Chierchia S et al: Relative roles of preload increase and coronary constriction in ergonovine-induced myocardial ischemia in stable angina pectoris, *Am J Cardiol* 60:238, 1987.

60. Katz LN: The role played by ventricular relaxation process in filling the ventricle, *Am J Physiol* 95:542, 1930.

61. Brecher GA, Kissen AT: Relation of negative intraventricular pressure to ventricular volume, *Cardiovasc Res* 5:157, 1957.

62. Suga H, Goto Y, Igarashi Y: Ventricular suction under zero source pressure for filling, *Am J Physiol* 251:H47, 1986.

63. Udelson JE, Bacharach SL, Cannon RO et al: Minimum left ventricular pressure during beta adrenergic stimulation in human subjects. Evidence for elastic recoil and diastolic suction in the normal heart, *Circulation* 82:1174, 1990.

64. Katz AM: The descending limb of the Starling curve and the failing heart, *Circulation* 32:871, 1965.

65. Monroe RG, Gamble WJ, LaFarge CG et al: Left ventricular performance at high end-diastolic pressures in isolated, perfused dog hearts, *Circ Res* 26:85, 1970.

66. Guyton AC: *The pumping ability of the heart as expressed by cardiac function curves*. In Guyton AC, Jones CE, Coleman TG, eds: *Circulatory physiology: cardiac output and its regulation*, Philadelphia, 1973, WB Saunders.

67. White HD, Norris RM, Brown MA et al: Left ventricular end-systolic volume as the major determinant of survival after recovery from myocardial infarction, *Circulation* 76:44, 1987.

68. Pfeffer MA, Pfeffer JM: Ventricular enlargement and reduced survival after myocardial infarction, *Circulation* 75(Suppl IV):IV-93, 1987.

69. Fuster V, Gersh BJ, Giuliani ER et al: The natural history of idiopathic dilated cardiomyopathy, *Am J Cardiol* 47:525, 1981.

70. Sokolow M, Perloff D: The prognosis of essential hypertension treated conservatively, *Circulation* 23:697, 1961.

71. Hammermeister KE, Chikos PM, Fisher L et al: Relationship of cardiothoracic ratio and plain film heart volume to late survival, *Circulation* 59:89, 1979.

72. Eaton LW, Weiss JL, Bulkley BH et al: Regional cardiac dilatation after acute myocardial infarction. Recognition by two-dimensional echocardiography, *N Engl J Med* 300:57, 1979.

73. Erlenbacher JA, Weiss JL, Weisfeldt ML et al: Early dilation of the infarct segment in acute transmural myocardial infarction: role of infarct expansion in acute left ventricular enlargement, *J Am Coll Cardiol* 4:201, 1984.

74. Mitchell GF, Lamas GA, Vaughan DE et al: Infarct expansion does not contribute to late left ventricular enlargement, *Circulation* 80(SupplII):II-589, 1989.

75. Lamas GA, Pfeffer MA: Left ventricular remodeling after acute myocardial infarction: clinical course and beneficial effects of angiotensin-converting enzyme inhibition, *Am Heart J* 121:1194, 1991.

76. Jacob R, Gulch RW: Functional significance of ventricular dilatation. Reconsideration of Linzbach's concept of chronic heart failure, *Basic Res Cardiol* 83:461, 1988.

77. Schlant RC, Sonnenblick EH: In Hurst JW, ed: *The heart, arteries and veins*, New York, 1986, McGraw-Hill.

78. Zelis R, Flaim SF, Liedtke AJ: Cardiocirculatory dynamics in the normal and failing heart, *Annu Rev Physiol* 43:455, 1981.

79. Hoffman JL: Transmural myocardial perfusion, *Prog Cardiovasc Dis* 29:429, 1987.

80. Krayenbuchl HP, Hess OM, Schneider J: Physiologic or pathologic hypertrophy, *Eur Heart J* 4(Suppl A):29, 1983.

81. Murphy ML: The pathology of the right heart in chronic hypertrophy and failure, *Cardiovasc Clin* 17:159, 1987.

82. Mulvaugh SL, Roberts R, Schneider MD: Cellular oncogenes in cardiovascular disease, *J Mol Cell Cardiol* 20:657, 1988.

83. Simpson PC: Proto-oncogenes and cardiac hypertrophy, *Annu Rev Physiol* 51:189, 1989.

84. Abboud FM, Heistad DD, Mark AL et al: Reflex control of the peripheral circulation, *Prog Cardiovasc Dis* 18:371, 1976.

85. Higgins CB, Vatner SF, Eckberg DL et al: Alterations in the baroreceptor reflex in conscious dogs with heart failure, *J Clin Invest* 51:715, 1982.

86. Creager MA, Hirsch AT, Dzau VJ et al: Baroreflex regulation of regional blood flow in congestive heart failure, *Am J Physiol* 258:H1409, 1990.

87. Chidsey CA, Braunwald E, Morrow AG: Catecholamine excretion and cardiac stress of norepinephrine in congestive heart failure, *Am J Med* 39:442, 1965.

88. Thomas JA, Marks BH: Plasma norepinephrine in congestive heart failure, *Am J Cardiol* 41:223, 1978.

89. Cohn JN: Abnormalities of peripheral sympathetic nervous system control in congestive heart failure, *Circulation* 82(Suppl I):I-59, 1990.

90. Cohn JN, Levine TB, Olivari MT et al: Plasma norepinephrine as a guide to prognosis in patients with congestive heart failure, *N Engl J Med* 311:819, 1984.

91. Hasking GJ, Esler MD, Jennings GL et al: Norepinephrine spillover to plasma in patients with congestive heart failure: evidence of increased overall and cardiorenal sympathetic nervous activity, *Circulation* 73:615, 1986.

92. Hasking GJ, Esler MD, Jennings GL et al: Norepinephrine spillover to plasma during steady-state supine bicycle exercise. Comparison of patients with congestive heart failure and normal subjects. *Circulation* 78:516, 1988.

93. Leimbach WN, Wallin BG, Victor RG et al: Direct evidence from intraneural recordings for increased central sympathetic outflow in patients with heart failure, *Circulation* 73:913, 1986.

94. Feldman MD, Copelas L, Gwathmey JK et al: Deficient production of cyclic AMP: pharmacologic evidence of an important cause of contractile dysfunction in patients with end-stage heart failure, *Circulation* 75:331, 1987.

95. Pfeffer JM, Pfeffer MA, Braunwald E: Influence of chronic captopril therapy on the infarcted left ventricle of the rat, *Circ Res* 57:84, 1985.

96. Sharpe N, Smith H, Murphy J et al: Treatment of patients with symptomless left ventricular dysfunction after myocardial infarction, *Lancet* 1:255, 1988.

97. Lamas GA, Pfeffer MA: Increased left ventricular volume following myocardial infarction in man, *Am Heart J* 111:30, 1986.

98. Ostman-Smith I: Cardiac sympathetic nerves as the final common pathway in the induction of adaptive cardiac hypertrophy, *Clin Sci* 1:265, 1981.

99. Starksen NF, Simpson PC, Bishopric N et al: Cardiac myocyte hypertrophy is associated with c-myc protooncogene expression, *Proc Natl Acad Sci* 83:8348, 1986.

100. Ikeda U, Tsuruya Y, Yaginuma T: Alpha-1-adrenergic stimulation is coupled to cardiac myocyte hypertrophy, *Am J Physiol* 260:H953, 1991.

101. Rona G, Chappel CI, Balazs T et al: An infarct-like myocardial lesion and other toxic manifestations produced by isoproterenol in the rat, *Arch Pathol* 67:443, 1959.

102. Fleckenstein A, Janke J, Doring HJ et al: Ca overload as the determinant factor in the production of catecholamine-induced myocardial lesions, *Rec Adv Stud Card Struct Met* 2:455, 1973.

103. Daly PA, Sole MJ: Myocardial catecholamines and the pathophysiology of heart failure, *Circulation* 82(Suppl I):I-35, 1990.

104. Lefkowitz RJ, Stadel JM, Cardon MG: Adenylate cyclase-coupled beta-adrenergic receptors: structure and mechanisms of activation and desensitization, *Annu Rev Biochem* 52:159, 1983.

105. Hirsch AT, Dzau VJ, Creager MA: Baroreceptor function in congestive heart failure: effect on neurohumeral activation and regional vascular resistance, *Circulation* 75(Suppl IV):IV-36, 1987.

106. Vogel JHK, Jacobwitz D, Chidsey CA: Distribution of norepinephrine in the failing bovine heart, *Circ Res* 24:71, 1969.

107. Bristow MR, Ginsburg R, Minobe W et al: Decreased catecholamine sensitivity and beta-adrenergic receptor density in failing human hearts, *N Engl J Med* 307:205, 1982.

108. Bristow MR, Ginsburg R, Umans V, et al: Beta 1 and beta 2 adrenergic-receptor subpopulations in nonfailing and failing human ventricular myocardium; coupling of both receptor subtypes to muscle contraction and selective beta 1 receptor down-regulation in heart failure, *Circ Res* 59:297, 1986.

109. Heillbrunn SM, Shah P, Bristow MR et al: Increased beta-receptor density and improved hemodynamic response to catecholamine stimulation during long-term metoprolol therapy in heart failure from dilated cardiomyopathy, *Circulation* 79:483, 1989.

110. Homcy CJ, Vatner SF, Vatner DE: Beta-adrenergic receptor regulation in the heart in pathophysiologic states: abnormal adrenergic responsiveness in cardiac disease. *Annu Rev Physiol* 53:137, 1991.

111. Gilman AG: G proteins: transducers of receptor-generated signals, *Annu Rev Biochem* 56:615, 1987.

112. Feldman AM, Cates AE, Veazey WB et al: Increase of the 40,000-mol wt pertussis toxin substrate (G protein) in the failing human heart, *J Clin Invest* 82:189, 1988.

113. Feldman AM, Cares AE, Bristow MR et al: Altered expression of alpha-subunits of G proteins in failing human hearts, *J Mol Cell Cardiol* 21:359, 1989.

114. Reid IA, Schrier RW, Earley LE: An effect of beta adrenergic stimulation on the release of renin, *J Clin Invest* 51:1861, 1972.

115. Eckberg DL, Drabinsky M, Braunwald E: Defective cardiac parasympathetic control in patients with heart disease, *N Engl J Med* 285:877, 1971.

116. Vatner SF, Higgins CB, Braunwald E: Sympathetic and parasympathetic components of reflex tachycardia induced by hypotension in conscious dogs with and without heart failure, *Cardiovasc Res* 8:153, 1974.

117. Condorelli M, Volpe M: Endocrine function of the heart in cardiac disease, *Acta Cardiol* 44:203, 1989.

118. Richards AM, Cleland JGF, Tonolo G et al: Plasma alpha natriuretic peptide in cardiac impairment, *Br Med J* 293:409, 1986.

119. Singer DRJ, Shore AC, Markandu ND et al: Atrial natriuretic peptide levels in treated congestive heart failure, *Lancet* 1:851, 1986.

120. Kortas C, Bichet DG, Rouleau JL et al: Vasopressin in congestive heart failure, *J Cardiovasc Pharmacol* 8(Suppl 7):S107, 1986.

121. Francis GS, Benedict C, Johnstone DE et al: Comparison of neuroendocrine activation in patients with left ventricular dysfunction with and without congestive heart failure, *Circulation* 82:1724, 1990.

122. Riegger GAJ, Liebau G, Kochsiek K: Antidiuretic hormone in congestive heart failure, *Am J Med* 72:49, 1982.

123. Liard JF: Cardiovascular effects of vasopressin: some recent aspects, *J Cardiovasc Pharmacol* 8(Suppl 7):S61, 1986.

124. Macho P, Perez R, Huidobro-Toro JP et al: Neuropeptide Y (NPY): a coronary vasoconstrictor and potentiator of catecholamine-induced vasoconstriction, *Eur J Pharmacol* 167:67, 1989.

125. Corr LA, Aberdeen JA, Milner P et al: Sympathetic and non-sympathetic neuropeptide Y-containing nerves in the rat myocardium and coronary arteries, *Cardiovasc Res* 66:1602, 1990.

126. Zukowska-Grojec Z, Marks ES, Haas M: Neuropeptide Y is a potent vasoconstrictor and cardiodepressant in rat, *Am J Physiol* 251:H1234, 1987.

127. Wahlestedt C, Edvinsson E, Ekblad E et al: Neuropeptide Y potentiates noradrenaline-evoked vasoconstriction: mode of action, *J Pharmacol Exp Ther* 234:735, 1985.

128. Maisel AS, Scott NA, Motulsky HJ et al: Elevation of plasma neuropeptide Y levels in congestive heart failure, *Am J Med* 86:43, 1989.

129. Sigrist S, Franco-Cereceda A, Muff R et al: Specific receptor and cardiovascular effects of calcitonin gene-related peptide, *Endocrinology* 119:381, 1986.

130. Shekhar YC, Anand IS, Sarma R et al: Effects of prolonged infusion of human alpha calcitonin gene-related peptide on hemodynamics, renal blood flow and hormone levels in congestive heart failure, *Am J Cardiol* 67:732, 1991.

131. Lerman A, Hildebrand FL, Margulies KB et al: Endothelin: A new cardiovascular regulatory peptide, *Mayo Clin Proc* 1990.

132. Margulies KB, Hildebrand FLJ, Lerman A et al: Increased endothelin in experimental heart failure, *Circulation* 82:2226, 1990.

133. SOLVD Investigators: Effect of enalapril on survival in patients with reduced left ventricular ejection fractions and congestive heart failure, *N Engl J Med* 325:293, 1991.

134. Dzau VJ: Renal and circulatory mechanisms in congestive heart failure, *Kidney Int* 31:1402, 1987.

135. Merrill AJ, Morrison JL, Brannon ES: Concentration of renin in renal venous blood in patients with heart failure, *Am J Med* 1:468, 1946.

136. McDonald KM, Linas SL, Schrier RW: *Disorders of the renin-angiotensin-aldosterone system.* In Schrier RW, ed: *Renal and electrolyte disorders,* Boston, 1980, Little, Brown.

137. Peach MJ: Renin-angiotensin system: biochemistry and mechanisms of action, *Physiol Rev* 57:131, 1977.

138. Kastner PR, Hall JE, Guyton AC: Control of glomerular filtration rate: role of intrarenally formed angiotensin II, *Am J Physiol* 246:F897, 1991.

139. Hirsh AT, Pinto YM, Schunkert H et al: Potential role of the tissue renin-angiotensin system in the pathphysiology of congestive heart failure, *Am J Cardiol* 66:22D, 1990.

140. Blantz RC, Konnen KS, Tucker BJ: Angiotensin II effects upon the glomerular microcirculation and ultrafiltration coefficient of the rat, *J Clin Invest* 57:419, 1976.

141. Schuster VL, Kokko JP, Jacobsen HR: Angiotensin II directly stimulates sodium transport in rabbit proximal convoluted tubules, *J Clin Invest* 73:507, 1984.

142. Gimbrone RW, Alexander RW: Angiotensin II stimulation of prostaglandin production in cultured human vascular endothelium, *Science* 189:219, 1975.

143. Yamaguchi K, Nishimura H: Angiotensin II-induced relaxation of fowl aorta, *Am J Physiol* 255:R591, 1988.

144. Brooks VL, Keil LC, Reid IA: Role of the renin-angiotensin system in the control of vasopressin secretion in conscious dogs, *Circ Res* 58:829, 1986.

145. Itoh H, Nakao K, Tamada T et al: Brain renin-angiotensin. Central control of secretion of atrial natriuretic factor from the heart, *Hypertension* 11(Suppl 1):1-57, 1988.

146. Malik KJ, Nasjletti A: Facilitation of adrenergic transmission by locally generated angiotensin II in rat mesenteric arteries, *Circ Res* 38:36, 1976.

147. Kawasaki K, Cline WH Jr., Su C: Involvement of the renin-angiotensin system in beta adrenergic receptor mediated facilitation of vascular neurotransmission in spontaneously hypertensive rats, *J Pharmacol Exp Ther* 231:23, 1984.

148. Roth RH: Action of angiotensin on adrenergic nerve endings: enhancement of norepinephrine biosynthesis, *Fed Proc* 31:1358, 1972.

149. Khairellah PA: Action of angiotensin on sympathetic nerve endings. Inhibition of norepinephrine uptake, *Fed Proc* 31:1351, 1972.

150. Field LS, McGowen RA, Dickenson DP et al: Tissue and gene specificity of mouse renin expression, *Hypertension* 6:597, 1984.

151. Lynch KR, Simnad VT, Ben-Ari VT, et al: Localization of preangiotensin messenger RNA sequences in rat brain. *Hypertension* 8:540, 1986.

152. Hirsch AT, Pinto YM, Schunkert H et al: Potential role of the tissue renin-angiotensin system in the pathophysiology of congestive heart failure, *Am J Cardiol* 66:22D, 1990.

153. Watkins LJ, Burton JA, Haber E et al: The renin-aldosterone system in congestive heart failure in conscious dogs, *J Clin Invest* 57:1606, 1976.

154. Dzau VJ, Collucci WS, Hollenberg NK et al: Relation of renin-angiotensin-aldosterone system to clinical state in congestive heart failure, *Circulation* 63:645, 1981.

155. Ichikawa I, Pfeffer JM, Pfeffer MA, et al: Role of angiotensin II in the altered renal function of congestive heart failure, *Circ Res* 55:669, 1984.

156. Skorecki KL, Brenner BM: Body fluid homeostasis in congestive heart failure and cirrhosis with ascites, *Am J Med* 72:323, 1982.

157. Eiskjaer H, Bagger JP, Danielesen H et al: Mechanisms of sodium retention in heart failure: relation to the renin-angiotensin-aldosterone system, *Am J Physiol* 260:F883, 1991.

158. Rouse D, Williams S, Suki W: Clonidine inhibits fluid absorption in the rabbit proximal tubules, *Kidney Int* 38:80, 1990.

159. DiBona G: Neural control of renal function: cardiovascular implications, *Hypertension* 13:539, 1989.

160. Kon V, Yared A, Ichikawa I: Role of renal sympathetic nerves in mediating hypoperfusion of renal cortical microcirculation in experimental congestive heart failure and acute extracellular fluid volume depletion, *J Clin Invest* 76:1913, 1985.

161. Ritz E, Fliser D: The kidney in congestive heart failure, *Eur Heart J* 12(Suppl C):14, 1991.

162. Murray JF: The lungs and heart failure, *Hosp Pract* 70:55, 1985.

163. Staub NC: Pulmonary edema, *Phys Rev* 54:679, 1974.

164. Franciosa JA, Cohn JN: Effect of isosorbide dinitrate on response to submaximal and maximal exercise in patients with congestive heart failure, *Am J Cardiol* 43:1009, 1979.

165. Jennings GL, Elser MD: Circulatory regulation at rest and exercise and the functional assessment of patients with congestive heart failure, *Circulation* 81(Suppl II):II-5, 1990.

166. Kumada T, Himura Y, Iwata T: Liver function in congestive heart failure: abnormal elevation of serum hepatic enzymes and hepatic venous flow velocity, *Jpn Circ J* 53:165, 1989.

167. Shibayama Y: On the pathogenesis of hepatic dysfunction and necrosis following acute circulatory failure, *Pathol Res Pract* 182:817, 1987.

168. Shibayama Y: The role of hepatic venous congestion and endotoxemia in the production of fulminant hepatic failure secondary to congestive heart failure, *J Pathol* 151:133, 1987.

169. Klatt EC, Koss MN, Young TS: Hepatic hyaline globules associated with passive congestion, *Arch Pathol Lab Med* 112:510, 1988.

170. Abe K, Shimoda T, Shikata T: Cytoplasmic blood plasma inclusions of canine hepatocytes: demonstration by immunoperoxidase labelling method, *Am J Vet Res* 41:1507, 1980.

171. Kannel W: Epidemiological aspects of heart failure, *Cardiol Clinics* 7:1, 1989.

172. McKee PA, Castelli WP, McNamara PM et al: The natural history of congestive heart failure: the Framingham study, *N Engl J Med* 26:1441, 1971.

172a. Schocken DD, Arrieta MI, Leaverton PE et al: Prevalence and mortality rate of congestive heart failure in the United States, *J Am Coll Cardiol* 20:301, 1992.

173. Smith WM: Epidemiology of congestive heart failure, *Am J Cardiol* 55:3A, 1985.

174. Kannel WB, Hjortland M, Castelli WP: Role of diabetes in congestive heart failure: the Framingham study, *Am J Cardiol* 34:29, 1974.

175. Zarich SW, Nesto RW: Diabetic cardiomyopathy, *Am Heart J* 118 (5 Part 1):1000, 1989.

176. Kannel WB, Savage D, Castelli WP: *Cardiac failure in the Framingham Study: twenty year follow-up.* In Braunwald E, ed: *Congestive heart failure: current research and clinical applications,* New York, 1982, Grune & Stratton.

177. Eriksson H, Svardsudd K, Larsson B et al: Risk factors for heart failure in the general population: the study of men born in 1913, *Eur Heart J* 10:647, 1989.

Chapter 17

DISORDERS OF BLOOD VESSELS

Robert J. Siegel

Vasculitis
    Predominantly large to medium vessels
        Giant cell (temporal) arteritis
        Takayasu arteritis
    Predominantly medium and small vessels
        Polyartertis nodosa group
        Wegener granulomatosis
        Kawasaki disease
        Thromboangiitis obliterans (Buerger disease)
        Angiocentric immunoproliferative lesions
        Behçet disease
        Associated with collagen vascular disorders
    Predominantly small vessels
Aneurysms
    Atherosclerotic aneurysms
    Aortic dissection
    Infectious aneurysms
    Vasculitic aneurysms
    Berry aneurysms
Fibromuscular dysplasia
Disorders of veins
    Varicose veins
    Thrombophlebitis
    Veno-occlusive disease
Vascular malformations
Vascular tumors
    Benign vascular tumors
    Neoplasms of intermediate malignancy
    Malignant vascular neoplasms
Disorders of lymphatics
    Lymphedema and lymphangiectasia
    Lymphangitis
    Miscellaneous vascular disorders
    Idiopathic arterial calcification of infancy
    Human Immunodeficiency Virus-related vascular disease
    Cardiac Transplant Arteriosclerosis
    Progressive arterial occlusive disease (Kohlmeier-Degos)
    Others

Hardly any disease can be named that does not affect the vasculature in some way. The intent of this chapter, however, is to discuss the major disorders that primarily represent inflammatory, degenerative, developmental, or neoplastic processes of vascular origin. Although many of these disorders are idiopathic, investigations into their pathogenesis and pathophysiology have yielded important insights into basic disease mechanisms. An emphasis on this aspect of vascular biology will be attempted throughout.

VASCULITIS

Simply defined, *vasculitis* refers to inflammation of blood vessels. In practice, the term conjures up a confusing array of conditions of uncertain pathogenesis and overlapping clinical and pathologic features. Although blood vessels may be secondarily affected by inflammation of adjacent tissue, the entities considered in this section are the primary vasculitides in which vascular inflammation is not readily attributable to any local tissue injury.

The vasculitides differ from each other in the size of vessels involved, organ systems affected, type of inflammatory infiltrate, age and sex distribution of patients, course and prognosis, implicated pathogenic mechanisms, and treatment. In spite of this diversity of clinical and pathologic features, the vasculitis syndromes have eluded a completely satisfactory classification scheme. Perhaps the best-known system, based primarily on clinical features, was proposed by Fauci.[1] Various morphology-based classification schemes also have been offered.[2,3] Because the clinical vasculitic syndromes tend to segregate by size of vessel involved, this parameter serves as a rational basis for classification. A modified version of such a classifica-

Vasculitis syndromes, classified by size of vessel involved

I. Predominantyly large to medium (aorta and major branches)
   A. Syphilitic arteritis
   B. Giant cell (temporal) arteritis
   C. Takayasu arteritis
II. Predominantly medium to small
   A. Polyarteritis nodosa group of systemic necrotizing vasculitis
      1. Polyarteritis nodosa
      2. Churg-Strauss syndrome
      3. Overlap syndrome
   B. Wegener granulomatosis
   C. Kawasaki disease
   D. Thromboangiitis obliterans (Buerger disease)
   E. Angiocentric immunoproliferative lesions
   F. Behçet disease
   G. Vasculitis associated with collagen vascular disorders
III. Predominantly small (arterioles, venules, capillaries)
   A. Hypersensitivity (leukocytoclastic) vasculitis associated with drugs, malignancy, cryoglobulinemia, collagen vascular disorders, serum sickness
   B. Henoch-Schonlein purpura

Table 17-1. Probable immunologic mechanisms in selected vasculitic syndromes

Vasculitis	Mechanism				
	IC	CMI	ANCA:MPO	ANCA:SP	CEA
Leukocytoclastic	+				
PAN group	+	+	+		
WG		+		+	
GCA		+			
TA		+			
KD	+	+			+

Abbreviations: ANCA:MPO: antineutrophil cytoplasmic antibodies, myeloperoxidase activity; ANCA:SP: antineutrophil cytoplasmic antibodies, serine protease activity; CEA: cytotoxic antiendothelial antibodies; CMI: cell-mediated immunity; GCA: giant cell (temporal) arteritis; KD: Kawasaki disease; PAN group: polyarteritis nodosa, Churg-Strauss syndrome, and overlap syndrome; TA: Takayasu arteritis; WG: Wegener granulomatosis.
Note: The mechanisms are not mutually exclusive; see text for details.

tion published by Lie[3] appears below (see Box).

It seems that classification based on pathogenic mechanism would be desirable; although this has been attempted,[4,5] the current state of knowledge of these mechanisms is still incomplete. A summary of the most likely mechanisms involved in selected vasculitic syndromes is given in Table 17-1; the mechanisms are considered in more detail in the relevant portions of the text. Classification by etiologic agent is not particularly helpful because putative agents are largely unknown, and even when one is identified, a single agent (e.g., hepatitis B virus) may cause vasculitis with different clinical and pathologic features in different patients.

In this chapter the author does not attempt to review exhaustively every known vasculitic syndrome, but rather to give a brief account of the clinical and pathologic features of the best-described syndromes, with an emphasis on current concepts of pathophysiology and pathogenesis of these largely idiopathic disorders.

Predominantly large to medium vessels

Included in this group are blood vessels the size of the aorta and its major muscular arterial branches. Although *syphilitic aortitis* is placed in this category, it is discussed in the section on aneurysms.

Giant cell (temporal) arteritis

Clinical features. Giant cell (temporal) arteritis (GCA) is a vasculitis that affects individuals usually 50 years of age or older. The designations *temporal* or *cranial* have been applied, indicating a predilection for muscular arteries of the head and neck. Headache is the most common symptom, but jaw claudication, scalp tenderness, facial pain, and visual disturbances are other local manifestations of the disease.[6] Systemic manifestations include fever, constitutional symptoms, and polymyalgia rheumatica (PR), a syndrome of aching and stiffness in proximal joints that occurs in one third to one half of patients.[7,8] Marked elevation of the erythrocyte sedimentation rate is an almost universal finding. Blindness is an important complication, and is preventable with corticosteroid therapy.

GCA is unique among the vasculitides affecting larger vessels in that the artery commonly involved (temporal) is readily accessible to biopsy. Although a negative biopsy does not exclude the diagnosis, biopsy is an important means of confirming the diagnosis and differentiating GCA from other disorders that may affect the temporal artery. Palpable nodular abnormalities, if present, are helpful in directing the surgeon to the appropriate area for biopsy.

Morphologic findings. The histopathologic changes encompass three patterns of vascular injury: classic (typical, granulomatous) arteritis; atypical (nongranulomatous) arteritis; and predominantly intimal hyperplasia with little active inflammation.[3] The typical form is characterized by the presence of an inflammatory infiltrate composed of lymphocytes, plasma cells, mononuclear histiocytes, and histiocytic multinucleated giant cells.

This infiltrate is centered on the internal elastic lamina, which typically becomes disrupted and fragmented (Fig. 17-1). The inflammation usually is segmental and mostly involves the inner media and intima; however, it may be

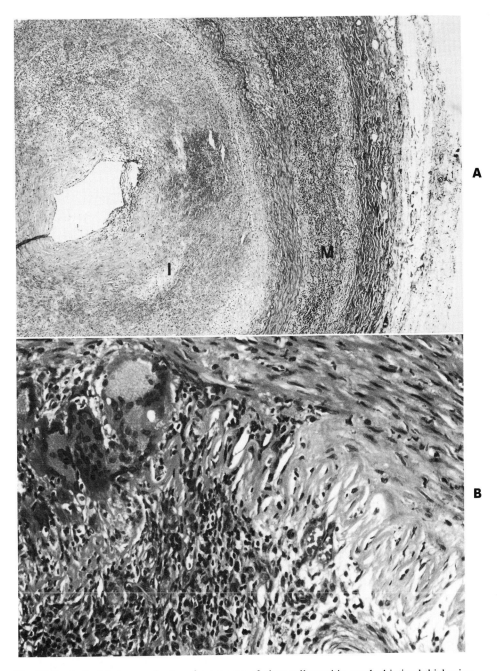

Fig. 17-1. A, In this temporal artery from a case of giant cell arteritis, marked intimal thickening *(I)* is present, and an infiltrate of mononuclear cells partly obscures the media *(M)*. Significant luminal narrowing is noted. **B,** This high power view demonstrates lymphocytes and multinucleated histiocytic giant cells (upper left) surrounding the internal elastic lamina. The intimal infiltrate is predominantly lymphocytic (lower left and center).

circumferential and transmural. The giant cells that lend their name to the condition may be difficult to find, requiring the examination of multiple sections, or may be absent, leading to the designation of *atypical* or *nongranulomatous* arteritis. Intimal proliferation commonly is present in all forms of GCA, and is an important cause of luminal obstruction, leading to local ischemia and probably accounting for the local complications of the disease (Fig. 17-1). In some cases of GCA, intimal proliferation may be the predominant finding. Some interpret this finding, together with intimal and medial fibrosis and fragmentation of internal elastic lamina, to represent evidence of healed arteritis.[9]

Etiology and pathogenesis. Any comprehensive theory of pathogenesis of GCA would have to take into account a number of disparate observations, such as genetic predisposition (association with HLA DR4[10,11]), racial predilection (GCA is less common in nonCaucasians[6]), predominance of CD4+ T-lymphocytes and HLA DR+ macrophages demonstrated by immunohistochemical analysis of tissue sections,[12-14] occasional presence of circulating immune complexes,[15] and the frequent finding of depletion and activation of CD8+ lymphocytes in peripheral blood.[16,17]

Such a comprehensive theory does not exist, and although the etiology of GCA remains unknown, substantial evidence points to a cell-mediated immune reaction. In the classic view of cell-mediated immunity leading to granuloma formation, T-cells are activated by the presence of specific antigen in association with HLA DR presented by macrophages.[18] Cytokines released by lymphocytes, macrophages, and other cells then lead to proliferation of immunocompetent cells. In particular, interleukin-1 (IL-1) released by activated macrophages induces B-cell proliferation and antibody production, as well as T-cell production of other lymphokines such as interleukin-2 (IL-2).[18] IL-2 receptors appear on activated T-cells, and the binding of IL-2 to these receptors leads to clonal expansion of T-cells that have already responded to a specific antigenic stimulus, thus amplifying the immune response.[19] Further amplification occurs because gamma-interferon released by activated T-cells increases class II histocompatibility antigen (HLA DR) expression on macrophages, thus facilitating presentation of antigen to other T-cells.[18] The presence of activated macrophages (as indicated by HLA DR positivity) and helper/inducer T-cells in lesions of GCA is consistent with the presence of such a process. The release of hydrolytic enzymes from macrophages and other cells also is enhanced by inflammatory mediators such as alpha-interferon and other cytokines, causing local tissue damage. Finally, the release of IL-1 and tumor necrosis factor/cachectin in inflammation is associated with systemic symptoms, fever, and the acute phase response, which is appreciated clinically as an elevated ESR. Interleukin-6 (IL-6), an important mediator of the hepatic synthesis of

acute phase reactants, also is released in inflammation, and recently has been observed to be elevated in patients with active PR or GCA.[20] Successful treatment produced a decline in IL-6 activity in many of these patients.[20]

The consistent finding of destruction of the internal elastic lamina in GCA has led to speculation that this material can in some way become the antigenic stimulus for the reaction described above in genetically predisposed individuals. An increased prevalence of HLA DR4 has been noted in patients with GCA; it appears that this increase is limited to the subset of GCA patients who also have polymyalgia rheumatica.[10,11] HLA DR4 positivity also is associated with other autoimmune diseases, especially rheumatoid arthritis, in which cell-mediated immunity is thought to play a pathogenic role.[21] Interestingly, the expression of DR4 in RA patients is particularly associated with those having vasculitic complications,[22] and DR4 expression also has been noted in Takayasu arteritis.[23]

While a cell-mediated immune mechanism explains many of the findings in GCA, some remain unexplained, such as the presence of immunoglobulin and complement in the arterial lesions[24] and circulating immune complexes in the serum of some patients.[15] The observation of increased cytotoxic activity directed against human endothelial cells in GCA patients' serum[25] suggests the potential role of endothelial damage as a primary event, allowing for immune complex localization in the arterial wall.[25] Several investigators have noted the presence of anticardiolipin antibodies in GCA.[26,27] These antibodies are seen in a variety of conditions characterized by microvascular damage and thrombosis, including systemic lupus erythematosus (SLE) and other rheumatic disorders.[28,29] Their association with severe vascular injury in GCA may indicate a primary pathogenic role,[27] but it also could be a manifestation of vascular damage.[28]

The low circulating number of CD8+ (suppressor/inducer) T-cells is an unexplained but consistent finding in GCA.[16] One study suggests that in patients with suspected GCA who have negative or inconclusive biopsies, CD8 count may help differentiate those with probable GCA from those who probably do not have GCA.[17]

Pathophysiology. The pathophysiologic derangements in GCA are somewhat easier to understand than the etiology. Whatever the cause of the vascular inflammation, its presence leads to blood vessel damage and luminal compromise with resulting local ischemic effects. Extracranial arteries occasionally are involved, and GCA has been recognized as a cause of aortic arch arteritis in elderly individuals.[30] The possibility of aortic regurgitation as a late complication of aortic root involvement has been noted.[31]

Takayasu arteritis. Takayasu arteritis (TA) is credited with more synonyms (more than two dozen by one account[32]) than almost any other condition, partly because of protean manifestations. The disease is an inflammatory fibrosing arteritis affecting predominantly the aorta and its major branches, and occurring predominantly in young women (80% to more than 90% of cases[33-35]). Although it was originally described and studied in Japan, where it still is more common, TA has a worldwide distribution.[32,33]

Clinical features. Clinically, the onset of symptoms occurs before 30 years of age in most patients.[34,35] In around one half of cases, the presentation is that of an acute inflammatory condition with fever, joint symptoms, and elevated erythrocyte sedimentation rate.[34] Cardiovascular and neurologic manifestations that may be present initially or develop subsequently include heart failure, systemic arterial hypertension, palpitations, bruits, headaches, and syncope.[34] Fundoscopic examination reveals vascular abnormalities in a substantial number of patients. Pulmonary artery involvement is common but generally does not lead to clinical problems related to pulmonary arterial flow. Diminished pulses were noted in 96% of patients in one study.[34] The acute phase is followed by a long chronic phase in which disease flare-ups may occur.[34]

TA has been classified into several pathologic types depending on the distribution of arteries affected. In the majority of cases, some involvement of the aortic arch branches is noted, with or without disease of the arch itself.[33,34] Cases limited to the abdominal aorta or pulmonary arteries are described, and in many cases the aorta and its major branches are extensively involved.[33,34]

Morphologic findings. Histologic findings in affected arteries include intimal, medial, and adventitial changes. The intima shows a varying degree of fibrocellular prolif-

eration and accumulation of extracellular material; usually, an inflammatory infiltrate is not observed to any significant extent.[33,36] Intimal proliferation causing luminal narrowing is seen in advanced lesions from longstanding cases.[3]

In active lesions, inflammation is centered within the media and may be granulomatous or nongranulomatous. Nasu[33] has proposed the progression from a granulomatous stage to one characterized by a lymphoplasmacytic infiltrate accompanied by proliferating blood vessels and fibrous tissue, to a fibrotic or cicatricial stage (Fig. 17-2).[33] In the adventitia, one observes a concentric fibrosis and often obliterative changes in the vasa vasorum.[33] In some cases of inflammatory aortitis, the histopathologic changes are nondiagnostic, and the designation *nonspecific aortitis* is applied (Fig. 17-3). In such cases, clinical and radiographic features can be helpful in making a more secure diagnosis of TA.

Pathophysiology. A combination of cellular processes in all three layers of the vessel conspire to alter the normal architecture. The pathophysiology of TA involves two major consequences of this inflammatory and fibrosing process: reduction of luminal diameter and aneurysm formation. The former is responsible for the pulselessness for which TA is best known. The adverse effects of such luminal compromise obviously depend on the segment of artery affected and the degree of narrowing, and are mitigated to the extent that collateral circulation has been established. Cerebral and visual manifestations result from ischemia in the distribution of relevant arteries involved. Ischemic heart disease caused by either narrowing of coro-

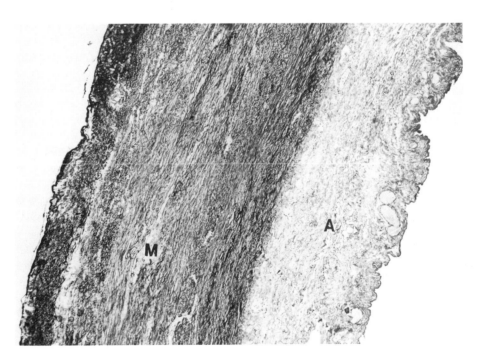

Fig. 17-2. Late noninflammatory stage of Takayasu arteritis. There is marked medial disorganization *(M)*, adventitial fibrous thickening *(A)*, and mild intimal hyperplasia.

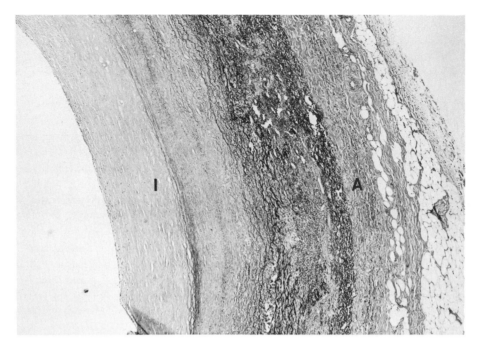

Fig. 17-3. In a case of nonspecific aortitis, a mononuclear infiltrate is seen within a disorganized media. The infiltrate is sparse in the adventitia *(A)*. Marked intimal thickening is seen *(I)*.

nary ostia or involvement of coronary arteries themselves is well described.[36,37] When TA involves the renal arteries, hypertension often results, as it does in fibromuscular dysplasia, and TA must be considered in the differential diagnosis of renovascular hypertension in young women. Systemic hypertension has been noted in 50% to 88% of patients with TA;[34-36] renal or abdominal aortic stenosis probably accounts for much of this high prevalence. Other possible causes include decreased aortic elasticity and aortic valvular insufficiency.[35]

Aneurysm formation in TA results from weakening of the vascular wall, and was encountered in 32% of 113 patients studied angiographically.[38] The ascending aorta was the most common site, and involvement of the aortic valve ring often led to aortic insufficiency. These aneurysms occasionally rupture.

Pathogenesis. The pathogenesis of TA is unknown, but three factors have received the most attention as potentially important in this regard: a relationship to tuberculosis (TB), genetic influences, and immunologic mechanisms. Because of the presence of granulomatous inflammation with Langhans-type giant cells in many cases of TA, and the frequent coexistence of TA with pulmonary or extrapulmonary TB, this organism naturally has been suspected of playing a role in the arteritis. Numerous investigators have addressed this question. In summarizing these studies, Pantell et al[32] found a reported range of tuberculin positivity of 85% to 100%, and evidence of active TB in 21% to 70%. A high endemic prevalence of TB in the reporting countries should be noted; even so, rates of active

TB in TA patients were many times more than expected. The absence of mycobacterial organisms in arteritic lesions in these patients, and the lack of response to antituberculous therapy[39] suggest that hypersensitivity to the organism, rather than direct mycobacterial invasion, must be considered as one potential pathogenic mechanism.

Geographic distribution of TA, with a high prevalence in Japan and Korea, suggests that genetic factors are probably important in pathogenesis. Several authors have examined the frequency of various HLA antigens in TA patients. In Japanese patients, associations with HLA-Bw52,[40,41] HLA-DR2,[41,42] HLA-A10 and HLA-B5[43] have been noted, whereas in a study from the National Institutes of Health including predominantly nonAsian individuals, HLA-DR4 was most closely associated.[44] Interestingly, those authors cited a study linking HLA-DR4 to the immune response of T-cells in vitro.[45] As mentioned during the discussion of GCA, increased prevalence of HLA-DR4 also has been noted in patients with that type of arteritis.

Because of rheumatic-type complaints in many TA patients, the relationship between TA and various autoimmune and collagen vascular disorders (rheumatoid arthritis, systemic lupus erythematosus, ankylosing spondylitis, and rheumatic fever) has been examined. Although the mechanism has not been clarified, it can be stated that immunopathogenic mechanisms probably are important in TA. In view of the lack of fibrinoid necrosis or infiltrate of neutrophils in arteritic lesions, it is not surprising that immune complexes have not been implicated in pathogenesis. However, increased serum immunoglobulins and the presence of antiaorta antibodies[34,39] indicate that humoral immune mechanisms cannot be dismissed. Alternatively, these antibodies may represent an epiphenomenon, a result rather than cause of aortic wall damage.

Cellular immune mechanisms are likely to be more intimately involved in TA. An immunofluorescence study in one patient demonstrated that the overwhelming number of infiltrating lymphocytes were T-cells of suppressor/cytotoxic phenotype (CD8-positive), and that peripheral blood lymphocytes, but not serum, from this patient showed in vitro cytotoxicity against endothelial cells.[46] Interestingly, low circulating CD8 cells, as noted in this patient, also characterizes GCA, in which cellular immune mechanisms are implicated in pathogenesis.[16]

Predominantly medium and small vessels

Polyarteritis nodosa group. Fauci et al[1] pointed out that within the large group of patients with systemic necrotizing vasculitis, some had clinical and pathologic manifestations of the relatively well-defined syndromes *polyarteritis nodosa* (PAN) and *Churg-Strauss syndrome* (CSS), whereas others had overlapping features, thus defying classification. He designated this latter entity the *overlap syndrome* and combined all three disorders into the *polyarteritis nodosa group of systemic necrotizing vasculitis*. In the following discussion, classic PAN and CSS will be described, but it should be borne in mind that cases sharing some features of both do occur.

Polyarteritis nodosa

CLINICAL FEATURES. Polyarteritis nodosa (PAN) is a systemic necrotizing vasculitis with a sufficiently distinctive set of clinical and pathologic features to warrant consideration as a clinicopathologic entity. It occurs most commonly in adults, especially after the fourth decade, and is more common in men than women. Signs and symptoms are referable either to the widespread vascular inflammation or to local complications resulting from compromise of vascular supply.[47] Nonspecific generalized complaints (fever, weight loss, malaise) often precede more localized manifestations of the disease.[47] Most patients manifest renal involvement, and hypertension, proteinuria, and hematuria are common.[1,47] Peripheral neuropathy and especially mononeuritis multiplex are characteristic neurologic findings, and central nervous system involvement in the form of encephalitis, focal neurologic defects, or seizures has been described.[48] Gastrointestinal vasculitis may cause nonspecific abdominal complaints or catastrophic gut injury in the form of gastrointestinal bleeding or bowel infarction with a high mortality.[49] The incidence of skin involvement varies with criteria used for the diagnosis of PAN; it was reported in 58% of patients in a study that did not attempt to separate PAN from hypersensitivity (small-vessel, leukocytoclastic) vasculitis.[49] An estimate of 5% to 15% probably is more accurate.[2] Allergic history, eosinophilia, and lung or splenic involvement are not characteristic of classic PAN, although difficulties in separating PAN from other systemic necrotizing vasculitides accounts for the variable incidence cited for these features.[1]

Laboratory evaluation of patients with PAN reveals nonspecific indicators of inflammation (e.g., elevated erythrocyte sedimentation rate or leukocytosis), and frequently evidence of renal dysfunction. Angiographic demonstration of multiple aneurysms of medium arteries, especially in those in the kidney and liver but also in vessels of other visceral organs, is an important clue to the diagnosis.[1]

MORPHOLOGIC FINDINGS. Pathologically, affected vessels are small and medium muscular arteries, with only occasional venous involvement. A predilection for branching sites has been noted. Fibrinoid necrosis, which refers to a brightly eosinophilic appearance on hematoxylin and eosin-stained sections, is characteristic of active lesions, and typically a transmural mixed inflammatory reaction infiltrates in and around the vessel wall (Fig. 17-4). "Blow-out" aneurysms form in vascular segments weakened by this process. Intimal proliferation is encountered in the healing or subacute phase, and "healed" blood vessels may have significant fibroobliterative sclerosis (Fig. 17-5). Mononuclear inflammatory cells replace neutrophils in healing and healed stages.[50]

A remarkable focal involvement characterizes the vascular lesions of PAN, in terms of both spatial and temporal distribution. A single blood vessel may show active fibrinoid necrosis in one area and a normal appearance in an adjacent serial section.[51] Palpable nodularity of blood vessels, which led to the designation *nodosa,* reflects this segmental involvement. The presence at the same time of active, healing, and healed lesions also is characteristic.

For the clinical diagnosis of PAN, histologic confirmation may be obtained from rectal, sural nerve, skeletal muscle, kidney, liver, or testicular biopsy; skin biopsy is less helpful because only small vessels usually are present, and because dermal vasculitis does not necessarily imply systemic disease.[50]

Two terms that have led to some confusion regarding PAN as a distinct entity are *infantile polyarteritis* and *microscopic polyarteritis*. The former can be considered primarily as a synonym for Kawasaki disease.[52] Although PAN of the usual type can occur in children, the marked predilection for coronary artery involvement, as well as other features of Kawasaki disease, differ substantially from typical PAN. "Microscopic polyarteritis" refers to a renal-limited variant in which primary crescentic and nonnecrotizing glomerulonephritis is believed to represent expression of small-vessel (glomerular capillary) vasculitis in the kidney.[53]

PATHOGENESIS. The pathogenesis of PAN almost certainly involves an immunologic mechanism, although over the years the relationship between hepatitis, hepatitis B surface antigen (HBsAg), immune complexes, and pol-

Text continued on p. 525.

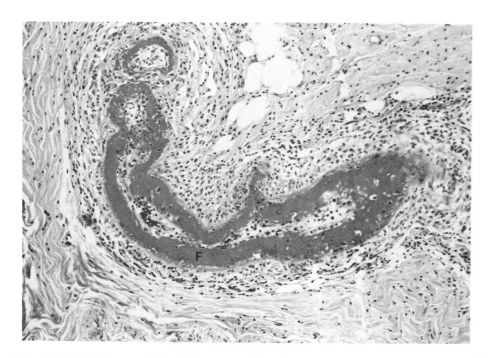

Fig. 17-4. Fibrinoid necrosis *(F)* of the type seen in active lesions of polyarteritis nodosa extensively involves a small muscular artery, which also demonstrates a transmural infiltrate of mixed inflammatory cells.

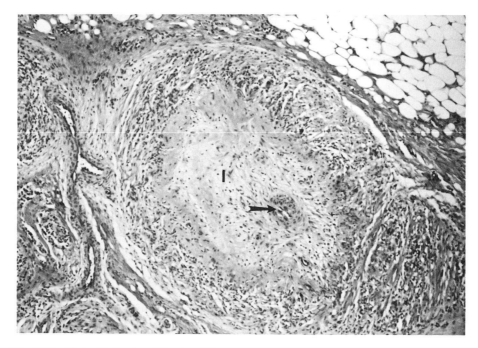

Fig. 17-5. Marked intimal proliferation *(I)* in a muscular artery has reduced the lumen to pinpoint size *(arrow)* in a "healing" lesion of polyarteritis nodosa. Inflammatory cells still are present in all layers of the vessel wall.

yarteritis has remained elusive. Hepatitis B surface antigenemia has been noted in one third to over half of patients with PAN,[54] and HBsAg, immunoglobulin, and complement have been identified in arterial lesions of such patients.[55] No clear relationship between the presence of circulating HBsAg-containing complexes and vasculitis has been found.[56] However, the coexistence of HBsAg and antihepatitis B surface antigen (HBsAb) or aggregated viral particles identified by electron microscopy in patients with active vasculitis suggests a pathogenic role for these immune complexes.[54] It may be that a particular size, amount, or antigen/antibody proportion is necessary to induce immunologic injury.[54]

Besides HBsAg, other associations with PAN have included various infectious agents, drugs, autoimmune disorders, and malignancies.[47] Several cases of PAN have appeared either following[57] or preceding[58] the diagnosis of hairy cell leukemia. Impaired reticuloendothelial clearance of antigen caused by massive splenic infiltration of hairy cells was offered as a possible explanation for this association.[57]

Vasculitic syndromes resembling those encountered in humans are difficult to induce in experimental animals. However, a strain of mice (SL/Ni) spontaneously develops a necrotizing arteritis that is histologically similar to PAN.[59] The findings of budding murine leukemia viral particles from medial smooth muscle cells, and binding of IgG and C3 to these cells before the appearance of a significant inflammatory infiltrate suggest a role for cytotoxic antibodies to an endogenous viral agent rather than immune complex deposition as a possible pathogenic mechanism for this model.[59]

The association and possible role of antineutrophil cytoplasmic antibodies in PAN is discussed in the section on Churg-Strauss syndrome.

Churg-Strauss Syndrome. In 1951, Jacob Churg and Lotte Strauss[60] reported 13 asthmatic patients with a systemic vasculitis characterized by fever, eosinophilia, and extravascular granulomas. These symptoms comprise the typical features of what has come to be called the *Churg-Strauss Syndrome* (CSS), or allergic angiitis and granulomatosis.

CLINICAL FEATURES. Characteristic clinical findings are a history of asthma, often with other allergic phenomena, peripheral blood hypereosinophilia, and lung involvement in up to half of the cases,[61] with age of onset in the third or fourth decade of life.[62] Mild renal disease is common but renal failure is not.[62,63] Neurologic manifestations (especially mononeuritis multiplex), myalgias, and arthralgias also are frequent.[62,63] Involvement of the heart is usual, and may take the form of congestive heart failure, pericardial disease, myocardial infarction, or valvular dysfunction.[60,64]

MORPHOLOGIC FINDINGS. Pathologic examination has centered on three characteristic findings: necrotizing arteritis,

granulomatous inflammation, and tissue infiltrate of eosinophils. The vasculitis affects primarily small and medium vessels, and may be similar to that seen in PAN or hypersensitivity vasculitis.[61] Fibrinoid necrosis is common. A prominent infiltrate of the blood vessel wall by eosinophils has been noted.[63,65] The extravascular granulomatous inflammation (the "Churg-Strauss granuloma") has a central core of necrotic eosinophilic fibrinoid material with a surrounding array of histiocytes, lymphocytes, and multinucleated histiocytic giant cells.[60] Eosinophils, either intact or fragmented, were described as a prominent feature of these lesions by the original authors.[60] These granulomas may be seen in close proximity to or within blood vessel walls.[60] Tissue infiltrate of eosinophils also may be seen separate from the granulomatous or vascular lesions.

PROBLEMS IN DIAGNOSIS AND CLASSIFICATION. Diagnostic criteria for CSS have emphasized various clinical and/or pathologic features. Lanham et al[62] stressed a relatively broad-minded approach, maintaining that a strict reliance on classic histopathologic features would inappropriately exclude many cases of what they would consider CSS. They proposed the presence of three criteria for the clinical recognition of CSS: a history of asthma, peripheral blood eosinophilia of at least 1.5×10^9/L, and systemic vasculitis involving two or more extrapulmonary organs.[62] Additional features incorporated into a recently proposed set of criteria for CSS are nonfixed pulmonary infiltrates, abnormality of paranasal sinuses, neuropathy, and extravascular eosinophils.[65]

Difficulties in classification of CSS and related disorders arise because of overlapping clinical and pathologic expression of what may broadly be called "hypersensitivity." Three major histologic manifestations of this state are granulomatous inflammation, tissue infiltration by eosinophils, and vasculitis. Any one of these may occur in a relatively pure form, with respective examples being sarcoidosis, Loeffler pneumonitis, and PAN. It should not be surprising that these forms of tissue injury are not mutually exclusive, and therefore may be seen in the same patient. Differences in tissue response may be explained only in part by etiologic agent, for we know that even the same agent (for example, hepatitis B antigen) may be associated with small vessel leukocytoclastic vasculitis in some individuals and PAN in others.[66] The existence of overlapping manifestations in the vasculitides, as codified by Fauci in his widely used classification of vasculitis,[1] is well known.

The problem of relating clinical vasculitis syndromes to histopathologic and/or immunopathologic findings lends itself to a Venn diagram approach.[5,62,67] A modified version of the diagram published by Suen and Burton[67] appears in Fig. 17-6. Thus classic CSS, in its strictest histopathologic sense, includes cases where all three patterns are identified in tissue, whereas Wegener granulomatosis (WG) is characterized by the combination of vasculitis and extravascular granulomatous inflammation. Other combinations of

Hypersensitivity Disorders

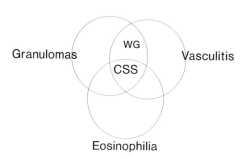

Fig. 17-6. Histopathologic manifestations of "hypersensitivity" include vasculitis, granuloma formation, and tissue eosinophilia. These may be observed alone or in any combination. In classic Churg-Strauss syndrome (CSS), all three are present, whereas Wegener granulomatosis (WG) is characterized by vasculitis and granulomatosis. (Modified from Suen KC and Burton JD Hum Pathol 10:31-43, 1979.)

these three patterns represent various overlap syndromes, and each may occur independently.

PATHOGENESIS. The pathogenesis of CSS is unknown, but immunologic mechanisms obviously are important. The findings of asthma and eosinophilia certainly suggest allergic phenomena. As one would expect, IgE levels have been found to be elevated, and immune complexes containing IgE have been identified.[68] As in other vasculitic syndromes, a decreased number of circulating CD8+ (suppressor/cytotoxic) T-lymphocytes with increased helper/suppresor ratio has been found, suggesting activation of cellular immunity.[61]

The demonstration in 1985 of antineutrophil cytoplasmic antibodies (ANCA) in patients with WG[69] has fostered a new approach to understanding potential pathogenic mechanisms not only in that disorder, but also in CSS and the other vasculitides in the "polyarteritis nodosa" group of systemic necrotizing vasculitis. Morphologic features common to these ANCA-associated vasculitides are focal distribution, necrosis, and infiltrate of neutrophils.[5] ANCA also are found in more than 80% of cases of glomerulonephritis without systemic vasculitis and without evidence of immune complex deposition.[5]

These antibodies are directed against constituents of lysosomes in neutrophilic primary (azurophilic) granules. Two major specificities of ANCA have been described. Those associated with Wegener granulomatosis seem to be directed against a 29 kilodalton serine protease,[70,71] whereas those encountered in CSS and PAN have activity against myeloperoxidase (MPO).[72] By indirect immunofluorescence, these correspond respectively to cytoplasmic (c-ANCA) and perinuclear (p-ANCA) patterns.[73] The ANCA found in Wegener granulomatosis have a relatively high sensitivity and specificity for that disease, and are

closely related to disease activity, suggesting a pathogenic role.[74] ANCA of MPO specificity are common in CSS and PAN with visceral organ involvement, but not in PAN limited to skin and muscle.[73] Interestingly, of patients in the PAN group of systemic necrotizing vasculitis, those with asthma or eosinophilia tend to have MPO antibodies, whereas those with nasal inflammation and glomerulonephritis tend to have ANCA of serene protease specificity.[73] Thus these antibodies have potential for clinical applicability in aiding in classification of vasculitic syndromes, indicating likely organ involvement, and monitoring disease activity.[5,73]

The exact pathogenic role of these antibodies has not been elucidated, but several possible mechanisms have been proposed. First, they might activate neutrophils by binding to their respective antigens. This could occur either by internalization of the antibody or by surface expression of these lysosomal antigens, presumably occurring in neutrophils "primed" by cytokines.[75] Immune complexes could be formed from ANCA reacting with degranulated neutrophils.[76] ANCA also could interfere with inactivation of released lysosomal enzymes.[76] Thus a complex interaction of cellular and humoral immunopathogenic mechanisms could be operative in individuals with ANCA-associated vasculitis.

Wegener granulomatosis. In its classic form, Wegener granulomatosis (WG) is recognized by the clinicopathologic triad of systemic necrotizing vasculitis, necrotizing granulomatous inflammation of upper and lower respiratory tract, and glomerulonephritis. Limited WG consists of the respiratory lesions without renal involvement. Although WG is a systemic disease in its full-blown expression, patients who have the condition may present with a localized destructive process in the upper respiratory tract (nose and paranasal sinuses), accounting for some cases of what previously was known as lethal midline or malignant granuloma.[77]

Clinical features. Patients generally are adults (mean age around 44 years.[78,79] with a slight male predominance. Presenting symptoms often are nonspecific and include upper respiratory complaints, arthralgias, cough, and hemoptysis. The absence of upper respiratory disease is unusual, seen in only 5 of 85 patients in one series.[79] Systemic manifestations (e.g., fever, weight loss) also are common. Involvement of skin, central nervous system, and other anatomic sites has been reported. Cardiac involvement is present in approximately one third of patients, either as coronary arteritis, pericarditis, or pancarditis; granulomas in the heart also have been observed.[78]

Pulmonary infiltrates and sinusitis were most common in one series, accounting for 71% and 67%, respectively, of presenting signs or symptoms.[79] Lung infiltrates typically are bilateral, nodular, and often cavitary.[79] Renal involvement is manifested by renal failure and nephritic syndrome (hematuria, proteinuria, and casts).[80]

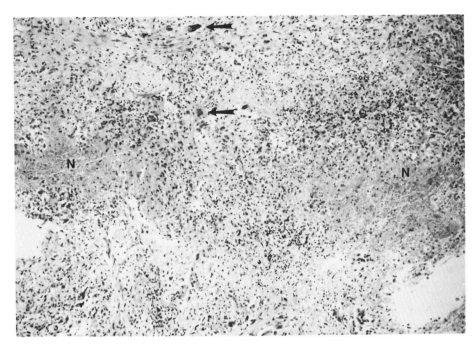

Fig. 17-7. Geographic areas of necrosis *(N)* are surrounded by inflammation in this lung biopsy from a patient with Wegener granulomatosis. Numerous multinucleated giant cells can be seen *(arrows)*.

Routine laboratory studies reveal nonspecific abnormalities indicative of inflammation, including leukocytosis, thrombocytosis, anemia of chronic disease, and marked elevation of erythrocyte sedimentation rate; antinuclear antibodies are not identified.[78] Laboratory evidence of renal dysfunction also is usual.

The natural history of WG without treatment is progressive renal and/or pulmonary impairment with a high mortality rate: a mean survival of 5 months was estimated in one early review.[77] A dramatic increase in overall survival has been obtained with modern treatment regimens including cyclophosphamide and prednisone, with a complete response rate of 93% and long-term remission in many patients.[79]

Morphologic findings. Histologically, the most distinctive feature is necrotizing inflammation of the respiratory tract that led to the term *granulomatosis*. This lesion consists of large, "geographic" areas of necrosis in which granular basophilic material is present, often surrounded by palisading histiocytes and multinucleated histiocytic giant cells (Fig. 17-7).[81] Suppurative necrosis with microabscesses formation also is common.[81] This inflammatory process may or may not be distinctly angiocentric. Distinction must be made from infectious diseases by appropriate stains and cultures, and from other entities in the "pulmonary angiitis and granulomatosis" category, including necrotizing sarcoid granulomatosis, Churg-Strauss syndrome, and angiocentric immunoproliferative lesions (AIL, discussed later in this chapter). The prominence of

neutrophils and relative paucity of lymphocytes help differentiate WG from AIL.[82]

The vasculitis in WG is notable for its morphologic variability, both in terms of the vessels affected (small to medium arteries or veins), and in the type of inflammatory infiltrate, which may be granulomatous or nongranulomatous, necrotizing or nonnecrotizing, or acute or chronic.[81] A pattern similar to leukocytoclastic vasculitis may be noted. In the lung, the presence of neutrophilic debris with associated necrosis and hemorrhage involving alveoli has been considered to represent a vasculitis of alveolar septal capillaries or "capillaritis".[83]

The typical renal lesion is a focal and segmental proliferative glomerulonephritis that varies in its intensity and extent (Fig. 17-8).[84] Other patterns described include vasculitis of parenchymal renal vessels and a periglomerular granulomatous response.[80] Immunofluorescence demonstrated glomerular C_3 deposition in 12 and IgG or IgM in 13 of 13 cases with severe renal disease.[84] Weiss and Crissman[85] emphasized glomerular necrosis and thrombosis rather than immune complex deposition in cases of WG.

Pathogenesis. Because of the coexistence of vasculitis and granulomatous inflammation, and the response to immunoregulatory agents, immunologic mechanisms have long been suspected to play a part in the pathogenesis of WG. The exciting discovery of antineutrophil cytoplasmic antibodies (ANCA) in WG patients[69] introduced a new potential pathogenic mechanism for WG as well as other vas-

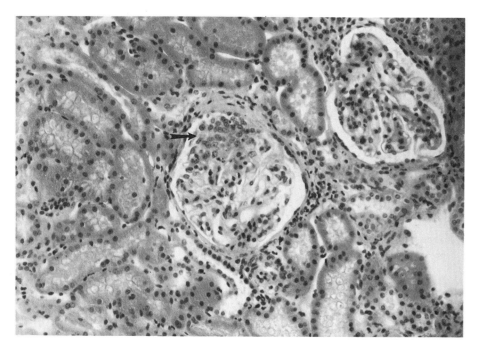

Fig. 17-8. Focal segmental proliferative glomerulonephritis *(arrow)* is a common manifestation of systemic vasculitis, including Wegener granulomatosis.

culitic syndromes; this topic is addressed in the discussion of Churg-Strauss syndrome. It should be reemphasized here that the association of WG with ANCA of serine protease specificity (cytoplasmic immunofluorescence pattern) is quite strong, and correlates with disease activity.[74] Experimental evidence suggests that the target antigen is proteinase 3, a component of azurophil granules of granulocytes and some monocytes.[86] The presence of ANCA may allow for earlier diagnosis of WG. Boudes et al[87] recently proposed recognition of a new form of WG called *microscopic Wegener disease,* in which cytoplasmic ANCA are present in association with renal or pulmonary capillary vasculitis, but without more traditional manifestations of full-blown WG. A microangiopathic hemolytic anemia and consumptive coagulopathy may be observed. Further evaluation will be necessary to determine the proper classification and natural history of this disease variant.

Kawasaki disease

Clinical features. Kawasaki disease (KD) is an acute febrile illness occurring in infancy and early childhood (mean age 2 years) that was named after the Japanese physician who described the condition in 1967.[88] The disease manifests clinically as a fairly distinctive syndrome in which the presence of five of the following six features secures the diagnosis: fever; conjunctival injection; oral changes such as erythema, fissuring, or "strawberry" tongue; extremity changes such as induration of hands and feet, or erythema of palms and soles; erythematous rash; and lymphadenopathy.[89] The synonym "mucocutaneous lymph node syndrome" denotes several of the characteristic clinical features. The disease described as "infantile polyarteritis nodosa" generally is thought to be clinically and pathologically indistinguishable from KD.[52] KD was first recognized in Japanese and other Oriental groups, but subsequently has been encountered in individuals of diverse ethnic and geographic origin.[89]

Morphologic findings. It is not surprising that a systemic vasculitis underlies the multiorgan dysfunction in KD. Pathologic studies have documented a predictable sequence of vascular changes over time.[90,91] In the first week of illness, a vasculitis affects primarily the smallest vessels (capillaries, arterioles, venules).[91] A variety of endothelial alterations have been described in early lesions, such as swelling, hyperplasia, and disruption of endothelial cells.[90] At this stage, inflammatory involvement of epicardial coronary arteries is limited to a "perivasculitis" of adventitia, vasculitis of vasa vasorum, and endarteritis of intima.[91] The infiltrate is edematous and contains neutrophils, lymphocytes, and some eosinophils. Myocardium and endocardium also may be affected.

The second to third weeks of illness are characterized by a panarteritis of medium muscular arteries in many organs, but particularly affecting the major coronary arteries. A mixed inflammatory infiltrate involves all layers, but unlike classic PAN, fibrinoid necrosis is not a prominent feature (Fig. 17-9).[91] Aneurysm formation is notable (Fig. 17-10), and thrombotic occlusion or rupture of a coronary artery aneurysm is an important cause of death at this stage. Among larger musculoelastic arteries, the iliac arteries are most commonly and most severely involved.[92] Veins also are affected.

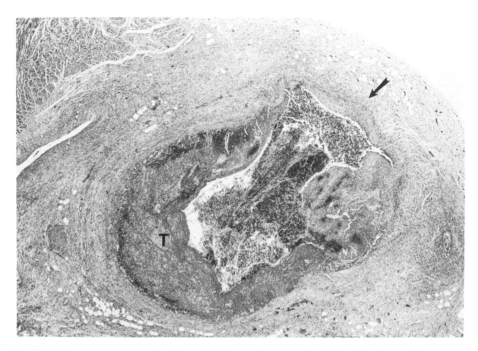

Fig. 17-9. A coronary artery in Kawasaki disease shows marked distortion by an inflammatory infiltrate, aneurysm formation *(arrow),* and luminal thrombus (T).

After around 1 month of illness, organization of thrombi and marked intimal proliferation are observed, whereas small vessel vasculitis is no longer present.[91] Subsequent vascular changes involve mural scarring, calcification, and luminal stenosis, which may lead to chronic ischemic heart disease.

Etiology. The etiology of KD is unknown, and although several features have suggested an infectious cause (periodic epidemics, seasonal occurrence, clinical similarity to some infectious diseases), the putative agent remains elusive. The finding of reverse transcriptase in peripheral blood mononuclear cell culture from KD patients has led to speculation of a retroviral agent.[93,94] However, not all groups have corroborated this finding.[95]

Pathogenesis. An immunologic reaction has been implicated in the pathogenesis of KD, and the following immunologic abnormalities have been described: transient decrease in T-suppressor/cytotoxic (CD8+) lymphocytes and increase in T-helper/inducer (CD4+) lymphocytes,[96]; increased proportion of activated CD4+ lymphocytes[97]; increased B-cell antibody production with elevated serum immunoglobulin levels;[97,98] circulating immune complexes;[99] and increased levels of several cytokines (e.g., IL-1 and TNF).[100,101] It is known that cytokines can activate endothelial cells and induce the expression of endothelial-leukocyte adhesion molecules (ELAM).[102] Leung et al[102] made the intriguing observation that acute serum from KD patients was cytotoxic to cytokine-treated endothelial cells, suggesting the presence of antibodies directed against new endothelial antigens induced by an inflammatory response

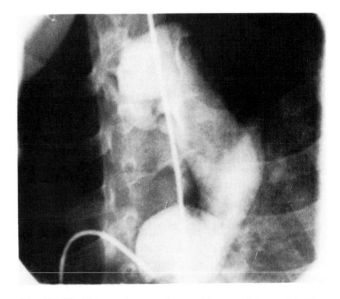

Fig. 17-10. This angiogram from a 7-year-old boy with Kawasaki disease shows marked aneurysmal dilatation of the proximal, mid, and distal left anterior descending coronary artery. For size comparison, the angiographic catheter is 3 mm in diameter.

to some as-yet-unknown agent. Pathologic studies showing endothelial damage in very early lesions lend some support to this possibility.[90] The importance of immunologic mechanisms in pathogenesis is underscored by the fact that several of the immunologic abnormalities are especially prevalent in patients with coronary artery aneurysm formation[96,101] (see Table 17-2, which summarizes the time

Table 17-2. Kawasaki disease: Idealized time course of selected histopathologic (H), immunologic (I), and clinical (C) manifestations

	Manifestation		Time Course	
	Stage I* (0-9 days)	Stage II (12-25 days)	Stage III (28-31 days)	Stage IV (>40 days)
H	Microvascular vasculitis with endothelial injury; pericarditis, endocarditis, myocarditis	Panvasculitis, coronary artery aneurysms with intimal proliferation	Organization of thrombi, coronary artery intimal thickening, absence of small vessel angiitis	Arterial scarring, calcification, stenosis of coronary arteries
I	Cytotoxic Ab to cytokine-induced endothelial Ag; IL-1 and Ig from PBMC; increased TNF; decreased CD4 and CD8 T-cells; CIC	Increased CD4, decreased CD8 cells in those with aneurysms, normal in others; increased TNF, especially with aneurysms; CIC peak 20-30 days		Normal CD4 and CD8 cell counts
C	Acute (1-2 weeks) Acute febrile illness: rash, conjunctival injection, oral mucosal and extremity changes, leukocytosis, elevated ESR, thrombocytosis	Subacute (2-3 weeks) Defervescence, arthritis, desquamation, marked thrombocytosis	Convalescent High risk of sudden death and ischemic heart disease	

*Pathologic stages I-IV as defined by Fujiwara et al[91] abbreviations: Ab: antibodies; Ag: antigens; CIC:circulating immune complexes; ESR: erythrocyte sedimentation rate; Ig: immunoglobulins; IL-1: interleukin-1; PBMC: peripheral blood mononuclear cells; TNF: tumor necrosis factor.

course of several pathologic, immunologic, and clinical features of KD).

Pathophysiology. Cardiac dysfunction is the most feared complication of KD. Early deaths in stage I appear to be caused by myocarditis, whereas later mortality results from coronary artery aneurysm rupture or ischemic heart disease.[103] In the era before effective treatment, mortality was around 2%, with most of these being sudden cardiac deaths, whereas approximately 20% of patients developed coronary artery aneurysms.[104] With modern treatment (aspirin and intravenous immunoglobulin), mortality has decreased to around 0.5%, and the incidence of coronary artery abnormalities is down to less than 5%.[89,104] Even after they are formed, aneurysms have been observed to regress with treatment.[104] Although the mechanism of this success is not fully understood, clearly modulation of the immune response somehow mitigates the destructive process.[105]

Thromboangiitis obliterans (Buerger disease). Through a checkered history of enthusiastic acceptance leading to overdiagnosis followed by vehement dismissal leading to underdiagnosis, thromboangiitis obliterans (TAO, or Buerger disease) has emerged as a well-defined clinical and pathologic entity.[106-108]

Clinical features. The disease classically was recognized as an inflammatory thrombosing process of blood vessels in distal extremities of young men (onset usually less than 40 years of age) leading to severe ischemic effects, including gangrene. Rarely, blood vessels of visceral organs or brain are affected. A strong association with cigarette smoking has been a consistent feature: the condition is rare in nonsmokers, and only cessation of smoking can arrest the disease activity.[109] A certain ethnic and geographic predilection has been noted; TAO is rare in blacks and more commonly is encountered in the Orient, Israel, India, and Asia than in Western countries.[108] The early impression that the disease occurred exclusively in Jews apparently was related to the presence of a predominantly Jewish patient population served by the hospital in which Leo Buerger worked.[108] Subsequently, a twofold increased incidence in Jewish patients has been surmised.[110]

The demographics of TAO have changed somewhat in recent years. The disease is being recognized more frequently in women, possibly paralleling an increase in smoking among women, even as the total number of cases is declining in the United States.[108,109,111] Some investigators also have noted an increase in upper extremity involvement.[109]

Morphologic findings. TAO predominantly involves small and medium arteries and veins. From a pathologic perspective, acute, intermediate, and chronic stages have been described. Early lesions are characterized by marked angiitis of these vessels, with or without thrombosis.[112] Unlike the usual bland thrombi encountered in severe atherosclerosis or in hypercoagulable states, those in TAO contain prominent inflammatory infiltrates that often are suppurative, with formation of microabscesses, and may have a granulomatous component with multinucleated histiocytic giant cells.[112] These features, along with integrity of the internal elastic lamina, are important in differentiating TAO from other vasculitides and thrombotic processes.

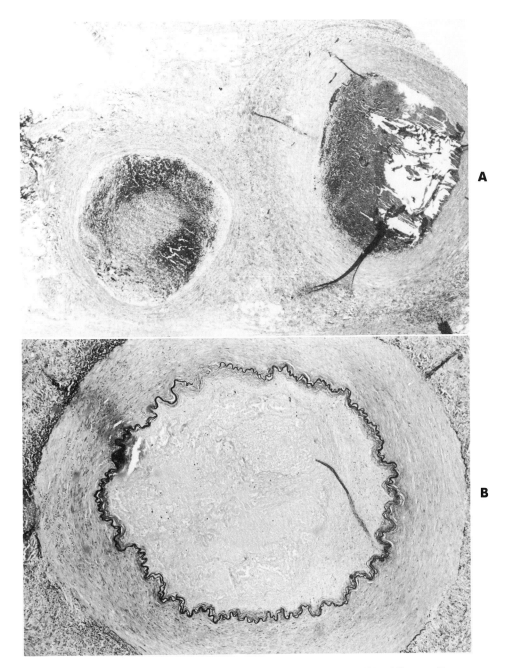

Fig. 17-11. A, Thrombosed vein (left) and artery (right) in thromboangiitis obliterans (Buerger disease). **B,** Elastic stain demonstrates intact internal elastic lamina in a muscular artery in thromboangiitis obliterans. The lumen is occluded by thrombus.

In intermediate stage lesions, organization of these thrombi occurs, and is accompanied by a mixed inflammatory infiltrate (Fig. 17-11). Late lesions show organized recanalized thrombi and fibrosis of the surrounding neurovascular bundle, presumably secondary to ischemia. Residual inflammatory activity may persist even at this stage, aiding in histopathologic detection of TAO even in late lesions.[112]

Pathogenesis. The pathogenesis of TAO is unknown. As in many of the vasculitides, an infectious agent has been sought but not conclusively demonstrated. The close association with cigarette use has been mentioned, but the exact component or components responsible have not been identified. Interestingly, a case of TAO has been reported in a heavy user of chewing tobacco.[113]

Thrombosis and inflammation are the hallmarks of the disease, but the precise roles played by abnormalities in thrombogenicity and abnormalities in immune function are not clearly defined. Circulating immune complexes have been identified by some investigators,[114] but their significance is uncertain. Gulati et al[115] demonstrated decreased total hemolytic complement and antibodies to human arterial antigen in TAO patients. Subsequently, the same group reported deposition of immunoglobulin and complement in involved vessel walls.[116] Adar et al[117] found cell-mediated immunity directed against type I and or III collagen, as well as anticollagen antibodies in TAO patients. Thus evidence points toward activation of both cellular and humoral arms of the immune system.

Abnormalities in platelet function have been detected by Pietraszek et al,[118] with the finding of enhanced response to serotonin-induced platelet aggregation in TAO. The known thrombogenic propensity in cigarette smokers[119] certainly could exacerbate other abnormalities in platelet function peculiar to TAO. Also, the close association between the inflammatory response and coagulation and thrombosis is well known.

In summary, TAO appears to represent a complex interaction of immunologic and thrombogenic mechanisms that is in some way initiated or exacerbated by cigarette smoking in genetically susceptible individuals.

Angiocentric immunoproliferative lesions. A group of lesions that will be considered under the rubric of "angiocentric immunoproliferative lesions" (AIL) blur the distinction between inflammatory and neoplastic vascular disorders. The prototype of lesions in this category is lymphomatoid granulomatosis (LYG), described by Liebow et al[120] in 1972. Characteristics of that disorder were nodular pulmonary infiltrates, frequent skin and central nervous system involvement, and unlike Wegener granulomatosis, lack of intrinsic glomerular disease. Histologic examination revealed *granulomatosis,* a term meant to indicate extensive necrosis with surrounding cellular inflammatory infiltrate, in which histiocytic multinucleated giant cells (as seen in true granulomatous inflammation) may or may not be found. A peculiar and notable feature of this process, and possibly responsible for the necrosis, was angiocentric distribution of the cellular proliferation, which tended to infiltrate blood vessel walls. The cellular population was polymorphous and contained varying numbers of large and/or atypical lymphoid cells. Fibrinoid necrosis of vessels was not a feature of this process. Untreated, the disease had a poor prognosis.

Subsequent to the description of LYG, Saldana et al[82] reviewed their experience with pulmonary angiitis and granulomatosis, and reported a group of cases that they termed *benign lymphocytic angiitis* and granulomatosis (BLAG). These differed from LYG in having less frequent necrosis, less extrapulmonary involvement, and a vascular infiltrate consisting of a more benign-appearing population of small lymphocytes, plasma cells, and plasmacytoid lymphocytes with few large cells.

The observation by Liebow et al[120] that 13% of LYG patients developed malignant lymphoma led to investigation into the possible premalignant or lymphoproliferative

nature of the disease process. In a prospective study of 15 patients with LYG, progression to malignant lymphoma occurred in 7 (47%).[121] On this basis, and because of the recognition of progression from BLAG to LYG, Fauci et al[121] proposed that these diseases were not separate entities, but represented a spectrum from benign to malignant lymphoproliferative disorders.

This concept has been extended and a histologic grading system proposed[122] with grade I AIL encompassing BLAG, grade II AIL including most cases of LYG, and grade III AIL describing cases of frank malignant lymphoma with an angiocentric pattern. Lipford et al[122] consider these to represent a spectrum of postthymic T-cell proliferation, analogous to follicular center cell lymphomas of B lymphocytes, which range from clinically indolent to aggressive diseases. (*Angiocentric* lymphoma is to be distinguished from *angiotrophic* lymphoma, in which lymphoma cells fill and distend intravascular spaces.)

In some cases of AIL, clonal populations of cells containing Epstein-Barr viral genomes have been identified, whereas T-cell receptor gene rearrangement, as expected in T-cell lymphomas, was found in only 1 of 8 cases.[123] These investigators proposed an analogy between AIL and Epstein-Barr virus-related lymphoproliferative disorders encountered in immunosuppressed individuals, in which a malignant clone eventually develops in the background of a polyclonal lymphoid proliferation.

DeRemee et al[124] recognized the similarity between LYG and a disease called *polymorphic reticulosis,* which was a destructive process involving the upper respiratory tract and encompassing many cases of so-called lethal midline granuloma. As was the case for LYG, the T-cell lymphoproliferative nature of this entity was suggested,[125] and this disorder generally is considered in the same spectrum as AIL.[122] An example of AIL occurring in an extrapulmonary location (lip) appears in Fig. 17-12.

Behçet disease. Behçet disease (BD) is a multisystem disorder in which vasculitis is thought to underlie most of the pathologic manifestations. Because vessels of any dimension may be affected, the vasculitis is difficult to classify based on size of vessel involved.

Clinical features. Originally identified by the clinical triad of aphthous stomatitis, genital ulcers, and relapsing iridocyclitis, BD now is recognized to encompass a variety of neurologic, gastrointestinal, ophthalmic, urogenital, pulmonary, and cardiovascular abnormalities.[126] Oral ulcers are present in almost all cases, and represent one of the major criteria for diagnosis, the other three being typical ocular symptoms, genital ulcers, and certain skin lesions (including erythema nodosum).[127] BD is most common in Japan and Mediterranean countries, occurs more frequently in men than women, and usually presents in the third or fourth decade of life.

Based on predominant organ system involvement, three subtypes of BD are distinguished: neuro-Behçet, entero-

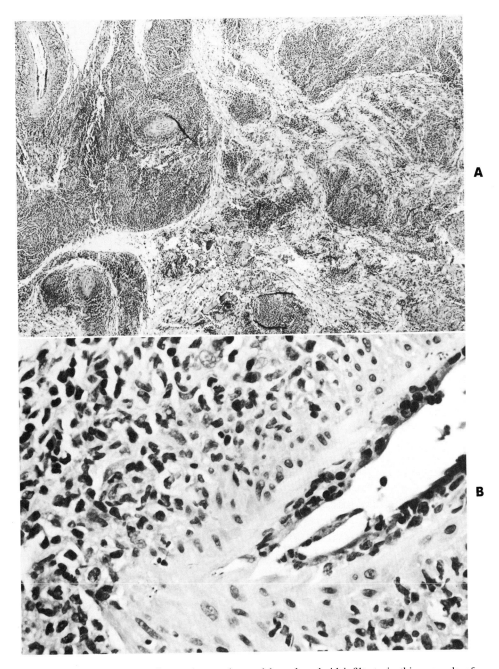

Fig. 17-12. A, Multiple small vessels are obscured by a lymphoid infiltrate in this example of angiocentric immunoproliferative lesion from the lip. **B,** High power photomicrograph of small vessel from same case as Fig. 17-12A shows atypical lymphoid cells within and around the vessel wall.

Behçet, and vasculo-Behçet disease. The latter is defined by the presence in large vessels of aneurysms, venous occlusions, or arterial occlusions, and represents 4% to 24% of patients with BD in various series.[128] Venous occlusions, presumably secondary to thrombophlebitis, may involve venae cavae, hepatic, femoral, or mesenteric veins.[126] Arterial aneurysms usually are saccular and most commonly affect the abdominal aorta or major arteries of the extremities.[126,128]

Morphologic findings. In active large arterial lesions, an inflammatory infiltrate of mixed type is seen in the media and adventitia, along with proliferation of vasa vasorum.[128] Degenerative medial changes, including loss of elastic fibers and fibrosis, are common, and a late scarred stage with little inflammation may be encountered.[128] Occasionally, changes indistinguishable from Takayasu arteritis may be seen in active aortitis. Pulmonary vascular involvement affecting arteries and veins of all sizes has been described, and may lead to massive hemoptysis, pulmonary hypertension, and other respiratory complications, which frequently are listed as the cause of death.[126,129]

Etiology and pathogenesis. The etiology of BD is unknown, and its pathogenesis is not clearly delineated. Various infectious agents, especially viruses, have been implicated but not proven to be causative. An association with streptococcal infections has been noted, and some investigators have found decreased titers of antistreptococcal antibodies in patients with BD compared to controls, suggesting the possibility that these patients cannot form sufficient antibody to neutralize streptococcal antigens.[127]

As with several other vasculitic disorders, racial and geographic distribution suggests a genetic component. Various HLA associations relating to ethnic background and disease manifestations have been noted.[130]

Immunologic investigations have been numerous and sometimes contradictory. One relatively consistent observation has been increased polymorphonuclear leukocyte activity, which may be mediated by lymphokines.[127] Circulating immune complexes have been identified in many patients, and are thought by some to play a pathogenic role via complement activation.[130] Cell-mediated immune mechanisms probably also are important. Abnormal B-cell function, decreased natural killer cell activity, and decreased T-cell response to interleukin 2 have been observed.[131]

Vasculitis associated with collagen-vascular disorders. Vasculitis of medium and small vessels may be seen in systemic lupus erythematosus and rheumatoid arthritis, as well as in other collagen-vascular disorders. The vasculitis may resemble PAN both morphologically and clinically, or may be of leukocytoclastic type (described below).

Predominantly small vessels

Leukocytoclastic vasculitis. Leukocytoclastic vasculitis (LCV), also referred to as *hypersensitivity, allergic,* and *small-vessel vasculitis,* may occur as a pure syndrome, but often is seen in the setting of collagen vascular disorders (especially systemic lupus erythematosus and rheumatoid arthritis), malignancies, infections, or exposure to drugs or toxins. Of patients with pathologically documented LCV, an associated condition was recognized in 20 of 54 (37%) in one study[132] and in 38 of 82 (46%) in another.[133] The importance of initiating a search for such an underlying condition in patients presenting with cutaneous lesions of LCV should be stressed.

Clinical features. Clinically, the skin is most prominently affected, and LCV is recognized by the classic "palpable purpura" on dependent parts, especially lower legs. Urticarial, nodular, and ulcerative lesions also have been described.[132] Arthralgias are common, and fever, malaise, and myalgias may occur.

The clinical course and prognosis depend primarily on the underlying disease, if any, and the presence and extent of visceral organ (especially kidney) involvement. In many patients, LCV is a relatively minor dermatologic accompaniment of a more serious condition; in a few, LCV may cause disabling multiorgan dysfunction or death, usually from renal failure.[132,134] Evidence of visceral organ dysfunction was present in 16 of 54 patients in Hodge's series.[132] Systemic signs or symptoms were recorded in 42 of 82 (51%) patients studied in a private practice setting; in order of decreasing frequency, these consisted of musculoskeletal, renal, gastrointestinal, pulmonary, neurologic, and other manifestations.[133]

The vasculitis encountered in *Henoch-Schonlein (or anaphylactoid) purpura* also is of the leukocytoclastic type, but the eponym is retained because the disorder is recognized as a distinct syndrome. In addition to the findings of skin lesions (palpable purpura) and LCV, this disorder, which occurs primarily in children, is characterized by abdominal signs and symptoms and renal abnormalities.[135] Skin and the intestinal tract are the organs predominantly involved by the small-vessel vasculitis.

Morphologic findings. LCV affects the smallest microscopic blood vessels, including capillaries, arterioles, and venules; electron microscopic observations have suggested that postcapillary venules are most notably involved.[134] The name derives from the characteristic finding of fragmentation of neutrophils that infiltrate the vasculature (Fig. 17-13). Fragments of nuclear debris are strewn within the vessel wall and in the surrounding tissue. Luminal microthrombi, endothelial swelling, and fibrinoid necrosis often are present, and disruption of these small vessels leads to extravasation of erythrocytes. The combination of these features often distorts the microvasculature to such an extent that the vessels themselves are difficult to identify in histologic sections.

Pathogenesis. Abundant evidence supports the contention that immune complexes (IC) are involved in the pathogenesis of LCV. Experience with animal models, reviewed by Cochrane,[136] has shown that injection of anti-

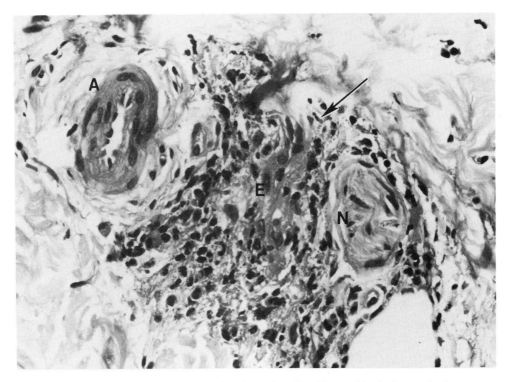

Fig. 17-13. A small vessel in the center has been virtually obliterated by leukocytoclastic vasculitis; hyperplastic endothelial cells *(E)* and neutrophilic nuclear debris *(arrow)* can be seen. An arteriole *(A)* and small nerve twig *(N)* are unaffected.

gen can cause soluble IC to appear in circulation; IC can become deposited in blood vessel walls, a process aided by vasoactive amine-mediated increase in vascular permeability; and local platelet aggregation and release of vasoactive amines may dictate the precise localization of IC deposition. As summarized by Sams et al,[134] the following mechanism is proposed. Immune complexes activate complement, leading to the production of chemotactic factors that attract neutrophils to the blood vessel wall (type III immunopathologic mechanism or Arthus reaction). After reaching the wall, these cells phagocytize the IC and release lysosomal enzymes that damage the vessel wall and lead to disintegration of neutrophils, accounting for the characteristic leukocytoclastic picture.

Evidence supporting various aspects of this proposed pathogenic sequence exists in humans. For example, Mackel and Jordon[137] found circulating IC in the serum of 28 of 39 (72%) patients with LCV, and showed a rough correlation between their concentration in serum and disease activity. Breedveld et al[138] demonstrated that in patients with rheumatoid arthritis and associated LCV, IC present in serum caused neutrophil-mediated injury to human endothelial cells in culture. Immunofluorescence occasionally demonstrates immunoglobulin and/or complement in affected vessels, but results are variable and highly dependent on the time of biopsy with respect to the evolution of the lesions.[134] In vascular and glomerular le-

sions of Henoch-Schonlein purpura, IgA deposition has been noted.[139] Low levels of complement in serum are not detected in the majority of cases of LCV, but may be seen in association with collagen vascular diseases[140] and are characteristic in a subtype of LCV known as *hypocomplementemic vasculitis.*[141]

Specific antigens targeted for immune complex formation can be demonstrated in a few patients with vasculitis. Examples are hepatitis B surface antigen[55] and streptococcal antigen.[142] In patients with cryoglobulinemia associated with LCV, the immunoglobulin/immunoglobulin complexes are presumed to be the offending agent. The putative antigen(s) responsible for LCV associated with malignancy have not been identified. In some cases of LCV, no etiologic agent is apparent. Instead of the IC mechanism described above, it is possible that some cases of LCV involve antineutrophil cytoplasmic antibodies[5] (see p. 526); this question has not been evaluated fully.

Although many drugs have been implicated as a cause of LCV, among them penicillins and other antibiotics, aspirin, and phenacetin, their association may be fortuitous in some cases. Interestingly, a clinicopathologic study of 30 cases of drug-related vasculitis indicated that the histologic appearance of the vasculitis was that of an infiltrate of eosinophils and mononuclear cells without fibrinoid necrosis or changes characteristic of LCV.[143] It is likely that drugs and toxins can cause different patterns of vascular injury in different patients.

Types of aneurysms

Atherosclerotic
Aortic dissection
Infectious
   Syphilitic
   Nonsyphilitic
      Mycotic (associated with infectious endocarditis)
      Secondarily infected aneurysms
      Microbial arteritis (hematogenous or direct extension)
Vasculitic
Berry (? acquired vs congenital)
Traumatic
Others

ANEURYSMS

A true aneurysm may be defined as a dilatation of a segment of blood vessel in which all three vascular layers are present in the distended area. Aneurysms more commonly arise in arteries than in veins, and may be classified by morphology (e.g., saccular, a sac-like outpouching from a small orifice; or fusiform, a spindle-shaped swelling) or etiology (see Box above). Aneurysms usually form when the arterial wall, weakened by some inflammatory or degenerative process, gives way locally to systemic pressure. Because most of the strength of an artery resides in its tunica media, the pathogenesis of most aneurysms involves damage to this layer.

Atherosclerotic aneurysms

Few diseases have been as thoroughly studied as atherosclerosis. Yet, like the atherogenic process itself, the pathogenesis of aneurysm formation in atherosclerotic arteries remains incompletely understood.

Clinical features. Atherosclerotic aneurysms occur more commonly in men than women, and although the most common location is in the abdominal aorta below the origin of the renal arteries (Fig. 17-14), they may be found anywhere along the aorta or its major branches (Fig. 17-15). They may cause symptoms by compression of or erosion into adjacent structures, and are disturbingly prone to rupture. Mural thrombus accumulation is common (Fig. 17-16), and may lead to luminal compromise or occlusion of local arterial branches. Embolization of thrombotic or atheromatous material into distal vessels also may occur. Unfortunately, most cases are asymptomatic until they are discovered radiographically or until they rupture, usually with catastrophic results.[144] The best predictors of this occurrence appear to be the size of the aneurysm and the presence of diastolic hypertension.[144]

Pathogenesis. The exact mechanism whereby atherosclerosis "causes" aneurysms is not clear, and some researchers have questioned the association. Nevertheless, it has been shown that the well-known risk factors for ath-

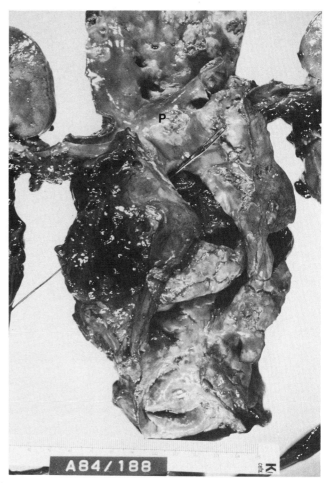

Fig. 17-14. This atherosclerotic aneurysm arose just distal to the renal arteries. A metallic probe passes through the site of rupture, and blood clot is present in periaortic tissue. Atherosclerotic plaques *(P)* mar the intimal surface.

erosclerosis (systemic arterial hypertension, smoking, and high serum cholesterol) also are risk factors for aortic aneurysms, and the vast majority of patients with nondissecting aortic aneurysms have severe diffuse atherosclerosis.[145] Although factors such as smoking and hypertension could lead to aneurysm formation by other mechanisms,[146] it still is prudent at present to consider the atherogenic process itself as the most likely "cause" of the common aortic aneurysm.

Aneurysm formation in atherosclerotic vessels generally is ascribed to impingement on the tunica media by the expanding intimal atheroma, with subsequent medial thinning and weakening of the vessel wall. Either pressure-induced atrophy or dissolution of media by hydrolytic enzymes could be envisioned in this process. Local and systemic hemodynamic factors then would dictate the site and degree of aneurysm formation. Measurement of medial thickness in surgically resected aneurysmal segments shows medial attenuation in some[147] but not all studies.[148]

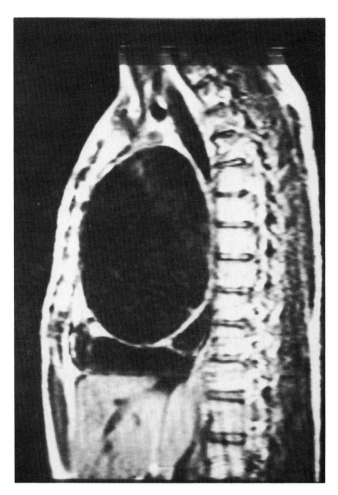

Fig. 17-15. A huge thoracic aortic aneurysm is visualized by magnetic resonance imaging (MRI) scan. (Photo courtesy of Dr. Louis Martin.)

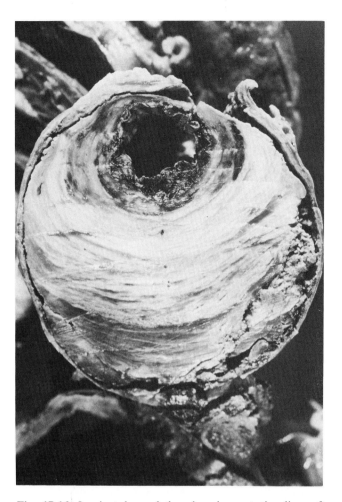

Fig. 17-16. Laminated mural thrombus demonstrating lines of Zahn fills the lumen in this cross-section of an atherosclerotic aortic aneurysm.

The observation that inflammatory infiltrates commonly are seen in pathologic specimens of atherosclerotic aneurysms suggests the possible role of an immune response in the pathogenesis of this disease. In some cases (approximately 10%[149]), in which the surgeon encounters adherence of the aneurysm to adjacent structures, and the pathologist recognizes a predominantly lymphocytic infiltrate in media and adventitia with marked adventitial fibrous thickening, the designation *inflammatory aneurysm* has been applied (Fig. 17-17). The intensity of inflammation may be such that constitutional symptoms such as fever, malaise, and weight loss appear.[150] Operative mortality is high, but may be related to attempts at excessive dissection of the aneurysm from vital structures.[151] Although a characteristic set of clinical and pathologic features defines "inflammatory" aneurysms, most authors favor the interpretation that these represent an extreme end of the spectrum of inflammation that may be seen in any atherosclerotic aneurysm.[150-152]

The significance of the inflammation in relation to

pathogenesis is somewhat more controversial. An immunohistochemical analysis using fresh frozen aortic tissue revealed an increase in inflammatory cells, especially CD4+ T helper/inducer lymphocytes, with the highest levels in "inflammatory aneurysms," an intermediate number in other abdominal aortic aneurysms, and the lowest number in aortas showing only occlusive atherosclerosis.[148] These cells were particularly numerous in the adventitia and media. Adventitial B-lymphocytes were seen in 75% of abdominal aneurysms and in 99% of inflammatory aneurysms, but were rare in atherosclerotic aortas without aneurysm formation. Macrophages similarly increased in number, reflecting the overall degree of mural inflammation. These authors theorized that the interaction of T-helper cells, antigen-presenting macrophages, and B-cells, with resulting local production of antibodies and lymphokines could be important in the pathogenesis of these lesions. However, the case can be made that the inflammation is a result, rather than cause, of aneurysm formation in advanced atherosclerosis.[150,152] Antibodies to

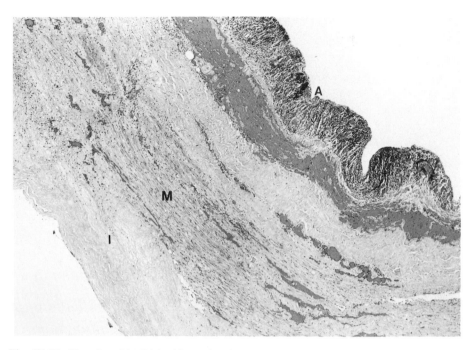

Fig. 17-17. The adventitia *(A)* in this section from the wall of an "inflammatory" atherosclerotic aneurysm displays an intense lymphocytic infiltrate. Sparse inflammatory cells also are present in the damaged media *(M)* overlying a thickened intima *(I)*.

components of atheromatous material have been demonstrated in patients with inflammatory aneurysms or periaortitis.[153] In atherosclerotic aneurysms, thinning of the media may allow leakage of atheromatous substances into adventitial tissues, where they might incite an inflammatory reaction.[150] Impingement on abdominal lymphatics by an expanding aneurysm also may explain periadventitial fibrosis in some cases.[150]

Aortic dissection

In aortic dissection (AD), the artery is widened by a column of blood that enters and separates the tunica media. Although also called dissecting aneurysms these are not true aneurysms because all layers of the wall are not expanded; *dissecting hematoma* would be a more accurate designation (Fig. 17-18).

Clinical features. Most patients with AD are adults, and the disorder is more common in men than in women in most age groups. Clinical presentation usually is dramatic, and AD should be considered in the differential diagnosis of severe chest or back pain of sudden onset. Mortality is extremely high if left untreated, whereas early survival is greater than 90% with early recognition and modern surgical intervention.[154]

AD has been classified into three major morphologic types, depending on the localization of the dissected segment: type I involves the ascending aorta and usually extends to involve both the distal thoracic and abdominal aorta; in type II, dissection is limited to the ascending

aorta; and in type III, the dissection begins at or distal to the left subclavian artery. Clinical relevance of this classification includes not only differences in expected symptoms and complications, but also a different therapeutic approach, in that type I and II dissections generally require surgical repair, whereas initial management of type III dissection is medical.[154]

Pathogenesis. The mechanism of blood entry into the media has been a point of controversy. In most cases, an intimal tear that communicates with the medial hematoma is recognized (Fig. 17-19). This tear, typically located 1 cm to 2 cm above the aortic valve in type I and II dissections, has been detected around 90% of the time, but was found in 100% of 161 cases carefully studied at autopsy.[155] The other possible site of entry, implicated especially in cases without an intimal tear, is from ruptured vasa vasorum.[156]

The pathogenesis of AD may be visualized as a two-step process: *initiation*, which allows entry of blood into the media, and *promotion*, which allows for propagation of the dissecting column within the media. Although overlapping to some extent, different factors probably play a role in these two processes.

Foremost among the factors favoring initiation of dissection is systemic arterial hypertension, noted in 60% to 70% of cases.[153,155,157] Occasionally, a sudden hypertensive crisis is identified surrounding, and presumably initiating, the acute dissection. It is possible to envision shear stress of sufficient magnitude in the ascending aorta of

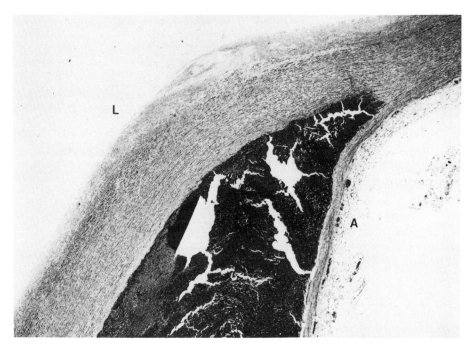

Fig. 17-18. In aortic dissection, a column of blood (dark area) splits the outer portion of media. L: lumen; A: adventitia.

such patients to cause an intimal tear, especially if the aorta was previously weakened. Other local hemodynamic factors involving turbulence or other disturbance of blood flow may be important in individual cases. *Traumatic dissection* may result from steering wheel impact in motor vehicle accidents, in which stress at the vulnerable aortic isthmus overwhelms intimal integrity at that site.[158] Iatrogenic intimal injury from catheter insertion is another mechanical cause of arterial dissection.

An association of AD with pregnancy has been noted: around one half of cases in women less than 40 years of age occur in late pregnancy.[159] Interestingly, many of these women also are hypertensive (25% to 50%[155]), and some have other lesions known to predispose to dissection, such as bicuspid aortic valve, coarctation, or Marfan syndrome. The gravid state is characterized by increased blood volume, which might add hemodynamic stress to the aorta, and a variety of biochemical and mechanical changes in arteries have been described experimentally in pregnancy.[159] These could be important either in initiation or promotion of AD.

Atherosclerosis generally is not considered a risk factor for AD; in fact, Roberts[158] has emphasized that the medial scarring often associated with severe atherosclerosis actually tends to limit the extent of dissection. However, complex atheromatous plaques may serve as an entry point for initiation of an intimal tear, especially in dissection of the distal aorta (type III).[155] Occasionally, an atheromatous plaque will ulcerate, leading to an intramural or extramural

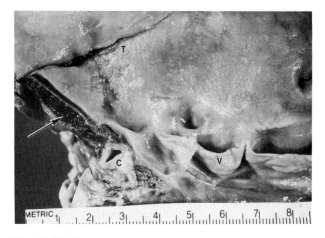

Fig. 17-19. Transverse intimal tear *(T)* is identified in the ascending aorta in a proximal aortic dissection, 3 cm above the aortic valve cusps *(V)*. The dissecting column can be seen *(arrow)* and extends in retrograde fashion toward a coronary artery *(C)*.

hematoma, with pseudoaneurysm formation or rupture. This process, termed the *penetrating aortic ulcer,* is seen in elderly hypertensive patients. Like most cases of AD, it requires surgical intervention.[160]

After blood enters the media, the hematoma will be propagated along the vessel to a varying degree depending on the arterial pressure and the underlying integrity of the medial tissue. In some instances, these factors are such that the aorta simply ruptures without dissection, or dissects only to a limited extent. Clues to this aspect of the pathogenesis of dissection have been sought in histologic examination of the media. Histopathologic medial changes identified in cases of AD include "cystic medial necrosis," elastic fragmentation, fibrosis, and "laminar necrosis."[155,157,161,162] The first of these is best known, and refers to the accumulation of vacuolated extracellular material separating muscle fibers; there is no actual tissue necrosis and no true cyst formation. None of these changes is particularly sensitive to or specific for the presence of dissection. Careful studies have indicated that these changes are found in aortas from patients without AD, are related to aging, and are not qualitatively different in pathologically dilated or dissected aortas compared with normal age-matched aortas.[162,163] The concept is gaining acceptance that these histologic findings reflect wear and tear and smooth muscle cell metabolic activity, all of which result from hemodynamic stresses endured over time.[164,165] Weakening of the aortic wall may result from such stresses, and may predispose certain individuals to dissection, or to aneurysmal dilatation without dissection. In a study of surgically resected thoracic aortic aneurysms, severe cystic medial degeneration was the most common histologic finding.[166]

Aside from aging and hemodynamic injury, as would be expected in hypertensive individuals, other acquired or hereditary abnormalities may weaken the tunica media. Marfan syndrome is well known for its predisposition to AD. An inherited disorder of connective tissue, Marfan syndrome appears to be caused by abnormalities in fibrillin, a component of microfibrils associated with elastin; recently, mutations in the fibrillin gene have been found in this condition.[167,168] Histopathologically, in dilated aortas with or without dissection, one sees marked cystic medial degeneration, often with extensive fragmentation of elastic lamellae.[166] AD also occurs in Ehlers-Danlos syndrome, another inherited disorder of connective tissue. Interestingly, it has been proposed that smooth muscle cell metabolic activity itself may be under genetic control, and that such activity can lead to structural weakness in the media.[164]

AD has been noted in association with several congenital heart lesions, particularly aortic valve abnormalities and aortic isthmic coarctation. Bicuspid aortic valves are reported in 7% to 13% of cases of AD, and of patients with bicuspid aortic valve, AD occurs in around 5%.[169] In one autopsy study, the incidence of bicuspid or unicuspid aortic valve in patients with AD was increased tenfold and twenty-two fold, respectively, over their incidence in the general population.[155] These valves are not necessarily dysfunctional, and the associated dissections involve the proximal aorta (types I and II). Severe loss of elastic fibers in the ascending aorta probably underlies the dissection in most of these cases.[169] Aortic isthmic coarctation also is associated with AD, but many of these cases have an abnormal aortic valve as well. Additionally, elevated arterial

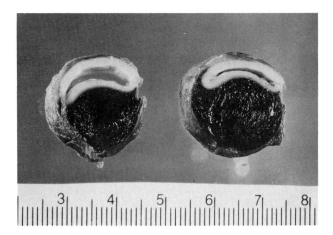

Fig. 17-20. Brachiocephalic trunk shows luminal compression by aortic dissection that has extended along the aortic arch branches.

pressure proximal to the coarctation is a contributing factor to dissection.[158]

Pathophysiology. The pathophysiologic consequences of AD are a direct result of the particular anatomic and hemodynamic features in a given case. Because the column of blood typically is located in the outer media, the outer wall (between hematoma and adventitia) is thinner than the inner wall of the false channel, making external rupture much more likely than reentry into the true aortic lumen (see Fig. 17-18).[158] Usually, the site of rupture is in the ascending aorta, and hemopericardium results, but rupture into pleural or abdominal cavities also is possible. Without urgent surgical intervention, death from exsanguination or cardiac tamponade is likely. A discussion of extensive experience with many potential complications of surgical repair is presented by Crawford.[153] In cases without external rupture, reentry of blood through a second intimal tear (occurring in around 10% of cases) creates a true double barrel aorta, and survival is more probable.[156,158] Healing of such a channel accounts for most cases of "chronic dissection."

In addition to rupture, dissection can compromise blood supply by a variety of means. Extension of hematoma around aortic branches can compress the lumen leading to ischemic effects; aortic arch branches commonly are so affected (Fig. 17-20). Compression of renal arteries may exacerbate the hypertensive state, and coronary artery compression from retrograde extension of the dissection may cause myocardial ischemia. The dissecting column may shear off smaller arterial branches, or may lead to occlusive thrombosis.

Dysfunction of the aortic valve apparatus may occur by several mechanisms. Extension of the dissection toward the aortic root may cause compression and functional aortic stenosis; the aortic outflow also may be obstructed by

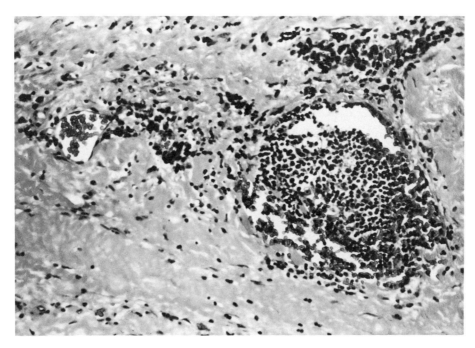

Fig. 17-21. In this example of syphilitic aortitis, a branch of vasa vasorum (to right of center) is obscured by a dense mononuclear infiltrate.

the intimal flap itself. Finally, loss of commissural support for the aortic valve may lead to aortic insufficiency.[158]

Infectious aneurysms

Syphilitic aortitis. Cardiovascular manifestations of syphilis occur as a late (tertiary) complication in around 10% of untreated cases.[170] In the primary infection, *Treponema pallidum* organisms gain rapid access to blood vessels and undergo hematogenous dissemination. Both the chancre characteristic of primary syphilis and the maculopapular cutaneous eruption of secondary syphilis are highly infectious, and organisms can be identified either by darkfield or fluorescence microscopy,[171] or in tissue sections by appropriate silver impregnation stains. A latency period follows, and in the early part (first 12 months), relapse of infectious mucocutaneous lesions may occur.[171] Cardiovascular lesions of tertiary syphilis are seen many years (8 to 30 in one study[172]) after the primary infection; often the primary infection was unrecognized.

Morphologic findings. Syphilitic aortitis and its complications account for virtually all of what is considered syphilitic cardiovascular disease. Pathologically, the hallmark of this process is *endarteritis obliterans* of the vasa vasorum, in which proliferative thickening of the wall of these small vessels leads to luminal narrowing. A lymphoplasmacytic infiltrate is seen in a perivascular distribution (Fig. 17-21). Presumably, medial changes present in affected aortas (patchy destruction of smooth muscle and elastic tissue with replacement by neovascularized scar tissue) represent ischemic injury in areas corresponding to

the distribution of the nutrient vasa vasorum. The resulting medial weakening underlies aortic dilatation and aneurysm formation. Intimal wrinkling overlying the scarred media causes the characteristic but not pathognomonic "tree-bark" gross appearance of affected aortas.

Pathophysiology. Based on an autopsy study of 100 cases, Heggtveit[173] recognized four categories of syphilitic cardiovascular disease: uncomplicated syphilitic aortitis, or syphilitic aortitis complicated by aortic insufficiency, coronary ostial stenosis, or aneurysm formation. Of these complications, *aneurysm formation* was most common, occurring in 40% of the 100 cases. The ascending aortic arch was most frequently involved, followed by the descending and transverse arch (Fig. 17-22). Occasionally, sinus of valsalva aneurysms occur. As emphasized by Silber, aneurysms of the ascending arch have prominent physical manifestations but few symptoms; those of the transverse arch frequently are symptomatic because of compression of adjacent structures, and those of the descending arch usually are discovered radiographically.[174] Symptoms from compression of the trachea, esophagus, recurrent laryngeal nerve, vertebrae, sympathetic nerves, or superior vena cava may signal the presence of an aortic arch aneurysm. Before effective treatment of syphilis, luetic aneurysm was as common a cause of superior vena cava syndrome as malignancy.[175] Radiographically, the findings of dilatation of the ascending aorta together with fine, linear dystrophic calcification is highly suggestive of syphilitic aortitis.[176] Rupture is, of course, the dreaded complication, and accounts for most of the mortality in syphilitic heart disease.

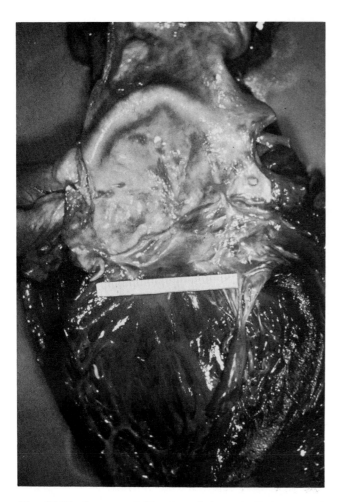

Fig. 17-22. Aneurysmal dilatation of the ascending aorta and aortic valve ring in a case of syphilitic aortitis. Wrinkling of the intimal surface also can be seen.

Aortic insufficiency may occur either as a consequence of aortic valve ring dilatation or widening of the valve commisures from syphilitic valvulitis, or both.[173] Some researchers believe that commissural widening always is secondary to the valve ring dilatation. The medial scarring with intimal wrinkling is responsible for *coronary ostial stenosis,* which may be further exacerbated by the usual atherosclerotic process. Myocardial infarcts may result from the syphilitic coronary ostial narrowing itself, but usually at least moderate atherosclerosis of the coronary arteries is superimposed.[173]

Pathogenesis. It is unusual to find treponemal organisms in the lesions of syphilitic aortitis. However, direct spirochetal invasion of *vasa vasorum,* with attendant immune response, is the proposed mechanism for the vasculitis. The pathogenesis of syphilis involves attachment of organisms via receptors both on *T. pallidum* and on host cells.[177] Spirochetes attach preferentially to endothelial cells, and may invade through endothelial intercellular junctions, aided by their unique shape and motility, into

surrounding tissue.[178] Organisms widely disseminate via lymphatic and vascular routes within hours of infection,[177] and could find their way to the ascending aortic adventitia by means of lymphatic drainage from mediastinal nodes and surrounding tissue.

Why so many years elapse between the initial infection and its eventual consequences is uncertain. Controversy surrounds the question of whether the immune response in syphilis is muted, or whether the organism itself is poorly immunogenic.[177] Soluble extracts from spirochetes of the oral cavity have been shown to inhibit the lymphocyte proliferative response in vitro,[179] and a reduction of lymphocyte reactivity has been observed in patients with secondary syphilis.[180] An additional explanation for latency and relapse may be that although most organisms in syphilis are extracellular, a small intracellular pool of spirochetes could serve as a reservoir for smoldering disease.[177]

Syphilitic heart disease certainly has decreased in prevalence since antiquity; however, it cannot be ignored even today as a cause of cardiovascular morbidity and mortality. In a Japanese population of more than 2000 adults over 60 years of age, the prevalence of a positive serologic test for syphilis was 17%, and aortic insufficiency was 4 to 10 times more frequent in these patients compared to those with negative syphilis serology.[181] With the presently increasing incidence of syphilis as well as other venereal diseases, one should expect to see a resurgence in late complications in the future.

Nonsyphilitic arterial infections
Mycotic aneurysms. Infectious agents can gain access to the blood vessel wall by a variety of mechanisms. The term *mycotic aneurysm,* as used by Osler, referred to aneurysms resulting from the embolization of septic thrombi originating from lesions of infectious endocarditis.[182] Although the term often is used more loosely to indicate any arterial infection, the original meaning will be retained in this discussion. These aneurysms, occurring in an estimated 18% of cases of infectious endocarditis,[182] often affect multiple arteries in visceral and/or peripheral locations. They may be detected on physical examination by the presence of a pulsatile tender mass. In spite of the term *mycotic,* most cases involve bacterial infection, with Gram-positive cocci accounting for the majority of pathogenic organisms.[182] The pathogenesis involves lodging of septic emboli within the vessel, and resulting extension of the infectious process and accompanying inflammation with weakening of the vessel wall. In larger arteries, the emboli may lodge instead in vasa vasorum, leading to spread of the infection from the adventitial side of the vessel.[182]

Secondarily infected aneurysms. Secondary infection of a preexisting, usually atherosclerotic aneurysm most often occurs outside the setting of infectious endocarditis, and may result from seeding of blood from a variety of primary sites; often, the source of infection is unknown.[182]

The abdominal aorta most commonly is affected, and local infection may account for rupture in many cases of atherosclerotic aneurysm. Presumably, the abnormal intimal surface, especially with an adherent mural thrombus, provides a nidus for infection. Most cases are caused by bacteria, especially Gram-positive cocci, but in a significant proportion salmonella or other Gram-negative bacilli are implicated.[182]

Microbial arteritis. With the advent of successful and earlier treatment of infectious endocarditis, fewer cases of true mycotic aneurysms have been seen. Wilson[182] proposed the term *microbial arteritis* for the occurrence of direct bacterial invasion of nonaneurysmal blood vessels. These usually are atherosclerotic, but congenital abnormalities such as coarctation also predispose to infection. Organisms involved most commonly are salmonella, staphylococci, and E. coli.[182] Like infected aneurysms, and unlike mycotic aneurysms, microbial arteritis tends to involve single rather than multiple vessels, and mortality is high. Arterial infection also may occur by contiguous spread from an adjacent septic focus such as osteomyelitis, abscess, or pancreatitis.[182]

Vasculitic aneurysms

Aneurysmal dilatation of blood vessels may occur in a number of the vasculitic syndromes, but are most characteristic of polyarteritis nodosa. These are discussed under the appropriate vasculitis headings.

Berry aneurysms

Berry aneurysm is the somewhat fanciful name applied to saccular aneurysms with a peculiar predilection for the cerebral arteries of the circle of Willis. They are, by some accounts, the most common aneurysm found in humans.[183] However, their pathogenesis remains poorly understood.

Clinical features. These aneurysms occur in adults, rarely before the age of 20 years,[184] and mostly between 40 to 70 years of age.[183,184] Most are found in the anterior half of the circle of Willis, with a tendency to involve bifurcation points. They may cause neuropsychiatric symptoms by mass effect, but are most notorious for sudden rupture leading to massive subarachnoid hemorrhage and often death (Fig. 17-23).

Pathogenesis. The intracranial distribution of berry aneurysms may be related to differences in normal morphology between cerebral and extracerebral arteries. The former are characterized by relatively thin media and adventitia, and concentration of the elastic tissue in the internal elastic lamina.[183] Two theories regarding pathogenesis have been debated in the literature. One holds that a congenital defect in the arterial wall predisposes to aneurysm formation, and the other postulates that these are acquired lesions. Occasional familial occurrence and association with other congenital abnormalities lend some support to

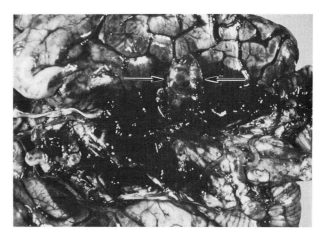

Fig. 17-23. Massive subarachnoid hemorrhage at base of brain obscures the circle of Willis in this case of ruptured berry aneurysm. An intact aneurysm can be seen between arrows.

the congenital origin theory.[185] In established aneurysms, absence of elastic tissue has been noted, but this does not prove a congenital defect in elastic fibers. Apparently, proposed congenital defects in the muscular wall or weakness in areas of persistent vestigial vessels have not been substantiated histologically.[183,185] Although berry aneurysms occur in disorders of connective tissue such as Marfan and Ehlers-Danlos syndromes, the vast majority of cases are seen outside of these settings.

Acquired factors that have been implicated in the pathogenesis of berry aneurysms include hypertension, atherosclerosis, and alterations of cerebral blood flow caused by local anatomic variations in the cerebral vessels. In one autopsy study of 170 patients, systemic arterial hypertension, cerebral atherosclerosis, and marked asymmetry of arteries of the circle of Willis were identified as risk factors for the presence of these aneurysms.[184] A combination of such factors may lead to mural thinning and dilatation at hemodynamically stressed points, with eventual rupture. Because wall stress increases with both pressure and radius (law of Laplace), the larger the aneurysm and the higher the arterial pressure, the more likely rupture is to occur. One group of investigators has noted that many of the risk factors identified, including long-term analgesic use, are associated with reduced levels of prostaglandin E.[184] Prostaglandin E causes a vasoconstriction-mediated reduction in cerebral blood flow, thus reduced levels may exacerbate other hemodynamic stresses by increasing arterial flow.[184]

It is possible that congenital and acquired factors work in concert to produce these aneurysms. One study has demonstrated a decrease in reticulin fibers in cerebral arterial media in patients younger than 50 years of age with ruptured berry aneurysm compared with control group patients.[185] This anatomic abnormality may predispose certain individuals to aneurysm formation, given the appropriate hemodynamic stress over time.

Table 17-3. Pathologic classification of fibromuscular dysplasia

Subtype	Morphologic abnormalities	Frequency*
Intimal fibroplasia	cellular intimal proliferation	1-5%
Medial fibroplasia	fibromuscular ridges alternate with aneurysmal areas of thinned media, leading to "string of beads" on angiogram	60-95%
Perimedial fibroplasia	variable fibrous proliferation in outer portion of media	15-25%
Medial hyperplasia	hyperplasia of medial smooth muscle	<5%
Periarterial fibroplasia	fibrous proliferation with sparse inflammation surrounds adventitia	<1%

*Approximate percentage of cases of idiopathic renal artery stenosis. Data from Luscher TF: Mayo Clinic Proc 62:931-952, 1987. and Harrison EG McCormack LJ: Mayo Clin Pro 46:161-167, 1971.

Before concluding the discussion of aneurysms, the importance of systemic arterial hypertension in the formation of several types of aneurysms should be noted. If hypertension were controlled, the considerable morbidity of dissecting, atherosclerotic, and berry aneurysms would be greatly diminished.

FIBROMUSCULAR DYSPLASIA

A group of disorders is characterized by abnormalities in the intimal, medial, or adventitial architecture of arteries. Called *fibromuscular dysplasia* (FMD) or *fibromuscular hyperplasia,* these disorders are classified according to the major morphologic abnormality present (Table 17-3). They may occur in any age group but most commonly are encountered clinically as a treatable form of renovascular hypertension in young adult women.

FMD affects predominantly medium and small muscular arteries. Approximately three quarters of cases occur in renal arteries; the majority of the remainder are cerebrovascular.[186,187] Lesions of FMD also have been reported in other sites including visceral arteries (mesenteric, splanchnic) and proximal arteries of upper and lower extremities. Often patients with extrarenal FMD have involvement of renal arteries as well; of 70 patients with renal FMD, 10 (14%) also had extrarenal involvement.[188]

Clinicopathologic and angiographic features

Clinicopathologic features of the various subtypes of FMD differ; they will be discussed in order of frequency. Accounting for the majority of cases (60% to 95%), *medial fibroplasia* is characterized histologically by the luminal protrusion of fibromuscular ridges, alternating with aneurysmal areas of medial thinning, leading to a "string of beads" pattern on angiographic study (Fig. 17-24).[187,189] This process tends to affect the distal two thirds of the renal arteries[187] and is the most common type of FMD encountered in extrarenal locations and in pediatric patients.[190] In *perimedial fibroplasia,* a variable proliferation of fibrous tissue occupies the outer portion of the media. A predilection for involvement of the right renal artery in women under the age of 30 years has been noted.[187] An-

giographically, "beads" are present but are less prominent than in medial fibroplasia. *Medial hyperplasia* refers to concentric muscular thickening of the tunica media causing relatively smooth arterial stenoses. *Intimal fibroplasia,* accounting for 1% to 5% of FMD, is characterized by cellular intimal proliferation that may be concentric or eccentric. Interestingly, a female sex predilection is not apparent in this subtype.[187] In the rarest type of FMD, *periarterial fibroplasia,* a fibrous proliferation with sparse inflammatory cells surrounds the adventitia. Some investigators[190] consider these cases more akin to idiopathic fibrosing disorders such as retroperitoneal fibrosis rather than as part of the FMD spectrum.

Pathophysiology

Pathophysiologic derangements resulting from FMD depend on the artery involved, the degree of luminal compromise, and presence of any local vascular complications such as dissecting hematoma, aneurysmal rupture, or thromboembolic events. Stenosis of a renal artery leads to hypertension of the Goldblatt type, with stimulation of the renin-angiotensin-aldosterone system. Although renovascular hypertension accounts for only approximately 4% of all hypertensive disease,[191] it remains an important cause because it is treatable by surgical techniques or percutaneous transluminal angioplasty. FMD is responsible for 20% to 50% of cases of renovascular hypertension;[187] the rest are primarily caused by atherosclerotic renal artery stenosis. In young women with renovascular hypertension, Takayasu arteritis is an important differential consideration. An abdominal or flank bruit from perturbation in renal artery flow may be a clue to the presence of renal artery stenosis, and is noted in over half of patients with renal FMD.[192] Indications of a "significant" renal artery lesion include stenosis of at least 75% diameter, presence of collateral vessels, decreased kidney size, and increased renal vein renin of 1.5 times in the involved side compared with the uninvolved side.[187] If renal artery stenosis is severe, impaired renal function may result, but this is uncommon.

Cerebrovascular FMD may cause a variety of neuro-

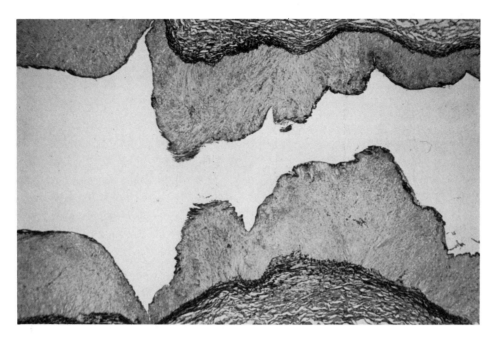

Fig. 17-24. Longitudinal section of a renal artery demonstrates fibromuscular ridges protruding into the lumen, alternating with areas of medial thinning. (Photo courtesy of Dr. William D. Edwards.)

logic signs and symptoms;[187] mechanisms include intracerebral hemorrhage caused by rupture of an aneurysm, infarcts from a thromboembolic mechanism, and ischemia resulting from gradual reduction in luminal cross-sectional area. Headaches are frequent (present in over 90%), and have been attributed to vasoactive substances released by platelets that aggregate in the abnormal vascular segments.[193] Lesions of FMD also may be found incidentally during angiography for unrelated conditions; determination of the significance of such lesions is occasionally problematic.

Pathogenesis and etiology

The etiology of FMD is unknown, but factors that have been implicated include hormonal, genetic, mechanical, toxic, ischemic, autoimmune, and developmental influences on affected vessels. The overwhelming female predominance (over 90% in most subtypes) has led to speculation regarding the role of estrogens in the pathogenesis of FMD. Estrogen can stimulate smooth muscle cells to synthesize extracellular material,[194] and intimal hyperplasia has been associated with oral contraceptive use.[195] However, no significant difference in parity or oral contraceptive use has been noted between cases and control groups[196] and FMD is rare in the general female population. Obviously, estrogen levels alone are insufficient to explain the female predominance in FMD. Because several autoimmune disorders are more prevalent in women, an abnormality in immune function has been sought in pa-

tients with FMD, but convincing evidence is lacking.

Early observations on the predilection for right over left renal artery involvement lead to the theory that mechanical stress might induce changes of FMD. Traction on the right renal artery associated with renal ptosis, and stretching of the internal carotid arteries over the upper cervical vertebrae, could induce continued mechanical injury to these arteries over time.[190] The exact mechanism whereby this injury might lead to FMD is unclear. In one case-controlled study, neither renal mobility, measured sonographically, nor renal artery length, measured angiographically, was significantly increased in FMD patients.[196]

It has been noted that the arteries typically involved by FMD are relatively sparse in vasa vasorum. This factor, possibly combined with extra mechanical trauma in these areas, could cause ischemic damage to the vessels.[190] Morphologic abnormalities of blood vessels have been induced experimentally by occlusion of vasa vasorum, and the occurrence of fibroplasia limited to outer but not inner media would be consistent with injury of an ischemic origin.[187]

Familial cases of FMD have been described, and an autosomal dominant inheritance pattern with variable penetrance has been suggested.[197] Predilection for white rather than nonwhite individuals also suggests genetic influences. An increased prevalence of HLA-DRw6 has been noted.[196]

Toxic injury has received little attention as a potential contributing factor to FMD. An increased prevalence of cigarette smoking has been noted in FMD patients with renovascular hypertension.[198] In a case-controlled study, a significant dose-related association between cigarette smoking and FMD was seen, with an eightfold increased prevalence in those who smoked at least 10 pack-years of cigarettes.[196] Potentially injurious vascular effects of tobacco include stimulation of platelet-derived growth factors,[199] endothelial damage, increased thrombogenicity, and altered rheologic properties.[119]

Intimal proliferation in FMD and other disorders

The intimal fibroplasia subtype of FMD differs sufficiently from the others to consider separate etiologic factors. As has already been mentioned, the marked female predominance seen in other subtypes is lacking, thus hormonal factors probably are not important. Intimal thickening is a common vascular response to a variety of agents such as deendothelialization,[200] chemical injury (e.g., homocystinemia[201] and arsenic exposure[202]), and autoimmune insults as seen in the arteriopathy of heart transplant rejection.[203] Histologically similar intimal proliferation has been noted in association with neurofibromatosis[204] and congenital rubella infection.[205] It appears that under a variety of influences, medial smooth muscle cells are induced to migrate into the intima, to "modulate" from a contractile to a synthetic state (myofibroblast), and to proliferate, leading to intimal thickening.[206] This proposed sequence represents the cornerstone of one of the major theories of atherogenesis.[207] The precise etiologic factor or factors responsible for this process in an individual case may not be apparent.

DISORDERS OF VEINS
Varicose veins

The pathogenesis of esophageal varices is well understood in relation to portal hypertension and portosystemic shunting of venous blood. It is ironic that the same cannot be said for the much more ubiquitous and accessible varicose veins of the lower extremities seen so commonly in older individuals. Obviously, local hemodynamic influences affecting venous blood flow or stasis must be important, but factors such as obesity, venous obstruction, and posture (prolonged standing) do not explain all cases. Two theories have dominated the conventional wisdom of pathogenesis of these lesions. The first theory maintains that valves in the saphenous venous system are incompetent or reduced in number, and the second postulate holds that degenerative changes in the vessel wall leads to venous dilatation.[208,209] Anatomic evidence supporting these contentions is lacking: the number of venous valves does not decrease with age, and degenerative alterations in the venous wall appear to be secondary phenomena.[209,210] More recent evidence has implicated precapillary arteriovenous shunts in the pathogenesis of this condition. As reviewed by Haimovici,[209] such shunts were shown to exist

in the saphenous venous system in the 1940s and 1950s, and increased oxygen saturation in variceal veins was demonstrated even earlier. This latter observation has been confirmed,[208] and direct surgical observation as well as angiographic data support the presence of such shunts.[209] The shunting of arterial blood into veins could lead to their dilatation over time; more study is needed to clarify the role of this purported mechanism in varix formation.

Thrombophlebitis

The reader hardly needs to be reminded that deep venous thrombosis, especially of the lower extremities and pelvic plexes, underlies the vast majority of cases of pulmonary thromboembolism, and that congestive heart failure, prolonged bed rest, neoplasia, pregnancy, and the postoperative state are the most common predisposing conditions.[211] Oral contraceptive use, obesity, and trauma also have been identified as risk factors. The triad of influences bearing Virchow's eponym still remain as a reminder of the principal components mediating venous thrombosis: alterations in blood flow, in coagulability, and in the blood vessel wall. A review of these factors is beyond the scope of this discussion, but a few recent observations will be noted.

The endothelial cell plays a pivotal role in vascular thrombogenicity, and injury to venous endothelium, either by stasis-induced anoxia or other mechanisms, may initiate the thrombogenic process.[212] Histologically, most venous thrombi are associated with mural inflammation (hence the term *thrombophlebitis*), and certainly thrombosis is seen in veins adjacent to inflammatory processes. Cytokines can induce endothelial cell activation, as discussed under Kawasaki disease, and also increase endothelial thrombogenicity.[213] This mechanism may be important in some cases of venous thrombosis.

In recent years, a greater recognition of the importance of hypercoagulable states has been attained. Laboratory methods for assay of protein C, protein S, and antithrombin-III have led to the recognition of hereditary deficiencies of these fibrinolytic mediators. Acquired defects in the fibrinolytic activity of blood have been noted in obesity and in the postoperative period, with a number of mechanisms proposed to explain these observations.[212] Anticardiolipin antibodies, associated with the lupus anticoagulant, may be seen in systemic lupus erythematosus, as well as in a variety of infectious and neoplastic conditions. The presence of these substances has been associated with thrombosis and fetal loss.[214] The mechanism is not certain, but probably is related to antiphospholipid activity.[214]

Complications of venous thrombosis include embolic events, infection, and obstruction. Secondary infection of thrombi from bacteremia or local suppurative processes may lead to further dissemination of the infectious process. The consequences of obstruction depend on the site of venous occlusion. Such occlusion obviously has more

Table 17-4. Vascular malformations of the gastrointestinal (GI) tract

Lesion	Site	Onset
Type 1: angiodysplasia	Right colon	Age over 55 years, acquired
Type 2: arteriovenous malformation	Small intestine	Age under 50 years, ? congenital
Type 3: angiomatosis	Multiple in GI tract, skin	Symptoms around puberty, familial
Other: Dieulafoy lesion	Stomach	Any age, congenital

important local effects in a visceral organ (e.g., Budd-Chiari syndrome from hepatic vein thrombosis) than in an extremity.

Venoocclusive disease

Venoocclusive disease refers to sclerosis of hepatic venules (central veins) in the liver, producing clinical findings similar to those in Budd-Chiari syndrome.[215] An association with chemotherapeutic drugs, immunosuppressive agents, irradiation, and other conditions has been noted.[215]

VASCULAR MALFORMATIONS

Vascular malformations are hereditary or acquired abnormalities of blood vessels which, although probably not true neoplasms, often present as expansile tumors. They may occur in numerous sites, but are most common in the gastrointestinal tract, skin, soft tissue, and central nervous system.

Vascular malformations of the gastrointestinal tract

Terminology of vascular malformations of the gastrointestinal tract has been confusing; a classification proposed by Moore et al[216,217] will be adopted for this discussion, and appears in modified form in Table 17-4). Type 1 malformations are better known as *angiodysplasia,* and are a common cause of lower gastrointestinal bleeding in elderly patients. They are acquired degenerative lesions and are identified histologically as dilated congested vessels within the submucosa, often with extension into the lamina propria (Fig. 17-25). An association with aortic stenosis has been suggested but subsequently questioned.[217,218] Type 2 malformations, for which the term AVM is applied, occur as probable congenital lesions of the small intestine that cause gastrointestinal bleeding in young individuals. Compared with type 1 lesions, these are less common, and are more likely to be visible grossly as areas of large, abnormal vessels (Fig. 17-26). Type 3 malformations *(angiomatosis)* are the multiple telangiectasias seen in hereditary hemorrhagic telangiectasia (Osler-Weber-

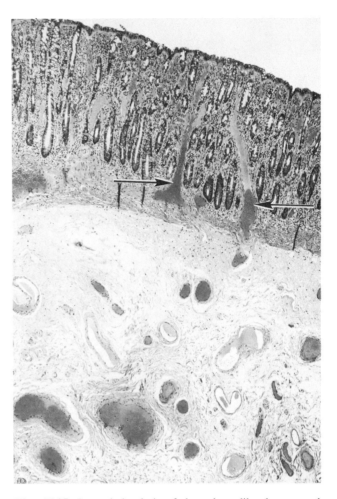

Fig. 17-25. In angiodysplasia of the colon, dilated congested blood vessels are seen in the submucosa (lower half of photograph) and extend into the lamina propria *(arrows).*

Rendu) syndrome. They involve multiple skin and mucosal sites, and histologically consist of telangiectatic vessels, which are indistinguishable from those in type 1 malformations.

Rarely, gastric bleeding is caused by a vascular anomaly known as *Dieulafoy's erosion.*[219] This lesion is described as an abnormally large artery that protrudes into the mucosa, where it is prone to ulceration and rupture. Other authors have termed this defect the *caliber persistent artery,* arguing that the abnormality is failure of the normal tapering of the vessel as it approaches the mucosa.[220]

Vascular malformations of skin

Dilated vessels, or *telangiectasias,* are seen in a variety of clinical settings. The "spider" hemangioma actually represents a form of acquired vascular ectasia noted in liver disease, pregnancy, and other states of physiologic or pathologic hormonal imbalance. The *port-wine stain (nevus flammeus)* is a large congenital vascular ectasia which, when occurring in trigeminal nerve distribution on the face

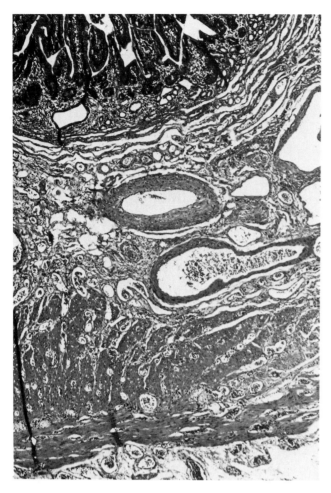

Fig. 17-26. In this arteriovenous malformation of small intestine, blood vessels of many sizes are present within the submucosa (center) and muscularis externa (lower portion of photograph). The lamina propria and intestinal villi are seen at upper left.

and associated with leptomeningeal and retinal vascular lesions, is a manifestation of *Sturge-Weber syndrome*.[221] Nevus flammeus associated with hemihypertrophy and varicosities comprise the *Klippel-Trenaunay syndrome*.[221]

Vascular malformations of soft tissue

Outside the gastrointestinal tract, the term *arteriovenous malformation* (AVM) has been used to describe a number of unrelated lesions. AVM of soft tissue, also known as *arteriovenous hemangioma* or *cirscoid aneurysm,* is an abnormal conglomeration of arteries, veins, and blood vessels of indeterminate type, which is found mostly in the head and neck region or lower extremities of young patients.[221] A bruit or thrill over the mass may give a clue as to its vascular nature.

Vascular malformations of the central nervous system

A lesion similar to the AVM of soft tissue occurs in the brain and spinal cord, and may cause compressive symp-

toms or may rupture, leading to intracerebral or subarachnoid hemorrhage.

A rare vascular anomaly in the base of the brain, causing massive cerebral hemorrhage, is known as *Moyamoya disease*. Pathologically, vessels of the circle of Willis display fibrotic stenoses, and the hemorrhage may result from rupture of collateral arteries.[222]

VASCULAR TUMORS

A comprehensive clinical or pathologic review of all known vascular neoplasms is beyond the scope of this chapter. Instead, the intent is to address salient features of selected tumors, with particular reference to biologic behavior. For purposes of this discussion, "vascular tumors" will include proliferations thought to arise from or differentiate toward endothelium, and that form structures resembling blood vessels or lymphatics (i.e., possessing "vasoformative" properties). Such features are usually obvious, but occasionally special studies are needed to document vascular differentiation. Endothelial cells are characterized by staining for factor VIII-related antigen and *Ulex europaeus* agglutinin; ultrastructurally, blood vessel endothelial cells, but not those of lymphatic vessels, contain structures known as Weibel-Palade bodies, in which factor VIII-related antigen is concentrated.[223] Clinically, the most important aspect of this group of tumors is their biologic behavior, and the full spectrum from innocuous to highly malignant is represented by these lesions (Fig. 17-27).

Benign vascular tumors

Papillary endothelial hyperplasia. Papillary endothelial hyperplasia is a reactive (nonneoplastic) proliferation of endothelial cells, possibly representing an unusually exuberant endothelial response in an organizing thrombus (Fig. 17-28).[224] *Hemangiomas* are common benign vascular neoplasms that have several morphologic subtypes, including cavernous (Fig. 17-29), capillary, and juvenile. In spite of its name, *pyogenic granuloma* also is a form of capillary hemangioma that occurs most commonly in the oral cavity and skin. Histologically, hemangiomas contain a proliferation of vascular spaces lined by a single layer of flattened endothelial cells, and usually containing blood. *Lymphangiomas,* most commonly encountered clinically as the cystic hygroma of the neck, are histologically similar to cavernous hemangiomas except that the spaces contain proteinaceous fluid rather than blood, and lymphoid aggregates often are seen in the walls (Fig. 17-30). Cavernous hemangiomas are associated with several syndromes. In *blue rubber bleb nevus syndrome*, pedunculated hemangiomas of the skin occur with hemangiomas of the gastrointestinal tract.[225] *Maffucci syndrome* is the combination of multiple hemangiomas and enchondromas.[216] Hemangiomas also occur in *von Hippel-Lindau disease*, and affect retina and brain in addition to skin.

One of the most peculiar entities among the vascular tu-

Vascular Tumors
Spectrum of Biologic Behavior

Benign

Malignant

Papillary Endothelial Hyperplasia

Hemangioma/Lymphangioma

Epithelioid Hemangioma

Epithelioid Hemangioendothelioma

Kaposi's Sarcoma

Angiosarcoma/Lymphangiosarcoma

Fig. 17-27. Vascular tumors range in their biologic behavior from hyperplastic and benign neoplastic conditions, to neoplasms of intermediate malignancy (epithelioid hemangioendothelioma), to frankly malignant sarcomas.

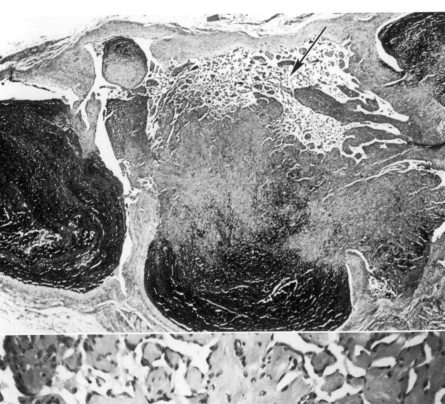

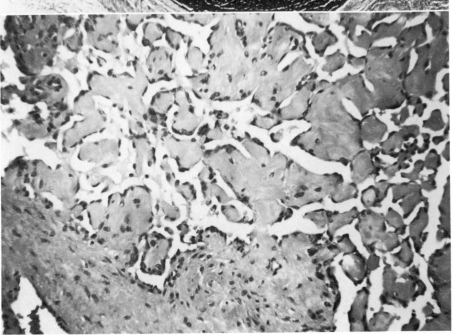

Fig. 17-28. A, A large vein contains unorganized thrombus (dark material, left and center), and papillary endothelial hyperplasia in an area of organizing thrombus *(arrow)*. Fig. 17-28 **B,** High-power photomicrograph from same case as Fig. 17-28 **A,** demonstrates papillary fibrous structures lined by endothelial cells.

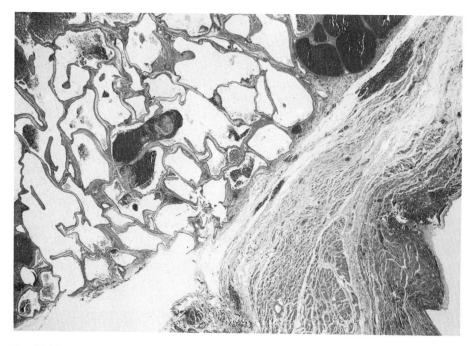

Fig. 17-29. Multiple thin-walled vascular spaces, some filled with blood, characterize this cavernous hemangioma that occurred in the heart.

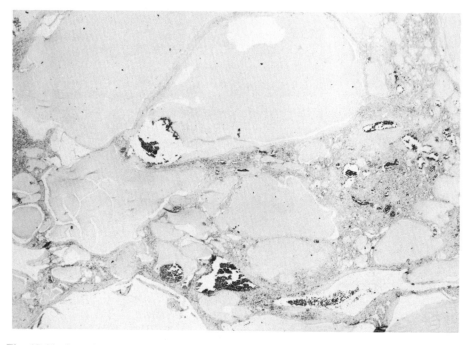

Fig. 17-30. Lymphangiomas are histologically similar to cavernous hemangiomas, except that the thin-walled spaces contain proteinaceous fluid rather than blood, and lymphoid aggregates often are present.

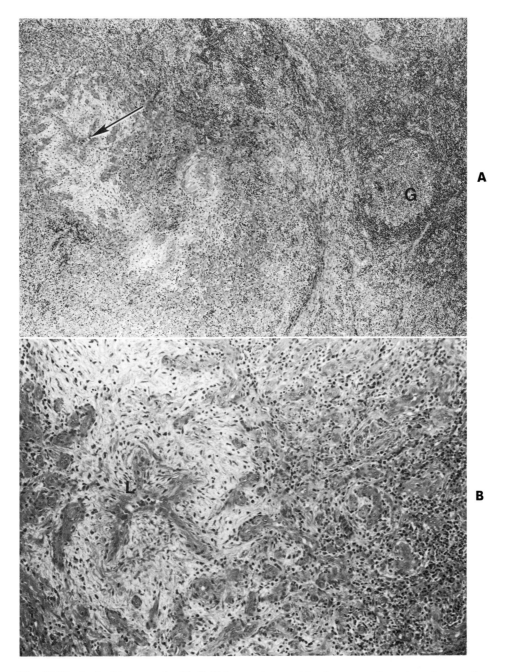

Fig. 17-31. A, In this case of epithelioid hemangioma arising in a muscular artery, the vessel lumen has been reduced to pinpoint size *(arrow),* and the wall has been obscured by an intense inflammatory infiltrate and proliferating endothelial channels. Just outside the vessel, a lymphoid aggregate with germinal center *(G)* is noted. **B,** In a high power view from the same case as Fig. 17-31A, capillary-sized vascular channels lined by plump endothelial cells appear to radiate from the central lumen *(L).* Numerous inflammatory cells are admixed.

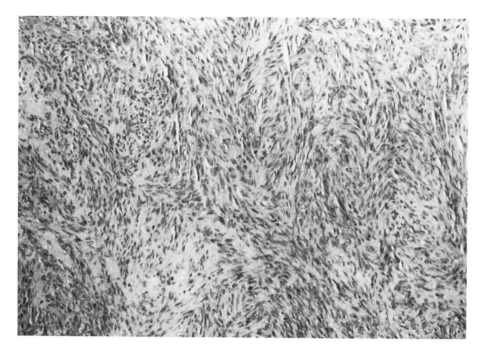

Fig. 17-32. This photomicrograph demonstrates the dense spindle cell proliferation and intervening slit-like spaces characteristic of Kaposi sarcoma.

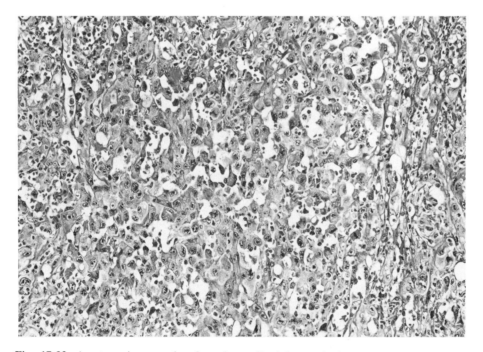

Fig. 17-33. Anastomosing vascular channels are lined by cytologically malignant endothelial cells in this angiosarcoma.

mors is known variously as angiolymphoid hyperplasia with eosinophilia, Kimuras disease, histiocytoid hemangioma, or the currently favored term *epithelioid hemangioma* (EH).[226-229] The characteristic morphologic feature is the appearance of the proliferating endothelial cell, which is plump rather than flattened, and resembles an epithelial or histiocytic cell (thus *epithelioid* or *histiocytoid*). Additional findings are a variable lymphoid infiltrate, usually with germinal center formation, and eosinophils (Fig. 17-31). The neoplastic versus reactive nature of this process has been debated. Most cases are probably neoplastic, and although benign, local recurrence is seen in around one-third.[229] It may be that cases described in the Orient as Kimura disease, with pronounced lymphadenopathy and peripheral blood eosinophilia, represent a different, more likely immunoreactive process.[227,229]

Neoplasms of intermediate malignancy

Epithelioid hemangioendothelioma. Epithelioid hemangioendothelioma (EHE) shares with EH the appearance of epithelioid endothelial cells, but differs in several important respects. First, vascular differentiation is more subtle and may be overlooked. Second, intracellular lumina give a vacuolar appearance to the endothelial cells, which may be mistaken for mucin-containing signet-ring cells of an adenocarcinoma. Third, EHE often occur in soft tissue, bone, liver, or lung, compared with EH, which tends to arise in the head and neck region. Fourth, EHE has a definite metastatic ability.[229] Thus these are considered to represent true neoplasms of low malignant potential. The lesion described in the lung as intravascular bronchioloalveolar tumor (IVBAT) actually represents pulmonary EHE.[229,230]

Malignant vascular neoplasms

Kaposi sarcoma. Kaposi sarcoma (KS) usually is seen today in association with AIDS, but sporadic cases in elderly nonimmunosuppressed individuals occasionally are encountered. The histologic appearance is identical in both clinical settings, and is characterized by a spindle-cell proliferation with intervening slit-like vascular spaces, extravasated erythrocytes, and PAS-positive eosinophilic globules of uncertain histogenesis (Fig. 17-32). Although it is usually thought of as a fully malignant neoplasm possessing the properties of local tissue infiltration and metastatic potential, some investigators entertain the possibility that KS may represent an unusual reactive hyperplasia.[231] There is some doubt regarding the endothelial nature of the proliferating cell itself; smooth muscle cells, other mesenchymal cells, and dermal dendrocytes (Langerhans-like cells) are other possible progenitor cells.[232]

The exact role of the human immunodeficiency virus (HIV) in pathogenesis of KS is uncertain. An indirect role based on HIV-induced secretion of several growth factors and cytokines by infected cells has been proposed. Although genomic HIV sequences have been difficult to identify in lesions of KS, one group was able to find HIV RNA transcripts in three of eight biopsies from HIV-infected individuals.[232] Thus the pathogenesis of HIV-associated KS may involve both direct and indirect mechanisms.

Angiosarcoma. Angiosarcoma is the unequivocally malignant soft tissue sarcoma with histologic and immunohistochemical evidence of vascular differentiation. As opposed to benign vasoformative neoplasms, the endothelial cells that line the anastomosing vascular channels are cytologically malignant (Fig. 17-33). Angiosarcomas may be seen in any age group, and occur in skin, soft tissue, or parenchymal organs.

Although the etiology of most vascular tumors is unknown, angiosarcomas of the liver have been related to exposure to arsenic, thorium dioxide (Thorotrast), and gaseous vinyl chloride used in manufacturing the plastic polyvinyl chloride.[233] Premalignant changes in hepatic tissue have been identified in some cases.[233] Another etiologic association is recognized for *lymphangiosarcoma*, a sarcoma of presumed lymphatic origin. This malignant neoplasm occurs rarely in the axillary region of women who have had a previous mastectomy, and is thought to be induced in some way by chronic lymphatic obstruction.[234]

In addition to their ability to cause morbidity by mass effect, local tissue infiltration, and metastasis, vasoformative tumors may cause unique pathophysiologic derangements by virtue of their vascular properties. Large cavernous hemangiomas, especially in relatively small individuals (infants and children), can be associated with thrombocytopenia and consumptive coagulopathy from activation of platelet aggregation and the coagulation cascade within the abnormal vascular channels (Kasabach-Merritt syndrome[235]). High output heart failure rarely can be seen if significant arteriovenous shunting is present. Such shunting, which may occur with large arteriovenous malformations (especially of deep soft tissue), also may cause "Branham's sign" (slowing of heart rate with compression) and increased venous oxygen saturation.[221]

DISORDERS OF LYMPHATICS
Lymphedema and lymphangiectasia

Lymphatic vessels are thin-walled endothelial-lined channels that carry protein-rich fluid from extracellular tissue spaces back into the bloodstream. Lack of tight junctions between lymphatic endothelial cells permits entry of particulate and cellular matter from the interstitial fluid. The movement of lymph, which eventually enters the central venous system by way of the thoracic duct and right lymphatic trunk, is aided by skeletal muscle contraction, arterial pulsation, respiratory activity, and the presence of one-way valves.[236]

Lymphedema, an accumulation of protein-rich fluid in the interstitial space, results from mechanical obstruction,

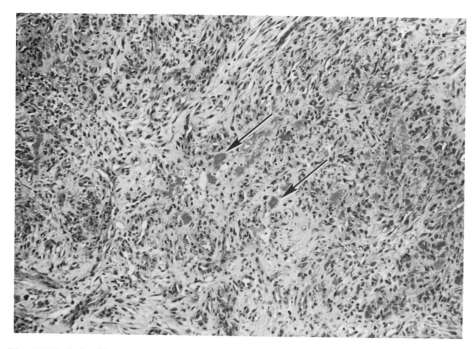

Fig. 17-34. In bacillary angiomatosis, proliferating capillaries give the appearance of a capillary hemangioma or pyogenic granuloma; however, clumps of bacteria *(arrows)* and a characteristic inflammatory component allow for the correct diagnosis.

maldevelopment, overload of lymphatic vessels, or unknown causes. Malignant tumors, radiation-induced changes, and posttraumatic or postsurgical interruption of lymphatics are clinically important conditions predisposing to lymphedema. Lymphangiosarcoma developing in the setting of chronic lymphedema has been mentioned previously. Worldwide, filariasis is a major cause of massive lymphedema of the extremities known as *elephantiasis;* the pathogenesis involves chronic lymphatic obstruction by inflammation and fibrosis surrounding adult worms of genus *Wuchereria* or *Brugia.*[237]

Lymphedema is considered *primary* when it results from maldevelopment or dysfunction of lymphatics without any specific associations such as those listed above.[236] Lymphedema of this type commonly manifests as edematous enlargement of a lower extremity. Several classification schemes exist based on various clinical or lymphangiographic features. Some cases are hereditary, for example Milroy disease (chronic lymphedema occurring from at or near the time of birth), whereas others are sporadic. Age of onset also varies: in *lymphedema praecox* onset is before 35 years of age, usually in adolescence, whereas onset in *lymphedema tarda* is after 35 years of age.[236] By lymphangiographic studies, aplasia, hypoplasia, or hyperplasia of lymphatic vessels have been described.[236]

Developmental abnormalities or obstruction of lymphatic vessels in the gastrointestinal tract is identified histologically as *lymphangiectasia,* a dilatation of lymphatics in the superficial gut mucosa. In severe cases, intraluminal loss of lymphatic contents may lead to a protein-losing enteropathy, particularly in children.[238] Lymphangiectasia also may occur in extraintestinal sites.

Lymphangitis

Lymphangitis usually is identified clinically as painful red streaks on an extremity, representing inflamed lymphatic channels. Bacterial organisms, especially group A streptococci, most commonly are implicated. Spread of infection to draining lymph nodes results in *lymphadenitis;* histopathologically, a suppurative and occasionally necrotizing inflammatory process is seen. Dissemination of infection may occur.

MISCELLANEOUS VASCULAR DISORDERS
Idiopathic arterial calcification of infancy

This is an uncommon disease that causes myocardial ischemia and infarction in early infancy, with most deaths occurring in the first 6 months of life, and only rare survival past the first year.[239] Marked intimal proliferation, without atheromatous change, is seen in the coronary arteries, and calcification along the internal elastic lamina is characteristic. The condition is not an arteritis because inflammatory infiltrates are not observed. Calcification, which is not always present, actually may be a secondary phenomenon, whereas intimal proliferation may be the principal pathologic abnormality.[240]

Human immunodeficiency virus-related vascular disease

Several vascular disorders are associated with HIV infection. Kaposi sarcoma (KS) already has been discussed under the heading of vascular tumors, and is the best known of these. A peculiar vascular proliferation, which may be mistaken for KS or other vascular tumors, occurs in association with bacterial organisms similar or identical to the cat-scratch bacillus and is called *bacillary angiomatosis*.[241] The vascular proliferation in this usually cutaneous hemangioma-like lesion appears to represent a response to infection by the organism (Fig. 17-34), and the condition responds to antibacterial therapy. In children with acquired immune deficiency syndrome (AIDS), Joshi et al[242] have described an *arteriopathy* characterized by intimal fibrosis, calcification, and occasional aneurysm formation, with involvement of multiple systemic organs.[242] Pathogenesis is uncertain, and whether the disorder is caused by HIV itself or is a manifestation of injury resulting from repeated opportunistic infections is not clear.[242]

Cardiac transplant arteriosclerosis

In spite of advances in management of patients with cardiac transplantation, vascular disease in the coronary arteries continues to be a major problem limiting long-term success. This lesion differs from typical atherosclerosis in that it progresses relatively rapidly, occurs diffusely along the coronary arteries into the intramyocardial branches, and causes concentric rather than eccentric intimal thickening.[203] Pathogenesis is uncertain, but obviously must involve immunological mechanisms. A cytotoxic T-cell-mediated endothelialitis has been implicated.[243] Expression of class II HLA antigens, which can be induced in endothelial cells by cytokines, may underlie a T-cell response against the foreign blood vessel endothelium. Elaboration of cytokines and growth factors in the vessel wall might lead to neointimal proliferation in this condition.[244]

Progressive arterial occlusive disease (Kohlmeier-Degos Disease)

In this rare disorder, fibrointimal proliferation involves small and medium arteries of skin and the gastrointestinal tract. Dermal vascular thrombosis often is noted.[245] Most cases have occurred in young men, and the skin eruption, which is seen early in the course of disease, apparently is pathognomonic.[246] Death often results from peritonitis or gastrointestinal hemorrhage. The disease has been considered by different authors to represent a coagulopathy, a vasculitis, or a primary mucinosis; the evidence for these various theories of pathogenesis is extensively reviewed by Magrinat.[245]

Others

Vascular lesions characterized predominantly by intimal hyperplasia are seen in neurofibromatosis, arsenic toxicity, homocystinemia, and rubella syndrome; these are mentioned in the discussion of the intimal hyperplasia subtype of fibromuscular dysplasia.

REFERENCES

1. Fauci AS, Haynes BF, Katz P: The spectrum of vasculitis: clinical, pathologic, immunologic, and therapeutic considerations, *Ann Intern Med* 89:660-676, 1978.
2. Gilliam JN, Smiley JD:Cutaneous necrotizing vasculitis and related disorders, *Ann Allergy* 37:328-339, 1976.
3. Lie JT: The classification and diagnosis of vasculitis in large and medium-sized blood vessels, *Pathol Annu* 22:125-162, 1987.
4. Ledford DK, Espinoza LR: Immunologic aspects of cardiovascular disease, *JAMA* 258:2974-2982, 1987.
5. Jennette JC: Antineutrophil cytoplasmic autoantibody-associated diseases: a pathologist's perspective, *Am J Kidney Dis* 18:164-170, 1991.
6. Hunder GG: Giant cell (temporal arteritis, *Rheum Dis Clin North Am* 16:399-409, 1990.
7. Machado EBV, Michet CJ, Ballard DJ et al: Trends in incidence and clinical presentation of temporal arteritis in Olmsted County, Minnesota, 1950-1985, *Arthritis Rheum* 31:745-749, 1988.
8. Huston KA, Hunder GG, Lie JT et al: Temporal arteritis: a 25-year epidemiologic, clinical, and pathologic study, *Ann Intern Med* 88:162-167, 1978.
9. Allsop CJ, Gallagher PJ: Temporal artery biopsy in giant-cell arteritis, *Amer J Surg Pathol* 5:317-323, 1981.
10. Richardson JE, Gladman DD, Fam A et al: HLA-DR4 in giant cell arteritis: association with polymyalgia rheumatica syndrome, *Arthritis Rheum* 30:1293-1297, 1987.
11. Cid MC, Ercilla G, Vilaseca J et al: Polymyalgia rheumatica: a syndrome associated with HLA-DR4 antigen, *Arthritis Rheum* 31:678-682, 1988.
12. Banks PM, Cohen MD, Ginsburg WW et al: Immunohistologic and cytochemical studies of temporal arteritis, *Arthritis Rheum* 26:1201-1207, 1983.
13. Andersson R, Jonsson R, Tarkowski A et al: T cell subsets and expression of immunological activation markers in the arterial walls of patients with giant cell arteritis, *Ann Rheum Dis* 46:915-923, 1987.
14. Cid MC, Campo E, Ercilla G et al: Immunohistochemical analysis of lymphoid and macrophage cell subsets and their immunologic activation markers in temporal arteritis: influence of corticosteroid treatment, *Arthritis Rheum* 32:884-893, 1989.
15. Papaioannou CC, Gupta RC, Hunder GG et al: Circulating immune complexes in giant cell arteritis and polymyalgia rheumatica, *Arthritis Rheum* 23:1021-1025, 1980.
16. Dasgupta B, Duke O, Timms AM et al: Selective depletion and activation of CD8 + lymphocytes from peripheral blood of patients with polymyalgia rheumatica and giant cell arteritis, *Ann Rheum Dis* 48:307-311, 1989.
17. Elling P, Olsson A, Elling H: CD8+ T lymphocyte subset in giant cell arteritis and related disorders, *J Rheumatol* 17:225-227, 1990.
18. Johnston RB: Current concepts: Immunology. Monocytes and macrophages, *N Engl J Med* 318:747-752, 1988.
19. Cohen S: Physiologic and pathologic manifestations of lymphokine action, *Hum Pathol* 17:112-121, 1986.
20. Dasgupta B, Panayi GS: Interleukin-6 in serum of patients with polymyalgia rheumatica and giant cell arteritis, *Br J Rheumatol* 29:456-458, 1990.
21. Klareskog L, Forsum U, Scheynius A et al: Evidence in support of a self-perpetuating HLA-DR-dependent delayed-type cell reaction in rheumatoid arthritis, *Proc Natl Acad Sci USA* 79:3632-3636, 1982.
22. Westedt ML, Breedveld FC, Schreuder GMT et al: Immunogenetic heterogeneity of rheumatoid arthritis, *Ann Rheum Dis* 45:534-538, 1986.

23. Fauci AS, Lane HC, Volkman DJ: Activation and regulation of human immune responses: Implications in normal and disease states, *Ann Intern Med* 99:61-75, 1983.

24. Liang GC, Simkin PA, Mannik M: Immunoglobulins in temporal arteries: an immunofluorescent study, *Ann Intern Med* 81:19-24, 1974.

25. Bocanegra TS, Germain BF, Saba HI et al: In vitro cytotoxicity of human endothelial cells in polymyalgia rheumatica and giant cell arteritis, *Rheumatol Int* 2:133-136, 1982.

26. McHugh NJ, James IE, Plant GT: Anticardiolipin and antineutrophil antibodies in giant cell arteritis, *J Rheumatol* 17:916-922, 1990.

27. Espinoza LR, Jara LJ, Silveira LH et al: Anticardiolipin antibodies in polymyalgia rheumatica-giant cell arteritis: association with severe vascular complications, *Am J Med* 90:474-478, 1991.

28. Alarcon-Segovia D: Pathogenetic potential of antiphospholipid antibodies, *J Rheumatol* 15:890-893, 1988.

29. Fort JG, Cowchock FS, Abruzzo JL et al: Anticardiolipin antibodies in patients with rheumatic diseases, *Arthritis Rheum* 30:752-760, 1987.

30. Perruquet JL, Davis DE, Harrington TM: Aortic arch arteritis in the elderly: an important manifestation of giant cell arteritis, *Arch Intern Med* 146:289-291, 1986.

31. Costello JM, Nicholson WJ: Severe aortic regurgitation as a late complication of temporal arteritis, *Chest* 98:875-877, 1990.

32. Pantell RH, Goodman BW Jr: Takayasu's arteritis: the relationship with tuberculosis, *Pediatr* 67:84-88, 1981.

33. Nasu T: Takayasu's truncoarteritis: Pulseless disease or aortitis syndrome, *Acta Pathol Jpn* 32(Suppl. 1):117-131, 1982.

34. Lupi-Herrera E, Sánchez-Torres G, Marcushamer J et al: Takayasu's arteritis. Clinical study of 107 cases, *Am Heart J* 93:94-103, 1977.

35. Ishikawa K: Natural history and classification of occlusive thromboaortopathy (Takayasu's disease), *Circulation* 57:27-35, 1978.

36. Rose AG, Sinclair-Smith CC: Takayasu's arteritis: a study of 16 autopsy cases, *Arch Pathol Lab Med* 104:231-237, 1980.

37. Cipriano PR, Silverman JF, Periroth MG et al: Coronary arterial narrowing in Takayasu's aortitis, *Am J Cardiol* 39:744-750, 1977.

38. Matsumura K, Hirano T, Takeda K et al: Incidence of aneurysms in Takayasu's arteritis, *Angiology* 42:308-315, 1991.

39. Nakao K, Ikeda M, Kimata S et al: Takayasu's arteritis: clinical report of eighty-four cases and immunological studies in seven cases, *Circulation* 35:1141-1155, 1967.

40. Isohisa I, Numano F, Maezawa H et al: Hereditary factors in Takayasu's disease, *Angiology* 33:98-104, 1982.

41. Moriuchi J, Wakisaka A, Aizawa M et al: HLA-linked susceptibility gene of Takayasu disease, *Hum Immunol* 4:87-91, 1982.

42. Kodama K, Kida O, Morotomi Y et al: Male siblings with Takayasu's arteritis suggest genetic etiology, *Heart Vessels* 2:51-54, 1986.

43. Numano F, Isohisa I, Maezawa H et al: HL-A antigens in Takayasu's disease, *Am Heart J* 98:153-159, 1979.

44. Volkman DJ, Mann DL, Fauci AS: Association between Takayasu's arteritis and a B-cell alloantigen in North Americans, *N Engl J Med* 306:464-465, 1982.

45. Solinger A, Stobo J: Immune response gene control of T cell reactivity to collagen in man: association of unresponsiveness with suppressive T cells, *Clin Res* 26:531A, 1981 (abstract).

46. Scott DGI, Salmon M, Scott DL et al: Takayasu's arteritis: a pathogenic role for cytotoxic T lymphocytes?, *Clin Rheumatol* 5:517-522, 1986.

47. Verztman L: Polyarteritis nodosa, *Clin Rheum Dis* 6:297-317, 1980.

48. Rosenberg MR, Parshley M, Gibson S et al: Central nervous system polyarteritis nodosa, *West J Med* 153:553-556, 1990.

49. Cohen RD, Conn DL, Ilstrup DM: Clinical features, prognosis, and response to treatment in polyarteritis, *Mayo Clin Proc* 55:146-149, 1980.

50. Lie JT: Systemic and isolated vasculitis: a rational approach to classification and pathologic diagnosis, *Pathol Annu* 24:25-114, 1989.

51. Lie JT, Hunder GG, Arend WP et al: Illustrated histopathologic classification criteria for selected vasculitis syndromes, *Arthritis Rheum* 33:1074-1087, 1990.

52. Landing BH, Larson EJ: Are infantile periarteritis nodosa with coronary artery involvement and fatal mucocutaneous lymph node syndrome the same? Comparison of 20 patients from North America with patients from Hawaii and Japan, *Pediatrics* 59:651-662, 1977.

53. Croker BP, Lee T, Gunnells JC: Clinical and pathologic features of polyarteritis nodosa and its renal-limited variant: primary crescentic and necrotizing glomerulonephritis, *Hum Pathol* 18:38-44, 1987.

54. Trepo CG, Zuckerman AJ, Bird RC et al: The role of circulating hepatitis B antigen/antibody immune complexes in the pathogenesis of vascular and hepatic manifestations in polyarteritis nodosa, *J Clin Pathol* 27:863-868, 1974.

55. Goecke DJ, Hsu K, Morgan C et al: Vasculitis in association with Australia antigen, *J Exp Med* 134:330s-336s, 1971.

56. Prince AM, Trepo C: Role of immune complexes involving SH antigen in pathogenesis of chronic active hepatitis and polyarteritis nodosa, *Lancet* 1:1309-1312, 1971.

57. Elkon KB, Hughes GRV, Catovsky D et al: Hairy-cell leukaemia with polyarteritis nodosa, *Lancet* 2:280-282, 1979.

58. Goedert JJ, Neefe JR, Smith FS et al: Polyarteritis nodosa, hairy cell leukemia and splenosis, *Am J Med* 71:323-326, 1981.

59. Miyazawa M, Nose M, Kawashima M et al: Pathogenesis of arteritis of SL/Ni mice: possible lytic effect of anti-gp70 antibodies on vascular smooth muscle cells, *J Exp Med* 166:890-908, 1987.

60. Churg J, Strauss L: Allergic granulomatosis, allergic angiitis, and periarteritis nodosa, *Am J Pathol* 27:277-294, 1951.

61. Lie JT: The classification of vasculitis and a reappraisal of allergic granulomatosis and angiitis (Churg-Strauss syndrome), *Mt Sinai J Med* 53:429-439, 1986.

62. Lanham JG, Elkon KB, Pusey CD et al: Systemic vasculitis with asthma and eosinophilia: a clinical approach to the Churg-Strauss syndrome, *Medicine* 63:65-81, 1984.

63. Chumbley LC, Harrison EG, DeRemee RA: Allergic granulomatosis and angiitis (Churg-Strauss Syndrome): report and analysis of 30 cases, *Mayo Clin Proc* 52:477-484, 1977.

64. Hasley PB, Follansbee WP, Coulehan JL: Cardiac manifestations of Churg-Strauss syndrome: report of a case and review of the literature, *Am Heart J* 120:996-999, 1990.

65. Masi AT, Hunder GG, Lie JT et al: The American College of Rheumatology 1990 criteria for the classification of Churg-Strauss syndrome (allergic granulomatosis and angiitis), *Arthritis Rheum* 33:1094-1100, 1990.

66. McCluskey RT, Fienberg R: Vasculitis in primary vasculitides, granulomatoses, and connective tissue diseases, *Hum Pathol* 14:305-315, 1983.

67. Suen KC, Burton JD: The spectrum of eosinophilic infiltration of the gastrointestinal tract and its relationship to other disorders of angiitis and granulomatosis, *Hum Pathol* 10:31-43, 1979.

68. Manger BJ, Krape FE, Gramatzki M et al: IgE-containing circulating immune complexes in Churg-Strauss vasculitis, *Scand J Immunol* 21:369-373, 1985.

69. van der Woude FJ, Lobatto S, Permin H et al: Autoantibodies against neutrophils and monocytes: tool for diagnosis and marker of disease activity in Wegener's granulomatosis, *Lancet* 1:425-429, 1985.

70. Goldschmeding R, van der Schoot CE, ten Bokkel Huinink D et al: Wegener's granulomatosis autoantibodies identify a novel diisopropylfluorophosphate-binding protein in the lysosomes of normal human neutrophils, *J Clin Invest* 84:1577-1587, 1989.

71. Niles JL, McCluskey RT, Ahmad MF et al: Wegener's granulomatosis antoantigen is a novel neutrophil serine protease, *Blood* 74:1888-1893, 1989.

72. Falk RJ, Jennette JC: Anti-neutrophil cytoplasmic autoantibodies with specificity for myeloperoxidase in patients with systemic vasculitis and idiopathic necrotizing and crescentic glomerulonephritis, *N Engl J Med* 318:1651-1657, 1988.

73. Tervaert JWC, Limburg PC, Elema JD et al: Detection of autoantibodies against myeloid lysosomal enzymes: a useful adjunct to classification of patients with biopsy-proven necrotizing arteritis, *Am J Med* 91:59-66, 1991.

74. Nölle B, Specs U, Lüdemann J et al: Anticytoplasmic autoantibodies: their immunodiagnostic value in Wegener granulomatosis, *Ann Intern Med* 111:28-40, 1989.

75. Ewert BH, Jennette JC, Falk RJ: The pathogenic role of antineutrophil cytoplasmic autoantibodies, *Am J Kidney Dis* 18:188-195, 1991.

76. Kallenberg CGM, Tervaert JWC, van der Woude FJ et al: Autoimmunity to lysosomal enzymes: new clues to vasculitis and glomerulonephritis?, *Immunol Today* 12:61-64, 1991.

77. Walton EW: Giant-cell granuloma of the respiratory tract (Wegener's granulomatosis), *Br J Med* 2:265-270, 1958.

78. Fauci AS, Wolff SM: Wegener's granulomatosis: studies in eighteen patients and a review of the literature, *Medicine* 52:535-561, 1973.

79. Fauci AS, Haynes BF, Katz P et al: Wegener's granulomatosis: prospective clinical and therapeutic experience with 85 patients for 21 years, *Ann Intern Med* 98:76-85, 1983.

80. Pinching LJ, Lockwood CM, Pussell BA et al: Wegener's granulomatosis: observations on 18 patients with severe renal disease, *Q J Med* 208:435-460, 1983.

81. Travis WD, Hoffman GS, Leavitt RY et al: Surgical pathology of the lung in Wegener's granulomatosis. Review of 87 open lung biopsies from 67 patients, *Am J Surg Pathol* 15:315-333, 1991.

82. Saldana MJ, Patchefsky AS, Israel HL et al: Pulmonary angiitis and granulomatosis. The relationship between histological features, organ involvement, and response to treatment, *Hum Pathol* 8:391-409, 1977.

83. Myers JL, Katzenstein A: Wegener's granulomatosis presenting with massive pulmonary hemorrhage and capillaritis, *Am J Surg Pathol* 11:895-898, 1987.

84. Horn RG, Fauci AS, Rosenthal AS et al: Renal biopsy pathology in Wegener's granulomatosis, *Am J Pathol* 74:423-440, 1974.

85. Weiss MA, Crissman JD: Renal biopsy findings in Wegener's granulomatosis: segmental necrotizing glomerulonephritis with glomerular thrombosis, *Hum Pathol* 15:943-956, 1984.

86. Braun MG, Csernok E, Gross WL et al: Proteinase 3, the target antigen of anticytoplasmic antibodies circulating in Wegener's granulomatosis, *Am J Pathol* 139:831-838, 1991.

87. Boudes P, Andre C, Belghiti D et al: Microscopic Wegener's disease: A particular form of Wegener's granulomatosis, *J Rheumatol* 17:1412-1414, 1990.

88. Kawasaki T: Acute febrile mucocutaneous syndrome with lymphoid involvement with specific desquamation of the fingers and toes in children (Japanese), *Japan J Allergol* 16:178-222, 1967.

89. Melish ME, Hicks RV: Kawasaki syndrome: Clinical features. Pathophysiology, etiology and therapy, *J Rheumatol* 17(suppl 24):2-10, 1990.

90. Amano S, Hazama F, Hamashima Y: Pathology of Kawasaki disease: I. Pathology and morphogenesis of the vascular changes, *Jpn Circ J* 43:633-643, 1979.

91. Fujiwara H, Hamashima Y: Pathology of the heart in Kawasaki disease, *Pediatrics* 61:100-107, 1978.

92. Amano S, Hazama F, Hamashima Y: Pathology of Kawasaki disease: II. Distribution and incidence of the vascular lesions, *Jpn Circ J* 43:741-748, 1979.

93. Burns JC, Geha RS, Schneeberger EE et al: Polymerase activity in lymphocyte culture supernatants from patients with Kawasaki disease, *Nature* 323:814-816, 1986.

94. Shulman ST, Rowley AH: Preliminary communication: does Kawasaki disease have a retroviral etiology, *Lancet* 2:545-546, 1986.

95. Melish ME, Marchette NJ, Kaplan JC et al: Absence of significant RNA-dependent DNA polymerase activity in lymphocytes from patients with Kawasaki syndrome, *Nature* 337:288-290, 1989.

96. Terai M, Kohno Y, Niwa K et al: Imbalance among T-cell subsets in patients with coronary arterial aneurysms in Kawasaki disease, *Am J Cardiol* 60:555-559, 1987.

97. Leung DYM, Siegel L, Grady S et al: Immunoregulatory abnormalities in mucocutaneous lymph node syndrome, *Clin Immunol Immunopathol* 23:100-112, 1982.

98. Goldsmith RW, Gribetz D, Strauss L: Mucocutaneous lymph node syndrome (MLNS) in the continental United States, *Pediatrics* 57:431-434, 1976.

99. Mason WH, Jordan SC, Sakai R et al: Circulating immune complexes in Kawasaki syndrome, *Pediatr Infect Dis J* 4:48-51, 1985.

100. Leung DYM, Kurt-Jones E, Newburger JW et al: Endothelial cell activation and high interleukin-1 secretion in the pathogenesis of acute Kawasaki disease, *Lancet* 2:1298-1302, 1989.

101. Maury CPJ, Salo E, Pelkonen P: Elevated circulating tumor necrosis factor-alpha in patients with Kawasaki disease, *J Lab Clin Med* 113:651-654, 1989.

102. Leung DYM, Collins T, LaPierre LA et al: IgM antibodies present in the acute phase of Kawasaki syndrome lyse cultured vascular endothelial cells stimulated by gamma interferon, *J Clin Invest* 77:1428-1435, 1986.

103. Fujiwara T, Fujiwara H, Hamashima Y: Frequency and size of coronary arterial aneurysm at necropsy in Kawasaki disease, *Am J Cardiol* 59:808-811, 1987.

104. Takahashi M, Mason W, Lewis AB: Regression of coronary aneurysm in patients with Kawasaki syndrome, *Circulation* 75:387-394, 1987.

105. Shulman ST: IVGG therapy in Kawasaki disease: Mechanism(s) of action, *Clin Immunol Immunopathol* 53:S141-S146, 1989.

106. Wessler S, Ming SC, Gurewich V et al: A critical evaluation of thromboangiitis obliterans: the case against Buerger's disease, *N Engl J Med* 262:1149-1160, 1960.

107. Barker NW: The case for retention of the diagnostic category "Thromboangiitis obliterans", *Circulation* 25:1-4, 1962.

108. Lie JT: The rise and fall and resurgence of thromboangiitis obliterans (Buerger's disease), *Acta Pathol Jpn* 39:153-158, 1989.

109. Olin JW, Young JR, Graor RA et al: The changing clinical spectrum of thromboangiitis obliterans (Buerger's disease), *Circulation* 82(Sup IV):IV-3-IV-8, 1990.

110. Kjeldsen K, Mozes M: Buerger's disease in Israel, *Acta Chir Scand* 135:495-498, 1969.

111. Lie JT: Thromboangiitis obliterans (Buerger's disease) in women, *Medicine* 65:65-72, 1986.

112. Lie JT: Thromboangiitis obliterans (Buerger's disease) revisited, *Pathol Annu* 23(pt 2):257-291, 1988.

113. O'Dell JR, Linder J, Markin RS et al: Thromboangiitis obliterans (Buerger's disease) and smokeless tobacco, *Arthritis Rheum* 30:1054-1056, 1987.

114. de Albuquerque RR, Delgado L, Correiga P et al: Circulating immune complexes in Buerger's disease. Endarteritis obliterans in young men, *J Cardiovasc Surg* 30:821-825, 1989.

115. Gulati S, Singh KS, Thusoo TK et al: Immunological studies in thromboangiitis obliterans (Buerger's disease), *J Surg Res* 27:287-293, 1979.

116. Gulati SM, Madhra K, Thusoo TK et al: Autoantibodies in thromboangiitis obliterans (Buerger's disease), *Angiology* 33:642-651, 1982.

117. Adar R, Papa MZ, Halpern Z et al: Cellular sensitivity to collagen in thromboangiitis obliterans, *N Engl J Med* 308:1113-1116, 1983.

118. Pietraszek MH, Choudhury NA, Koyano K et al: Enhanced platelet response to serotonin in Buerger's disease, *Thromb Res* 60:241-246, 1990.

119. Krupski WC: The peripheral vascular consequences of smoking, *Ann Vasc Surg* 5:291-304, 1991.

120. Liebow AA, Carrington CRB, Friedman PJ: Lymphomatoid granulomatosis, *Hum Pathol* 3:457-558, 1972.

121. Fauci AS, Haynes BF, Costa J et al: Lymphomatoid granulomatosis: prospective clinical and therapeutic experience over 10 years, *N Engl J Med* 306:68-74, 1982.

122. Lipford EH, Margolick JB, Longo DL et al: Angiocentric immunoproliferative lesions: a clinicopathologic spectrum of post-thymic T-cell proliferations, *Blood* 72:1674-1681, 1988.

123. Medeiros LJ, Peiper SC, Elwood L et al: Angiocentric immunoproliferative lesions: a molecular analysis of eight cases, *Hum Pathol* 22:1150-1157, 1991.

124. DeRemee RA, Weiland LH, McDonald TJ: Polymorphic reticulosis, lymphomatoid granulomatosis: Two diseases or one? *Mayo Clin Proc* 53:634-640, 1978.

125. Ishii Y, Yamanaka N, Ogawa K et al: Nasal T-cell lymphoma as a type of so-called "lethal midline granuloma", *Cancer* 50:2336-2344, 1982.

126. Lakhanpal S, Kenji T, Lie JT et al: Pathologic features of Behcet's syndrome: a review of Japanese autopsy registry data, *Hum Pathol* 16:790-795, 1985.

127. Mizushima Y: Recent research into Behcet's disease in Japan, *Int J Tissue React* 10:59-65, 1988.

128. Matsumoto T, Uekusa T, Fukuda Y: Vasculo-Behcet's disease: a pathologic study of eight cases, *Hum Pathol* 22:45-51, 1991.

129. Lie JT: Cardiac and pulmonary manifestations of Behcet syndrome, *Pathol Res Pract* 183:347-355, 1988.

130. James DG: Behcet's syndrome, *N Engl J Med* 301:431-432, 1979.

131. Lombard C: Letter to the case: Behcet's disease, *Pathol Res Pract* 183:352-354, 1988.

132. Hodge SJ, Callen JP, Ekenstam E: Cutaneous leukocytoclastic vasculitis: correlation of histopathological changes with clinical severity and course, *J Cutan Pathol* 14:279-284, 1987.

133. Ekenstam E, Callen JP: Cutaneous leukocytoclastic vasculitis: clinical and laboratory features of 82 patients seen in private practice, *Arch Dermatol* 120:484-489, 1984.

134. Sams WM, Thorne EG, Small P et al: Leukocytoclastic vasculitis, *Arch Dermatol* 112:219-226, 1976.

135. Mills JA, Michel BA, Bloch DA et al: The American College of Rheumatology 1990 criteria for the classification of Henoch-Schonlein purpura, *Arthritis Rheum* 33:1114-1121, 1990.

136. Cochrane CG: Mechanisms involved in the deposition of immune complexes in tissues, *J Exp Med* 134:75s-86s, 1971.

137. Mackel SE, Jordon RE: Leukocytoclastic vasculitis: a cutaneous expression of immune complex disease, *Arch Dermatol* 118:296-301, 1982.

138. Breedveld FC, Heurkens AHM, Lafeber GJM et al: Immune complexes in sera from patients with rheumatoid vasculitis induce polymorphonuclear cell-mediated injury to endothelial cells, *Clin Immunol Immunopathol* 48:202-213, 1988.

139. Giangiacomo J, Tsai CC: Dermal and glomerular deposition of IgA in anaphylactoid purpura, *Am J Dis Child* 131:981-983, 1977.

140. Soter NA, Austen KF, Gigli I: The complement system in necrotizing angiitis of the skin: analysis of complement component activities in serum of patients with concomitant collagen-vascular diseases, *J Invest Dermatol* 63:219-226, 1974.

141. McDuffie FC, Sams WM, Maldonado JE et al: Hypocomplementemia with cutaneous vasculitis and arthritis: possible immune complex syndrome, *Mayo Clin Proc* 48:340-348, 1973.

142. Parish WE: Studies on vasculitis I. Immunoglobulins, beta-1C, C-reactive protein, and bacterial antigens in cutaneous vasculitis lesions, *Clin Exp Allergy* 1:97-109, 1971.

143. Mullick FG, McAllister HA Jr, Wagner BM et al: Drug related vasculitis: clinicopathologic correlations in 30 patients, *Hum Pathol* 10:313-325, 1979.

144. Crawford ES, Hess KR: Abdominal aortic aneurysm, *N Engl J Med* 321:1040-1042, 1989.

145. Reed D, Reed C, Stemmermann G et al: Are aortic aneurysms caused by atherosclerosis, *Circulation* 85:205-211, 1992.

146. Tilson MD: Aortic aneurysms and atherosclerosis, *Circulation* 85:378-379, 1992.

147. Pennell RC, Hollier LH, Lie JT et al: Inflammatory abdominal aortic aneurysms: a thirty-year review, *J Vasc Surg* 2:859-869, 1985.

148. Koch AE, Haines GK, Rizzo RJ et al: Human abdominal aortic aneurysms: immunophenotypic analysis suggesting an immune-mediated response, *Am J Pathol* 137:1199-1213, 1990.

149. Walker DI, Bloor K, Williams G et al: Inflammatory aneurysms of the abdominal aorta, *Br J Surg* 59:609-614, 1972.

150. Lie JT: Inflammatory aneurysm of the aorta or chronic periaortitis: A nosologic quandry, *Cardiovasc Pathol* 1:75-77, 1992.

151. Sterpetti AV, Hunter WJ, Feldhaus RJ et al: Inflammatory aneurysms of the abdominal aorta: incidence, pathologic, and etiologic considerations, *J Vasc Surg* 9:643-649, 1989.

152. Imakita M, Yutani C, Ishibashi-Udea H et al: Atherosclerotic abdominal aortic aneurysms: comparative data of different types based on the degree of inflammatory reaction, *Cardiovasc Pathol* 1:65-73, 1992.

153. Parums DV, Brown DL, Mitchinson MJ: Serum antibodies to oxidized low-density lipoprotein and ceroid in chronic periaortitis, *Arch Pathol Lab Med* 114:383-387, 1990.

154. Crawford ES, Svensson LG, Coselli JS et al: Aortic dissection and dissecting aortic aneurysms, *Ann Surg* 208:254-272, 1988.

155. Larson EW, Edwards WD: Risk factors for aortic dissection: a necropsy study of 161 cases, *Am J Cardiol* 53:849-855, 1984.

156. Gore I, Hirst AE Jr.: Dissecting aneurysm of the aorta, *Cardiovasc Clin* 5:239-259, 1973.

157. Wilson SK, Hutchins GM: Aortic dissecting aneurysms: causitive factors in 204 subjects, *Arch Pathol Lab Med* 106:175-180, 1982.

158. Roberts WC: Aortic dissection: anatomy, consequences, and causes, *Am Heart J* 101:195-214, 1981.

159. Snir E, Levinsky L, Salomon J et al: Dissecting aortic aneurysm in pregnant women without Marfan disease, *Surg Gynecol Obstet* 167:463-465, 1988.

160. Cooke JP, Kazmier FJ, Orszulak TA: The penetrating aortic ulcer: pathologic manifestations, diagnosis, and management, *Mayo Clin Proc* 63:718-725, 1988.

161. Klima T, Spjut HJ, Coelho A et al: The morphology of ascending aortic aneurysms, *Hum Pathol* 14:810-817, 1983.

162. Schlatmann TJM, Becker AE: Pathogenesis of dissecting aneurysm of the aorta: comparative histopathologic study of significance of medial changes, *Am J Cardiol* 39:21-26, 1977.

163. Schlatmann TJM, Becker AE: Histologic changes in the normal aging aorta: implications for dissecting aortic aneurysm, *Am J Cardiol* 39:13-20, 1977.

164. Hartman JD, Eftychiadis AS : Medial smooth-muscle cell lesions and dissection of the aorta and muscular arteries, *Arch Pathol Lab Med* 114:50-61, 1990.

165. Hirst AE, Gore I: Is cystic medionecrosis the cause of dissecting aortic aneurysm?, *Circulation* 53:915-916, 1976.

166. Pomerance A, Yacoub MH, Gula G: The surgical pathology of thoracic aortic aneurysms, *Histopathology* 1:257-276, 1977.

167. Lee B, Godfrey M, Vitale E et al: Linkage of Marfan syndrome and a phenotypically related disorder to two different fibrillin genes, *Nature* 352:330-339, 1991.

168. Dietz HC, Cutting GR, Pyeritz RE et al: Marfan syndrome caused by a recurrent *de novo* missense mutation in the fibrillin gene, *Nature* 352:337-339, 1991.

169. Roberts CS, Roberts WC: Dissection of the aorta associated with congenital malformation of the aortic valve, *J Am Coll Cardiol* 17:712-716, 1991.

170. Clark EG, Danbolt N: The Oslo study of the natural course of untreated syphilis: an epidemiologic investigation based on a re-study of the Boeck-Brusgaard material, *Med Clin North Am* 48:613-623, 1964.

171. Horowitz CA: Labatory investigation of syphilis, *Postgrad Med* 68:71-80, 1980.

172. Herrera H: Luetic aortitis in El Salvador, *Path Microbiol* 43:147-149, 1975.

173. Heggtveit HA: Syphilitic aortitis: a clinicopathologic autopsy study of 100 cases, 1950 to 1960, *Circulation* 29:346-355, 1964.

174. Silber EN: *Miscellaneous disorders affecting the heart*. In Silber EN, ed: *Heart disease*, ed 2, New York, 1987, Macmillan.

175. Phillips PL, Amberson JB, Libby DM: Syphilitic aortic aneurysm presenting with the superior vena cava syndrome, *Am J Med* 71:171-173, 1981.

176. Lande A, Berkmen YM: Aortitis: pathologic, clinical, and arteriographic review, *Radiol Clin North Am* 14:219-240, 1976.

177. Fitzgerald TJ: Pathogenesis and immunology of *Treponema pallidum*, *Annu Rev Microbiol* 35:29-54, 1981.

178. Thomas DD, Navab M, Haake DA et al: Treponema pallidum invades intercellular junctions of endothelial cell monolayers, *Proc Natl Acad Sci USA* 85:3608-3612, 1988.

179. Shenker BJ, Listgarten MA, Taichman NS: Suppression of human lymphocyte responses by oral spirochetes: monocyte-dependent phenomenon, *J Immunol* 132:2039-2045, 1984.

180. Friedmann PS, Turk JL: A spectrum of lymphocyte responsiveness in human syphilis, *Clin Exp Immunol* 21:59, 1975.

181. Shibata H, Matsuzaki T, Shichida K et al: Syphilis and its cardiovascular complications in the elderly, *Jpn Heart J* 17:452-458, 1976.

182. Wilson SE, Van Wagenen P, Passaro E Jr.: Arterial infection, *Curr Probl Surg* 15:1-89, 1978.

183. Stehbens WE: Pathology and pathogenesis of intracranial berry aneurysms, *Neurol Res* 12:29-34, 1990.

184. de la Monte SM, Moore GW, Monk MA et al: Risk factors for the development and rupture of intracranial berry aneurysms, *Am J Med* 78:957-964, 1985.

185. Hegedus K: Some observations on reticular fibers in the media of the major cerebral arteries: a comparative study of patients without vascular diseases and those with ruptured berry aneurysms, *Surg Neurol* 22:301-307, 1984.

186. Luscher TF, Keller HM, Imhof HG et al: Fibromuscular hyperplasia: extension of the disease and therapeutic outcome; results of the University Hospital Zurich Cooperative Study on Fibromuscular Hyperplasia, *Nephron* 44(Suppl 1):109-114, 1986.

187. Luscher TF, Lie JT, Stanson AW et al: Arterial fibromuscular dysplasia, *Mayo Clin Proc* 62:931-952, 1987.

188. Wylie EJ, Binkley FM, Palubinskas AJ: Extrarenal fibromuscular hyperplasia, *Am J Surg* 112:149-155, 1966.

189. Harrison EG, McCormack LJ: Pathologic classification of renal arterial disease in renovascular hypertension, *Mayo Clin Proc* 46:161-167, 1971.

190. Stanley JC, Gewertz BL, Bove EL et al: Arterial fibrodysplasia: histopathologic character and current etiologic concepts, *Arch Surg* 110:561-565, 1975.

191. Wollam GL, Hall WD: The diagnosis and management of renovascular hypertension, *Weekly Update: Cardiol* 1:2-7, 1978.

192. Simon N, Franklin SS, Bleifer KH et al: Clinical characteristics of renovascular hypertension, *JAMA* 220:1209-1218, 1972.

193. Mettinger KL, Ericson K: Fibromuscular dysplasia of the brain: observations on angiographic, clinical and genetic characteristics, *Stroke* 13:46-52, 1982.

194. Ross R, Klebanoff SJ: The smooth muscle cell. I. In vivo synthesis of connective tissue proteins, *J Cell Biol* 50:159-171, 1971.

195. Irey NS, Manion WC, Taylor HB: Vascular lesions in women taking oral contraceptives, *Arch Pathol Lab Med* 89:1-8, 1970.

196. Sang CN, Whelton PK, Hamper UM et al: Etiologic factors in renovascular fibromuscular dysplasia: a case-control study, *Hypertension* 14:472-479, 1989.

197. Rushton AR: The genetics of fibromuscular dysplasia, *Arch Intern Med* 140:233-236, 1980.

198. Nicholson JP, Teichman JH, Alderman MH et al: Cigarette smoking and renovascular hypertension, *Lancet* 2:765-766, 1983.

199. Oberai B, Adams CWM, High OB: Myocardial and renal arteriolar thickening in cigarette smokers, *Atherosclerosis* 52:185-190, 1984.

200. Liu MW, Roubin GS, King SB: Restenosis after coronary angioplasty: potential biologic determinants and role of intimal hyperplasia, *Circulation* 79:1374-1387, 1989.

201. Harker LA, Ross R, Slichter SJ et al: Homocystine-induced arteriosclerosis: the role of endothelial cell injury and platelet response in its genesis, *J Clin Invest* 58:731-741, 1976.

202. Rosenberg HG: Systemic arterial disease and chronic arsenicism in infants, *Arch Pathol Lab Med* 97:360-365, 1974.

203. Billingham ME: Cardiac transplant ateroclerosis, *Transplant Proc* 4(suppl 5):19-25, 1987.

204. Greene JF Jr, Fitzwater JE, Burgess J: Arterial lesions associated with neurofibromatosis, *Am J Clin Pathol* 62:481-487, 1974.

205. Fortuin NJ, Morrow AG, Roberts WC: Late vascular manifestations of the rubella syndrome, *Am J Med* 51:134-140, 1971.

206. Campbell GR, Campbell JH, Manderson JA et al: Arterial smooth muscle: a multifunctional mesenchymal cell, *Arch Pathol Lab Med* 112:977-986, 1988.

207. Ross R: The pathogenesis of atherosclerosis—an update, *N Engl J Med* 314:488-500, 1986.

208. Baron HC, Cassaro S: The role of arteriovenous shunts in the pathogenesis of varicose veins, *J Vasc Surg* 4:124-128, 1986.

209. Haimovici H: Role of precapillary arteriovenous shunting in the pathogenesis of varicose veins and its therapeutic implications, *Surgery* 101:515-522, 1987.

210. Leu HJ, Vogt M, Pfrunder H: Morphological alterations of non-varicose and varicose veins (a morphological contribution to the discussion on pathogenesis of varicose veins), *Basic Res Cardiol* 74:435-444, 1979.

211. Cotran RS, Kumar V, Robbins SL: *Blood vessels*. In Cotran RS, Kumar V, Robbins SL, ed: *Robbins Pathologic Basis of Disease*, ed 4, Philadelphia, 1989, WB Saunders.

212. Nadrowski LF: Deep venous thrombosis: recent advances in pathogenesis and treatment, *Surg Annu* 23(pt 1):147-173, 1991.

213. Bevilacqua MP, Pober JS, Majeau GR et al: Recombinant tumor necrosis factor induces procoagulant activity in cultured human vascular endothelium: characterization and comparison with the actions of interleukin 1, *Proc Natl Acad Sci USA* 83:4533-4537, 1986.

214. McHugh NJ, Moye DA, James IE et al: Lupus anticoagulant: clinical significance in anticardiolipin positive patients with systemic lupus erythematosus, *Ann Rheum Dis* 50:548-552, 1991.

215. Woods WG: Fatal veno-occlusive disease of the liver following high dose chemotherapy, irradiation, and bone marrow transplantation, *Am J Med* 68:285, 1980.

216. Moore JD, Thompson NW, Appleman HD et al: Arteriovenous malformations of the gastrointestinal tract, *Arch Surg* 111:381-389, 1976.

217. Katz AJ: Weekly clinicopathological exercises: Case 24-1991, *N Engl J Med* 324:1726-1732, 1991.

218. Mehta PM, Heinsimer JA, Bryg RJ et al: Reassessment of the association between gastrointestinal arteriovenous malformations and aortic stenosis, *Am J Med* 86:275-277, 1989.

219. Juler GL, Labitzke HG, Lamb R et al: The pathogenesis of Dieulafoy's gastric erosion, *Am J Gastroenterol* 79:195-200, 1984.

220. Miko TL, Thomazy VA: The caliber persistent artery of the stomach: a unifying approach to gastric aneurysm, Dieulafoy's lesion, and submucosal arterial malformation, *Hum Pathol* 19:914-921, 1988.

221. Enzinger FM, Weiss SW: *Benign tumors and tumorlike lesions of blood vessels.* In Enzinger FM, Weiss SW ed: *Soft tissue tumors,* ed 2, St Louis, 1988, CV Mosby Co.

222. Oka K, Yamashita M, Sadoshima S et al: Cerebral haemorrhage in Moyamoya disease at autopsy, *Virchows Arch A Pathol Anat Histopathol* 392:247-261, 1981.

223. Pearson JM, McWilliam LJ: A light microscopical, immunohistochemical, and ultrastructural comparison of hemangiomata and lymphangiomata, *Ultrastruct Pathol* 14:497-504, 1990.

224. Clearkin KP, Enzinger FM: Intravascular papillary endothelial hyperplasia, *Arch Pathol Lab Med* 100:441-444, 1976.

225. Hagood MF, Gathright JB: Hemangiomas of the skin and gastrointestinal tract: report of a case, *Dis Colon Rectum* 18:141, 1975.

226. Reed RJ, Terazakis N: Subcutaneous angioblastic lymphoid hyperplasia with eosinophilia (Kimura's disease), *Cancer* 29:489-497, 1972.

227. Ishikawa E, Tanaka H, Kakimoto S et al: A pathological study on eosinophilic lymphofolliculoid granuloma (Kimura's disease), *Acta Pathol Jpn* 31:767-781, 1981.

228. Rosai J, Gold J, Landy R: The histiocytoid hemangiomas: a unifying concept embracing several previously described entities of skin, soft tissue, large vessels, bone, and heart, *Hum Pathol* 10:707-730, 1979.

229. Weiss SW, Ishak KG, Dail DH et al: Epithelioid hemangioendothelioma and related lesions, *Semin Diagn Pathol* 3:259-287, 1986.

230. Dail D, Liebow A: Intravascular bronchioloalveolar tumor, *Am J Pathol* 78:6a, 1975 (abstract).

231. Auerbach HE, Brooks JJ: Kaposi's sarcoma: neoplasia or hyperplasia? *Surg Pathol* 2:19-28, 1989.

232. Mahoney SE, Duvic M, Nickoloff BJ et al: Human immunodeficiency virus (HIV) transcripts identified in HIV-related psoriasis and Kaposi's sarcoma lesions, *J Clin Invest* 88:174-185, 1991.

233. Popper H, Thomas LB, Telles NC et al: Development of hepatic angiosarcoma in man induced by vinyl chloride, Thorotrast, and arsenic, *Am J Pathol* 92:349-369, 1978.

234. Woodward AH, Ivins JC, Soule EH: Lymphangiosarcoma arising in chronic lymphadematous extremities, *Cancer* 30:562-572, 1972.

235. Straub PW, Kessler S, Schreiber A et al: Chronic intravascular coagulation in Kasabach-Merritt syndrome, *Arch Intern Med* 129:475-478, 1972.

236. Lewis JM, Wald ER: *Lymphedema praecox, J Pediatr* 104:641-648, 1984.

237. Grove DI: Selective primary health care: Strategies for the control of disease in the developing world. VII. Filariasis, *Rev Infec Dis* 5:933-944, 1983.

238. Abramowski C, Hupertez V, Kilbridge P et al: Intestinal lymphangiectasia in children: a study of upper gastrointestinal endoscopic biopsies, *Pediatr Pathol* 9:289-297, 1989.

239. Moran JJ: Idiopathic arterial calcification of infancy: a clinicopathologic study, *Pathol Annu* 10:393-417, 1975.

240. Witzleben CL: Idiopathic infantile arterial calcification—a misnomer?, *Am J Cardiol* 26:305-309, 1970.

241. LeBoit PE, Berger TG, Egbert BM et al: Bacillary angiomatosis: the histopathology and differential diagnosis of a pseudoneoplastic infection in patients with human immunodefficiency virus disease, *Am J Surg Pathol* 13:909-920, 1989.

242. Joshi VV, Pawal B, Connor E et al: Arteriopathy in children with acquired immune deficiency syndrome, *Pediatr Pathol* 7:261-275, 1987.

243. Hruban RH et al: Accelerated arteriosclerosis in heart transplant recipients is associated with a T-lymphocyte-mediated endothelialitis, *Am J Pathol* 137:871, 1990.

244. Berman JW, Calderon TM: The role of endothelial cell adhesion molecules in the development of atherosclerosis, *Cardiovasc Pathol* 1:17-28, 1992.

245. Magrinat G, Kerwin KS, Gabriel DA: The clinical manifestations of Degos' syndrome, *Arch Pathol Lab Med* 113:354-362, 1989.

246. Strole WE, Clark WH Jr., Isselbacher KJ: Progressive arterial occlusive disease (Kohlmeier-Degos): A frequently fatal cutaneosystemic disorder, *N Engl J Med* 276:195-201, 1967.

INDEX

A